Oral and Maxillofacial Pathology

A Rationale for Diagnosis and Treatment

Oral and Maxillofacial
PATHOLOGY

A Rationale for Diagnosis and Treatment

Robert E. Marx, DDS

Professor of Surgery and Chief
Division of Oral and Maxillofacial Surgery
University of Miami
School of Medicine
Miami, Florida

Diane Stern, DDS

Clinical Professor of Surgery
Division of Oral and Maxillofacial Surgery
University of Miami
School of Medicine
Miami, Florida

Quintessence Publishing Co, Inc

Chicago, Berlin, Tokyo, Copenhagen, London, Paris, Milan, Barcelona,
Istanbul, São Paulo, New Delhi, Moscow, Prague, and Warsaw

Library of Congress Cataloging-in-Publication Data

Marx, Robert E.
  Oral and maxillofacial pathology : a rationale for diagnosis and
treatment / Robert E. Marx, Diane Stern.
           p. ; cm.
Includes bibliographical references and index.
  ISBN 0-86715-390-3 (hardcover)
  1. Mouth--Pathophysiology. 2. Face--Pathophysiology.
  [DNLM: 1. Face--pathology. 2. Jaw--pathology. 3. Mouth--pathology.
4. Jaw Diseases--pathology. 5. Mouth Diseases--pathology. WU 140
M392o 2002] I. Stern, Diane. II. Title.
  RK301 .M216 2002
  617.5'2--dc21

                                              2002005048

The authors and the publisher of this work have made every effort to provide information that is reliable and complete. However, because of the possibilities of human error and new developments in the field, neither the authors nor the publisher of this work guarantees that the information contained herein is in every respect accurate or complete. Readers are encouraged to confirm the information contained herein with other sources, and they are advised to be aware of all pertinent governmental regulations and to review the manufacturer's information.

All histologic slides are stained with hematoxylin & eosin unless otherwise noted.

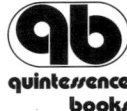

quintessence
books

© 2003 Quintessence Publishing Co, Inc

Quintessence Publishing Co, Inc
551 Kimberly Drive
Carol Stream, Illinois 60188
www.quintpub.com

Editor: Lisa C. Bywaters
Production: Susan Robinson
Cover design: Eric M. O'Malley

Printed in Hong Kong

Dedication

Sir Isaac Newton, the founder of modern physics, which has made possible the air and land travel that we take for granted today, as well as computers, the Internet, space travel, and very much more, uttered these words in 1722: "If I have seen further, it is because I sat on the shoulders of giants." His remarkable contributions and the humility that he showed are models for us today. Inspired by his words, we would like to dedicate this book to those "giants" of oral and maxillofacial surgery and oral and maxillofacial pathology who, through their efforts, not only set the foundation for this book but instilled pride in these two great specialties of dentistry. An incomplete list of those individuals, with apologies to any that have been inadvertently omitted, would look something like this:

Charles C. Alling
Harry S. Archer
S. Elmer Bear
William H. Bell
Joseph L. Bernier
James Bertz
Philip Boyne
Lester R. Cahn
R. Bruce Donoff
Leon Eisenbud
Bruce N. Epker
Raymond J. Fonseca
Benjamin J. Gans
Robert J. Gorlin
Thomas Gunning

Walter C. Guralnick
Eric Hjörting Hansen
James R. Hayward
John F. Helfrick
Fred A. Henny
Robert P. Johnson
James F. Kelly
John N. Kent
Donald A. Kerr
Stuart N. Kline
Daniel M. Laskin
Charles A. (Scotty) McCallum
Irving Meyer
Alec Monheim
Kursheed Moos
Hugo Obwegeser

Donald B. Osbon
Jens J. Pindborg
David Poswillo
Hamilton B.G. Robinson
William Shafer
Robert B. Shira
Emil Steinhauser
Orion R. Stuteville
Bill C. Terry
Kurt Thoma
Daniel Waite
Charles A. Waldron
Robert V. Walker
Terence G. Ward
Larry M. Wolford

Students of dentistry, residents in each specialty, and practicing clinicians alike owe these individuals a debt of gratitude for taking an interest in "hospital dentistry" and recognizing a unique need in health care, which they have built into two thriving professions that serve the conditions of mankind in a way that no other specialty of medicine or dentistry can serve.

Preface

This book is intended to be a clinically oriented and forward-looking guide for oral and maxillofacial surgeons and other advanced dental and medical specialists who deal with pathologies in the oral cavity, midface, and neck. It focuses on the mechanism of each disease and how that dictates its clinical and radiographic presentation as well as the serious considerations on a sample differential diagnosis. It then progresses to specific treatment recommendations that the authors use or have researched as the most beneficial. Treatments avoid such vague phrases as "a wide local excision" and instead provide specific margins and anatomically based techniques. Generic medication protocols also are avoided for those conditions not treated with surgery; instead, specific drugs, doses, routes of administration, length of treatment, and alternative treatments are described in the context of how each works to affect the natural course of the disease. Discussion of each disease or condition concludes with the prognosis after treatment.

This book challenges some of the established concepts and dogmas currently prevailing in oral and maxillofacial pathology and surgery. It also is likely to challenge the reader's acceptance of dental and medical school teaching, which too often consists of a rushed and superficial presentation of these pathologies. It is the authors' hope that the evidence and rationales presented in this text are convincing of this change and of this approach to learning. This book is also specifically intended to simplify and streamline terminology. The reader will note numerous terminology changes from the past—changes that generally use only one name to describe and identify the specific underlying cause of each condition. This is reinforced in the last chapter of the book, "Where Have All the Great Terms Gone?," a concise review and explanation of why the original name for some diseases is inappropriate today.

Readers may use this text as a cover-to-cover course in clinical and histopathologic oral and maxillofacial pathology; as a reference text on a chapter-by-chapter basis to review the specifics of each disease category; or as a case reference to refresh their knowledge about a specific disease or the specific presentation of a new patient. In any case, it is the fond hope of both authors that clinicians will increase their knowledge and ability to care for their patients, who in turn will receive more accurate diagnoses and better treatment.

No book is created by its authors alone. The numerous individuals who have referred patients and biopsy material to our practices must be acknowledged, although their numbers preclude individual mention. These include our present and past hard-working and scientifically curious residents in oral and maxillofacial surgery whose "great cases" appear in the book. A specific and certainly sentimental acknowledgment must be given to our mentors: Stuart N. Kline and Robert P. Johnson, the mentors of Robert Marx; and Lester R. Cahn and Leon Eisenbud, the mentors of Diane Stern. Their teaching and self-sacrifice have not only advanced our knowledge but motivated us throughout our careers and personal lives. We have acknowledged the source of all illustrations that are not our own. It is possible that with the passage of time there may have been some whose source we no longer recall. If this is the case, we humbly apologize.

Photomicrographs require the work of several individuals. There is the histology technician who prepares the microscopic slide; many of these are the work of Maureen Frazel, ART. Others were prepared by the late Sarah Spector. Then there is the photographer who captures the microscopic image on film; the majority of these have been the work of Leroy Ivey of the Veterans Administration Medical Center, Miami. The drawings were executed by Hans Neuhart. Maria Ruiz typed the manuscript with her characteristic efficiency and good humor, to the benefit of everyone involved. To these skilled, dedicated, and patient individuals, our sincere thanks. Thanks also to Carlos Valdes, MD, whose generosity in sharing his dermatopathology material is greatly appreciated. We are most grateful to our publisher, represented by Tomoko Tsuchiya, who made the creation of this book as smooth and pleasant as is humanly possible; Susan Robinson, who handled the physical production of the book with true professionalism and grace; and Lisa Bywaters, our editor, whose infinite patience, knowledge, and understanding guided us to the final result. We are indeed fortunate to have been able to work with her.

Our families have sustained us with their love, support, and encouragement despite the considerable infringement that this book has made on their time.

Finally, without the patients we have treated in the past, this book could not have been written. We hope that it will ultimately benefit those who are patients today and in the future.

Table of Contents

3 Immune-Based Diseases

4 Conditions of Developmental Disturbances

5 Hyperplasias, Hamartomas, and Neoplasms

6 Benign Epithelial Tumors of Mucosa and Skin

7   Premalignant and Malignant Epithelial Tumors of Mucosa and Skin

8   Management of Irradiated Patients and Osteoradionecrosis

13 Odontogenic and Nonodontogenic Cysts

14 Odontogenic Tumors: Hamartomas and Neoplasms

15 Pigmented Lesions of Mucosa and Skin

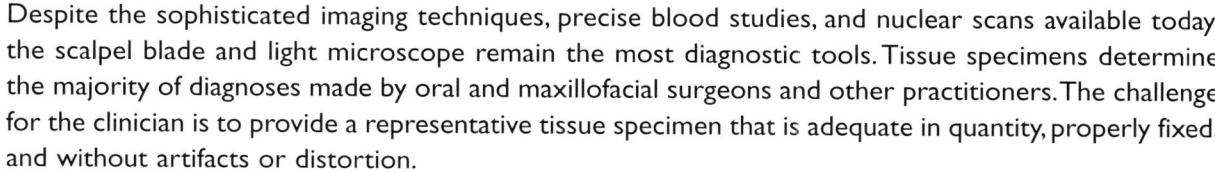

Biopsy Principles and Techniques

▶ "As is your pathology, so is your practice."
—*Sir William Osler*

▶ "As goes your technology and your skills, so goes your practice."
—*Robert E. Marx and Diane Stern*

Despite the sophisticated imaging techniques, precise blood studies, and nuclear scans available today, the scalpel blade and light microscope remain the most diagnostic tools. Tissue specimens determine the majority of diagnoses made by oral and maxillofacial surgeons and other practitioners. The challenge for the clinician is to provide a representative tissue specimen that is adequate in quantity, properly fixed, and without artifacts or distortion.

The approach to a biopsy depends somewhat on the size, shape, location, and type of disease the practitioner anticipates.

Brush Biopsy As a Screening Tool for Oral Cancer

Exfoliative cytology has not been a very diagnostic or useful screening method for oral cancer because hyperkeratosis and keratin itself interfere with cell obtainment and a greater proportion of diagnostic cells are below the surface (most at the basement membrane level) (Fig 1-1a). Today, the preferred screening tool is the brush biopsy technique, which enables a transepithelial capture of cells. With this method, a brush is rotated against the tissue until slight bleeding is observed, indicating that the brush has reached the basement membrane (Figs 1-1b and 1-1c). The cellular aggregate on the brush is transferred to a glass slide, fixed, and then analyzed by computer scans and pathologists trained specifically in oral brush biopsy interpretation. This method is preferred over an exfoliative biopsy because its simplicity and practicality allow its use by all practitioners regardless of whether they have surgical training. Therefore, the technique can be applied to a wider segment of the population. However, it must be remembered that the brush biopsy technique is only a screening tool; "positive" biopsies or atypical cell identification require a follow-up incisional biopsy.

Incisional Versus Excisional Biopsy

The clinician's conundrum about whether to remove the entire lesion (excisional biopsy) or to sample it (incisional biopsy) is common, yet the decision can be straightforward. If the differential diagnosis includes as the four most realistic possibilities lesions that are "curable" by a local excision or enucleation procedures, an excisional biopsy is recommended. Should the excised specimen turn out to be a more aggressive lesion or tumor than was anticipated by the differential diagnosis and not curable by the excisional biopsy, the excisional biopsy becomes an incisional biopsy and a curative surgery is planned. If, on the other hand, the four most realistic possibilities of the differential diagnosis include a mixture of lesions that are usually curable by different treatments or degrees of surgery, an incisional biopsy is recommended to obtain a diagnosis for which the best treatment choice can be made.

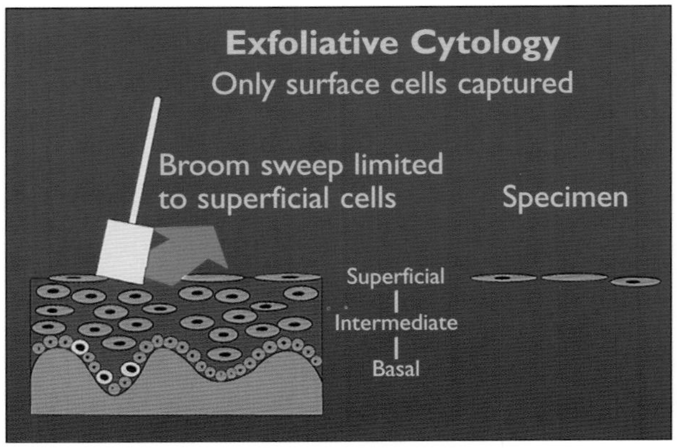

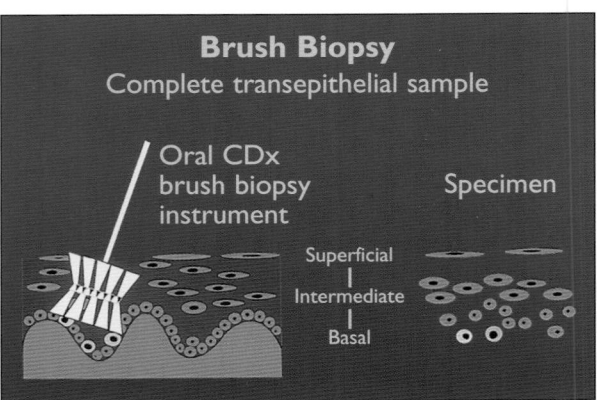

Fig 1-1a Traditional exfoliative cytology is inadequate for sampling potentially dysplastic cells. (Courtesy of Oral Scan Labs, New York.)

Fig 1-1b The firm brush is able to capture deeper cells to the level of the basement membrane. (Courtesy of Oral Scan Labs, New York.)

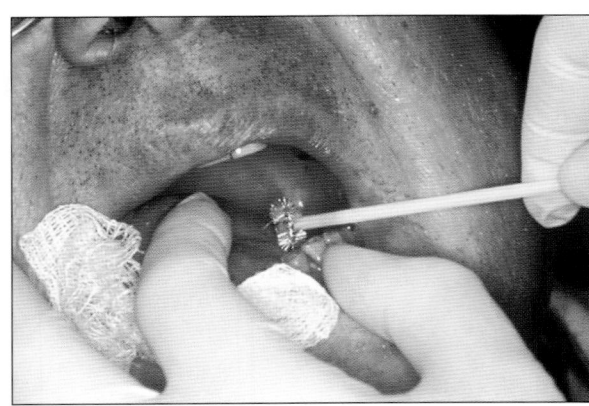

Fig 1-1c Brush placed and rotated to capture epithelial cells.

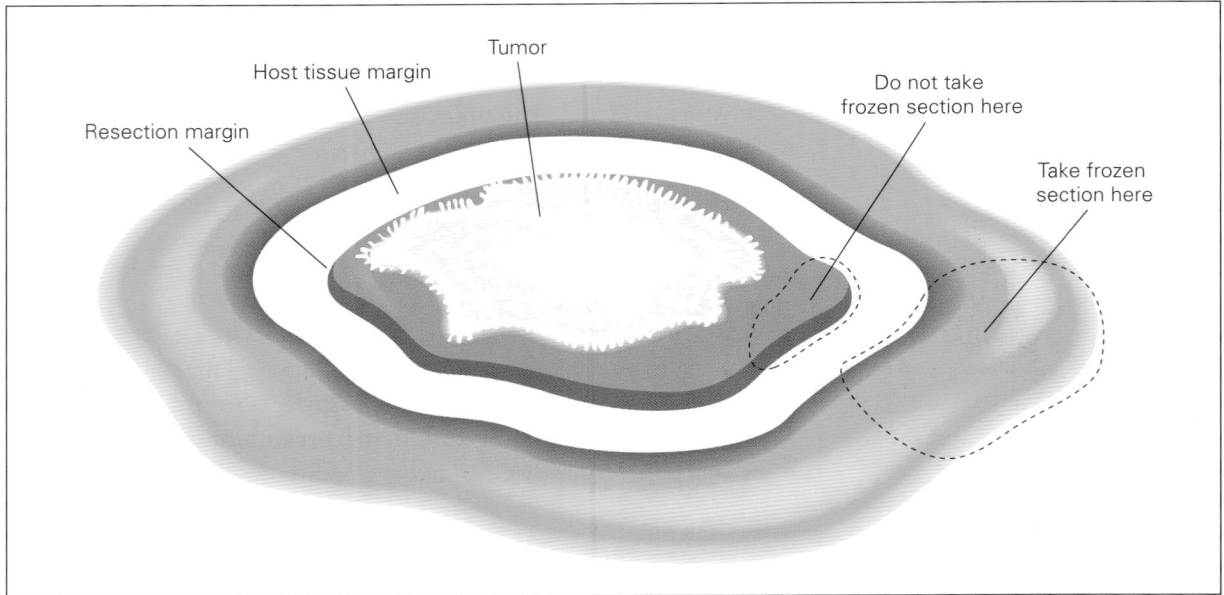

Fig 1-2 Frozen sections should be taken from the host tissue edge rather than from the specimen tissue edge.

Principles of Frozen Section Specimens

Frozen sections are used during surgery mainly to assess the margins of resected tissue for residual or proximal tumor. They can also be used to confirm a suspected diagnosis or relate to the surgeon a type of tissue, eg, nerve vs scar. When assessing margins, it is important to submit a tissue specimen outside the resection periphery. If a tissue specimen is taken from the main resection specimen itself, it will appear on the permanent sections that the tumor was closer to the resection margin than it actually was (Fig 1-2). This will be recorded on the final pathology report and may precipitate additional treatment recommendations unnecessarily.

When frozen sections of the main specimen are required, the specimen should be marked with sutures, or the edge should be inked to direct the pathologist to areas of concern (Fig 1-3a). In addition, clearly noted orientation should be included on the pathology request, noting anterior, superior, medial, and lateral edges. Dental terms such as *mesial, distal* (meaning dental distal rather than the opposite

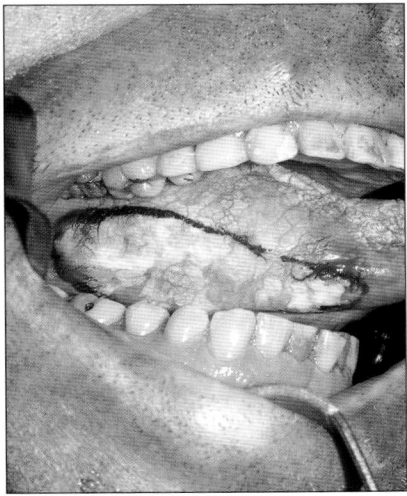

Fig 1-3a Excision of a surface lesion should be guided by outlining the excisional periphery with a sterile marking pen.

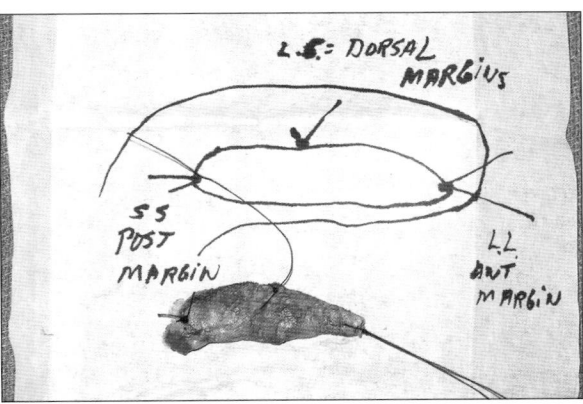

Fig 1-3b The excised specimen should be adequately tagged at reference margins and annotated to the pathologist. A diagram such as this to accompany the specimen is ideal.

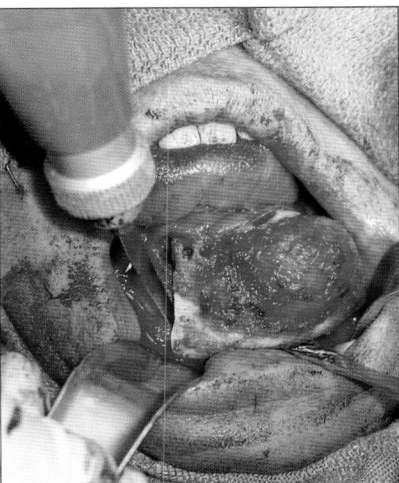

Fig 1-4a The resection margin of a benign tumor in bone is based on a knowledge of the tumor's invasive properties, the radiographic and/or CT scan margin, and the clinical observation of the tumor's edge.

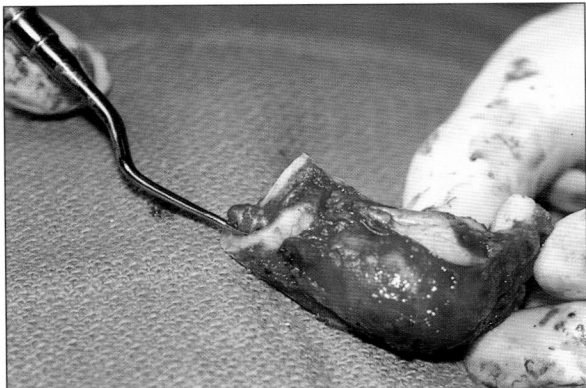

Fig 1-4b Since both benign and malignant tumors advance further within the marrow space than in the cortex, curettings from the marrow space can be used as frozen sections or for cytology.

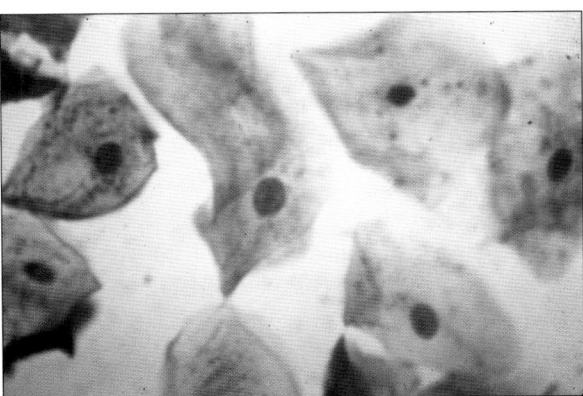

Fig 1-4c Cytology of normal-appearing epithelial cells. Note the small nuclei, abundant cytoplasm, and regular cell outlines.

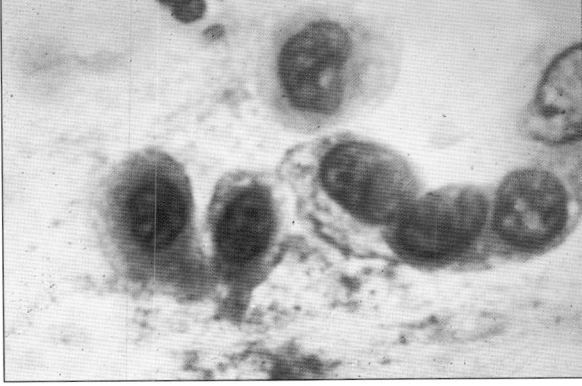

Fig 1-4d Cytology of abnormal cells with large nuclei, resulting in a reversal of the nuclear-cytoplasmic ratio.

of proximal), *lingual, buccal,* and *labial* should be avoided. These terms are unfamiliar and confusing to general pathologists, and although oral and maxillofacial pathologists understand them, they are rarely the ones involved in interpreting frozen sections; anatomic orientations more consistent with all surgical specimens are preferred. It is also useful to provide a sketch of the specimen with the same orientation sutures or inked edges on the drawing. This can be accomplished without violating sterile scrub by using a sterile marking pen and the paper in which sterile gloves are packaged (Fig 1-3b).

Frozen sections also may be obtained from a margin in bone even though hard tissue requires decalcification before processing. Because most tumors advance through bone within the marrow cavity, this area rather than the cortex is the preferred area to sample (Fig 1-4a). A frozen section can, therefore, be obtained by curetting the marrow cavity from the native bone at each resection margin (Fig 1-4b). This is almost always a fibrofatty tissue that does not require decalcification (Fig 1-4c). If the pathologist believes that the curettings are still too "gritty" to microtome without decalcification, then at least a touch preparation or cytologic slide (Figs 1-4c and 1-4d) can be prepared from the specimen.

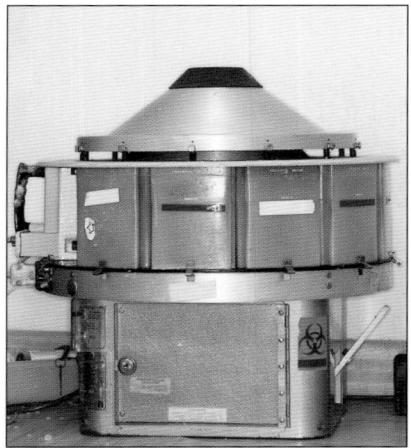

Fig 1-5a The Autotechnicon (Miles), one of the automatic tissue processors available.

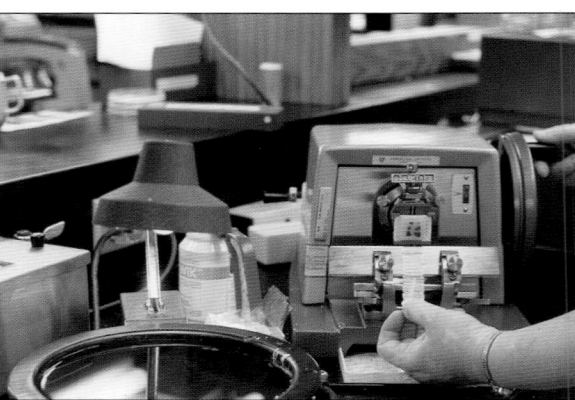

Fig 1-5b The microtome with the paraffin block in place. The handle of the microtome moves the block up and down against the knife to produce the paraffin ribbon.

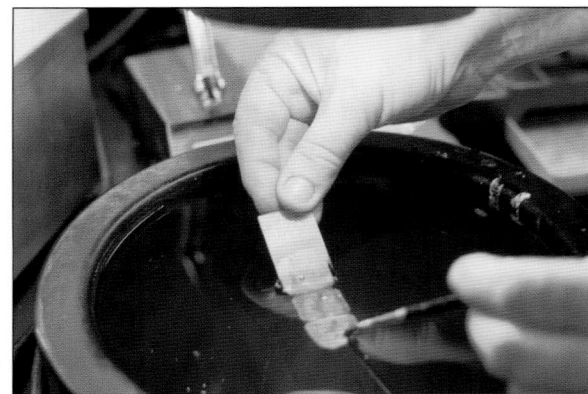

Fig 1-5c The ribbon is floated on a bath of warm water, and the slices are picked up on a clean glass slide.

Processing of Biopsy Specimens

Although many sophisticated techniques are available to assist in tissue diagnosis, the standard method remains the preparation of a paraffin block from which serial sections of tissue are prepared. This technique has been in use since Klebs introduced chloroform paraffin in 1881. The sections are then stained with hematoxylin & eosin (H&E) stain. It is on this basis that most diagnoses are made.

The excised tissue must be "fixed" to prevent autolysis and make the tissue rigid for easier handling. Fixing also kills microorganisms. The fixative most frequently used is 10% buffered formalin, which should be about 20 times the volume of the specimen. Large specimens should be sectioned to allow for optimum fixation; 0.5 cm is suggested. The tissue should remain in the fixative for a minimum of 8 hours, and longer for larger specimens.

After fixation and gross examination, the specimen is prepared by passing it through a series of graded alcohols (from 70% to absolute) to dehydrate the tissue, followed by immersion in xylene or similar substance to remove the alcohol, followed by immersion in liquid paraffin. This sequence is typically accomplished overnight in a machine such as the Autotechnicon (Miles) (Fig 1-5a), which automatically moves the tissue from one container to another. The specimen itself is contained in a plastic cassette. Newer technology enables the tissues to remain in a fixed position while the different solutions are passed over them.

In the morning, the histotechnologist removes the tissue and embeds the specimen in liquid paraffin, which is contained in a metal mold. This is a challenging task in which the tissue must be oriented appropriately so that, for example, a mucosal specimen will be cut at right angles to the surface rather than tangentially. The base of the plastic cassette is placed on top of the mold, the whole is chilled on ice, the mold is removed, and the paraffin block is trimmed and placed in the microtome. The microtome works much like a meat slicer and cuts serial sections of the paraffin block at a preset thickness, which for most routine purposes is 5 to 6 μm (Fig 1-5b). The ribbon of paraffin containing the tissue is then floated on a bath of warm water, so that the paraffin and tissue can spread out to provide a flat, unwrinkled specimen. It is then mounted onto a clean glass slide to which the tissue immediately adheres (Fig 1-5c). This slide is called a "blank." These slides are then warmed to a temperature beyond the melting point of paraffin (60°C).

The next step is tissue staining. While there are many "special" histochemical stains available, nearly all tissues are initially stained with H&E. The hematoxylin, which is basophilic, stains nuclei blue. Eosin, which is acidophilic, stains collagen, muscle, and nerve red. Because H&E is an aqueous stain, the paraffin present within the tissue must be removed. This is accomplished by passing the slides back through the xylene and graded alcohols, but in reverse order. This process takes approximately 10 minutes and is done by hand or machine. The slides are then dipped in a series of staining dishes, after which the tissues are again placed briefly in alcohol to dehydrate the specimen and allow for the placement of the coverglass by a plastic mounting medium. This affords an airtight seal and protects the tissue, allowing the slide to remain as a permanent record.

The technique described is appropriate for soft tissue. Calcified tissue is handled in the same manner, but an additional step is required after fixation and before processing in the Autotechnicon. This is the decalcification process, which is necessary to allow the tissue to be sectioned by the microtome knife. The tissue is placed in an acid, usually hydrochloric acid. The time necessary varies considerably—from 1 or 2 hours to several days or even a week or more—depending on the size and degree of calcification of the specimen. Care must be taken not to overdecalcify, as this can cause complete disintegration of the tissue. Additional types of stains can be used subsequently as needed, including stains for microorganisms (Brown and Brenn or acid-fast), or for tissue products such as mucin (mucicarmine or periodic acid–Schiff). It is important to understand, however, that this old tried and true method with the use of H&E is still the basis for histologic diagnosis. As has been said, "Special stains make what you don't know a different color."

A well-made slide can last indefinitely. At this time, laboratories are required to retain slides for a minimum of 10 years. If over time the stain should fade, it is possible to remove the coverglass and restain the slide. The paraffin blocks are also retained. At this time, the minimum time is 2 years. If additional slides are ever needed, the block can be retrieved and new sections made.

Approach to Histologic Interpretation

Although new modalities have been developed, routine light microscopy using sections cut from a paraffin block and stained with H&E is still the primary method for the diagnosis of biopsy and surgical material. This method of identifying tissue and cells by the patterns they make, the substances they produce, and their shape and size is essentially a morphologic science. The relationship of the pathologic tissue to the surrounding normal tissue is also diagnostically important. At the low-power view, this relationship and the overall pattern can be assessed. A stratified squamous epithelium that is not maturing properly and that has a disturbed pattern can be recognized by this means; a tumor that is encapsulated or infiltrative can also be appreciated. The low-power view gives a sense of the problem. At higher powers, the impressions can be confirmed or rejected, and attention can be focused on individual cells. There are many cells that can be easily recognized by their morphology. As long as a cell is sectioned through its center, we can probably identify it, but if it is sectioned through its tip, it may be unrecognizable. Hence it may not be possible to identify all cells on any given slide. In the same way, one can easily recognize a picture of the Eiffel Tower (Fig 1-6a); however, if the Eiffel Tower is viewed from an unusual angle, recognition may not be so easy (Fig 1-6b).

The importance of viewing the whole rather than a part can be appreciated when looking at a photo of the Statue of Liberty (Fig 1-6c). Immediately one assumes the picture was taken in New York harbor. But a broader and wider view of the photo (Fig 1-6d) shows the Eiffel Tower in the background, indicating that the location shown in the photo is actually Paris. One must likewise remember that a Langhans giant cell by itself does not justify a diagnosis of tuberculosis; a Reed Sternberg cell without the proper background does not constitute Hodgkin lymphoma. The importance of putting everything together—the clinical picture, the history, the low-power and high-power views of biopsy and surgical material, and the radiographs, when appropriate—cannot be overemphasized. Indeed, histopathologic interpretation is like a jigsaw puzzle in that all of the various pieces of evidence must fit together.

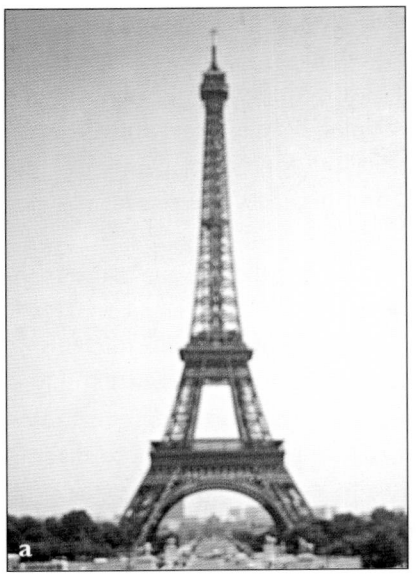
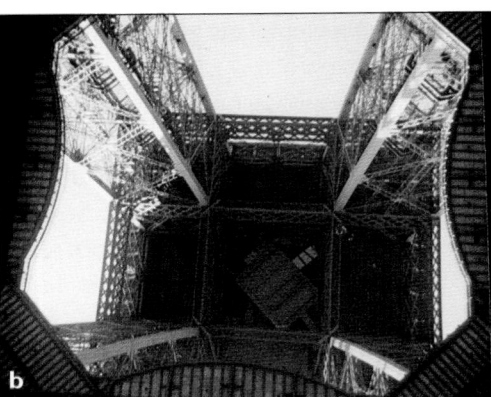
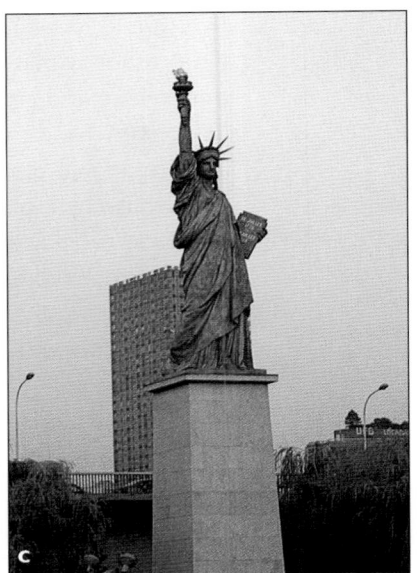
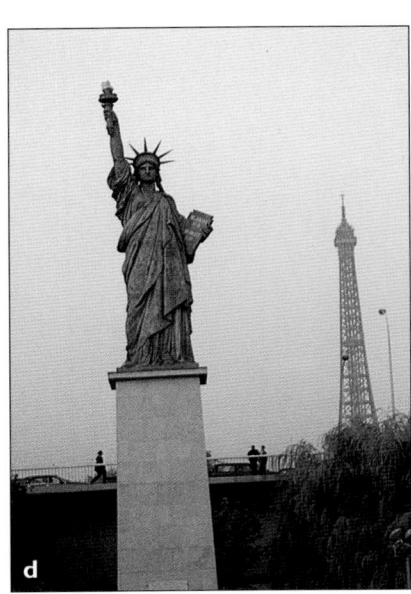

Figs 1-6a and 1-6b Viewing histopathology or the Eiffel Tower from two different perspectives will change the view greatly and may suggest that the viewer is looking at two different structures. (Photo shown in Fig 1-6a courtesy of Michael Sard.)

Figs 1-6c and 1-6d Viewing histopathology or the Statue of Liberty without considering the background can guide the viewer to the wrong assumptions.

Immunofluorescence Testing

Immunofluorescence techniques serve as an important diagnostic tool in several areas of oral pathology. The techniques are directed toward but not limited to immune-based diseases and find use primarily in the area of chronic autoimmune vesiculobullous disease. There are two basic techniques. With direct immunofluorescence testing, an attempt is made to identify the presence and location of various immunoreactants within tissue. The specimen is usually taken from perilesional tissue immediately adjacent to a new vesiculobullous lesion, and is incubated with fluorescein-labeled antibodies against human immunoglobulins, complement, and fibrin. If the immunoreactant is present in the specimen, it will react with the labeled antibody and its presence and location can be visualized under the microscope with ultraviolet light (Fig 1-7). For this test, fresh tissue or tissue that is held in a special fixation medium is necessary. One of the more frequently employed media is Michel's fixative. This is composed of ammonium sulphate, N-ethyl malemide, and magnesium sulfate in a citrate buffer. The antibodies used are typically from rabbits that have been immunized with immunoglobulins taken from human myelomas.

With indirect immunofluorescence testing, the presence and concentration of circulating antibodies within the patient's serum are assayed. The serum is incubated with a tissue substrate that may be human or from another species. Specific substrates are chosen for specific diseases. Often this is human lip or monkey esophagus. The antibodies from the patient's serum that target specific antigens in the substrate will then bind to the substrate. The next step is to add a fluorescein-labeled anti-human immunoglobulin so that the bound immunoglobulins can be seen under the fluorescence microscope. Antibody titers can be obtained by serial dilution of the patient's serum.

Because direct immunofluorescence is the more sensitive test and has diagnostic significance, it has wider application. With indirect immunofluorescence, antibody titers can be measured. In some instances, as in pemphigus, this may be useful in monitoring disease activity and response to treatment. In other diseases, however, the level of antibody and disease activity have no correlation.

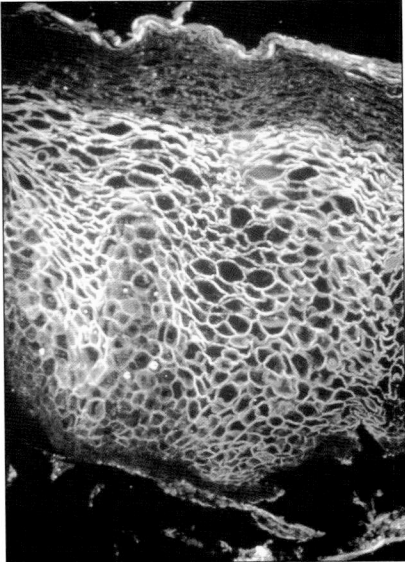

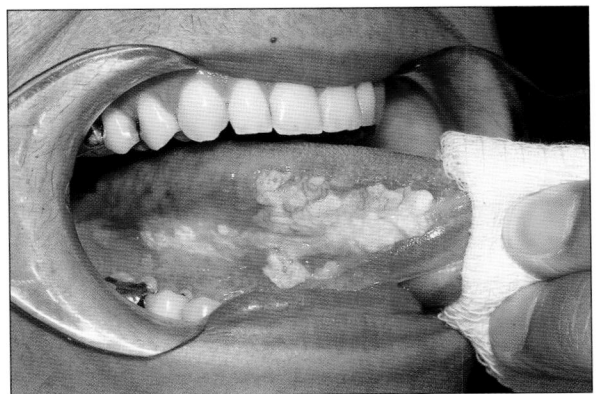

Fig 1-7 Direct immunofluorescence of a portion of mucosa from a patient with pemphigus vulgaris shows the intercellular deposition of IgG.

Fig 1-8 This lesion can be excised for a complete histopathologic examination. However, if incisional biopsies are used, areas of erythroplakia, atrophy, or indurations are the best sites for sampling.

Erythroleukoplakia of Oral Mucosa

A biopsy of a clinical erythroleukoplakia is made to determine whether dysplasia or invasive carcinoma is present. Because a biopsy is an invasive procedure that may cause inflammatory lymphadenopathy, which would confuse a later TNM (primary tumor, regional nodes, and metastases) classification if carcinoma is found, a brief clinical staging using the TNM classification is done before the biopsy. The biopsy may be taken using local anesthesia, but a nerve block or field block technique is recommended. Although injecting local anesthetic into the lesion will not spread or seed tumor cells because of the thin needle gauge, the solution volume itself will distort tissue and create artifacts.

The most yielding areas for biopsy are the erythroplakic areas, areas of atrophy, or areas where induration is palpated. Often multiple areas are biopsied and, when practical, the entire clinical lesion excised (Fig 1-8). The experienced clinician may not require biopsy site aids, but toluidine blue may be used to determine the most yielding site for an incisional biopsy. This aid may be of particular value in the biopsy of a clinically homogeneous lesion. Toluidine blue is a vital dye that binds to DNA and sulfated mucopolysaccharides in all tissues. However, because actively replicating tissues such as dysplasias and cancers contain elevated levels of each, the blue dye will concentrate in these tissues, thus guiding the clinician to the best site for biopsy (Figs 1-9a and 1-9b). The technique uses a 1% aqueous solution of toluidine blue, which is applied to the lesion and allowed to remain for 1 minute. It is then "decolorized" with 1% acetic acid. The areas of persistent toluidine dye staining are recommended for biopsy.

The area of biopsy should remain within the confines of the clinical lesion. Taking a margin of normal-appearing tissue for this type of biopsy will not assist the microscopic assessment and will only risk extending a tumor margin into uninvolved areas. The biopsy should be sufficiently deep to include underlying muscle. Should a carcinoma in situ or an invasive carcinoma be found, determining the integrity of the basement membrane and the depth of invasion, possibly into muscle tissue, will be important.

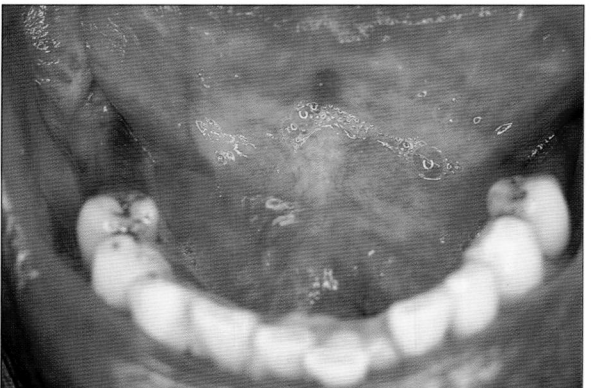

Fig 1-9a Suspicious floor-of-the-mouth lesion.

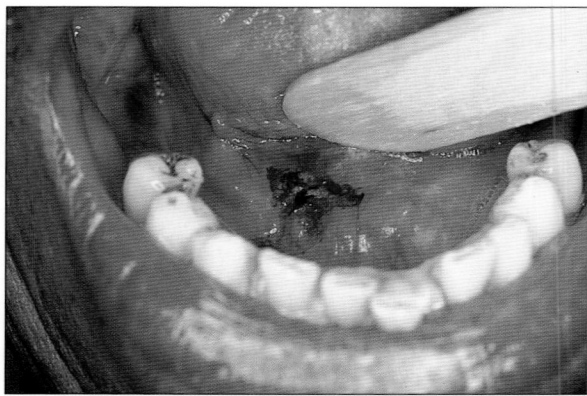

Fig 1-9b Increased uptake of 1% toluidine blue, implying a greater DNA turnover, indicates the preferred site for an incisional biopsy.

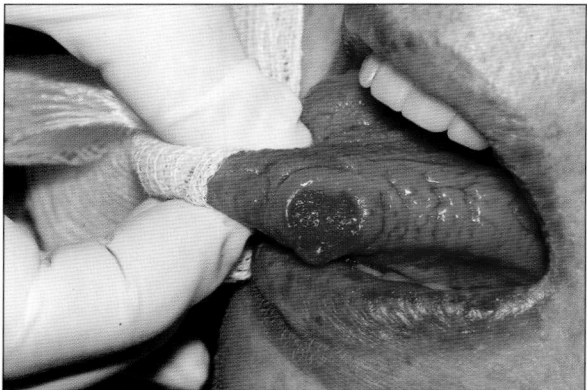

Fig 1-10 An incisional biopsy of a lesion suspicious for carcinoma should include the ulcer's edge and base without extension into normal tissues. It should also be sufficiently deep so as to include some muscle for assessment of muscle invasion.

Unless the pathologist states a preference for a different fixative, 10% formalin (4% formaldehyde) in a neutral-buffered solution is best. If the specimen is shipped in winter, it should be labeled, "Do not allow to freeze," because freezing will induce artifacts.

Ulcerative Lesions of the Oral Mucosa

If the ulcerative lesion is suspected to represent a carcinoma or an infectious or specific fungal disease rather than an immune-based disease such as pemphigus or lichen planus, the biopsy should include the edge of the ulcer and the ulcer base without extending into normal tissues (Fig 1-10). The ulcer base and edge will be representative of carcinomas, infections, and specific fungal diseases. Secondary infections or colonizations by the oral flora will not usually obscure these types of histopathologic features. Biopsy of the ulcer's base is required to determine the greatest depth of invasion. Biopsy of the edge of the ulcer is required because this area is most likely to harbor organisms and, if the lesion represents carcinoma, show the best cellular definition without either inflammation or necrosis obscuring the picture. If an underlying muscle layer is present, it must also be included in the biopsy.

Immune-Based Vesicles and Ulcers

Autoimmune diseases such as pemphigus, lichen planus, the spectrum of pemphigoids, and systemic lupus erythematosus affect the entire mucosa. The areas of vesicles and/or ulcers tend to be more advanced localizations of a process occurring subclinically throughout the mucosa in a histologically specific manner for each disease. However, areas of ulcers or ruptured vesicles become secondarily colonized with the oral flora and develop a nonspecific inflammatory response that may obscure the specific histopathologic characteristics of that disease. Therefore, for cases in which immune-based diseases are suspected, a biopsy should avoid ulcers and ruptured vesicles. The target areas for this type of biopsy are clinically involved areas with an intact surface and some adjacent normal-appearing tissue (Fig 1-11). Because direct immunofluorescence may be needed to confirm the diagnosis, either one large biopsy specimen that can be separated into two specimens or two separate tissue specimens should be taken (Fig 1-12). One specimen is fixed in 10% neutral-buffered formalin for routine H&E-stained sections and the other specimen fixed in Michel's medium (or fresh frozen as an alternative) for direct immunofluorescence studies.

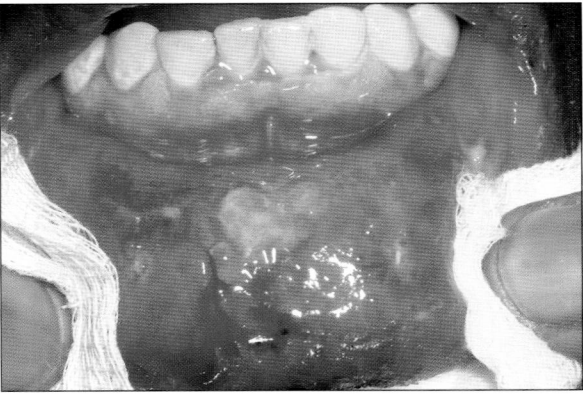

Fig 1-11 Ulcers, vesicles, or erythematous lesions suspicious for immune-based diseases like pemphigus, pemphigoid, and lichen planus should include clinically normal-appearing adjacent tissue.

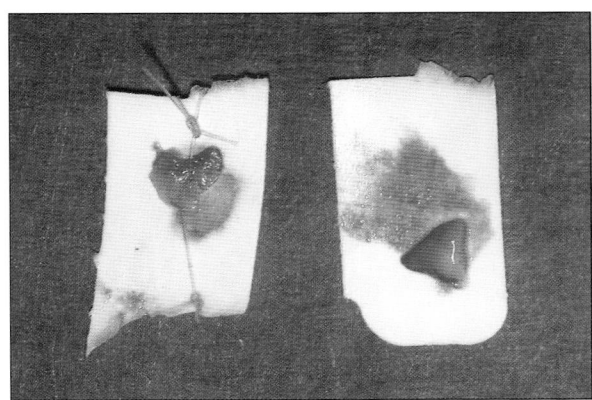

Fig 1-12 Specimens from lesions suspected to be immune based should be divided into two specimens so that both H&E and direct immunofluorescent staining can be accomplished. Suturing the specimens to the suture pack cardboard will prevent them from curling up in the fixative.

Radiolucent Lesions in Bone

Radiolucent lesions in bone may represent idiopathic bone cavities, infections, cysts, and cystic or solid tumors (Fig 1-13). Aspiration of most radiolucent lesions is done before biopsy to assess for potential bleeding that may occur during the biopsy. Aspiration should be accomplished with a 20-gauge or larger needle. The lesion should also be aspirated in three areas by directing the needle tip to three locations within the lesion from a single entrance point. This maneuver is recommended because many lesions are compartmentalized into solid and fluid spaces. A 10-mL syringe containing 1 mL of saline is used. The clinician should observe the first component of the aspirate. If bubbles of air or a serosanguineous fluid precede blood, an idiopathic bone cavity is likely. Aspirated blood does not confirm an arteriovenous hemangioma (Fig 1-14). Lesions of lower vascular pressure such as cavernous hemangiomas, central giant cell tumors (including what was formerly called "aneurysmal bone cysts"), and idiopathic bone cavities will return blood upon aspiration. If blood is returned, it is useful to disconnect the syringe barrel from the needle. Low-pressure vascular lesions, which will not represent a significant clinical bleeding concern, will yield blood flow from the needle hub but stop within 1 minute. High-pressure vascular malformations will result in spurting blood from the needle hub.

In addition to these maneuvers that provide information about the risks of entering a lesion that returns blood, a portable Doppler ultrasound is useful (Fig 1-15). Low-pressure lesions will produce an echoing sound resembling wind blowing through a tunnel. High-pressure lesions suggestive of arteriovenous hemangiomas will produce harsh arterial sounds identical to a reference sounding of the carotid or radial pulse. If either a harsh arterial sound is heard by Doppler, or a spurting type of blood return is observed with the syringe barrel disconnected, the clinician should withdraw the needle, seal the entry (usually with bone wax or oxidized cellulose [Surgicel, Ethicon]), and plan for diagnostic angiography with embolization as a possibility.

If a fluid other than blood is returned, it is not necessary to chemically analyze the fluid or to perform cytologic studies. Neither undertaking has proven to produce reliable diagnostic information.

The incisional biopsy is best performed through a midcrestal incision. Such an incision will not compromise the incisional approach at a later definitive surgery and will provide the surgeon maximum flexibility for extending or modifying the incision to gain access to the intrabony tissue (Fig 1-16). Wide access is recommended because the incisional biopsy is also somewhat of an exploration. The clinician should observe whether the lesion has a lumen, the thickness of any lining, material within the lesion,

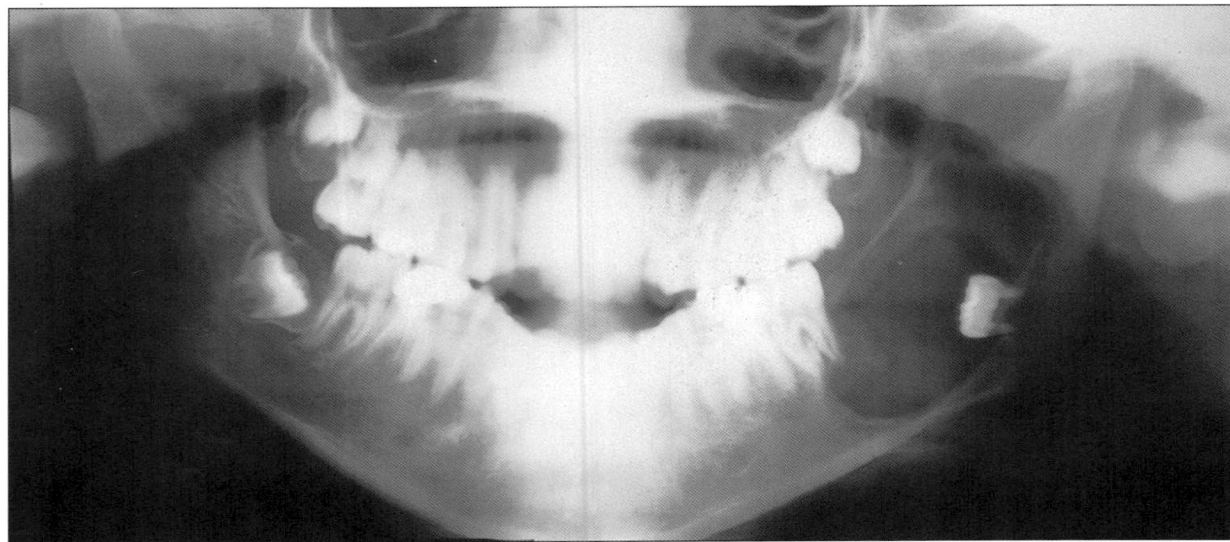

Fig 1-13 Radiolucent lesions are recommended for aspiration prior to biopsy to assess for possible high-pressure bleeding that may complicate the procedure.

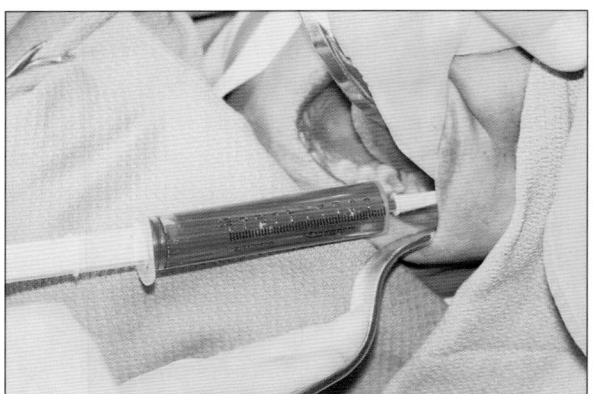

Fig 1-14 Blood filled this syringe upon drawing back the plunger. This lesion was an idiopathic bone cavity.

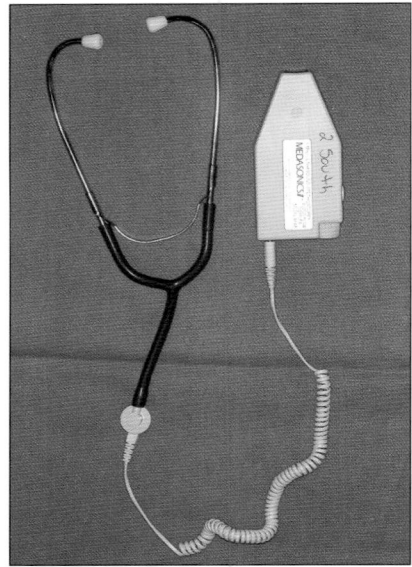

Fig 1-15 A simple, portable Doppler is useful to assess for arterial sounds within bone prior to biopsy. Harsh arterial sounds and a withdrawal of blood on aspiration indicate the necessity for a pre-biopsy arteriogram.

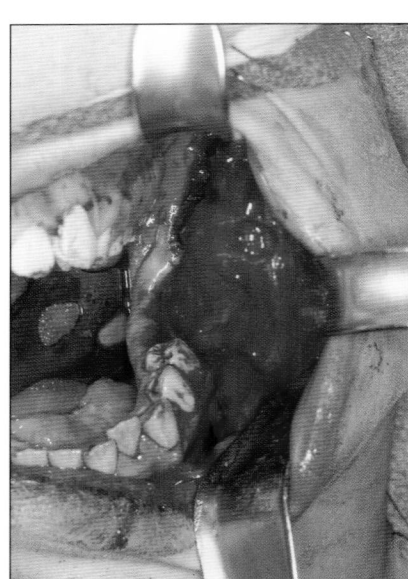

Fig 1-16 An incisional biopsy should also include a wide access to allow for visualization of the area and the most representative biopsy sampling.

color and texture of the lesion, and whether it is a solid multiloculated or a unilocular lesion. To be most representative, tissue specimens should be taken from the center of the lesion and from deep in the lesion. The incisional access should be closed with suture and without packing material unless packing is necessary to control hemorrhage.

The tissue specimen should be fixed in 10% neutral-buffered formalin. However, if an infectious disease is suspected, a portion of the lesion should be submitted for Gram staining and appropriate cultures before placing in formalin.

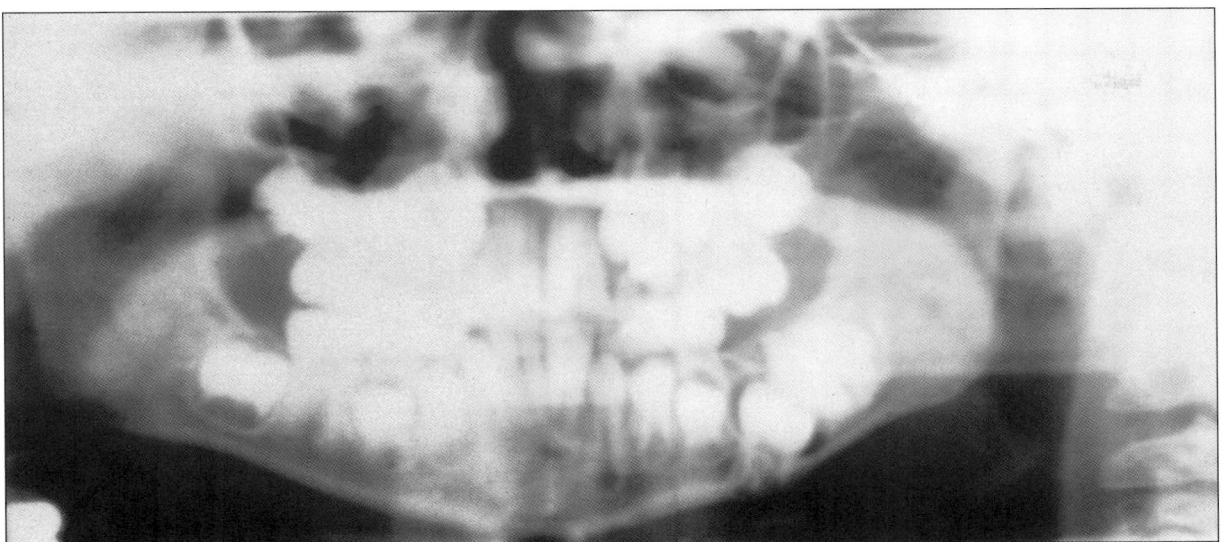

Fig 1-17 This radiopaque lesion shows a density greater than bone. Its similar density to that of adjacent teeth suggests tooth product formations, as was the case in this ameloblastic fibro-odontoma.

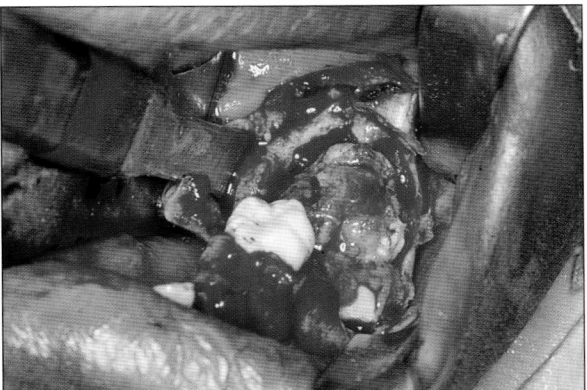

Fig 1-18 A midcrestal incision for access is the best and most versatile biopsy approach.

Radiopaque Lesions in Bone

Lesions are radiopaque because they produce either tumor bone or reactive bone or some calcified dental product, enamel, dentin, or cementum (Fig 1-17). Many radiographically obvious lesions such as odontomas may be enucleated at biopsy. However, most radiopaque lesions suggest a diverse differential diagnosis, including an osteomyelitis, fibro-osseous diseases, benign bone tumors, some vascular lesions, mixed odontogenic tumors, and osteosarcoma as well as other malignancies in bone, and therefore require an incisional biopsy. Because osteosarcomas, in particular, and many benign tumors in bone stimulate reactive bone responses at their periphery, it is especially important to obtain tissue from the lesion's center.

Unless the location of the lesion indicates a better entry area, a midcrestal incision usually provides the best access (Fig 1-18). Obtaining a tissue specimen from deep within the lesion's center may require osteotomes or a saw for removal. If there is associated soft tissue in the lesion, some of this should be included for histopathologic studies, including Gram stain and culture. Hard tissue specimens may be divided into two specimens. One specimen should be treated with a rapid decalcifying solution, which will provide a faster diagnosis but will result in lost cellular definition and may make the diagnosis less certain. The second specimen should be treated with a slower-acting decalcifying solution, which may take several weeks or more but will preserve cellular detail maximally for the best histopathologic assessment. The biopsy area should be sutured without packing the bony cavity unless packing is necessary for hemorrhage control.

Biopsy of a Mass at the Junction of the Hard and Soft Palate Mucosa

Mass lesions at the junction of the hard and soft palate mucosa are usually minor salivary gland tumors. Although other conditions and tumors such as neural tumors, non-Hodgkin lymphoma, and palatal abscesses are possible, they may be diagnosed with the same biopsy principles.

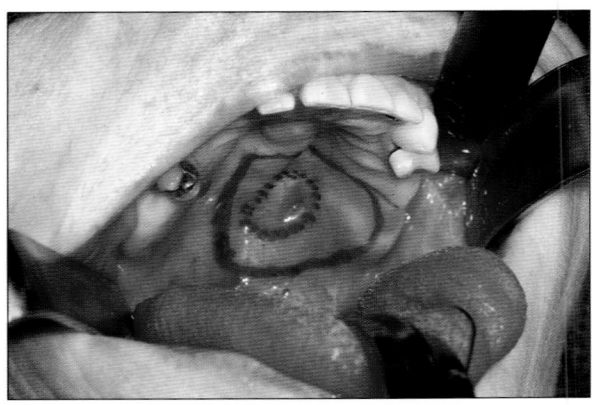

Fig 1-19 The palpable tumor mass is outlined with the solid line. The incisional biopsy outlined by the dotted line includes a sufficient amount of tissue for a histopathologic assessment with multiple cuts and sufficient tissue for reviews by consultants if necessary.

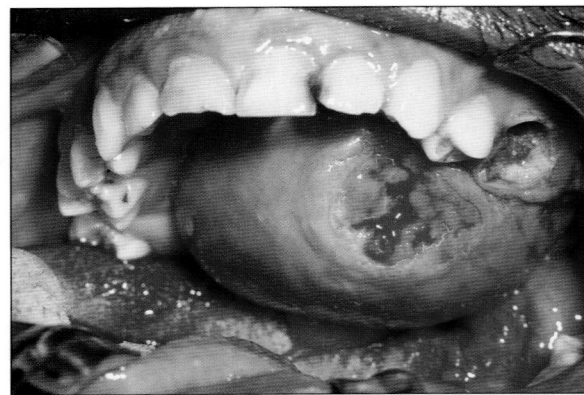

Fig 1-20 Incisional biopsies of a large tumor mass do not necessarily require a closure.

Anesthesia for this area should be a peripheral field block of local anesthesia. Direct injection of solution into the lesion, which could create artifacts, should be avoided. The biopsy should include an ellipse of overlying mucosa and a sample from the center of the mass (Fig 1-19). Because salivary gland histopathologic diagnoses are often overlapping and controversial, a large biopsy specimen is recommended to allow for multiple sections and special stains, and possibly outside consultation on slides or even tissue blocks. With adequate quantities of biopsy specimens, equivocal or uncertain diagnoses can be studied further and consultations can be made. The biopsy should approach the periosteum but need not include the periosteum or bone. If the lesion is ulcerated, some of the ulcer, its edge, and normal-appearing mucosa should be included as long as the biopsy does not violate the clinical borders of the mass. The resultant wound need not be sutured; it may be left open until definitive surgery is performed (Fig 1-20).

Nodules in the Lip or Cheek

Freely movable masses in the lip or cheek usually represent mucoceles, mucus cysts, minor salivary gland tumors, or diseased lymph nodes. If the mass is freely movable, it is simply excised with a straightforward pericapsular excision. Removal of overlying mucosa is not necessary. However, if the lesion approaches overlying mucosa, the mucosa may need to be included in the biopsy (Figs 1-21a and 1-21b). In most cases, this excisional biopsy is diagnostic and curative. If the mass is fixed or indurated, an inflammatory process or a malignancy is suggested. In such cases, it is best to perform an incisional biopsy (see Figs 1-21a and 1-21b).

Lesions of the Lower Lip Vermilion

Lesions of the lower lip vermilion are usually sun damage–related lesions, such as slow-growing squamous cell carcinomas, keratoacanthomas, and actinic keratoses, or lesions related to potential salivary gland diseases, such as mucoceles or minor salivary gland tumors. Mass lesions that involve the vermilion surface are best excised with 5-mm margins and frozen section control (Figs 1-22a and 1-22b). If this is not feasible, a preliminary incisional biopsy is also acceptable. In such cases, the biopsy incision should be placed vertically in the mass rather than horizontally, which would extend the margin into uninvolved

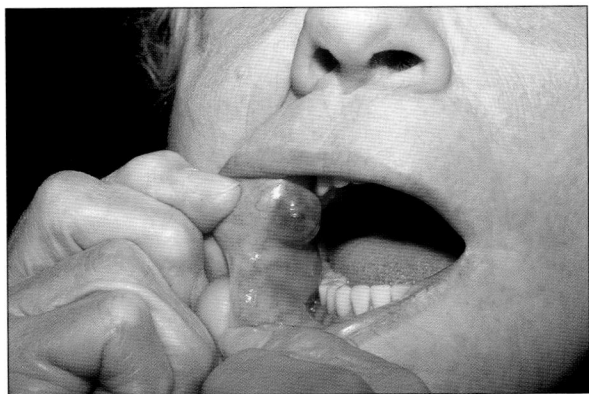

Fig 1-21a Biopsy of a movable mass in the buccal mucosa should be excisional with 1- to 2-mm margins. If indurated, the potential for a malignancy increases and an incisional biopsy is preferred.

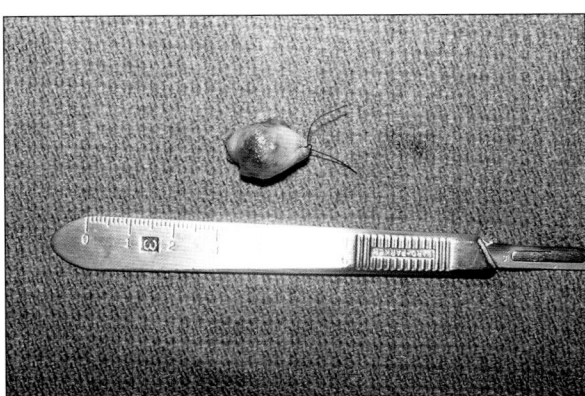

Fig 1-21b This pericapsular excisional biopsy and specimen would be curative for a fibroma, schwannoma, canalicular adenoma, or basal cell adenoma, but not for other salivary gland neoplasms, neurofibromas, or malignancies. In such cases, the specimen becomes an incisional rather than an excisional biopsy.

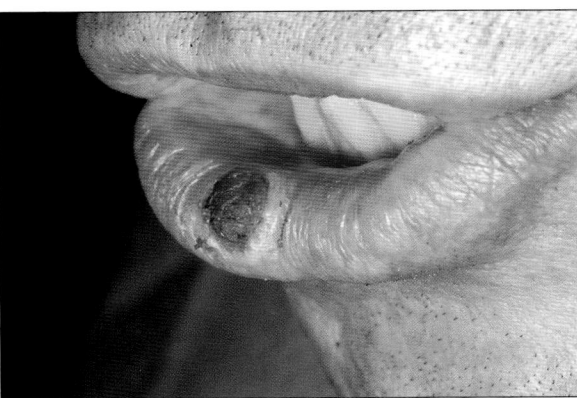

Fig 1-22a This exophytic mass of the lower lip vermilion most likely represents an exophytic lip carcinoma or a keratoacanthoma. Both are best treated for diagnosis and cure by an excisional biopsy.

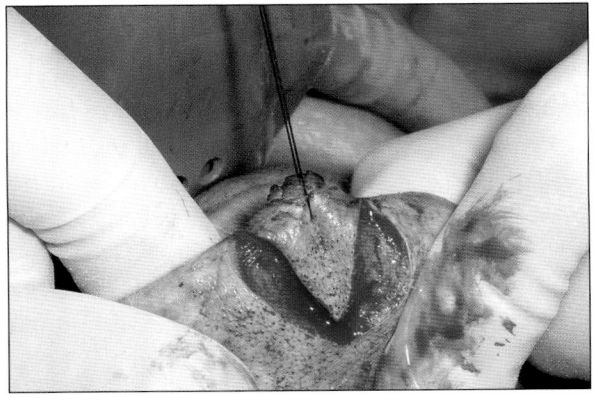

Fig 1-22b Small to moderate exophytic masses of the lower lip are excised with a V-excision using 5-mm margins. Traction sutures are useful in making precise 90-degree incisions.

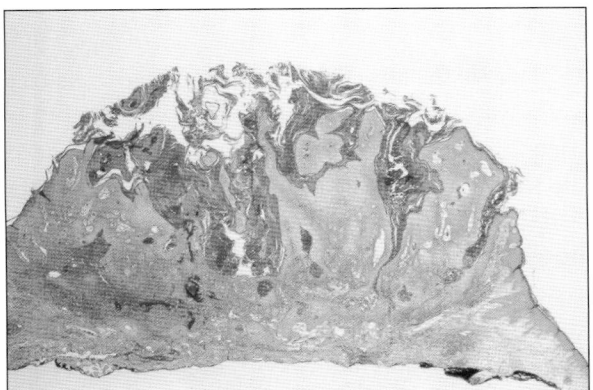

Fig 1-22c The lesion shown in Figs 1-22a and 1-22b was consistent with a keratoacanthoma; it is best diagnosed by this complete excisional specimen slide.

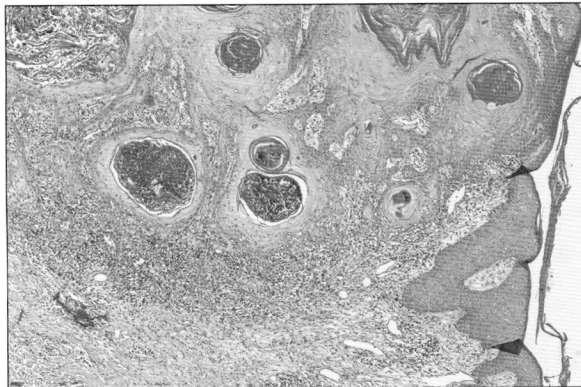

Fig 1-22d An incisional biopsy of the keratoacanthoma in Fig 1-22c shows the lesion's relationship to normal tissues and is consistent with a keratoacanthoma but is more equivocal than the full specimen seen in Fig 1-22c.

vermilion. Because keratoacanthoma, which is diagnosed by noting the normal epithelium at the edge of the mass rapidly plunging to form the keratoacanthoma base (Figs 1-22c and 1-22d), is included in the differential diagnosis, the biopsy specimen should include the edge of the mass and a small amount of normal tissue at the edge. The vertical placement of the incision keeps the biopsy site within the definitive excision specimen.

If a mass lesion of the vermilion is excised with 5-mm margins and clear frozen sections are produced, the lip can undergo a direct primary closure without creating a significant microstomia if the defect occupies 40% or less of the vermilion. If greater than 40% is excised, the lip will require flap reconstruction with either a Karapandzic flap or a modified Estlander flap.

Biopsy of a nodule in the substance of the lower or upper lip that does not involve the vermilion surface is best accomplished as a pericapsular dissection, which will resolve mucoceles, minor salivary gland stones, and some minor salivary gland tumors such as the canalicular adenoma and basal cell adenoma. Should a more aggressive tumor be diagnosed histopathologically, this original biopsy would be considered an incisional biopsy, and the biopsy area, marked by a nonresorbable suture, would be excised in a manner appropriate for the diagnosis.

Cervical Lymph Node Biopsies

The deep cervical lymph node chain is in the drainage pathway of many infectious and malignant diseases. The lymph nodes themselves are often the diseased organ, as it is in Hodgkin and non-Hodgkin lymphomas, cat-scratch disease, and sarcoidosis, among others. Therefore, a cervical lymph node biopsy can be a very useful diagnostic tool.

Before performing a cervical lymph node biopsy, the clinician should make an effort to rule out metastatic squamous cell carcinoma. This is done by the usual thorough oral examination, either an indirect or direct laryngoscopy or fiberoptic nasopharyngoscopy, and a fine-needle biopsy of the mass. If no primary carcinoma focus is found and the fine-needle biopsy fails to show atypical epithelial cells, a cervical mass–lymph node biopsy is indicated. This preliminary work-up is necessary to avoid violating the anatomic planes if cancer is found in the neck. Although removing a lymph node involved with metastatic carcinoma and treating the disease appropriately after resection have not been shown to promote recurrences or reduce survival, it is better to avoid the potential of seeding tumor cells in the neck and committing the patient to radiotherapy.

The goal of a cervical lymph node biopsy is to provide the pathologist with a large, representative specimen with an intact capsule that is well fixed to avoid autolysis; a touch preparation; and a culture specimen. The surgeon should choose the largest and deepest lymph node if several are involved (Fig 1-23a). Smaller superficial lymph nodes are too often reactive nodes overlying the actual area of pathology. The use of intravenous sedation or general anesthesia is recommended so that the largest and deepest lymph node can be removed without tearing the capsule and introducing artifacts into the specimen (Fig 1-23b). Before biopsy, a courtesy call to the receiving pathologist is advised. Some pathologists prefer to receive the specimen fresh or fresh frozen and make arrangements for shipping or courier delivery. If not, the pathologist should be asked if he or she wants the specimen or a portion of the specimen placed in a particular fixative. Some pathologists request 95% alcohol for best preservation of lymph node architecture, Michel's medium or B-5 for fine cytologic organelle and nuclear preservation, or glutaraldehyde for electron microscopy. If there is no preference, 10% neutral-buffered formalin is a good all-purpose choice.

The surgeon will need to remove the lymph node using a dissection that is deep to the platysma. The diseased lymph node will be doughy or rubbery and usually oblong (Fig 1-23c). The lymph node, which will lie on or adjacent to the internal jugular vein, should be removed with a pericapsular dissection. The surgeon should have an electrocautery available to coagulate small vessels, preventing bleeding that may obscure view of the dissection. The main reasons lymph node specimens are returned by the pathologist as nondiagnostic are lack of hemorrhage control and insufficient anesthesia. In these cases, the surgeon often damages the specimen because of obscured vision and a desire to expedite the procedure.

After the lymph node is removed and assuming the pathologist did not request the specimens fresh or fresh frozen, the surgeon should do a touch preparation first. This is done by slicing the lymph node specimen in half through its smaller circumference. Like a rubber stamp, the cut edge is pressed lightly on a dry glass slide without a twisting motion (Fig 1-23d). Two such imprints can be placed on one slide. The slide is then placed into either formalin or 95% alcohol. The touch preparation will provide a monolayer of cells and thus allow the pathologist a better visualization of cellular and nuclear detail (Fig 1-23e). The remaining specimen is sliced into 2-mm-thick sections, like a loaf of bread (Fig 1-23f). A central section is further cut into smaller sections for various cultures. The remaining sections can then be placed into the requested fixative. The fixative volume should be 10 times the volume of the specimen. Lymph nodes have very little stroma and are, therefore, prone to autolysis, which can make the specimen nondiagnostic. Cutting 2-mm sections and using a high fixative-to-specimen volume ratio will prevent such autolysis.

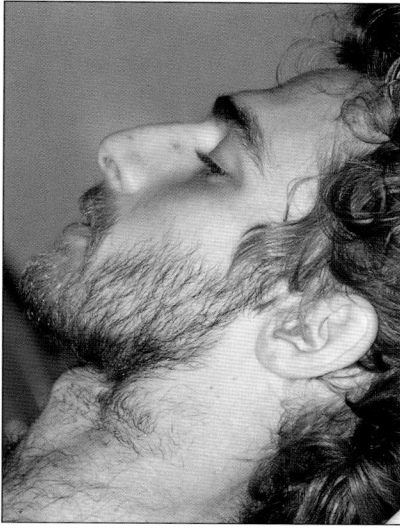

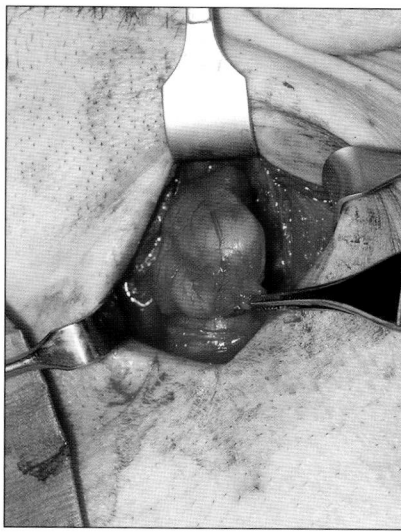

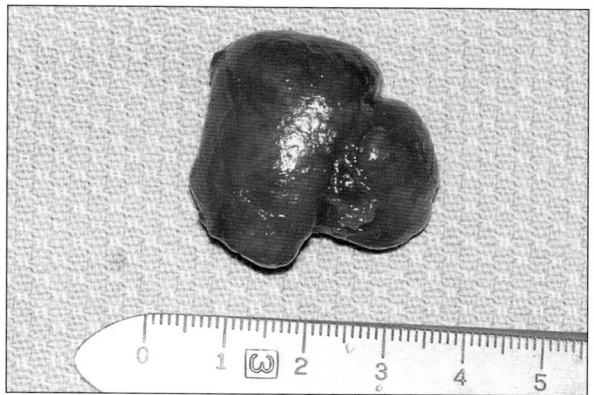

Fig 1-23a Two clinically enlarged cervical lymph nodes. The largest and deepest lymph node is usually more diagnostic and is therefore the preferred one to be removed for diagnosis.

Fig 1-23b The lymph node should be removed without entering the node and with the capsule intact. Tissue forceps should engage the pericapsular fat rather than the capsule.

Fig 1-23c Pathologic lymph nodes are oblong rather than the normal oval shape. It is not uncommon for two lymph nodes to be fused together, as seen here.

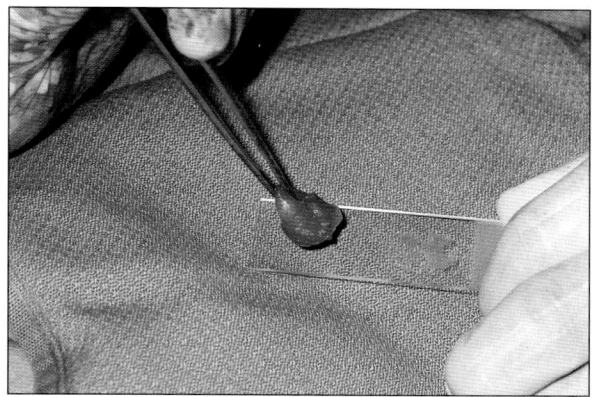

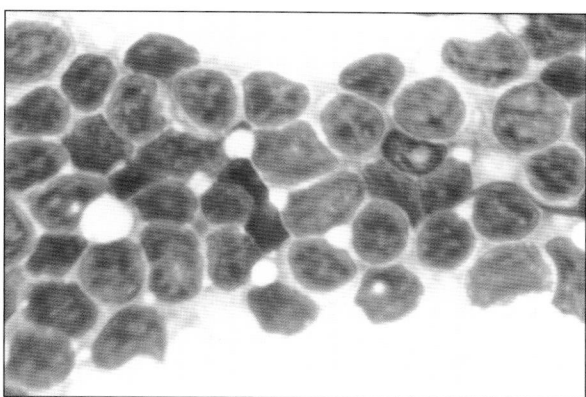

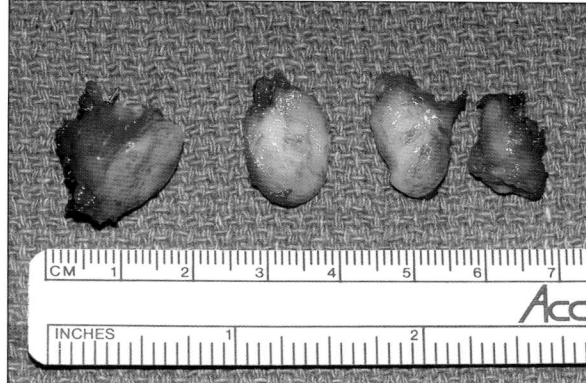

Fig 1-23d A "touch prep" can be accomplished by sectioning the lymph node and imprinting the cut edge on a clean, dry glass slide.

Fig 1-23e The single layer of cells obtained from a touch preparation allows for greater clarity of cellular detail that would otherwise be masked by additional cell layers.

Fig 1-23f It is best to slice lymph nodes into 2-mm-thick slices. One slice should be subdivided and sent for various cultures and the other placed into the fixative or fixatives preferred by the pathologist.

Specimens removed and submitted in this manner will allow for a more rapid and unequivocal diagnosis and, therefore, early treatment. Repeated biopsy of lymph nodes can be virtually eliminated. Because the newer classifications of lymphoma rely heavily on cytologic detail and nuclear shape, well preserved, representative tissue specimens are especially critical.

Inflammatory, Reactive, and Infectious Diseases

▶ *"The desire to take medicine is perhaps the greatest feature that distinguishes man from animals."*

—William Osler

Inflammation and Repair

Inflammation and repair are fundamental processes that pervade the spectrum of pathology. They represent a continuum of constant change, so that any given microscopic view represents only a "freeze-frame" in the evolution of any inflammatory lesion.

Inflammation is the reaction of vascular tissue to injury, be it physical, chemical, bacterial, or immunologic in nature. The result is a dilation of capillaries (Fig 2-1a), swelling of endothelium, margination of polymorphonuclear leukocytes (Fig 2-1b), and subsequent migration of neutrophils, followed by plasma, through the vessel wall (ie, a vascular change followed by exudation). This is characteristic of the acute phase of inflammation. The neutrophils remove and digest the inciting agent. Repair may follow with the formation of granulation tissue, which is the result of ingrowth by capillaries and fibroblasts (Fig 2-1c).

The inflammatory process may resolve completely with no adverse effect on the host. Alternatively, there may be a "walling off" with focal destruction of tissue secondary to the action of the neutrophils. This may result in abscess and/or scar formation (Fig 2-1d). If there is failure to eliminate the injurious agent, the more prolonged state of chronic inflammation occurs, which typically results in fibrosis and scarring (Fig 2-1e). Although inflammation and repair are sequential in acute inflammation, in chronic inflammation they are simultaneous. The short-lived neutrophils are reinforced and eventually replaced by the much hardier macrophages with the addition of lymphocytes and plasma cells, and the inflammatory process hence acquires an immunologic component.

In some specific cases, the inciting agent persists; it may be sequestered within macrophages, where, if it exists in particulate form or in high concentrations, it can stimulate the formation of a granuloma in which the "wandering" macrophage becomes immobile and mature (Fig 2-2a). If it induces a strong delayed hypersensitivity response, the macrophages may develop into so-called epithelioid cells (Fig 2-2b). These cells are not really epithelial cells but mature macrophages from the blood monocyte lineage that vaguely take on an appearance resembling an epithelial cell. There may also be cytoplasmic fusion of macrophages with the resultant formation of multinucleated giant cells. Granulomas may show necrosis if the inciting agent is highly toxic or if it induces a marked delayed hypersensitivity reaction. There may also be a superimposed infiltration of neutrophils, eosinophils, and/or lymphocytes. Once destruction of the injurious agent has occurred, the macrophage dies, disperses, or reverts to a less mature form. The granuloma then resolves to form fibrosis (scar).

Many factors influence the specific inflammatory picture. Trauma-induced inflammation tends to have a sparser cellular component than that caused by microorganisms. The type of agent may alter the nature of the cellular component, as for example the marked eosinophilic response that is seen secondary to parasites.

Inflammation itself also acts as a stimulus to repair. Platelets begin the repair process by secreting platelet-derived growth factors (PDGFaa, PDGFab, PDGFbb), which induce cellular proliferation and capillary angiogenesis, as well as several transforming growth factor-betas (TGF-betas), which promote not

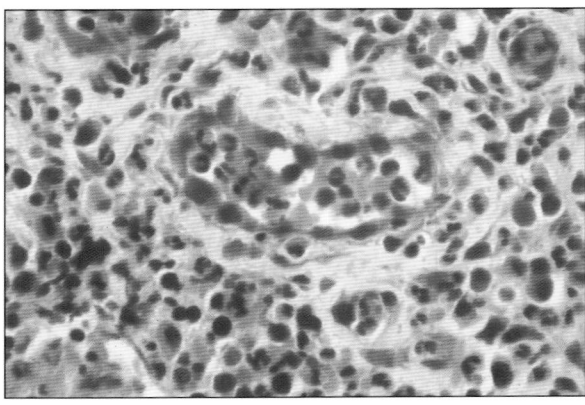

Fig 2-1a A capillary lined by swollen endothelial cells in the center of the field. Neutrophils migrate between the endothelial cells into the surrounding tissue (diapedesis).

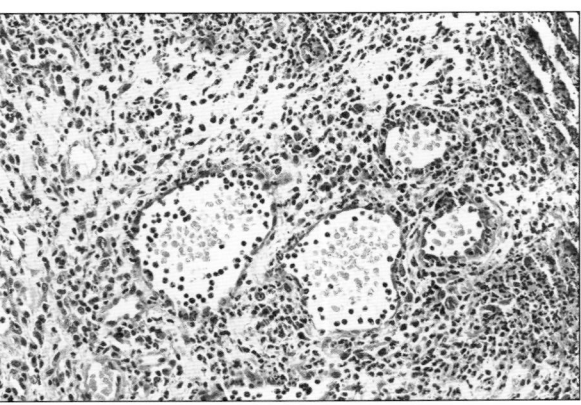

Fig 2-1b Dilated capillaries showing margination of neutrophils.

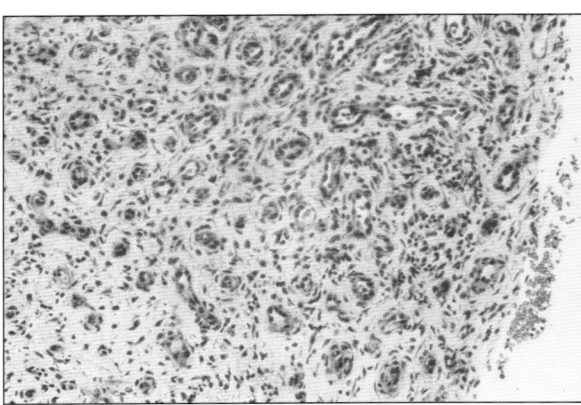

Fig 2-1c Numerous capillaries in a background of fibrous tissue with some inflammatory cells, typical of granulation tissue.

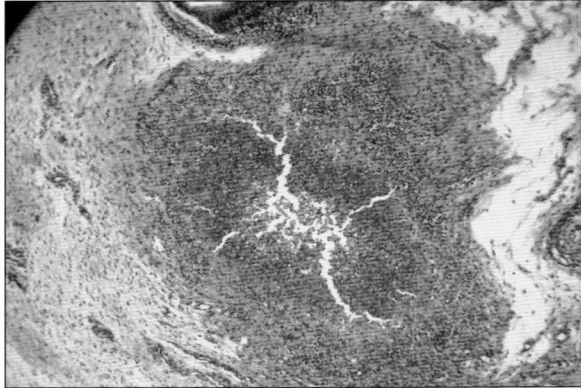

Fig 2-1d An abscess showing liquefaction and an influx of neutrophils in the center. Beyond that are chronic inflammatory cells and fibrous tissue.

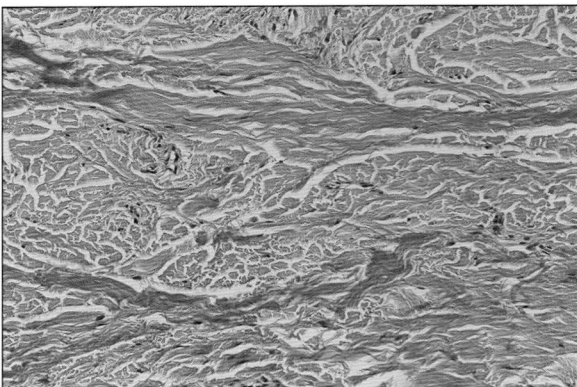

Fig 2-1e Densely collagenized, sparsely cellular tissue, characteristic of scar tissue.

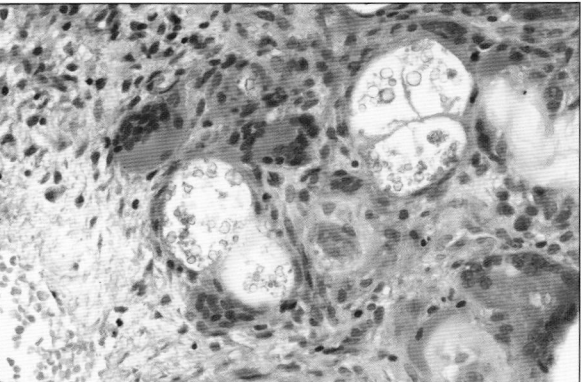

Fig 2-2a A foreign body granuloma in which the exogenous material is surrounded by multinucleated giant cells. The cells contort themselves around the foreign body. Additional giant cells and inflammatory cells are seen. The giant cells develop by cytoplasmic fusion of macrophages.

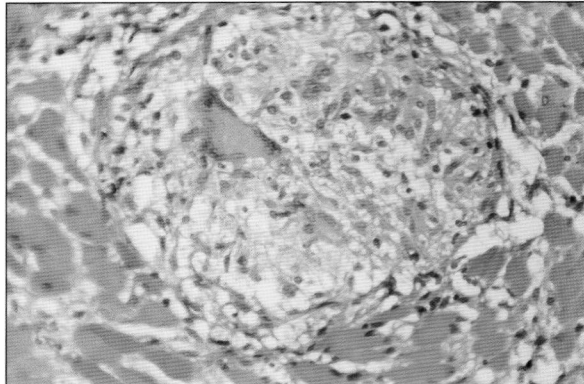

Fig 2-2b A so-called epithelioid granuloma in which there is an organized cluster of immunologically altered macrophages (epithelioid cells) with some lymphocytes and a multinucleated giant cell of the Langhans type (peripherally located nuclei).

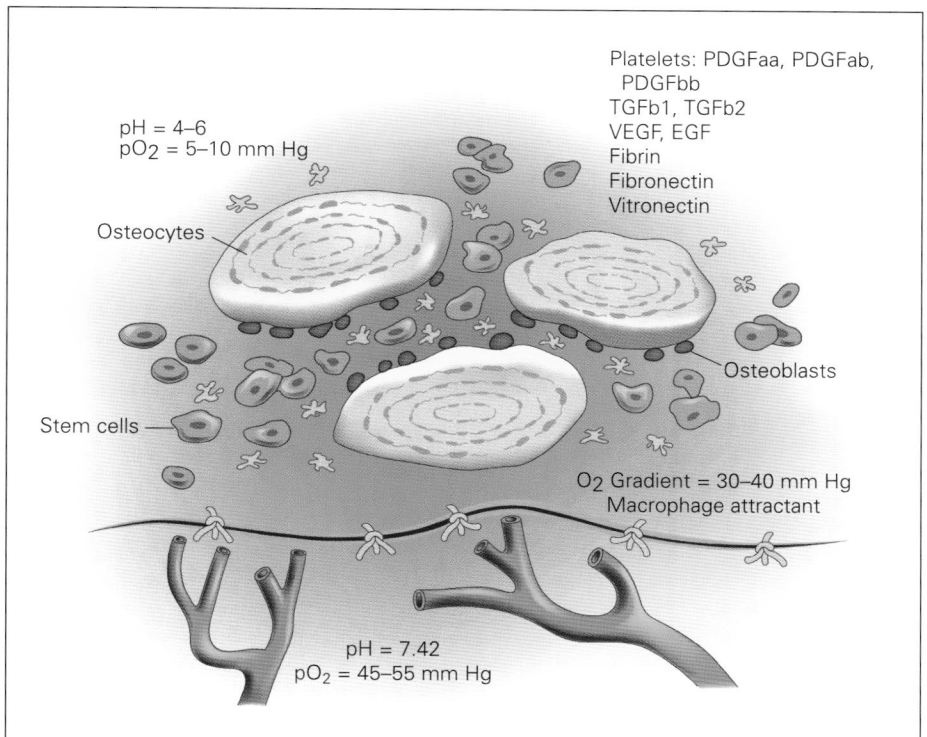

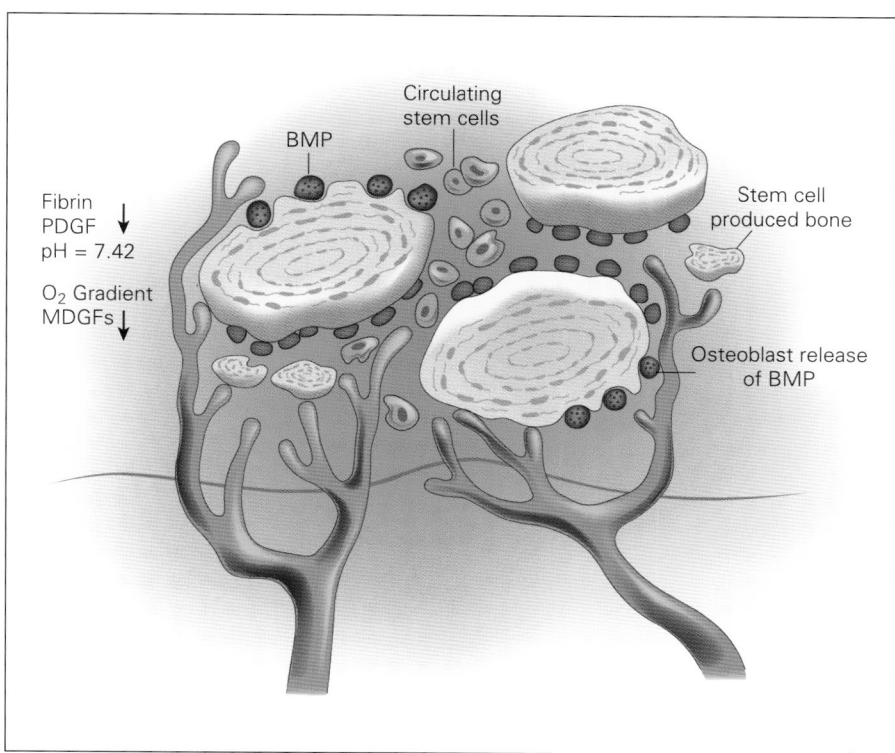

Fig 2-3a As shown in this illustration of a bone graft, platelets are the initiators of wound healing. They secrete at least seven different growth factors (cytokines) that stimulate and direct the healing process. Their effect continues for about 7 days, after which the macrophage takes over wound-healing direction and stimulation by secreting its own growth factors.

Fig 2-3b Revascularization of the wound prevents overexuberant cellular proliferation by normalizing the oxygen gradient, thereby down regulating macrophage function. Revascularization also allows the osteoclast access to resorb nonviable bone, if present, or to remodel viable bone.

only cellular proliferation and angiogenesis but connective tissue differentiation. They also secrete vascular endothelial growth factor (VEGF), which promotes capillary angiogenesis, and epithelial growth factor (EGF), which promotes epithelial proliferation to cover an open wound. When platelets are exhausted, macrophages take over repair modulation after 7 to 10 days. The platelets arrive at the injured site via the ubiquitous blood clot from vascular injury. The macrophages arrive in the area via migration in response to hypoxia in the wound. The macrophages then secrete PDGFs and various TGF-betas, as well as other growth factors to modulate repair (Figs 2-3a and 2-3b). When revascularization is nearly complete (about 21 days), the reversal of the wound hypoxia causes the macrophages to down regulate their growth-factor secretions and leave the area. Consequently, the wound repair slows to a final completion and does not progress indefinitely as does a tumor.

Under certain circumstances, this process becomes overexuberant or induces reactive changes. Examples of this may be found in the first group of lesions presented in this chapter.

Inflammatory and Reactive Diseases

Inflammatory Fibrous Hyperplasia

The oral mucosa is subjected to many inflammatory stimuli, and the consequence of repeated low-grade insults with reparative fibrous reactions may lead to common, nonspecific lesions that histologically are inflammatory fibrous hyperplasias. Two lesions with specific clinical features are discussed here.

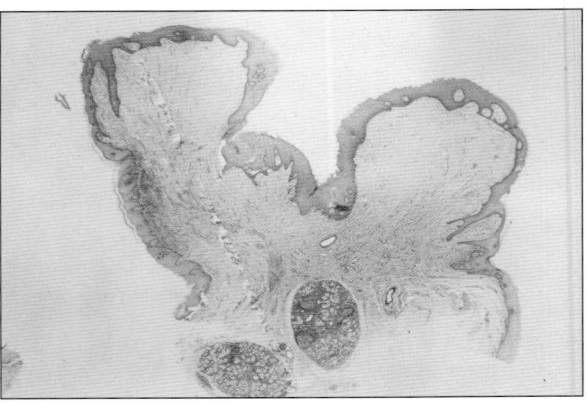

Fig 2-4 Low-power view of an epulis fissuratum. The central depression corresponds to the groove formed by the denture flange. The specimen shows a fibrous hyperplasia. There are some inflammatory foci, predominantly adjacent to the epithelium but also apparent within the mucous glands at the base.

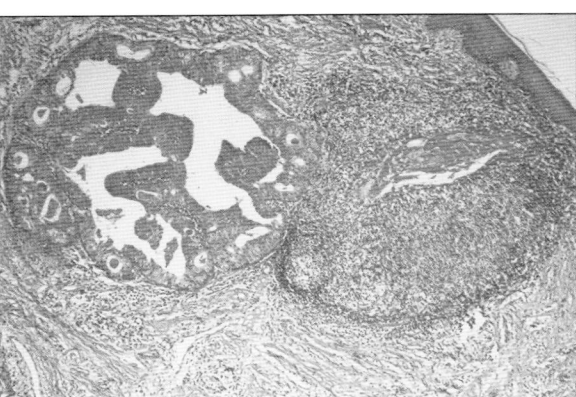

Fig 2-5 High-power view of changes in a salivary duct located within an epulis fissuratum. The ductal epithelium has proliferated in a papillary pattern, and hyperplasia of lymphoid tissue is seen adjacent to the duct. The picture is reminiscent of a Warthin tumor.

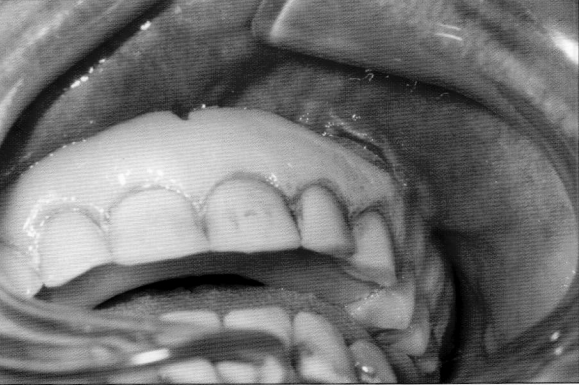

Fig 2-6a Ill-fitting denture with what seems to be an epulis fissuratum around the flange.

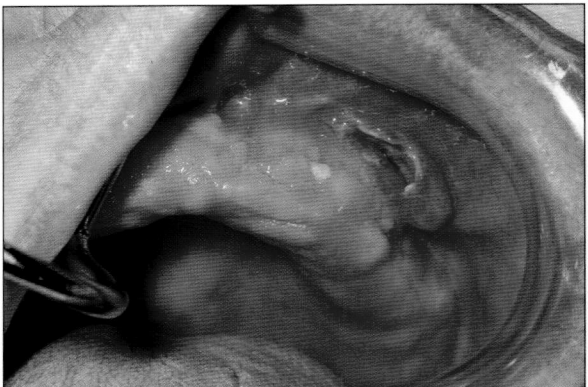

Fig 2-6b With the denture removed, the tissue excess and ulcer can be better visualized. A biopsy of the lesion revealed a squamous cell carcinoma.

Epulis Fissuratum

Epulis fissurata are inflammatory fibrous hyperplasias that are found most commonly in the mucolabial and mucobuccal folds and arise secondary to irritation from a denture flange. Typically, a central groove is present within the mass, corresponding to the margin of the denture. Although often covered by an intact mucosa, the lesions may sometimes be ulcerated.

Histologically, the lesions are composed of an increased quantity of fibrous tissue with varying numbers of chronic inflammatory cells, which are predominantly plasma cells (Fig 2-4). Changes in the underlying minor salivary glands, ranging from a nonspecific chronic sialadenitis to a papillary oncocytic ductal hyperplasia, are often seen (Fig 2-5).

The most significant feature of the epulis fissuratum is that it may actually represent a squamous cell carcinoma that has proliferated around a denture flange (Figs 2-6a and 2-6b). Therefore, a suspected epulis fissuratum is managed by excision and biopsy to eradicate the lesion and to rule out a possible malignancy and by relining or remaking the prosthetic appliance that was presumably the inciting agent of the inflammation.

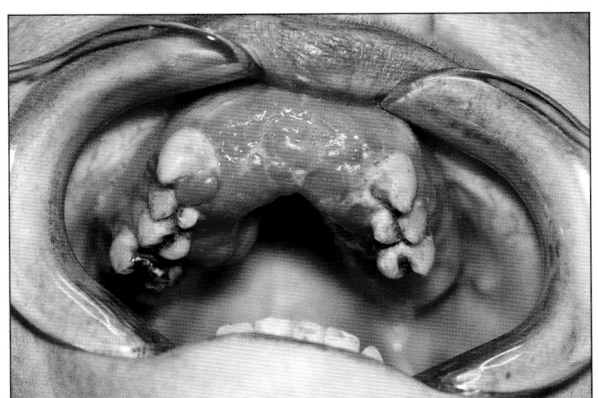

Fig 2-7a Inflammatory papillomatosis outlining the exact coverage of an ill-fitting, porous partial denture.

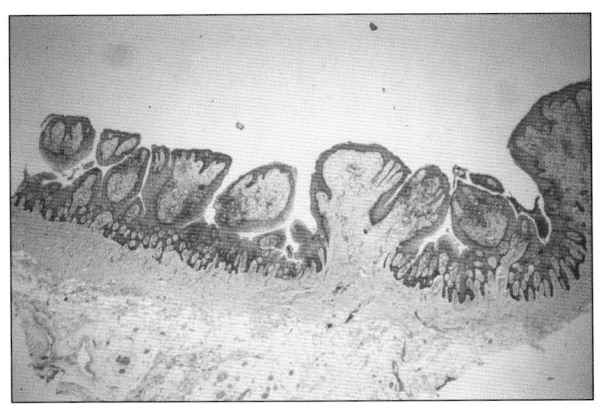

Fig 2-7b Inflammatory papillomatosis often has a multinodular surface that is the result of a fibrous hyperplasia. Inflammatory cells can be seen below the epithelium.

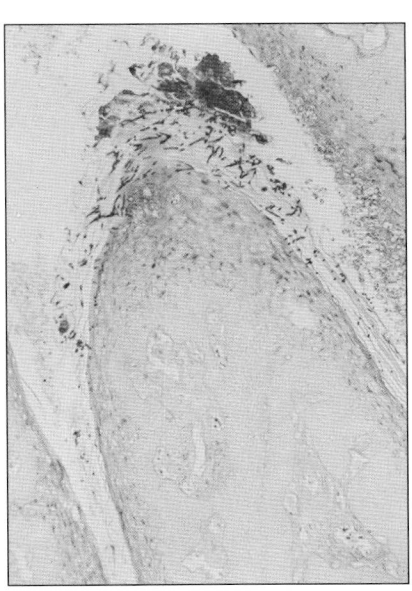

Fig 2-7c The crevices formed by the projections in papillomatosis are a good environment for proliferation of candidal organisms. Here the hyphae can be seen (periodic acid–Schiff [PAS] stain).

Inflammatory Papillomatosis

Although papillomatosis may occasionally be seen in other areas, the maxilla, gingiva, and hard palate are by far the most common sites. In almost all cases, it is associated with an ill-fitting denture. The palatal vault is commonly involved and it has a granular, multinodular appearance that is erythematous (Fig 2-7a).

Histologically, the multinodular surface is covered by a usually intact parakeratinized epithelium. The nodules or papillary projections consist of fibrous tissue with varying degrees of chronic inflammation (Fig 2-7b). The surface crypts may sometimes harbor candidal organisms, which may also have a stimulatory action on this lesion (Fig 2-7c). The clinical management of this common condition is usually nonsurgical. The denture must be rebased or relined and the infection treated with anticandidal drugs. Nystatin oral suspension 100,000 U/mL, a white tasteless solution, 5 mL (1 tsp), is used four times daily as a swish and swallow and also placed under the denture. In addition or as an alternative, nystatin powder 100,000 U/g may be placed under the denture. Persistent cases may require the addition of fluconazole (Diflucan, Pfizer US), 100 mg daily, to a nystatin regimen.

Pyogenic Granuloma

CLINICAL PRESENTATION AND PATHOGENESIS ▶

Given that these lesions are neither pus-producing nor granulomatous, the term *pyogenic granuloma* actually represents a double misnomer. However, the term is universally understood, and any attempts to change it are likely to cause confusion.

A pyogenic granuloma will present as a soft, fleshy, easily bleeding red mass. It will often be found on the skin and particularly on the face. Pyogenic granulomas are also common in the oral cavity, where they are usually found arising from the interdental gingiva (Fig 2-8a). They occur at any age and are often stimulated by a foreign object such as the sharp margin of a restoration, calculus, or a foreign body within the gingival crevice. Typically, these are red-purple in color and may be ulcerated with a fibrinopurulent covering. They also occur infrequently on the lips, tongue, or buccal mucosa and then only in association

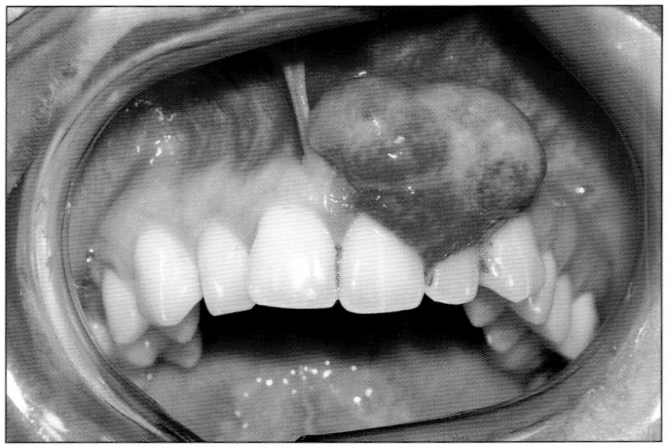

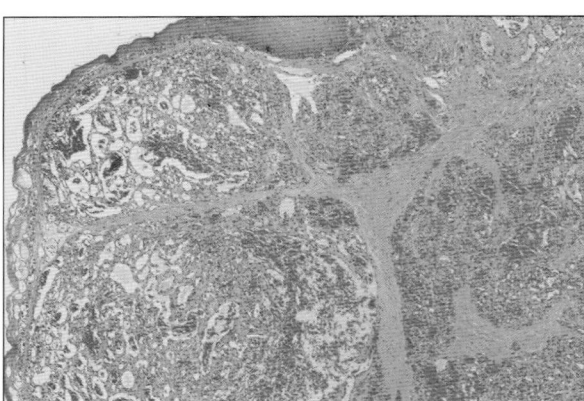

Fig 2-8a A large pyogenic granuloma (in this case, a so-called pregnancy tumor) that persisted for 1 year after childbirth and required excision.

Fig 2-8b The lobular pattern is apparent in this pyogenic granuloma.

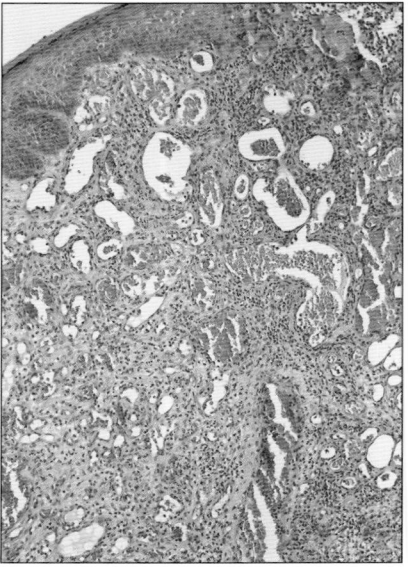

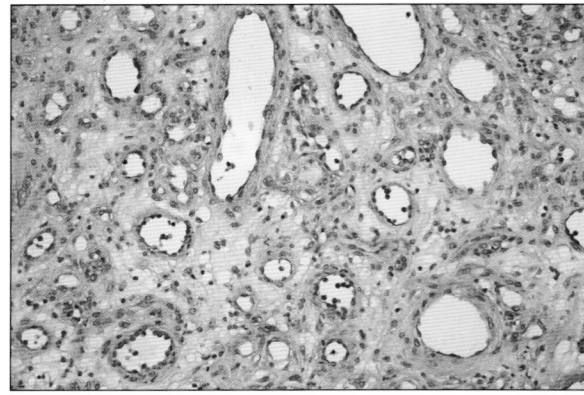

Fig 2-8c The pyogenic granuloma contains numerous capillaries. Some are widely dilated while others have very small lumina. An inflammatory infiltrate is present within the supporting fibrous tissue.

Fig 2-8d High-power view of a pyogenic granuloma showing the prominent endothelial cells lining the dilated capillaries.

with a puncture wound or foreign body. They often undergo initial rapid growth and then remain static in size. They bleed readily when traumatized.

The pyogenic granuloma represents inflammation and repair attempts that are stymied due to ongoing etiologic stimulation. It, therefore, amounts to hyperplastic granulation tissue.

DIFFERENTIAL DIAGNOSIS ▶

A pyogenic granuloma is clinically indistinguishable from a *peripheral giant cell proliferation*. A *peripheral ossifying fibroma* will also resemble a pyogenic granuloma, except that the latter is usually more firm and not as red. Of greatest importance, however, is its clinical resemblance to a *primary or metastatic malignancy*. *Squamous cell carcinoma, fibrosarcoma, leukemia, non-Hodgkin lymphoma,* and *metastatic foci from the breast, lung, kidney, prostate,* etc, have been known to seed bone and proliferate a soft tissue mass, mimicking a pyogenic granuloma.

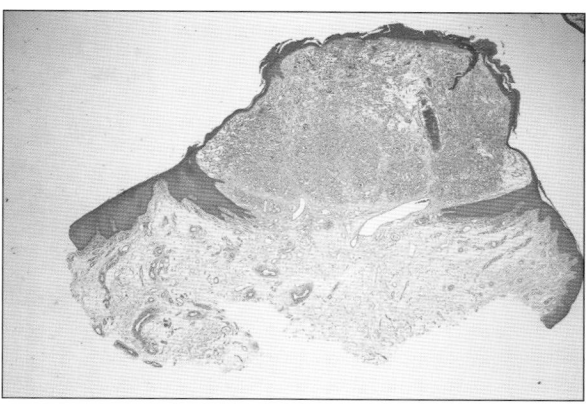

Fig 2-9 Low-power view showing the obvious exophytic nature of this pyogenic granuloma and the collarette of epithelium that develops below the lesion. A feeding vessel can be seen in the center of the field.

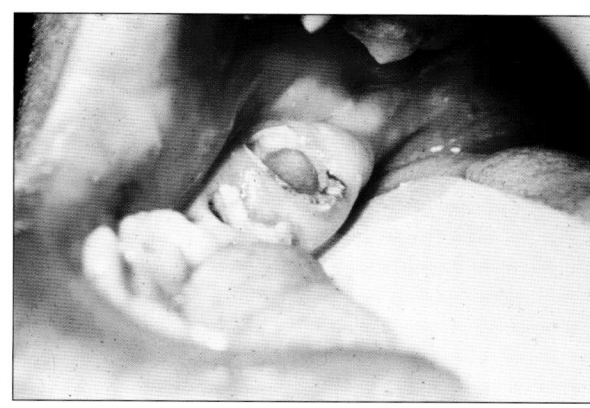

Fig 2-10 A so-called pulp polyp can be seen in this open caries lesion in a permanent first molar.

DIAGNOSTIC WORK-UP ▶

A pyogenic granuloma is a lesion of clinical recognition. However, a periapical or panoramic radiograph is advised to rule out bony destruction suggestive of malignancy or to identify a foreign body or sharp restorative margin that would need to be removed with the lesion.

HISTOPATHOLOGY ▶

These lesions, which are not actually granulomas, consist of exuberant granulation tissue, sometimes in a lobular arrangement (Fig 2-8b). There is a marked proliferation of endothelial cells. The capillary channels tend to be dilated and lined by prominent endothelial cells (Figs 2-8c and 2-8d). The stroma is fibrillar and often edematous. Inflammatory cells will be present and may include neutrophils, lymphocytes, and plasma cells. Sometimes an underlying collarette of epithelium will be seen (Fig 2-9). Because of the inflammatory nature of these lesions, their histologic appearance may vary, with evidence of fibrosis indicating a reparative phase. This may eventuate in the formation of a fibroma.

The so-called pregnancy tumor is nothing more than a pyogenic granuloma that appears to arise more readily in the hormonally primed gingiva. The "pulp polyp" also is a pyogenic granuloma that occurs in children or young adults with open caries lesions and large pulp openings that have a rich vascular supply. Thus primary molars and the first permanent molars are the sites of predilection (Fig 2-10).

TREATMENT ▶

A pyogenic granuloma should be excised with 2-mm margins at its clinical periphery and to a depth to the periosteum or to the causative agent. Any foreign body, calculus, or defective restoration should be removed as part of the excision.

PROGNOSIS ▶

Recurrence is rare and is almost always related either to a failure to remove the stimulating factor or to the so-called pregnancy tumor, which may continue or recur because of ongoing hormonal stimulation.

Peripheral Ossifying Fibroma

CLINICAL PRESENTATION AND PATHOGENESIS ▶

The peripheral ossifying fibroma is one of a triad of lesions that present as a gingival mass, usually emerging from interdental gingiva and seemingly from the periodontal ligament (Fig 2-11). The other two lesions are the pyogenic granuloma, which may represent an early immature form of the peripheral ossifying fibroma, and the peripheral giant cell proliferation. The peripheral ossifying fibroma will be more firm and have a less friable nature than the other two lesions.

The mass will usually have a broad base, but it may also have a pedunculated appearance. It is slightly more common in young adults, in women, and in the anterior quadrant of either arch. A close examination of the base will identify an emergence from the periodontal ligament space. The associated teeth are usually not mobile.

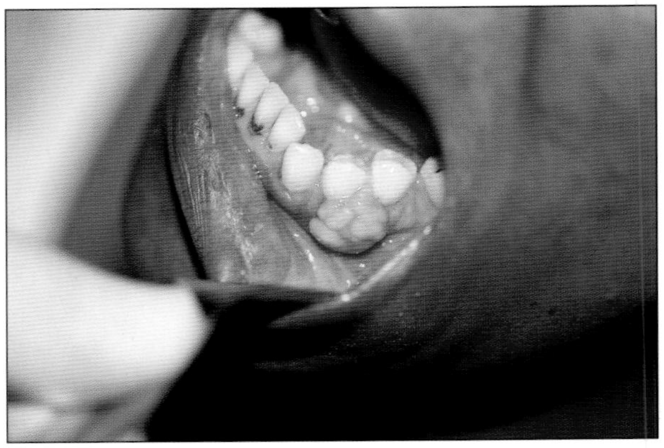

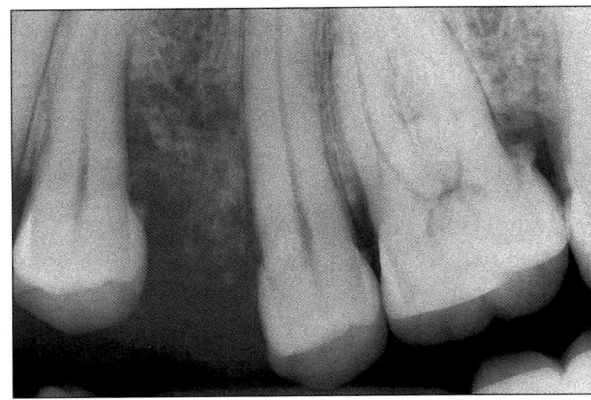

Fig 2-11 A peripheral ossifying fibroma is firm and will arise from the periodontal membrane space.

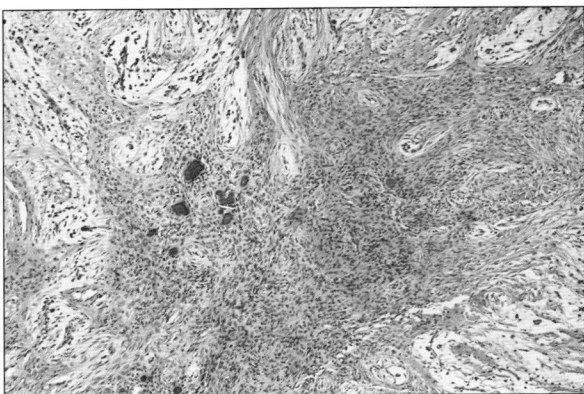

Fig 2-12 In some cases, the ossifications within a peripheral ossifying fibroma are sufficiently dense to be seen on a periapical radiograph.

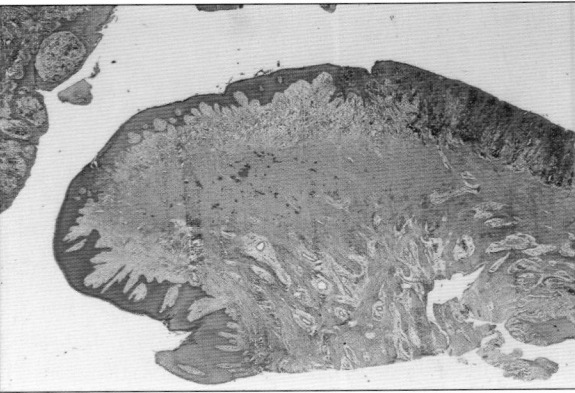

Fig 2-13a Peripheral ossifying fibroma showing an exophytic gingival mass consisting essentially of dense cellular fibrous tissue containing some small scattered ossifications. Inflammatory cells also can be seen.

Fig 2-13b Higher-power view of Fig 2-13a showing the cellularity of the dense fibrous tissue, the ossifications, and the inflammatory cells, which are predominantly plasma cells, in the looser stroma.

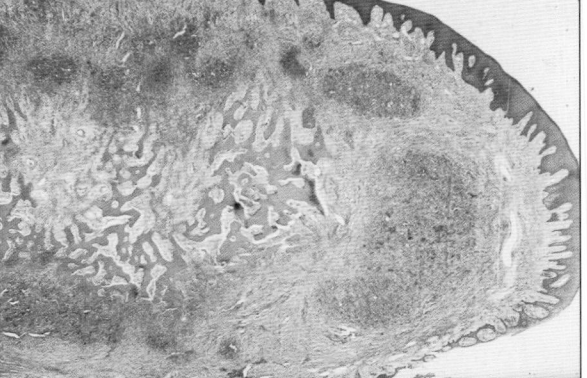

Fig 2-14a Two areas can be seen within this mass, one representing a peripheral giant cell proliferation and the other containing osseous trabeculae consistent with a peripheral ossifying fibroma.

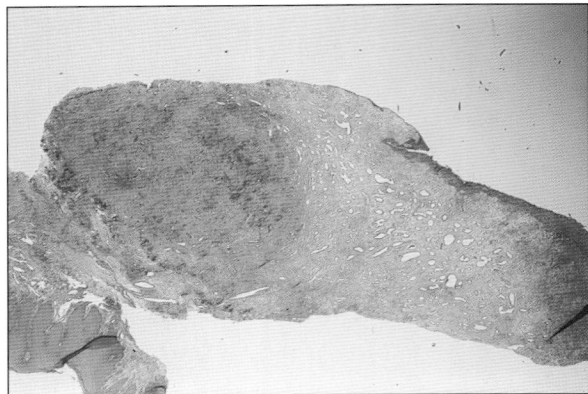

Fig 2-14b This mass shows an area of peripheral giant cell proliferation on the left and pyogenic granuloma on the right.

The fact that this lesion emerges from the periodontal ligament and is not seen in edentulous areas suggests its origin to be the connective tissue elements of the periodontal ligament. The fact that ossifications are found in these lesions is, therefore, not surprising since cementum and lamina dura are part of the periodontal ligament complex. The variant that shows odontogenic epithelium within it, ie, the peripheral odontogenic fibroma, is also not surprising, since rests of Malassez are rather abundant in the periodontal ligament and can easily become incorporated into lesions arising from the periodontal ligament.

DIFFERENTIAL DIAGNOSIS ▶

A peripheral ossifying fibroma must be distinguished histologically from a *pyogenic granuloma* or a *peripheral giant cell proliferation*. In addition, gingival masses, particularly those arising from deeper tissues, should suggest a possible *primary malignant lesion* or even a *metastatic malignancy*.

RADIOGRAPHIC FINDINGS ▶

A periapical radiograph may or may not detect the small foci of ossifications in these lesions. In those with a great amount of ossification, radiopaque flecks will be apparent on routine periapical radiographs (Fig 2-12) and may even appear on a panoramic radiograph. In the more usual case, the lesion will contain only small amounts of ossifications and will not be visible on a periapical radiograph because of the other mineral-dense structures in the field, such as teeth, restorations, and alveolar bone. Therefore, in cases where a peripheral ossifying fibroma is high on the differential list, a radiograph of the excised specimen is recommended. It will show subtle radiopacities that would otherwise not be evident.

HISTOPATHOLOGY ▶

The peripheral ossifying fibroma is yet another reactive lesion found on the gingiva, despite the nomenclature that suggests a neoplasm. The lesion consists of very cellular fibrous tissue with areas of more delicate fibrovascular tissue that often contain an inflammatory component rich in plasma cells (Fig 2-13a). Within the cellular areas, ossifications are usually present (Fig 2-13b). These vary considerably both in quality and quantity. Small, rounded calcific deposits may be seen, or, at the other extreme, broad osseous trabeculae lined by active osteoblasts may be formed. Sometimes ossification is such that the specimen requires decalcification before sectioning. Multinucleated giant cells may sometimes be present but are not a prominent component. The mass is not encapsulated.

In a differential diagnosis of surgically excised gingival masses, the pyogenic granuloma, peripheral giant cell proliferation, and peripheral ossifying fibroma are considered together, although each appears to be a distinct clinicopathologic entity. They may overlap, and the histologic features of more than one entity may occur within a single lesion (Figs 2-14a and 2-14b). Present knowledge indicates that these are all reactive lesions.

TREATMENT ▶

The peripheral ossifying fibroma is treated by local excision with surgical margins at the periphery of the lesion and deep margins to include its periodontal ligament origin. Failure to excise the periodontal ligament origin will predispose to recurrence, which has been reported to be as high as 20%.

Peripheral Giant Cell Proliferation

CLINICAL PRESENTATION AND PATHOGENESIS ▶

A peripheral giant cell proliferation will present as a soft, fleshy, broad-based, and easily bleeding mass (Fig 2-15). Like the pyogenic granuloma, it will arise from the gingiva, but unlike the pyogenic granuloma, it may also arise from an edentulous ridge and not from extragingival sites such as the lips, tongue, or buccal mucosa. Also, like the pyogenic granuloma, some peripheral giant cell proliferations are associated with failing dental restorations, sharp tooth edges, or foreign bodies. Some will attain sizes of 5 to 7 cm and may develop superficial ulcerations with a fibrin base, mimicking a fungating tumor. There is a slight female predilection.

The peripheral giant cell proliferation is an enigmatic lesion that seems to arise from the periosteum or periodontal ligament and contains granulation tissue with osteoclasts. The presence of such giant cells (osteoclasts) and its designation as a giant cell lesion should not raise concerns about hyperparathyroidism. There is no known association between these lesions and primary, secondary, or tertiary hyperparathyroidism.

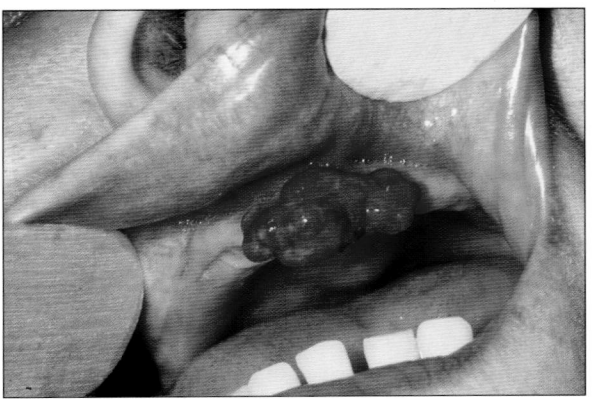

Fig 2-15 The peripheral giant cell proliferation is an exophytic red friable mass that often arises from a source of inflammation such as a root tip, a foreign body, a sharp crown margin, etc.

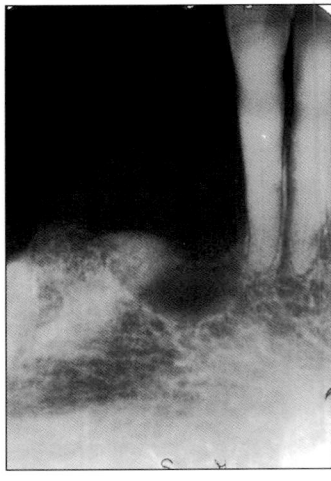

Fig 2-16a Periapical radiograph showing the typical cupped-out resorption of the alveolar crest by a peripheral giant cell proliferation.

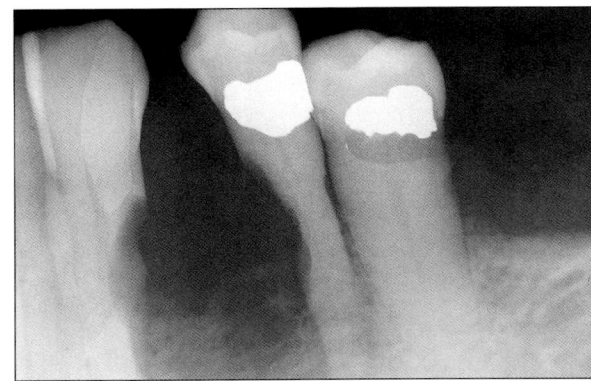

Fig 2-16b The resorptive capacity of a peripheral giant cell proliferation is illustrated by the destruction of the teeth adjacent to the mass.

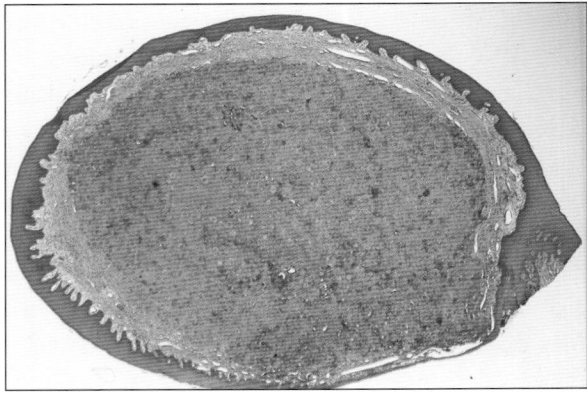

Fig 2-17a Low-power view of a peripheral giant cell proliferation showing a well-demarcated mass that stands out against the normal subepithelial connective tissue.

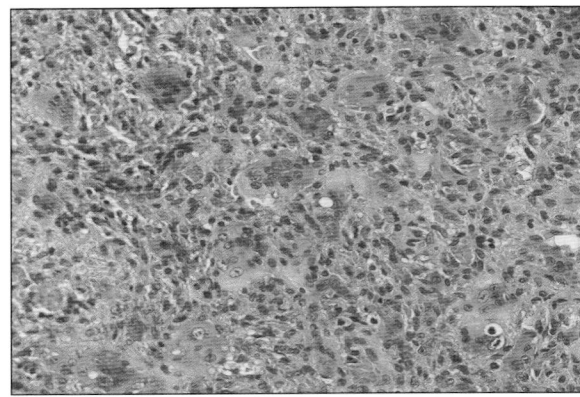

Fig 2-17b Higher-power view of Fig 2-17a showing a cellular fibrous stroma with numerous multinucleated giant cells and erythrocytes.

RADIOGRAPHIC FINDINGS ▶

Seen best in edentulous areas, a peripheral giant cell proliferation will characteristically show a cupped-out resorption of the alveolar crest and sometimes of root surfaces (Figs 2-16a and 2-16b). The resorptive pattern is well demarcated and is not suggestive of a destructive or an infiltrating lesion.

DIFFERENTIAL DIAGNOSIS ▶

Where lesions associated with teeth arise, the peripheral giant cell proliferation bears the closest resemblance to the *pyogenic granuloma* followed by the *peripheral ossifying fibroma*. The clinician must also differentiate such presentations from a *primary* or *metastatic malignancy*.

HISTOPATHOLOGY ▶

Histologically, a discrete tumor mass is usually seen (Fig 2-17a). The covering mucosa may sometimes be ulcerated. Whether or not this is the case, there will be numerous capillaries and an inflammatory infiltrate with prominent plasma cells. The mass itself is very cellular and consists of spindle cells with numerous multinucleated giant cells of varying size and some extravasated blood (Fig 2-17b). Hemosiderin, usually more prominent at the periphery, may be present.

The histogenesis of the component cells has been controversial. Based on the elegant studies of Flanagan et al, it would seem that the multinucleated giant cells are indeed osteoclasts. They may be brought in through the circulation or formed on site. The stromal cells may be a mixed population that

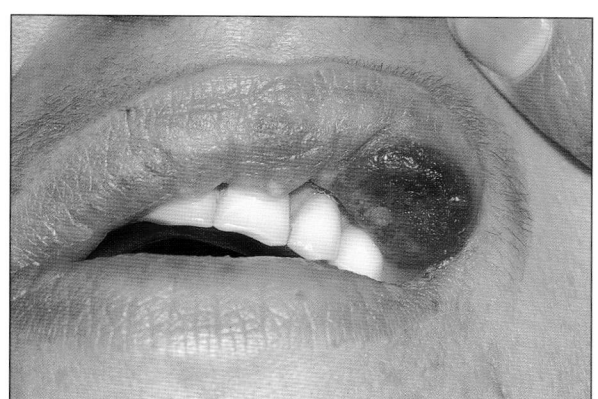

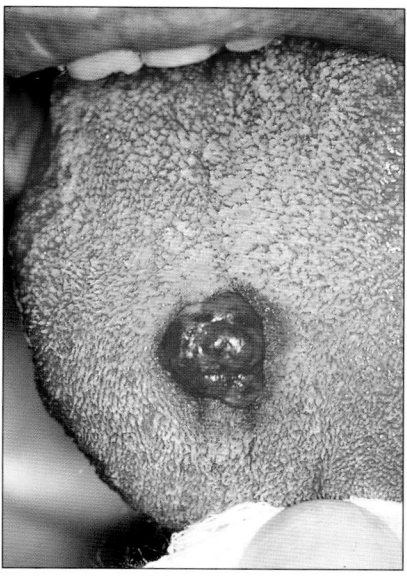

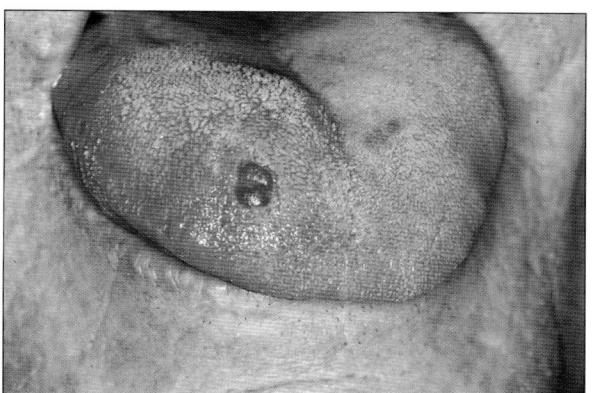

Fig 2-18a Although these lesions have sometimes been called traumatic eosinophilic granulomas of the tongue, they can occur in other areas overlying skeletal muscle.

Fig 2-18b This traumatic eosinophilic granuloma exhibited a more exophytic red mass.

Fig 2-18c A typical traumatic eosinophilic granuloma will be ulcerative with induration and may have a friable red base.

includes macrophages. Some stromal cells are alkaline phosphatase–positive and form woven bone, which indicates that they are osteoblasts.

TREATMENT ▶

Peripheral giant cell proliferations should be excised with surgical margins at the periphery of the clinical lesion, and the excision should include the periosteum and/or periodontal ligament from which they are thought to arise. If there is an apparent stimulating etiology such as a failing restoration, foreign body, etc, it should be removed with the lesion. The resultant defect is left to heal by secondary intention if a primary approximation of tissues is impossible.

PROGNOSIS ▶

Excision of the lesion and removal of any stimulators resolves the lesions without recurrence.

Traumatic Eosinophilic Granuloma

CLINICAL PRESENTATION AND PATHOGENESIS ▶

The traumatic eosinophilic granuloma is a rare ulcerated condition of uncertain pathogenesis. It is mostly seen in adults older than 30 years and is almost exclusively seen in the tongue or, more rarely, in the lip. It is presumed to be a condition initiated by a traumatic injury to the skeletal muscle in one of these two sites. The muscle injury itself stimulates a chemotaxis of eosinophils, which infiltrate and efface the local muscle fibers. The traumatic incident is a single injury rather than a chronic repetitive trauma and is usually of a puncture type.

Lesions on the lip will be ulcerated and crusted (Fig 2-18a). Such ulcerated lesions will have an indurated base and periphery, giving the strong impression of a squamous cell carcinoma (Fig 2-18b). This impression may be reinforced by a history of excision with local recurrence. The ulcer is usually small (less than 2 cm) and may have an exophytic protrusion similar to that of a pyogenic granuloma (Fig 2-18c). The lesion itself is only mildly painful or asymptomatic. Most patients seek care because of its long duration without healing or recurrence after an initial excision.

DIFFERENTIAL DIAGNOSIS ▶

The indurated ulcer presentation of the traumatic eosinophilic granuloma of the tongue or lip may indeed be identical to that of a *squamous cell carcinoma*. In those that have an exophytic bulge of muscle or red mass of friable granulation tissue, a *pyogenic granuloma* or a fungal ulceration such as *histoplasmosis* or *coccidioidomycosis* are considerations. If the trauma is constant and repetitive, such as that from a

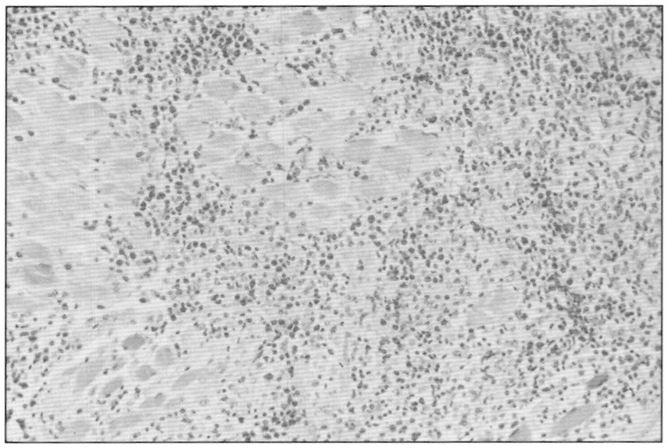

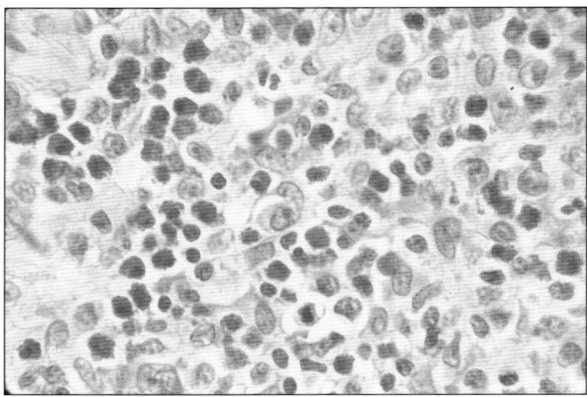

Fig 2-18d Infiltration of skeletal muscle by inflammatory cells in a traumatic eosinophilic granuloma.

Fig 2-18e Higher-power view of Fig 2-18d showing that the infiltrating cells are predominantly eosinophils and histiocytes.

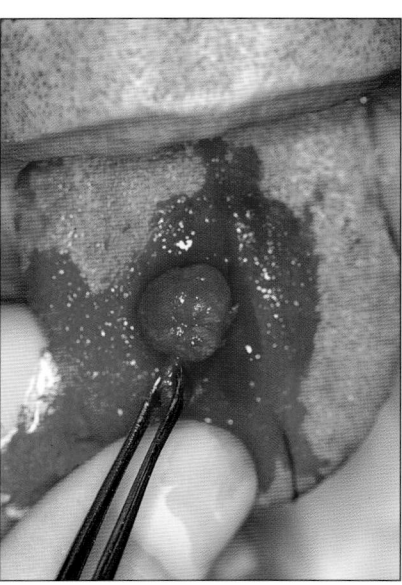

Fig 2-18f A traumatic eosinophilic granuloma should be excised with 0.5-cm margins with particular attention to the deep margin.

sharp dental restoration or a habit, a *nonspecific traumatic ulcer* should be suspected. In addition, other mild to severe, painful, single ulcerative conditions, such as a *syphilitic chancre* or a *tuberculosis ulcer*, must also be considered.

DIAGNOSTIC WORK-UP ▶

Unless an obvious source of chronic trauma is evident, these tumors should be biopsied without hesitation. Even if a source of chronic trauma is found and removed, no more than 14 days should be allowed for the area to show unequivocal signs of healing before a biopsy is accomplished. There are no specific radiographic or blood studies that will confirm a diagnosis of traumatic eosinophilic granuloma, and no peripheral blood eosinophilia is seen with this diagnosis.

HISTOPATHOLOGY ▶

This reactive lesion is usually ulcerated. The most striking feature is the presence of numerous histiocytes and eosinophils, which infiltrate deeply into skeletal muscle (Figs 2-18d and 2-18e). Varying numbers of neutrophils and plasma cells will also be seen, with the heaviest concentrations in the area of the ulcer. Degeneration of skeletal muscle fibers is often noted. These lesions have been reproduced experimentally following injury to rat tongue muscle.

TREATMENT AND PROGNOSIS ▶

Once an incisional biopsy has ruled out the other ulcerative lesions on the differential diagnosis and hopefully established the diagnosis of a traumatic eosinophilic granuloma, the lesion should be excised with 0.5-cm peripheral margins (Fig 2-18f). Although common, recurrences are usually the result of an inadequate depth of excision rather than positive margins at the surface. Therefore, excision with frozen section guidance and close follow-up are recommended. Recurrent lesions should be re-excised with particular attention to the deep margins and controlled with frozen sections, and the histopathology should be carefully reviewed to be certain that one of the other lesions on the differential list is not present.

Frey Syndrome

CLINICAL PRESENTATION AND PATHOGENESIS ▶

Frey syndrome is a condition of faulty tissue repair and regeneration in which transsected postganglionic parasympathetic fibers become misdirected to innervate sweat glands and vasomotor receptors, producing sweating and flushing (vasodilation) of the involved area of the face. This condition was described by others, but it was Lucja Frey who, in 1923, brought it to the attention of the medical community.

Individuals with Frey syndrome experience a focal area of facial sweating, flushing, and sometimes a sense of warmth or pain when eating or just thinking about foods that provoke a strong salivary stimulation. The syndrome usually develops as a result of parotid tumor surgery or direct parotid trauma; it has also resulted as a complication of temporomandibular joint surgery and open reduction of a ramus fracture. Most cases go unrecognized or are accepted by patients without complaint. Therefore, this syndrome is underreported. If tested for, it may be seen in 20% of individuals who have undergone superficial parotidectomy surgery.

Frey syndrome development begins with a surgical or traumatic transsection of sympathetic fibers to sweat glands and to the precapillary vasomotor smooth muscle cells, which control vasoconstriction and vasodilation. Postganglionic parasympathetic fibers from the otic ganglion to the parotid gland are also transsected. Since these types of fibers and the injury to them primarily involve the auriculotemporal nerve, Frey syndrome has previously been termed *auriculotemporal syndrome*. However, this is not accurate since the skin areas innervated by the greater auricular nerve and occipital nerve may also be involved. During nerve regeneration, the parasympathetic fibers grow randomly and become misdirected along sympathetic pathways to innervate sweat glands and vascular smooth muscle. The facial sympathetic system is unique in that its neurotransmitter is acetylcholine (and not the usual norepinephrine), which allows the cholinergic parasympathetic fibers to functionally excite these normally sympathetic receptors to produce sweating and flushing. This process takes 2 months to 2 years; however, patients may not become aware of the facial sweating for several more years.

DIFFERENTIAL DIAGNOSIS ▶

Frey syndrome is often readily apparent by its symptoms. However, it should not be confused with more generalized facial sweating in response to very spicy foods or after sympathectomy surgery.

DIAGNOSTIC WORK-UP ▶

The diagnosis of Frey syndrome can be confirmed and the area of involvement mapped for surgical correction with a starch-iodine test. This is a simple clinical test requiring wheat starch or corn starch powder (available from any grocery store) and tincture of iodine (I_2), which cannot be substituted (eg, betadine, an iodinate organic molecule, will not work as well) (Fig 2-19a). The tincture of I_2 is painted on the involved side of the face and allowed to dry (Fig 2-19b). Next, the dry starch powder is dusted onto the area (Fig 2-19c). Salivation is then best stimulated by a tart candy or chewing gum, although 10 mg of intravenous edrophonium (Tensilon, ICN), a parasympathomimetic drug, will also stimulate salivary flow. If Frey syndrome is present, the sweating will solubilize the I_2 and the starch, which will allow them to react and produce a blue color (Fig 2-19d).

TREATMENT AND PROGNOSIS ▶

Frey syndrome is only a social and practical annoyance and therefore may be accepted by the patient without the need for correction. The most complete and predictable resolution of Frey syndrome is via surgery. However, temporary or ongoing treatment with 3% scopolamine cream or 1% glycopyrrolate cream can offer a nonsurgical means of control in some cases.

Some cases have been treated by transsection of the auriculotemporal nerve trunk. However, this is not recommended because nerve regeneration may reinitiate the Frey syndrome and raise the risk for development of a painful C-fiber neuroma. Instead, the standard and most effective surgery involves the development of an anterior-based skin flap at the dermal-subcutaneous or SMAS level beneath the area of involvement (Fig 2-19e). This retranssects the nerve fibers to the sweat glands and vasculature in the area (Fig 2-19f). A sheet or barrier tissue—usually autogenous fascia lata or freeze-dried allogeneic dura from any tissue bank certified by the American Association of Tissue Banks—is placed beneath the flap before it is reapproximated and closed (Figs 2-19g and 2-19h). Either of these dense collagenous barriers will become incorporated into the subcutaneous tissue, thereby preventing regeneration of the aberrant fibers and permanently resolving the syndrome.

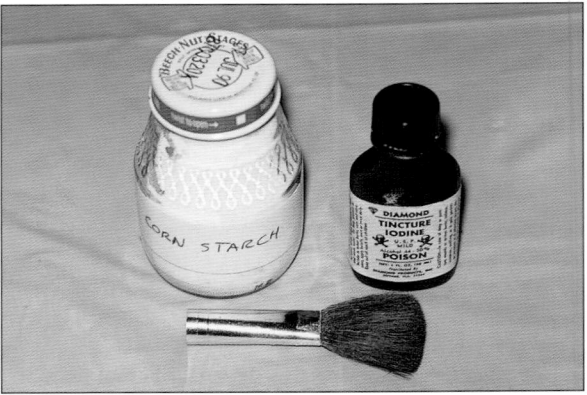

Fig 2-19a The presence of and area involved with gustatory sweating can be determined with the starch-iodine test. Here corn starch, a brush, and tincture of iodine (I_2) are gathered.

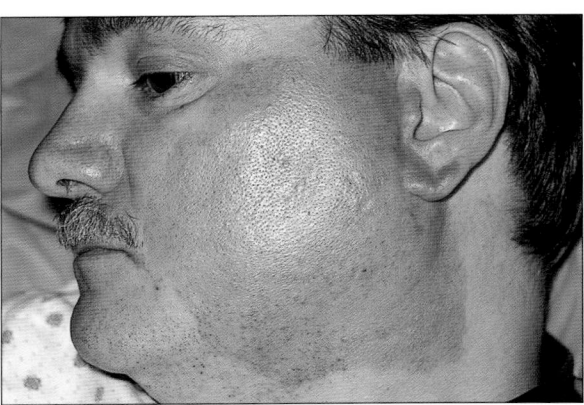

Fig 2-19b The tincture of I_2 is applied and allowed to dry.

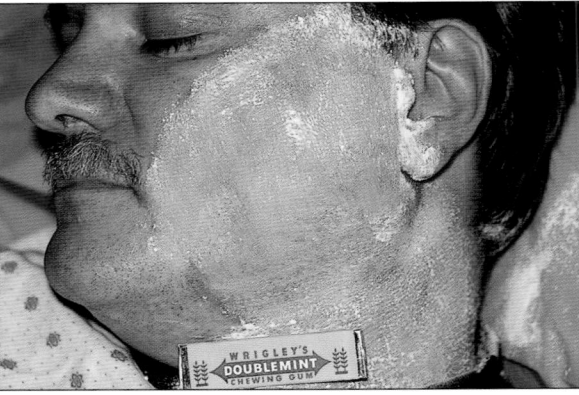

Fig 2-19c The powdered starch is applied to the dried tincture of I_2, and salivation is then stimulated. Here standard chewing gum is used.

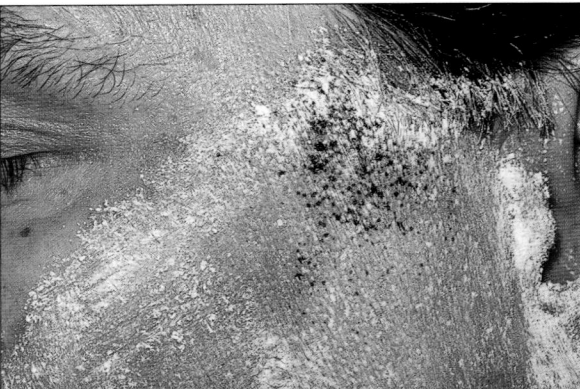

Fig 2-19d As sweating occurs the moisture mixes the starch and I_2 in a solution that appears blue.

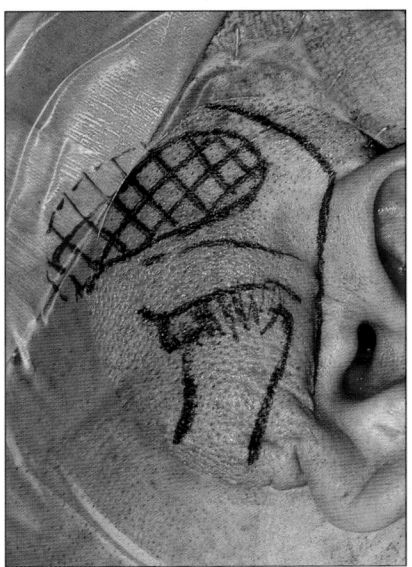

Fig 2-19e The area of sweating can be photographed or marked for surgical correction in the exact area of the misdirected parasympathetic fibers.

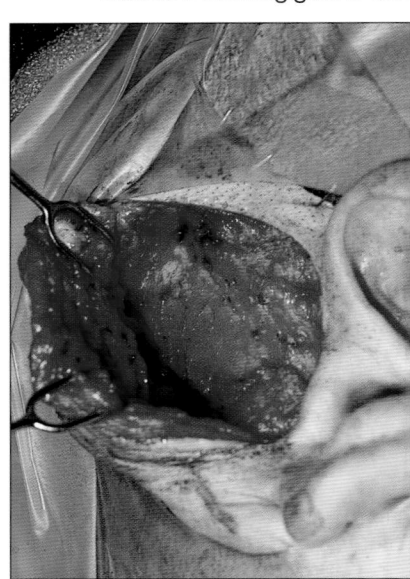

Fig 2-19f Correction of Frey syndrome requires an anterior-based skin flap that transsects the misdirected parasympathetic fibers.

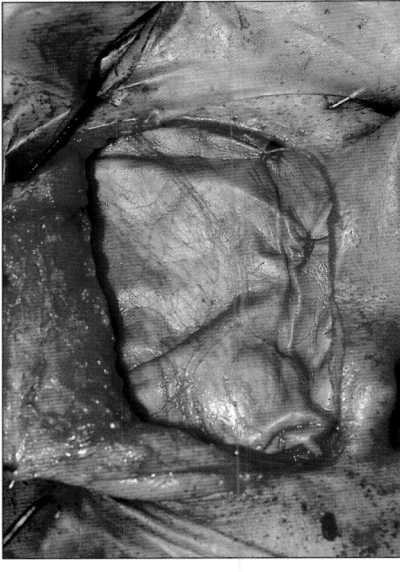

Fig 2-19g To prevent a second regeneration of misdirected fibers, a separating tissue—here, freeze-dried ethylene oxide–sterilized allogeneic dura—is placed.

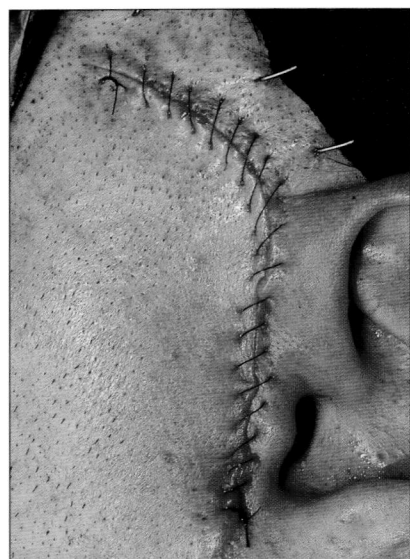

Fig 2-19h The skin flap is closed over the separating tissue, which becomes incorporated into the subcutaneous tissue plane.

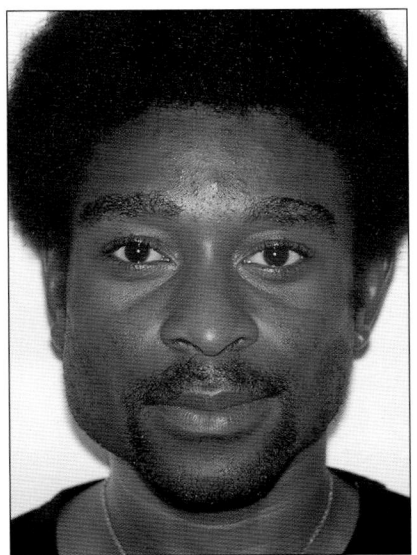

Fig 2-20a Benign masseteric hypertrophy is most often unilateral and may be confused with a parotid enlargement or parotid tumor.

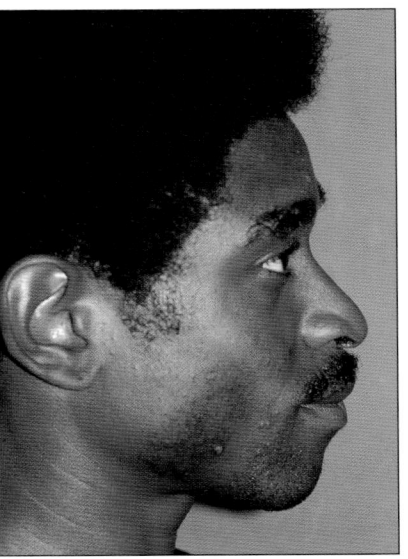

Fig 2-20b Benign masseteric hypertrophy can be distinguished from parotid tumors by palpation of the masseter muscle and the outline of the muscle as the patient clenches the teeth.

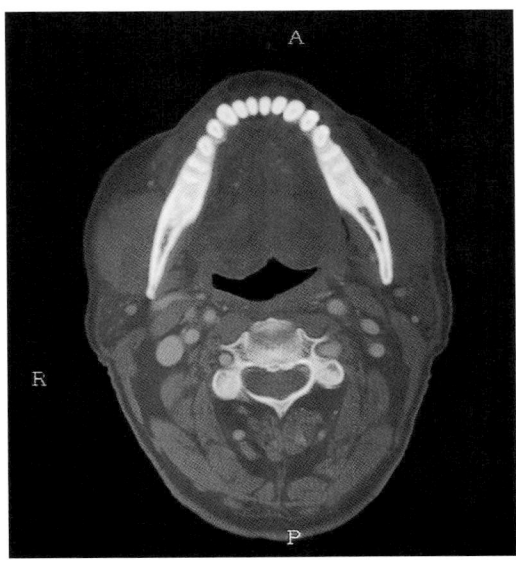

Fig 2-20c Benign masseteric hypertrophy can be readily confirmed with a CT scan, which will show a uniform enlargement of the masseter muscle.

Benign Masseteric Hypertrophy

CLINICAL PRESENTATION AND PATHOGENESIS ▶

Benign masseteric hypertrophy is the clinical enlargement of one or sometimes of both masseter muscles related to a teeth-clenching or gum-chewing habit. In such cases, the muscle undergoes a type of repetitive isometric exercise that induces the hypertrophy. It occurs somewhat more frequently in men and is ipsilateral in 85% of cases.

The most common presentation is the appearance of an asymptomatic unilateral swelling in the preauricular area that may be confused with parotitis, a tumor of the mandibular ramus, or a fascial space abscess (Fig 2-20a). Several cases have undergone parotid surgery for the mistaken diagnosis of a parotid tumor. In all cases, the condition can be confirmed by palpation while the individual clenches his or her teeth. In some cases, the area of insertion of the masseter on the mandibular ramus will respond by forming a bone projection that may be palpable or seen on an anteroposterior radiograph. Presumably, this is due to the tension created by the masseter muscle during these contractions, which produces a periosteal reaction and activity.

DIFFERENTIAL DIAGNOSIS ▶

The initial clinical impression of a firm mass over the ramus of the mandible may indeed be that of a *parotitis* or a *parotid tumor*. In addition, an *odontogenic tumor* or a *bone tumor* in the ramus of the mandible will present in a near-identical fashion. If the pain and erythema of a *cellulitis* or *abscess involving the pterygomasseteric space* is mild, each would also be a consideration.

DIAGNOSTIC WORK-UP ▶

The prudent clinician should examine the dentition thoroughly. Benign masseteric hypertrophy is caused by teeth clenching, not teeth grinding or bruxism. Therefore, the respective teeth in each arch will not have flattened working cusps. A dentition with minimal wear facets and a palpable muscle bulge upon clenching should confirm the diagnosis (Fig 2-20b). The expectation of a benign masseteric hypertrophy to be bilateral or symmetrical is misguided; as with most oral habits, one side of the mouth is favored. In this case, the habit of clenching or, in rare instances, excessive gum chewing, is usually focused on only one side.

In equivocal cases or those in which another professional opinion suggests a tumor or an infection, a computed tomography (CT) scan or magnetic resonance imaging (MRI) scan will definitively show an enlargement of one masseter muscle and rule out the presence of other pathologies (Fig 2-20c).

HISTOPATHOLOGY ▶

There is no pertinent histopathology. In cases where a portion of the muscle is removed for contouring, the muscle is normal-appearing and striated.

TREATMENT AND PROGNOSIS ▶

There is often a desire by the patient and the surgeon to accomplish a surgical reduction of the masseter for contouring correction. However, this should be delayed until after the teeth-clenching habit has been treated, which may require patient counseling, anti-anxiety medications, occlusal equilibrations, splint therapy, and/or behavior modification. Even then, resection of a portion of the masseter may not eventuate in the anticipated normalization of contours because of postsurgical fibrosis and/or rehypertrophy of the muscle by a continuation or reinitiation of the teeth-clenching habit.

If a masseter muscle recontouring is accomplished, it is best to reflect the masseter from the lateral ramus and resect a medial wedge from the insertional area and lower one third of the muscle. The resultant thinned muscle is then sutured to the pterygomasseteric sling. This approach avoids risk to the marginal mandibular branch of the facial nerve, which courses within the fascia over the lower lateral portion of the muscle, and reduces the potential for rehypertrophy from its detachment of the muscle.

Use of botulino toxin-A (Botox-A, Allergan) to atrophy this muscle has not been attempted and is not recommended because of the very large size of the hypertrophied muscle and the current lack of approval for this type of application.

Traumatic Myositis Ossificans

CLINICAL PRESENTATION AND PATHOGENESIS ▶

Most individuals presenting with traumatic myositis ossificans will be children or young adults (approximately 40 years or younger), usually with a history of penetrating trauma or a crush injury of the involved muscle. Because the masseter is most commonly affected, most will seek attention due to limited jaw opening (Fig 2-21a). Other muscles can also be affected, either separately or simultaneously with the masseter (Fig 2-21b). If the muscle involved is a superficial one, such as the masseter or sternocleidomastoid muscle, a firm bony hardness can be palpated.

The usual mechanism of traumatic myositis ossificans is the implantation of active periosteum into a muscle, hence the increased incidence in younger individuals and those with penetrating injuries. Following a crush injury to muscle, muscle fascia, and perimysium, bone is formed from mesenchymal stem cells, which retain their ability to differentiate along bone-forming lines. Such crush injuries can establish a local environment capable of stimulating these cells into actual bone formation or in some cases a combination of true bone formation and dystrophic calcification or even calcified chondroid matrix.

Another mechanism of traumatic myositis ossificans is the overproduction of bone morphogenetic protein-4 (BMP-4) in response to injury. In such cases, either the cells within the muscle fascia or the muscle cells themselves elaborate this morphogen.

DIFFERENTIAL DIAGNOSIS ▶

A limited jaw opening associated with radiographic ossifications/calcifications in soft tissue should alert the clinician to a possible bone tumor. Both *osteosarcoma* and *chondrosarcoma* can form tumor-related opacifications (osteosarcoma via tumor bone formation and chondrosarcoma via calcified tumor cartilage or distracted periosteum). If the lesion seems to emanate from a bony surface as do most lesions of traumatic myositis ossificans, *osteoblastoma* is also a realistic consideration. Diffuse opacities seemingly in muscle may also represent mature *venous hemangiomas with multiple phleboliths*.

DIAGNOSTIC WORK-UP ▶

A CT scan or a model developed from a CT scan are the most valuable means of assessing the location of the lesion, its relationship to host bone, and the possible presence of other lesions (Figs 2-21b and 2-21c). Radiographs will show a fluffy radiopacity within the muscle, which can often be traced to a bony surface.

HISTOPATHOLOGY ▶

Traumatic myositis ossificans is a reactive lesion that occurs within skeletal muscle. Typically, there is a central cellular zone that may contain pleomorphic fibroblasts with mitoses and numerous capillaries. This zone is surrounded by osteoid trabeculae with proliferative osteoblasts. Maturation of the osseous tissue is usually seen. Chondroid proliferation and myxoid areas may be present. Degenerating skeletal

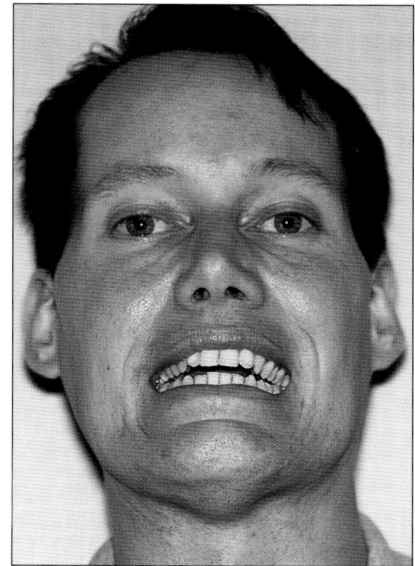

Fig 2-21a Traumatic myositis ossificans often presents with limited jaw opening. This individual's maximum interincisal opening is 3 mm.

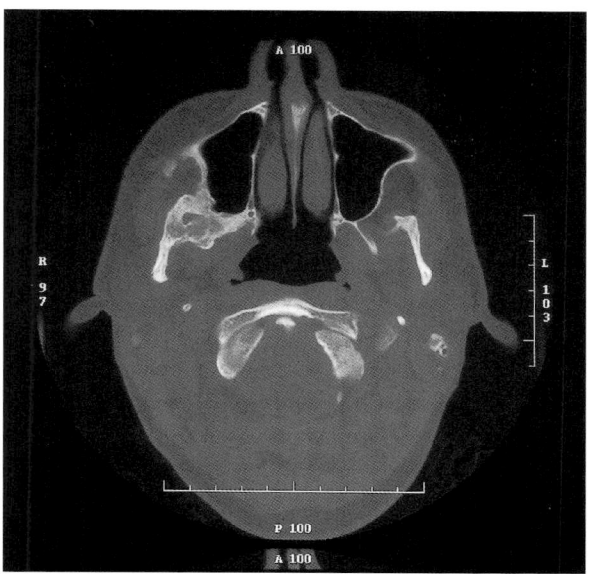

Fig 2-21b Ossifications in the lateral pterygoid and temporalis muscles in traumatic myositis ossificans.

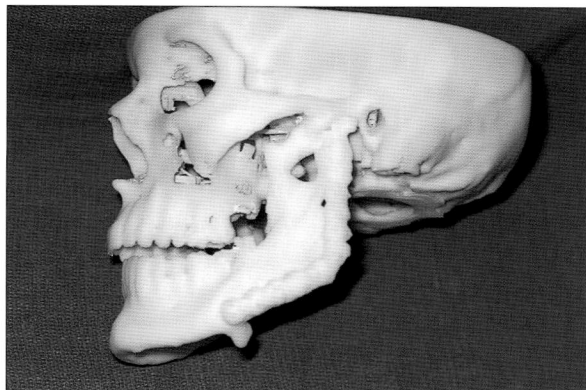

Fig 2-21c Traumatic myositis ossificans is seen here to form a bridge of bone in the temporalis muscle. It limits jaw opening by fusing the anterior ramus to the posterior maxilla, pterygoid plate, and zygomatic arch.

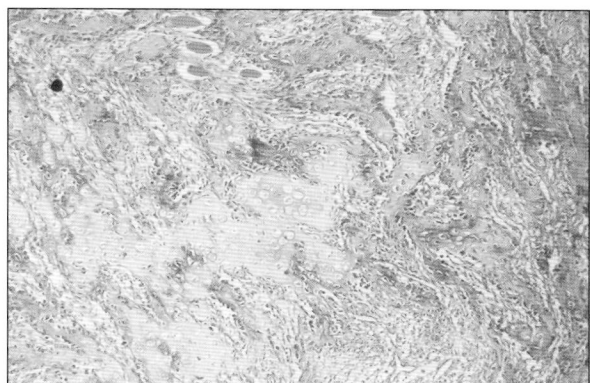

Fig 2-21d Within this traumatic myositis ossificans, disruption of skeletal muscle can be seen along with proliferation of chondroid and osteoid tissue. Skeletal muscle fibers are visible at the top of the field.

muscle is apparent. This rapidly growing tissue with an atypical appearance may suggest sarcoma, but the zoned character of the lesion indicates otherwise (Fig 2-21d).

TREATMENT AND PROGNOSIS

Traumatic myositis ossificans, unlike myositis ossificans progressiva (see below), responds to surgical excision. Surgical excision followed by aggressive physical therapy will remove the lesion and restore most but not all of the jaw motion. In cases that express a temporomandibular joint ankylosis, an arthroplasty with biologic interpositional materials (temporal fascia, fascia lata, allogeneic fresh-frozen cartilage, or allogeneic dura) rather than alloplastic interpositional materials (Silastic, Proplast, Proplast-Teflon, etc) will result in a much more permanent increase in jaw mobility with fewer complications (Figs 2-21e to 2-21j). At times, a reconstruction plate fixated to the ramus with a condylar replacement that articulates against one of the biologic interpositional materials in the fossa will be needed. This approach is indicated if the bony removal in the ramus is significant and the resultant loss of ramus vertical dimension would produce a malocclusion.

Since both mechanisms of traumatic myositis ossificans involve reactive bone-producing cells, recurrent and/or persistent cases may require radiotherapy. Immediately following surgical extirpation of al-

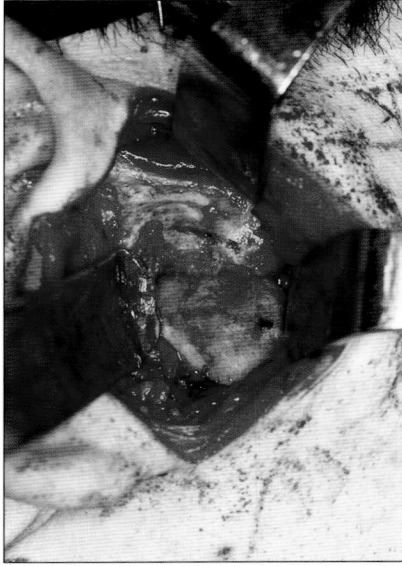

Fig 2-21e Traumatic myositis ossificans may produce a large amount of heterotopic bone. Here, complete bony ankylosis is seen.

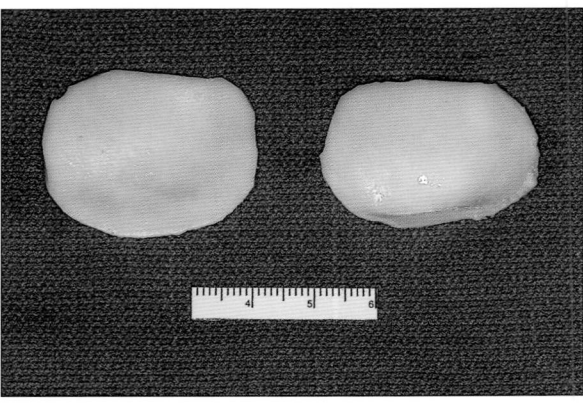

Fig 2-21f Fresh frozen allogeneic cartilage is often placed into the temporal fossa. Its subchondral bone side will fuse to the temporal fossa and its hyaline cartilage surface will remodel into fibrocartilage and thus resist re-ankylosis.

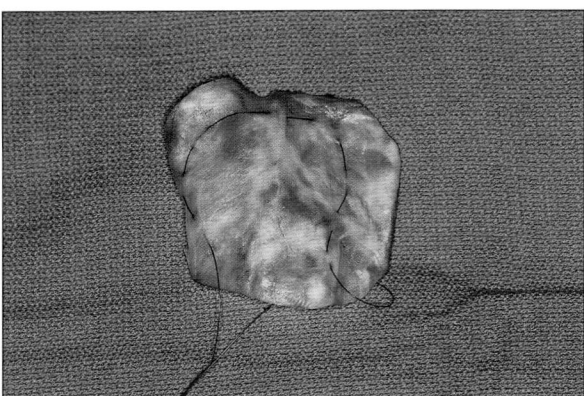

Fig 2-21g Freeze-dried allogeneic dura is often used to cover the ramus resection edge. It can be draped over and sutured to the cut ramus stump via bur holes to serve as another barrier to re-ankylosis.

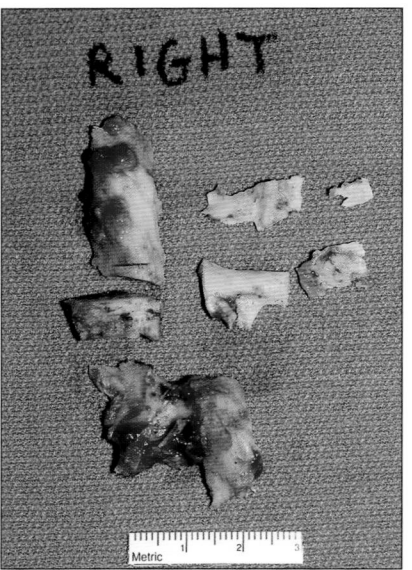

Fig 2-21h Release of ankylosis induced by traumatic myositis ossificans often requires the removal of a large quantity of bone.

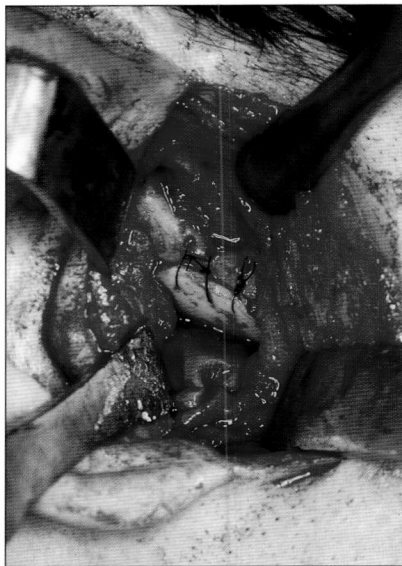

Fig 2-21i After the heterotopic bone has been removed, the allogeneic cartilage is sutured to the temporal fossa and the allogeneic dura to the ramus stump.

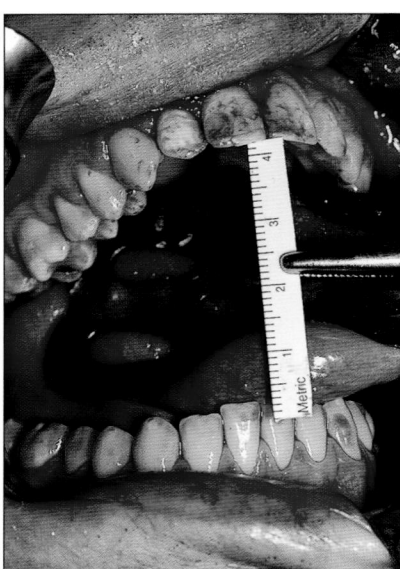

Fig 2-21j Complete removal of the heterotopic bone and coronoidectomies will allow the patient to regain maximum jaw opening.

ready formed bone, external beam radiotherapy can be used in dosages between 800 cGy and 2,000 cGy. Such radiotherapy is reserved for those who have not responded to surgery alone; however, these individuals must be counseled concerning the potential carcinogenic effects of radiotherapy on reactive bone processes.

Surgical excision and physical therapy usually provide a long-term, stable result. The final jaw opening is usually about two thirds to three quarters that of normal.

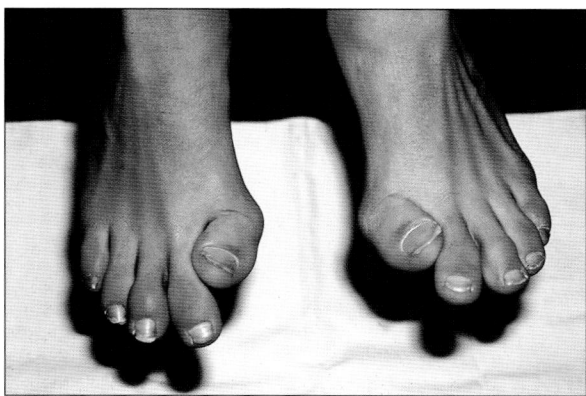 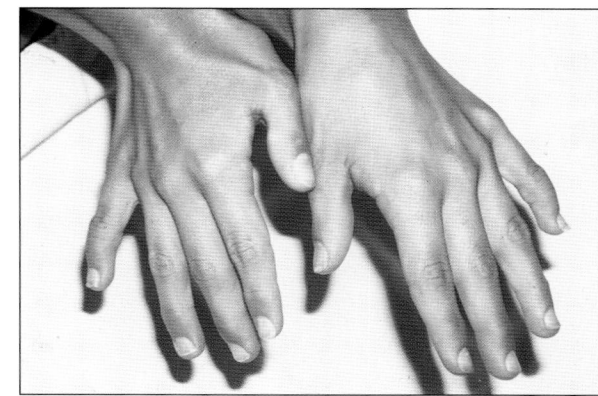

Figs 2-22a and 2-22b Congenital hallux valgus of the feet and hands is often an early sign of myositis ossificans progressiva.

Myositis Ossificans Progressiva

CLINICAL PRESENTATION AND PATHOGENESIS ▶

The individual presenting with myositis ossificans progressiva is usually a preteen or teenager, often with a vague history of a "stiff gait" or limited extremity and jaw movements. A history of a congenital bilateral hallux valgus is common and is an early indication of this autosomal-dominant disease (Figs 2-22a and 2-22b).

Examination will show limited motion of most joints. Among the most prominent may be wrist calcifications, jaw openings of less than 5 mm interincisally, foreshortening and malformation of the metatarsals and phalanges of the great toe (hallux valgus), and an inability to bend the trunk due to paraspinous ossifications.

Myositis ossificans progressiva, also termed *fibrodysplasia ossificans progressiva*, is a complete connective tissue maldevelopment that affects tendons, aponeuroses, and muscle fascia to the same degree that it affects muscle itself. The disease may be transmitted as an autosomal-dominant trait, but most cases are believed to represent new mutations.

Initially, the areas of involvement undergo a fibrous cellular proliferation that progresses through the stages of endochondral ossification into mature lamellar bone. The areas of earliest involvement are the metatarsals and phalanges and the paraspinous areas around the vertebral bodies.

DIAGNOSTIC WORK-UP ▶

A CT scan is appropriate for assessing the location and degree of involvement in certain muscle groups. Otherwise, plain radiographs can reveal their presence or absence in most areas. The lesions will appear as feathery radiopaque collections within a muscle (early in the disease course) or as irregular masses (late in the disease course) (Fig 2-23a).

Myositis ossificans progressiva remains a history-related clinical diagnosis. There is no known specific laboratory abnormality.

HISTOPATHOLOGY ▶

Systemic or progressive myositis ossificans shows skeletal muscle replaced by fibrous tissue, which undergoes osteoid formation with mineralization. Chondroid areas may or may not be present, and muscle fibers entrapped within bone are seen.

TREATMENT ▶

The surgeon should resist the impulse to try to increase motion via surgical excision of the ossifications in all but the most unusual circumstances. Areas of surgical excision have been noted to reossify and limit mobility even further (Fig 2-23b). Additionally, attempts to slow the progression of ossifications with drugs also have been unsuccessful. Trials of isotretinoin (13-*cis*-retinoic acid) (Accutane, Roche), corticosteroids, and disodium etidronate (Didronel, Procter and Gamble) have each been ineffective. There is currently no known mechanism to halt or correct this genetically driven muscle and tendon ossification process.

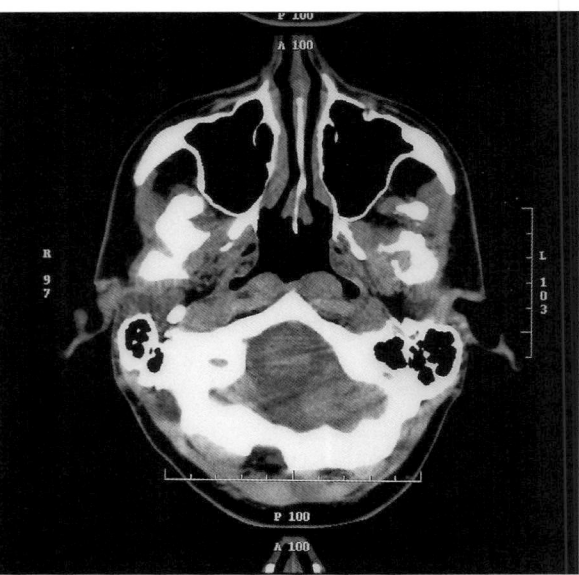

Fig 2-23a When myositis ossificans progressiva affects the muscles of mastication, it often affects bilateral muscle groups and will produce a bony ankylosis.

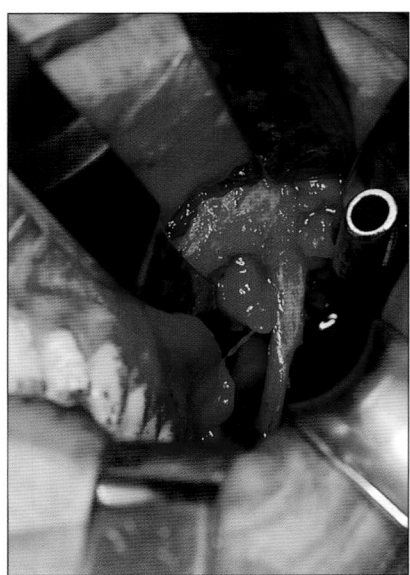

Fig 2-23b Complete replacement of the temporalis muscle by heterotopic bone may be part of myositis ossificans progressiva.

Since myositis ossificans progressiva involves reactive bone–producing cells, radiotherapy may be required in recurrent and persistent cases. Dosages between 800 cGy and 2,000 cGy of external beam radiotherapy can be used and should immediately follow surgical extirpation of already formed bone. Such radiotherapy is reserved for those who have not responded to surgery alone. However, these individuals must be counseled concerning the potential carcinogenic effects of radiotherapy on reactive bone processes.

PROGNOSIS ▶

Individuals progress to a plateau of disability determined by their individual genetic expression. Longevity is reduced by immobility, which often affects the intercostal muscles and diaphragm and leads to respiratory failure. Rare instances of starvation deaths from complete jaw immobility have been reported.

Drug-Induced Avascular Necrosis of Bone

CLINICAL PRESENTATION AND PATHOGENESIS ▶

Patients with drug-induced avascular necrosis of bone will present with exposed white- or yellow-colored bone, either in the maxilla or the mandible, that is obviously nonvital (Fig 2-24). It will be painless or only mildly painful. Larger areas of exposed bone may be secondarily infected, resulting in inflammation, pus, and a greater degree of pain. In edentulous individuals, the mylohyoid ridge and the crestal bone are the more commonly affected sites, apparently because of denture pressure. In dentate areas, any of the teeth may be involved in what will look like advanced periodontal disease. When such teeth are removed, the bone often fails to heal and remains exposed, as occurs in osteoradionecrosis, osteopetrosis, and in focal areas of severe florid cemento-osseous dysplasia. Attempts to cover the bone with local flaps often fail, eventuating in a further exposure of bone and loss of overlying soft tissue.

The majority of patients will be older than 40 years and will usually be undergoing maintenance therapy for controlled multiple myeloma. Because of improvements in chemotherapy, which allow longer survival (currently up to 10 years) for patients with multiple myeloma, drug-induced avascular necrosis of bone is essentially a new disease entity of the twenty-first century (previously, survivals had been limited to 2 to 3 years).

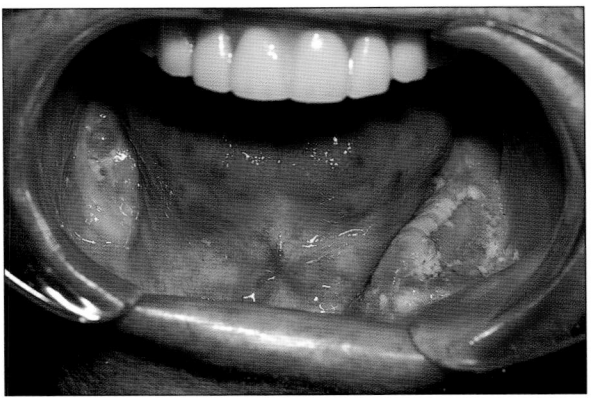

Fig 2-24 Bilateral exposure of avascular bone due to Aredia therapy for multiple myeloma.

Today the bisphosphonates are widely used in the treatment of osteoporosis and other bone-losing metabolic diseases. The most common bisphosphonates used for osteoporosis, such as alendronate, risedronate, and etidronate, are without serious bone necrosis complications when used according to their recommended dosages. However, pamidronate (Aredia, Novartis), used to treat hypercalcemia related to malignancies in the dosage range of one 60- to 90-mg dose intravenously every 1 week to 1 month, produces a significant incidence of exposed nonvital bone in the mandible and/or maxilla. This is most often seen when Aredia is used in combination with dexamethasone or other steroids in the long-term treatment of multiple myeloma.

The bisphosphonates in general are a class of drugs that inhibit osteoclasts. Therefore, their use in hypercalcemic states is very effective and their maintenance of bone mass works against osteoporosis. However, osteoclastic function is part of the normal bone-turnover cycle, where osteocytes live out their life spans (about 150 days); their mineral matrix is resorbed by osteoclasts, which release BMP and insulin-like growth factors (IGFs), which in turn induce local stem cells to differentiate into osteoblasts and form new bone. This cycle is critical to maintaining bone stocks and the viability of bone. If osteoclastic function is too severely impaired, dead and dying osteocytes are not replaced and the capillary network in the bone is not maintained. The end product is avascular bone necrosis. This process is analogous to that of osteopetrosis (Albers-Schönberg or marble bone disease), in which an autosomal-dominant inheritance defect in osteoclast development also eventuates into exposed nonviable bone almost exclusively in the jaws.

DIFFERENTIAL DIAGNOSIS ▶

Only a few diseases produce nonviable exposed bone in the jaws: *osteoradionecrosis*, *osteopetrosis*, a severe localized area of *florid cemento-osseous dysplasia*, and *chronic osteomyelitis*. Most of these can be ruled out by a thorough history and simple radiographs.

DIAGNOSTIC WORK-UP ▶

While it is prudent to obtain a panoramic radiograph and a CT scan to assess the potential degree of involvement and to rule out some of the diseases on the differential list, a drug-induced avascular necrosis of bone often produces a normal radiographic or CT scan picture because of its maintenance of bone mineral, which is what these studies identify. Instead, the patient's history and a clinical examination are the most important factors in establishing a diagnosis. Those who have been taking Aredia for more than 1 year and those on concomitant steroids are at highest risk. If the individual has residual multiple myeloma or another malignancy, hypoproteinemia, or renal impairment from disease or drugs, or is currently taking other chemotherapy agents, the risk and probability of an avascular necrosis of bone increases further.

HISTOPATHOLOGY ▶

The histopathology of a drug-induced avascular necrosis of bone is nonspecific. It will, of course, show bone with empty lacunae and Haversian systems. There will be no Howship lacunae and sparse, if any, osteoblastic rimming. Occasionally, some inflammatory cells and bacterial colonies on bone surfaces may be seen, which is consistent with bone exposed to the oral environment.

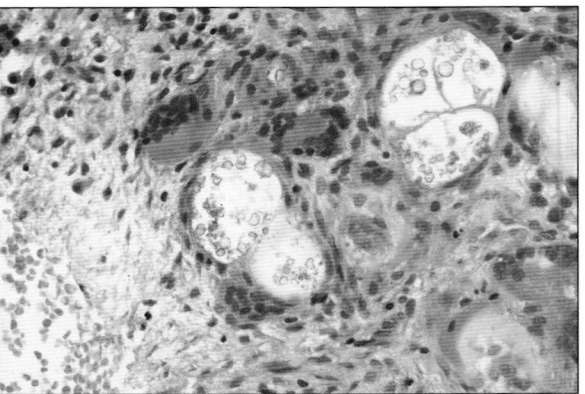

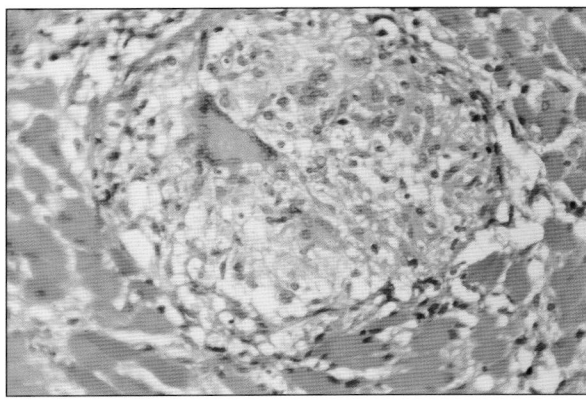

Fig 2-25a In this foreign body granuloma, exogenous material is surrounded by multinucleated giant cells (fused macrophages) and mixed chronic inflammatory cells.

Fig 2-25b This epithelioid granuloma, which is more compact, consists of a defined mass of pale-staining macrophages (epithelioid cells). A Langhans type of giant cell also is visible.

TREATMENT AND PROGNOSIS ▶

This disease presents a serious treatment dilemma for the oral and maxillofacial specialist. Since Aredia and the other bisphosphonates, if given in very high doses, affect the entire skeleton, the surgeon cannot debride to an uninvolved bone margin. In addition, many individuals must continue with Aredia therapy and/or other chemotherapies to maintain multiple myeloma control. Therefore, a common option is a combination of 0.12% chlorhexidine oral rinses, denture relief and reline if needed, intermittent courses of antibiotic therapy to treat secondary infections, and analgesics to treat painful episodes.

To resolve the disease, Aredia or the offending drug must be discontinued for at least a 2-month period prior to debridement surgery and flap advancements for a primary closure and must not be restarted for at least another 2 months. This will, of course, require the consultation and cooperation of the medical oncologist. In addition, the patient's blood studies and nutritional balance should be optimized to support healing in these compromised individuals.

Hyperbaric oxygen does not play a significant role in the treatment of this disease, and antibiotics by themselves are indicated only to treat secondary infection. These patients are also not candidates for dental implants, and the wearing of dentures must be closely monitored to prevent pressure areas from exposing the drug-altered bone.

Granulomatous Diseases

Granulomas may be defined as focal collections of macrophages that aggregate for the purpose of phagocytosis. There are two major types of granulomas: *foreign body granulomas,* which consist of immature macrophages that accumulate because of the presence of concentrated inert material such as silica or talc (Fig 2-25a); and *epithelioid granulomas,* which consist of activated or mature macrophages and typically develop through the action of T cells in a delayed hypersensitivity reaction. Often this is the consequence of infection by certain microorganisms, such as *mycobacterium tuberculosis* (Fig 2-25b).

Oral Tuberculosis and Scrofula

CLINICAL PRESENTATION AND PATHOGENESIS ▶

Oral lesions of tuberculosis (TB) will present as painful, ragged ulcers, mostly on the posterior aspect of the oral tongue, pharyngeal tongue, or palate (Fig 2-26a). They are almost always secondary to active pulmonary tuberculosis, which seeds the oral site from coughed-up sputum. The lesions are painful because, by definition, they are infected ulcers. Occasionally, further invasion into bone may create a TB-related osteomyelitis. Statistically, since 1990, there has been a declining incidence of mucosal ulcers from the vocal cords to the lips.

About 26,000 new cases of active TB are diagnosed in the United States each year. The incidence is higher within densely populated areas, areas of lower socioeconomic status, aged populations, HIV-infected individuals, and others with immunocompromise. The incidence of all forms of TB skyrocketed beginning in 1986 in relation to the HIV/AIDS epidemic. TB cases in the US rose from 1,700 per year to 26,000 per year and have been between 22,000 and 26,000 per year since. In addition, resistant TB strains have emerged; in the US, there is a 2% overall incidence of "multidrug-resistant" TB in the HIV-negative population and a 19% incidence in the HIV-positive population.

Transmission occurs via aerosolized droplets, which seed organisms into the lungs that persist viably within macrophages after ingestion. These organisms and macrophages become contained or "walled off" within a granuloma. Often called the primary infection, this site is asymptomatic. The focus of dormant but viable organisms in the lung has been called the *Simon focus*; when calcified and apparent on a chest radiograph, it has been called the *Ghon focus*. Active tuberculosis develops as a reactivation of this primary disease either by reinfection or a change in the individual's immune status. Active lung destruction (usually cavitary lesions) develops, and lymphatic or hematogenous spread can occur.

DIFFERENTIAL DIAGNOSIS ▶

Oral TB will closely mimic several other important and well-known diseases, the most important of which is *squamous cell carcinoma*. In addition, the chancres of *primary syphilis* and the oral lesions of pulmonary fungal diseases such as *histoplasmosis, coccidioidomycosis*, and *blastomycosis* will have a similar appearance. If there is a history of *trauma* or a suspiciously sharp tooth edge exists, it is important to remember that trauma is still the leading cause of oral ulcers and should be included in the differential diagnosis.

DIAGNOSTIC WORK-UP ▶

All suspected or proven cases of oral or pulmonary TB should be reported to local and state public health departments. Suspected oral TB ulcers require biopsy to rule out carcinoma and the fungal lesions that will show suspicious organisms on high-power or oil immersion. A tissue specimen should be sent fresh for acid-fast staining (eg, Ziehl-Neelsen stain) and for culture in Löwenstein-Jensen media. Another tissue specimen should be sent for hematoxylin and eosin (H&E) histopathology. The Ziehl-Neelsen stain is accomplished as follows:

1. A thin smear is made of the deepest portion of the ulcer.
2. The smear is air dried for 30 seconds and heat fixed for 15 seconds.
3. The smear is stained with carbolfuchsin (a red cytoplasmic dye) for 20 seconds and washed with water.
4. A solution of 0.6 N HCl and 95% ethanol is applied for 20 seconds and washed in an attempt to decolorize cells.
5. The smear may be counterstained with either brilliant green or methylene blue.

The acid-fast organisms (nearly all mycobacteria species along with some others) will appear as red bacilli (Fig 2-26b), located within the cytoplasm of macrophages ("epithelioid cells"). Non–acid-fast organisms will appear either blue or green. Retention of the carbolfuchsin dye in the cell (acid fastness) is due to a thick, waxy protein-phospholipid cell wall that resists not only acid dissolution but also macrophage intracytoplasmic digestion, explaining to some degree the chronicity of this disease.

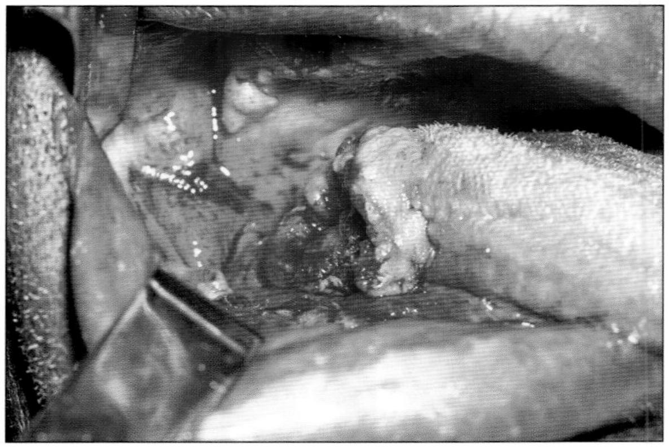

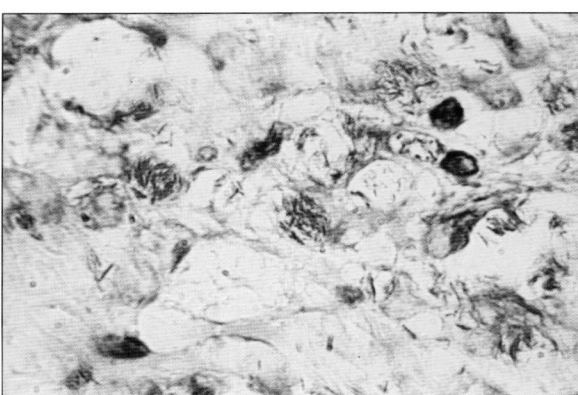

Fig 2-26a A tuberculous ulcer of the tongue is usually deep, ragged-edged, and painful.

Fig 2-26b An acid-fast stain identified acid-fast bacilli in the ulcer shown in Fig 2-26a, raising suspicion of a tuberculous etiology (Ziehl-Neelsen stain).

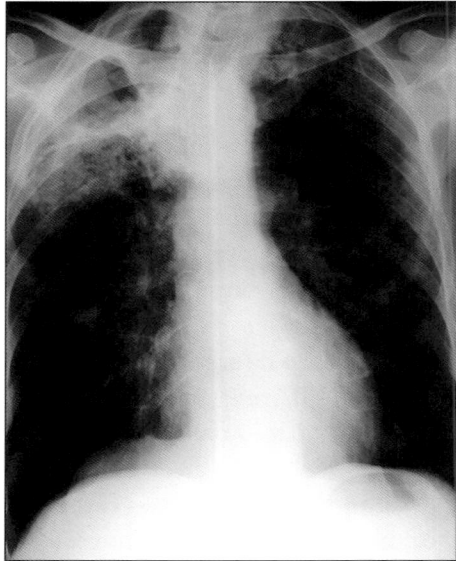

Fig 2-26c Tuberculosis of the lungs involving a right apical cavitary lesion, mediastinal/hilar lymph nodes, and focal involvement of the lower lung field.

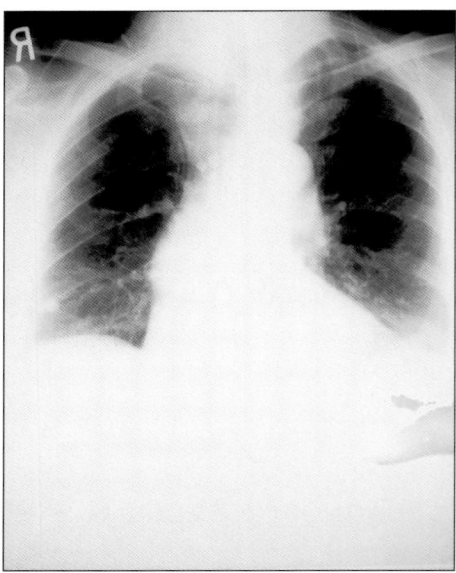

Fig 2-26d Bibasilar pleural thickening and a right apical infiltrate were the chest radiographic findings in this pulmonary tuberculosis.

Because oral TB is secondary to pulmonary TB, a chest radiograph should be taken. Active TB will most likely show a cavitary lesion in an apical lobe, since mycobacteria are obligate aerobes and the oxygen gradient is greatest in the lung apices (Fig 2-26c). More subtle pulmonary foci of TB may show lower-lobe cavitation or pleural thickenings (Fig 2-26d). In some cases, overt signs and symptoms such as fatigue, weight loss, fever, apical rales, and night sweats may further suggest active pulmonary disease. If a chest radiograph is suspicious and/or the oral lesion biopsy specimen shows granulomatous disease, sputum collection for acid-fast staining and culture, preferably by transtracheal irrigation and aspiration, is recommended.

The purified protein derivative (PPD), also called the *tine TB test*, and a variant of this test called the *Mantoux test*, are intradermal skin tests utilizing tubercle bacillus PPD. It is used in a dose of 5 tuberculin units (TU) in a saline solution as the antigen. An erythematous reaction greater than 2 mm with induration after 48 hours indicates that an individual has been exposed to the tubercle bacillus and has

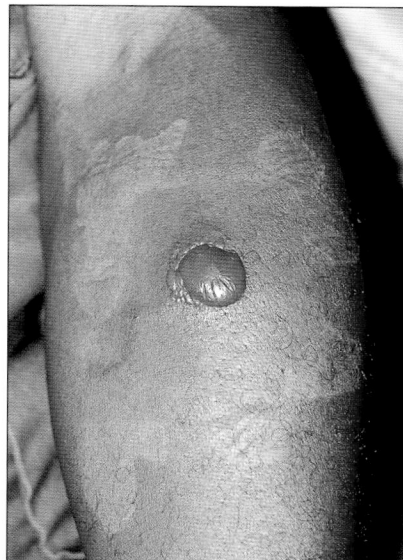

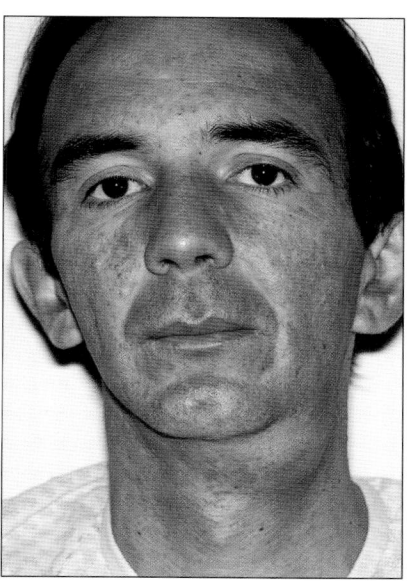

Fig 2-27a Painful blistering response to a PPD skin antigen test placed on an individual with a history of successfully treated tuberculosis.

Fig 2-27b Tuberculous lymphadenitis (scrofula) in the neck, which had no lung involvement and was limited to the lymphatics. Cultures grew out *M scrofulateum.*

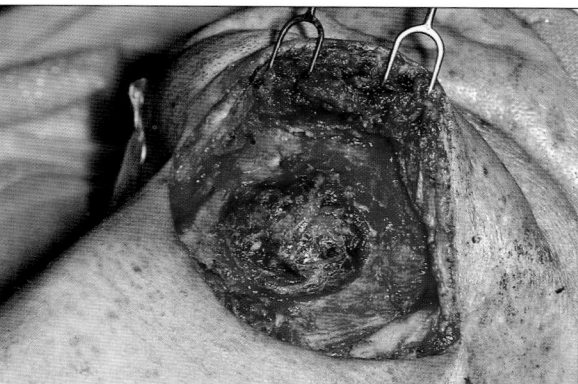

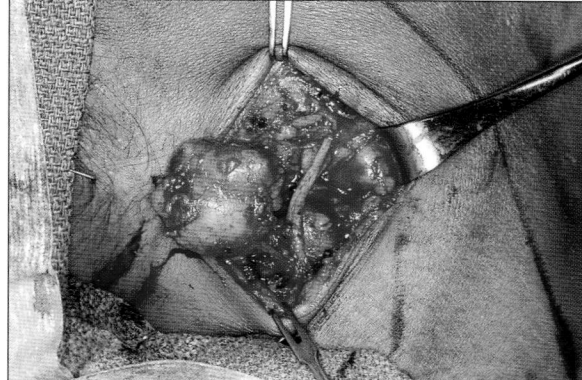

Fig 2-27c Excision of tubercular lymph nodes may reveal large necrotic nodes filled with caseous necrosis, as shown here. Others may reveal multiple smaller, nonnecrotic lymph nodes.

Fig 2-27d This tubercular lymph node was one of several firm, freely movable lymph nodes.

cell-mediated hypersensitivity to the antigen. This test has no usefulness in a clinically overt case with oral and pulmonary lesions and confirmatory staining or culture. In fact, it is not advisable to administer a PPD test if the history includes a TB diagnosis. In such cases, an exuberant response to the PPD may occur, causing a painful blistering and skin slough (Fig 2-27a). A reactive PPD denotes prior exposure and a competent immune response, not necessarily active disease.

Scrofula may be due to *Mycobacterium scrofulateum* as an independent cervical lymphadenitis, or it may be due to pulmonary tuberculosis from coughed-up sputum with either *M tuberculosis* or *M scrofulateum* draining into the cervical lymphatics through the oral mucosa. Many will present with one or two large, indurated, fixed nodes with a suspicion of fluctuation due to necrosis (Figs 2-27b and 2-27c). Others will present as several smaller, firm nodes that are freely movable (Fig 2-27d). Cervical lymph node excision will diagnose and resolve the involved node, but the other cervical lymph nodes may be infected in earlier stages of the disease or may harbor mycobacteria. Therefore patients require the same systemic drug regimens as for oral or pulmonary tuberculosis. In addition, a chest radiograph and a thorough survey for other areas of tuberculosis are warranted.

HISTOPATHOLOGY ▶

Tuberculosis is a disease that epitomizes the formation of so-called epithelioid granulomas. In the initial infection in an unsensitized host, the organisms multiply freely and there is a proliferation of neutrophils with necrosis. The bacteria are subsequently picked up by macrophages, where they proliferate intracellularly, since mycobacteria, with their thick, protein-phospholipid, hydrophilic, and lysosomal enzyme-resistant cell wall, are well protected. These immature macrophages cannot initially destroy them. Over a 3- to 6-week period, cell-mediated immunity develops, stimulated at least in part by the mycobacterial cell wall. Sensitized T cells secrete lymphokines, which promote the influx of macrophages into the area, immobilize them at the site, and then stimulate them to develop into mature macrophages, which have increased phagocytic ability and higher levels of lysosomal enzymes. Continued stimulation transforms these macrophages into epithelioid cells, which have abundant eosinophilic cytoplasm. These cells are mainly secretory and have greatly decreased phagocytic ability. Their function appears to be digestion of the organisms and foreign material. Multinucleated giant cells develop by fusion of macrophages. Their function is similar to that of the epithelioid cells. The giant cells have intensely eosinophilic cytoplasm and more frequently will have nuclei rimming the cell in a horseshoe arrangement (Langhans giant cell), although some may show clumping of nuclei (foreign body giant cell). The center of the granuloma may undergo caseous necrosis. This process is one in which the necrotic mononuclear cells persist as eosinophilic debris, devoid of cell outlines. Grossly it is soft, white, and cheesy, hence the term *caseous*. It is thought to be a result of the action of the peptidoglycolipids that comprise the waxy wall of the mycobacterium. Once the immune system begins to prevail, reparative features become apparent, including fibrosis and calcification. Residual bacilli may persist to give rise to a reinfection at some future time.

The typical histology of tuberculosis then is effacement of the normal architecture by numerous granulomas, which are often confluent (Fig 2-28a). The granulomas consist of macrophages, epithelioid cells, and multinucleated giant cells usually of the Langhans type, with peripheral lymphocytes, plasma cells, and fibroblasts (Figs 2-28b and 2-28c). The center of the granuloma may show caseous necrosis (Fig 2-28d). This is not usually seen in intraoral lesions but may be an important component in lymph node involvement and in the lung.

TREATMENT ▶

Oral TB lesions are treated with the same drug regimens used to treat pulmonary TB, except that treatment lasts for a duration of 9 months rather than 6 months because the lesions are considered extrapulmonary foci. Before the mid-1980s, oral as well as pulmonary TB in adults and children 12 years or older was treated with oral isoniazid (INH), 300 mg daily, and oral rifampin, 600 mg daily, for 9 months. This regimen had a cure rate of 97% in compliant individuals and remains the preferred regimen in the HIV-negative patient with culture-proven sensitivity to these drugs. However, HIV-positive individuals, patients with known exposure to multidrug-resistant strains, and high-risk individuals such as medical personnel, drug abusers, and lower-body-weight persons are candidates for a four-drug regimen. That regimen is oral isoniazid (INH), 5 mg/kg (300 mg maximum) daily; oral rifampin, 10 mg/kg (600 mg maximum) daily; oral pyrazinamide, 15 to 30 mg/kg (2 g maximum) daily; and oral ethambutol, 15 mg/kg daily, or intramuscular streptomycin, 20 to 30 mg/kg per day (1 g maximum).

INH is bactericidal to mycobacteria that have been engulfed by macrophages. It is also bactericidal to extracellular organisms. INH is exceedingly effective, but resistant mutations will arise in organism populations greater than 1×10^7, hence the need for double-, triple-, and even quadruple-drug therapy. INH also may produce a drug-induced neuritis or hepatitis due to its metabolic breakdown product, hydralazine.

The incidence of both INH-induced neuritis and hepatitis increases after the age of 35 years. Therefore, oral pyridoxine, 10 mg daily, is often used to prevent neuritis. Liver function tests (aspartate aminotransferase [AST]/alanine aminotransferase [ALT]) should be used to assess for possible hepatitis,

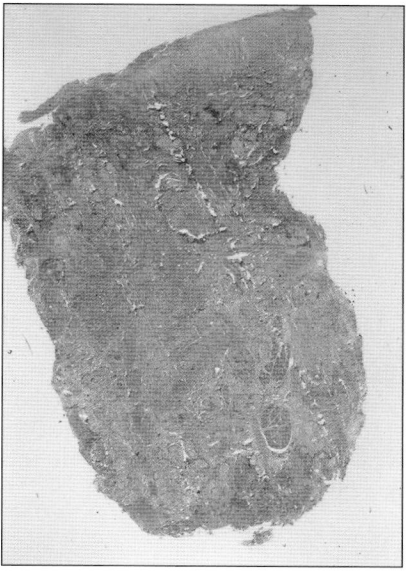

Fig 2-28a Low-power view of the tongue showing effacement of the normal muscular architecture. It is caused by replacement of the normal tissue by the granulomatous process of tuberculosis.

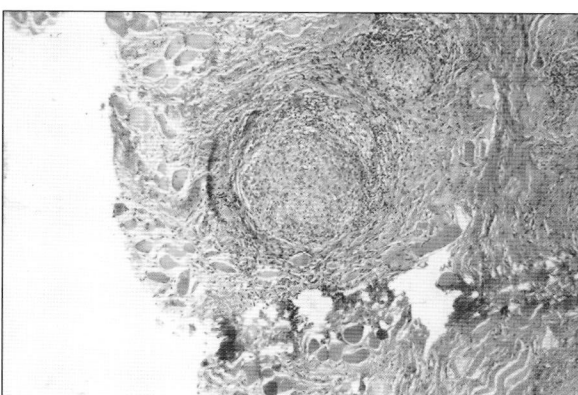

Fig 2-28b Higher-power view of Fig 2-28a showing a focal aggregate of macrophages (epithelioid cells) with peripheral lymphocytes.

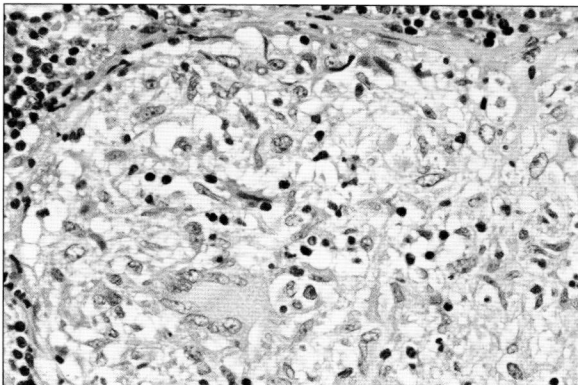

Fig 2-28c High-power view of a granuloma in tuberculosis showing pale epithelioid cells (the morphology of the nuclei demonstrates their histiocytic origin), a Langhans-type giant cell with peripherally placed nuclei, and some lymphocytes.

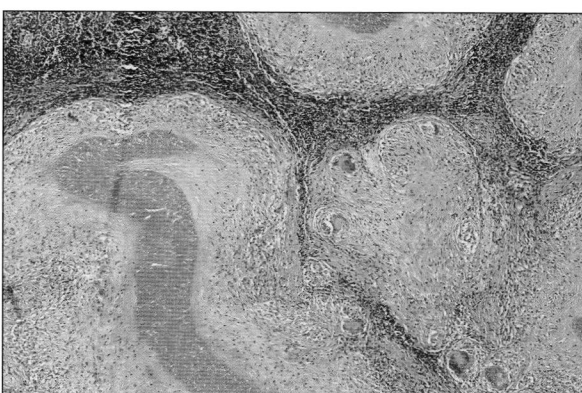

Fig 2-28d Epithelioid granulomas in tuberculosis with lymphocytes at the periphery. On the left is a granuloma containing a central area of caseous necrosis, which stains intensely with eosin.

which may require INH withdrawal. Rifampin is similarly bactericidal both to extracellular and intracellular organisms and may also produce a drug-induced hepatitis. Pyrazinamide is bactericidal to intracellular organisms only. If either of these drugs must be discontinued, oral ethambutol, which is bacteriostatic but still very effective, is substituted at a dose of 15 mg/kg (2.5 g maximum) daily.

PROGNOSIS ▶ A responding patient will have a reduction in pain associated with the oral lesion and evidence of healing. The pulmonary lesion will heal with a dense scarring, which causes a "white-out" area of the lung in the location of the previous cavitary radiolucency and usually a deviation of the trachea to the involved side (Fig 2-29). Response rates are over 95% in all individuals with drug-sensitive organisms. The less than 5% of cases that relapse are due to noncompliance. Household members and other close contacts of the treated patient should undergo PPD testing. Those who test reactive should receive INH, 300 mg

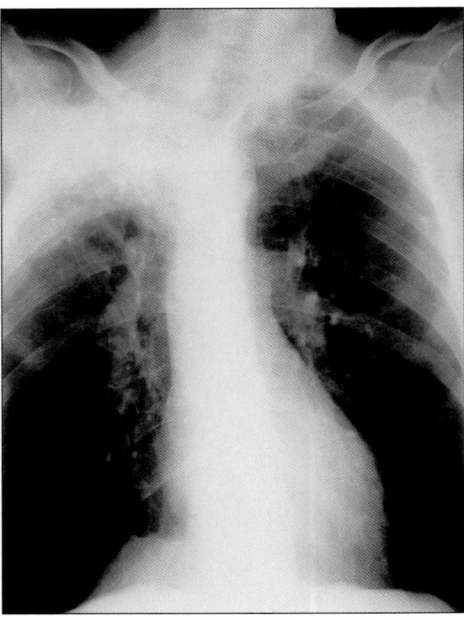

Fig 2-29 Healed pulmonary tuberculosis, evidenced by a "white-out" of the previously radiolucent area. Also noteworthy is a tracheal deviation toward the previously involved side. Both observations are due to scar formation as the result of healing.

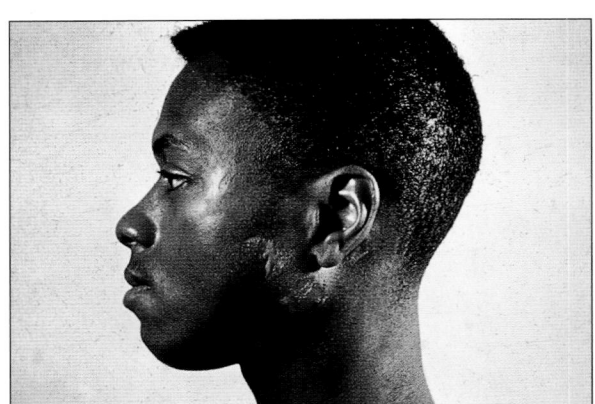

Fig 2-30 Tuberculosis of the skin (lupus vulgaris) is very rare today. It presents as a single set or multiple sets of skin ulcers with rolled margins.

daily for adults and 10 to 14 mg/kg for children, over a 12-month period. Because these patients are exposed or infected with organism inoculums significantly less than 1×10^7, INH is effective as a single prophylactic drug without a significant incidence of drug resistance.

Tuberculosis of the Skin

The oral and maxillofacial specialist should recognize that in very rare instances TB may also present as a primary skin infection. In medieval times, it was referred to as *lupus vulgaris* because of the wolf-like appearance of the face. TB of the skin is almost always independent of pulmonary TB. It will present as a chronic ulcerative involvement of the skin with rolled margins (Fig 2-30) and may resemble the lesions of sarcoidosis, discoid lupus erythematosus, or early leprosy. Caseation is usually mild or absent. Once granulomas are identified by skin biopsy and cultures reveal *M tuberculosis*, treatment with the same drug regimens as are used for pulmonary TB is indicated.

Leprosy

CLINICAL PRESENTATION AND PATHOGENESIS ▶

Individuals with the lepromatous form of leprosy will often show disfiguring, erythematous, malignant-looking plaques and nodules, particularly around cooler tissues of the body: skin, nose, eyes, oral mucosa (Fig 2-31), pharynx, testicles, and superficial nerves. Symmetric involvement of superficial nerves by direct infiltration and a thickening response of the nerve itself results in anesthesias, paresthesias, and pain in various areas. Moreover, the anesthesia often complicates the course by causing unrealized trauma, leading to ulcers, secondary infections, and necrosis.

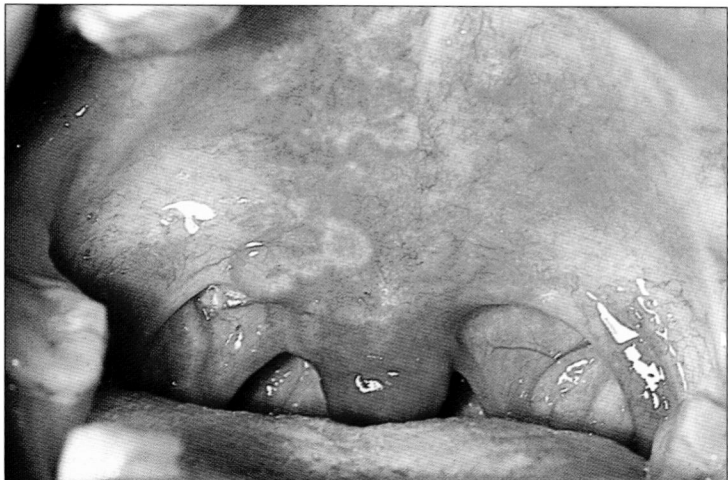

Fig 2-31 Mucosal lesions involving the palate in lepromatous leprosy. (Reprinted from Bork K et al, *Diseases of the Oral Mucosa and the Lips*, with permission from WB Saunders Co.)

Individuals with the tuberculoid form of leprosy, in contrast, have skin lesions that are more benign and less progressive. The same distribution of skin lesions occurs, but the lesions are macular rather than plaque-like and nodular. The nerve involvement may be of sudden onset, but its distribution is more asymmetric and less severe than in the lepromatous form.

Historically, epidemiologic control of leprosy has been attempted without much success. This is probably because the early stage of leprosy, when it may either go undetected or be confused with other disease entities, is the stage of highest transmissibility. Today, segregation of those with leprosy, either in the home or in voluntary institutions such as the National Leprosarium in Carville, Louisiana, is common. Isolation during active treatment is, however, unnecessary. The mode of transmission seems to be respiratory and requires prolonged exposure during childhood. Adults rarely contract the disease even in the tropical and subtropical areas of Asia, Africa, the Pacific, and Central America, where the disease is endemic.

DIFFERENTIAL DIAGNOSIS ▶

Disfiguring facial skin lesions with sensory neurologic changes are also seen in *mycosis fungoides* (a cutaneous lymphoma), *sarcoidosis, chronic skin lichen planus, discoid lupus erythematosus,* and the other known mycobacterial skin disease, *tuberculosis of the skin* (lupus vulgaris).

DIAGNOSTIC WORK-UP ▶

Lepromatous leprosy occurs in individuals with defective cellular immunity. Therefore, their clinical course is progressive and debilitating. Lesions will contain abundant numbers of the acid-fast bacillus *Mycobacterium leprae*. Because of patients' inherent reduced cellular immunity, the lepromin skin antigen test is nonreactive. In the tuberculoid type, cellular immunity is intact, thereby limiting the severity and progression of the disease and reducing the number of organisms present in lesions. The lepromin skin antigen test is reactive in this type of leprosy.

Confirmation of the diagnosis requires identification of acid-fast bacilli from scrapings or smears obtained from skin, oral, or nasal lesions. An acid-fast stain such as Ziehl-Neelsen is used in the manner described in the tuberculosis section (see above). Skin biopsy specimens that include cutaneous nerves will show a thickened nerve due to a granulomatous reaction and fibrosis. Cultures on artificial media will not support the growth of *M leprae* colonies. With some effort, transmission to the foot pad of mice or the nine-banded armadillo is possible, but this remains a research model more than a diagnostic technique.

HISTOPATHOLOGY ▶

The histologic spectrum of leprosy is a wonderful illustration of the cellular changes that are a reflection of the immune response.

In tuberculoid leprosy, the patient has a strong, competent cellular immune response to *M leprae*. Thus, just as in tuberculosis, epithelioid granulomas are formed with some Langhans giant cells and peripheral lymphocytes. The granulomas closely resemble those of sarcoidosis. However, acid-fast organ-

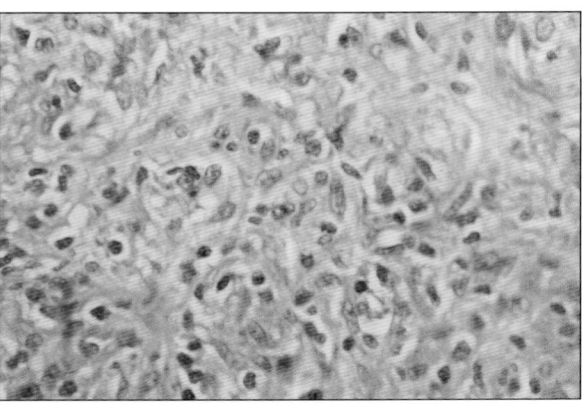

Fig 2-32a Lepromatous leprosy showing sheets of pale-staining macrophages.

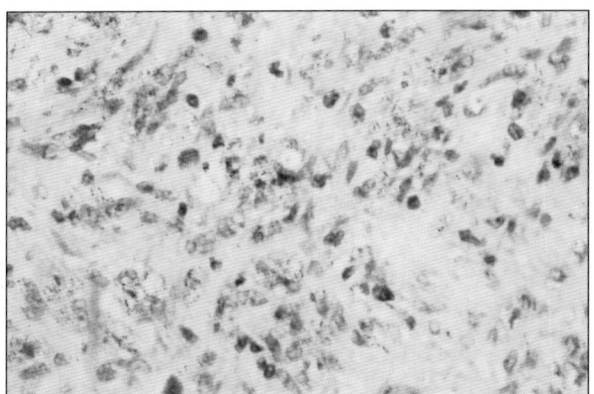

Fig 2-32b Ziehl-Neelsen stain demonstrating the large number of acid-fast organisms (*M leprae*) present in lepromatous leprosy.

isms, although sparse and often absent, may sometimes be identified. *M leprae*, like *M tuberculosis*, have thick protein-phospholipid cell walls so that both organisms are well protected, grow slowly, and are acid fast. Since leprosy affects nerve, some of this tissue may be seen within the granuloma.

At the other extreme is lepromatous leprosy, in which the patient shows no cell-mediated immune response to the organism. This appears to be a specific immunodeficiency to the organism, for these patients are otherwise immunocompetent. The consequence is that there is no granuloma formation. Instead, there is a proliferation of macrophages (Fig 2-32a), most of which contain lipid and have a foamy appearance (lepra cells). They frequently contain large numbers of organisms that can be identified by an acid-fast stain such as a Ziehl-Neelsen or Fite stain (Fig 2-32b). Lymphocytes are sparse, and the macrophages are separated from overlying epithelium by a band of normal fibrous tissue (grenz zone).

The intermediate forms of leprosy show an intermediate histologic picture and reflect an intermediate immunologic response.

▶ TREATMENT

Combination antibiotic therapy is required for all types of leprosy because single-drug therapy rapidly leads to the emergence of resistant strains. For the lepromatous type, in which there is little natural host defense, and for those types that may be intermediate between the lepromatous and tuberculoid types, triple-drug therapy is recommended. The most effective regimen is dapsone, 50 to 100 mg daily, clofazimine (Lamprene, CibaGeneva), 50 mg daily, and rifampin, 10 mg/kg per day up to a maximum of 600 mg. All of these drugs are given orally and are continued indefinitely or until toxicity develops. Ethionamide (Trecator-SC, Wyeth-Ayerst), 250 to 375 mg daily, may be substituted for clofazimine if toxicity develops.

For the tuberculoid type, which has a contribution from host defenses, a double-drug regimen of dapsone and rifampin in the same doses is used for 6 months, followed by dapsone alone for up to 5 years.

A phenomenon called *erythema nodosum leprosum* is known to occur as a response to drug therapy. This is caused by the eradication of numerous *leprae*, which results in the dispersion of antigens systemically. Antigen-antibody complexes thus form and become deposited in the skin and other tissues. The skin lesions and nerve involvements will temporarily seem to worsen. The patient may also develop fever, fatigue, and myalgia. This reaction may be reduced with oral prednisone, 40 to 80 mg daily, for 1 to 2 weeks, but the leprosy therapy should not be discontinued. As an alternative to prednisone, thalidomide (Thalomid, Celgene), 300 mg daily, can be used initially for a few days followed by a tapering dosage to 100 mg daily at bedtime for 3 weeks. Of course, thalidomide, which has the potential for mutagenesis in sperm and eggs as well as in the developing fetus, is contraindicated in pregnancy and even in those in childbearing years, including men who do not use condoms.

▶ PROGNOSIS

The tissue destruction of skin and nerve is irreversible, leading to scars and tissue contraction as devastating as the original lesion. Relapse is common because of the slow turnover rate of the organism, which gives the false clinical impression of control or cure, and to breaks in therapy due to the tedium of continued multidrug therapy.

Sarcoidosis

CLINICAL PRESENTATION AND PATHOGENESIS ▶

Sarcoidosis is known to present with any of a wide range of manifestations or with none at all. In the head and neck area, the most commonly seen manifestations include soft parotid enlargements, cervical lymphadenopathy, maxillary sinus masses with bone destruction, enlargement of submandibular or sub-lingual glands, and nodular mucosal lesions. In North America, blacks have a much higher incidence than whites (6:1), and black women are affected more than black men. In Europe, whites are more commonly affected without a sex predilection. In both groups, disease signs or symptoms usually begin in the 20s or early 30s.

Although oral and maxillofacial specialists are attuned to the head and neck manifestations of sarcoidosis, it is important to remember that sarcoidosis is a systemic disease with a 90% incidence of lung involvement. Other organ involvements include liver (50%), skin (25%) (usually as disfiguring facial skin lesions called *lupus pernio*), and bone (5%). Symptoms also are variable; the most common symptom is fatigue or easy fatigability.

Sarcoidosis remains a disease of unknown etiology, but theories abound. Originally, pine pollens and beryllium were suspected causes but are now discounted. Viral and autoimmune causes have been suggested, but without any real evidence. Most recently, the identification of mycobacterial DNA and RNA in sarcoid tissue has strongly suggested either an atypical mycobacterial infection or an altered reaction to mycobacterial tuberculosis.

DIFFERENTIAL DIAGNOSIS ▶

In the clinical presentation manifesting parotid enlargement, the clinician must distinguish sarcoidosis from other lesions known to cause diffuse parotid enlargements, such as *Sjögren syndrome, sialosis, parotid lymphoma,* and a *benign lymphoepithelial lesion.* In those cases that present instead as a cervical lymph node enlargement, sarcoidosis must be distinguished from both *Hodgkin* and *non-Hodgkin lymphoma, cat-scratch disease,* the generalized *lymphadenopathy stage of HIV infection, TB adenitis,* and the many other causes of lymph node enlargement. In those cases that present as erosive maxillary sinus masses, consideration must be given to *maxillary sinus squamous cell carcinoma, malignant salivary gland tumors,* and *osteomyelitis of the maxilla.*

DIAGNOSTIC WORK-UP ▶

Because of the protean nature of the actual and potential manifestations of sarcoidosis, a suspected case requires a comprehensive work-up.

History

Look for complaints of chronic fatigue, lethargy, visual changes, anorexia, and reduced exercise tolerance or reduced daily activity level.

Review of Systems

Erythema nodosum, which are purple, elevated, nontender skin plaques, may occur on the extremities (Fig 2-33a). On the facial skin, similar lesions infiltrate the nose, cheek, and ears (Fig 2-33b). Mucosal nodules may be found on the lips and buccal mucosa. Ocular field cuts, scotomas, and reduced visual acuity may occur. The lacrimal glands may also be enlarged (Fig 2-34a). Cases in which parotid glands are also enlarged have been called *uveo-parotid fever* or *Heerfordt syndrome,* indicative of choroid, retinal, and parotid replacement by sarcoid granulomas (Fig 2-34b). Other findings include lymphadenopathy, hepatomegaly, splenomegaly, and decreased breath sounds.

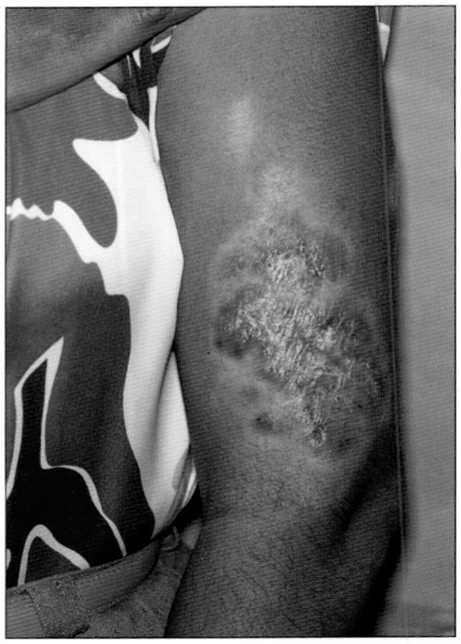

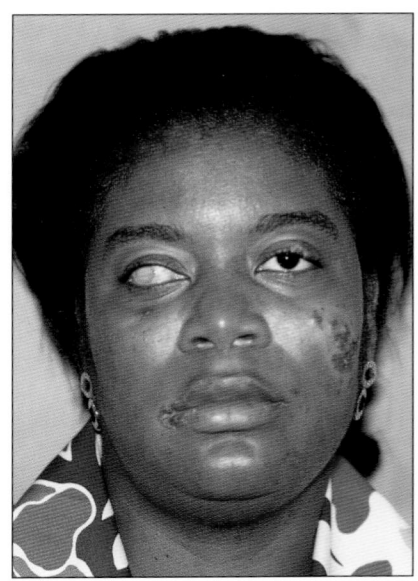

Fig 2-33a Cutaneous sarcoidosis will form large areas of rolled margins and pigment changes around a central area of either thinned skin or overt ulceration (erythema nodosum).

Fig 2-33b Cutaneous sarcoidosis of the face (lupus pernio) and right eye is evident in this individual as a deforming condition that resulted in loss of vision in the affected eye.

Radiographs

A chest radiograph is often expected to show hilar adenopathy. However, this is only one possible radiographic picture, and it is the least advanced. One may see bilateral hilar adenopathy (Stage I), bilateral hilar adenopathy with parenchymal involvement (Stage II), or parenchymal involvement alone (Stage III). The parenchymal involvement represents pulmonary fibrosis, which produces hypoxemia and is a troubling finding indicative of advanced disease (Fig 2-34c). Other radiographs may show erosive or punched-out bony lesions, particularly of the maxilla or distal phalanges.

Laboratory Tests

A complete blood count (CBC) may show leukopenia and/or eosinophilia. An erythrocyte sedimentation rate (ESR) is expected to be elevated. About 10% of cases will show hypercalcemia, which is indicative of advanced disease. Arterial blood gases may show hypoxemia (PaO_2 in the range of 50 to 80 mm Hg) and normocarbia indicative of pulmonary fibrosis in advanced disease. Anergy (absence of a delayed hypersensitivity response) exists in 70% of sarcoid patients. A negative response to skin tests with dinitrochlorobenzene (DNCB) as well as mumps, PPD, or *Candida* is consistent with, but not confirmatory of, sarcoidosis.

As a diagnostic test, the Nickerson-Kveim test was popular prior to 1985. It used human spleen or lymph node preparations from confirmed sarcoid patients as a source of antigen. The material was injected intradermally and observed for 4 to 6 weeks. If a nodule emerged, it was excised and considered confirmatory for sarcoidosis if it demonstrated noncaseating granulomas. Its positivity level was 80% to 85% if radiographic pulmonary lesions were present. It is no longer used today because of the concern about transmitting other diseases such as HIV or hepatitis from donor to test recipient.

Additionally, assessment of angiotensin-converting enzyme (ACE) levels has been advanced as a diagnostic test. ACE is a biochemical known to be found within the cell membranes of macrophages com-

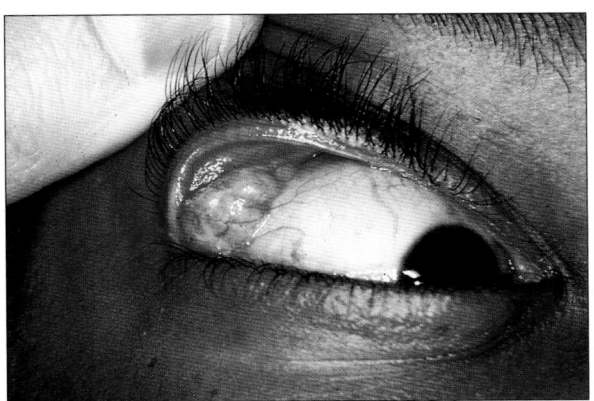

Fig 2-34a Enlarged lacrimal gland due to sarcoidosis. Sarcoidosis may involve the parotid or other salivary glands as well as the lacrimal gland.

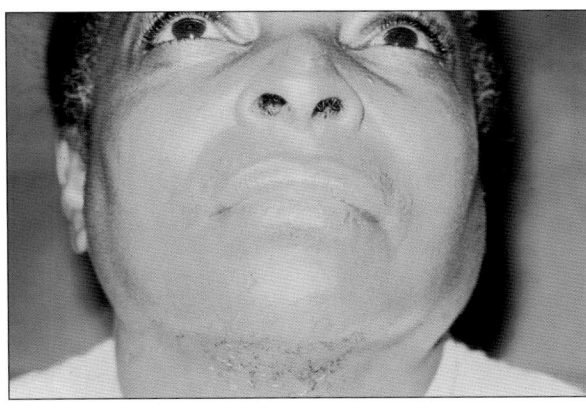

Fig 2-34b Bilateral diffuse enlargement of the parotids is a sign of sarcoidosis. This individual also had lacrimal gland involvement, lung involvement, and involvement of the uveal and retinal areas of both eyes consistent with Heerfordt syndrome.

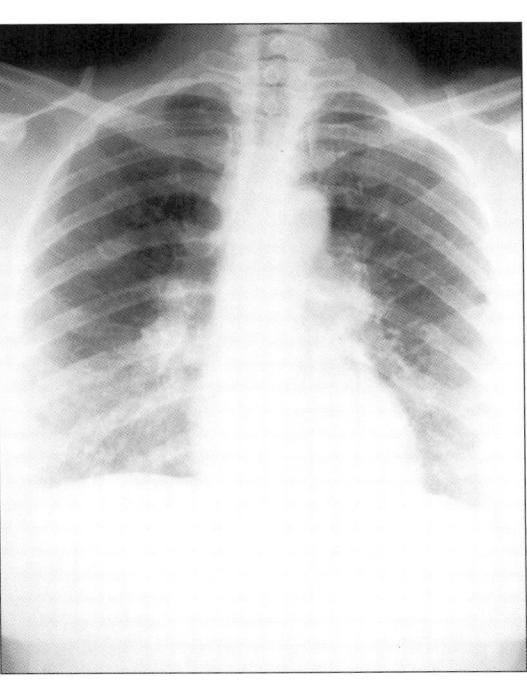

Fig 2-34c The lung involvement of the individual shown in Fig 2-34b included hilar adenopathy and interstitial fibrosis. Her PaO_2 was 67 mm Hg.

posing sarcoid granulomas. However, elevated levels of ACE are seen in many other diseases that have macrophage responses. In addition, only 40% to 80% of known sarcoid patients have elevated ACE levels. Since neither its specificity nor its sensitivity is reliable, it has little diagnostic value but can nevertheless be used as an indicator of the activity level of already-diagnosed disease.

Biopsy

Currently, the most yielding diagnostic approach is through either an incisional parotid gland biopsy or a transbronchial biopsy using a fiberoptic scope. The parotid has been found to have early involvement in sarcoidosis, making it a readily accessible biopsy site even in suspected cases that show no parotid enlargement. Incisional parotid biopsy has been shown to produce a 93% positive yield in early and subclinical sarcoidosis (Figs 2-35a and 2-35b). In cases where obvious lung involvement is observed and a parotid biopsy cannot be performed, transbronchial biopsies have produced a 70% yield. Minor salivary gland biopsy has shown a 40% to 50% yield, but only in advanced and already diagnosed cases. It is not a very yielding diagnostic step in early or less severe cases.

HISTOPATHOLOGY ▶

Sarcoidosis is another of the classic epithelioid granuloma–producing diseases. The most significant difference between sarcoidosis and tuberculosis is that sarcoidosis lacks caseous necrosis and acid-fast organisms.

The inciting agent remains unknown, but the response is the formation of compact granulomas consisting of epithelioid cells with scattered multinucleated giant cells, usually of the Langhans type (Fig 2-35c). Peripheral lymphocytes, plasma cells, and fibroblasts are usually present, and there may be formation of dense collagen. Within the granulomas, inclusion bodies may be seen. These may be asteroid bodies, reddish stellate protein structures, or Schaumann bodies, which are concentrically arranged,

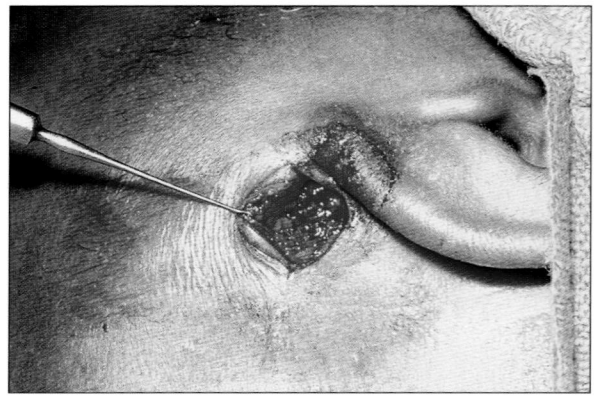

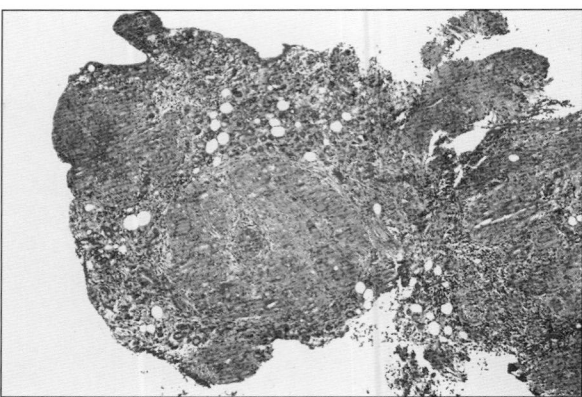

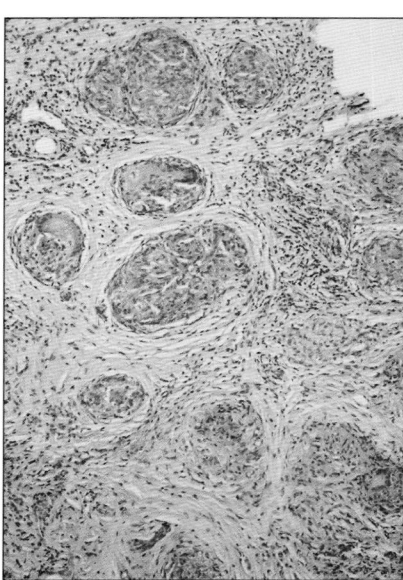

Fig 2-35a An individual suspected to have sarcoidosis undergoing an incisional parotid biopsy, which represents the most accurate and specific diagnostic approach to non-neoplastic parotid disease.

Fig 2-35b The incisional parotid biopsy of the individual shown in Figs 2-34a to 2-34c and 2-35a reveals effacement of the parotid acini by noncaseating granulomas with Langhans giant cells diagnostic for sarcoidosis.

Fig 2-35c Sarcoid granulomas composed of macrophages (epithelioid cells) and Langhans type of giant cells. Peripheral lymphocytes may be seen but are not always prominent.

lamellar, oval basophilic proteinaceous structures that contain calcium salts. Hamazaki-Wesenberg bodies, which contain giant lysosomes, may be found beyond the granulomas. The center of the granuloma does not undergo caseation, but fibrinoid necrosis is occasionally seen. Immunoglobulins can be demonstrated within the granulomas.

TREATMENT ▶

Some patients will undergo spontaneous remissions and others will continue with mild, nonprogressive disease, which requires no specific treatment. However, those with certain organ involvements or disease manifestations require corticosteroid therapy, usually prednisone. The indicators for prednisone therapy include: (*1*) Heerfordt syndrome or signs of iritis or uveitis; (*2*) disfiguring cutaneous lesions; (*3*) central nervous system sarcoidosis; (*4*) sarcoid hepatitis; (*5*) pulmonary fibrosis; (*6*) bony or joint sarcoidosis; (*7*) hypercalcemia; and (*8*) renal or cardiac sarcoidosis.

The dosage of prednisone varies with each case. Generally, loading doses are in the range of 40 mg of oral prednisone daily, which is gradually reduced by 5 mg daily every 2 weeks to the lowest dose that continues to control the disease. Usual maintenance doses are 10 to 15 mg daily for 8 months before further reductions of the daily dose by 2.5 mg per month are attempted.

PROGNOSIS ▶

Cases requiring prednisone management usually show improvement, but periodic exacerbations occur and not all symptoms are alleviated. In addition, these patients often must deal with the long-term side effects of continual corticosteroid management, such as weight gain, hypertension, fat deposits, muscle loss, osteoporosis, increased risk for cataracts, and adrenal suppression.

Pulmonary fibrosis, the most ominous finding, is associated with the worst prognosis. About 5% to 8% of all sarcoid patients succumb to respiratory failure despite prednisone therapy.

Cheilitis Granulomatosis

CLINICAL PRESENTATION AND PATHOGENESIS ▶

Individuals with cheilitis granulomatosis will present with diffuse enlargement of the lips, most notably the lower lip (Figs 2-36a and 2-36b). The enlargement resembles edema, is nonpitting and painless, and increases over several months. The vermilion may show some fissuring if the enlargement is extensive,

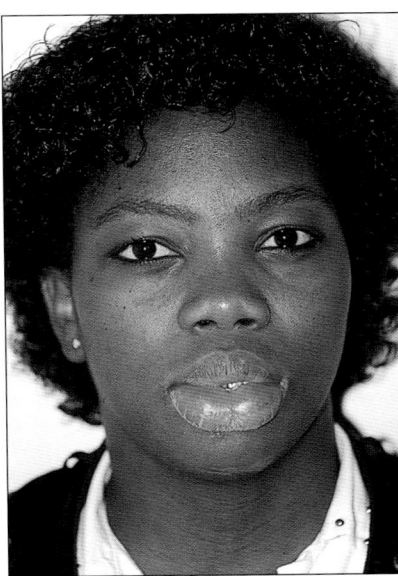 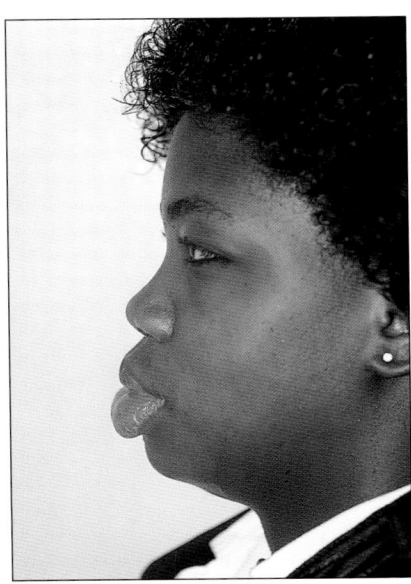

Figs 2-36a and 2-36b The clinically enlarged lower lip developed spontaneously and evidenced noncaseating granulomas. Without any signs of sarcoidosis or Melkersson-Rosenthal syndrome, this finding can be termed *cheilitis granulomatosis*.

but the skin and mucosa remain intact. As an individual entity, it must be histologically confirmed to have sarcoid-like noncaseating granulomas without other findings. If such granulomas are noted together with a fissured tongue or facial paralysis, it is considered part of the Melkersson-Rosenthal syndrome (see Chapter 3).

The pathogenesis of cheilitis granulomatosis remains unknown. It may represent a variant of sarcoidosis. As a single entity, it may even represent a forme fruste of the Melkersson-Rosenthal syndrome.

DIFFERENTIAL DIAGNOSIS ▶ The clinical presentation will suggest *angioneurotic edema, cheilitis glandularis* (an inflammatory hyperplasia of labial minor salivary glands without granuloma features), or *Melkersson-Rosenthal syndrome.*

DIAGNOSTIC WORK-UP ▶ Tissue biopsy is indicated to assess the presence or absence of sarcoid-like granulomas. Tissue biopsy specimens should include minor salivary glands and adjacent submucosa. It is recommended to consider a biopsy in the midline of the lower lip, which will be well hidden and will avoid small sensory nerve branches to the vermilion from the mental nerve.

HISTOPATHOLOGY ▶ Cheilitis granulomatosis is yet another disease process characterized by the presence of noncaseating epithelioid granulomas, resembling sarcoidosis. The granulomas are usually small with occasional Langhans giant cells. They may encroach on or obstruct the lumen in a perivascular location. Superficial edema of the connective tissue with perivascular lymphocytic infiltrates also is often seen.

TREATMENT ▶ If untreated, the disease will last for many years. Some cases will diminish slowly with time. A reduction cheiloplasty is often used to reduce drooling and improve speech. The cheiloplasty usually takes the form of a wedge resection of surface and deep mucosa paralleling the lip vermilion–cutaneous line and located in the oral-labial mucosa. As the wound is closed, the everted lip is rotated orally. If sufficient submucosa is excised, the lip bulk will approach a more normal contour. In some cases, a two-stage reduction cheiloplasty is required because of the excessive bulk and distortion of the lip.

PROGNOSIS ▶ Even with a reduction cheiloplasty, the lower lip remains somewhat enlarged and everted. This may result from an inability to remove the precise amount of submucosa required or from redevelopment of the granulomatous cheilitis.

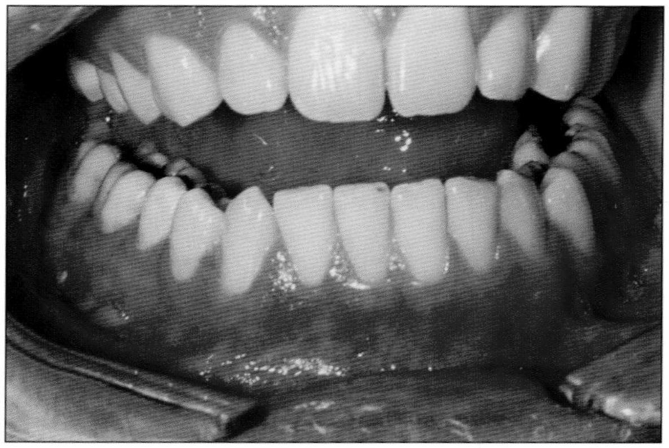

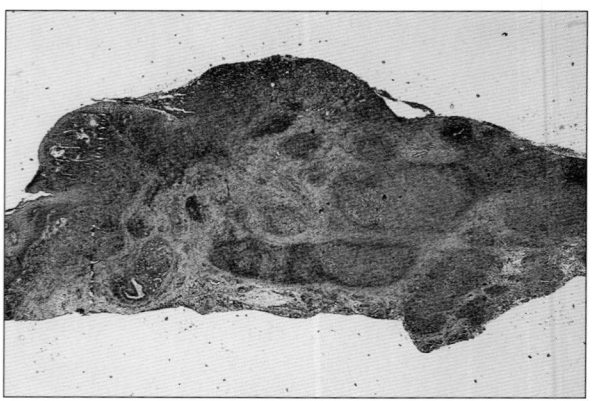

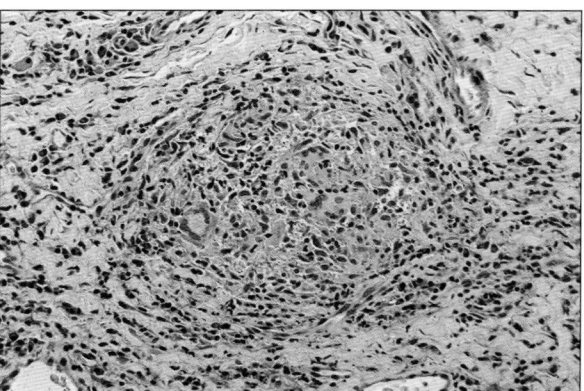

Fig 2-37a Crohn disease may present as painful submucosal nodules with or without ulceration.

Fig 2-37b Gingival biopsy specimen from a patient with Crohn disease showing numerous areas of granulomatous inflammation, many of which are deeply placed.

Fig 2-37c High-power view of Fig 2-37b showing a loose aggregate of macrophages, lymphocytes, and Langhans giant cells.

Crohn Disease

CLINICAL PRESENTATION AND PATHOGENESIS ▶

Because Crohn disease is primarily a transmural (ie, involves all depths of the mucous membrane) granulomatous colitis, most signs and symptoms will be related to the gastrointestinal system. The disease infrequently involves oral mucous membranes with granulomatous nodules and ulcers. Some patients will be identified early by recognition and biopsy findings of the oral lesions without specific signs or symptoms related to their developing colitis. Diarrhea is the most common symptom of Crohn disease, followed by abdominal cramps and weight loss. Severe cases will frequently result in bowel perforation and fistula formation. Oral lesions are uncommon, but perianal lesions are common. The oral lesions may be asymptomatic but will often be recognized by the patient because of pain. The lesions will present as focal edema, small aphthous ulcers, linear ulcers, hyperplastic gingivitis, or small polypoid cobblestone papules. Oral lesions occur mostly on lips, gingiva, and the vestibules of the mouth (Fig 2-37a).

The cause of Crohn disease remains an enigma. Theories suggesting immune disorders, nutritional imbalance, folate deficiency, infections, and even toothpaste-related hyperimmune reactivity have been proposed, but nothing has been documented.

DIFFERENTIAL DIAGNOSIS ▶

The presentation with oral ulcers will strongly suggest the vasculitis now recognized as part of *aphthous stomatitis*. Other painful conditions with such oral lesions may suggest *Behçet syndrome* or possibly *pemphigus vulgaris*. Mild or painless lesions may mimic *reactive arthritis* or a nonspecific *periodontal inflammation*.

DIAGNOSTIC WORK-UP ▶

The oral lesions should undergo biopsy to confirm their granulomatous nature consistent with Crohn disease. The patient should undergo a complete gastrointestinal fiberoptic visual evaluation with biopsy as well as a complete upper and lower gastrointestinal radiographic series with contrast. Distinguishing Crohn disease from ulcerative colitis can be difficult. However, two serum tests are useful. Serum testing for antineutrophil cytoplasmic antibodies with perinuclear staining (p-ANCA) is 70% positive in ulcerative colitis but rarely positive in Crohn disease. Conversely, a test for antibodies to the yeast *Saccharomyces cerevisiae* (ASCA) is positive in 70% of cases of Crohn disease but rarely positive in ulcerative colitis.

HISTOPATHOLOGY ▶

The oral lesions of Crohn disease share the same histologic characteristics as lesions at other sites. They consist of noncaseating epithelioid granulomas with multinucleated giant cells of the Langhans type. Schaumann and asteroid bodies also may be seen, as in sarcoidosis. The overlying epithelium is infiltrated by lymphocytes and plasma cells, and a mononuclear perivascular infiltrate is usually present. Ulceration

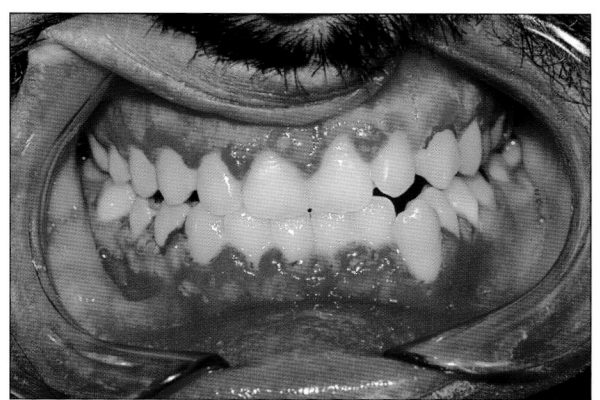

Fig 2-38 Acute necrotizing ulcerative gingivitis is a severe inflammation limited to the gingiva with ulcerations and necrosis of the interdental papillae.

of the epithelium may occur. The granulomas tend to be deeply placed and loosely arranged (Figs 2-37b and 2-37c). The mucosal thickenings consist of a fibrous hyperplasia. The connective tissue may be edematous.

TREATMENT ▶

Crohn disease is incurable. The objectives of treatment are disease control, prevention of complications such as bowel perforation and enterocutaneous fistulae, and limitation of disease progression. The core of treatment is systemic corticosteroids. Oral prednisone beginning at 60 mg daily in divided doses is usually given for 2 weeks. The prednisone is tapered by 5 mg per day each week if improvement is noted. A maintenance dose of 5 mg daily is often maintained for 6 months in a drug-induced remission. Exacerbations may require maintenance doses of more than 5 mg daily. In cases that are somewhat refractory to prednisone or exacerbate frequently, oral azathioprine (Imuran, Glaxo Wellcome), 50 mg 2 or 3 times daily, can be used as a substitute for or in addition to prednisone.

PROGNOSIS ▶

Oral lesions of Crohn disease respond well to prednisone or to azathioprine. However, the patient often undergoes progression and frequent exacerbations of the symptomatic phase. Most require lifelong medication and develop some of the complications and stigmata associated with long-term corticosteroid use.

Bacterial Diseases

Acute Necrotizing Ulcerative Gingivitis

CLINICAL PRESENTATION AND PATHOGENESIS ▶

Acute necrotizing ulcerative gingivitis (ANUG) is a rapid onset, painful bacterial infection of the gingiva caused primarily by the *Fusobacterium* species, probably in combination with oral spirochetes. As the name implies, it is acute (a rapid onset); necrotizing (the interdental gingival papillae necrose into a crater-like shape); ulcerative (the necrosis causes surface ulcerations); and a gingivitis (limited to the gingiva without progressing beyond the mucogingival line) (Fig 2-38). In the acute stage it does not affect the underlying alveolar bone, although pre-existing periodontitis may give the impression of alveolar bone loss.

Individuals will present with a complaint of pain and a noticeably fetid odor to their breath. The gingiva will be red and friable, the interdental gingival papillae will be lost, and a gray pseudomembrane of fibrin will be present. The gingiva will bleed readily if probed. The teeth will have some plaque and may also show calculus indicative of long-standing neglect. Individuals are most often young, that is, between the ages of 15 and 30 years. Most will have mild lymphadenopathy, and a few may be febrile.

The causative *Fusobacterium* species are gram-negative, obligate, anaerobic, rod-shaped organisms. Although there are 16 known species of fusobacterium, *F nucleatum* is the main organism found in the oral cavity. It is postulated that the temporary establishment of a specific anaerobic environment allows

Fusobacterium and the normal oral spirochetes to synergistically multiply, producing this infection. In the past, associations with emotional stress and smoking have been suggested as causal, but these remain only coincidental findings.

Acute painful gingival lesions with a foul odor in young individuals are also characteristic of *acute herpetic gingivostomatitis*, one of the few infectious diseases that presents in a like manner. Otherwise, immune-related diseases such as *pemphigus vulgaris, erosive lichen planus*, and *lichenoid drug reactions* are also serious considerations.

No specific test or histopathologic picture is diagnostic of ANUG. However, the clinician should carefully examine the lesions for characteristic cratering and loss of interdental papillae as well as gray surface fibrin accumulations. The presence of vesicles would focus the attention on *primary herpetic gingivostomatitis* or *pemphigus*. The involvement of oral sites other than the gingiva, particularly the tongue or buccal mucosa, will focus the attention on *erosive lichen planus* or a *lichenoid drug reaction*.

Treatment generally consists of local debridement and irrigation coupled with oral antibiotics. Initially, the teeth should undergo a light scaling to remove superficial plaque and calculus and irrigation with a solution of 3% hydrogen peroxide mixed 1:1 with saline. Local or topical anesthesia may be required to accomplish these procedures. In addition, home care plaque control instructions should be provided, and oral rinses with either the same hydrogen peroxide solution or 0.12% chlorhexidine (Peridex, Procter and Gamble) should be used. Oral antibiotics are effective, and penicillin remains the drug of choice. In the non–penicillin-allergic patient, oral phenoxymethyl penicillin (Pen Vee K, Wyeth-Ayerst), 500 mg four times daily for 7 to 10 days, is recommended. For the penicillin-allergic patient, erythromycin ethyl succinate, 400 mg twice a day for 7 to 10 days, or doxycycline, 100 mg once daily for 7 to 10 days, are good second choices.

Suppurative Osteomyelitis

Suppurative osteomyelitis can be defined as an infection of the medullary portion of bone that includes the production of pus. It is thus distinct from an osteitis such as alveolar osteitis, which is a colonization of organisms on the surface of bone, or sclerosing osteomyelitis, which does not produce pus but instead produces a thickened trabecular bone network from the endosteum.

Patients will variably present with some or all of the signs of inflammation, including swelling, limited motion, erythema, and warmth of the overlying tissues. Most will have pain. Most will be afebrile and have a normal white cell count unless the infection is severe. In such cases, a leukocytosis with a slight left shift toward immature neutrophils is seen.

The two most common causes are an extension of a dentoalveolar infection or a complication of a fracture. Another common cause is an incomplete or failed root canal treatment (Figs 2-39a and 2-39b). Some are also related to infections from extraction sockets from the removal of infected and sometimes even noninfected teeth or other pathologies such as cysts. Rare cases are related to bloodborne pathogens (Figs 2-40a and 2-40b). The mandible is affected much more than is the maxilla. Occasionally, oral cutaneous, oral-antral, or oronasal fistulae result (Fig 2-41). In some cases, bacteria-induced vessel thrombosis will create an ischemic neuropathy, causing lip paresthesias.

An early osteomyelitis may show a normal radiographic appearance. If the infection continues or progresses, an irregular radiolucent pattern with ragged borders develops, indicative of bone necrosis and pathologic resorption (Fig 2-42). Some radiographs will show a portion of bone separated from the parent bone. This has been termed a *sequestrum*, and the radiolucent band separating it from the parent bone an *involucrum*. Extensive bone infection will lead to a pathologic fracture.

Infection within the jaws and/or facial bones is usually apparent both clinically and radiographically. However, the clinician needs to be aware that malignancies such as *squamous cell carcinoma, Ewing sarcoma, non-Hodgkin lymphoma of bone, osteosarcoma*, and *multiple myeloma*, among others, can be destruc-

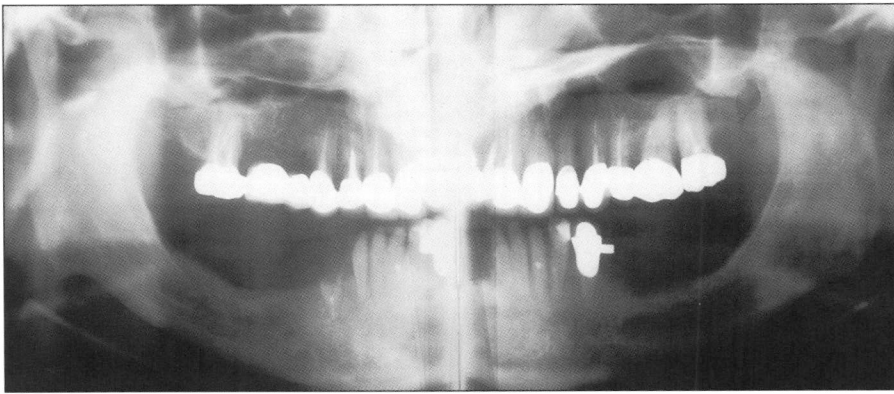

Fig 2-39a The residual root tip with an old, inadequately filled root canal is a source of microorganisms into the mandible.

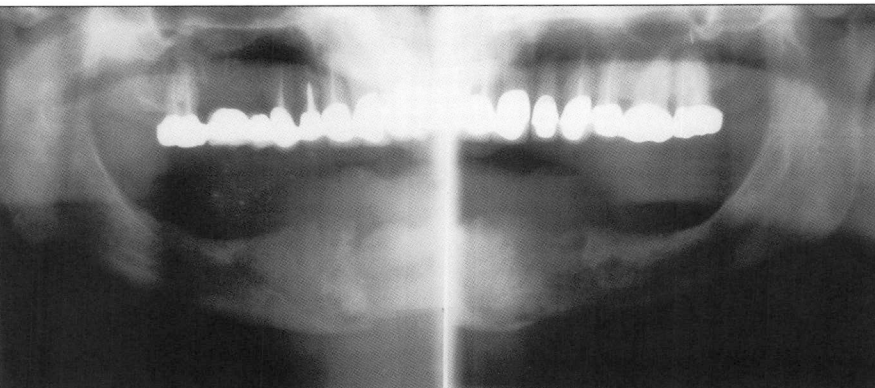

Fig 2-39b Despite removal of the root tip and other nonsalvageable teeth, a significant suppurative osteomyelitis with sequestra and osteolysis ensued.

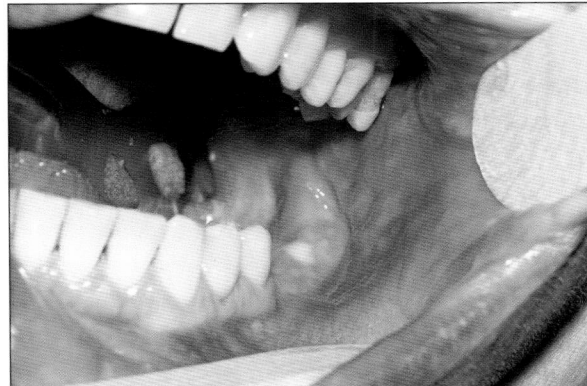

Fig 2-40a Infected tooth socket with suppuration suspicious for an osteomyelitis.

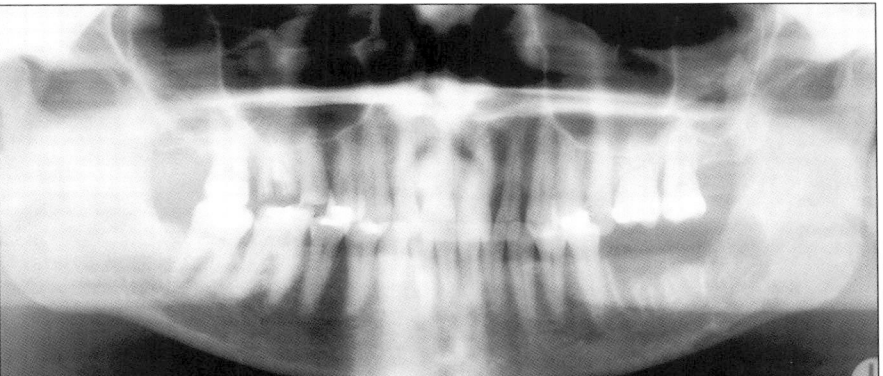

Fig 2-40b Panoramic radiograph of the same patient showing osteolysis at the inferior border, confirming an osteomyelitis.

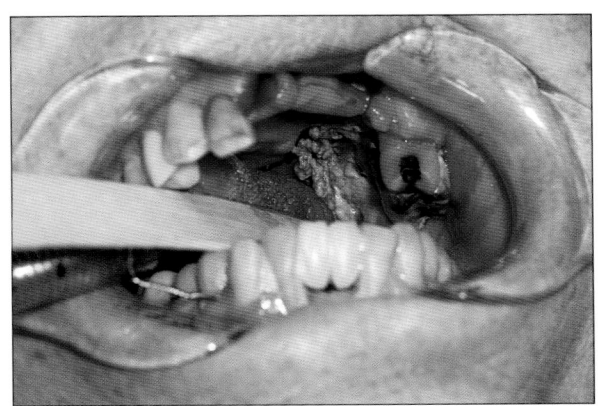

Fig 2-41 Osteomyelitis of the maxilla with significant necrotic bone and soft tissue.

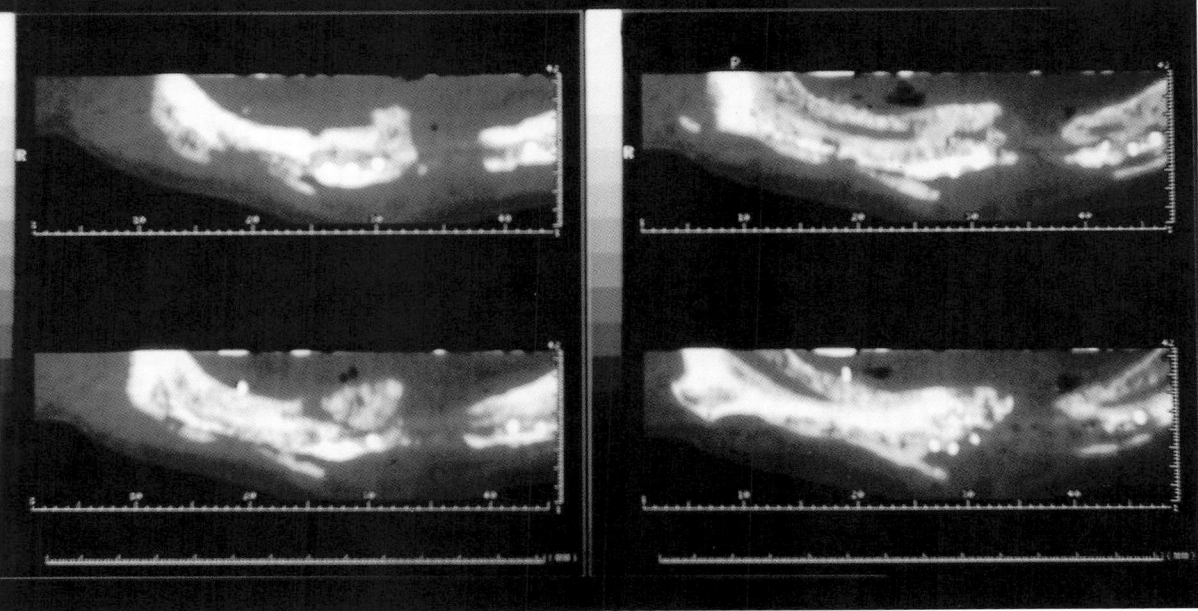

Fig 2-42 Osteomyelitis of the mandible with extensive osteolysis and numerous sequestra.

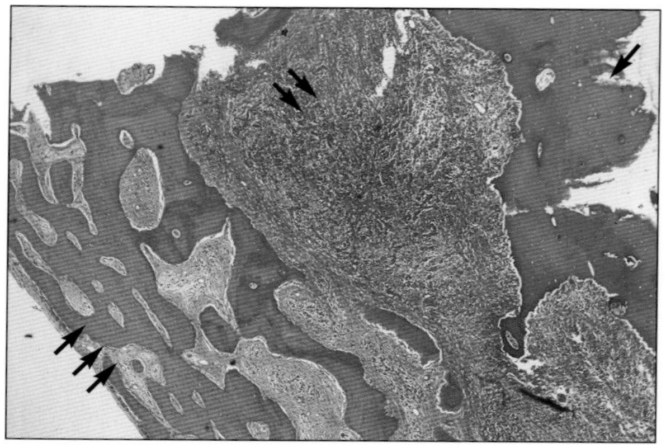

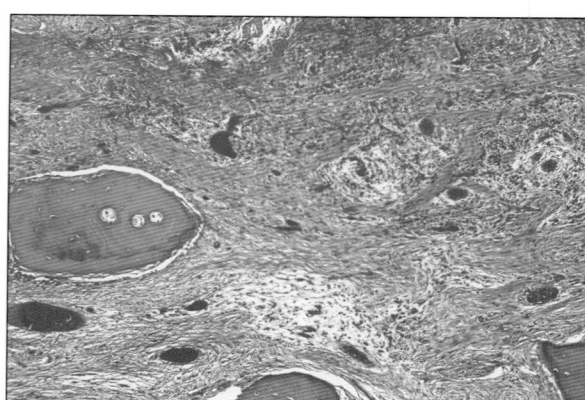

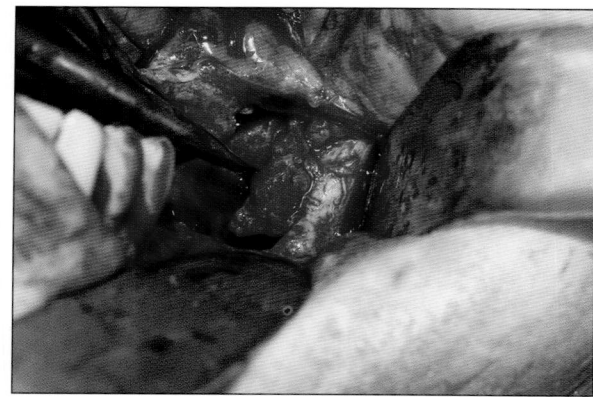

Fig 2-43a All the histopathologic features of osteomyelitis can be seen in this specimen: necrotic bone (*single arrow*), internal marrow inflammation with vascular thrombosis (*double arrows*), and attempts at reactive new bone formation (*triple arrows*).

Fig 2-43b Multiple vascular thrombi with necrotic bone. The vessel thrombosis results in a lowered tissue P_{O_2}, which supports anaerobic microorganisms.

Fig 2-44 Debridement of granulation tissue and necrotic bone is required to resolve a suppurative osteomyelitis.

tive of bone in a similar pattern and produce enough tumor-related necrosis to mimic osteomyelitis. Indeed, in those cases of osteomyelitis that present with a paresthesia, malignancy is even more likely to be suspected.

HISTOPATHOLOGY ►

Histologically, the marrow contains an inflammatory exudate consisting essentially of neutrophils. There is an accompanying loss of osteoblasts with increased bone resorption by osteoclasts. Sometimes a portion of necrotic bone with no viable cells forms (Fig 2-43a).

Within the spectrum of inflammation, a chronic osteomyelitis may supersede the acute disease, or the chronic form may result de novo from a low-grade infection. Organisms are often difficult to identify in cases of chronic disease. The histologic pattern is variable. The inflammatory component, predominantly lymphocytes and plasma cells, may be extremely sparse. The stroma is fibrous. Venous thrombosis is frequently seen (Fig 2-43b). Osteoblastic activity indicative of attempts at bone regeneration and osteoclastic activity may be seen together, often causing the bone to demonstrate prominent resting lines. When the inflammatory component is minimal, the microscopic appearance is often similar to that of fibro-osseous diseases.

DIAGNOSTIC WORK-UP AND TREATMENT ►

The approach to all suppurative infections should begin with a search for the focus of infection and a plan for removing it. If the source of the infection is a tooth, foreign body, necrotic bone, cyst, etc, failure to remove it will result in continued infection or initial recovery followed by a reinfection. At the time the infection's source is removed, all necrotic tissue should also be debrided and tissue samples taken for Gram staining, aerobic culture, and anaerobic culture before antibiotics are administered (Fig 2-44). After culture specimens are taken, empiric antibiotics, chosen by the surgeon based on his or her experience and the clinical impression of the wound, can be administered.

If the osteomyelitis is in the mandible, immobilization with maxillomandibular fixation or external skeletal pins is recommended. Internal fixation plates are not recommended in such infected tissue beds unless a resection type of debridement is undertaken. If there is abundant necrotic bone and soft tissue, an irrigating drain for 2 to 5 days can be helpful. Physiologic irrigants such as normal saline or Ringer's lactate are as effective as antibiotic irrigations. However, if residual necrotic tissue remains, debriding irrigant solutions such as one-fourth strength Dakin's solution (2.5% NaOCl and 10% $NaHCO_3$), 9-aminoacridine, or one-half strength 3% hydrogen peroxide will assist tissue debridements.

Definitive antibiotic choices should take the culture and sensitivity data into consideration, but a change of antibiotic is not warranted if the clinical course shows response to current therapy. Hyperbaric oxygen is a useful adjunct only in cases that have been refractory to aggressive treatment and to culture-specific antibiotics. These refractory cases benefit from hyperbaric oxygen's ability to oxygenate hypoxic

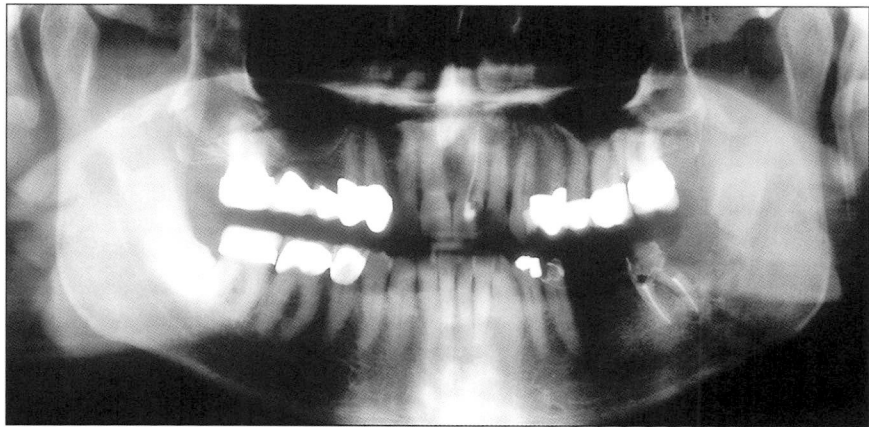

Fig 2-45a This osteomyelitis, which resulted from a failed root canal, shows significant osteolysis, including the inferior border.

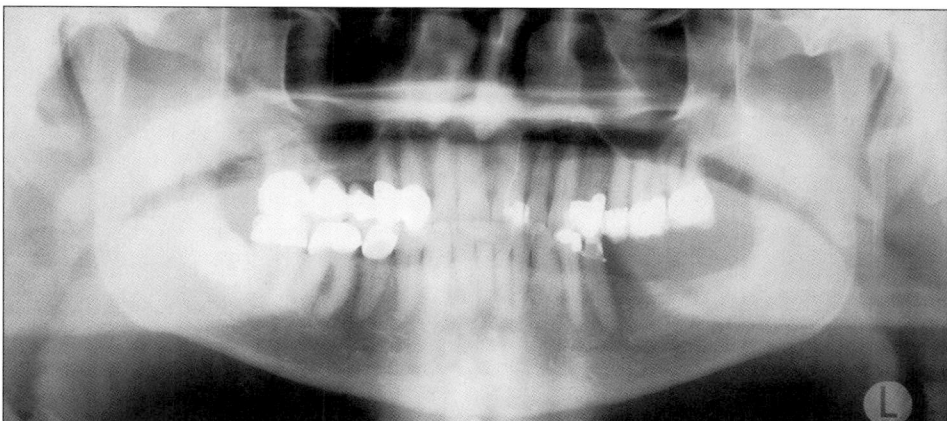

Fig 2-45b Radiographic evidence of a resolved osteomyelitis will be seen as re-formation of bone in the osteolytic areas and re-development of a distinct inferior border.

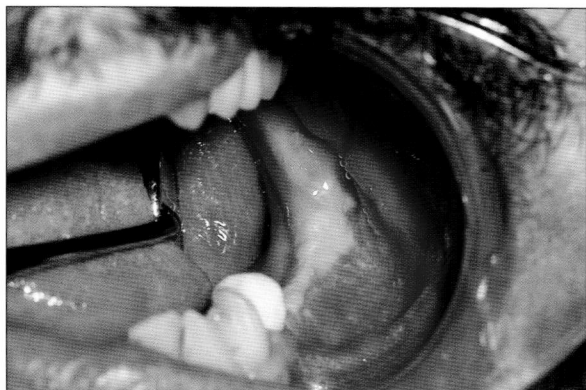

Fig 2-45c Clinical evidence of a resolved osteomyelitis will be seen as a mature soft tissue covering over all bone with no erythema, swelling, or drainage.

osteomyelitic bone and enhance neutrophil and macrophage microbial killing ability. The protocol of hyperbaric oxygen in these cases begins just after tissue debridement and is continued along with the antibiotic therapy until the osteomyelitis is clinically reversed and healing occurs. Hyperbaric oxygen is given at a dose of 2.4 atmospheres of absolute pressure (ATA) for 90 minutes, 100% oxygen, once or twice daily.

PROGNOSIS ▶

Suppurative osteomyelitis usually resolves with treatment. The bone shows signs of remodeling by the rounding off of edges and a return of a trabecular bone pattern (Figs 2-45a and 2-45b). The overlying soft tissue heals (Fig 2-45c). If signs of osteomyelitis persist, three distinct possibilities must be considered: (*1*) residual nonviable bone, a tooth fragment, or a foreign body exists within the wound or within the remaining host bone; (*2*) the organism is resistant to the antibiotic used or the true pathogen did not grow in culture (*Actinomyces* species, methicillin-resistant *Staphylococcus aureus, Eikenella corrodens*, and some *Bacteroides* species are notoriously persistent); or (*3*) a subtle malignancy mimicking an osteomyelitis is the cause.

Chronic Sclerosing Osteomyelitis

CLINICAL PRESENTATION AND PATHOGENESIS ▶

Chronic sclerosing osteomyelitis (CSO) is a sclerosing intramedullary bone infection caused by one of the *Actinomyces* species in a mutualism with *E corrodens* (Fig 2-46). The hallmark of CSO is persistent intense pain. There are periods of more intense pain, mild expansion of the mandible, and even soft tissue swelling "active exacerbations," but there remains a background of constant pain. The mandible is involved mostly in the body, angle, and ramus area. Suggestive similar cases have been seen in the maxilla but in much fewer numbers. The mandible may be tender to palpation, particularly at the buccal cortex. No suppuration or drainage is noted.

CSO has a 2:1 predilection for women and an average course of nearly 5 years before diagnosis. The disease can occur at any age but has a peak onset in the 30s. There is no racial predilection, although some believe that one should exist because florid cemento-osseous dysplasia, for which CSO is often mistaken, has a predilection for blacks.

The combination of an *Actinomyces* species and *E corrodens* produces a sclerosis in bone analogous to the fibrosis that these organisms are known to produce in soft tissue. Normal inhabitants of the oral flora, they become pathogens upon gaining a portal of entry into bone, where they establish and maintain an anaerobic environment via sclerosis and fibrosis. Their portal of entry may be via pulpal infection, endodontic therapy, or local hematogenous spread from periodontal disease.

DIFFERENTIAL DIAGNOSIS ▶

The diffuse sclerotic nature of a panoramic radiograph will mimic fibro-osseous diseases and some abnormalities of bone remodeling. If the patient is older than 40 years, *Paget disease* is a distinct consideration. In younger patients, a *Garré osteomyelitis* and *fibrous dysplasia* may show a similar radiographic picture. In addition, a well-differentiated *osteosarcoma* that produces dense tumor bone may also initially present a similar picture.

RADIOGRAPHIC FINDINGS ▶

A panoramic radiograph will show a poorly demarcated, increased trabecular bone density, which will diffusely involve alveolar bone, basilar bone, and/or the ramus (Fig 2-47a). That is, it will not be limited to the tooth-bearing alveolar bone as is florid cemento-osseous dysplasia. The mandibular canal will appear to be widened. Occlusal radiographs and especially an axial CT scan are highly recommended. CSO will characteristically show a prominent endosteal sclerosis without prominent cortical bone loss and with minimal or no periosteal bone formation (Fig 2-47b).

DIAGNOSTIC WORK-UP ▶

A panoramic radiograph, an occlusal radiograph, and a CT scan are recommended. The mandible requires medullary bone exploration for biopsy and cultures (Fig 2-47c). Because *Actinomyces* species, in particular, are very difficult to grow, a specific specimen and culture protocol should be strictly followed.

Specimen procurement and handling are as follows:

1. Discontinue antibiotic or hyperbaric oxygen therapy for 1 week prior to obtaining specimens.
2. Obtain a bone biopsy specimen for cultures from the medullary space.
3. Transport the specimen to the microbiology laboratory within 15 minutes.
4. In a tissue grinder, grind the specimen in thioglycolate broth.
5. Culture anaerobic specimens using a CO_2-enriched gas pouch.
6. Use CDC anaerobic blood agar and chocolate blood agar after initial colony growth in thioglycolate.
7. Hold plates for observation for at least 7 days before specific biochemical identification is accomplished.

Such rigid microbiologic detail has identified the pathogenic species of *Actinomyces* to be any one of the known species: *A viscosus, A naeslundii, A israelii, A meyerii,* or *A odontolyticus* combined with *E corrodens*. Occasionally, *Arachnia propionica*, which is similar to *Actinomyces* organisms, will be cultured instead of an *Actinomyces* organism, and various other oral organisms may be part of the culture yield.

HISTOPATHOLOGY ▶

The histologic picture is one related to a chronic inflammatory process with reactive and reparative features. Thus the marrow will appear fibrous, and varying quantities of inflammatory cells, predominantly lymphocytes and plasma cells, will be seen, sometimes with admixed neutrophils. Irregular, thick, osseous trabeculae are seen with increased resting lines (Fig 2-47d). Sometimes colonies of organisms are seen on the bone trabeculae (Figs 2-47e and 2-47f). The sclerotic component is dense bone with prominent resting lines.

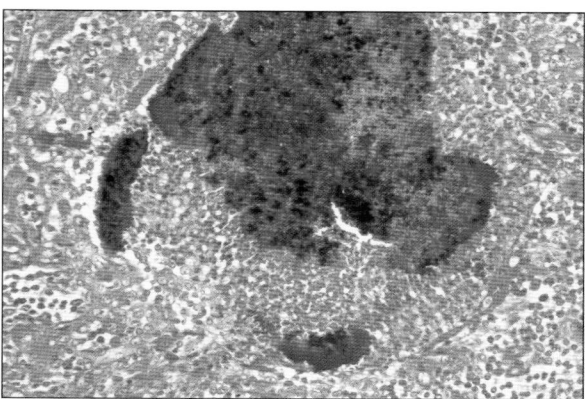

Fig 2-46 An *Actinomyces* colony (sulfur granule). The dark areas represent gram-positive *Actinomyces* while the smaller, more subtle pink rods represent *E corrodens* (Brown and Brenn stain).

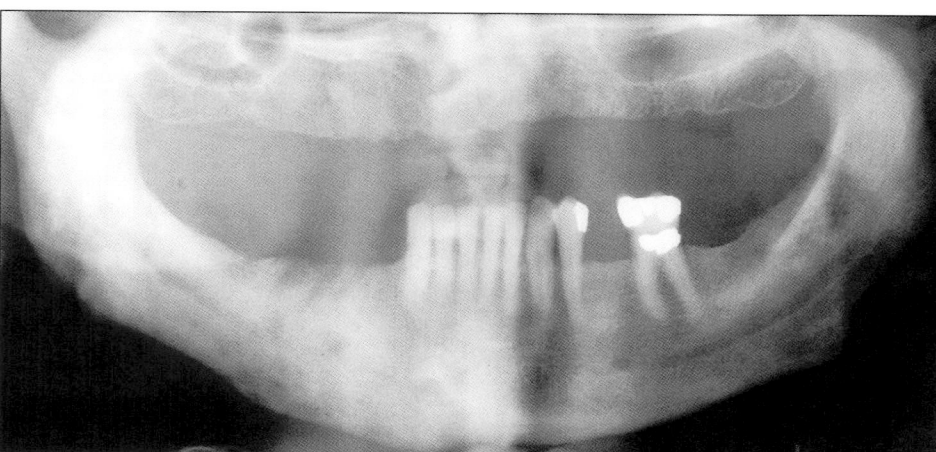

Fig 2-47a Chronic sclerosing osteomyelitis in the right hemimandible is evidenced by diffuse radiopacity, elimination of the inferior border cortex, and the process partially obscuring the widened mandibular canal outline.

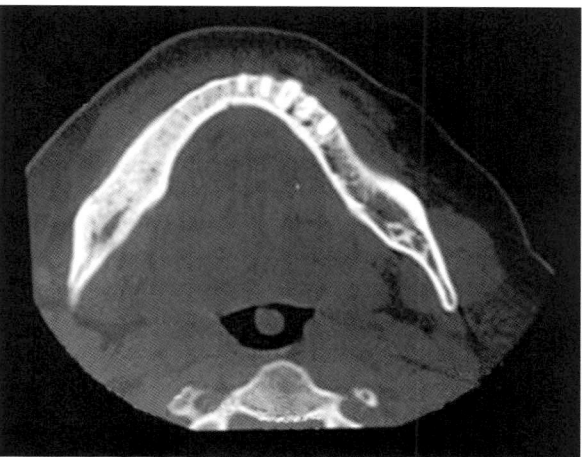

Fig 2-47b A CT scan of chronic sclerosing osteomyelitis will reveal endosteal sclerosis with some marrow space radiolucencies and usually no or little extracortical bone formation or cortical destruction.

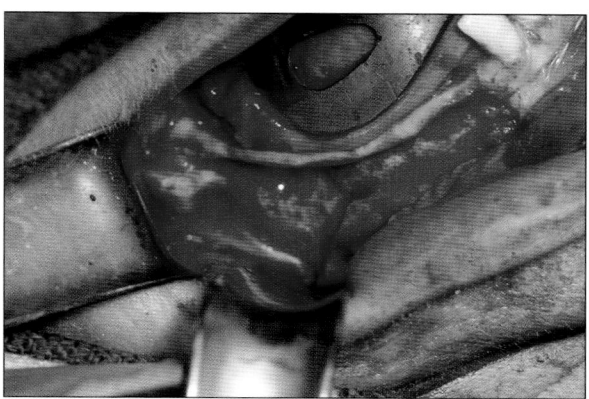

Fig 2-47c Exploration of a mandible with chronic sclerosing osteomyelitis will reveal dense medullary bone. Biopsies and cultures are more yielding if taken from the areas of radiolucency within the marrow space.

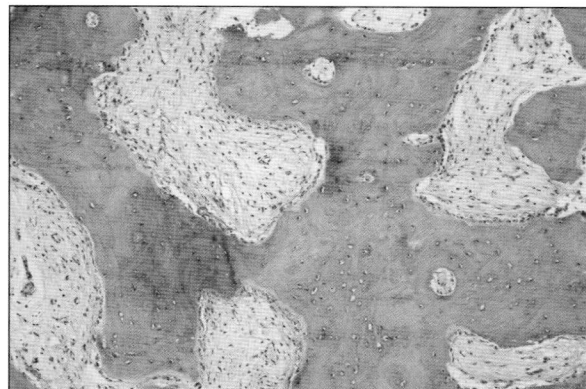

Fig 2-47d Biopsies in the more sclerotic portions of the marrow space will show thickened trabecular bone and marrow fibrosis.

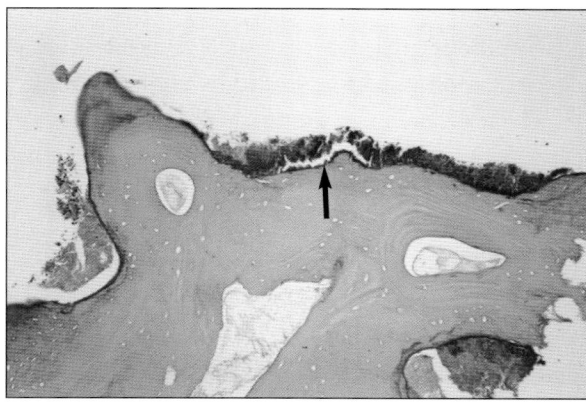

Fig 2-47e Biopsies in the more radiolucent areas of the sclerotic marrow space may identify microorganisms on the surface of thickened bony trabeculae. Here *Actinomyces* can be seen on the trabecular surface (*arrow*).

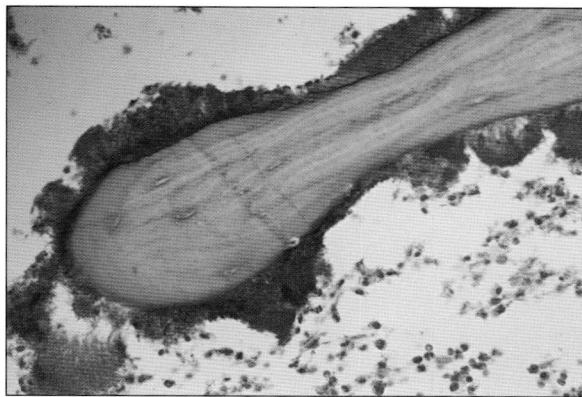

Fig 2-47f Close-up view of trabecular bone showing the elongated mycelia of *Actinomyces* organisms, one of the main pathogenic organisms in chronic sclerosing osteomyelitis.

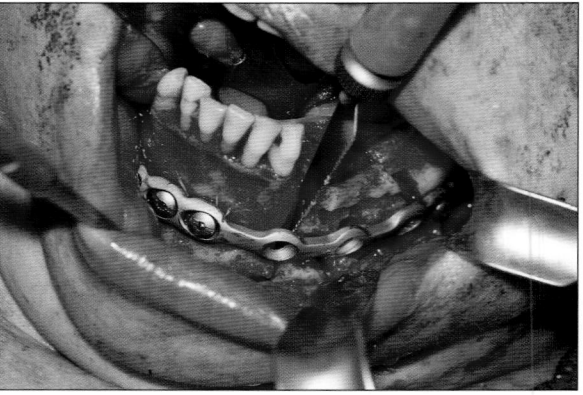

Fig 2-48a Osteomyelitis that is refractory to local debridements and antibiotics often indicates more extensive necrotic bone and may require a resection to achieve resolution.

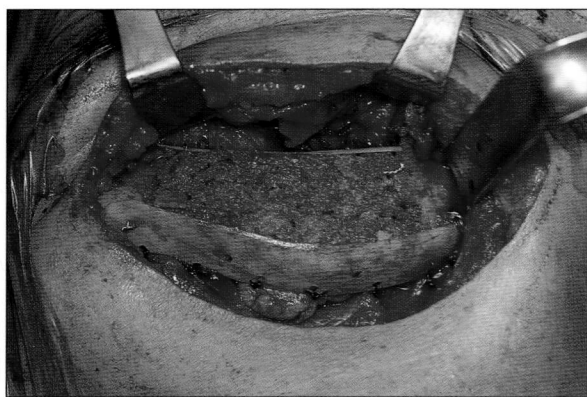

Fig 2-48b Once the osteomyelitis is resolved and an infection-free, contamination-free tissue is developed, standard bone-grafting techniques can be employed to reconstruct the defect.

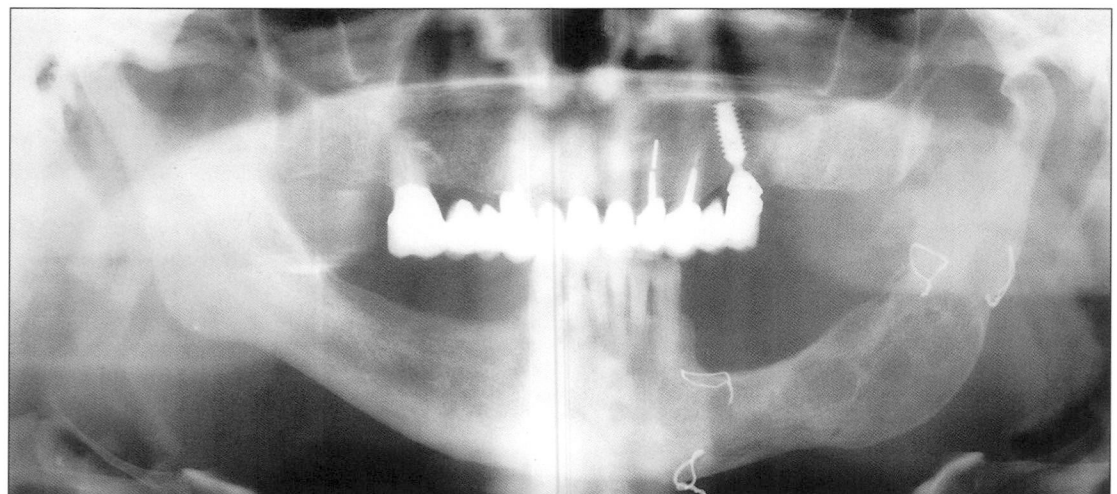

Fig 2-48c The outcome of an osteomyelitis-related continuity defect reconstruction should be a full return of continuity and alveolar bone height.

TREATMENT ▶

Antibiotic treatment is usually not curative but alone or in combination with hyperbaric oxygen and decortication reduces symptoms and may hold the disease in remission. The drug of choice is penicillin, to which *Actinomyces* species and *E corrodens* are both sensitive. In patients allergic to penicillin, doxycycline (Vibramycin, Pfizer US) is the drug of choice. Clindamycin is somewhat effective against *Actinomyces* species, but *E corrodens* is always resistant.

The most effective treatment is high-dose aqueous penicillin at 3 million U every 4 hours via a Port-a-Cath (Bard Access Systems) system for 1 month followed by 1 million U every 4 hours for another 5 months. This usually requires home health-care assistance. If oral penicillin must be used after the first month, a dose of 1 g four times daily is recommended.

Even with intensive high-dose antibiotic regimens, the majority of patients exacerbate and return with symptoms once the antibiotics are discontinued. In severe cases, resection of the affected bone has eradicated the disease. The surgeon must judge the location of the resection margins based on CT scan evidence relating the extent of endosteal sclerosis. The continuity defect created by a resection can be reconstructed at the same time with a reconstruction plate (Fig 2-48a). However, definitive bony reconstruction is best deferred approximately 6 months to complete antibiotic treatment and gain a sterile host tissue. In such cases, reconstruction accomplished after a 6-month postresection antibiotic course has successfully restored mandibular continuity (Figs 2-48b and 2-48c).

PROGNOSIS ▶

Patients may exacerbate from an antibiotic-induced remission because the bone sclerosis limits drug penetrance and because of the slow turnover rate of *Actinomyces* species and the protective nature of *Actinomyces* sulfur granules. Physical debridement would be the treatment of choice and provides an improved prognosis, but the extent of mandibular involvement often requires a resection of a hemimandibular nature or greater.

Osteomyelitis with Proliferative Periostitis (Garré Osteomyelitis)

CLINICAL PRESENTATION AND PATHOGENESIS ▶

Osteomyelitis with proliferative periostitis is a clinical-radiographic variant of a chronic osteomyelitis found in young individuals because of their high resistance, increased local blood supply, and greater bone regenerative capabilities. It has been termed *Garré osteomyelitis with proliferative periostitis* and more recently *periostitis ossificans* because of the associated formation of new paracortical bone. Osteomyelitis with proliferative periostitis presents most often in a child or teenager (although sporadic cases have been reported in patients in their 20s and 30s) associated with an apical infection in a mandibular posterior tooth. It does not seem to occur in the maxilla. The expansion is bone hard and not usually painful or tender to palpation. There is no pus, drainage, or erythema.

In 1893, Karl Garré first described a similar entity as a noted bone production and reaction in a case of acute tibial osteomyelitis. Pell, in 1955, was the first to completely describe this entity in the mandible; he correctly identified the chronic nature of the disease as well as the periosteal new bone formation. It is he who coined the term *Garré osteomyelitis*. In 1988, Nortje and coworkers reapplied Gorman's 1951 term of *periostitis ossificans* to the formation of extracortical new bone formation. They quarrel with the term *Garré osteomyelitis*, noting that Garré did not actually describe a periosteal bone reaction and that his case was actually an acute suppurative infection. *Periostitis ossificans*, however, is also not an ideal term because the periosteum does not become ossified; it merely deposits new bone as infection-induced inflammation lifts it off the cortex. The periosteum remains and will be one of the mechanisms of bone remodeling once the inflammation subsides.

DIFFERENTIAL DIAGNOSIS ▶

Osteomyelitis with proliferative periostitis is not a serious disease and will readily respond to removal of the source of infection. However, *Ewing sarcoma* also is seen in this age group and has been noted to produce a periosteal bone reaction termed an "onionskin" appearance. In addition, *endosteal* and *parosteal osteosarcomas* can produce a similar clinical radiographic presentation, as, more rarely, can *chondrosarcoma* and *monostotic fibrous dysplasia*. Therefore, in presentations in which the source of the infection is not obvious or the radiographic picture is not typical of osteomyelitis with proliferative periostitis, a bone biopsy is recommended.

RADIOGRAPHIC FINDINGS ▶

Because osteomyelitis with proliferative periostitis is primarily a clinical-radiographic diagnosis, good right-angled radiographs or sometimes CT scans are valuable. One should look for a tooth with pulpal invasion by caries and/or a periapical radiolucency suggestive of pulpal-periapical infection. One should also look for what clinically seems to be an expanded cortex but is not. Instead, it is the deposition of extracortical new bone outside an existing intact cortex (Figs 2-49a and 2-49b). The extracortical bone often appears to have a trabecular cancellous bone pattern but may have a layering appearance typical of the onionskin pattern. This is produced by inflamed and stimulated periosteum laying down new bone. If it lays down new bone in an alternating pattern of new bone formation–rest–new bone formation, the onionskin pattern will usually result. Otherwise, a trabecular-cancellous bone pattern will result. This phenomenon of extracortical new bone formation outside an intact cortex helps to differentiate osteo-

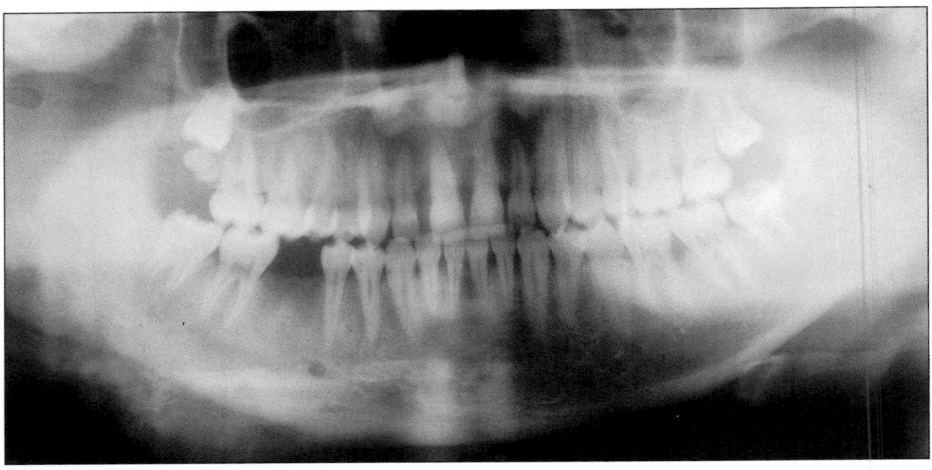

Fig 2-49a Extracortical bone formation may be seen as part of osteomyelitis with proliferative periostitis, which developed from an infected first molar that had just been removed.

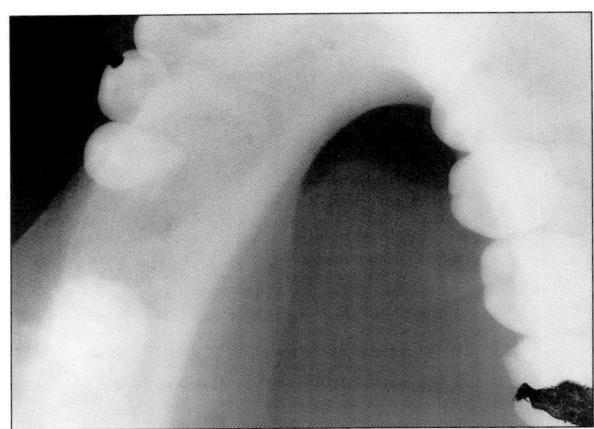

Fig 2-49b Osteomyelitis with proliferative periostitis will present radiographically with a smooth outline of regular extracortical bone formation. The cortex should be intact except around the involved tooth, and a layered "onionskin" effect may be seen within the extracortical bone.

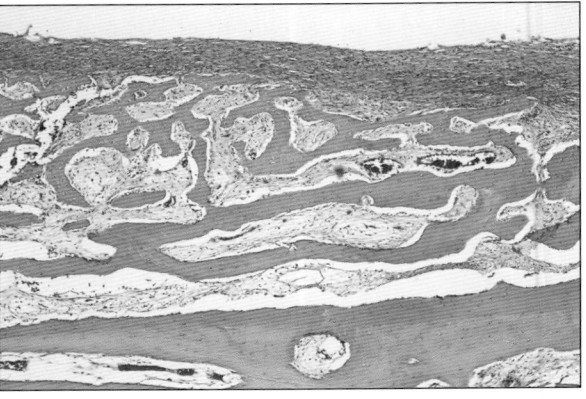

Fig 2-49c The histopathology of osteomyelitis with proliferative periostitis is distinct. Here an intact cortex can be seen below layered trabecular bone that mostly appears parallel to the cortex. The overlying periosteum has a significant inflammatory infiltrate.

myelitis with proliferative periostitis from Ewing sarcoma and osteosarcoma, wherein the cortex is usually destroyed and intramedullary radiopacities often exist. It also helps to distinguish osteomyelitis with proliferative periostitis from chronic sclerosing osteomyelitis, wherein there is no or little periosteal new bone formation but rather endosteal sclerosis, and from fibrous dysplasia, wherein there is no well-defined cortex but a homogeneous trabecular pattern throughout. The extracortical new bone formation will have reactive woven bone in parallel layers to the cortex connected by bridges perpendicular to the cortex (Fig 2-49c).

HISTOPATHOLOGY ▶ Histologically, the marrow is fibrous with scant chronic inflammatory cells. The bony mass consists of reactive new bone with the trabeculae running parallel to the cortex (see Fig 2-49c). There is usually prominent osteoblastic activity and inflammation within the periosteum, often within the extracortical new bone.

TREATMENT ▶ Treatment is straightforward: removal of the source of infection, which is usually a pulpal periapical infection, by either extraction or root canal therapy. A 10-day course of empiric antibiotics, such as penicillin, tetracyclines, or erythromycin, has justification but is not needed in every case.

PROGNOSIS ▶ The lesions usually resolve with new bone formation, but complete recontouring may take 3 to 4 months. Any progression of bony expansion should alert the clinician to the possibility of a malignancy or a more serious infection. In such cases, cultures and biopsy should be performed.

Actinomycosis

Actinomycosis is a specific chronic infection caused by any one of the five *Actinomyces* species pathogenic to humans. It may involve only soft tissue or bone (actinomyces osteomyelitis) or the two together. The classic description of a cervicofacial actinomycosis is that of a chronic, persistent infection with induration and nodularity due to fibrosis, and intermittent, spontaneously occurring drainage tracts (Fig 2-50a). This presentation is often termed the "lumpy jaw" presentation after a similar disease in cattle caused by *Actinomyces bovis*, which is not pathogenic in humans. A variation of this description is another presentation in which the most prominent finding is limited jaw opening often months or years after removal of a posterior tooth or after some trauma. In this situation, the limited jaw opening is most often attributable to fibrosis within one of the muscles of mastication or from a chronic, deep-seated focus of infection (Fig 2-50b).

A israelii is often thought to be the sole or most important pathogen in actinomycosis. However, this species is neither more common nor more frequently associated with clinical disease than the other four *Actinomyces* species common to the oral flora: *A viscosus, A naeslundii, A odontolyticus*, and *A meyerii*. All are capable of becoming pathogens by entry into injured deep tissue, where they can establish and maintain an anaerobic environment through tissue necrosis and fibrosis. It is the great degree of necrosis and fibrosis that is unique to *Actinomyces* species. Therefore, high doses of antibiotics are required to penetrate this barrier. The *Actinomyces* organisms are actually exquisitely sensitive to penicillin in low doses.

Actinomyces organisms colonize into so-called sulfur granules only in vivo, where they are mostly observed histologically and only rarely clinically. These organisms are also difficult to positively identify histologically because they do not always form sulfur granules and frequently evade detection by appearing as 1-μm-diameter gram-positive branching filaments or by dispersing into coccoid forms and thus resembling routine gram-positive streptococci. All of the *Actinomyces* species are facultative anaerobes (ie, they grow best anaerobically but are somewhat aerotolerant) with the exception of *A meyerii*, which is the only true obligate anaerobe.

The differential diagnosis should include *infections* or *infectious conditions* with some reason for chronicity. Examples include mixed infections related to foreign bodies such as Proplast, metal plates, Silastic, or wire. It should include infections caused by organisms known to be resistant such as methicillin-resistant *Staphylococcus aureus, E corrodens*, and *Pseudomonas* species. It may include *mixed infections* in patients with compromised host immunity, such as diabetes, HIV infection, or radiation tissue injury from radiotherapy.

The focus of the infection may be difficult to locate. Plain radiographs such as a panoramic radiograph often need to be supplemented by a CT scan or MRI (see Fig 2-50b). In a few cases, a scan using [67]gallium, which is taken up by inflammatory cells, or a scan using [99]technetium methylene diphosphonate, which is taken up by osteoblasts, will locate a focus of infection that CT scans and plain radiographs cannot.

The treatment of actinomycosis is focused on surgical debridement. Surgical debridement, including the source of the infection, is required to reduce the numbers of organisms and more importantly to change the anaerobic environment that is so important for survival of these organisms. In soft tissue, the debridement takes the form of excising necrotic tissue or, at times, lymph nodes (Fig 2-50c). In bone (ie, an *Actinomyces* suppurative or sclerosing osteomyelitis), the debridement may take the form of a curettage, decortication, or saucerization depending on the location and extent of bony involvement. At times, refractory or long-standing cases will require a continuity resection. At the time of debridement, tissue specimens should be taken for Gram staining and aerobic and anaerobic cultures before initiating antibiotics. If actinomycosis is suspected, a specific culture protocol must be followed. The steps are:

1. The specimen should be delivered to the microbiology laboratory within 15 minutes.
2. The specimen should be ground in a tissue grinder with thioglycolate broth.

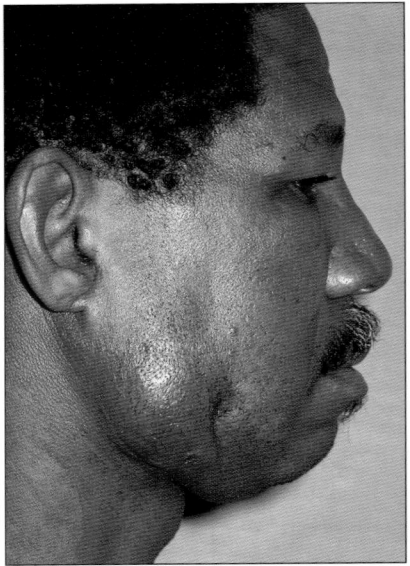

Fig 2-50a An actinomycosis infection produced this "lumpy jaw" appearance with abscess, fibrosis, and a depressed scar from a healed fistula.

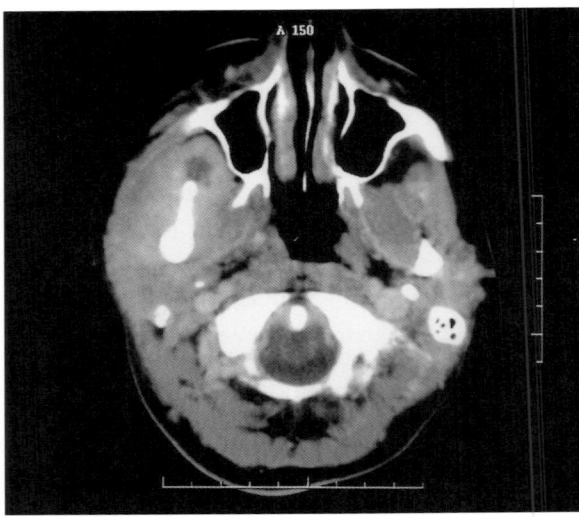

Fig 2-50b A CT scan suggestive of actinomycosis by virtue of the fibrosis seen in the masseter and temporalis muscle as well as a central abscess in the temporalis tendon area.

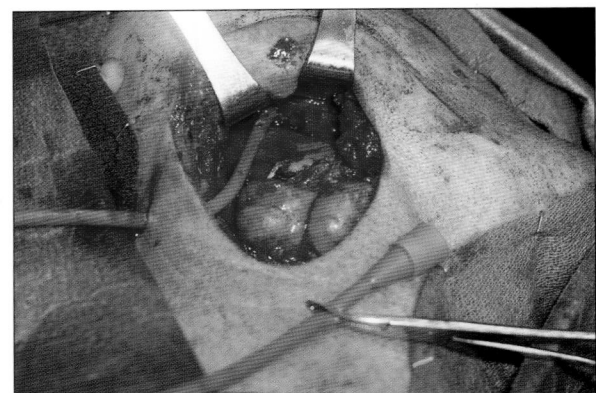

Fig 2-50c Debridement of actinomycotic infections is designed to reverse the anaerobic environment by removing necrotic tissue and microorganisms. Irrigating drains continue this concept in the postoperative phase.

3. The culture should be prepared using a CO_2 concentration greater than 5% and an O_2 concentration less than 2% in a 37°C environment.
4. Cultures can continue in routine plate media after initial colony formation in thioglycolate. CDC anaerobic blood agar plates and chocolate agar plates yield *Actinomyces* colonies very well.
5. Anaerobic culture plates should be retained for a minimum of 7 days because of the slow colony growth of *Actinomyces* organisms.

Irrigating drains are another method of reversing the anaerobic environment of actinomycosis infections (see Fig 2-50c). If there is an abundance of necrotic tissue, a debriding irrigant may be used for the first 72 hours. Irrigation solutions that are known to debride necrotic tissue are one-fourth strength Dakin's solution (2.5% NaOCl and 10% $NaHCO_3$), 9-aminoacridine, and one-half strength of 3% hydrogen peroxide. After 72 hours, normal irrigating solutions such as normal saline or Ringer's lactate may be used for another 3 to 5 days.

If actinomycosis is confirmed, penicillin G is the drug of choice. Eighteen million units of intravenous aqueous penicillin G are given daily, usually as 3 million units every 4 hours. This dose and route should continue to be followed for 1 month, which often requires home health-care assistance. After 1 month of intravenous penicillin G, this therapy is replaced with oral phenoxymethyl penicillin at 1 g every 6 hours for 5 months. Reduced doses and shortened antibiotic courses lead to a higher incidence of recurrent infection. In penicillin-allergic patients, intravenous imipenem/cilastatin (Primaxin, Merck) is effective, as is clindamycin (Cleocin, Pharmacia and Upjohn), 600 mg intravenously, three times daily. When a transition to oral antibiotics is acceptable, oral sulfamethoxazole (Gantanol, Roche), 2 to 4 g daily in divided doses, is effective, as is oral clindamycin, 300 mg three times daily, and doxycycline (Vibramycin, Pfizer US), 100 mg daily. No drug, however, is as completely effective as penicillin.

HISTOPATHOLOGY ▶

Actinomycosis differs from the previously described granulomatous lesions in that abscesses are the predominant finding. Purulent loculations develop, within which granules of varying size may be found (Fig 2-50d). The granules consist of colonies of *Actinomyces*. Although almost always only a histologic observation, if large enough to be seen macroscopically, they will have a yellow color, hence the descriptive term *sulfur granule* (Fig 2-50e). Macroscopic sulfur granules are rare. Surrounding the sea of neutrophils,

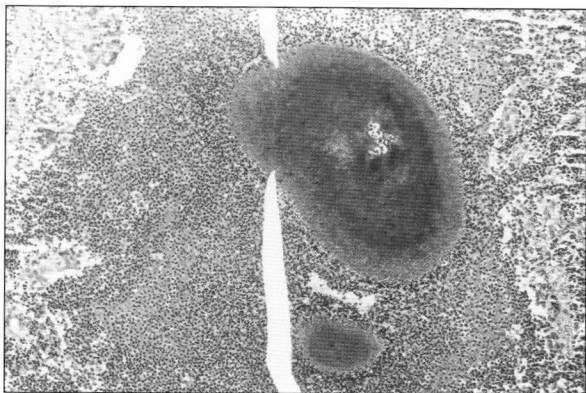

Fig 2-50d A large expanse of neutrophils, which is characteristic of actinomycosis, together with a sulfur granule.

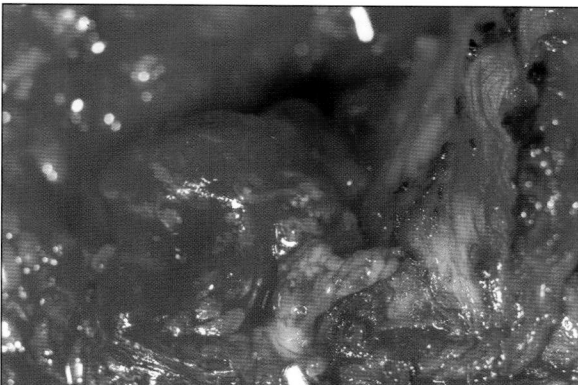

Fig 2-50e Small yellow specks representing sulfur granules from an *Actinomyces* infection. It is unusual to see sulfur granules clinically; they are usually visible only under light microscopy.

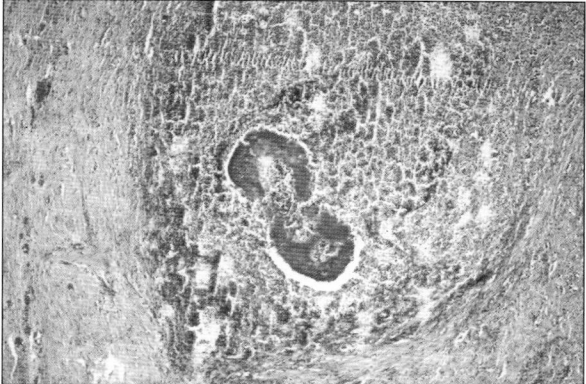

Fig 2-50f A classic sulfur granule (colony of *Actinomyces* organisms) surrounded by a ring of necrosis, which in turn is surrounded by fibrosis. This is a good example of how actinomycosis evades the immune system and why antibiotics cannot penetrate to the organisms.

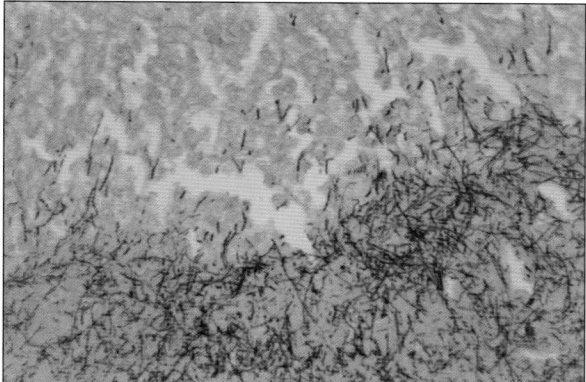

Fig 2-50g Gram staining allows identification of the gram-positive (blue) filamentous and sometimes coccoid organisms within the sulfur granule (Brown and Brenn stain, a tissue Gram stain).

granulation tissue is usually found with fibrous tissue, capillaries and plasma cells, lymphocytes, and an occasional foamy macrophage. Older lesions show more fibrosis with a decrease in the inflammatory component. This walling off prevents antibodies, oxygen, and antibiotics from reaching the organisms (Fig 2-50f).

The granules are round to oval, often indurated basophilic structures consisting of intertwined filamentous organisms (Fig 2-50g), the ends of which are frequently encased by eosinophilic material, giving them a club-shaped appearance (Splendore-Hoeppli phenomenon). This radiating pattern has led to the designation *ray fungus*, an obvious misnomer because *Actinomyces* are true bacteria. The granules are usually homogeneous but may show some central degeneration with loss of basophilia. Their average diameter is 290 µm. The organisms themselves cannot be demonstrated by H&E but are clearly evident with Gram stain, where they are gram-positive (see Fig 2-50g). The clubs and granule matrix are gram-negative, periodic acid–Schiff (PAS) stain variable, and methenamine-silver negative. The *Actinomyces* average 1 µm in width and 13 µm in length. They appear beaded because of alternative gram-positive staining and nonstaining segments. They are branching, filamentous bacteria that can break into bacillary and coccoid forms (see Fig 2-50g). The organisms themselves stain blue with Giemsa and gray to black with methenamine silver. They are not acid fast and usually are PAS positive. Their clustering arrangement is probably a protective action, defending the organisms against the offensive actions of oxygen, antibodies, and antibiotics. This, in combination with a fibrous wall, leads to the chronicity of the disease process.

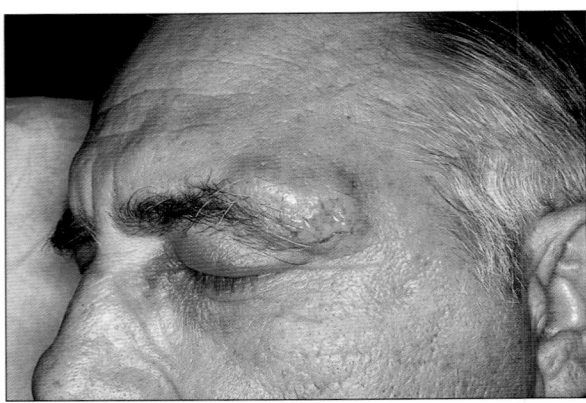

Fig 2-51 Abscessing skin nodule of nocardiosis in a farmer who had a pulmonary focus of nocardia.

Actinomyces organisms that are not pathogenic form colonies that are loosely arranged, lack clubbing, and have no surrounding inflammatory component.

The diagnosis of actinomycosis requires the identification of granules that show clubbing as well as gram-positive branching bacilli in tissue secretions, exudates, or on culture. Granules may be very scarce, as was demonstrated by Brown in his series of 181 patients. One quarter of his cases showed only a single granule. Thus multiple sections of tissue specimens should be examined.

PROGNOSIS ▶ Surgical debridement and a 6-month course of antibiotic therapy, preferably penicillin, usually result in disease resolution. In refractory cases, a reassessment for residual necrotic tissue and additional surgical debridement are more yielding than is extending the antibiotic therapy.

Nocardiosis

CLINICAL PRESENTATION AND PATHOGENESIS ▶ Nocardia lesions will be seen in the maxillofacial subcutaneous tissues as a rare dissemination focus from a primary pulmonary infection. *Nocardia asteroides* and *Nocardia brasiliensis* are aerobic, gram-positive, filamentous bacteria that bear a close histologic resemblance to *Actinomyces* species. In fact, the clinical lesions caused by *Nocardia* species resemble those of actinomycosis because of their fibrotic nature and tendency to drain. However, the similarity that *Nocardia* has to *Actinomyces* has been overstated. *Nocardia* is a separate genus; the organisms are aerobic and not a normal part of the oral flora as are those of *Actinomyces*. *Nocardia* organisms are soil bacteria that produce disseminated skin nodules (Fig 2-51) due to hematogenous spread after establishing an aerobic chronic lung infection. Most patients will have an exposure to soil or soil products. *Nocardia* is a weak pathogen; many patients have histories of chronic steroid use, immune deficiency states, or chronic illness.

DIFFERENTIAL DIAGNOSIS ▶ Because there may be one or more firm infected skin nodules, *cervicofacial actinomycosis, diffuse skin metastasis from a primary malignancy,* and *sebaceous cysts* should be considered in addition to other disseminated infections that arise from the lungs, such as *histoplasmosis* or *coccidioidomycosis.*

DIAGNOSTIC WORK-UP ▶ The clinical examination should assess for decreased breath sounds, purulent sputum production (which should be cultured aerobically), and fever. Historically, weight loss, malaise, and night sweats are consistent with most types of pulmonary infections. A chest radiograph may show infiltrates and/or a pleural effusion.

The skin lesion should be excised if small or drained if too large to excise, and tissue specimens should be submitted for culture.

HISTOPATHOLOGY ▶ This is another disease in which there is abscess formation with abundant suppuration. The organisms, which are found in the areas of suppuration, are gram-positive filamentous bacteria but do not typically form granules. Instead, they fragment into bacillary structures, which resemble *M tuberculosis*. In addition, *Nocardia* organisms are weakly acid fast. Unlike mycobacterium, however, they are methenamine-silver positive.

Facial, scalp, or neck lesions of *Nocardia* are only a small part of diffuse and disseminated nocardiosis. Nocardiosis requires intravenous trimethoprim-sulfamethoxazole (Bactrim IV, Roche), 15 mL (240 mg trimethoprim/1,200 mg sulfamethoxazole) every 6 hours in 375 mL of D5W. Other diluents have not been tested and are not recommended. Intravenous drug therapy should continue for 1 month followed by 5 months of oral trimethoprim-sulfamethoxazole, one tablet (trimethoprim 160 mg/sulfamethoxazole 800 mg) (Bactrim DS, Roche) twice daily.

Response to therapy is slow because of the slow turnover rate of *Nocardia* organisms. Disease resolution is related to compliance and promptness of treatment.

Diphtheria

Diphtheria initially presents with the classic diphtheritic pseudomembrane in the oropharynx. At that time, constitutional symptoms of fever, pain, and malaise may not be present or may be just emerging. Within a few days, the patient's condition worsens, with fever, cervical lymphadenopathy, and extensive weakness. Upper airway or bronchial obstruction may occur.

Corynebacterium diphtheriae is transmitted by air-water droplets from infected patients or healthy carriers. The incubation period after contact is 2 to 7 days. The organism's virulence is attributable to its exotoxin, the action of which produces the oropharyngeal pseudomembrane as well as the myocarditis and cranial nerve neuropathy complication. The exotoxin inhibits an elongation factor, which is required in protein synthesis, thus causing cell death.

Active immunization is part of childhood immunization programs (diphtheria-pertussis-tetanus [DPT]). Immunity is not directed against the organism but against the toxin, by stimulation of the IgG and IgA classes of antibodies. Neutralizing the toxin with antibodies (antitoxin) protects against primary infection by preventing bacterial adherence to cells. Booster immunization of toxoid is required, particularly in exposed persons. The degree of immunity can be evaluated with the Schick test, in which diphtheria toxin and a control are injected intradermally and the reactions assessed.

Sore throat, fever, lymphadenopathy, and a pharyngeal exudate should generate considerations of *streptococcal pharyngitis, infectious mononucleosis,* and *adenovirus-related pharyngitis*. However, diphtheria is a life-threatening disease. Clinically suspicious cases are best treated without ruling out other lesions on a differential list and without waiting for laboratory confirmation.

Treatment is begun as throat cultures are taken to identify the causative organism, *C diphtheriae*.

The organisms attach to the epithelium of the upper respiratory tract but do not penetrate it. There is an acute inflammatory response characterized by hyperemia, edema, focal hemorrhages, and an infiltrate of neutrophils. Considerable amounts of fibrin are formed. A few days after the acute inflammatory response, the epithelium becomes necrotic and, with the debris of inflammation, becomes enmeshed within the fibrin, forming a membrane that is bound to the underlying inflammatory tissue. In areas of stratified squamous epithelium, such as the pharynx, the membrane is tenacious. In areas of thinner respiratory epithelium, such as the nasopharynx, it is more easily separable. The membrane is subsequently coughed up or resorbed.

Horse serum antitoxin, 40,000 to 60,000 U, should be given as soon as possible after conjunctival or skin tests for horse serum hypersensitivity are completed. If the patient is hypersensitive to horse serum, desensitization must be accomplished and antitoxin administration delayed. Diphtheria equine antitoxin can be obtained from the Centers for Disease Control and Prevention (Atlanta, Georgia). Simultaneously, aqueous penicillin G, 2 million U intravenously every 6 hours, or oral potassium penicillin V, 500 mg four times daily for 10 days, should be started. In the penicillin-allergic patient, erythromycin, 1 g intravenously

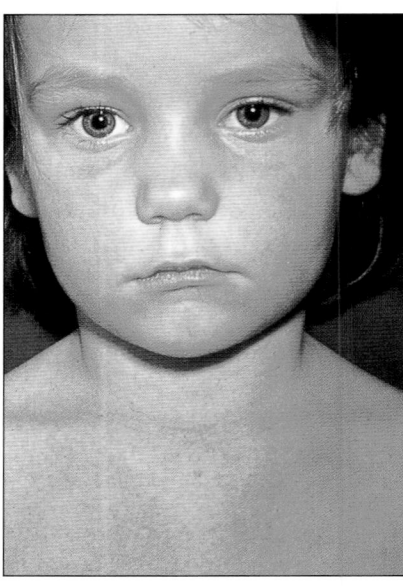

Fig 2-52 A striking red (scarlet) macular skin rash in a child with scarlet fever. (Reprinted from Strassburg M and Knolle G, *Diseases of the Oral Mucosa*, with permission from Quintessence Publishing Co.)

every 6 hours, or oral erythromycin, 500 mg four times daily for 10 days, is used. In cases that are diagnosed late or in extensive disease, 100,000 U of horse serum antitoxin are given in addition to the antibiotics.

In cases where the pseudomembrane causes obvious upper airway obstruction, removal by direct laryngoscopy or fiberoptic nasopharyngoscopy is useful. If it cannot be removed, intubation is required. If intubation is not possible, a tracheostomy may be necessary.

PROGNOSIS ▶ Early recognition and treatment lead to disease resolution and the prevention of complications. Myocarditis and cranial nerve neuropathies are the two most common complications. Myocarditis can cause arrhythmias, heart failure, and cardiovascular shock. The cranial nerve complication may produce dysphagia, diplopia, slurred speech, and ocular strabismus.

Scarlet Fever

CLINICAL PRESENTATION AND PATHOGENESIS ▶ Children and young adults with scarlet fever develop a sudden onset of fever and sore throat. There may also be headaches, malaise, irritability, and nausea. The pharynx will appear red and swollen, and the cervical lymph nodes will be tender and swollen. At the time of presentation or shortly thereafter, a red macular skin rash will develop, starting on the chest and spreading outward (Fig 2-52). The rash will be most intense in the axillas and groin areas. The rash blanches on pressure, and some petechiae may form. The rash lasts 4 to 5 days. The face is characteristically red with a circumoral pallor. The tongue develops a white coat within which reddened and swollen fungiform papillae stand out ("strawberry tongue"). As the disease progresses, the skin erythema fades and the white coating on the tongue is lost, leaving a swollen, irregular, beefy tongue ("raspberry tongue").

Scarlet fever itself is caused by group A ß-hemolytic streptococci, as are other cases of so-called strep throat that do not exhibit all the features of classic scarlet fever. Transmission is via air-water droplet dissemination or infected secretions. The scarlet skin rash is caused by an erythrogenic exotoxin that damages capillary endothelium, which is the cause of the poststreptococcal complications of rheumatic fever and glomerulonephritis. Rheumatic fever usually requires several episodes of group A streptococcal infections; glomerulonephritis requires only a single infection.

The rash of scarlet fever is due to the elaboration of an erythrogenic toxin by the streptococci, which causes injury to endothelium and dilation of small blood vessels with hyperemia. During recovery, the formation of antibodies neutralizes the toxin.

DIFFERENTIAL DIAGNOSIS ▶

The initial presentation of a febrile pharyngitis with cervical lymphadenitis is suggestive of *infectious mononucleosis* and of *nonstreptococcal pharyngitis*, usually attributable to adenoviruses. *Diphtheria* will have a similar clinical presentation, as will *pseudomembranous candidiasis of the pharynx.*

DIAGNOSTIC WORK-UP ▶

The bacterial nature of scarlet fever and streptococcal pharyngitis can be confirmed by a white blood cell count. Streptococcal sore throat will show a leukocytosis with a left shift toward immature forms. Viral pharyngitis, including mononucleosis, will show a leukopenia with an absolute or a relative lymphocytosis. In some cases, atypical lymphocytes are present.

The diagnosis should be confirmed with a throat culture. Throat culture in a single blood agar plate has a sensitivity of 70% to 80%. Throat cultures in a two-plate system, one blood agar and the other trimethoprim-sulfamethoxazole (Bactrim, Roche) blood agar to eliminate nonstreptococcal competitors, are almost 100% sensitive. Antistreptolysin O antibody titers are elevated in 80% of cases but are more useful for follow-up than for diagnosis.

TREATMENT ▶

Antibiotics have a minimal effect on symptoms; their role is to shorten the disease course and eradicate the organism to prevent complications. Oral potassium penicillin V, 500 mg four times daily for 10 days, is effective. However, compliance is often a problem because symptoms dissipate in 4 to 5 days and a full 10-day course is needed to prevent complications. Therefore, penicillin G benzathine (Bicillin LA, Wyeth-Ayerst), 1.2 million U intramuscularly as a single dose, is an effective alternative. For penicillin-allergic patients, oral erythromycin, 500 mg four times daily or 40 mg/kg per day for 10 days, is recommended.

PROGNOSIS ▶

The prognosis is excellent, and complications can be avoided if antibiotics are begun early and the full course is taken. If not, there is a high incidence of otitis media, sinusitis, mastoiditis, and peritonsillar abscesses.

Necrotizing Fasciitis

CLINICAL PRESENTATION AND PATHOGENESIS ▶

In the oral and maxillofacial area, necrotizing fasciitis will present as a rapidly progressive dissecting subcutaneous infection in the neck. There will most likely be a history of a recent surgery, trauma, or odontogenic infection. Frequently, the individual is diabetic.

The neck will be crepitant as a result of the infection dissecting along the platysma. The skin will be mottled and blue due to venous stasis secondary to small vessel thrombosis. Other areas of the skin (most likely at the advancing edge of the infection) will be erythematous (Fig 2-53). The skin will be painful but may also have a notable paresthesia. Areas of skin breakdown will occur, which usually include necrosis of the subcutaneous fascia and the platysma. In most cases, fever and tachycardia accompany the local findings.

Necrotizing fasciitis represents a true synergistic infection, that is, an infection in which the combined effect of two or more organisms is greater than the sum of the individual effects of each. In most cases affecting the head and neck, anaerobic streptococci produce spreading factors such as hyaluronidase and streptokinase, which results in vessel thrombosis leading to ischemia. *Bacteroides* species and other like species maintain and enhance the anaerobic environment by their own metabolism and the production of insoluble gases such as nitrogen and hydrogen.

DIFFERENTIAL DIAGNOSIS ▶

Necrotizing fasciitis is recognized by history and clinical appearance.

DIAGNOSTIC WORK-UP ▶

Tissue for Gram stains and cultures from nonnecrotic tissue should be obtained and submitted for aerobic and anaerobic cultures. Routine blood counts will show a leukocytosis with a shift to the left indicative of immature neutrophils. Blood glucose should be assessed, urinalysis performed, and blood urea nitrogen (BUN) and creatinine measured to assess potential ketoacidosis and dehydration. Soft tissue radiographs of the head and neck are valuable. Hydrogen and nitrogen gas formation by anaerobic organisms will not only produce the clinical picture of crepitus but will often show gas-bubble formation on a radiograph (Fig 2-54).

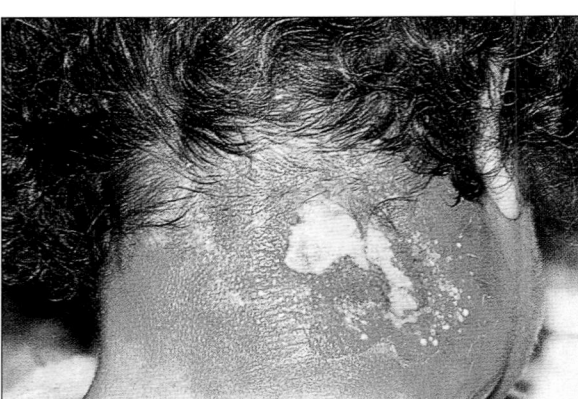

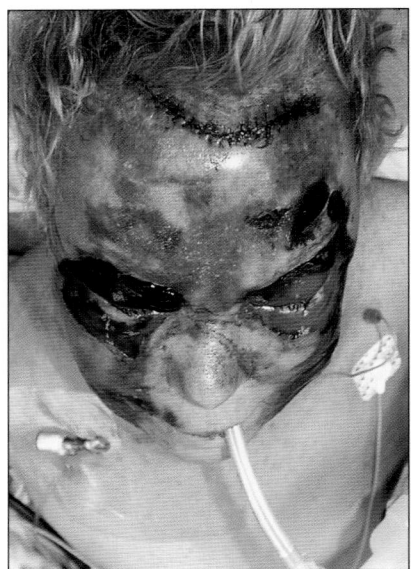

Fig 2-53 Necrotizing fasciitis with a central area of necrosis and a large area of rapidly advancing erythema.

Fig 2-54 Necrotizing fasciitis with mottled and discolored skin along with some areas of frank necrosis and epithelial slough. The ballooning-out of the skin is due to gas formation. (Courtesy of Dr Curt Schalit.)

The cultures should identify a mixed aerobic-anaerobic infection. In the neck, anaerobic *Peptostreptococcus*, *Bacteroides*, and *Fusobacterium* species are the main pathogens, accounting for 50% to 60% of cases. Aerobic species, particularly *Streptococcus pyogenes*, *Staphylococcus aureus*, and *Enterobacteriaceae*, have also been reported.

HISTOPATHOLOGY ▶ Tissue changes include edema, widespread inflammation, and necrosis of fascia and subcutaneous tissue.

TREATMENT ▶ Necrotizing fasciitis is a severe and serious infection. Nearly every patient loses some tissue, hence the lay term *flesh-eating bacteria*. Most require some type of reconstructive surgery, and about 30% die. When it affects other body areas (particularly the male genital area, in a condition called *Fournier disease*), mortality can reach 60%.

Each patient is aggressively treated with aqueous penicillin, 2 million U intravenously every 4 hours, and clindamycin, 600 mg intravenously every 8 hours. In addition, an initial debridement followed by hyperbaric oxygen at 2.4 ATA, 90-minute exposures twice daily, is indicated. The intravenous antibiotics should be continued until the clinical signs of infection have been reversed and granulation tissue begins to develop in the wound areas. Hyperbaric oxygen should continue until a nearly complete granulation tissue base has formed across these areas. In the penicillin-allergic patient, erythromycin, 1 g intravenously every 6 hours, may be substituted for penicillin.

PROGNOSIS ▶ Mortality and morbidity can be reduced by early and aggressive treatment. Resultant wounds usually undergo skin grafting after a granulation tissue base develops and quantitative cultures reveal fewer than 1×10^5 organisms/g of tissue. Smaller areas can be left to epithelialize secondarily, and larger wounds may require either a myocutaneous flap or a free vascular flap.

Noma

CLINICAL PRESENTATION AND PATHOGENESIS ▶ The classic picture of a noma patient is a child or teenager with a gangrenous, black tissue slough of oral mucosa and skin who has another debilitating infection such as dysentery, pneumonia, severe anemias, severe malnutrition, or a leukemia with ongoing chemotherapy. Some cases occur in adults. Most are associated with chemotherapy or immunosuppressive drugs.

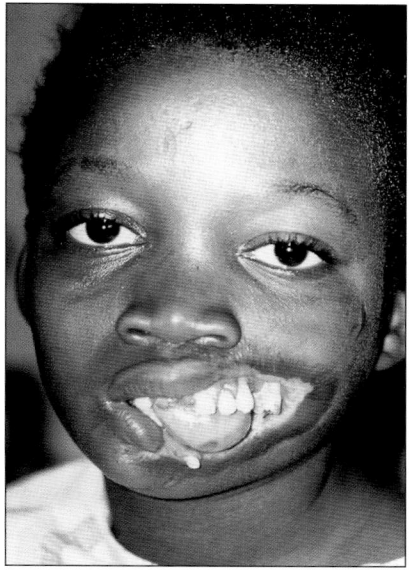

Fig 2-55a Noma will cause significant tissue loss, creating a functional compromise and a deformity.

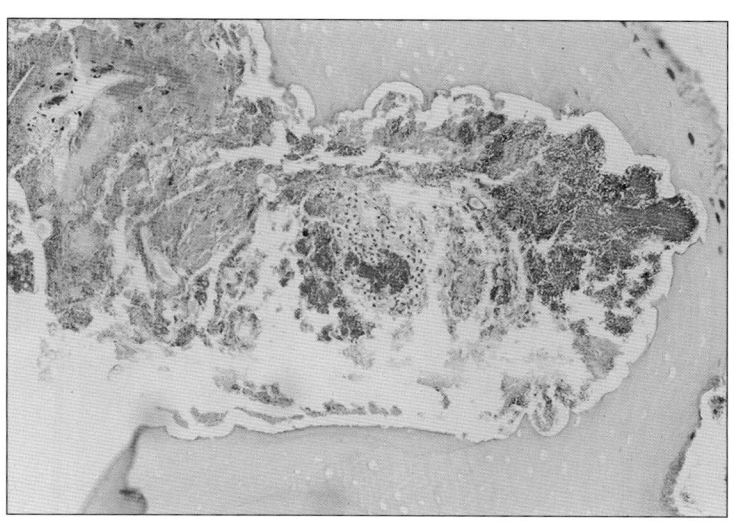

Fig 2-55b Necrosis involving bone in a patient with noma.

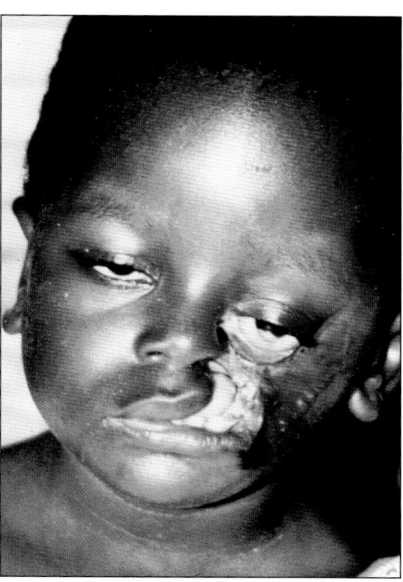

Fig 2-55c Although noma may begin in the perioral area, it can extend into contiguous areas. Here a portion of the nose has been necrosed and the lower eyelid is severely retracted because of scarring.

The lesion often begins as a painful ulcer from trauma or from spontaneous tissue breakdown. The ulcer rapidly extends as inflammation progresses to tissue necrosis, often lysing sufficient mucosa and skin to expose underlying bone, which may also become necrotic. Before the tissue slough, the ulcer will blacken, suggesting ischemic necrosis (Fig 2-55a). A sour odor is often noted during this process. As the disease progresses, a sharp line of demarcation develops, separating necrotic tissue from adjacent healthy, well-perfused tissue.

Noma is not a primary disease but a secondary complication of another disease. It is rare in developed countries except when related to chemotherapy and immunosuppression because of the epidemiologic prevention and frequent intervention when debilitating conditions occur. The organisms take advantage of host tissue compromise and produce a progressive tissue destruction. Although unproven, it has been suggested that the tissue destruction is caused by bacterial enzymic digestion or via progressive vascular thrombosis, leading to ischemic tissue necrosis. In some areas of Africa, noma is a frequent complication of childhood measles.

DIFFERENTIAL DIAGNOSIS ▶

The most important disease from which to distinguish noma is a rapidly progressing malignancy, particularly entities such as *immunoblastic lymphoma* and *leukemias*. In addition, *necrotizing fasciitis*, which is an analogous disease but localized to fascial planes, may in its early stages resemble noma.

DIAGNOSTIC WORK-UP ▶

The diagnosis of noma is based on knowledge of the underlying condition that predisposes tissue to necrosis and the clinical identification of progressive ischemic changes with necrosis. Cultures from the edge of the necrotic tissue in front of and adjacent to seemingly healthy tissue often identify Vincent spirochetes and fusiform bacilli, making this disease somewhat analogous to acute necrotizing ulcerative periodontitis.

HISTOPATHOLOGY ▶

Initially, there is acute inflammation with edema and neutrophils; this is followed by extensive necrosis (Fig 2-55b). Granulation tissue may develop around foci of necrosis, but this tissue becomes infected and also undergoes necrosis. Masses of bacteria are readily identified. The mechanism for the massive necrosis has not been elucidated. Thrombosis of larger vessels is not seen in these lesions.

TREATMENT ▶

The two most important aspects of treatment are the reversal of the underlying predisposing condition and surgical debridement. In addition, aggressive supportive care in the form of nasogastric high-calorie–

high-protein feedings and intravenous fluids is useful. Antibiotics are of course used but play a secondary role to debridement and improvement of systemic health. Both Vincent spirochetes and fusiform bacilli are sensitive to penicillin. Aqueous penicillin G 1 to 2 million U is given every 4 hours intravenously until the debrided wound shows evidence of healing. Therapy then changes to oral penicillin, 500 mg four times daily, until resolved. For the penicillin-allergic patient, erythromycin 1 g intravenously every 6 hours then converted to 500 mg by mouth four times daily is useful. Hyperbaric oxygen, if available, may also be used in an attempt to preserve as much unaffected tissue as possible. It will oxygenate the nonnecrotic but is-chemic tissue and enhance leukocyte microbial killing ability, limiting tissue loss.

PROGNOSIS ▶

Today, noma is resolvable with the treatment described. The tissue loss requires reconstruction when possible to prevent scar retraction from further distorting tissues and limiting function (Fig 2-55c). The soft tissue loss is often so great that a myocutaneous flap or a free microvascular transfer is necessary. Bone loss requires bone graft reconstruction. However, in the past and in areas where access to care is not available, significant mortality occurs.

Syphilis

CLINICAL PRESENTATION AND PATHOGENESIS ▶

The clinical presentation of syphilis varies with the disease stage. The chancre of primary syphilis is an ulcer with elevated, rolled edges, which emerges at the site of inoculation of *Treponema pallidum*. Chancres occur mostly around the genitals of either sex or on the lips, tongue, and other oral mucous membranes (Figs 2-56a to 2-56d). There is usually regional lymphadenopathy; the nodes are mildly ten-der, smooth, and freely movable (Fig 2-56e).

Untreated chancres will involute, and the regional lymphadenitis will dissipate in 1 to 3 months. Many individuals thus believe the problem has "gone away" and will not seek treatment. After a latency period of another 1 to 3 months, the secondary stage emerges: a reddish brown, uncomfortable skin rash (Fig 2-57a) or painless or mildly painful oral lesions. The oral lesions may take the form of broad patches (mu-cous patches) (Fig 2-57b); or diffuse, mucoid, white, crusty, and hemorrhagic ulcers (Figs 2-58a to 2-58d); or broad-based, elevated, white plaques called *condyloma latta* (not to be confused with *condyloma acumi-nata*, which are wart-like papillomatous lesions caused by another sexually transmitted DNA virus). During this stage, the *T pallidum*, which were formerly confined to the chancre and perhaps to the re-gional lymph nodes, are now found in large numbers throughout the body and bloodstream. This results in widespread skin involvement due to capillary endarteritis as well as retinal hyperemia, which causes photophobia and visual disturbances. The primary and secondary stages are termed *early syphilis* and can be treated in the same manner. In early syphilis, about 30% of patients also present with concomitant gonorrhea, confusing the clinical picture with the additional symptoms of dysuria, pyuria, and sometimes foul-smelling urine.

Untreated, the lesions of secondary syphilis will enter a prolonged latency period in which the anti-body arm of the immune system slowly eradicates the organisms; 65% of patients never advance to the tertiary stage. The 35% who develop tertiary syphilis can develop any one of a number of manifestations resulting from endarteritis and its ischemic destruction of tissues. The cardiovascular and nervous sys-tems seem to be the primary targets. Aneurysms of the aorta, paralysis, and ataxic gait (tabes dorsalis) are some of the more well-known tertiary manifestations. In the oral cavity, gummas of the palate may produce a large oronasal communication (Fig 2-59), or the tongue may develop a thickened, hard im-mobility (interstitial glossitis) (Fig 2-60).

Congenital syphilis results from a fetal spirochetemia (caused by the transplacental transmission of viable *T pallidum* into the circulation of the developing fetus). The baby is born with a secondary-stage form of the disease. If the infection is fulminant, the child may be stillborn. Otherwise, various manifes-tations resulting from a variety of organ involvements is possible. Among the more common congenital syphilis lesions are so-called Saber shins, caused by a tibial bowing resulting from anterior tibial periosteal

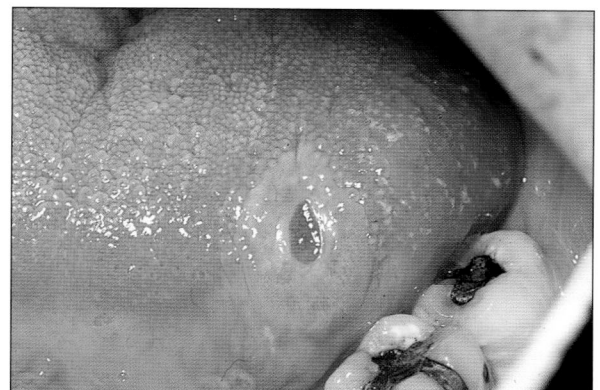

Fig 2-56a A chancre of primary syphilis may present as a clean painless ulcer with elevated and rolled margins.

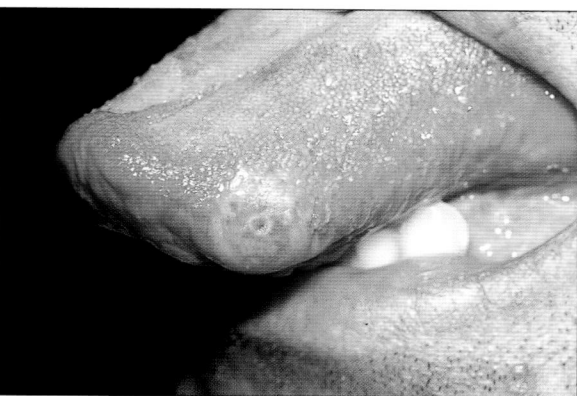

Fig 2-56b Appearance of the chancre in Fig 2-56a 1 week after receiving 1.2 million U of benzathine penicillin.

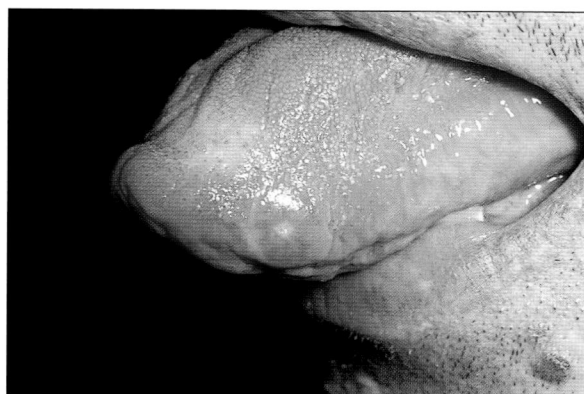

Fig 2-56c Two weeks after administration of 1.2 million U benzathine penicillin, the chancre is almost completely resolved and the disease is deemed nontransmissible.

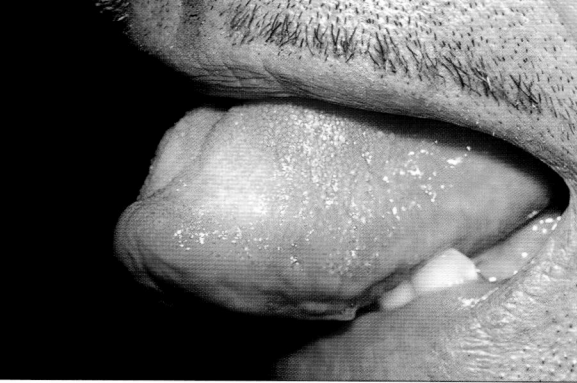

Fig 2-56d Four weeks after the administration of benzathine penicillin, the chancre is completely resolved.

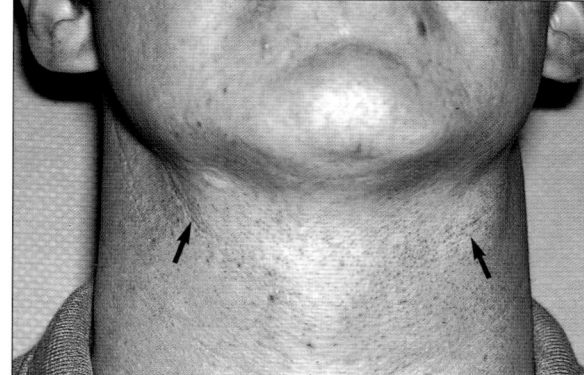

Fig 2-56e Along with a chancre of primary syphilis, a mildly tender lymphadenopathy is often found to be present (*arrows*).

new bone formation; a saddle nose deformity, caused by destruction of the vomer; perioral creases, called *rhagades* (Fig 2-61), caused by skin endarteritis with resultant scarring; interstitial keratitis, caused by active infection of the cornea and conjunctiva; Hutchinson teeth (Figs 2-62 and 2-63), caused by arrested enamel formation of the permanent molars and incisors; and eighth nerve deafness, caused by endarteritis and ischemia of the eighth nerve. Collectively, these last three entities have been termed *Hutchinson's triad*.

Historically, nonsyphilitic treponemal infections (yaws) were noted as early as 500 AD. However, true syphilis did not emerge in Western civilization until the fifteenth century. Some attribute this to the sailors who accompanied Christopher Columbus on his return from the New World. Nevertheless, syphilis spread rapidly throughout Europe and Asia and, of course, throughout the Americas as well. Prior to World War II, there were about 600,000 new cases being reported annually in the United States. As a result of intensive public health efforts during and after World War II and the common use of penicillin, the annual infection rate dropped to about 6,000 new cases by 1955. With the sexual revolution of the 1960s, an increase in new cases of syphilis, as well as all other sexually transmitted diseases, was noted. In the early 1980s a sharp increase occurred related particularly to a large increase in the men having sex with men group and in the transmission related to the drug-addicted populations. There then began a slight downturn in 1984 to 1985 as the population's concern over the AIDS epidemic reached its zenith, but since 1985 it has once again steadily increased. There are now about 52,000 new cases re-

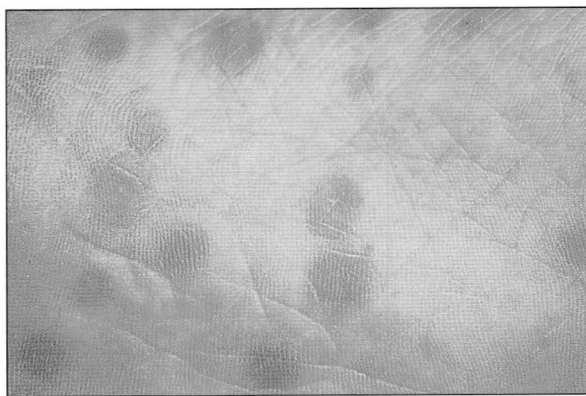

Fig 2-57a A macular eruption is frequently seen in secondary syphilis. This illustrates the hematogenous spread that occurs in the secondary stage.

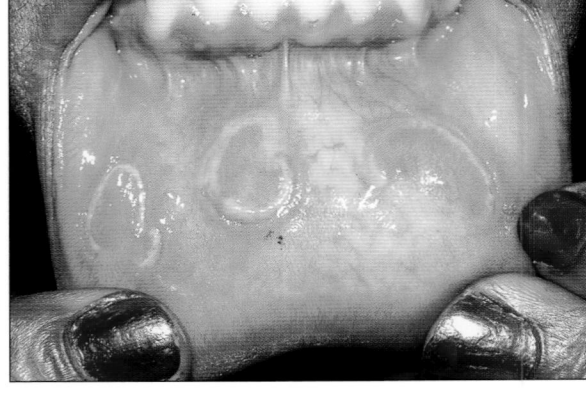

Fig 2-57b Oral lesions of secondary syphilis are referred to as *mucous patches*: discrete erythematous patches with a pale peripheral ring.

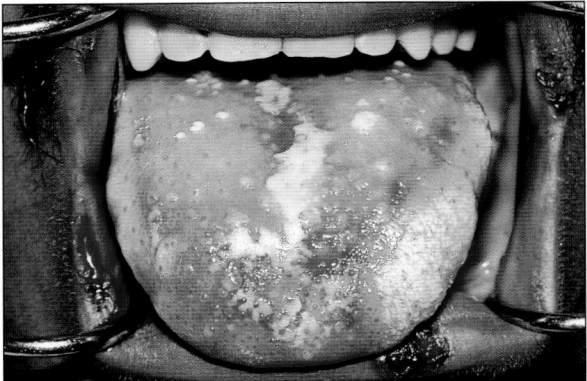

Fig 2-58a Painless oral lesions of secondary syphilis (mucous patches) may also mimic candidiasis or lichen planus.

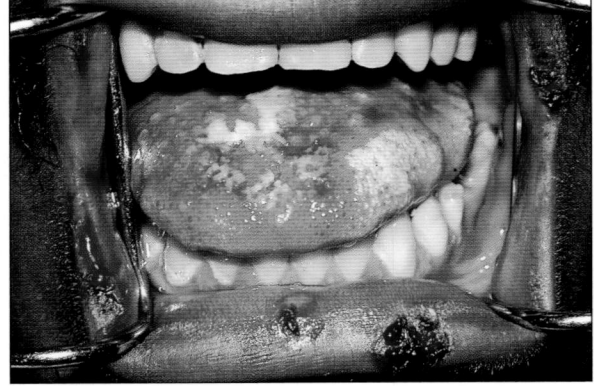

Fig 2-58b Secondary syphilis usually produces a macular skin rash. On occasion, the oral cavity and lips are involved without a skin rash.

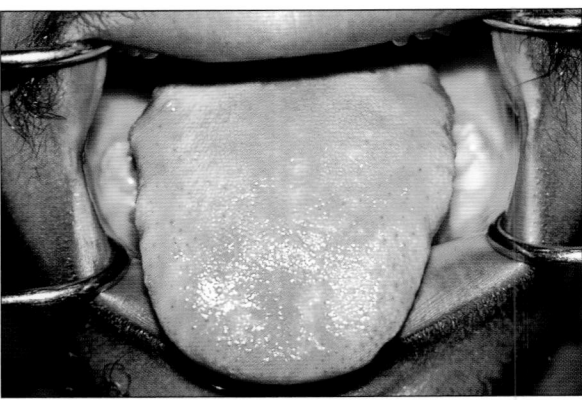

Fig 2-58c Two weeks after receiving 1.2 million U of benzathine penicillin, the tongue lesions of secondary syphilis have completely resolved.

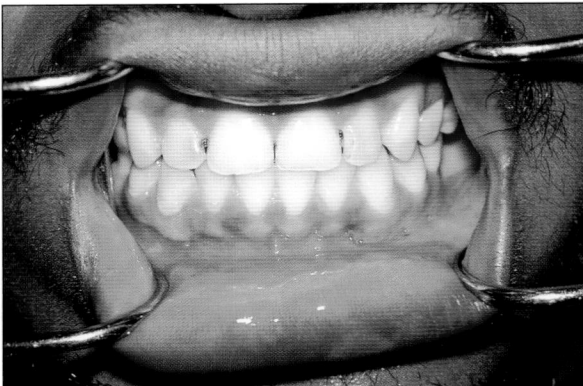

Fig 2-58d Two weeks after receiving 1.2 million U of benzathine penicillin, the lip lesions resolved as well.

ported annually, much of it attributed to "crack cocaine," which has resulted in a sex-for-drugs type of prostitution, a sex-for-money-for-drugs type of prostitution, and a transmission of syphilis to newborns as part of the "crack baby" syndrome.

DIFFERENTIAL DIAGNOSIS ▶

If a *traumatic ulcer* is ruled out, an oral primary chancre should suggest the possibility of other serious diseases presenting with oral ulcers, such as *squamous cell carcinoma*, *TB*, and systemic fungal diseases (particularly *histoplasmosis* and *coccidioidomycosis*).

The oral mucous patches of the secondary stage of disease, with and without the skin rash, may also mimic *reactive arthritis* (formerly known as Reiter syndrome) (particularly if photophobia is present and/or concomitant gonorrhea causes a dysuria mimicking the urethritis of reactive arthritis), *diffuse candidiasis, erythema multiforme*, and *lichen planus* at times.

The destruction of the palate seen in the rare cases of oral tertiary syphilis must be distinguished from the other entities known to cause palatal destruction: *peripheral T-cell lymphoma* (formerly known as *midline lethal granuloma*), *mucormycosis*, and a *nasopharyngeal carcinoma*.

DIAGNOSTIC WORK-UP ▶

Patients suspected of having syphilis should undergo a screening VDRL (Venereal Disease Research Laboratory) serologic test. The VDRL, like the RPR (rapid plasma reagin), is a nontreponemal flocculation test. It uses beef heart cardiolipin (a phospholipid), which has an antigenic similarity to treponemes and, therefore, will cross-react with formed antibodies (reagin) against treponemes as well as several other specific and nonspecific antibodies (the basis of the "biologic false-positive"). This test is quick, inexpen-

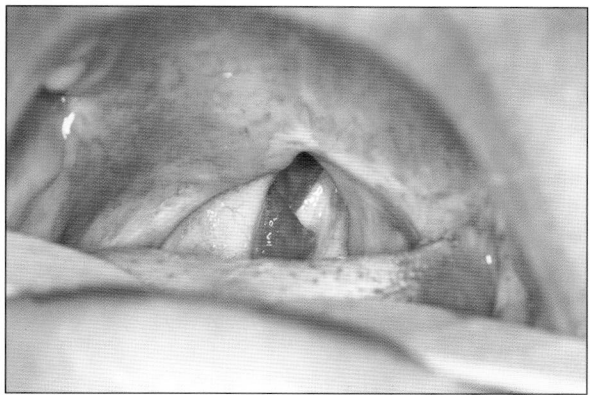

Fig 2-59 A gumma of the palate in tertiary syphilis, which has produced an oronasal fistula. (Courtesy of Dr Roman Carlos.)

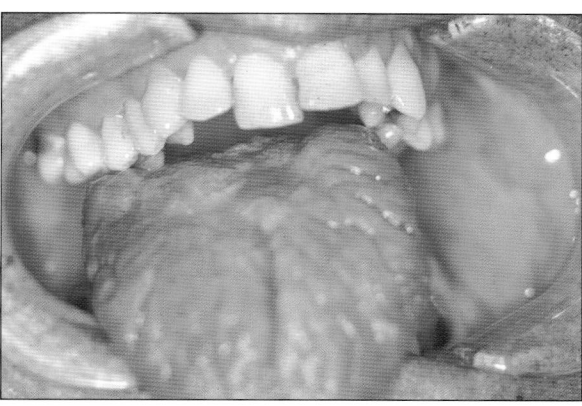

Fig 2-60 Interstitial glossitis in tertiary syphilis is rare today. The tongue will be fissured and firm to hard.

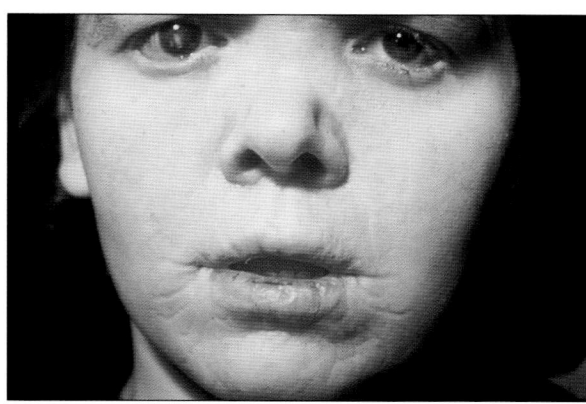

Fig 2-61 The facies of congenital syphilis in this patient includes interstitial keratitis of the right eye, a saddle nose, and rhagades.

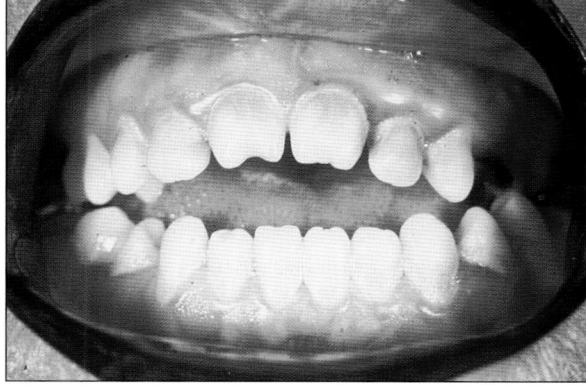

Fig 2-62 Hutchinson teeth in congenital syphilis with notching of the incisal edges of the permanent maxillary and mandibular incisors and tapering of the crowns (screwdriver shape).

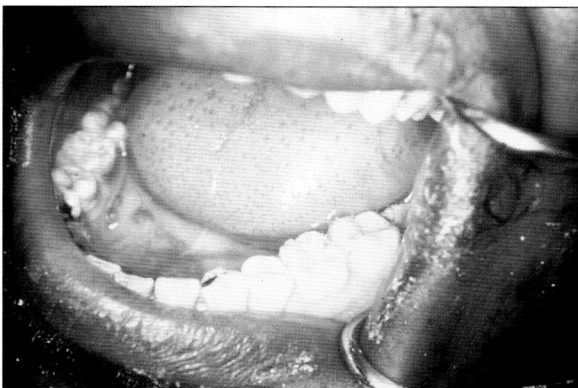

Fig 2-63 Enamel hypoplasia of the permanent first molars in congenital syphilis, also known as *mulberry molars*.

sive, and easy to perform and is, therefore, an ideal test for screening numerous blood samples. If quantitated by serial dilutions (VDRL quantitative), a titer baseline can be established against which follow-up testing can be compared for assessment of treatment response.

The VDRL is positive in 99% of secondary syphilis cases, but positive in only 70% to 75% of primary syphilis cases and in 75% of tertiary syphilis cases. In primary syphilis, a chancre may precede the peak of IgG antibody production by 1 week (chancre 2 weeks after inoculation, IgG peak 3 weeks after inoculation) and, therefore, be weakly positive or even negative. In tertiary syphilis, immune exhaustion causes 25% of these patients to be seronegative despite active disease. Tests not in use today (Wasserman and Kulmer) were also nontreponemal, but rather than causing a flocculation, they fixed complement. They are noted here for historical reference only.

Suspected cases that have a reactive VDRL must be confirmed with a fluorescent treponema antibody-absorption (FTA-ABS) serologic test. The FTA-ABS reaction tests for serum anti–*T pallidum* antibodies by using killed *T pallidum* as the specific antigen after absorbing (removing) other possible antitreponema antibodies with nonpathogenic treponemal organisms. The FTA-ABS is, therefore, highly specific, time-consuming, and somewhat expensive, but it will confirm the diagnosis of syphilis and rule out false-positive VDRL tests. The FTA-ABS test is positive in 85% to 95% of primary syphilis cases, 100%

Table 2-1 Percentage of syphilis patients with positive serologic test results

	Stage (%)		
	Primary	Secondary	Tertiary
VDRL	70–75	99	75
FTA-ABS	85–95	100	98

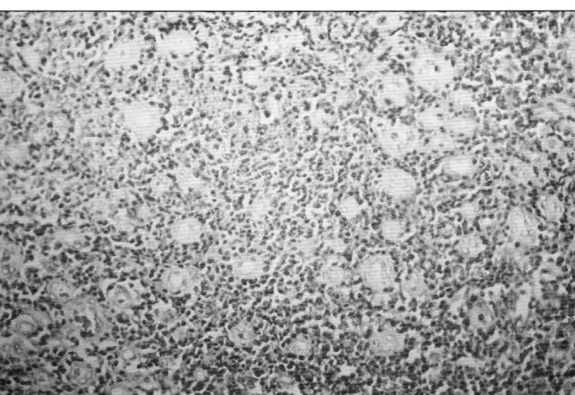

Fig 2-64 Endothelial proliferation and infiltration by predominantly plasma cells in a case of primary syphilis.

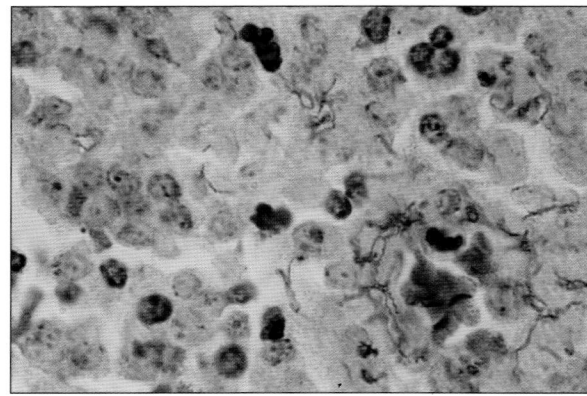

Fig 2-65 At very high magnification (×1,000) and by means of a Warthin-Starry stain, the treponemes can be seen as fine, black, thread-like organisms. Their mobility can be appreciated by their shape, which sometimes resembles a corkscrew.

of secondary syphilis cases, and 98% of tertiary syphilis cases (Table 2-1). Other diagnostic tests such as biopsy or dark-field examination are unreliable because of lack of specificity. However, all cases of secondary syphilis or latent syphilis not adequately treated in the second stage should be considered for a spinal tap and VDRL testing of cerebrospinal fluid (CSF). A positive VDRL result of CSF is considered neurosyphilis. A negative test result does not exclude neurosyphilis, and the test may need to be repeated after 3 weeks.

HISTOPATHOLOGY ▶ The fundamental changes in syphilis are vascular, exemplified by a proliferative endarteritis in which there is swelling and proliferation of endothelial cells, resulting in constriction of the vascular lumen.

The early stages of syphilis are characterized by dense perivascular infiltrations of plasma cells and lymphocytes, an immunologic reaction to treponemal antigen (Fig 2-64). In the chancre, the reaction may be so dense at the center of the lesion that clear identification of the cells and the endothelial proliferation may be made only more peripherally. Occlusion of vessels by the endothelium may cause necrosis and ulceration of the chancre, and the epithelial margins may show a reactive acanthosis. The treponemes can be identified within the tissue by means of a silver stain such as Warthin-Starry. They appear as narrow (0.25 μm), black, thread-like organisms, often with a corkscrew configuration (Fig 2-65). This, however, does not distinguish *T pallidum* from other treponemes such as *Treponema microdentium*. The organisms tend to concentrate around capillary walls and within the epithelium. Most are extracellular and are destroyed by phagocytosis. Some organisms appear to survive intracellularly, however.

Tertiary or late syphilis is characterized by epithelioid granuloma formation, a cellular immune response to reactivation of the treponemes, most likely the consequence of a decrease in circulating antibodies. Multinucleated giant cells are usually present. Caseation may or may not be seen, but is extensive in gummatous lesions. Vascular changes with obliterative endarteritis are also present in late syphilis. Organisms are sparse. Granulomas more typical of tertiary syphilis may sometimes be seen in secondary syphilis.

TREATMENT ▶

Early syphilis (ie, primary, secondary, and early latent syphilis, which is a relapsing form of secondary syphilis after lesions have disappeared) is treated once with 1.2 to 2.4 million U of benzathine penicillin (Bicillin LA, Wyeth-Ayerst) intramuscularly in the gluteal region. Benzathine penicillin is the drug of choice for all forms of syphilis because it maintains effective tissue levels for weeks, which is required in the treatment of spirochetal disease because of their prolonged turnover time (about 30 hours) (see Figs 2-56a to 2-56d and 2-58a to 2-58d).

For the penicillin-allergic patient, oral tetracycline, 500 mg four times daily, oral doxycycline, 100 mg twice daily, or oral erythromycin, 500 mg four times daily for 14 days, are effective. However, noncompliance is a problem because many patients will cut their course short of 14 days as the lesions start to disappear, hence the frequency of latent syphilis. Erythromycin is less effective than penicillin or tetracycline.

These same regimens are given to individuals who had sexual contact with the patient within the past 90 days and anyone who may have sexual relations with the patient within 14 days after treatment initiation. A diagnosed case of syphilis in any stage requires a reporting to the public health authorities for assistance in identifying and treating sexual contacts. It also requires an HIV test because of a higher incidence of treatment failures in the HIV-positive group and, therefore, the need for closer follow-up and retesting.

The Jarisch-Herxheimer reaction is a well-known reaction to initial therapy. It results from a massive spirochete kill, which releases large quantities of antigen into the bloodstream. Antigen-antibody complexes then lodge into almost all tissues, producing constitutional symptoms of fever, malaise, myalgia, and exacerbation of the syphilitic lesions. It is treated with reassurance, rest, and anti-inflammatory drugs. It usually begins within 24 hours of the treatment and subsides after another 24 hours.

Tertiary syphilis is treated with 2.4 million U of benzathine penicillin intramuscularly three times at 7-day intervals, or oral tetracycline, 500 mg four times daily, or oral doxycycline, 100 mg four times daily, for 28 days.

For established neurosyphilis, 2.4 million U of benzathine penicillin intramuscularly three times at 7-day intervals is administered with 2 to 4 million U of aqueous penicillin G intravenously every 4 hours for 14 days so that a higher CSF penetration can be obtained. In neurosyphilis, a penicillin-allergic patient is tested carefully for the degree of hypersensitivity. No effective alternative to penicillin is known for the treatment of neurosyphilis.

PROGNOSIS ▶

Recurrent syphilis results either from treatment failure (usually due to noncompliance by those using oral medications) or from reinfection. Treponemes have no ability to form resistance to penicillin. Follow-up should be both clinical and serologic. The quantitative VDRL should show a fourfold decrease within 3 months in early syphilis and within 6 months in latent and late syphilis.

Gonorrhea

CLINICAL PRESENTATION AND PATHOGENESIS ▶

Gonorrhea is a sexually transmitted genital infection that rarely affects the pharynx and even more rarely affects oral mucous membranes or the temporomandibular joint. Oropharyngeal gonorrhea is usually brought to the patient's attention by sore throat accompanied by mild cervical lymphadenitis. The throat and even parts of the oral cavity will have a diffuse erythema and possibly some small nonspecific ulcers.

In patients with concomitant genital gonorrhea, men will develop urethritis with dysuria and pyuria. Women may have dysuria and frequent vaginitis and swelling around the orifice of Bartholin glands. Either sex may be asymptomatic, but women are reported to be asymptomatic more often than men and are thus believed to be the more significant reservoir of disease.

Oropharyngeal gonorrhea is more commonly seen in women and homosexual men because of genital-oral transmission from fellatio and cunnilingus. The pharyngeal mucosa is more susceptible to infection than is the oral mucosa, hence the greater incidence of pharyngeal lesions than oral lesions.

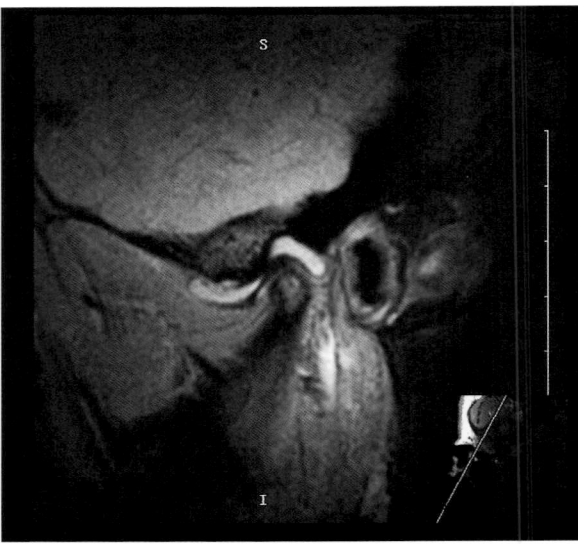

Fig 2-66 Septic temporomandibular joint due to gonococchal arthritis. This is demonstrated as enhanced water content evidencing a joint effusion within the entire joint space.

Gonorrhea is caused by *Neisseria gonorrhoeae*. It is, today, the most prevalent communicable disease reported in the US, with an estimated 2.5 million cases annually. Cases of gonorrhea showed a dramatic rise from 1965 to 1975 as the sexual revolution took hold and the drug-resistant strains imported from Vietnam became more widely disseminated in the US. Today, the fear of AIDS has affected sexual habits and sexual expressions; a reduction in the practice of fellatio is reducing the incidence of gonorrhea in homosexual men and in heterosexual women. Conversely, the prevalence of drug use continues to drive the incidence of gonorrhea upward as sex-for-drugs and sex-for-money-for-drugs activity continues.

DIFFERENTIAL DIAGNOSIS ▶ The oropharyngeal symptoms are nonspecific. *Streptococcal pharyngitis* is the most important differentiation to make. In addition, the features of oropharyngeal lesions coupled with genitourinary symptoms of dysuria suggest *reactive arthritis* (formerly known as Reiter syndrome) or *candidiasis*, possibly associated with HIV infection or other sexually transmitted diseases. Gonorrhea is also known to affect various joints, and gonococchal arthritis is occasionally seen as a secondary complication of genital infections. This may very occasionally be seen even in the temporomandibular joint, where it will present as a clinically swollen and painful joint with limited jaw opening, typical of septic arthritis. A T-2–weighted MRI will show a significant effusion in both the anterior and posterior compartments of the joint space (Fig 2-66).

DIAGNOSTIC WORK-UP ▶ Throat culture or cultures of oral lesions should show gram-negative diplococci on Gram staining, as will "clean-catch" urine Gram staining. Culture identification is possible on either Thayer-Martin or Transgrow media (Becton Dickinson).

HISTOPATHOLOGY ▶ On mucous membranes, the organisms attach to the epithelium and penetrate into the submucosa, provoking a mild acute inflammatory reaction with edema, hyperemia, and neutrophils. They are phagocytosed and found within the lysosomes of the neutrophils. In the event of a gonococcemia, a vasculitis secondary to the presence of the organisms within the vessels occurs.

TREATMENT ▶ The most effective treatment for oropharyngeal gonorrhea, even for resistant strains, is currently a single dose of ceftriaxone (Rocephin, Roche), 250 mg intramuscularly. As an oral alternative, trimethoprim 80 mg/sulfamethoxazole 400 mg (Bactrim SS, Roche), nine tablets daily for 5 days, is also effective. Other regimens that may also be effective but are less frequently used are single doses of the following: oral ciprofloxacin (Cipro, Bayer), 500 mg; oral cefixime (Suprax, Lederle), 800 mg; or spectinomycin (Trobicin, Pharmacia and Upjohn), 16 mg intramuscularly.

The clinician should be alert for other sexually transmitted diseases that may occur simultaneously with gonorrhea. Coexistent chlamydial infection is common and should be treated additionally with either oral erythromycin or oral tetracycline, 500 mg four times daily, for 7 days. Coexistent syphilis should

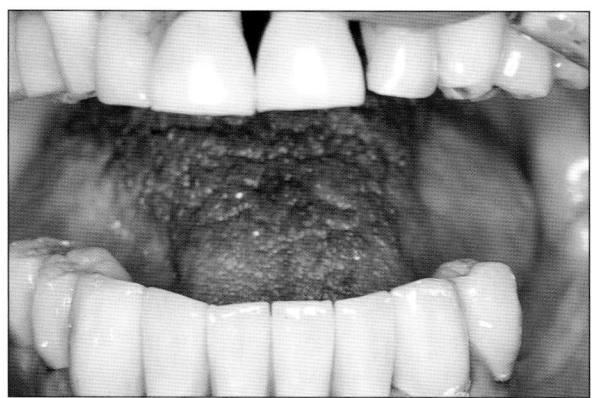

Fig 2-67 Black hairy tongue will initially seem like a removable dark stain on the tongue surface, but actually represents inflammation, elongated filiform papillae, and bacteria-produced black pigment.

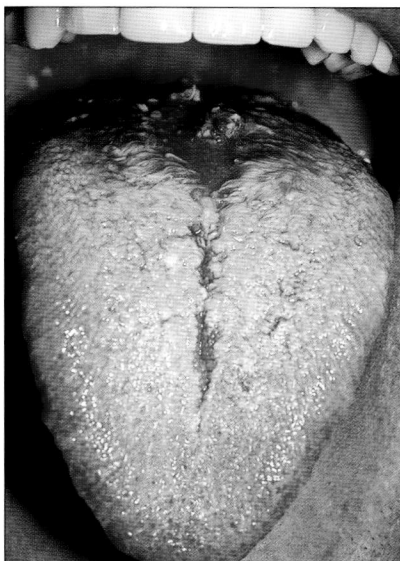

Fig 2-68a Black hairy tongue will also have some white areas and often will have a denuded area of obvious inflammation.

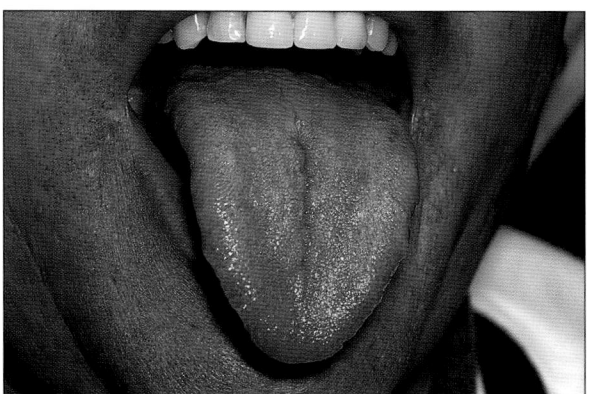

Fig 2-68b Resolution of black hairy tongue after penicillin therapy.

be assessed with a VDRL serologic test and followed by an FTA-ABS test if the VDRL is positive. Confirmed cases of concomitant syphilis need to be treated separately from gonorrhea using the regimens noted in the syphilis section (see above). Neither regimen will suffice to treat both diseases.

PROGNOSIS ▶

Treatment with ceftriaxone is almost 100% effective, even for ophthalmic gonorrhea. Recurrent disease is usually related to reinfection or treatment with other drugs, particularly penicillin, and the subsequent emergence of penicillin-resistant strains.

Black Hairy Tongue

CLINICAL PRESENTATION AND PATHOGENESIS ▶

As its name implies, black hairy tongue will present as a black area, along with some small red and white areas, on the dorsum of the tongue. The patient may complain of pain or a burning sensation on the tongue and also of pain on swallowing or a generalized pharyngitis.

Black hairy tongue actually represents a superficial bacterial infection of the tongue by pigment-producing microorganisms often called *chromogenic* bacteria (Fig 2-67). It is therefore a type of glossitis that may exist in isolation or as part of a pharyngitis or tonsillitis. Although *Candida* organisms may sometimes be found in the microorganismal mix that comprises black hairy tongue, it is not a primary *Candida* infection and will not respond to anti-*Candida* medications alone.

In addition to the elongated filiform papillae and the colonies of microorganisms formed upon an inflamed base (Fig 2-68a), which gives rise to the hairy appearance of the tongue, there may be a submandibular or cervical lymphadenopathy.

DIFFERENTIAL DIAGNOSIS ▶

Black hairy tongue is a clinically recognizable entity. *White hairy tongue*, which has been described by many, represents the same type of glossitis except the microorganisms do not produce as much pigment. Although most cases of black hairy tongue occur in otherwise normal individuals because of an unexplained overproliferation of certain microorganisms, the clinician should bear in mind that systemic steroid medications, overuse of certain antibacterial mouthwashes, smoking, immunosuppression, and systemic antibiotics or antifungal drugs may predispose individuals to this entity.

DIAGNOSTIC WORK-UP ▶

Since black hairy tongue is a clinically recognizable entity, no particular work-up is required. Cultures of the dorsum of the tongue are usually not very yielding. No specific microorganism has been consistently isolated; usually a nonspecific polymicrobic flora is seen.

TREATMENT AND PROGNOSIS ▶

Black hairy tongue is treated with oral antibiotics for 10 to 14 days and physical tongue brushing. The antibiotic of choice remains phenoxymethyl penicillin (Pen-Vee K, Wyeth-Ayerst), 500 mg four times per day. In the penicillin-allergic patient, erythromycin ethyl succinate (EES, Abbott), 400 mg three times per day, is effective. The tongue brushing can be accomplished with toothpaste or with 0.12% chlorhexidine (Peridex, Procter and Gamble) or with the bare brush alone. The use of hydrogen peroxide or other oxygenated mouthwashes is not recommended because of their potential to select out anaerobes. Also not recommended is the use of clindamycin because of its reduced effectiveness against several streptococcal species and *E corrodens*.

Such therapy usually resolves black hairy tongue (Fig 2-68b). However, recurrences are seen in about 10% to 20% of individuals because of predisposing factors and/or premature cessation of treatment.

Cat-Scratch Disease

CLINICAL PRESENTATION ▶

Cat-scratch disease usually presents as a painless, irregular, firm mass of matted lymph nodes. The nodes are initially nontender, although some cases present with painful lymphadenitis. They are fixed to surrounding tissues and often to the mandible if they arise in the submandibular or submental triangle. The nodes present in much the same fashion as one would expect in cervical lymph node metastases from oral squamous cell carcinoma (Fig 2-69).

The disease is almost always associated with cats and very rarely with dogs or other animals. Of particular note is that the cat itself is almost always less than 1 year old and that most patients are young: peak incidence is between the ages of 5 and 25 years. A physical cat scratch is observed in only 40% of cases. Even when a scratch is observed, only 33% of those individuals develop an infection at the site of the scratch. When lymph nodes become enlarged, they are not necessarily within the lymphatic drainage of the scratch site. The nodes will usually enlarge and achieve a size of 4 to 6 cm within a matter of 1 to 2 weeks. Symptoms of infection such as fever, erythema, and leukocytosis are only rarely seen. Most cases present as asymptomatic, firm lymph node masses.

DIFFERENTIAL DIAGNOSIS ▶

The rapid emergence of firm, fixed, and usually painless nodes should give the clinician some concern about *squamous cell carcinoma nodal metastasis* despite the young age of these patients. *Hodgkin lymphoma*, *HIV-related lymphadenopathy*, and *cervical TB adenitis* are also distinct considerations. If the nodes are indeed fixed to the mandible or to another bone, *desmoplastic fibroma* and *aggressive fibromatosis* become possibilities. In those patients who develop lymph node enlargement in the deep midcervical chain, a *branchial cyst* (benign cystic lymph node) also becomes a consideration.

DIAGNOSTIC WORK-UP ▶

The diagnosis of cat-scratch disease is a clinical patient-history diagnosis confirmed by serum antibody identification. The association with cats, the age of the cat, and the clinical quality of the nodes are the most important criteria. Standard laboratory data are not very useful. There is usually no leukocytosis, and other laboratory data are also within normal limits.

Before 1985, the Rose-Hanger skin antigen test was used. It was more than 90% specific and confirmed the diagnosis of cat-scratch disease in suspected cases without lymph node biopsy. Because the Rose-Hanger test used lymph node preparations from known cat-scratch tissue, however, concern about HIV and hepatitis transmission has forced this test out of use. Today, a serum cat-scratch antibody test, a test that most laboratories can perform, is used to confirm the diagnosis. This test was made possible by the culture identification of the causative organism, *Bartonella henselae,* in 1988. Previously, the organism was suspected to be *Afipia felis*, named after the Armed Forces Institute of Pathology, which first documented a bacterial etiology of cat-scratch disease with a Warthin-Starry stain of lymph nodes. To further confuse the matter, this causative organism was first classified as *Rochalimaea henselae*. Therefore,

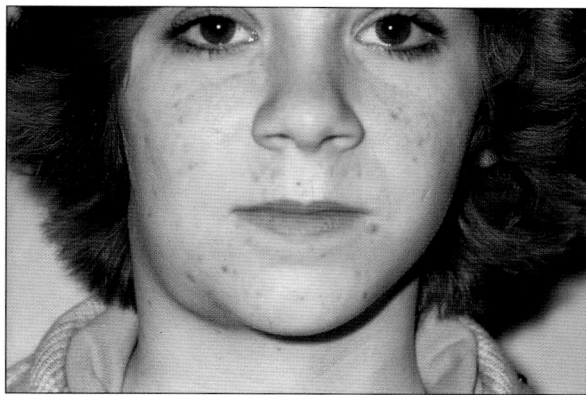

Fig 2-69 Cat-scratch disease associated with kittens but no reported scratch. These large, fixed, fused, and mildly tender lymph nodes appeared in just 2 weeks.

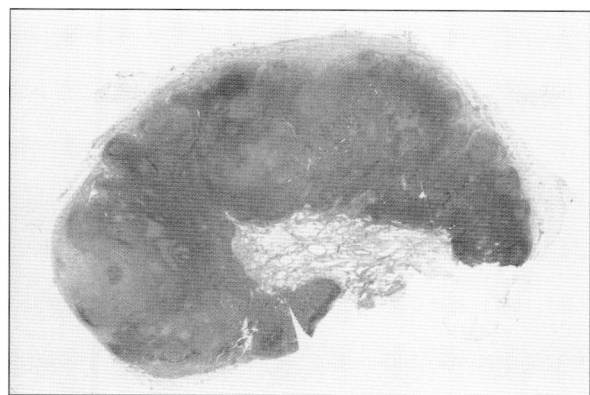

Fig 2-70a Low-power view of a cat-scratch–infected lymph node showing the enlargement of the node and the effacement of its normal architecture in most areas. The full spectrum of change was present in this node.

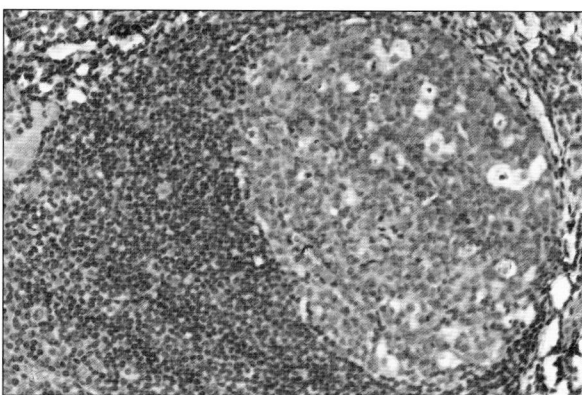

Fig 2-70b The follicular hyperplasia shows an enlarged germinal center containing pale-staining macrophages (tingible body macrophages).

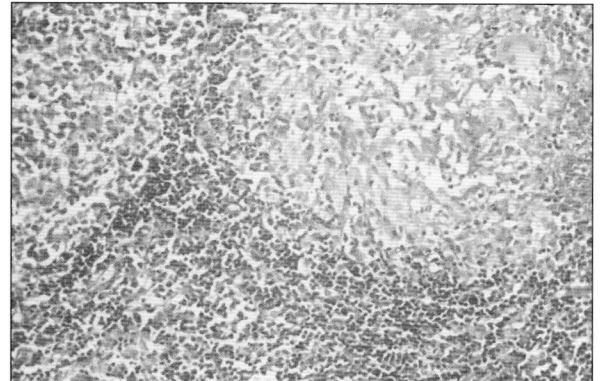

Fig 2-70c Within the same lymph node, granulomas with aggregates of macrophages (epithelioid cells) can be seen.

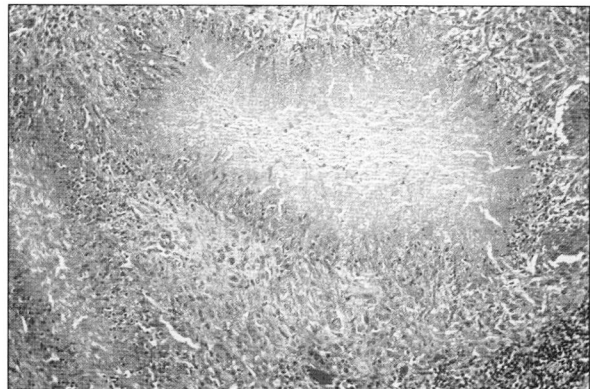

Fig 2-70d Another area of the same lymph node shows central necrosis, palisaded epithelioid cells, fibrin, and neutrophils.

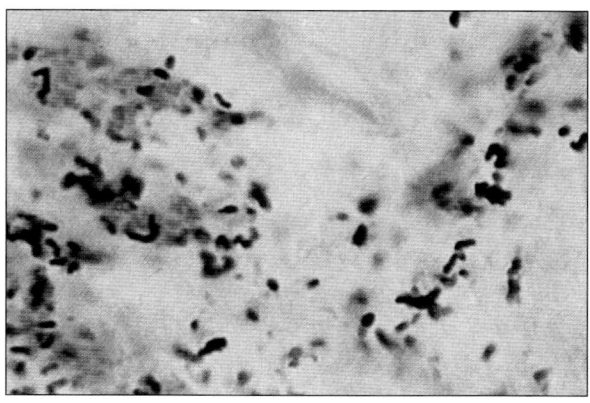

Fig 2-70e A Warthin-Starry stain reveals the presence of the small pleomorphic bacteria in cat-scratch disease (*B henselae*).

older literature and some reports may still refer to either *A felis* or *R henselae* rather than the actual causative agent, *B henselae*.

If the cat-scratch antibody test either cannot be accomplished or is equivocal, the diagnosis should be established by a lymph node biopsy, which should include Warthin-Starry staining in an attempt to identify the organism.

HISTOPATHOLOGY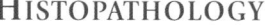

The histologic changes associated with cat-scratch disease represent a regional lymphadenitis. The spectrum of change within this inflammatory process can be broken down into three stages. Early changes show a nonspecific reactive follicular hyperplasia with prominent follicles of varied size. The sinuses may be distended, but there is little distortion of architecture. The follicles have peripheral small lymphocytes with prominent germinal centers within which mitotic and phagocytic activity are seen (Figs 2-70a and 2-70b). Inflammatory cells such as plasma cells and eosinophils are found between the follicles and are accompanied by endothelial proliferation.

This stage may be followed by granulomatous inflammation in which epithelioid granulomas with occasional Langhans giant cells may be found within the cortex and medulla (Fig 2-70c).

Ultimately, the granulomas may undergo central necrosis (Fig 2-70d). In this case, a focus of neutrophils, nuclear debris, and fibrin surrounded by palisaded epithelioid cells is seen. Granulomas and abscesses may be found in the capsule and may break out into the surrounding fat.

Identification of the small pleomorphic bacteria within damaged vessels and microabscesses of the lymph nodes can be accomplished by means of a Warthin-Starry stain (Fig 2-70e).

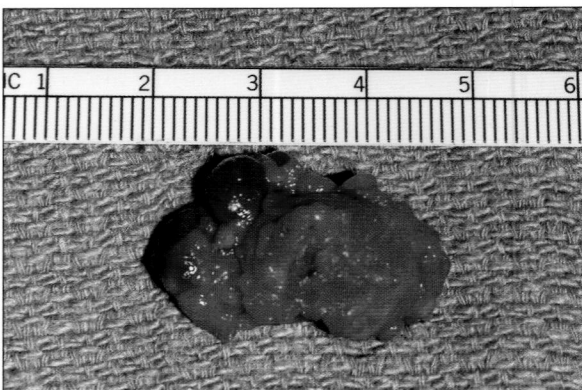

Fig 2-71 If cat-scratch lymph nodes are removed before resolution or breakdown into necrosis, they will be fibrosed together, darkened, and hyperemic.

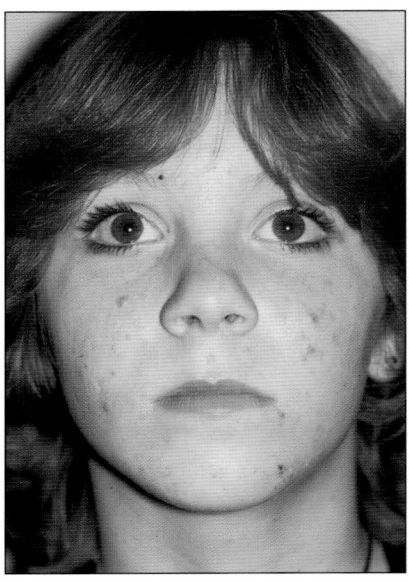

Fig 2-72 The cat-scratch disease shown in Fig 2-69 clinically resolved in 1 month without surgery or antibiotic treatment.

TREATMENT ▶

If the diagnosis is confirmed by a cat-scratch antibody test, no biopsy or surgery is necessary. If the diagnosis is confirmed by lymph node biopsy, further surgery is unnecessary. *B henselae* is a very small gram-negative aerobe that belongs to a class of organisms called *proteobacteria*, which are transitional forms between the more primitive rickettsia and true bacteria. It is an organism sensitive to tetracyclines, erythromycin, azithromycin, and clarithromycin, which allows the clinician to treat with a choice of antibiotics. However, 80% of cases will resolve spontaneously without treatment, making the value of antibiotic therapy questionable.

In about 10% of cases, the lymph node will undergo central necrosis and begin to show clinical fluctuance. If this course becomes evident, incision and drainage is to be avoided in favor of complete lymph node excision (Fig 2-71). In such cases, postexcision antibiotics, either tetracycline or erythromycin, should be given. When incision and drainage is carried out, the disease is often prolonged while the entire lymph node continues a slow necrosis and drainage, which eventually produces a large, retracted scar.

PROGNOSIS ▶

Although very rare cases of erythema nodosum, papular rashes, and even encephalitis have been reported as complications from cat-scratch disease, spontaneous involution or resolution after lymph node excision is the rule (Fig 2-72).

Tetanus

CLINICAL PRESENTATION AND
PATHOGENESIS ▶

Tetanus is a life-threatening infection caused by the microorganism *Clostridium tetani*, a ubiquitous inhabitant of soil. Its production of the neurotoxin tetanospasmin produces the hyperreactive muscle and actual muscle spasms of this disease.

Most cases occur in unvaccinated individuals. Newborns, the elderly, migrant workers, and intravenous (IV) drug users are at greatest risk. Although most cases are the result of a penetrating wound, any wound with nonvital tissues and anaerobic conditions may incubate *C tetani*.

C tetani is not especially invasive. In fact, it exists in an anaerobic wound as a vegetative growth, producing the tetanospasmin toxin, a metalloproteinase enzyme that cleaves synaptobrevin, which is a protein required for central spinal motor nerves to release neurotransmitters. The point of action of tetanospasmin appears to be the neurotransmission at spinal synapsis of the inhibitory neurons. The loss of inhibition results in overexcitatory impulses and muscle spasms from minor or even no stimuli. Once infected, it takes about 8 to 12 days to produce enough tetanospasmin for symptoms to develop.

The first symptoms that would be seen by the oral and maxillofacial specialist are limited jaw opening, stiff neck, diplopia, or dysphagia (Fig 2-73a). The site of infection may be normal in appearance or show the typical signs of infection. Pain and spasticity of the nearest muscle to the infection site may be noted as an early sign. The location of the infection site has no correlation with the location of the uncontrolled spasms once sustained spasms begin. As the disease progresses, the increased levels of tetanospasmin will progress, first involving muscles of higher power-to-size ratios (masseter, external ocular, neck muscles) and then involving muscles of lower power-to-size ratios (back muscles, leg muscles, and diaphragm), that is, the larger muscles. The cardiac muscle is not directly affected because of its autonomic innervation, which has no synapses in the spinal cord. As the disease progresses further, contractions of the facial muscles result in a so-called sardonic smile (Fig 2-73b), so named after the island of Sardinia, where the crowfoot plant is known to create the same type of facial muscle spasm. Later in the course, spasms in the back muscles will cause *opisthotonos*, an arching of the back resembling a wrestler's bridge position (Fig 2-73c). Although the extensors and flexors of the trunk are affected to the same degree, the back muscles (extensors) are stronger and more numerous. When the diaphragm and intercostal muscles become involved, apnea results and death follows unless the individual is placed on a ventilator and paralyzed with muscle relaxants.

DIAGNOSTIC WORK-UP ▶

The first step in diagnosing a case of tetanus is recognizing that tetanus can occur in modern society. Young individuals of lower socioeconomic status and recent immigrants often do not receive vaccination and are more likely to suffer the classic puncture injury (Fig 2-73d). Since no laboratory tests can aid in the diagnosis of tetanus, an index of suspicion gained from the immunization and social history are of great importance. Intravenous drug abusers will pose the greatest work-up challenge because they are at risk for identical symptoms from strychnine contamination in their IV drugs and from designer drugs that can cause unknown reactions, as well as from the potential for needle contamination with *C tetani*. All of these patients need to be treated as if their symptoms did arise from tetanus.

DIFFERENTIAL DIAGNOSIS ▶

In the early stages of tetanus, the jaw and neck stiffness as well as diplopia may suggest *meningitis*. As more obvious muscle spasms develop, *strychnine poisoning* or *phenothiazine overuse* may be suspected. It is important to note that street-grade heroin and similar drugs are often "cut" or diluted with additives such as strychnine, phenothiazines, talc, dental powders, etc, to stretch the stock. Therefore, IV drug abusers are at risk for any of these diseases as well as for tetanus. In addition, *severe hypocalcemia* also produces tetanus via a different mechanism and may on rare occasion result after parathyroidectomy or overdoses with bisphosphonates.

TREATMENT ▶

Once tetanus is diagnosed, time is of the essence, and therefore several measures need to be taken concurrently. All cases should receive 5,000 U of tetanus immune globulin intramuscularly (Hyper-Tet) (passive immunity). The concerning wound requires debridement, irrigation, and cultures. Intravenous aqueous penicillin, 20 million U per day in divided doses, is also required. The strategy of this treatment regimen is for the preformed antibodies (passive immunity) to neutralize the tetanospasmin, for the debridement to remove nonvital tissue and reverse the anaerobic environment, and for the penicillin to reduce the toxin-producing organisms.

In early cases, the patient needs to be sedated and placed on bed rest in a dark, quiet room with minimal external stimuli. However, respirations and oxygen saturation must be continuously monitored because progression of tetanus will lead to severe respiratory depression and apnea. Later cases or those showing progressive signs of respiratory failure require intubation or tracheostomy with paralysis and mechanical ventilation (Fig 2-73e).

PROGNOSIS ▶

The chances for survival are directly proportional to the amount of time taken to diagnose and treat tetanus. Cases that are recognized before respiratory failure begins and treated aggressively can be sal-

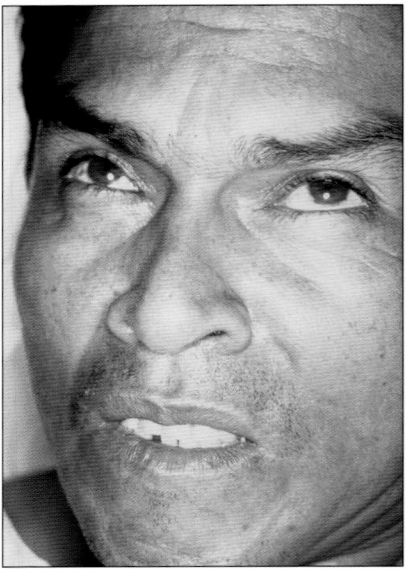

Fig 2-73a Tetanus may be seen by the oral and maxillofacial specialist first because of its early involvement of the facial muscles, extraocular muscles, and masseter. (Courtesy of Dr Clara Ardilla.)

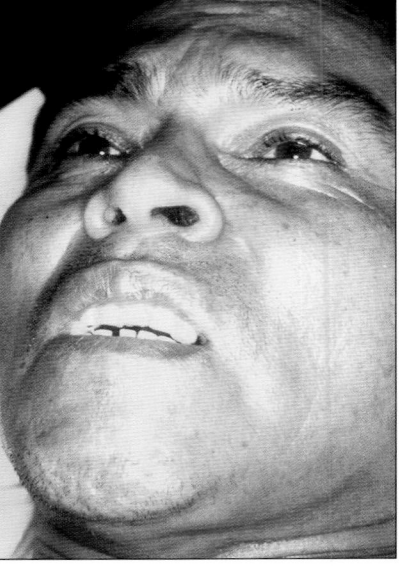

Fig 2-73b The contraction of the upper lip produces a smile or snarl appearance termed *risus sardonicus*. (Courtesy of Dr Clara Ardilla.)

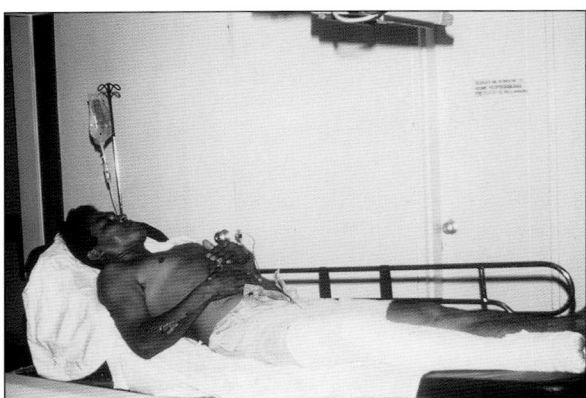

Fig 2-73c The spasm of the masseter can be seen by its bulging appearance. In addition, involvement of the extensors of the back may give the appearance of an arched positioning. (Courtesy of Dr Clara Ardilla.)

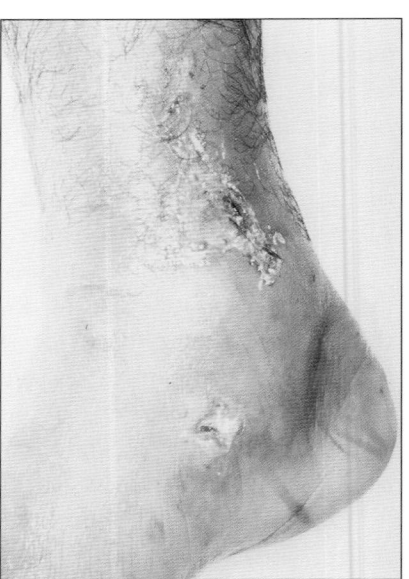

Fig 2-73d This tetanus arose from puncture wounds in the foot reportedly due to falling on rocks and a fishhook by the seashore. (Courtesy of Dr Clara Ardilla.)

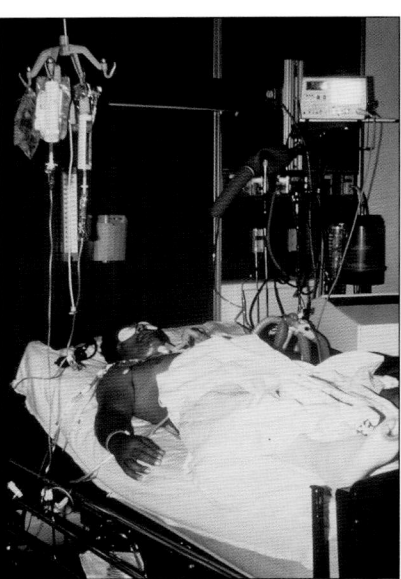

Fig 2-73e Tetanus is life threatening. In addition to tetanus immune globulin, tetanus toxoid, antibiotics, and wound debridement, intubations or a tracheostomy with ventilatory support under paralysis is necessary. (Courtesy of Dr Clara Ardilla.)

vaged. However, there remains an overall 40% mortality rate due to cases that remain unrecognized until late in their course or for whom access to medical care is delayed. It is important to note that contaminated wounds of the head and neck area are more dangerous than wounds elsewhere because of the abundant blood supply absorbing and systemically distributing a greater quantity of the toxin.

Rheumatic Fever–Rheumatic Heart Disease– Subacute Bacterial Endocarditis

Rheumatic fever is a systemic immune process that is initiated by a bacterial infection. It can lead to immunologically created heart valve damage (rheumatic heart disease), which in turn can lead years later to a bacterial infection of the damaged heart valve (subacute bacterial endocarditis [SBE]). This relationship is of significance not only to the oral and maxillofacial specialist but to all dentists because of the well-known risks associated with gingivitis, periodontitis, and dental or oral surgical procedures in precipitating an SBE. It is therefore important for the clinician to understand the pathophysiology of rheumatic fever, the nature of rheumatic heart disease, the means of assessing rheumatic heart disease, the recommended protocols for prevention of SBE, and the treatment for and life-threatening nature of SBE.

Rheumatic Fever

CLINICAL PRESENTATION AND PATHOGENESIS ▶

Rheumatic fever usually begins with a beta-hemolytic streptococcal pharyngitis in a child between 5 and 15 years of age. While some are severe, others are dismissed as nothing more than a "sore throat." However, antibodies develop to streptococcal protein toxins, especially to streptolysin O and streptodornase, and these in turn cross-react with and damage host connective tissues, particularly those in heart valves. If severe enough, this can lead to rheumatic heart disease.

Signs of rheumatic fever usually do not develop until sufficient antistreptolysin O and antistreptococcal DNA antibody titers rise, about 2 to 3 weeks after the onset of pharyngitis. The classic signs and symptoms of rheumatic fever historically are referred to as *Jones criteria* and are still employed today. A diagnosis of rheumatic fever can be made either when two major criteria or when one major criterion and one minor criterion are present.

CLINICAL PRESENTATION AND DIAGNOSTIC WORK-UP ▶

1. Major Criteria

A. Carditis

Pericarditis as identified by an auscultatory friction rub and substernal pain, cardiomegaly as seen on a chest radiograph, congestive heart failure as evidenced by venous distension and painful hepatomegaly, and mitral or aortic valvular regurgitation as heard via stethoscope auscultation or echocardiography.

B. Erythema Marginatum or Subcutaneous Nodules

These findings are indicative of the systemic antigen/antibody complexes provoking inflammation and fibrosis, the main pathophysiology of rheumatic fever. Erythema marginatum is the physical sign of a rapidly enlarging skin macule that will have a clear center and an irregular red ring at the periphery. Subcutaneous fibrous nodules, which are uncommon and seem only to occur in children, are less than 2 cm in diameter and will seem to be attached to underlying fascia or tendons.

C. Sydenham Chorea

These are rapid, jerky, involuntary movements primarily of the muscles of facial expression, the tongue, and the arms.

D. Arthritis

This will be a migratory polyarthritis in which the child will complain of a specific joint pain one day and then of a different joint pain or many joint pains the next day. The target joints are the larger joints such as the knee, elbow, and hip. These symptoms characteristically respond to aspirin or to nonsteroidal anti-inflammatory drugs, which serves as a diagnostic sign. Radiographs will show bony erosions that are reversible with treatment.

2. Minor Criteria

A. History of a streptococcal pharyngitis within the past 6 weeks

B. Fever

C. Polyarthralgia, ie, joint pains but no radiographic evidence of bony erosion

To complement the major and minor Jones criteria, infectious disease specialists will draw serial blood samples for antistreptolysin O antibodies and antistreptococcal DNA antibodies. Rising titers of these antibodies are consistent with rheumatic fever.

DIFFERENTIAL DIAGNOSIS ▶

The purpose of the Jones criteria is to establish an unequivocal diagnosis of rheumatic fever and to begin treatment quickly so as to prevent the permanent heart damage known as rheumatic heart disease. Jones criteria help the clinician distinguish rheumatic fever from the many childhood and early adult illnesses that may produce a similar picture, including *recurrent pharyngitis, meningitis, acute* and *subacute bacterial endocarditis, juvenile rheumatoid arthritis, osteomyelitis, sickle cell anemia*, and even *Lyme disease*.

HISTOPATHOLOGY ▶

In rheumatic fever, the acute involvement of the heart is a pancarditis (endocarditis, myocarditis, and pericarditis), of which the most significant component is the myocarditis. There is interstitial inflammation with the formation of Aschoff bodies, a perivascular fibrinoid necrosis with lymphocytes, plasma cells, and neutrophils. Ultimately, there can be fibrosis of the myocardium. The endocarditis affects mainly the valves with a verrucous appearance at the line of closure. There is focal collagen degeneration in the valve with inflammation and ulceration of the valve's endocardial surface. Fibrin may be deposited on the surface of the valve. In chronic rheumatic disease, which follows repeated episodes of rheumatic fever, the most significant aspect is the valvular damage, which is progressive in nature. The most common site of involvement is the mitral valve, in which there is irregular thickening and calcification of the leaflets. There may be fusion of the commissures and of the chordae tendinae, resulting in stenosis. The aortic valve is the second most frequently involved site; here there is fusion of the commissures with subsequent thickening and calcification of the cusps, resulting in stenosis or insufficiency. The other valves are rarely involved. The subcutaneous nodules consist of irregular but well-demarcated foci of palisaded histiocytes surrounding fibrin masses, which often contain neutrophils. Dense fibrosis occurs between the granulomas.

TREATMENT AND PROGNOSIS ▶

Rheumatic fever itself can be prevented with timely antibiotic treatment. Penicillin remains the drug of choice and is given once using the slow-absorption and long-lasting tissue-level form benzathine penicillin (Bicillin LA, Wyeth-Ayerst), 1.2 million U intramuscularly. As an alterative, 600,000 U of procaine penicillin G (Wycillin, Wyeth-Ayerst) may be given intramuscularly for 10 days, or 500 mg of oral phenoxymethyl penicillin may be given four times a day for 10 days. However, noncompliance with the latter two therapies is common and risks recurrent rheumatic fever episodes and rheumatic heart disease. In the penicillin-allergic patient, the drug of choice is erythromycin, 1 g intramuscularly or intravenously once daily for 10 days, or erythromycin ethyl succinate, 400 mg by mouth three times a day for 10 days. Along with antibiotics, aspirin, 650 mg every 6 hours, or the equivalent of a nonsteroidal anti-inflammatory drug should be used to reduce joint pains and fever. In addition, bed rest is recommended until the patient is afebrile.

Recurrent episodes of rheumatic fever commonly occur in about 20% of individuals, most of whom demonstrated the criterion of carditis. Since most recurrences occur within 5 years of the first episode, many infectious disease specialists will provide rheumatic fever prophylaxis for a period of 5 years or more in the form of benzathine penicillin, 1.2 million U intramuscularly once a month, or phenoxymethyl penicillin (Pen Vee K, Wyeth-Ayerst), 250 mg by mouth twice a day. For penicillin-allergic patients, erythromycin ethyl succinate, 400 mg by mouth twice a day, or sulfadiazine, 1 g by mouth daily, is used.

The incidence of rheumatic fever in the US has been reduced considerably through increased awareness of its potential and improved access to medical care dating back to the 1970s. However, the initial mortality rate remains at 1% and the 10-year death rate at 30%, primarily as the result of persistent carditis. Two thirds of the survivors will show some evidence of valvular damage (ie, rheumatic heart disease).

Rheumatic Heart Disease

Rheumatic heart disease is a complication of rheumatic fever that occurs in about 50% of all individuals who contract rheumatic fever and in 67% of all those still living after 10 years. Therefore, the oral and maxillofacial specialist should take seriously even a vague history of a possible rheumatic fever.

The valvular damage may consist of rigidity of the valves, fusion of the valve commissures, deformity of the cusp tips, or fusion and shortening of the chordae tendineae. Such damage is the result of fibrosis, or scar tissue, and will produce a valvular stenosis, insufficiency, or combination of the two. The target valve is the mitral valve, and it alone is involved in 50% to 60% of all cases. In another 20% of cases, the mitral valve is involved together with the aortic valve. The aortic and tricuspid valves are only rarely involved alone. The tricuspid valve is involved together with the mitral valve in 10% of cases.

Pertinent to the clinician is the fact that only 60% of patients with rheumatic heart disease recall or relate a history of rheumatic fever. The only sign that may raise suspicion of valvular damage is the identification of a heart murmur; therefore, all heart murmurs other than obvious systolic ejection murmurs should be taken seriously. For these patients, echocardiography should be considered because it will detect valve cusp thickening, stenosis, the presence and degree of regurgitation, and even early heart chamber enlargement.

Subacute Bacterial Endocarditis

CLINICAL PRESENTATION AND PATHOGENESIS ▶

Subacute bacterial endocarditis is a bacterial growth and invasive infection of one or more heart valves. It is a well-known complication caused by the seeding of oral microorganisms associated with existing gingivitis and periodontitis and further promoted by oral manipulations that can create a bacteremia. Other bacteremic sources that may produce SBE include tonsillitis, osteomyelitis, upper respiratory tract manipulations, and urogenital tract manipulations.

SBE can develop in undamaged heart valves as well as damaged or dysfunctional heart valves. While damaged heart valves from rheumatic fever are the most common predisposing factor, individuals with congenital heart deformities such as ventricular septal defects, patent ductus arteriosus, tetrology of Fallot or one of its components, and coarctation of the aorta are also at risk. Other valvular conditions known to be at risk for SBE are stenotic or calcified aortic valves in the elderly, mitral valve prolapse, hypertrophic subaortic stenosis, and bicuspid aortic valves. Undamaged valves that develop SBE are almost always the result of IV drug use or hospital in-patient–acquired infections from long-standing IV catheter and central lines.

Subacute bacterial endocarditis that results from oral cavity–associated bacteremias is associated with *Streptococcus viridans* 60% of the time, with *Staphylococcus aureus* 20% of the time, and with enterococci, other staphylococci, and a wide spectrum of various gram-positive, gram-negative, and rarely even *Candida* organisms the remaining 20% of the time.

Table 2-2 American Heart Association prophylaxis for bacterial endocarditis for dental and oral and maxillofacial surgery

I. Standard Regimen	
Able to take oral medication:	Amoxicillin 2 g by mouth 1 hour before procedure
Unable to take oral medication:	Ampicillin 2 g intramuscularly or intravenously within 30 minutes prior to the procedure
If penicillin allergic and able to take oral medications:	Clindamycin 600 mg by mouth, or cephalexin or cefadroxil 2 g by mouth, 1 hour before procedure. Also can use azithromycin or clarithromycin 500 mg by mouth 1 hour before procedure
II. Regimen for High-Risk Patients	
Patients not allergic to penicillin:	Ampicillin 2 g intramuscularly or intravenously plus gentamycin 1.5 mg/kg (maximum 120 mg) within 30 minutes prior to procedure and ampicillin 1 g intramuscularly or intravenously or amoxicillin 1 g by mouth 6 hours after procedure
High-risk patients and patients allergic to penicillin:	Vancomycin 1 g intravenously over 1 to 2 hours plus gentamycin 1.5 mg/kg (maximum 20 mg) infused completely within 30 minutes of procedure

Initially, the microbiology of SBE when a prosthetic heart valve is in place differs from the microbiology of SBE in a damaged native valve. If the prosthetic valve has been in place less than 3 months, staphylococcal and gram-negative organisms are the usual causative bacteria. After 3 months, the distribution of microorganisms is the same as for the damaged native valves.

In the IV drug user, the incidence of SBE associated with *S aureus* rises to 60% of cases.

HISTOPATHOLOGY ▶ At the site of valvular damage, *S viridans* organisms become enmeshed in a thrombus of fibrin, platelets, and erythrocytes. Within these vegetations, bacterial colonies are able to proliferate, as they are protected by the thrombus. The valves are avascular, so there is little acute inflammatory reaction to eliminate the bacteria. The vegetations are friable and form emboli, which can then cause infarction in the kidney, spleen, gastrointestinal tract, and brain.

PREVENTION ▶ The prevention of SBE is an established protocol of the American Heart Association (Table 2-2). The American Heart Association protocol evolves and changes in response to new clinical and bacteriologic information. Because of the life-threatening potential of SBE, the protocol cannot be studied via randomized double-blind clinical trials, and therefore it is not perfect. However, its rationale is sound in that it recognizes that ampicillin and amoxicillin have a better efficacy against *S viridans* and a wider spectrum, including *Haemophilus* species and *Actinobacillus actinomycetemcomitans*, and therefore are the drugs of choice. In the penicillin-allergic patient, each of the available choices has a shortcoming: clindamycin provides no coverage for *E corrodens*, while cephalexin and cefadroxil do not provide coverage for most anaerobes such as the *Bacteroides* species, and azithromycin/clarithromycin are not as effective against the streptococcal organisms. Therefore, the penicillin-allergic patient with a need for SBE prophylaxis must settle for a second-line antibiotic and is at greater risk for SBE.

In high-risk patients, a combination of ampicillin and gentamicin is an excellent empiric choice because of its wide-spectrum coverage that includes the so-called HACEK organisms (*Haemophilus aphrophilus*, *H parainfluenza*, *A actinomycetemcomitans*, *Cardiobacterium hominis*, *E corrodens*, and *Kingella kingae*). These organisms account for 5% to 10% of SBE. In the high-risk penicillin-allergic patient, vancomycin plus gentamicin provides coverage for *Staphylococcus aureus* risk (for which vancomycin is the drug of choice) and for the gram-negative aerobe risk of *Pseudomonas* and *Proteus* species as well as for enterococci (for which gentamicin is preferred).

The specialist in infectious diseases is responsible for the treatment of SBE. Blood cultures are mandatory. As an initial empirical treatment, most patients are started on ampicillin, 1.5 mg/kg every 4 hours, plus gentamicin, 1 mg/kg every 8 hours. In the penicillin-allergic patient, vancomycin, 15 mg/kg every 12 hours, is used to replace ampicillin.

As cultures are returned, single isolates of *S viridans* or other streptococcal species are treated with intravenous aqueous penicillin G, 2 to 3 million U every 4 hours for 4 weeks. In the penicillin-allergic patient, vancomycin, 15 mg/kg every 12 hours for 4 weeks, is used. If enterococci are isolated, ampicillin, 2 g intravenously every 4 hours, is used, and in the penicillin-allergic patient, vancomycin, 15 mg/kg every 12 hours, is used along with gentamicin, 1 mg/kg every 8 hours. Therapy is extended for 4 weeks.

If staphylococci that are not methicillin-resistant *S aureus* (MRSA) are isolated, oxacillin, 1.5 g every 4 hours for 4 to 6 weeks, is recommended. In the penicillin-allergic patient, this group is treated with cefazolin, 2 g every 8 hours, or vancomycin, 15 mg/kg every 12 hours. In the MRSA group, only vancomycin is effective and is used in a dose of 15 mg/kg every 12 hours.

If one or more of the HACEK organisms is cultured, the drug of choice is ceftriaxone (Rocephin, Roche), 2 g every day for 4 weeks or, alternatively, a combination of ampicillin, 2 g every 4 hours, together with gentamicin, 1 mg/kg every 8 hours for 4 to 6 weeks.

Subacute bacterial endocarditis remains a life-threatening disease. Mortality statistics in the 1950s and 1960s were over 80%, but today intensive antibiotic regimens and valve replacement surgery have reduced mortality to 20% to 30% of patients, most of whom succumb to congestive heart failure from valvular insufficiency.

Botryomycosis

Botryomycosis is not a fungal infection, as its name might imply, but an exceedingly rare and unusual bacterial infection that produces fungal-like structures histopathologically. Botryomycosis usually involves internal organs such as viscera, kidney, and lungs with a suppurative and granulomatous reaction. No specific causative organism has been identified, but botryomycosis has been associated with *S aureus* and to a lesser degree with *Pseudomonas aeruginosa*, *Escherichia coli*, as well as *Proteus* and *Bacteroides* species. The clinical picture is most often an individual who is aged, chronically ill, or debilitated. However, a case has been reported involving oral and facial soft tissues, including the mandible, in an individual who was 25 years old and otherwise healthy.

The few reported cases in the oral and maxillofacial area produced indurated soft tissue swellings with infiltrative growth and even paresthesia. The tissues become firm, simulating the nodular induration of actinomycosis.

The infiltrative nature of this infection will clinically suggest tumors such as *fibrosarcoma, osteosarcoma* if it involves bone, *desmoplastic fibroma*, and *aggressive fibromatosis*. It may also suggest other chronic granulomatous diseases such as *actinomycosis, TB adenitis* (scrofula), and even *sarcoidosis*.

Tissue specimens for histopathologic studies and for cultures are the only means of diagnosis.

Botryomycosis bears a close histologic resemblance to actinomycosis with areas of suppuration surrounded by granulation tissue. The suppurative foci contain granules of variable size that are basophilic (Figs 2-74a and 2-74b). A Gram stain shows the presence of gram-positive cocci and usually gram-negative rods. In culture, the organisms are usually *S aureus* and *P aeruginosa*. The granules may also show peripheral clubbing.

Surgical excision of affected tissue followed by long-term culture-specific antibiotics is the treatment of choice. Too few cases have been reported to gauge optimal length of treatment and prognosis, but botryomycosis seems to be a deep-seated chronic infection that warrants antibiotic therapy for at least 3

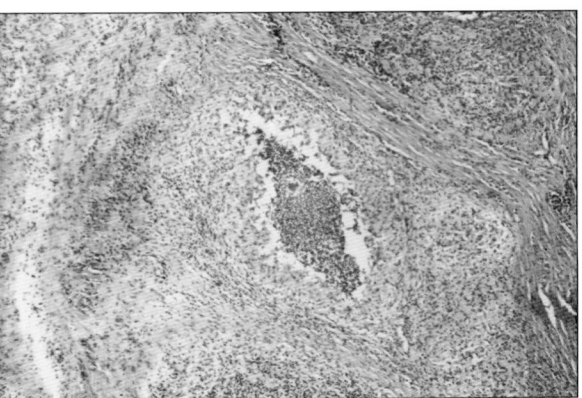

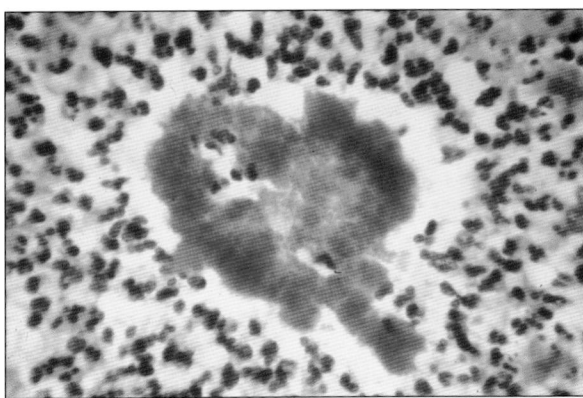

Fig 2-74a A central focus of neutrophils surrounding a colony of organisms is in turn surrounded by chronic inflammatory cells and dense fibrous tissue. This botryomycosis bears a striking resemblance to actinomycosis.

Fig 2-74b High-power view of Fig 2-74a showing the colony of organisms with adjacent neutrophils.

months. If the *S aureus* is not an MRSA strain, it may be treated with oral dicloxacillin or cephalexin, both at 1 g four times daily. In addition, oral rifampin, 300 mg twice daily, or oral ciprofloxacin (Cipro, Bayer), 750 mg twice daily, may also be used. If the organism is a true MRSA, then vancomycin (Vancocin, Eli Lilly), 500 mg intravenously twice daily, with home health-care assistance and a central venous catheter, is the best choice. Oral doxycycline (Vibramycin, Pfizer), 100 mg twice daily, may be used in MRSA infections but less effectively. The *P aeruginosa* may be treated with oral ciprofloxacin, 750 mg three times daily, or with gentamicin, 80 to 120 mg intravenously three times daily.

Fungal Diseases

Candidiasis

CLINICAL PRESENTATION AND PATHOGENESIS ▶

Oral candidiasis is usually caused by the normally present *Candida albicans* organism becoming pathogenic because of some alteration in the host's defense system. Table 2-3 indicates some of the host defense alterations (predisposing factors) associated with the development of candidiasis. The clinical presentations of candidiasis vary widely, since a different clinical expression may result with each predisposing factor and the stage of disease development at the time of patient examination. Table 2-4 lists the current clinical types of oral candidiasis.

C albicans is the most common cause of candidiasis. However, *Candida krusei, Candida tropicalis, Candida glabrata, Candida parapsilosis, Candida pseudotropicalis,* and *Candida guilliermondii* may in rare cases be causative pathogens; their identification is important because of their reduced sensitivity to fluconazole (Diflucan).

Candida organisms are unicellular yeasts of the Cryptococcaceae family. They are all weak pathogens that exist in any one of three forms: the oval yeast form (blastospores 1.5 to 5 μm in diameter), the elongated form (pseudohyphae 3 to 5 μm in diameter), and the thick rectangular form (chlamydospores 7 to 17 μm in diameter). Each of these forms is seen in invasive candidiasis, but the pseudohyphae are most recognizable. All exist in balance with the bacterium of the oral cavity and the series of human defenses, from saliva to the mucous membrane barrier to cell-mediated immunity to basic cellular integrity; they become pathogenic only when opportunity allows.

Table 2-3 Predisposing factors for *Candida* infection

A. Systemic	B. Local
Immunologic immaturity of infants	Ill-fitting dentures
Immunologic exhaustion of elderly	Reduced occlusal vertical dimension
Systemic corticosteroid therapy	Lip-licking habit
Systemic antibiotic therapy	Overuse of antiseptic or antibiotic mouth-washes
Systemic immunosuppression therapy	
Cancer-related chemotherapy	
Radiation-induced xerostomia	
Disease-induced xerostomia (eg, Sjögren syndrome)	
Drug-induced xerostomia	
Endocrinopathies:	
Diabetes mellitus	
Hypoparathyroidism	
Hypoadrenalism	
Chronic debilitating illnesses	
Malnutrition-malabsorption	
HIV infection and AIDS	

Table 2-4 Oral candidiasis classification

A. Systemic	B. Local
Mucocutaneous (oral, facial, skin, scalp, phalangeal skin, nails)	Pseudomembranous
Familial	Atrophic
Syndrome associated	Hypertrophic
Disseminated	

Pseudomembranous Candidiasis

The most common form of oral candidiasis is the pseudomembranous form often referred to as *thrush*. The most common predisposing factor is the concurrent or recent administration of systemic antibiotics or even a short course of antibiotics used for prophylaxis to cover a surgery. The affected mucosa becomes tender with red and white areas (Fig 2-75). The white areas are gelatinous plaques of cellular debris mixed with *Candida* organisms. The red areas are caused by organism invasion into the upper layers of the mucosa, resulting in loss of parakeratinization, atrophy, hyperemia, and inflammation. The white plaques characteristically can be scraped off, leaving small hemorrhagic areas behind. This pseudomembranous form also is the type seen in the very young and very old: infants often have immature host defenses, and the elderly often have immune exhaustion or chronic disease impairment of their host defenses (Fig 2-76). Similarly, patients with oral cancer and other more distant types of cancer develop candidiasis, presumably as a result of exhaustion of the cell-mediated arm of their immune system.

It is estimated that 5% of cancer patients, 10% of the institutionalized elderly, and 5% of newborns develop candidiasis. Patients with radiation xerostomia, a recent history of chemotherapy, a Sjögren syndrome–type of xerostomia, and leukemia develop candidiasis with an incidence approaching 70%. In addition, HIV-infected patients and those who have progressed to AIDS frequently develop candidiasis, indicative of their T-cell impairment.

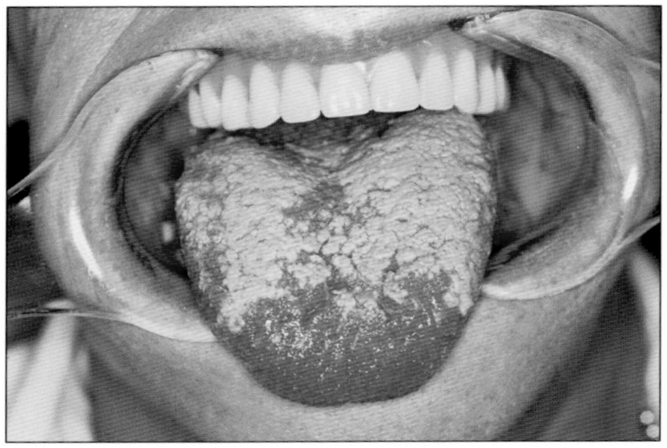

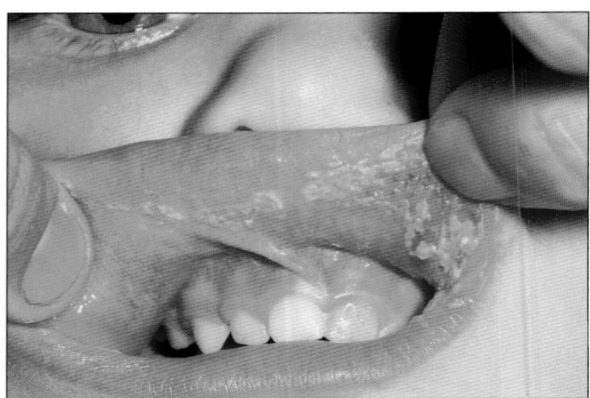

Fig 2-75 A presentation of candidiasis referred to as *thrush*. The white *Candida* colonies may be removed with a tongue blade; the remainder of the dorsal tongue surface is inflamed.

Fig 2-76 Candidiasis may develop unrelated to any syndrome in children with no immune compromise.

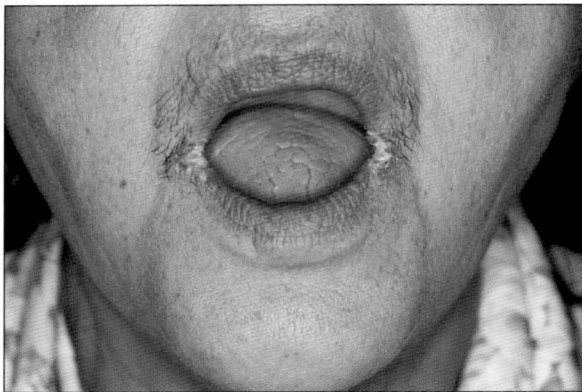

Fig 2-77 A presentation of candidiasis referred to as *perlèche*. White *Candida* ulcerations form in response to constant wetting of the commissure due to loss of occlusal vertical dimension secondary to tooth loss.

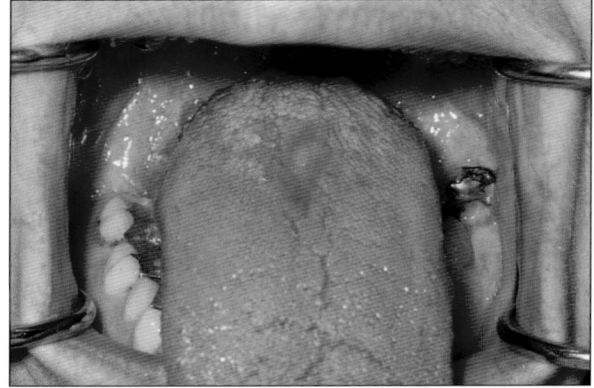

Fig 2-78a A presentation of candidiasis referred to as *median rhomboid glossitis*. A superficial *Candida* infection produces a focal inflammation and atrophy of the filiform papillae.

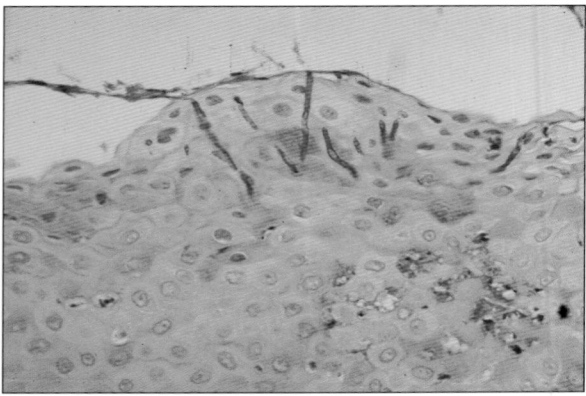

Fig 2-78b Median rhomboid glossitis biopsies stained with PAS stain will show elongated burrowing, PAS-positive, nonseptate, nonbranching organisms representative of *Candida* species.

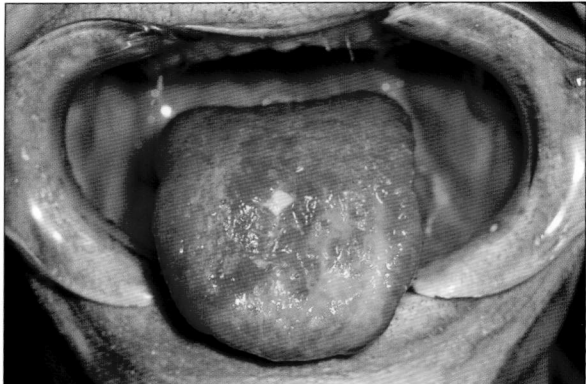

Fig 2-79 A presentation of candidiasis referred to as *atrophic glossitis*. In this case a large surface area of the tongue is affected, producing a diffuse loss of filiform papillae.

Atrophic Candidiasis

The most common clinical presentation of atrophic candidiasis is the red, velvet-like, tender palatal mucosa under a denture. Here the high-frequency, low-intensity trauma of a denture surface compressing the palatal mucosa during swallowing alters the barrier defense, allowing the normally innocuous *Candida* organisms to become pathogenic.

Another type of atrophic candidiasis is angular cheilitis (perlèche), which often begins when a loss of occlusal vertical dimension creates a constant moisture and cracking at the commissure and predisposes the tissue to *Candida* proliferation and invasion (Fig 2-77). In this form, the commissures are tender, fissured, and often crusted, and there may also be some skin erythema. A variant of this is found in individuals with a chronic lip-licking habit. It is also frequently seen as an extension of intraoral candidiasis. These individuals will develop a skin erythema due to their habitual wetting and maceration of skin and the subsequent invasion by *Candida* species. A form of atrophic candidiasis involving the dorsum of the tongue in a diamond-shaped pattern is often referred to as *median rhomboid glossitis* (Fig 2-78a). This entity was previously believed to be developmental, specifically a persistence of the tuberculum impar portion of the second branchial pouch. However, this lesion is always anterior to the foramen cecum, plac-

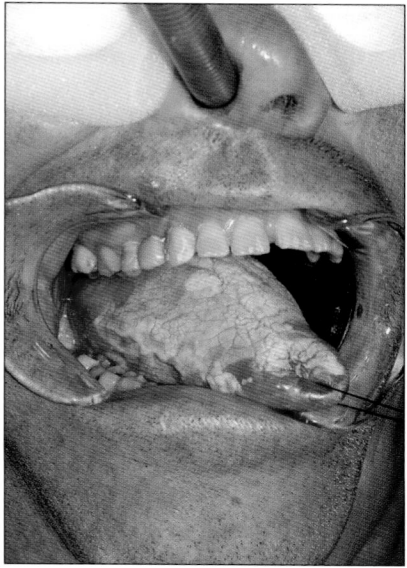

Fig 2-80 A presentation of candidiasis referred to as *hypertrophic candidiasis*. In this case a biopsy is planned to identify candidiasis and to rule out dysplasia or lichen planus.

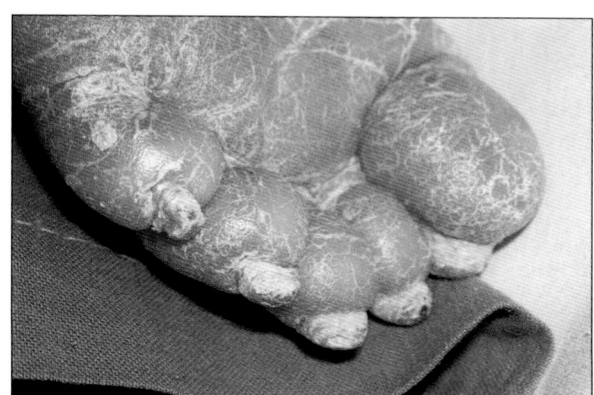

Fig 2-81 Systemic candidiasis in a young child, showing extensive skin and nail involvement.

ing it in a position that cannot be a second arch derivative. Additionally, it is not noted in young individuals, making it unlikely to be a persistence of any embryonic structure. Moreover, tissue biopsies will indicate vertically invading *Candida* organisms (Fig 2-78b). A more common diffuse form, known as *atrophic glossitis*, also involves the tongue and is frequently associated with burning pain (Fig 2-79).

Hyperplastic Candidiasis

Some cases of candidiasis will become hyperplastic and, therefore, elevated. Clinically, it will be less likely to be scraped off as it becomes associated with an acanthotic/hyperkeratotic response. Moreover, it will be less tender and will mimic a lichen planus, a verrucous carcinoma, or even a squamous cell carcinoma (Fig 2-80).

Mucocutaneous Candidiasis

Mucocutaneous candidiasis is the most serious form of candidiasis. It suggests a systemic distribution and a more extensive degree of host defense compromise. It will present with a pseudomembranous oral presentation but will also show skin, esophageal, and nail involvement (Fig 2-81). The nail involvement will be particularly prominent: The nail bed will be destroyed and the nails disfigured. Several etiologies of this form of candidiasis are recognized. One is a predisposition for the infection, which is the result of an autosomal-recessive inheritance; 50% of these are associated with an endocrinopathy consisting of either hypoparathyroidism, hypothyroidism, Addison type of adrenal cortical insufficiency, or diabetes mellitus. The remaining inherited forms include those related to cellular immune deficiencies and rarely to deficiencies of iron metabolism. The candidiasis seen in AIDS patients and those with HIV infection not yet progressed to AIDS is essentially a mucocutaneous form, which is often first seen on the oral mucosa but may become disseminated to involve skin and even internal organs.

Disseminated Candidiasis

Disseminated candidiasis is not commonly seen by the oral and maxillofacial surgeon. It may result from a mucocutaneous candidiasis that has invaded through skin or mucosa to seed the blood stream, a condition more probable in the immunocompromised patient. However, it is usually seen as a complication of a long-term in-dwelling catheter, such as a central intravenous line, a subcutaneous port, or even a urinary catheter.

DIFFERENTIAL DIAGNOSIS ▶

The pseudomembranous form of candidiasis will resemble the mucous patches of *secondary syphilis, mucosal chemical* or *heat burns*, and the spectrum of lesions of clinical leukoplakia such as *verrucous hyperplasia, verrucous carcinoma*, and *squamous cell carcinoma*. The median rhomboid glossitis presentation is also suggestive of *lichen planus*. The atrophic form, in which a pebbly, velvet-like, soft tissue enlargement of the palate develops, will at times suggest a *non-Hodgkin lymphoma*. It is also often termed *inflammatory hyperplasia of the palate*. The disseminated form will appear as a *bacterial septicemia* often with thrombophlebitis.

DIAGNOSTIC WORK-UP ▶

The most straightforward and least equivocal diagnostic approach is a tissue biopsy stained with a PAS stain. Lesion scrapings for a smear with 20% potassium hydroxide added to digest debris and sloughed epithelial cells (the so-called KOH prep) remains unreliable. The KOH preparation is often difficult to read because of residual mucosal cells and the vague outlines of organisms in an unstained preparation. The interpretation of nonseptate hyphae consistent with *Candida* organisms is also unreliable because their numbers are the only differentiation one can use between normal presence and overcolonization. Invasion cannot be assessed. A PAS-stained tissue specimen will better outline the organisms and show evidence of tissue invasion.

Candida organisms can and should be cultured as part of the diagnostic work-up, although the diagnosis is primarily achieved by microscopy. The organisms can be readily cultured on Sabouraud's media or routine blood agar plates. The culture has less diagnostic value than it has for treatment selection, since *C albicans* is very sensitive to fluconazole (Diflucan), whereas other species of *Candida* are usually not as sensitive.

HISTOPATHOLOGY ▶

In acute pseudomembranous candidiasis, the plaque represents a thickened parakeratinized layer, separated by edema and infiltrated by neutrophils. The neutrophils collect as microabscesses at the base of the plaque, enabling its ready separation. It also contains numerous hyphae, many of which lie perpendicular to the surface (Fig 2-82). The organisms are readily identified with PAS or silver stain. They are capable of invading the epithelial cytoplasm and existing as intracellular parasites. Beneath the plaque, the epithelium is acanthotic and usually free of inflammation. The underlying connective tissue, however, is infiltrated by lymphocytes, plasma cells, and macrophages.

In acute atrophic candidiasis, the hyphae tend to be sparser, but the inflammatory infiltrate in the lamina propria is denser.

In chronic as in acute forms of candidiasis, there is a thickened parakeratinized layer containing inflammatory cells and hyphae, although fewer in number. Because there is less inflammation and edema, the plaque does not separate. The acanthosis is more marked, and the connective tissue is densely inflamed (Fig 2-83). It has been demonstrated experimentally that *Candida* organisms are capable of inducing the epithelial hyperplasia that results in a clinical leukoplakic lesion. Some cellular atypia may also occur. Thus the question of whether chronic candidiasis may be a premalignant lesion has been raised. However, there is no proof that this is the case.

TREATMENT ▶

In all forms of candidiasis, an important prerequisite to treatment is reversal or withdrawal of the concomitant underlying factor when possible. Specific therapy for mild oral disease is nystatin oral suspension (Mycostatin, Westwood Squibb), 100,000 U/mL to be taken 5 mL (one teaspoon) at a time as an oral swish and spit or swish and swallow four times daily. For chronic, well-established candidiasis limited to the oral cavity and upper digestive tract, nystatin as noted above combined with clotrimazole

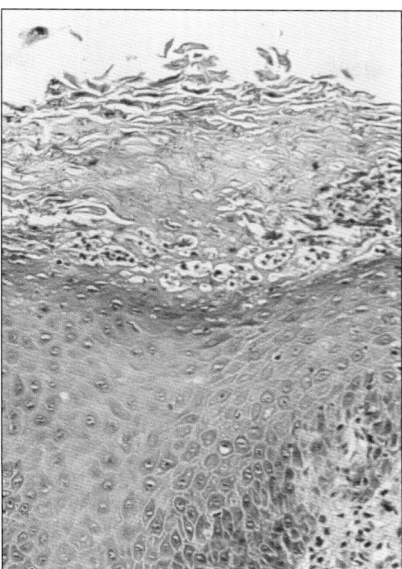

Fig 2-82 Thickened parakeratinized plaque-containing neutrophils and candidial hyphae in pseudomembranous candidiasis (PAS stain).

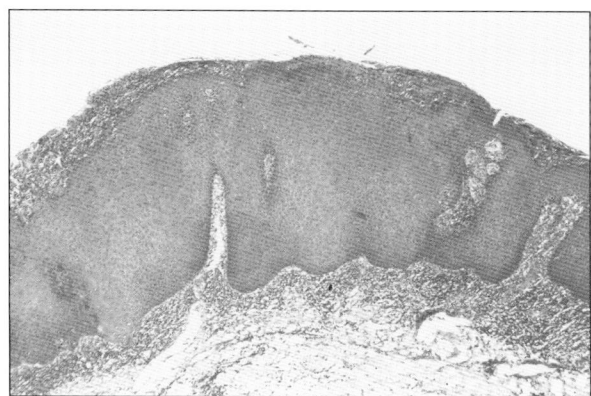

Fig 2-83 Acanthosis is apparent in chronic candidiasis. Neutrophils can be seen in the superficial layers of the epithelium, and a chronic inflammatory infiltrate is visible in the underlying fibrous tissue.

troches (Mycelex, Alza), 10 mg five times daily, or the vaginal suppositories used as an oral troche three times daily, is very effective. It should be noted that the clotrimazole troches contain sugars that in xerostomic patients, in particular, may stimulate active caries. For this reason, some clinicians prefer the nystatin vaginal suppositories combined with nystatin oral suspension.

In chronic, well-established candidiasis that is refractory to two topical agents or where there is a noted immunocompromise but no systemic dissemination, nystatin with the addition of fluconazole (Diflucan, Pfizer US), 100 mg daily, or ketoconazole (Nizoral, Janssen), 200 mg twice daily, or itraconazole, 100 mg daily, as an alternative will often resolve the infection.

In true disseminated candidiasis or severe mucocutaneous candidiasis, amphotericin B given intravenously with D5W at a rate of 50 mg per day to a total dose of 1 g is recommended. This sometimes must be combined with oral ketoconazole or fluconazole. If toxicity develops to amphotericin B, the more expensive lipid preparations can be used. This will reduce nephrotoxicity in particular as well as allow daily doses to be increased to 140 to 400 mg per day.

PROGNOSIS ▶

Candidiasis is resolvable if the underlying factor can be controlled. Where it cannot, long-term maintenance therapy is often required.

Benign Migratory Glossitis

CLINICAL PRESENTATION AND PATHOGENESIS ▶

Benign migratory glossitis is usually noted as an incidental examination finding or by patient recognition. While all surfaces of the tongue may be involved, the dorsum is the most common. The tongue will show alternating areas of normal texture and a whitish color due to filiform papillae and surface keratinization, contrasted with smooth red areas where the filiform papillae have flattened and a dekeratinization of the surface has occurred (Fig 2-84a). The confluent borders of these two areas are usually elevated, rolled, and more intensely white. The pattern and areas of involvement will change over a period of days. At times the tongue will revert to a normal texture and appearance, and at times it will exhibit almost a bald denudation. Usually the appearance will be somewhere in between.

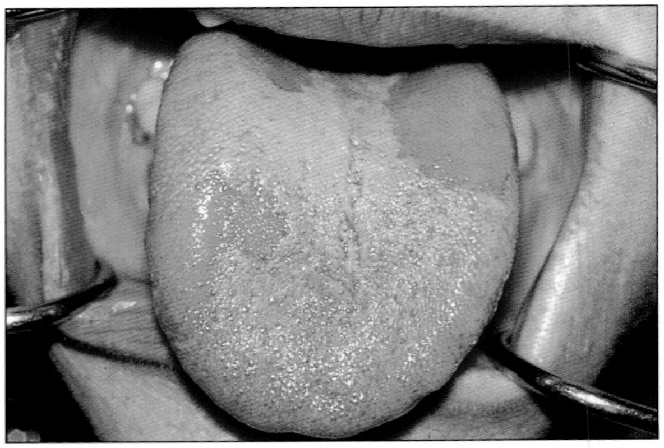

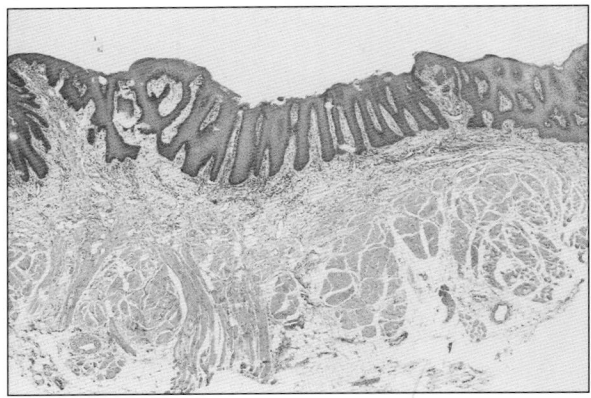

Fig 2-84a Benign migratory glossitis with smooth areas of flattened filiform papillae and white areas of either *Candida* or keratin buildup.

Fig 2-84b Narrow elongated rete ridges, thinning of the epithelium over the tips of the connective tissue papillae, and an inflammatory infiltrate are characteristic of the "psoriasiform" pattern in this example of benign migratory glossitis.

The lesions are innocuous and asymptomatic except on occasions when spicy foods or acidic citrus products are consumed. A small percentage of benign migratory glossitis cases will be accompanied by constant burning pain, known as the *glossopyrosis presentation*. These cases are usually related to invasive candidiasis and occasionally to erosive lichen planus. In fact, *Candida* colonization rather than true invasive infection may be the stimulus for benign migratory glossitis.

Although the disease is often referred to as "geographic tongue," it does occasionally appear in the floor of the mouth or buccal mucosa as a *benign migratory stomatitis*.

Benign migratory glossitis is an intermittent disease over many years in 2% of the US population. Adults are affected more than children and women slightly more than men. Countless theories related to etiology and associations have been advanced—for example, psoriasis, psychologic stress, nutritional deficiencies, reactive arthritis, insulin-dependent diabetes mellitus—none of which has been proved. In fact, if the disease occurs in as much as 2% of the population, coincidental associations with many diseases would be expected. There does seem to be a higher incidence in individuals with the trait of a fissured tongue, and some evidence has been presented relating the genetic tissue type HLA-B15 in atopic patients (those with allergic diseases) with benign migratory glossitis.

DIFFERENTIAL DIAGNOSIS ▶ Surface tongue lesions that are generally asymptomatic include *candidiasis, lichen planus*, and perhaps lesions related to both *systemic lupus erythematosus* and *discoid lupus erythematosus*. In addition, the clinician must be aware of the possibility of *premalignant dysplasia*.

DIAGNOSTIC WORK-UP ▶ Benign migratory glossitis is a diagnosis of clinical recognition. If clinical doubt exists or a burning tongue sensation accompanies the lesion, a biopsy is indicated to rule out the other entities on the differential list. A PAS stain is recommended to rule out *Candida* organisms.

HISTOPATHOLOGY ▶ Histologically, lesions of benign migratory glossitis resemble psoriasis, although no clinical correlation with this disease has been found. In the erythematous areas affecting the tongue, there is a loss of filiform papillae. The epithelium shows acanthosis with a downward extension of the rete ridges. Vascular and inflamed connective tissue papillae are seen beneath the overlying nonkeratinized epithelium (Fig 2-84b). The infiltrate consists of neutrophils, lymphocytes, and plasma cells. Neutrophils infiltrate the epithelium and may concentrate near the surface as microabscesses. The clinically white margins show hyperkeratosis and acanthosis. These changes are not unlike those of candidiasis, but hyphae are not present.

TREATMENT ▶ No specific treatment is indicated in asymptomatic cases. Emphasis on the innocuous nature of the condition and the fact that it is not malignant or premalignant is recommended. Symptomatic cases respond well to nystatin oral suspension, 100,000 U/mL given as 5 mL (1 teaspoon) oral swish and expec-

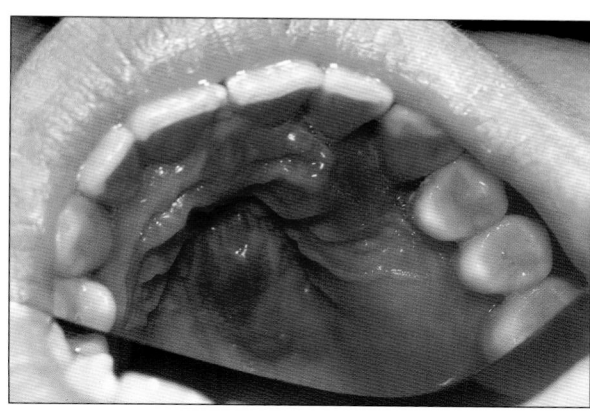

Fig 2-85a An oral lesion of histoplasmosis that presented as a fleshy red mass in the palatal mucosa and ulcerations around several teeth.

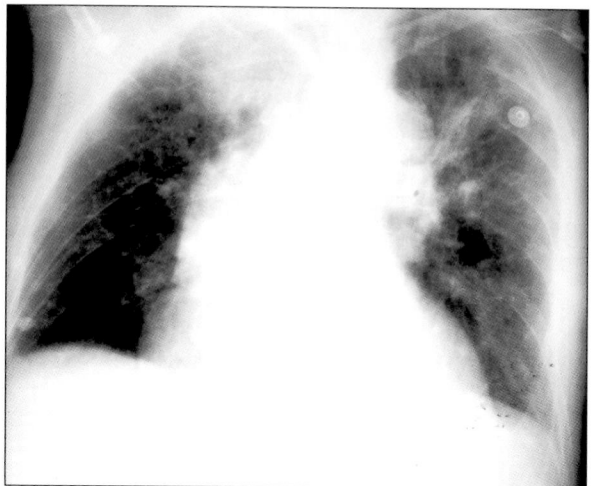

Fig 2-85b Oral histoplasmosis arises from hematogenous spread from the lungs. This chest radiograph shows histoplasmosis masses in the right apex, hilar adenopathy, and focal areas in the left lung.

torate four times daily, alone or combined with clotrimazole troches (Mycelex, Alza), 10 mg as a lozenge three times daily. Response to such therapy suggests the presence of *Candida* organisms.

Histoplasmosis

CLINICAL PRESENTATION AND PATHOGENESIS ▶

The most common oral and maxillofacial presentation of histoplasmosis is the appearance of single or multiple oral ulcers in an older person with chronic obstructive pulmonary disease. The oral ulcers are mildly painful or painless and will appear as fleshy, mildly elevated tissue masses (Fig 2-85a). This presentation is often referred to as *chronic progressive histoplasmosis* and exists as the result of a chronic lung infection that seeds the oral mucosa from coughed-up sputum or from hematogenous spread from lungs to oral mucosa. Such patients will often present with signs of chronic illness. They may be fatigued, weak, febrile, and dyspneic and complain of cough. They often will have a normochromic-normocytic anemia (anemia of chronic disease) and will be leukopenic. A chest radiograph may show only emphysematous changes or may show diffuse infiltrates (Fig 2-85b).

Histoplasmosis is endemic to the central and eastern United States (the Ohio and Mississippi valleys in particular), as well as eastern Canada, Mexico, Central America, and South America. It is a soil mold (true fungus) that causes a primary pulmonary infection from the inhalation of spores, which bud in the lung tissue. The budding *Histoplasma capsulatum* organisms are engulfed by macrophages in which they can remain viable because of their capsule, which resists enzymatic digestion. The organisms can then be transported hematogenously to other organs and are also frequently seeded into the larynx, pharynx, or oral cavity by coughed-up sputum.

DIFFERENTIAL DIAGNOSIS ▶

An oral ulcer in a person with a chronic lung illness should also suggest other so-called deep fungal infections, such as *coccidioidomycosis* and *blastomycosis*. In addition, such oral ulcers may suggest *squamous cell carcinoma*, a *syphilitic chancre*, or an *oral TB ulcer*.

DIAGNOSTIC WORK-UP ▶

The most diagnostic examination to confirm a suspected histoplasmosis is a biopsy of the oral ulcer area. The small PAS-positive organisms can be readily seen within the macrophages associated with the ulcer. Skin antigen tests are available but unreliable because acute histoplasmosis is a common unrecognized infection often resembling an upper respiratory tract infection, and many individuals test positive as a result of a long-ago exposure from which they carry convalescent antibodies (causing the positive

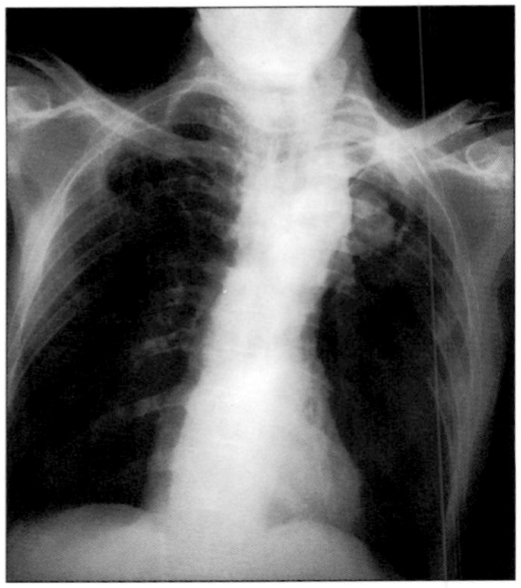

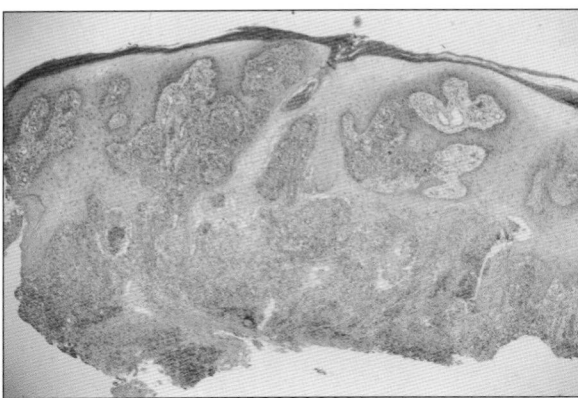

Fig 2-86 Calcified nodule in the apex of the left lung from a healed histoplasmosis lesion.

Fig 2-87a Noncaseating granulomas due to histoplasmosis in an oral biopsy.

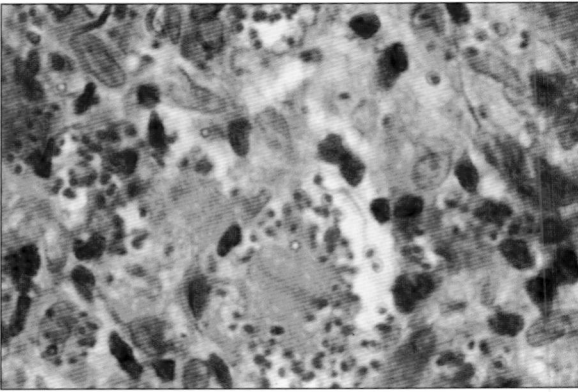

Fig 2-87b PAS stain showing the *H capsulatum* organisms within the cytoplasm of macrophages. Oral histoplasmosis is best diagnosed via a biopsy.

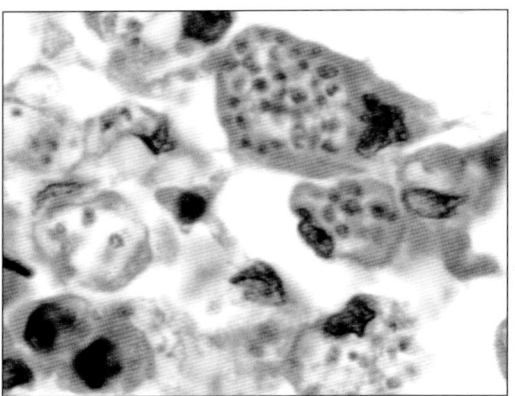

Fig 2-87c Oil immersion light microscopy will show *H capsulatum* within the cytoplasm of macrophages pushing the nucleus to one side. Note the clear halo around the *Histoplasma* organisms. This is characteristic but represents an artifact rather than its actual capsule. (Reprinted from Ramzy I, *Clinical Cytopathology and Aspiration Biopsy* 2nd ed, with permission from McGraw-Hill Co.)

reaction) but no active disease. In fact, small calcified foci seen as an incidental finding in routine chest radiographs are usually due to old, healed histoplasmosis lesions (Fig 2-86). Cultures are positive in only 50% of known histoplasmosis cases; cultures in Sabouraud's medium are recommended but not absolutely reliable.

HISTOPATHOLOGY ▶

The histologic and clinical spectrum of histoplasmosis reflects the immune competence of the host versus the yeast phase of *H capsulatum*. In the forms of the disease where there is strong cellular immunity, caseating or noncaseating epithelioid granulomas will be found (Fig 2-87a). However, in the disseminated form of the disease where the cell-mediated response is defective, the histologic picture is characterized by diffuse infiltration of mononuclear phagocytes. The cytoplasm of these cells is engorged with the yeast cells (Fig 2-87b). Other inflammatory cells also are usually present. In the most serious deficiencies, the organisms may lie extracellularly in a spectrum resembling that of leprosy.

The yeast is round to oval and measures 1 μm in diameter. It is surrounded by a clear space that does not represent the capsule and is most likely an artifact. The organisms stain with H&E, although Giemsa and Gram stains are more reliable, showing the clear halo to better effect. They are also PAS- and methenamine-silver–positive (Fig 2-87c).

TREATMENT ▶

For a nonimmunocompromised individual, the current drug of choice for histoplasmosis that does not involve the meninges is oral itraconazole (Sporanox, Janssen), 200 to 400 mg daily for 7 months. Response to itraconazole is about 80% and affords the patient the possibility of gaining a cure. Amphotericin B cholesteryl sulfate (Amphotec, Sequus) is reserved for those who are nonresponsive to itraconazole therapy, are immunocompromised, or have histoplasmosis meningitis.

Itraconazole inhibits the synthesis of ergosterol in the cell walls of susceptible fungi. This inhibition results in a cell wall that is not maintained by the fungus and therefore leaks, leading to organism death. Amphotericin B also inhibits ergosterol incorporation in the fungal cytoplasmic membrane and cell wall, causing it to leak intracellular components and killing the organism. Amphotericin B causes local phlebitis, pain at the infusion site, and histamine release. It is, therefore, given in graduated increments with 2,500 U of heparin and 50 mg of diphenhydramine (Benadryl, Warner Lambert). It is initiated with 5 mg in 100 mL of D5W infused over 1 hour. The dosage is then increased by 10 mg, adding another 100 mL of D5W until 50 mg is given in 500 mL of D5W in 1 day. Fifty milligrams of amphotericin B daily is considered the maximum dose and is given until a total dose of 2 to 3 g is administered or until toxicity forces a dose reduction.

Systemic toxicity of amphotericin B manifests primarily as bone marrow suppression and renal damage. Drug discontinuance or dose reduction is considered if the hematocrit falls below 25% or the BUN rises above 50 mg/dL (17.9 mmol/L). Toxicity is reversible if the drug is reduced or discontinued promptly. Lipid-based amphotericin B (Abelcet, Lipsome) may be used to reduce nephrotoxicity and permit higher dosages. Dosages between 2 and 6 mg/kg per day (140 to 400 mg per day for the average person) are possible with this more costly but less toxic lipid-based form of the drug.

PROGNOSIS ▶

If treatment is started promptly, death is rare. Most patients recover over several months, but relapses are not uncommon and are particularly high in HIV-related histoplasmosis. Therefore, for immunocompromised patients, lifelong maintenance with itraconazole, 200 to 400 mg daily, is usually administered as a suppressive therapy.

Coccidioidomycosis

CLINICAL PRESENTATION AND PATHOGENESIS ▶

Coccidioidomycosis in the oral and maxillofacial area occurs either on skin or on oral mucous membranes as a soft, fleshy mass or ulcerative lesion representing a disseminated focus from pulmonary disease (Fig 2-88a). The disease has a predilection for Filipinos and is 10 times more common in blacks than whites.

Of immunocompetent individuals who develop a pulmonary coccidioidomycosis, 99% recover after about 3 weeks. Most are not confirmed to be infected by *Coccidioides immitis* but rather are diagnosed with a nonspecific pneumonitis. In about 0.1% of white and 1% of nonwhite patients, organisms cannot be localized or eliminated. These patients instead continue to develop progressive pulmonary disease, which may lead to oral mucosa or facial skin lesions via hematogenous spread. When oral lesions appear as the only disseminated focus, they may be the result of coughed-up sputum.

Coccidioidomycosis results from the inhalation of the fungal organism *C immitis*, which is a soil mold found in the arid regions of the southwestern US (the so-called San Joaquin Valley), in Mexico, and in Central and South America. The organism may produce a pneumonitis with rash, but this is seen in only 40% of cases. The organism is usually engulfed and eliminated by macrophages and fixed phagocytic cells. In less than 1% of infected immunocompetent individuals and for reasons as yet unclear (possibly related to the number of inhaled organisms), the organisms proliferate and spread to other organs through the blood and sputum.

DIFFERENTIAL DIAGNOSIS ▶

In those with oral lesions, the ulcerative and sometimes indurated and often fleshy quality of the lesions suggests *squamous cell carcinoma* and other fungal diseases, particularly *histoplasmosis* and to some

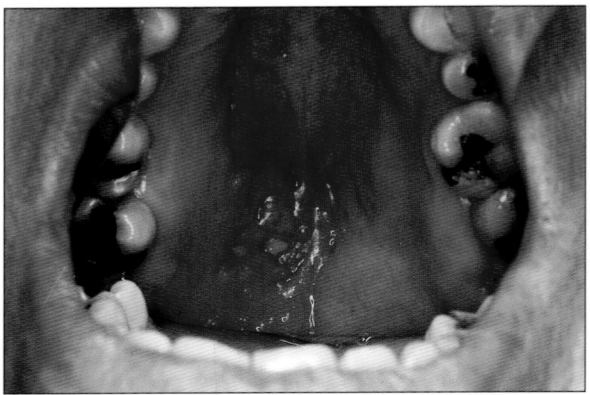

Fig 2-88a Coccidioidomycosis of the palate secondary to hematogenous spread from pulmonary coccidioidomycosis.

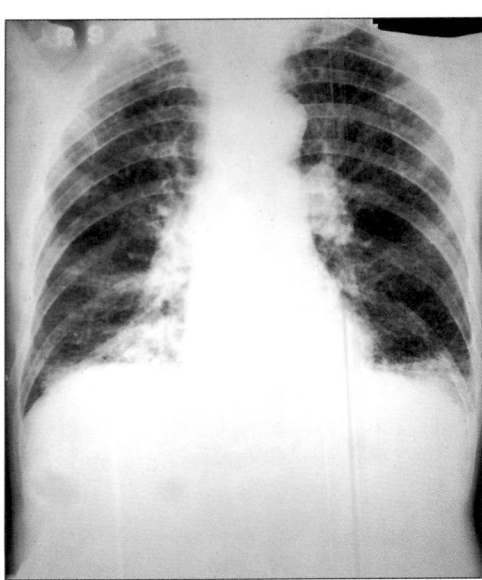

Fig 2-88b Hilar adenopathy and pleural effusions due to coccidioidomycosis.

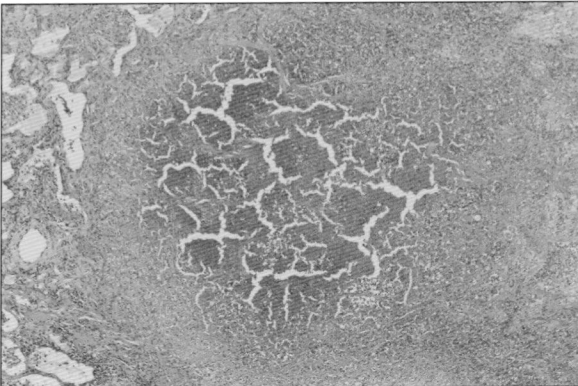

Fig 2-88c Within the lung, abscesses consisting predominantly of neutrophils are seen in coccidioidomycosis.

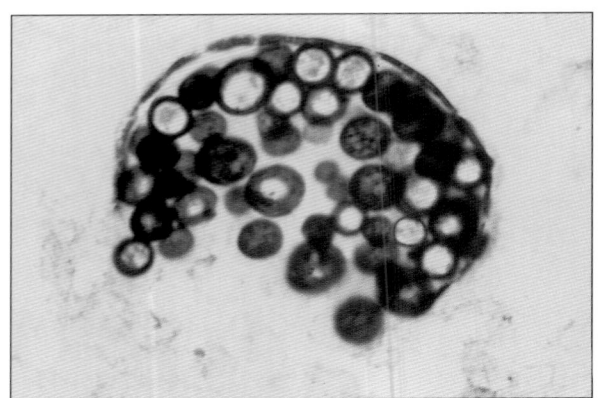

Fig 2-88d The large sporangia of coccidioidomycosis can easily be seen with a methenamine silver stain (magnification ×1,000). Here, the sporangia are dispersing many small endospores.

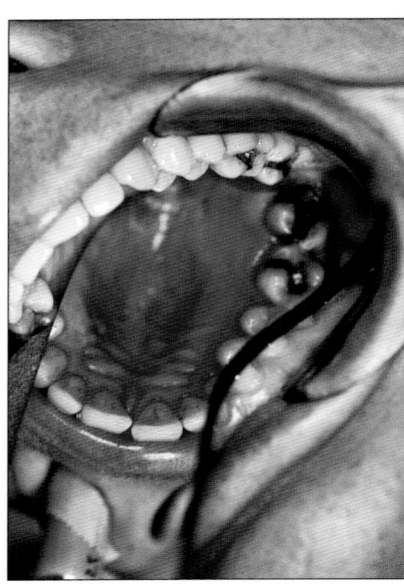

Fig 2-88e Healed palate after treatment with amphotericin B.

extent *blastomycosis*. If the lesions are painful and irregular around their borders, an *oral TB ulcer* should be considered. Palatal lesions may also resemble Wegener granulomatosis. In addition, a *chancre of primary syphilis* and even a *traumatic ulcer* with some secondary infection is possible.

DIAGNOSTIC WORK-UP ▶

Suspected cases of coccidioidomycosis call for a chest radiograph in addition to a routine complete blood count. Many cases will show a moderate leukocytosis and an eosinophilia. The chest radiograph most commonly shows nodular pulmonary infiltrates similar to those seen in histoplasmosis (see Fig 2-85b), but hilar adenopathy and pleural effusions may also be seen (Fig 2-88b). Coccidioidin skin antigen tests are not reliable.

The most important diagnostic measure is a tissue biopsy, which will show the large coccidiospore (sporangia) and the smaller endospores within them. Oral and/or facial lesions contain abundant colonies of *C immitis* and afford a readily accessible means of establishing a diagnosis.

HISTOPATHOLOGY ▶

Unlike many other infectious diseases in which the histologic picture reflects the sensitivity of the host to the organism, in coccidioidomycosis the histologic picture reflects the developmental stage of the organism. The arthrospores induce essentially a neutrophilic response, although eosinophils and some lymphocytes and plasma cells may be seen. Small abscesses may result (Fig 2-88c). Development into the spherule provokes an influx of monocytes and the formation of epithelioid granulomas. These will often show caseation and contain Langhans giant cells. With the release of the endospores, neutrophils are once again stimulated with the formation of microabscesses. These may become necrotic.

The organisms may be seen with H&E, but are more apparent with PAS or methenamine silver (Fig 2-88d). The sporangia, which are 30 to 60 μm in diameter, may be found free within necrotic tissue or within the epithelioid cells and giant cells of the granuloma. The endospores measure 1 to 5 μm.

TREATMENT ▶

Any fungal disease found in the oral cavity or on facial skin with concomitant lung infection represents a serious disseminated disease that must be treated aggressively. The current drug of choice for coccidioidomycosis remains amphotericin B (Amphotec, Sequus). This drug reacts with ergosterol molecules in the fungal cytoplasmic membrane and cell wall, causing it to leak intracellular components and killing the organism. Amphotericin B causes local phlebitis, pain at the infusion site, and histamine release. It is, therefore, given in graduated increments together with 2,500 U of heparin and 50 mg of diphenhydramine (Benadryl, Warner Lambert). It is initiated with 5 mg in 100 mL of D5W infused over 1 hour. The dosage is then increased by 10 mg, adding another 100 mL of D5W until 50 mg is given in 500 mL of D5W in 1 day. The maximum daily dose of amphotericin B, 50 mg, is given until a total dose of 2 to 3 g is administered or until toxicity forces a dose reduction.

Systemic toxicity manifests as bone marrow suppression and renal damage. Drug discontinuance or dose reduction is considered if the hematocrit falls below 25% or the BUN rises above 50 mg/dL (17.9 mmol/L). Toxicity is reversible if the drug is reduced or discontinued promptly. However, lipid preparations of amphotericin B will permit higher daily doses and total doses to be administered with reduced nephrotoxicity. Because coccidioidomycosis has a high relapse rate, these costly preparations become a strong consideration.

PROGNOSIS ▶

Cases with limited dissemination have complete recovery (Fig 2-88e). Extensive lung involvement with cavitation at the time of diagnosis is associated with recurrent, persistent pulmonary disease and often with coccidioides meningitis. In such cases, a partial or total pneumonectomy is often part of the therapy.

Blastomycosis

CLINICAL PRESENTATION AND PATHOGENESIS ▶

Blastomycosis is less common in the United States than either histoplasmosis or coccidioidomycosis. It nevertheless represents another "deep fungal" infection that has a primary pulmonary involvement that then disseminates via hematogenous routes to other organs, particularly skin and bones and to the oral cavity and pharynx via coughed-up sputum. The oral lesions are raised, fleshy verrucous lesions with mild or no pain (Figs 2-89 and 2-90). Skin lesions appear raised and are also verrucous with a rolled, sharply sloping border. The skin lesions resemble basal cell carcinomas and may become disfiguring.

Cough, sputum production, fever, chills, weight loss, and chest pain are found in most cases with well-established lung disease. In rare cases, pulmonary infection may be asymptomatic.

Blastomyces dermatitidis is a fungus associated with wet, decaying wood. The disease was first called the Chicago disease, as the first reported cases came from that area in 1894. Later, different North American and South American forms were distinguished. Today it is recognized that there is only one form of the disease with a single etiology. Sporadic outbreaks in the Midwest have clustered cases in areas where outdoor activities associated with wood were present. Although it has a slightly greater incidence in the Great Lakes region of the United States and Canada, blastomycosis has a near-worldwide distribution.

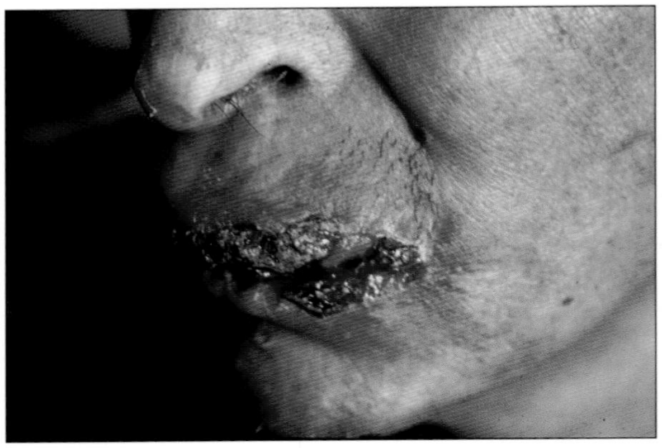

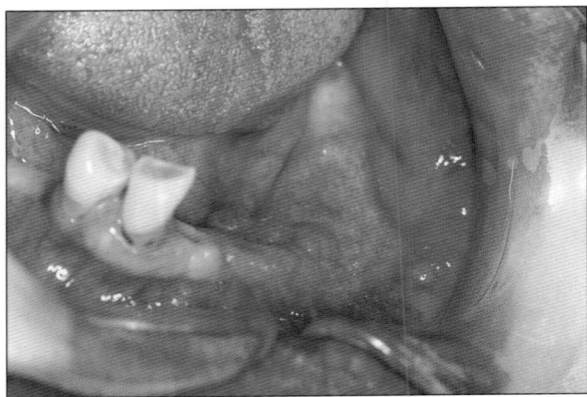

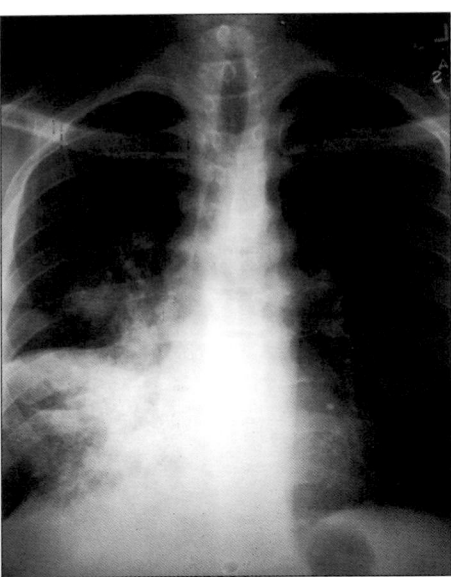

Fig 2-89 Lesions of blastomycosis are usually raised and verrucous in appearance. (Courtesy of Dr Roman Carlos.)

Fig 2-90 This mucosal blastomycosis lesion is red, fleshy, and verrucous. (Courtesy of Dr Roman Carlos.)

Fig 2-91 Blastomycosis of the lungs showing nodular lesions and a large infiltrate in the right base.

DIFFERENTIAL DIAGNOSIS ▶

In those rare cases with only oral and pulmonary lesions, the oral lesions are strongly suggestive of *squamous cell carcinoma, verrucous carcinoma,* or *verrucous hyperplasia*. In addition, the presence of pulmonary symptoms should give some credence to the possibilities of *histoplasmosis, coccidioidomycosis,* and an *oral TB ulcer.*

In those cases with skin lesions, the lesions may be similar to *skin squamous cell carcinoma* and *basal cell carcinoma* as well as *leprosy, sarcoidosis, lupus vulgaris* (TB of the skin), and other fungal diseases such as *histoplasmosis* and *coccidioidomycosis.*

DIAGNOSTIC WORK-UP ▶

The diagnosis is established by tissue biopsy of skin or mucosal lesions; the offending organism, *B dermatitidis,* is readily seen on histologic specimens. Skin antigen tests, chest radiographs (Fig 2-91), and blood studies are not specific.

HISTOPATHOLOGY ▶

The initial reaction in blastomycosis is suppuration with an influx of neutrophils and formation of small abscesses. This is followed by granuloma formation with epithelioid cells and multinucleated giant cells. Caseation is not a feature, however. Skin and mucosal lesions will often show pseudoepitheliomatous hyperplasia of the overlying adjacent epithelium.

The spores of *B dermatitidis* may be found free within abscesses or within giant cells. They are 8 to 15 μm in diameter with a thick, sharply defined "double-contoured" wall. They may show a single broad-based bud. The spores are most easily visualized with PAS or methenamine silver.

TREATMENT ▶

Oral itraconazole (Sporanox, Janssen), 100 to 200 mg daily for 3 months, is the treatment of choice. Response rates are over 80% with this regimen. Amphotericin B is used if itraconazole treatment fails. It is given intravenously with D5W to a maximum daily dose of 50 mg and then continued until a total dose of 2 g is given using the same delivery protocol as described for histoplasmosis and coccidioidomycosis.

PROGNOSIS ▶

Relapses are less common in blastomycosis than in histoplasmosis or coccidioidomycosis. However, 3- to 5-year follow-up is required. Relapses are seen more frequently in those cases in which the initial presentation included extensive skin or lung involvement.

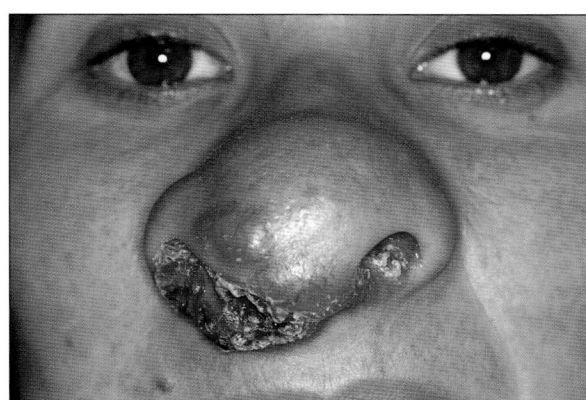

Fig 2-92a Early nasal involvement with rhinoscleroma showing a diffuse enlargement and formation of granulomatous nodules called the *Hebra nose*. (Courtesy of Dr Roman Carlos.)

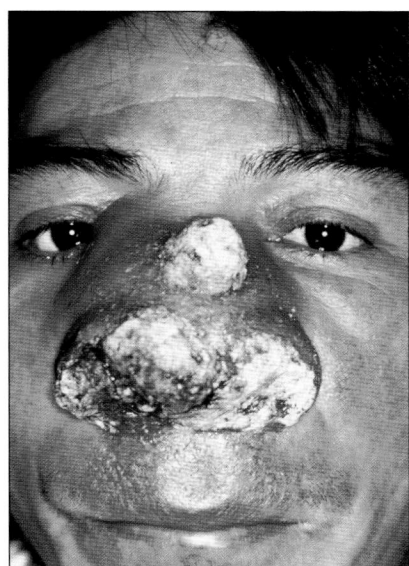

Fig 2-92b The nose may show further involvement and disfiguration due to nontreatment, foreshortened treatment, or resistance to treatment. (Courtesy of Dr Roman Carlos.)

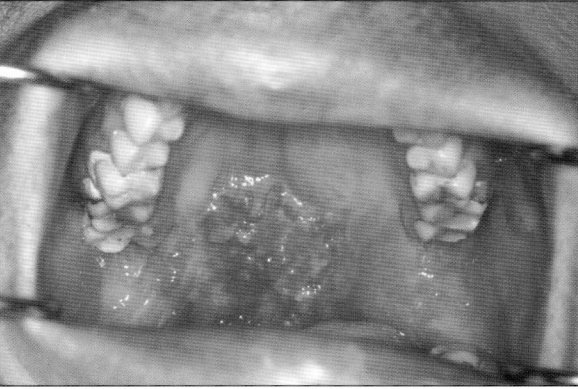

Fig 2-92c Firm nodular mass on the palate due to rhinoscleroma. (Courtesy of Dr Roman Carlos.)

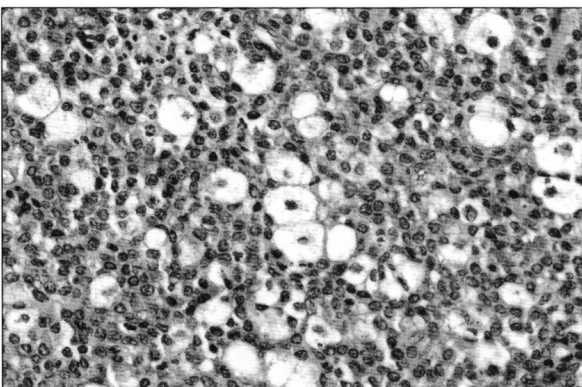

Fig 2-92d Amid a background of lymphocytes and plasma cells, foamy histiocytes (Mikulicz cells) can be seen in this case of rhinoscleroma. The *Klebsiella* are contained within the Mikulicz cells.

Rhinoscleroma

CLINICAL PRESENTATION AND PATHOGENESIS ▶

A typical patient with rhinoscleroma will present with nasal obstruction caused by granulomatous masses arising from the nasal mucosa as a result of infection with *Klebsiella pneumoniae rhinoscleromatis*. The nose will be diffusely enlarged and firm, a condition called the *Hebra nose* after Von Hebra, who first described this disease in 1870 (Figs 2-92a and 2-92b). Granulomatous masses may also concomitantly arise from the anterior gingiva, the maxillary sinuses, the palate, the vocal cords, and the trachea (Fig 2-92c). Specific symptoms of obstruction and dysfunction develop related to their site of occurrence.

The term *rhinoscleroma* is something of a misnomer, as it is found throughout the upper aerodigestive tract and into the ear (otoscleroma). It is extremely rare in the US and is found usually in immigrants or visitors from endemic areas such as Egypt, Central America, Indonesia, and Central Europe.

DIFFERENTIAL DIAGNOSIS ▶

Mass obstruction and enlargement of the nose suggest nasal tumors: a *nasopharyngeal angiofibroma* in the young and a *nasal or antral squamous cell carcinoma* or *lymphoepithelioma* in an older individual. It is also suggestive of sebaceous gland hyperplasia of the nasal skin, called a *rhinophyma*. In addition, *mucormycosis* may produce a sufficient granulation tissue response to cause nasal obstruction and, therefore, mimic a rhinoscleroma. However, rhinoscleroma is not specifically related to diabetes or immunosuppression as is mucormycosis.

DIAGNOSTIC WORK-UP ▶

Suspected cases should undergo biopsy and tissue culture to identify granulomatous disease, so-called Mikulicz cells, the characteristic subepithelial infiltrate, and the *K pneumoniae rhinoscleromatis* organism called the *Von Frisch bacillus*.

HISTOPATHOLOGY ▶

An initial infiltration of neutrophils, plasma cells, and macrophages is followed by granulomatous inflammation, which is characterized by numerous plasma cells and the presence of Russell bodies and Mikulicz cells. Russell bodies, which represent excess immunoglobulins produced by the plasma cells, are round to ovoid, homogeneous, eosinophilic, and up to 40 µm in diameter. They stain bright red with PAS. Mikulicz cells are large macrophages, 10 to 100 µm in diameter, with vacuolated cytoplasm within which are numerous gram-negative rods, 2 to 3 µm in length, that are *K pneumoniae rhinoscleromatis* (Von Frisch bacilli) (Fig 2-92d). They may be seen with H&E but are better visualized with Giemsa or silver stains. Overlying mucosa usually shows pseudoepitheliomatous hyperplasia, and over time, fibrosis becomes significant.

TREATMENT ▶

Early stages of the disease are best treated with antibiotics. Clofazimine (Lamprene, Ciba Geneva), a well-known antileprosy drug, is reasonably effective. It is given in the form of 100-mg capsules by mouth twice daily for an indeterminate period depending on clinical response. Alternative drugs include oral rifampin, 300 mg twice daily for 3 months, and topical rifampin in a 2% ointment applied directly to the granuloma.

In later stages, which are less responsive to antibiotics, the lesions become less cellular and more fibrotic. Excision of the masses with a carbon dioxide laser has been reported as effective in relieving nasal obstruction, improving swallowing, and improving vocal cord function. These excisions are associated with a low recurrence rate.

PROGNOSIS ▶

Relapse and recurrence of granulomatous masses are common. Many patients require repeated treatment or prolonged treatment courses. The disease is resistant to antibiotic therapy and even to surgery because of the induced fibrosis and slow turnover rate of the organism.

Mucormycosis

CLINICAL PRESENTATION AND PATHOGENESIS ▶

The most common presentation of mucormycosis is maxillary and orbital cellulitis in a person with inadequately controlled diabetes with ketoacidosis. It is caused by organisms of one of three genuses of the family Mucorales: *Absidia, Mucor*, and *Rhizopus*. All of these are usually nonpathogenic saprophytic soil fungi associated with decaying vegetable matter. The term *phycomycetes* is often used because it refers to a class of bread molds, of which the Mucorales is one family.

Mucormycosis is an opportunistic infection. Although the vast majority of those affected have uncontrolled diabetes, cases also sometimes occur in individuals undergoing transplant-related immunosuppressive therapy, AIDS patients, renal failure patients, leukemia patients, and even severe burn patients, all of whom have in common some loss of tissue integrity and compromised systemic immunity. Very rarely, mucormycosis will develop in an otherwise normal individual.

The nasal mucosa may ulcerate, exposing gray-black necrotic nasal cartilage, vomer, and ethmoid bones. The maxillary sinuses are usually filled with granulation tissue (Fig 2-93a), and bony sequestra may be present. Black necrotic bone is often visible (Fig 2-93b). Palatal ulcers frequently occur and will often progress to large oral-nasal-antral communications.

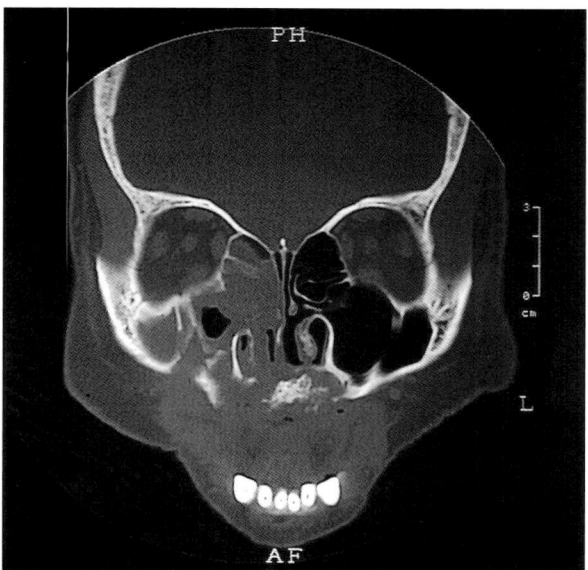

Fig 2-93a Mucormycosis may extend into the maxillary and ethmoid sinuses. Necrotic sequestra from the palate, alveolar ridge, and right nasal wall can also be seen here.

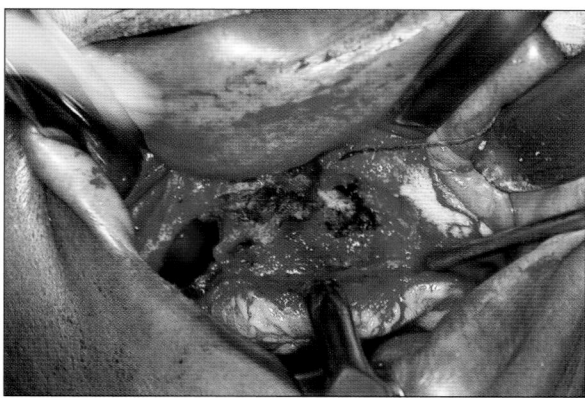

Fig 2-93b Extensive black-colored necrotic bone and soft tissue are seen in mucormycosis of the nasal cavity and paranasal sinuses.

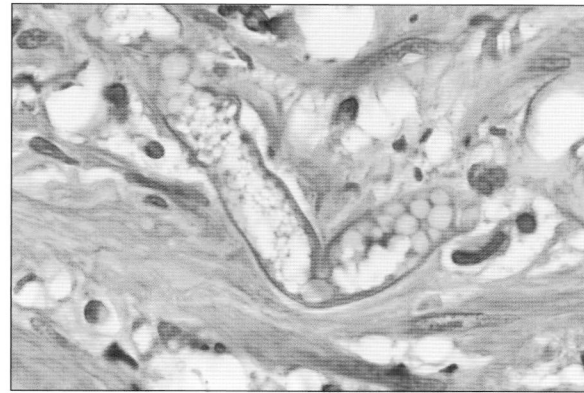

Fig 2-93c Hyphae showing right-angle branching in mucormycosis.

Ocular signs and symptoms of epiphora, blurred vision, ptosis, eye pain, headache, and periorbital paresthesias are common and suggest the possibility of impending cerebral extension.

Infection probably begins through airborne inhalation, which establishes an infection in only the compromised tissues of a compromised host. In the diabetic ketoacidotic patient, there is a high incidence of mucormycosis caused by *Rhizopus oryzae*, also known as *Rhizopus arrhizus* because they produce the enzyme ketoreductase, which allows them to utilize the patient's ketone bodies. It is also likely that the hyperglycemia stimulates fungal growth, and the diabetic reduction in chemotaxis and phagocytic efficiency permits these otherwise innocuous organisms to proliferate.

DIFFERENTIAL DIAGNOSIS ►

Destructive lesions of the palate and maxilla should suggest a *peripheral T-cell lymphoma* (formerly termed *midline lethal granuloma*), *nasopharyngeal carcinoma*, and *tertiary syphilis*. Some might be concerned about a Wegener granulomatosis, but this disease is limited to the palatal soft tissue and does not necrose the palate or maxilla.

DIAGNOSTIC WORK-UP ►

Suspicion of mucormycosis requires a CT scan of the maxilla, orbits, and brain. In particular, evidence of intracranial brain abscesses and orbital extensions is critical. Sinus and orbital extensions are recognized by membrane or periosteal thickenings as well as bony disruption (see Figs 2-93a and 2-93b).

Routine blood studies will show a leukocytosis in the 12,000 to 20,000/µL range and usually a left shift (Schilling shift to the left indicative of immature neutrophils). If the patient is diabetic, a full workup of serum glucose, electrolytes, blood chemistries, and blood gases is required.

Confirmation of the diagnosis is best obtained with a tissue specimen from the junction of necrotic and nonnecrotic tissue. Staining with methenamine silver or a PAS stain, in addition to H&E, will often show the organism in vessel walls or nerve bundles.

HISTOPATHOLOGY ►

These fungi can penetrate vessel walls, causing subsequent thrombosis and necrosis. The tissue infected by the organisms usually shows nonspecific acute and chronic inflammation with granulation tissue and necrosis. Granulomas are not seen. The large (up to 30 µm in diameter), long (100 to 200 µm), nonseptate hyphae, which demonstrate right-angle branching, may be seen with H&E (Fig 2-93c), but are better visualized with PAS or silver stains. They are found mostly in areas adjacent to clinical necrosis, especially within necrotic vessel walls.

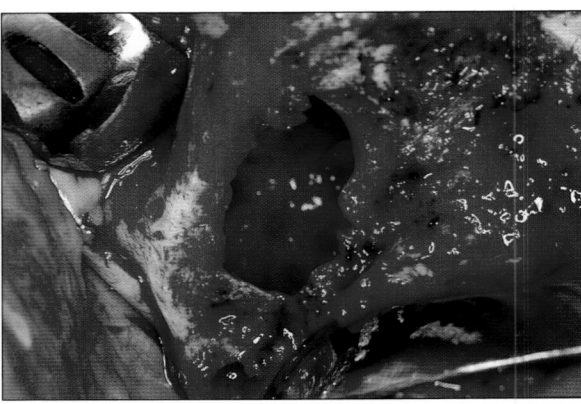

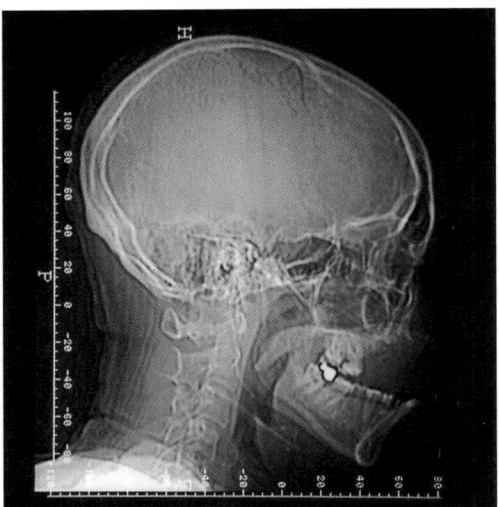

Fig 2-93d Extensive debridement to remove all necrotic tissue in combination with amphotericin B therapy is necessary to resolve a mucormycosis. Hyperbaric oxygen is also a useful adjunct.

Fig 2-93e The resultant deformity created by mucormycosis will resemble a partial or total maxillectomy.

TREATMENT ▶

Mucormycosis is a severe tissue-loss and life-threatening disease (Fig 2-93d). Aggressive control of the underlying disease and aggressive debridement are needed. Patients should undergo a resection type of debridement as soon as they are physiologically stable. This often takes the form of a partial or total maxillectomy (Fig 2-93e) and in some cases includes ethmoidectomy or frontal sinus or even orbital exenteration. The subsequent wound is best left open for care and irrigation but may be obturated with a removable prosthesis-obturator to support speech and feeding.

Amphotericin B therapy should also be initiated as soon as possible. It is usually given in D5W intravenously at a dose of 1.0 to 1.5 mg/kg daily. Adjunctive hyperbaric oxygen should also be used when available. Evidence now shows a better prognosis with the use of hyperbaric oxygen, probably because it reverses the hypoxia in local tissues and enhances neutrophil and macrophage killing ability.

PROGNOSIS ▶

The prognosis is directly related to the severity of the underlying disease, the extent of the disease when treatment begins, and the aggressiveness of the treatment. Death is a common outcome of this disease (30% to 50%). Hence, the general approach is to treat early, aggressively, and with all modalities available.

Aspergillosis

CLINICAL PRESENTATION AND PATHOGENESIS ▶

Aspergillosis infections are uncommon in individuals who are immunocompetent. In this group, the oral and maxillofacial specialist is most likely to see it in one of two clinical presentations. The first is an external otitis in which black colonies of *Aspergillus niger* or *Aspergillus fumigatus* develop as a result either of injury during cerumen removal or of repetitive ear cleanings or swimming in chlorinated water. In such cases, the protection of the cerumen is lost, permitting the colonization of *Aspergillus* and leading to a tender otitis externa. The second presentation is usually a chronic maxillary sinusitis, particularly when previous surgeries have disturbed the normal physiology and blood supply of the sinus and even more commonly when foreign bodies have been placed in the sinus. In such cases, the patient will complain of stuffiness in the nose and sinus, chronic pain, and intermittent nasal drainage. If the patient reports a black color to the drainage or the presence of black particles, the clinician should immediately be suspicious for aspergillosis or mucormycosis.

Aspergillosis infection in the oral and maxillofacial areas is much more common in the severely immunocompromised individual, particularly transplant patients and those with advanced HIV infection. Less commonly, aspergillosis infections develop in poorly controlled diabetics. In the severely immunocompromised, the aspergillosis may present as a necrotic black skin ulceration on the face or neck (Fig 2-94a) or as sinus infections, once again resembling mucormycosis. The black coloration of aspergillosis is due in part to the black coloration of most *Aspergillus* species and their thrombosis of blood vessels, causing local tissue infarction.

DIFFERENTIAL DIAGNOSIS ▶

In cases of otitis externa or chronic sinus infection, aspergillosis would not necessarily be the prime consideration. *Pseudomonas otitis externa* and other *nonspecific bacterial otitis externa* would be considered first. In a chronic sinusitis, *Pseudomonas sinusitis, Klebsiella sinusitis*, and even *Actinomyces sinusitis* may be considered as well.

In the immunocompromised individual, aspergillosis should be the prime consideration, along with *mucormycosis*. In addition, other fungal organisms may also colonize such vulnerable tissue so that almost any *mycotic* or *bacterial infection* may be suspected.

DIAGNOSTIC WORK-UP ▶

Blood cultures and even tissue cultures are not sufficiently yielding to have diagnostic value, nor is there a specific blood test or skin antigen test that can diagnose aspergillosis. The mainstay of diagnosis is a tissue biopsy that demonstrates branched septate hyphae in the tissue. Therefore, in suspected cases biopsies should sample the ulcer's edge where the black discoloration exists. The center of the ulcer usually consists only of necrotic tissue and is devoid of organisms. The *Aspergillus* prefer the ulcer's edge because of abundant substrate, reduced oxygen tension, and minimal immunocompetent cells. This histologic visualization can often be enhanced with a methenamine silver stain or a PAS stain to highlight the organisms as black or red, respectively.

If aspergillosis is strongly suspected or is confirmed by the oral and maxillofacial biopsy specimen, a chest radiograph and/or chest CT scan are of value. Pulmonary aspergillosis is life threatening and often requires a partial lung resection in addition to antifungal therapy.

HISTOPATHOLOGY ▶

The organisms appear as branching septate hyphae measuring 3 to 4 μm in diameter (Fig 2-94b). They invade blood vessels, causing occlusion and consequent necrosis. In the immunocompromised individual, necrosis may be extensive, whereas in patients with a normal immune system this process is limited by the granulomatous response the patient is able to mount against the organism.

TREATMENT AND PROGNOSIS ▶

Otitis externa due to aspergillosis responds well to acidified otic drops. Use of acetic acid/aluminum acetate (Domeboro Otic, Bayer), 4 to 6 drops in the affected ear, or acetic acid/propylene glycol (Vosol Otic, Wallace) 2% solution, 4 to 6 drops in the affected ear four times a day, will resolve an *Aspergillus* otitis externa as well as a *Pseudomonas* otitis externa.

In an immunocompetent individual, a chronic sinusitis due to *Aspergillus* is best treated with an exploration and debridement followed by dilute acetic acid (1% acetic acid) irrigations for 3 to 5 days, or longer in persistent cases. This is supplemented with itraconazole (Sporanox, Janssen), 200 mg by mouth twice a day for 2 weeks, or longer in persistent cases.

In the immunocompromised individual, aspergillosis requires restoration of the immune function to the greatest degree possible before any other therapy is likely to be of value. The tissues infected with aspergillosis require excision to a bleeding margin indicative of viable tissues (Fig 2-94c). This excision will resemble a tumor excision because of the fact that a nonbleeding edge must be excised until a bleeding edge is finally attained (Fig 2-94d). This should be followed by amphotericin B therapy. Pulmonary involvement often requires the highest dosage of amphotericin B short of major toxicity, which is usually the lipid amphotericin B preparation (Abelcet, Liposome) given as a 5- to 10-mg test dose over 30 minutes followed by 3 to 4 mg/kg per day intravenously at a rate of 1 mg/kg per hour. For the immunocompromised individual in whom there is no pulmonary involvement, the dosage can be adjusted downward from this point and titrated to the best response. The maximum dose of the lipid amphotericin B is not precisely known and will vary with each patient. However, it is thought to be between 3 and 5 g.

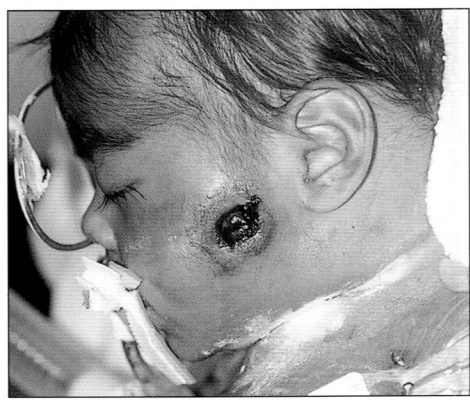

Fig 2-94a Black-colored ulceration typical of aspergillosis as seen here is a complication in an immunocompromised organ transplant patient.

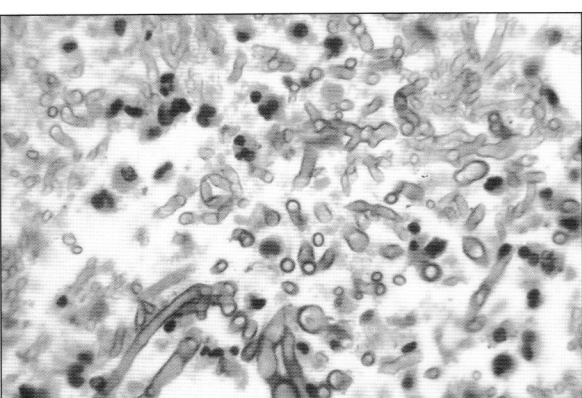

Fig 2-94b The septate hyphae of aspergillosis.

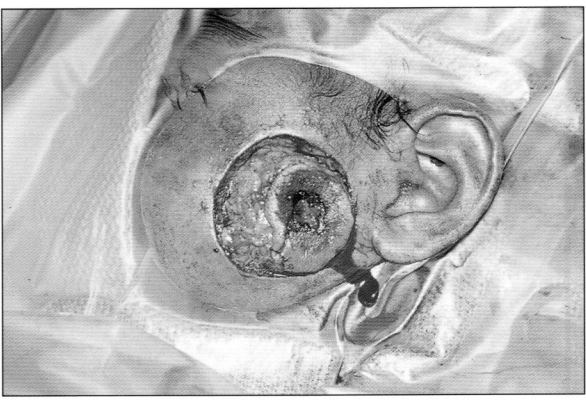

Fig 2-94c In addition to antifungal therapy and correcting the immune compromise, a wide surgical excision to bleeding tissue edges is required.

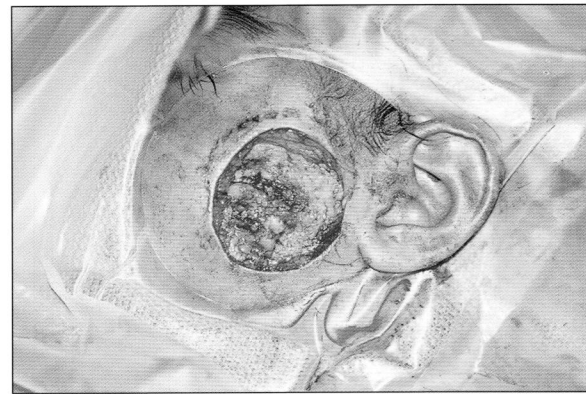

Fig 2-94d Assessment of the vascularity at the periphery after excision indicated a nonbleeding rim from the 9 o'clock to the 3 o'clock position. This area will require re-excision.

Parasitic Diseases

Leishmaniasis

CLINICAL PRESENTATION AND PATHOGENESIS ▶

Leishmaniasis is a collective term denoting a group of separate infections. Clinical presentations differ depending on the species involved, all of which are parasites transmitted by the bites of sandflies. The different *Leishmania* clinical presentations are:

1. **New World cutaneous leishmaniasis** caused by *Leishmania mexicana mexicana*. It is common in South and Central America as well as in Mexico. Rarely, cases are seen in the southern US. The disease will present with solitary ulcers and nodules, and less commonly vegetative growths, usually on the facial skin.
2. **Mucocutaneous leishmaniasis** (espundia) caused by *Leishmania braziliensis braziliensis*. This disease is found mostly in the forested lowlands of South America and Central America. Producing a set of severe oral and nasal ulcers, papillomatous growths, and nodules, it is destructive, resulting in disfiguring tissue loss (Figs 2-95a and 2-95b).

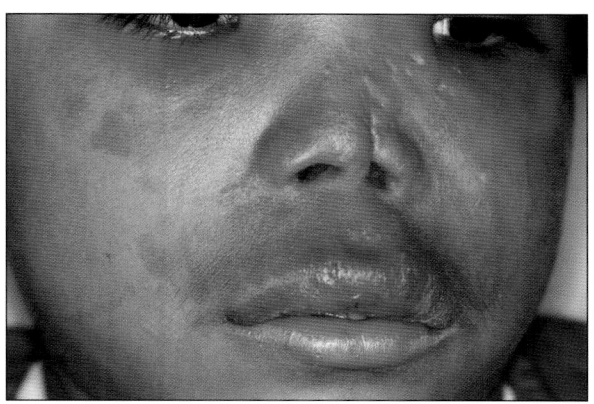

Fig 2-95a Oral, perioral, and nasal ulcerations in a mucocutaneous leishmaniasis (espundia). (Courtesy of Dr Roman Carlos.)

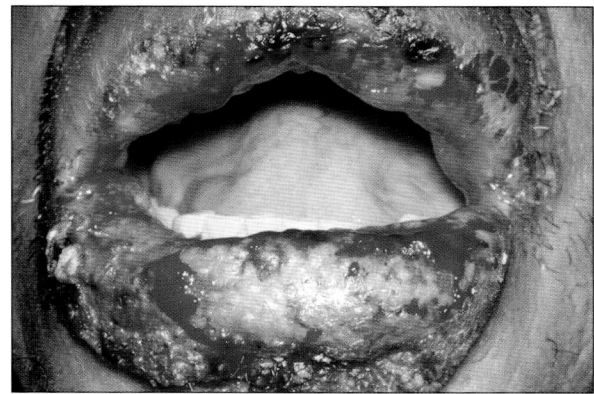

Fig 2-95b Severe cases of mucocutaneous leishmaniasis will exhibit more papillomatous features and be more destructive.

3. **Old World cutaneous leishmaniasis.** The three parasites involved are:

   - *Leishmania tropica*, which is found in the Middle East, south central Asia, and northern India as well as Greece, Italy, and France. This parasite produces a more benign presentation with skin papules that are single, dry, and only rarely ulcerate.
   - *Leishmania major*, which is found mainly in desert areas such as the Middle East, Arabian peninsula, Afghanistan, and the desert areas of Africa. The lesions are characteristically multiple, weeping ulcers that crust over.
   - *Leishmania aethiopica*, which occurs in Ethiopia and Kenya. It forms multiple nonulcerating papules that heal slowly over several years.

4. **Visceral leishmaniasis** (Kala-Azar), which is caused by *Leishmania donovani donovani*. It is found in India, Bangladesh, southeast Asia, China, Ethiopia, and Kenya. The patients develop twice-daily episodes of fever, sweats, and chills and exhibit weight loss, weakness, and diarrhea. Hepatosplenomegaly is common, as is prominent ascites. Skin hyperpigmentation may also be seen. Oral petechiae are noted along with gingival hemorrhage due to capillary fragility and liver dysfunction.

The bite of sandflies harbored in animals, both domestic and wild, results in transmission of the parasite in all forms of leishmaniasis except the visceral form (Kala-Azar), in which the parasites are transmitted from human to human.

In animals and in humans, the parasite is a small intracellular "mastigote" that exists within macrophages and blood monocytes. When a sandfly feeds on an infected host, the parasite is ingested along with these cells. Within the sandfly, the parasite develops into an extracellular flagellated "promastigote," which in turn is transmitted to another host through another sandfly bite, where it then repopulates macrophage-like cells to produce clinical disease in a new host. Over 1 million cases accompanied by 5,000 deaths are estimated to occur yearly.

DIFFERENTIAL DIAGNOSIS ▶ The rare cases seen in the US are either the New World cutaneous leishmaniasis or the more destructive mucocutaneous form of leishmaniasis called *espundia*. Either may bear a resemblance to *leprosy, lupus vulgaris* (cutaneous tuberculosis), or skin cancers such as *basal cell carcinoma* or *skin squamous cell carcinoma*. In addition, skin involvement associated with deep fungal infections such as *blastomycosis, histoplasmosis,* or *coccidioidomycosis* may also bear some resemblance.

DIAGNOSTIC WORK-UP ▶ The diagnosis of leishmaniasis is made by tissue biopsy or from scrapings in which the parasitic organisms can be readily identified using the Giemsa stain. The parasites can be cultured in Novy, MacNeal,

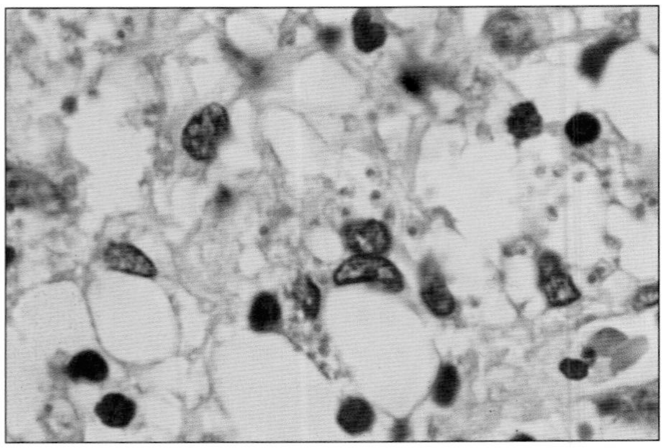

Fig 2-96 Leishmaniasis specimens will show enlarged macrophages containing round organisms (Giemsa stain).

and Nicolle (NNN) medium or Schneider's insect media if the organism cannot be identified by microscopy.

HISTOPATHOLOGY ▶ A spectrum of changes may be seen depending on the stage of disease and host response. In the early stage, there is infiltration by macrophages, which are enlarged because of the numerous leishmania organisms within the cytoplasm. The organisms lie free within the cytoplasm or within phagosomes (Fig 2-96). Lymphocytes and some plasma cells also are present. With time, the number of organisms decreases, and noncaseating, epithelioid granulomas with multinucleated giant cells develop.

The *Leishmania* protozoa have round to oval bodies, 2 to 4 μm in diameter, and are unencapsulated. Within each body is a 1-μm round basophilic nucleus and a small rod-like paranucleus (kinetoplast), which stain bright red with Giemsa. H&E also will show these structures, but less effectively.

TREATMENT ▶ The more benign Old World cutaneous form may resolve spontaneously. The New World forms, especially the mucocutaneous espundia, require aggressive treatment. Treatment takes the form of sodium antimony gluconate (sodium stibogluconate [Sb-5]), which is started with a 200-mg test dose followed by 20 mg/kg per day to a maximum daily dose of 850 mg. The drug is given intravenously in a solution form containing 100 mg/mL in three divided daily doses for 4 weeks.

Alternative drugs that may be used if intolerance to Sb-5 occurs are pentamidine, 2 to 4 mg/kg intramuscularly or intravenously daily for 15 days, or a course of amphotericin B similar to that used for histoplasmosis to a total dose of 30 mg/kg.

PROGNOSIS ▶ Treatment is prolonged and complex but usually effective. Recurrent disease is usually due to insufficient length of therapy. Scarring and disfigurement are noted, particularly in espundia.

Viral Diseases

Herpes Simplex Infections

Primary Herpetic Gingivostomatitis

CLINICAL PRESENTATION AND PATHOGENESIS ▶ Primary herpetic gingivostomatitis develops mostly in children and young adults. Painful vesicular lesions develop on all mucosal surfaces and rupture to produce foul-smelling ulcers (Figs 2-97a and 2-97b). The patient is usually febrile, drools, has significant malaise, "feels miserable," and will have tender cervical lymphadenopathy. The lesions and acute illness last about 10 days and resolve with scar formation.

The herpes simplex virus-1 (HSV-1) gains access to the patient via direct or airborne water-droplet transmission from an infected individual. The mucous membrane lesions represent direct viral infection at the site of inoculation. The clinical course is limited by the synthesis of viral-specific antibodies (IgM,

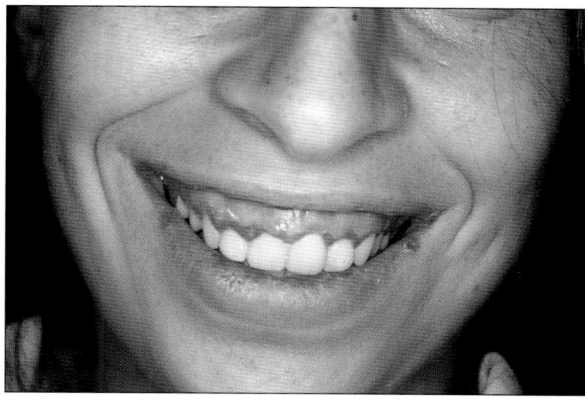

Fig 2-97a Gingival inflammation in primary herpetic gingivostomatitis.

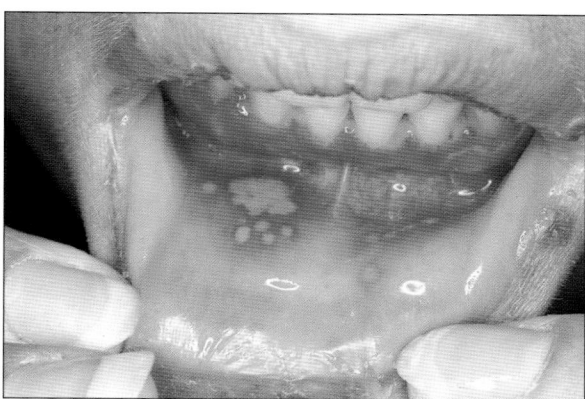

Fig 2-97b Clusters of ruptured vesicles, some of which have coalesced, in the patient shown in Fig 2-97a.

days 3 to 5; IgG, days 5 to 21). The virus is not completely eradicated, however, because residual viruses ascend proximally along the epineurium of the trigeminal nerve to the gasserian ganglion. In the gasserian ganglion, the virus is protected from further antibody attack by the blood-brain barrier and, therefore, develops a viable dormant existence within ganglion cell bodies.

Recurrent Herpes Infections

CLINICAL PRESENTATION AND PATHOGENESIS ▶

Recurrent herpes lesions may begin with a prodrome of burning, tingling, or pain without a visible lesion. Next, a vesicle may appear that will soon rupture into a moist ulcer, or an ulcer will emerge directly. Such secondary lesions have a predisposition for the vermilion and vermilion-skin edge of the lips; in the past, the condition has been termed *recurrent herpes labialis*. The lesions otherwise have a predisposition for the keratinized surfaces of the palate and gingiva.

Such recurrent lesions represent reactivation and migration of the virus. Stimulants such as sun exposure, cold temperatures ("cold sores"), and fevers from other diseases ("fever blisters") evoke HSV-1 activity by some unknown mechanism. Some viruses migrate distally down the epineural sheath of the trigeminal nerve, proliferate, and infect the epithelial tissue at the terminal nerve ending to generate vesicles and ulcers.

In immunosuppressed individuals, particularly bone marrow–transplant and HIV-infected patients, recurrent herpes is more serious. It tends to be more painful and destructive, and lesions may become secondarily infected, causing further destruction. The lesions are not limited to the lips, palate, and gingiva as they are in recurrent herpes in immunocompetent individuals.

Herpetic Whitlow

CLINICAL PRESENTATION AND PATHOGENESIS ▶

Herpetic whitlow has a history as an occupational hazard among dentists. Before the common use of examination gloves, dentists regularly contracted HSV-1 infection on their finger pads from infected patients (Fig 2-98). Herpetic whitlow mainly represents a primary HSV-1 infection, although it can be a recurrent secondary infection.

Emerging 2 to 10 days after contact, the lesions are painful red vesicles and pustules that rupture into ulcers. The lesions may last as long as 2 months, much longer than those of primary oral herpes. Some individuals develop axillary lymphadenitis and pain in the forearm, causing disability. Lesions may recur and will develop at the same site as the initial lesion.

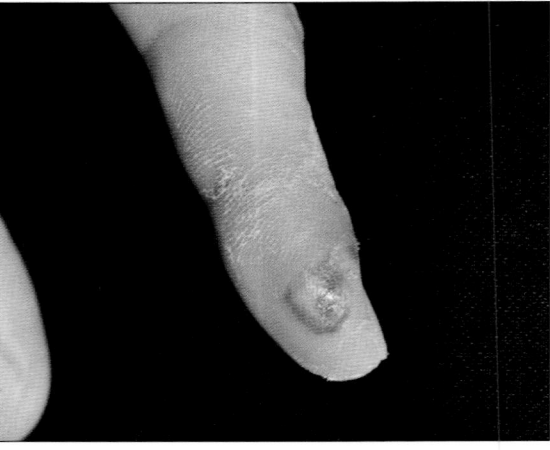

Fig 2-98 Painful red vesicles of herpetic whitlow related to direct contamination from an oral HSV-1 ulcer. (Reprinted from Pillsbury DM, *A Manual of Dermatology*, with permission from WB Saunders Co.)

Oral Versus Genital Herpes

HSV-1 is responsible for most cases of oral herpes. However, a small number of oral herpes cases are caused by HSV-2 secondary to oral sexual contact. HSV-2 is responsible for most of the more symptomatic and more debilitating cases of genital herpes, but a few cases are related to HSV-1 for the same reason. HSV-2 genital herpes has a similar pathogenicity involving the genital mucosa and sacral nerves. It is, however, more virulent.

Genital herpes, like oral herpes, forms more frequent and more intense recurrent secondary lesions within the first few years after the primary infection. As time passes, the episodes become less severe and the intervals longer. Transmission of genital herpes always occurs via sexual contact and may even arise from a lesion-free partner or a partner taking acyclovir. Viral shedding occurs mostly during the time of active lesions and is, therefore, the time of greatest transmissibility. However, viral shedding occurs to some degree at all times.

HSV-1 and HSV-2 have been suggested to be part of the inducer-promoter complex of cellular malignant transformation and are, therefore, possibly carcinogenic. There is a strong association of HSV-2 genital herpes to human cervical cancer and some evidence of a relationship of HSV-1 to oral cancer.

DIFFERENTIAL DIAGNOSIS ▶

The painful vesicular ulcerative lesions of acute herpetic gingivostomatitis may resemble *necrotizing ulcerative periodontitis* or *pemphigus vulgaris*. The oral lesions by themselves might be suggestive of *erythema multiforme*, but without concomitant skin lesions true erythema multiforme is not likely. In adults, *erosive lichen planus* is another consideration as is *streptococcal pharyngitis-mucositis* in younger patients.

Lesions of recurrent herpes simplex, particularly on the palate and gingiva, can be confusing. Intermittent episodes of "burning" lesions will occur. Their duration may be so brief that the practitioner and the patient miss the acute stage. *Aphthous ulcers* and *focal atrophic candida* lesions are other prime considerations. *Early herpes zoster* is also possible.

DIAGNOSTIC WORK-UP ▶

Laboratory evaluation to detect HSV circulating antibodies may be useful in children with suspected primary herpetic gingivostomatitis. However, it is not reliable in recurrent lesions or perhaps even in primary lesions because of the near universal exposure (over 90%) to HSV. Lesions can be scraped and smeared for cytologic studies, which may identify viral particles and multinucleated epithelial cells. Viral cultures from fresh tissue specimens may demonstrate cell death of human monolayered fibroblasts; studies using murine monoclonal antibodies against HSV may also be yielding. In addition, tissue biopsy specimens may show suggested viral particles on routine H&E staining. Otherwise, murine monoclonal antibody immunohistochemistry can identify the presence of intracellular HSV in formalin-fixed routine specimens.

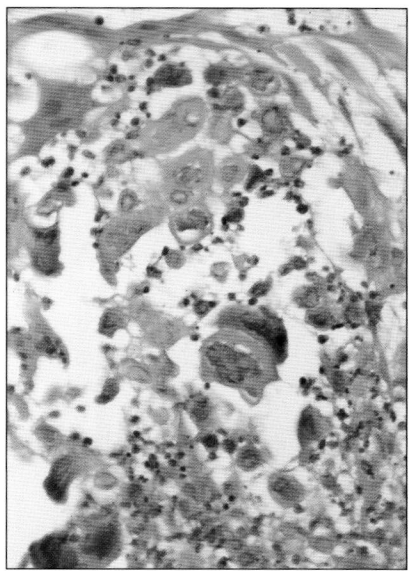

Fig 2-99 Amid a background of ruptured epithelial cells and neutrophils, acantholytic cells with pale steel-gray nuclei and margination of nuclear material can be seen.

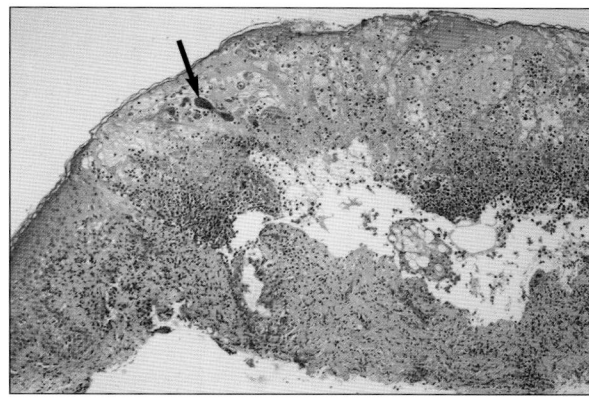

Fig 2-100 Low-power view of Fig 2-99 showing rupture of the vesicle into the connective tissue; the inflammatory infiltrate; ruptured epithelial cells; and multinucleated giant cells (*arrow*).

HISTOPATHOLOGY ▶

The essential histologic changes within skin and mucous membrane are the same for the three infections—herpes simplex, varicella, herpes zoster—caused by herpesvirus. As in all vesiculobullous lesions, the specific features may be seen only in early lesions; biopsy of long-standing and ruptured lesions should be avoided.

In these herpetic infections, the vesicle initially forms in the prickle cell layer secondary to degenerative changes induced by the virus. This takes two forms. Ballooning degeneration, which is seen mainly in the floor of the vesicle, causes expansion of the cell. The cell has an eosinophilic cytoplasm and a single nucleus or multiple nuclei. The nucleus is usually enlarged and may have an irregular contour. With H&E, it has a washed-out, steel-gray appearance and shows margination of the nuclear material (Fig 2-99). These cells lose their intercellular bridges, and this acantholytic process creates the vesicle. These cells may be identified by cytologic smears. The vesicle may "bottom out," so that it has a subepithelial rather than an intraepithelial location.

In reticular degeneration, which occurs essentially in the superior and lateral aspects of the vesicle, there is intracellular edema, such that the epithelial cells rupture, leaving strands from the cell walls to form a multilocular vesicle (Fig 2-100).

Eosinophilic inclusions (Lipschütz bodies), about 3 to 8 µm in diameter, may be seen within the nucleus. The underlying connective tissue shows an inflammatory reaction of varying intensity.

TREATMENT ▶

The two drugs most effective against HSV are systemic acyclovir and ganciclovir (Cytovene, Roche). Topical 5% acyclovir is not very useful in shortening the duration of secondary lesions or in aborting their course once developed. Unless the patient is immunocompromised, topical acyclovir should be withheld because of its potential to stimulate resistant viral strains in the face of very little therapeutic gain. Primary herpetic gingivostomatitis is self-limiting and should require only supportive care consisting of hydration, antipyretics, nutrition, and possibly antibiotics if secondary bacterial infections arise.

Recurrent oral herpes also does not necessarily warrant treatment. Mild clinical expressions are also self-limiting and their course can be endured over 1 week to 10 days. In those cases that present with multiple debilitating recurrent lesions and/or frequent extensive recurrences, oral acyclovir, 200 mg five

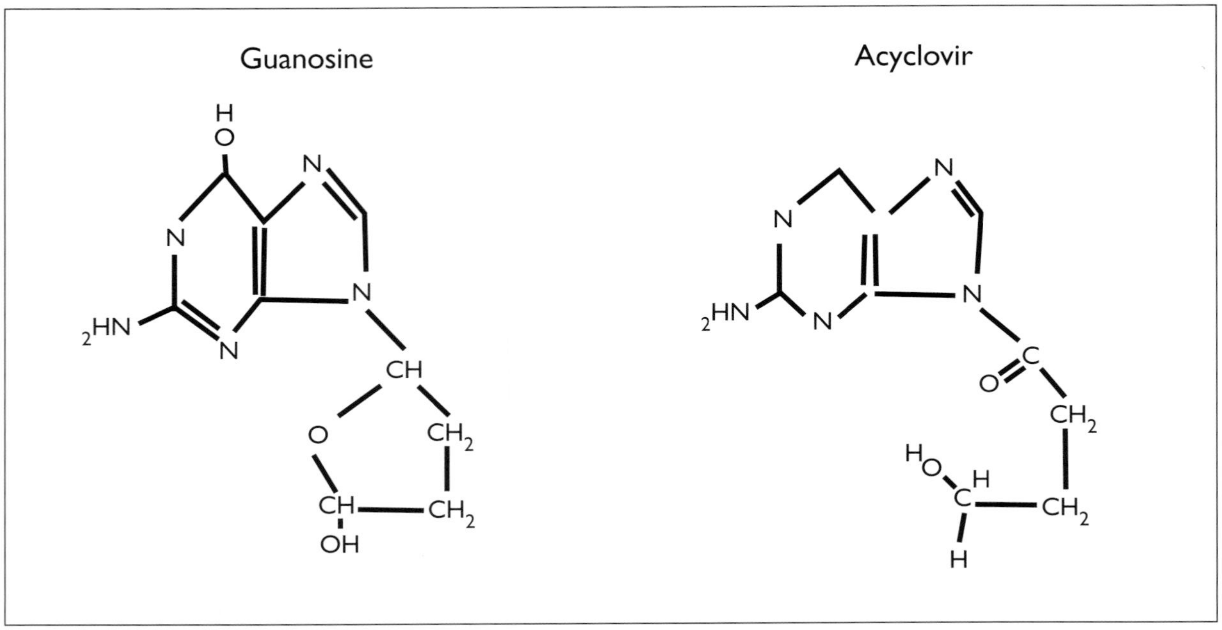

Fig 2-101 As its name suggests, acyclovir is an open ring analog of the purine guanosine in DNA. It acts to disrupt DNA synthesis and takes advantage of the fact that viral thymidine kinase is more efficient than the human enzyme in incorporating acyclovir into DNA.

times daily, is given for 10 days at the first sign of new lesions. To prevent frequent severe outbreaks, maintenance at 400 mg twice daily is recommended. If recurrences are infrequent but severe enough to warrant therapy, oral acyclovir, 200 mg five times daily, is used at each recurrence to shorten its course and limit disability.

Immunocompromised patients warrant acyclovir therapy at each episode. Some may require intravenous therapy, usually in divided dosages for a total of 30 mg/kg per day. As an alternative, ganciclovir, 500 mg orally three times daily, may be used as well. Continued prophylactic oral acyclovir is recommended in immunocompromised patients, usually at 400 mg twice daily.

Acyclovir is an analog of the purine guanosine. The five-member sugar moiety in guanosine is closed. In acyclovir it is open-ended, hence its name (Fig 2-101). Acyclovir disrupts viral and potentially human DNA polymerization by inhibiting viral DNA polymerase. It is selective for viruses because the viral enzyme thymidine kinase, which converts acyclovir to acyclovir monophosphate, is more efficient in this phosphate reaction than is human thymidine kinase. Therefore, only infected host cells—which add two more phosphates to acyclovir, thus converting it to acyclovir triphosphate—are affected. The acyclovir triphosphate is the actual false guanosine analog that ties up and halts the enzyme DNA polymerase as it progresses along the uncoiled DNA template strand to inhibit DNA synthesis and hence viral replication. Because human and most mammalian cells do not accomplish the first step of acyclovir monophosphate production as efficiently as do viral cells, they are protected from most of acyclovir's actions. Acyclovir-resistant strains of HSV-1 or HSV-2 are sometimes found in HIV-infected patients. In such cases, foscarnet (Foscavir, AstraZeneca) is either substituted for acyclovir or added to it at a dose of 40 to 60 mg/kg intravenously three times daily.

PROGNOSIS ▶ Acyclovir for those who warrant it is effective, particularly if started early in the disease course. Long-term acyclovir therapy in the immunocompromised patient is effective and safe. However, it does not prevent viral shedding in the symptomatic or asymptomatic patient and will, therefore, not prevent transmission of either HSV-1 or HSV-2 disease.

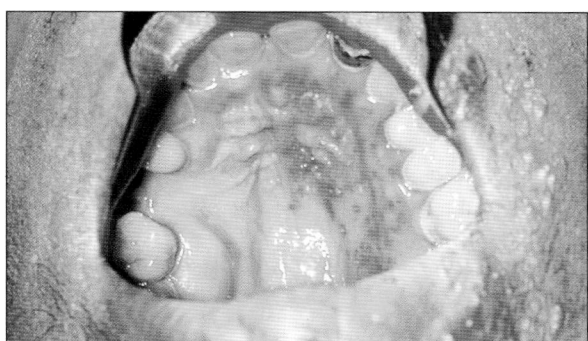

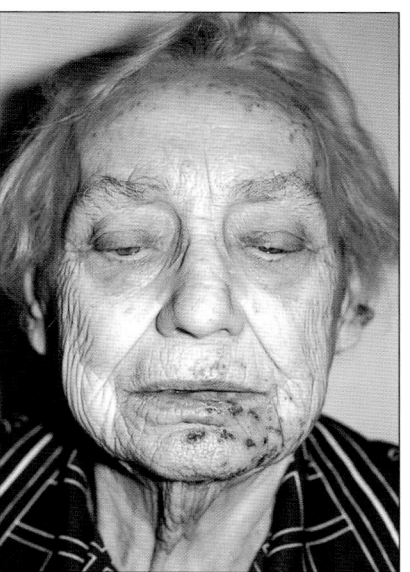

Fig 2-102a Painful palatal herpes zoster lesions following the distribution of the greater palatine nerve and abruptly stopping at the midline.

Fig 2-102b Herpes zoster lesions of the skin following the mental nerve distribution.

Herpes Zoster

CLINICAL PRESENTATION ▶ Herpes zoster is a disease of reactivated latent varicella zoster virus (VZV), which frequently occurs in older adults who have had some compromise in their immune status. Lesions that are pustular and vesicular form after a short prodrome of pain and itching sensations. The lesion will follow a peripheral nerve distribution precisely and stop abruptly at the midline (Figs 2-102a and 2-102b). The lesions will quickly ulcerate and become necrotic with crusting (Figs 2-103a to 2-103c). Pain is usually intense and constant. The most common immune status alterations are those related to lymphomas (particularly Hodgkin lymphoma and T-cell lymphomas) and leukemias. It is also seen in chronically ill patients and patients who are receiving chemotherapy, radiotherapy, or immunosuppressive drugs. It may also occur in otherwise normal individuals.

The dermatomes of the chest wall is the most common site for herpes zoster, but the areas of trigeminal nerve distributions, particularly the ophthalmic division, is the next most common site. If herpes zoster lesions involve a trigeminal nerve distribution plus one other cranial nerve distribution (most commonly the facial nerve producing a facial paralysis [see Figs 2-103a and 2-106d]), the condition is termed the *Ramsay Hunt syndrome* (after James Ramsay Hunt), and the lesions characteristically begin in the external ear and mimic a painful otitis externa (Fig 2-104). This syndrome may also produce symptoms related to other cranial nerve involvement: vertigo and deafness related to the vestibular-cochlear nerve (cranial nerve VIII), dysphagia, uvular deviation to the unaffected side related to the vagus nerve (cranial nerve X), and even paralysis of the ipsilateral tongue related to the hypoglossal nerve (cranial nerve XII).

DIFFERENTIAL DIAGNOSIS ▶ Herpes zoster is a diagnosis of clinical recognition rarely confused with other diseases. In the oral cavity and in its early stages, the presentation of burning and pain may be confused with recurrent *herpes simplex* lesions or perhaps a *focal atrophic candidiasis*.

DIAGNOSTIC WORK-UP ▶ In equivocal cases, immunoperoxidase testing using anti-VZV antibodies to identify VZV in fixed biopsy specimens may be needed. Otherwise, herpes zoster is a clinical diagnosis.

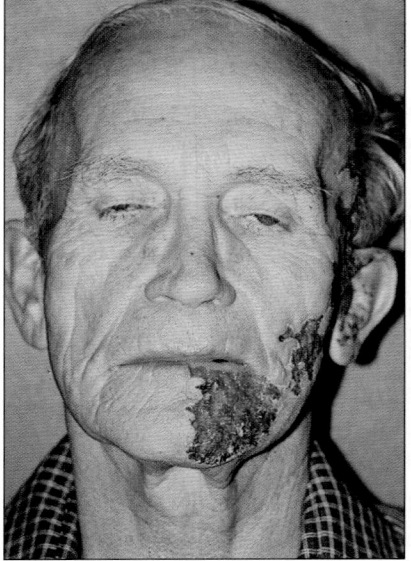

Fig 2-103a Crusted lesions end abruptly at the midline and follow the mandibular distribution of the trigeminal nerve. Note a slight paresis of the facial muscles, an early sign of the Ramsay Hunt syndrome.

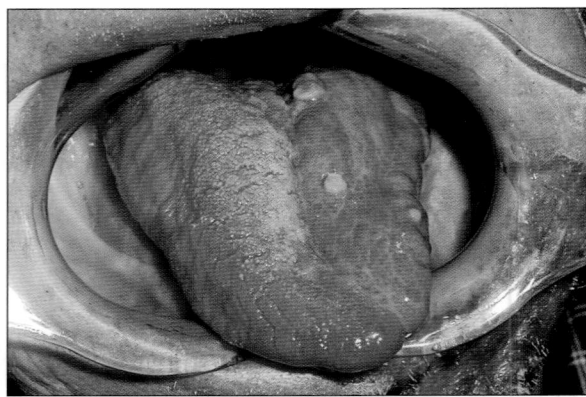

Fig 2-103b Loss of filiform papillae and ulcers of the tongue unilaterally in a herpes zoster infection.

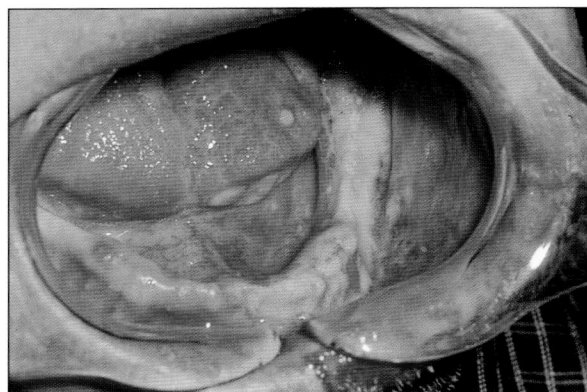

Fig 2-103c Denudation of bone in herpes zoster.

HISTOPATHOLOGY ▶

Changes beyond those within skin and mucosa may be seen and can be significant in this disease. With reactivation of the virus in the ganglion, the ganglion becomes edematous and there is infiltration by lymphocytes, plasma cells, and macrophages (Fig 2-105). Focal areas of necrosis may occur, and intranuclear inclusions may be found in the neurons. Following the attack, the ganglion returns to normal except for loss of neurons secondary to fibrous scarring. The varicella-zoster virus may also cause a lymphadenitis, which may resemble lymphoma because of its diffuse pattern, capsular involvement, and atypical immunoblasts.

TREATMENT ▶

Herpes zoster is a painful and debilitating disease that is destructive of tissue. Skin necrosis with severe scar formation often occurs, as does pain after the lesions have healed (a condition called *postherpetic neuralgia*). Lesions frequently become secondarily infected by bacteria, and there is a high incidence of encephalitis complications if the ophthalmic division is involved (Figs 2-106a to 2-106d). Treatment should begin as soon as possible and it should be aimed at shortening the disease course, preventing tissue loss, and reducing postherpetic neuralgia. Acyclovir, as much as 800 mg five times daily, is recommended, along with carbamazepine (Tegretol, Novartis), 200 mg three or four times daily, to reduce neuralgic pain. If oral lesions predominate, patients often will not be able to eat. In such cases, intravenous fluid management or nasogastric feedings may be needed.

In the immunocompromised patient, herpes zoster is even more serious. Intravenous acyclovir, 30 mg/kg per day in three divided doses, is used. Immunocompromised individuals exposed to herpes zoster are considered for the varicella-zoster immune globulin (VZIG) as discussed in the varicella (chickenpox) section, below.

Immunocompetent patients respond to acyclovir very well. Lesions remit, leaving scars and, in up to 40% of cases, postherpetic neuralgia. Postherpetic neuralgia is at its most intense early after a herpes zoster infection and will diminish with time. During this time, carbamazepine, 200 mg one to three times daily, will alleviate most of the pain. Postherpetic neuralgia is thought to be due to the predilection of herpesviruses for the cell bodies of the large myelinated A fibers. In the gate control theory of pain, the

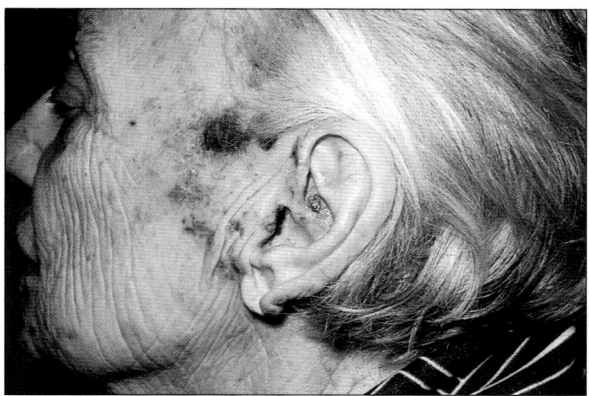

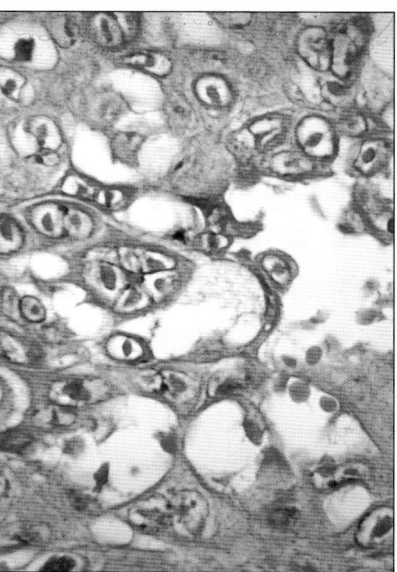

Fig 2-104 Early herpes zoster will often begin in the external ear canal or in the area of the pinna and will mimic an external otitis.

Fig 2-105 Edematous gasserian ganglion cells infected by the herpes zoster virus.

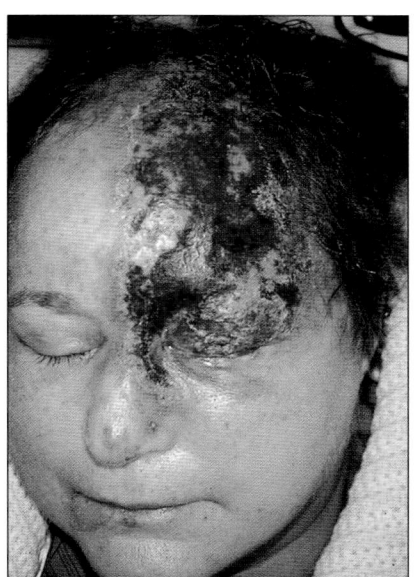

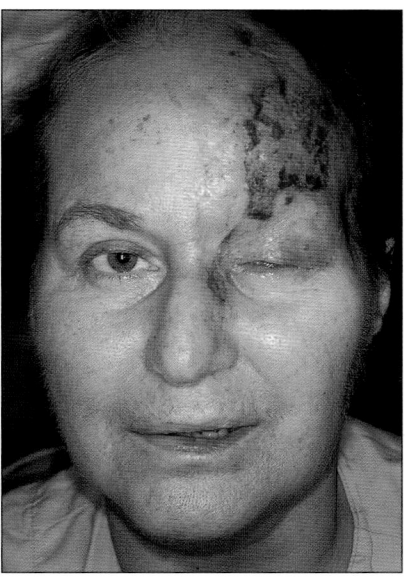

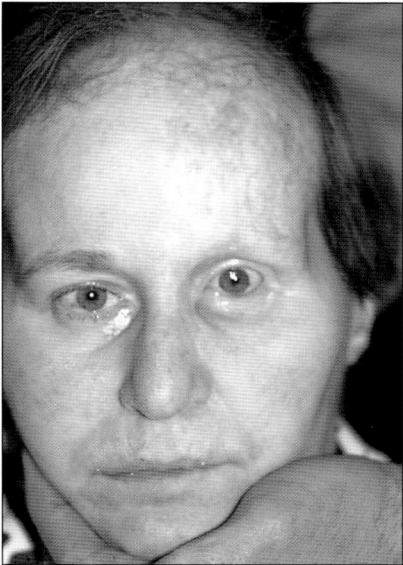

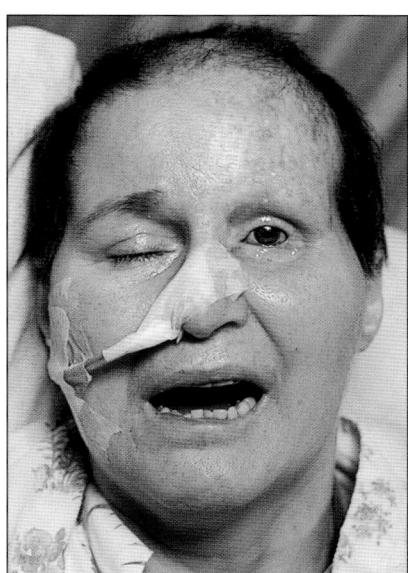

Fig 2-106a Herpes zoster of the ophthalmic division in Ramsay Hunt syndrome.

Fig 2-106b Although the acute herpes zoster lesions begin to subside, alopecia skin necrosis and an encephalitis developed.

Fig 2-106c Blindness, opthalmoplegia, facial paralysis, scarring, and alopecia resulting from this herpes zoster infection.

Fig 2-106d Severe disability with dysphagia and permanent facial paralysis due to herpes zoster in which an encephalitis eventuated.

large A fibers produce a dampening effect on the gating mechanism in the nucleus caudalis of the trigeminal nerve and the substantia gelatinosa of somatic nerves. Their selective destruction by herpesviruses leaves unopposed the small, unmyelinated C fibers, which are excitatory to the gate, thereby creating a clinical pain syndrome.

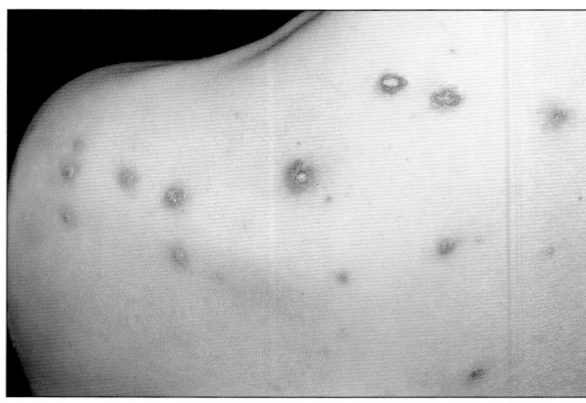

Fig 2-107 Painful pustules with a red periphery are characteristic of varicella. These will rupture to form crusting ulcers.

Varicella (Chickenpox)

Classic chickenpox is one of the usual childhood diseases for which vaccinations were not available until the late 1990s. A live attenuated viral vaccine is now recommended for all children over 12 months of age who have not had clinical chickenpox. It is also recommended that children receiving the vaccine not take aspirin for the following 6 weeks because of the possibility of Reye syndrome, a rare complication that may produce progressive hepatic failure and encephalopathy with a 30% mortality rate. While Reye syndrome may occur unrelated to any specific event, vaccinations are a recognized risk that increases with aspirin ingestion.

The child who develops varicella is usually between 4 and 10 years of age. Painful red pustules and vesicles develop mainly on the trunk and facial skin. The vesicles quickly rupture and form crusting lesions as they mature (Fig 2-107). The child is usually acutely ill with fever, chills, agitated behavior lapsing into malaise, and a complaint of headache. Successive formations of new lesions occur because of intermittent viremias, producing lesions in all stages of maturity. The oral mucosa may also show lesions, but they are fewer in number. The lesions are both pruritic and painful. Children often scratch them, creating secondary bacterial infections.

In adults, the lesions are identical, but complications are more frequent. Rare complications such as viral encephalitis and pneumonia have been noted. Varicella virus does cross the placenta and may cause fetal malformation.

Chickenpox is caused by the varicella-zoster virus (VZV), which is a type of herpesvirus; that is, it is a DNA virus with a protein capsid and a lipid envelope. VZV and HSV, therefore, have some antigenicity in common, and their mechanism of causing disease is similar. The VZV, like the HSV, is transmitted initially by direct water-droplet transmission. The VZV penetrates the epithelium and becomes engulfed by macrophages and other phagocytes. The virus proliferates within the phagocytes and egresses from them to be disseminated via the circulation, which is often called the *incubation* phase. The subsequent viremia-associated dissemination implants viruses throughout the skin, producing the characteristic skin lesions.

As the host defenses—consisting mainly of IgM and IgG antibody production and T cell–mediated reactions with interferon production—gain ground on the vast viral numbers, the lesions begin to heal and the constitutional symptoms dissipate. Like HSV, VZV will escape to the protection of the blood-brain barrier via proximal migration along the epineurium of sensory nerves to their respective ganglia. There they remain in a latent or dormant form and will, on certain stimuli or reductions in the level of immune surveillance, migrate outward toward the same nerve endings to produce the lesions of herpes zoster.

The main differential diagnoses of concern in a child with painful skin lesions with accompanying fever are the other childhood diseases such as *rubeola* (measles) and *rubella* (German measles). A developing *Stevens-Johnson form of erythema multiforme* is another possibility. Less common today, *scarlet fever* and, if

DIAGNOSTIC WORK-UP ▶

in the summer, *hand-foot-and-mouth disease* may also show skin rashes, associated fever, and constitutional symptoms.

Diagnosis is made by history and clinical examination only. Varicella is diagnosed by the onset, appearance, and locations of characteristic lesions.

HISTOPATHOLOGY ▶

The essential histologic changes within skin and mucous membrane are the same for the three infections caused by herpesvirus: herpes simplex, varicella, herpes zoster. As in all vesiculobullous lesions, the specific features may be seen only in early lesions; biopsy of long-standing and ruptured lesions should be avoided.

In these herpetic infections, the vesicle initially forms in the prickle cell layer secondary to degenerative changes induced by the virus. This takes two forms. Ballooning degeneration, which is seen mainly in the floor of the vesicle, causes expansion of the cell. The cell has an eosinophilic cytoplasm and a single nucleus or multiple nuclei. The nucleus is usually enlarged and may have an irregular contour. With H&E, it has a washed-out, steel-gray appearance and shows margination of the nuclear material. These cells lose their intercellular bridges, and this acantholytic process creates the vesicle. These cells may be identified by cytologic smears. The vesicle may "bottom out," so that it has a subepithelial rather than an intraepithelial location.

In reticular degeneration, which occurs essentially in the superior and lateral aspects of the vesicle, there is intracellular edema such that the epithelial cells rupture, leaving strands from the cell walls to form a multilocular vesicle.

Eosinophilic inclusions (Lipschütz bodies), about 3 to 8 µm in diameter, may be seen within the nucleus. The underlying connective tissue shows an inflammatory reaction of varying intensity.

TREATMENT ▶

Varicella is a self-limiting disease in the immunocompetent individual because of the formation of antivaricella antibodies. Supportive care consisting of hydration, analgesics, antipyretics, and rest is recommended during the course of the disease, which lasts from 10 to 21 days. Patients should be isolated until they are afebrile, the crust from skin lesions has disappeared, and the healing areas are dry. Immunocompromised individuals and HIV-infected individuals are at particularly high risk. In immunocompromised patients and pregnant women in the third trimester, acyclovir, 30 mg/kg per day in three intravenous doses for 7 to 10 days, is the treatment of choice. For cases refractory to acyclovir, foscarnet (Foscavir, AstraZeneca) may be administered at a loading dose of 20 mg/kg intravenously followed by 120 mg/kg intravenously three times daily for 2 weeks.

Varicella zoster immune globulin (VZIG) is effective in preventing varicella in exposed, susceptible individuals with no natural or vaccine-derived immunity. It is given at a dosage of 125 U/kg up to a maximum of 625 U with consideration for a repeat dose in high-risk individuals with continued exposure. However, VZIG is not to be used to treat an active case of varicella. Because VZIG binds directly to live attenuated virus in the varicella vaccine, they should not be used together.

PROGNOSIS ▶

In the immunocompetent individual, varicella is a self-resolving disease that may leave some residual scarring. In the immunocompromised individual, it can be a desperate situation requiring trials of potent antiviral drugs at high doses and may contribute to the individual's death.

Infectious Mononucleosis

CLINICAL PRESENTATION AND PATHOGENESIS ▶

Affected individuals are usually teenagers or young adults who present with a sore throat, fever, malaise, headache, and prominent tender cervical lymphadenopathy. The cervical lymphadenopathy is somewhat distinctive in that it involves both anterior and posterior lymph node chains equally. The pharynx is red with a gray-yellow exudate. Tonsillar and gingival inflammation frequently accompany the pharyngitis. A maculopapular rash is seen in 15% of cases. Some will even develop petechial hemorrhages, often noted on the palatal mucosa. If given ampicillin, 90% of patients will develop a rash or their current rash will worsen.

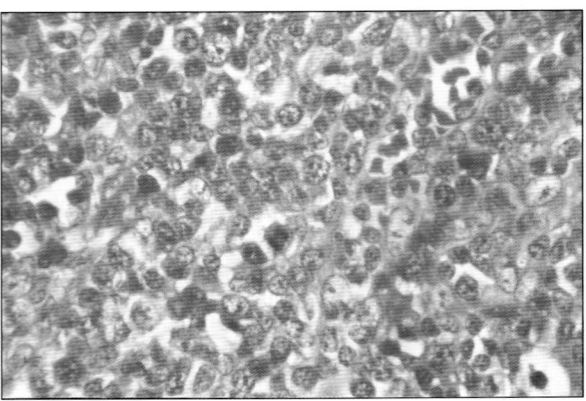

Fig 2-108 Mitoses are seen within the lymphadenitis of infectious mononucleosis.

The individual will appear acutely ill with prominent fatigue as a chief complaint. Often the individual will be anorexic and nauseated. Neck stiffness and photophobia are also frequently present, as is splenomegaly in 50% of cases.

Chronic fatigue syndrome, which became recognized in the 1980s, has been suggested to be a form of chronic mononucleosis. Indeed, these patients usually have elevated Epstein-Barr (EB) virus capsid and nuclear antibodies. However, no real cause and effect has been established. It may merely represent an unassociated immunologic finding.

There is also a possible association of EB virus with the development of Burkitt lymphoma and nasopharyngeal carcinoma. This may be a casual rather than a causal association.

The EB virus is a herpesvirus (human herpesvirus 4), which causes infectious mononucleosis. Transmitted via saliva by direct contact and primarily associated with the 15- to 40-year age group, infectious mononucleosis was called the "kissing disease" in the 1960s and sometimes appears in small epidemic forms. Once contact has occurred, incubation over 5 to 15 days results in inflammation at the sites of contact, which can and does spread to cervical lymph nodes or other organs.

DIFFERENTIAL DIAGNOSIS ▶

An exudative pharyngitis with cervical lymphadenitis should make the clinician consider *diphtheria* or an *adenovirus-related pharyngitis*. The common *streptococcal pharyngitis* and the less common *measles (rubeola)* and *gonococcal pharyngitis* are also possible.

DIAGNOSTIC WORK-UP ▶

Laboratory studies consisting of liver function tests in addition to routine blood counts will show elevation of serum aspartate aminotransferase (AST) and alanine aminotransferase (ALT) enzymes as well as neutropenia and an absolute lymphocytosis. Some of the lymphocytes will be extremely large, mimicking monocytes (hence the term *mononucleosis*, which is a misnomer because the cells are actually altered lymphocytes). Some will appear atypical, a hallmark of the disease.

The Monospot (Color Slide II, Seradyn) test or the heterophile antibody test will give a positive result by agglutinating the red blood cells of horse, sheep, or cow. Either test may be used as a screening test, although the Monospot is the more common. If the test is positive, specific titers for EB viral antigens (EB virus capsid antigen and EB virus nuclear antigen) are assessed with direct immunofluorescence and will confirm the diagnosis.

HISTOPATHOLOGY ▶

The lymphadenitis associated with infectious mononucleosis may show marked paracortical hyperplasia and follicular hyperplasia with irregularly shaped follicles because of the proliferating immunoblasts. Within the follicles, there may be numerous mitoses (Fig 2-108) and focal areas of necrosis with tingible body macrophages (macrophages with clear reticulated cytoplasm–containing nuclear debris). Occasional large hyperchromatic cells with multilobed nuclei and prominent nucleoli, resembling Reed-Sternberg cells, may be present. This, together with the other atypical features, may suggest Hodgkin disease.

In addition, the immunoblastic proliferation with loss of normal modal architecture can mimic non-Hodgkin lymphoma. Infectious mononucleosis does not have a pathognomonic histopathology and is notorious for mimicking lymphomas. Lymph node biopsy is thus not recommended for diagnosis.

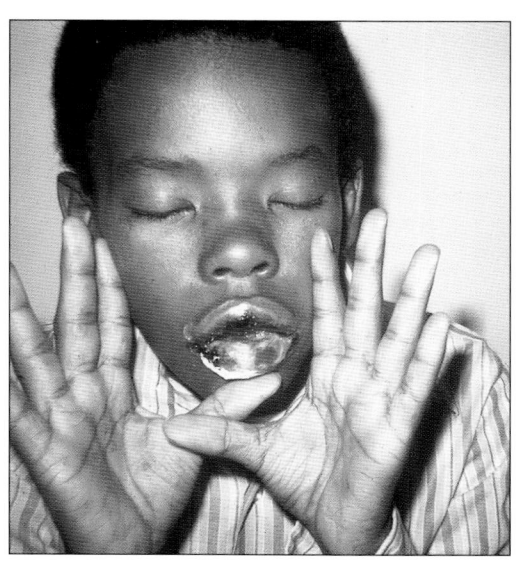

Fig 2-109 Vesicles on the lip and palms in a patient with hand-foot-and-mouth disease.

TREATMENT

No specific treatment is required. Acyclovir, which is effective against herpes infection, is ineffective against EBV and is not indicated. Supportive care consisting of hydration, long-term rest, analgesics, antipyretics, and often penicillin or erythromycin to prevent or treat secondary streptococcal pharyngitis is of value.

PROGNOSIS

In uncomplicated cases, the fever disappears within 10 days and the lymphadenopathy in 6 weeks. Fatigue and malaise often linger for 3 to 4 months.

Complicated presentations of mononucleosis do occur. A small percentage of patients develop a severe hemolytic anemia, hepatitis, myocarditis, or encephalitis. Overt splenomegaly to the point of splenic rupture has occurred, causing a life-threatening emergency requiring immediate splenectomy. Splenic rupture and encephalitis are the two complications accounting for the rare reports of death related to mononucleosis.

Hand-Foot-and-Mouth Disease

CLINICAL PRESENTATION AND PATHOGENESIS

Hand-foot-and-mouth disease will present in a child younger than 5 years during the summer. Uncomfortable but usually not severely painful oral lesions often will be the reason the parent seeks attention. The oral lesions begin as vesicles but may not be evident because of early rupture. More likely, yellow oral ulcers that will show a fibrinopurulent base surrounded by a red erythematous ring will be present. Similar target-like lesions already will be present or soon will develop on the fingers and hands as well as the toes and feet (Fig 2-109). Because skin epidermis is thicker than mucosa, the skin lesions will form visible vesicles of up to 1 cm in diameter before rupture. Constitutional symptoms are mild. The child is not usually as irritable as are those with most other childhood diseases.

Hand-foot-and-mouth disease is caused by coxsackievirus A16. Other coxsackieviruses, A5, A9, A10, B2, and B5, and enterovirus 71 have been but are not generally the cause of hand-foot-and-mouth disease. They do cause other diseases such as herpangina (A2–6, A8, and A10), epidemic pleurodynia (B1–5), and aseptic meningitis (A7, A9, and B5). Coxsackieviruses are called *picornaviruses* because they are small (pico) RNA viruses. They are named after Coxsackie, New York, a town where the virus was first identified. Coxsackie A and B groups have different behavioral characteristics.

Hand-foot-and-mouth disease is transmitted via airborne particles and possibly oral-fecal spread. The virus seems capable of penetrating mucous membranes, establishing a viremia, and becoming disseminated with a preference (probably due to cooler temperatures) for the hands, feet, and mouth.

DIFFERENTIAL DIAGNOSIS ▶

Early *varicella* (chickenpox), *rubeola* (measles), and *herpangina* will also present with concomitant oral lesions and skin lesions. In addition, one must be concerned about a developing *Stevens-Johnson syndrome variant of erythema multiforme*, although the course of hand-foot-and-mouth disease would be less rapid and the lesions less painful.

DIAGNOSTIC WORK-UP ▶

Hand-foot-and-mouth disease is a diagnosis of history and clinical findings. The pattern of lesions, the patient's young age, and the time of year (summer or warm-weather periods) contribute to the diagnosis.

HISTOPATHOLOGY ▶

Initially, intraepithelial vesicles are formed, and reticular degeneration may cause multilocular vesicles. In the deep epithelium, ballooning degeneration may occur. Intraepithelial vesicles may become subepithelial. Multinucleated giant cells and inclusion bodies are absent. A dense inflammatory infiltrate of neutrophils and mixed chronic inflammatory cells is present within the connective tissue and vesicles.

TREATMENT ▶

No specific treatment is required. Supportive care and reassurance to parents about the self-limiting nature of the disease are helpful.

PROGNOSIS ▶

Lesions and their symptoms dissipate within 2 weeks. Mild scarring may remain.

Herpangina

CLINICAL PRESENTATION AND PATHOGENESIS ▶

Herpangina is seen in children in the summer months with the primary findings of abrupt-onset high fever (104°F to 105°F range), a diffuse pharyngitis, 1- to 2-mm gray-white vesicles, and petechiae and ulcers of the soft palate and tonsillar fossa. The oral mucosa anterior to the anterior tonsillar pillars usually is not involved. Fever and dysphagia are usually the chief complaints. The lesions stand out as gray-white, discrete fibrinous lesions against a diffuse erythematous mucosa.

Like hand-foot-and-mouth disease, herpangina is a coxsackievirus disease caused by coxsackievirus A and B (A2–6, A8, A10, and unspecified B-type viruses); it is transmitted via direct salivary contact, aerosolized droplets, and possibly oral-fecal contamination. The viruses establish an infection by systemic viremia, hence the abrupt onset of fever and a selection for the oropharynx probably due to its optimal temperature.

DIFFERENTIAL DIAGNOSIS ▶

The finding of fever with lesions limited to the posterior oral cavity and oropharyngeal area should rule out diseases with prominent skin lesions such as *varicella* (chickenpox), and *hand-foot-and-mouth disease*. These findings should also distinguish it from diseases that are predominantly limited to the true oral cavity, such as *primary herpetic gingivostomatitis*. However, the presentation does initially resemble a *streptococcal pharyngitis* and *tonsillitis* and may be similar to early *diphtheria*.

DIAGNOSTIC WORK-UP ▶

Most cases are diagnosed by their clinical presentation. Equivocal cases may need confirmation by serum anticoxsackievirus determinations or by viral cultures from fresh lesions. It is important, however, to take bacterial throat cultures to rule out a primary streptococcal pharyngitis or a secondary streptococcal infection, which places the child at risk for rheumatic fever.

HISTOPATHOLOGY ▶

Because this is a mild disease of short duration affecting the most posterior aspects of the oral cavity, histology does not play a role in the diagnosis of herpangina. The oral lesions do form intraepithelial vesicles.

TREATMENT ▶

Herpangina requires no specific treatment other than parental reassurance and supportive care in the form of hydration, antipyretics, analgesics, and rest. If the disease is complicated by a streptococcal pharyngitis, oral phenoxymethyl penicillin (Pen-Vee K, Wyeth-Ayerst), 250 mg four times daily, is required for 10 days. In penicillin-allergic patients, oral erythromycin ethyl succinate (EES, Abbott) is a good substitute at 200 to 400 mg four times daily for 10 days. An alternative to penicillin, oral cefuroxime (Ceftin, Glaxo Wellcome), 125 mg twice daily for 10 days, is also effective.

PROGNOSIS ▶

Herpangina usually resolves as a result of host immune responses within 2 weeks.

HIV Disease and AIDS

**CLINICAL PRESENTATION AND
PATHOGENESIS** ▶

Human immunodeficiency virus (HIV) infection and acquired immunodeficiency syndrome (AIDS) represent two ends of a spectrum of one infectious disease that first became known to medical scientists in 1980. Between 1980 and 2000, the infectious agent, its mode of transmission, its mode of cellular entry, and its transmissibility were thoroughly documented, and potent antiretroviral medications were developed to control the effects of this disease. During the same period, a combination of preventive measures and lifestyle modifications reduced both individual risk and the rate of disease transmission. This is an amazing accomplishment in a short 20-year span.

Today, HIV infection is confirmed either by the identification of HIV antibodies in the serum or, more commonly, by measurement of viral load, which identifies the level of HIV RNA in copies/mL. The progression of HIV infection to AIDS is defined by CD4 cell counts of less than 200/mm^3, or about 14% of the usual number of CD4 T-helper lymphocytes.

Epidemiology of HIV

According to World Health Organization (WHO) estimates, more than 35 million people were infected with HIV as of January 1, 2000; about 20% of these were children and 45% were women. Statistics continue to show that individuals in the 15- to 49-year age group, who are among the most sexually active, are at highest risk, and that 1% of the individuals in this age group are already HIV positive. HIV/AIDS currently ranks as the seventh leading cause of death worldwide, immediately behind diarrheal diseases and not far behind better known causes such as heart disease, cancer, and trauma.

The WHO statistics, which were gathered in July of 1998, indicate that as part of the North American statistical group, the United States ranks fourth in the overall number of HIV infections reported, accounting for only 2% of cases worldwide; sub-Saharan Africa (67%) and South and Southeast Asia (20%) rank first and second, respectively (Table 2-5). It is estimated that 89% of the population of sub-Saharan Africa is HIV positive.

In the United States, 80% of all HIV transmissions are due to men having sex with men (MSM, 49%), injection drug use (IDU, 25%), or both (MSM and IDU, 6%) (Table 2-6). Other means of transmission include heterosexual sex (9.5%), hemophilia treatment (1%), transfusion (1%), and other/unknown (8%).

HIV/AIDS Infection and the Natural Disease Course

After gaining access to the bloodstream, viable HIV viruses initially become entrapped in the regional lymph nodes. In terms of size, the viral particles are 100 nm (or 0.1 μm), much smaller than bacteria, which are about 1 μm (10 times larger) or human lymphocytes, which are 15 μm (150 times larger). The presence of the virus evokes an antigenic stimulation, which activates the CD4 T-helper cell lymphocytes and macrophages. These cells secrete growth factors and other cytokines, such as tumor necrosis factor (TNF) and interleukin-6, leading to a multiplication of the CD4 cells. Paradoxically, this increases the number of cells vulnerable to the HIV virus, thereby increasing the viral load itself.

To infect the CD4 lymphocyte, the HIV virus adheres to its surface via interaction between the viral gp120 surface glycoprotein and a CD4 cell surface membrane receptor, which serves as the point of entry for the viral RNA. However, this surface interaction cannot occur without the stabilization effects of a coreceptor in the form of a transmembrane protein that was initially known as *fusin* but now is more accurately described as the chemokine receptor-5 or the CCR-5 receptor. Together, these two unique receptors to the CD4 cell permit the injection of single-strand HIV RNA into the CD4 cytoplasm. In addition, it is likely that the reverse transcriptase enzyme (RNA-dependent DNA polymerase) and transfer RNA (tRNA) are also injected into the CD4 cell to prime viral replication (Fig 2-110).

Table 2-5 Distribution of HIV/AIDS worldwide

No. of cases reported	Percentage	Region
22.5 million	67	Sub-Saharan Africa
6.7 million	20	South and Southeast Asia
1.4 million	4	Latin America
890,000	2	North America
560,000	1	East Asia and Pacific
500,000	1	Western Europe
330,000	0.9	Caribbean
270,000	0.01	Eastern Europe and Central Asia
210,000	0.06	North Africa and Middle East
12,000	0.01	Australia and New Zealand

Table 2-6 Vectors of HIV transmission in the United States

No. of cases reported	Percentage	Exposure categories (as of 7/31/98)
309,247	49	Male to male contact (MSM)
161,872	25	Injection drug user (IDU)
58,884	9.5	Heterosexual contact
40,594	6	MSM/IDU
8,214	1	Transfusion related
4,689	1	Hemophiliac
49,560	8	None of the above

Within 2 weeks, the HIV virus will have repeatedly replicated itself in the many CD4 cells that will have proliferated by means of the antigenic stimulus and migrated throughout the body. At first the CD4 cells will mount a humoral and cellular attack on the HIV virus, reducing its numbers in serum and partially controlling the infection. However, the continued replication of viruses in the lymph nodes will continue subclinically. Initially thought to represent a latency period, during which time the flu-like symptoms of HIV inoculation and lymphadenopathy cease, it is now known that viral numbers (viral load) actually increase during this period.

Viruses present in the plasma come from recently infected circulating CD4 cells that replicate HIV viruses in great numbers. They produce 93% of circulating viruses and are the driving force behind the disease. In addition, however, many noncirculating and slow-turnover cells, such as macrophages in lymph nodes, the central nervous system, testicles, and other tissues, also harbor viruses but are not stimulated to replicate, thereby serving as reservoirs of HIV. These so-called immunologic sanctuaries are an important factor in the treatment of HIV because of the difficulty of most antiretroviral drugs to penetrate such tissues.

After several years, the continuously high rate of HIV replication eventually destroys the lymph nodes, which until then had kept the virus relatively contained by means of the controlling effects of humoral (antibody) and cellular (cytokine and engulfment) responses that subdued viral reproduction. At this point the virus will reproduce itself unchecked, leading to an explosion of viral numbers (viral load increases) and a reduction in the number of CD4 cells. When the CD4 cell blood count falls below

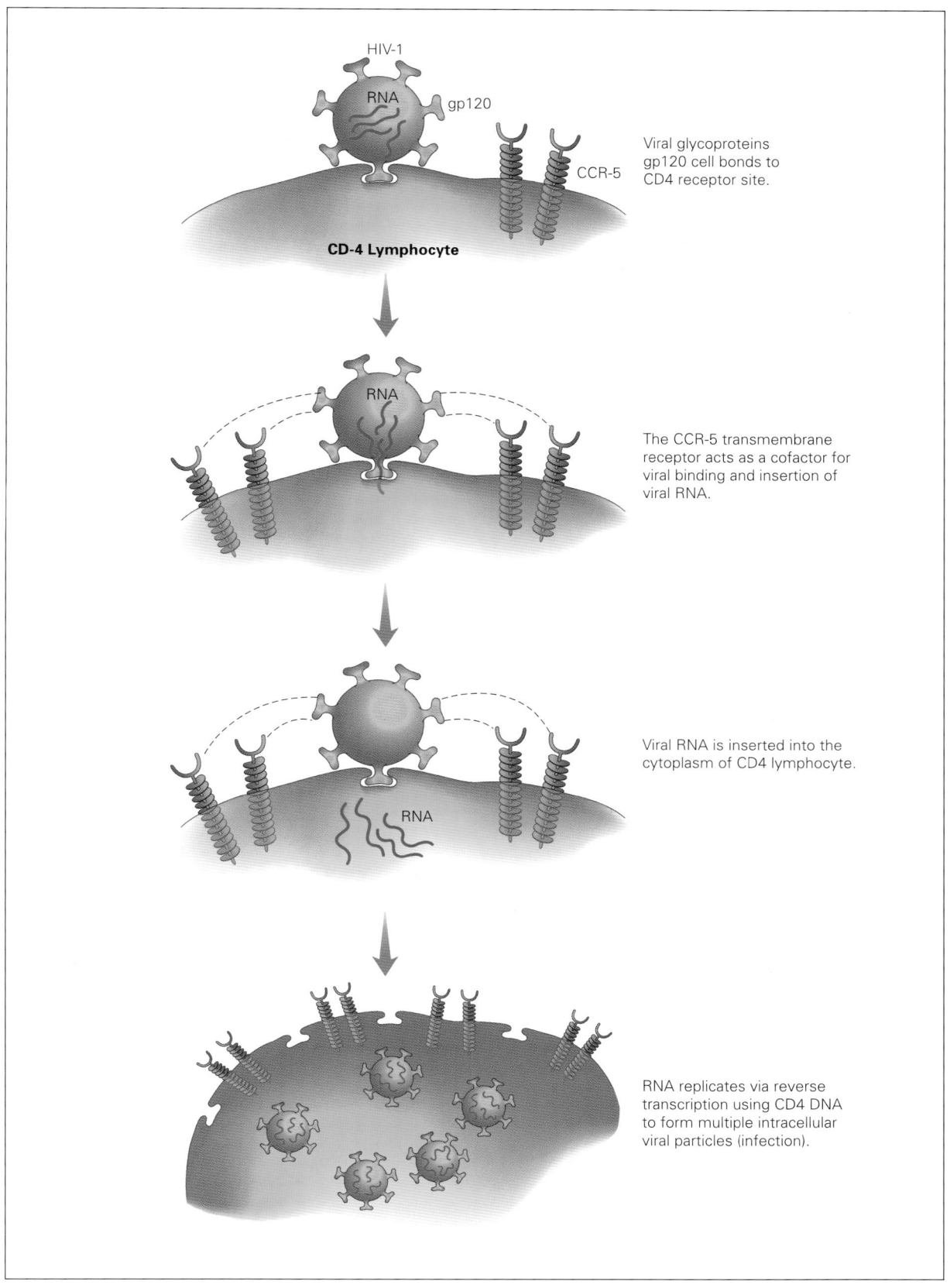

HIV-1

RNA   gp120

CCR-5

Viral glycoproteins gp120 cell bonds to CD4 receptor site.

CD-4 Lymphocyte

RNA

The CCR-5 transmembrane receptor acts as a cofactor for viral binding and insertion of viral RNA.

RNA

Viral RNA is inserted into the cytoplasm of CD4 lymphocyte.

RNA replicates via reverse transcription using CD4 DNA to form multiple intracellular viral particles (infection).

Fig 2-110 The mechanism by which the HIV virus inoculates a human CD4 lymphocyte involves direct binding of the gp120 proteins to the CD4 cell and stabilization of the viral binding by the CCR-5 coreceptor.

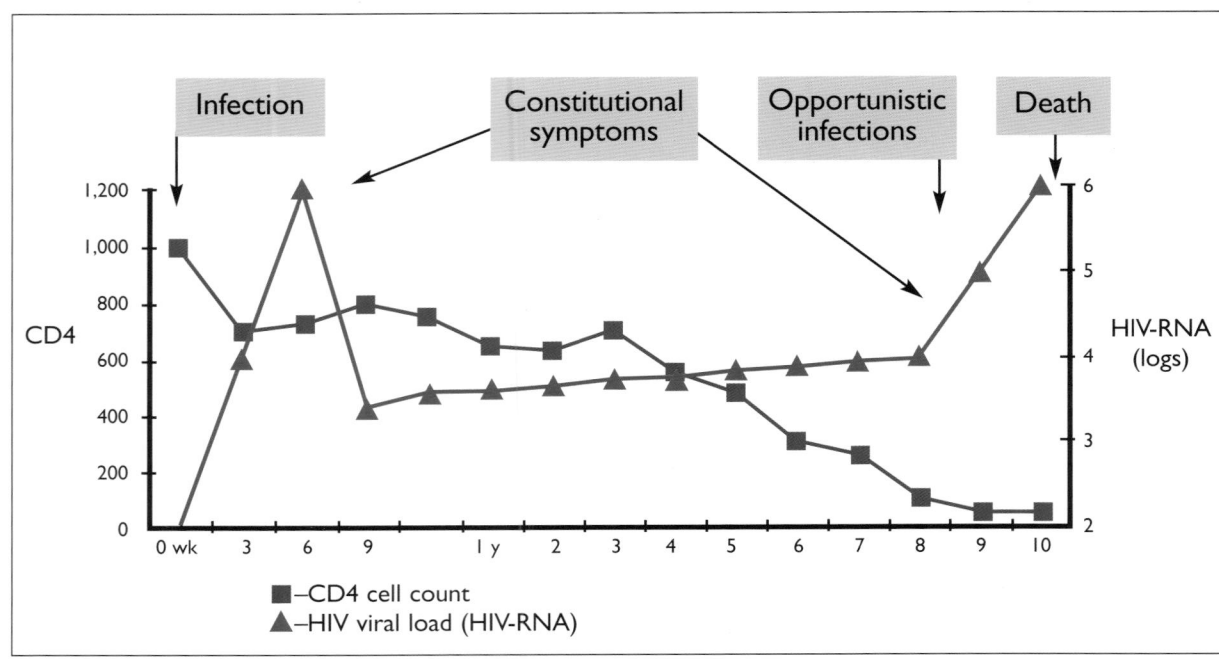

Fig 2-111 Approximate time chart of CD4 cell counts and viral load from initial infection to death in an untreated HIV infection.

200/mm³, the individual is diagnosed with AIDS, at which point secondary opportunistic infections, such as candidiasis, hairy leukoplakia, pneumocystis carinii pneumonia (PCP), and neoplasias begin to emerge. When left untreated, the course from HIV inoculation to AIDS takes about 7 to 10 years (Fig 2-111).

Position of Individuals in the HIV/AIDS Continuum

Normally, the oral and maxillofacial specialist will not be directly involved in the initial diagnosis or complex treatment of HIV-infected individuals. However, he or she will often manage HIV-related complications by providing therapies or accomplishing surgeries. This requires an assessment of the stage and degree of control of the HIV infection and can be accomplished with knowledge of two specific laboratory values—the viral load and the CD4 count—in addition to those commonly used to assess surgical/anesthetic risk. As stated earlier, the viral load refers to HIV RNA in copies/mL of blood and serves as an index of the rate of HIV progression. Viral load values should be assessed every 2 to 4 months to monitor any changes, since increasing viral loads imply a faster progression of HIV to AIDS, a lack of response to antiretroviral treatment, or a resistance to antiretroviral treatment, each of which will increase the risk of complications and death if surgery is accomplished. The CD4 cell count refers to the absolute number of CD4 cells and serves as a yardstick of the individual's progression toward AIDS and its related opportunistic infections and neoplasms, and of the severity of AIDS (if the count is under 200/mm³). The lower the CD4 count, the higher the risk of complications and death should surgeries become necessary. To better understand these values, they can be conceptualized by imagining the HIV-infected individual running toward a cliff (Fig 2-112). The speed at which the individual runs is represented by the viral load; when he or she reaches a CD4 cell count of 200 cells/mm³, a mile marker in the individual's path indicates actual AIDS. The point at which the individual reaches the cliff and falls to his or her death occurs soon after he or she passes the 200/mm³ milestone, somewhere around 50/mm³.

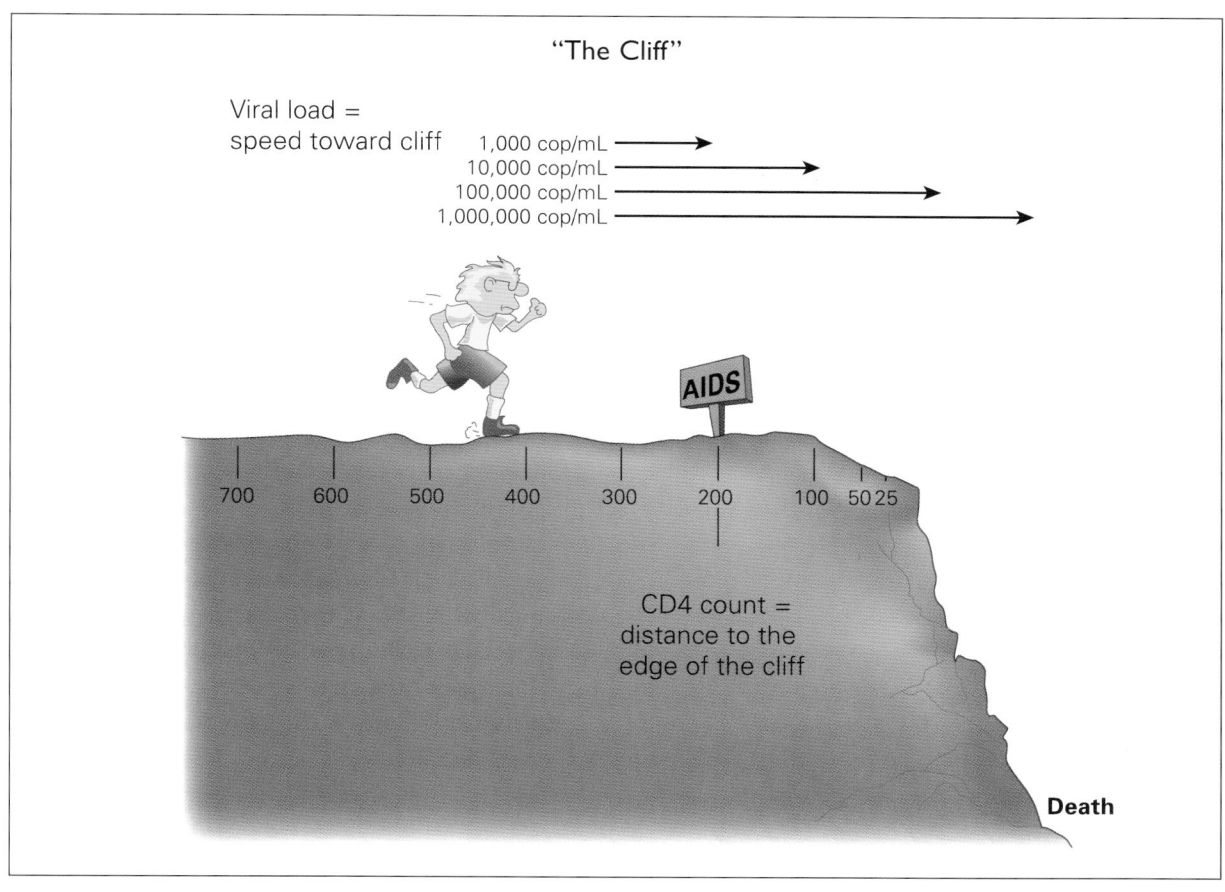

Fig 2-112 The advance of untreated HIV infection to AIDS and on to death can be conceptualized as an individual running to the edge of a cliff. The speed at which he or she runs is the viral load and a mile marker at 200 CD4 cells/mm³ is the signpost of actual AIDS.

Current HIV/AIDS Therapies

At the time of this writing, a catch phrase for treating HIV/AIDS is to treat with a lot of HAART, which stands for *highly active antiretroviral therapy* and refers to combinations of drugs that include a protease inhibitor and/or a non-nucleoside reverse transcriptase inhibitor (NNRTI). The goal of this therapy is to reduce the viral load to undetectable levels so that, at most, only those viruses in the immunologic sanctuaries remain. Combinations of three drugs—zidovudine (ZDV or AZT), lamivudine (3TC), and indinavir (IDV)—have produced undetectable viral loads in 75% to 80% of individuals, and this therapy remains encouraging.

The antiviral HIV drugs currently in use are:

1. Nucleoside analogs

These were the first drugs used to treat and prevent HIV infection. Represented by ZDV or AZT, zalcitabine (DDS), didanosine (DDI), and 3TC, these drugs competitively inhibit viral replication by competing with natural nucleosides when the HIV virus synthesizes proviral DNA using its reverse transcriptase enzyme. As a result, the faulty proviral DNA does not transcribe HIV RNA, and replication is blocked. However, their effectiveness is reduced by competitive inhibition, whereby the viral speed of reproduction incorporates natural nucleosides so quickly that it overcomes the drug. Effectiveness is also reduced by specific mutations to resistant forms.

2. Protease inhibitors

The protease inhibitors represented a revolution in antiretroviral therapy when they were introduced in 1995, and they remain a focal point of therapy today. Represented by saquinavir (SAQ), ritonavir (RIT), IDV, nelfinavir (NFV), and amprenavir (APV), these drugs are both competitive and noncompetitive inhibitors of HIV replication, acting on the HIV protease enzyme. The HIV protease enzymes are necessary for viral infectivity; they act in the later phases of virion maturity, when various glycoproteins necessary for infection are assembled. The protease inhibitors work by creating an immature noninfective virus that the immune system can destroy, and since the structure of HIV proteases is unique to retroviruses and differs significantly from that of human proteases, human toxicity is minor or nonexistent. However, used alone, even these potent antiretroviral drugs are not completely effective. Various mutations in the HIV proteases have already conferred resistance to some drugs, which explains initial responses followed by an increase in viral load.

3. Non-nucleoside reverse transcriptase inhibitors

The NNRTIs have received FDA approval only for the treatment of HIV infection in combination with other drugs of a different type, owing to the rapid emergence of drug resistance to NNRTIs when used alone. (This well-known microorganism response to a single drug recalls to mind the rapid emergence of resistant mycobacteria to isoniazid (INH) when used alone to treat tuberculosis.) Represented by nevirapine (NVP), delavirdine (DLV), and efavirenz (EFV), this group acts as noncompetitive inhibitors of the reverse transcriptase enzyme. Essentially, these agents bind directly and irreversibly to the active site of the enzyme to deactivate it and thus prevent the synthesis of proviral DNA.

Oral Manifestations of HIV and AIDS

The oral and maxillofacial specialist must be trained to recognize the oral and head-neck manifestations of HIV infection and AIDS (Fig 2-113). The following is a brief overview of the more common oral manifestations of AIDS and some palliative measures that can be taken. However, it is important to remember that the best controlling measure is systemic antiretroviral therapy to reduce the HIV viral load.

1. Candidiasis

Oral candidiasis is common in HIV infection and may be caused by several species. Active oral candidiasis is best treated with oral nystatin suspension, 500,000 U three times a day swish and spit or swish and swallow, combined with fluconazole (Diflucan, Pfizer), 100 mg by mouth daily. Diflucan can be discontinued if or when the oral lesions improve and if those at other sites are resolved.

2. HIV lymphadenitis

A generalized lymphadenopathy may be seen early or late in the HIV continuum. Later in the course of the disease lymph node biopsies may be necessary to rule out lymphoma or scrofula.

3. Kaposi sarcoma

Today, Kaposi sarcoma is much less pervasive in HIV/AIDS than it was in the 1980s. The explanation for this decline is unknown but is probably related to a mutation in the HIV virus or to improved control of secondary viral infections in the MSM group, which was virtually the only group to develop Kaposi lesions associated with HIV/AIDS. In HIV/AIDS, oral Kaposi lesions most commonly appear on the palate (Fig 2-114). They may first appear in the submucosa as a bluish macular area or develop into a reddish-purplish mass. While a reduction in the viral load will often reduce the size of the Kaposi lesions, direct therapy with intralesional injections of vinblastine (0.1 to 0.5 mg/mL) will produce this effect more directly. In addition, local radiotherapy of 1,800 cGy is effective, as well as local excision if the lesions are accessible to surgery. Systemic chemotherapy is a last resort, but graded responses are known with varying doses of doxorubicin (Adriamycin, Pharmacia and Upjohn).

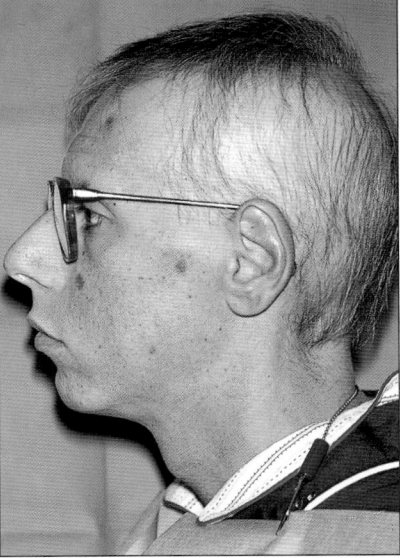

Fig 2-113 An individual with HIV/AIDS who has a CD4 count of 75. Weight loss, alopecia, and focal Kaposi sarcoma lesions of skin are evident.

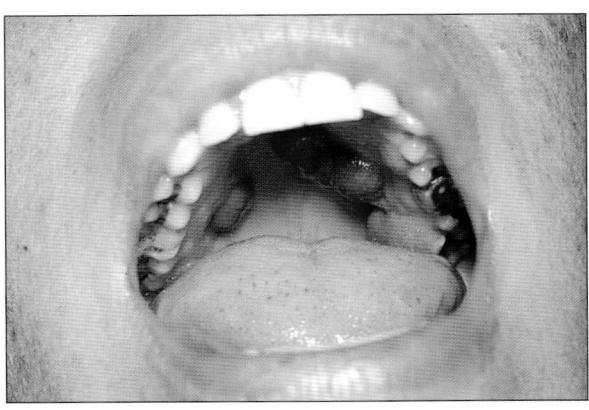

Fig 2-114 Oral Kaposi sarcoma lesions are commonly seen on the palate, are red-blue in color, and may appear either as an exophytic mass or as a submucosal lesion resembling ecchymosis.

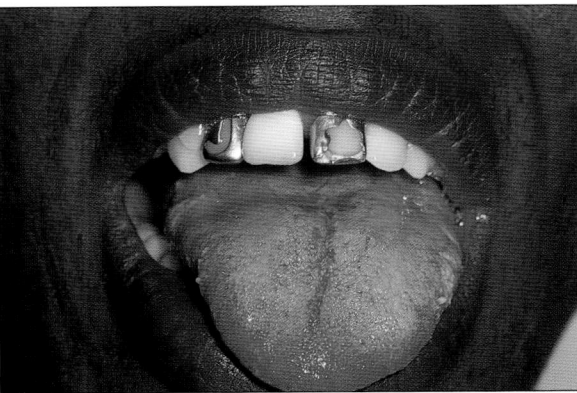

Fig 2-115 Hairy leukoplakia is seen as short, white, hair-like strands on the tongue in this individual.

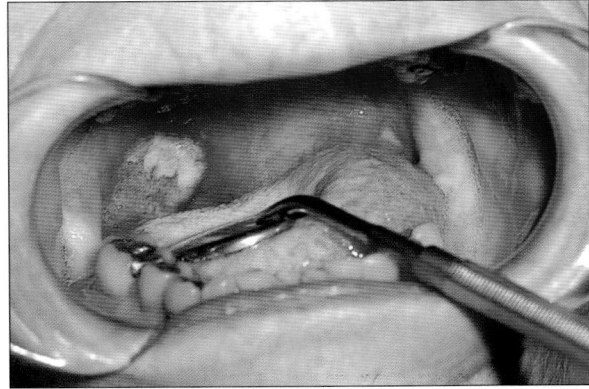

Fig 2-116 Numerous oral infections occur in HIV/AIDS individuals. Here a large aphthous-like ulcer is apparent on the soft palate—anterior tonsillar pillar.

4. Hairy leukoplakia

Hairy leukoplakia represents another opportunistic infection, in this case by the Epstein-Barr virus. The lateral border and dorsum of the tongue are the most commonly affected sites (Fig 2-115), although the floor of the mouth and the buccal mucosa may be involved as well. The lesions appear as short, white strands that project from the surface epithelium. Once thought to be an early sign of AIDS, hairy leukoplakia is now understood to be only one of many opportunistic infections that may develop as the CD4 count approaches 200/mm^3. There is no specific treatment for hairy leukoplakia other than systemic antiretroviral therapy.

5. Oral infections

A whole host of oral infections may be seen, and a more rapid advancement of each type has been reported. Those most commonly seen in HIV/AIDS are aphthous ulcers (Fig 2-116), so-called HIV gingivitis and HIV periodontitis, recurrent herpes simplex lesions, herpes zoster, cytomegalic virus infec-

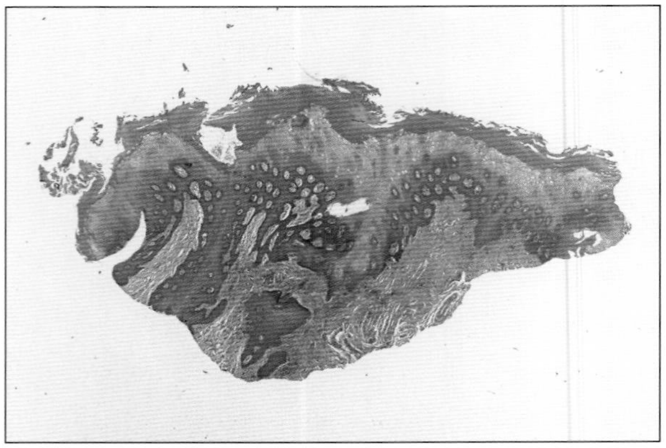

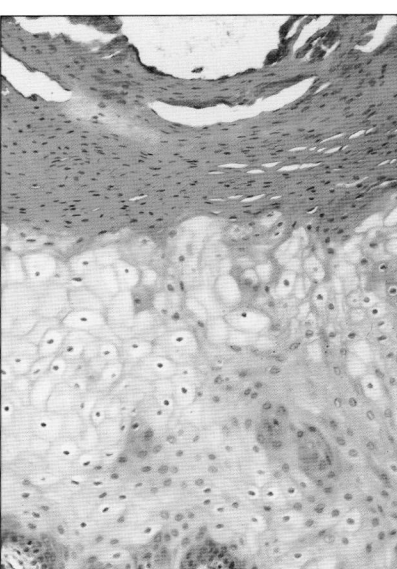

Fig 2-117 Low-power view of hairy leukoplakia showing an irregular surface, hyperparakeratosis, acanthosis, and a lack of underlying chronic inflammation.

Fig 2-118 High-power view of Fig 2-117 showing hyperparakeratosis. Below the parakeratin layers, epithelial cells with pyknotic nuclei and clear halos (koilocytic cells) are present. These are identified by the pale area in Fig 2-117.

tions, and even osteomyelitis. All are treated as they are in the non-HIV patient, but treatments may be more intensive and need to continue for longer durations.

6. HIV parotitis

This entity, which is discussed in detail in Chapter 11, represents the development of multiple lymphoepithelial cysts and generalized lymphocytic infiltrations of the parotids. It is usually expansile and painful and is treated with either superficial parotidectomies or with radiotherapy of 1,800 cGy to 2,400 cGy.

HISTOPATHOLOGY ▶

In hairy leukoplakia, the surface of the specimen is covered by a thick layer of parakeratin, which may have surface projections. Below the parakeratin are balloon cells with pyknotic nuclei surrounded by clear areas. Called *koilocytes* (hollow cells), they tend to be seen in viral infections. Some cells may show peripheral rimming of nuclear chromatin. The epithelium is also acanthotic. The corium is either free of inflammation or contains a minimal number of inflammatory cells (Figs 2-117 and 2-118). Many cases will also have candidal hyphae within the parakeratin. Ultrastructural and immunopathologic studies have confirmed the presence of Epstein-Barr virus. The histologic features of other entities are discussed elsewhere in this text.

Condyloma Acuminatum

CLINICAL PRESENTATION AND PATHOGENESIS ▶

The most common oral presentation of condyloma acuminatum, a viral, sexually transmitted disease, is that of a young man with soft, wart-like exophytic lesions of the oral commissure and tongue (Fig 2-119). Other oral lesions may also be present in the floor of the mouth, gingiva, or upper lip. The lesions will be asymptomatic but noticed by the patient. There is usually a concomitant penile lesion on either the shaft or the glans (Figs 2-120a and 2-120b). In women, who represent only 8% to 10% of oral condyloma acuminatum cases, there will be concomitant lesions on the labia and/or vulva. In either sex, there may be similar anal lesions. Homosexual men have a particularly high incidence of anal lesions.

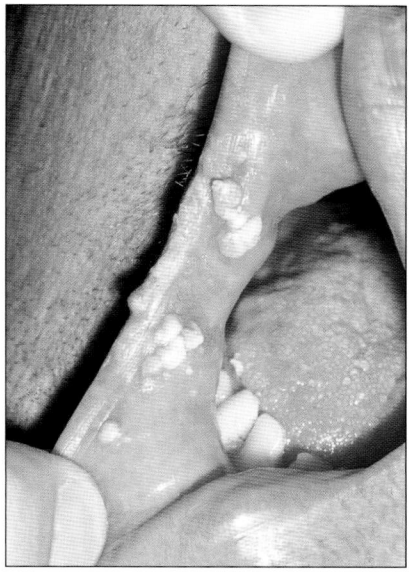 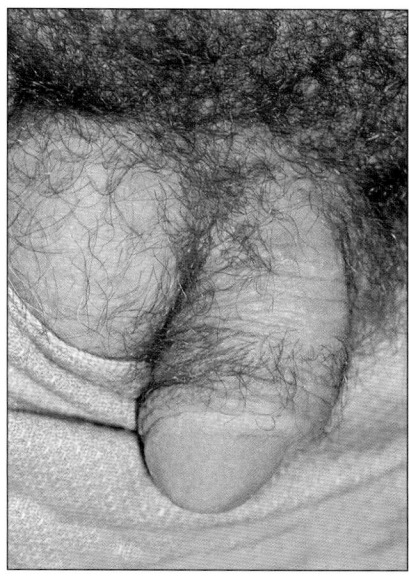 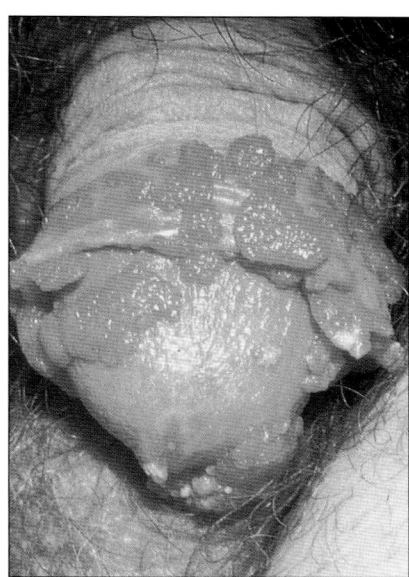

Fig 2-119 Warty lesions of condyloma acuminatum on the commissure, buccal mucosa, and tongue.

Fig 2-120a Subtle condyloma acuminatum lesion on the shaft of the penis.

Fig 2-120b Multiple condyloma acuminatum lesions on glans, shaft, and tip of the penis.

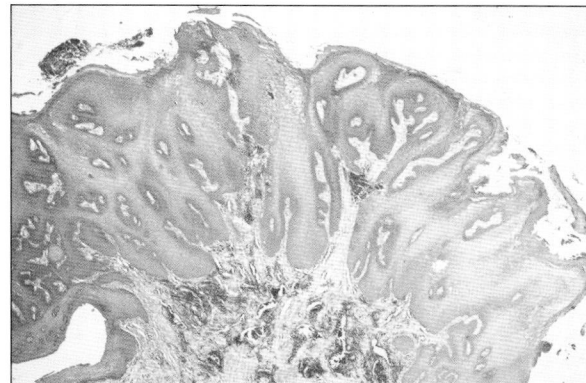

Fig 2-121 Condyloma acuminatum showing acanthosis.

Condyloma acuminatum is also called "venereal warts" or "genital warts." They represent true warts because of their viral etiology, which is the human papillomavirus (HPV) group, specifically subtypes 6 and 11. This DNA virus is highly transmissible. It penetrates the outer parakeratin or orthokeratin surfaces of moist, warm mucosa and skin areas. It infects the nucleus of squamous cells and produces a proliferation recognized as a condyloma or wart.

DIFFERENTIAL DIAGNOSIS ▶

Individual lesions will resemble a *squamous papilloma* or a *verrucous vulgaris* (oral wart). Multiple lesions may resemble a premalignant *verrucous hyperplasia*, a *verrucous carcinoma*, or even an *exophytic squamous cell carcinoma*. Condyloma acuminatum also bears a clinical resemblance to the focal epithelial thickenings seen in *focal epithelial hyperplasia* (*Heck disease*).

DIAGNOSTIC WORK-UP ▶

The diagnosis of condyloma acuminatum is made primarily by the appearance and location of characteristic lesions. Biopsy of the condyloma will rule out the other entities on the differential list and may or may not show enough evidence of intranuclear changes to confirm the diagnosis.

HISTOPATHOLOGY ▶

This verrucous lesion is characterized by marked acanthosis with elongation and broadening of the rete ridges (Fig 2-121). Hyperkeratosis or hyperparakeratosis is not usually present. Mitoses are frequent. Cells with pyknotic nuclei and perinuclear halos are typical and suggest viral involvement. However, mucosal epithelium often shows vacuolization under normal circumstances.

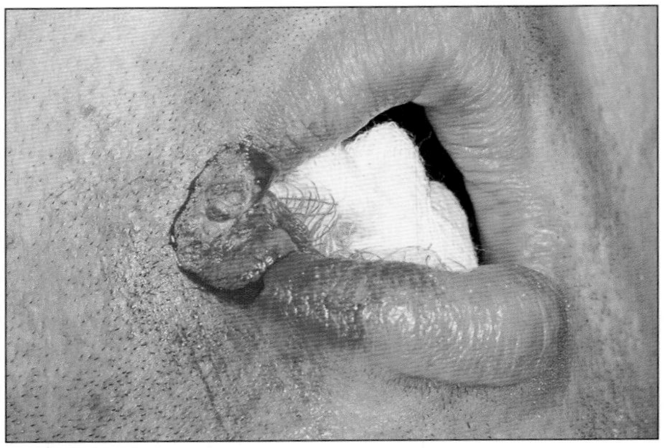

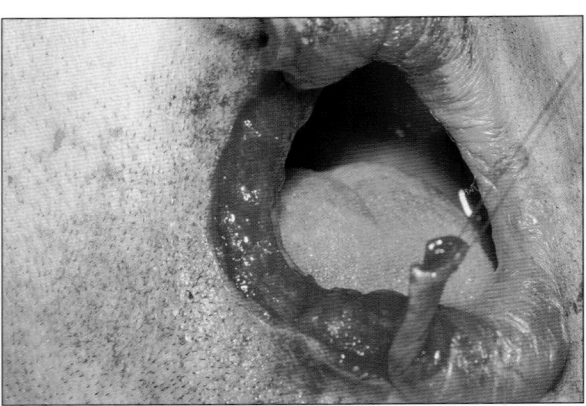

Fig 2-122a Local excision of oral lesion is the preferred treatment of condyloma acuminatum.

Fig 2-122b Excision of condyloma acuminatum will usually require local flap reconstruction. Here a vermilion advancement flap is developed.

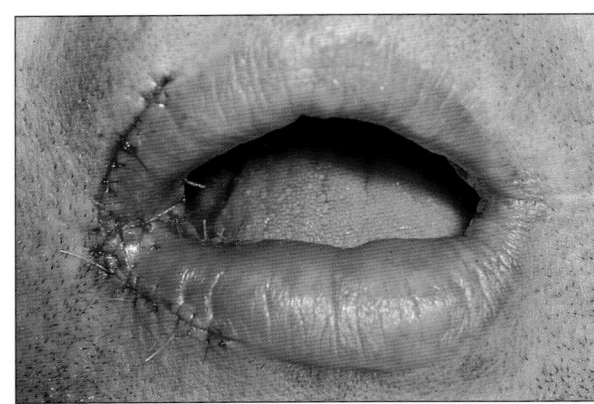

Fig 2-122c Reconstruction of the vermilion and right commissure after a condyloma acuminatum excision.

TREATMENT ▶

The oral and perioral lesions must be treated after the genital and anal lesions have been treated in order to prevent reinfection from hand to mouth transmission. In addition, the sexual partners of the patient must be treated concomitantly or a second round of transmission will occur. Oral and anal lesions are best treated with surgical excision (Figs 2-122a to 2-122c). Some surgeons prefer cryotherapy, the CO_2 laser, or electrodesiccation over scalpel excision. Each can be effective if all the lesions are removed.

The lesions are superficial and are, therefore, excised with peripheral margins at their base and to a depth within the submucosa. Penile and other genital lesions may also be excised but are more frequently treated with 25% podophyllum resin in a tincture of benzoin. Podophyllum resin is a 25% concentrate that may be applied every 2 to 3 weeks. The purified active compound of podophyllum, podofilox (Condylox, Oclassen), is available for application twice daily for three consecutive days per week for 4 to 6 weeks. Longer applications risk necrosis of normal tissues. In addition, podophyllum is not indicated in pregnant women.

An alternative topical application is 50% trichloroacetic acid (TCA), which can be effective, but treatment is painful and may damage surrounding tissues. Imiquimod (Aldara, 3M) is a 5% cream that induces local interferon as an antiviral cytokine. It is 75% effective in women but only 40% effective in men, presumably because of better tissue absorption through the thinner and moister tissue of the vulva and labial mucosa. It is applied once daily for three alternating days per week. Because of its high response rate in women, it is recommended for use in pregnancy over the riskier podophyllum.

PROGNOSIS ▶

Recurrent lesions are common with all treatment modalities. Some recurrent lesions arise from infected areas that are clinically normal appearing during treatment, since the virus incubates within cells. Other recurrences are due to reinoculations from infected sexual partners or from unrecognized and untreated genital or anal lesions.

Molluscum Contagiosum

CLINICAL PRESENTATION AND
PATHOGENESIS ▶

This viral-related skin disease presents with a single or perhaps several round, dome-shaped, waxy papules 2 to 5 mm in diameter. The lesion will be raised with circular rings (umbilicated) and will often contain a caseous plug (Fig 2-123). Early lesions are firm and flesh colored. As they mature, the lesions become light gray in color and develop their caseous center. Lesions will be seen on the face, hands, lower abdomen, and genitals.

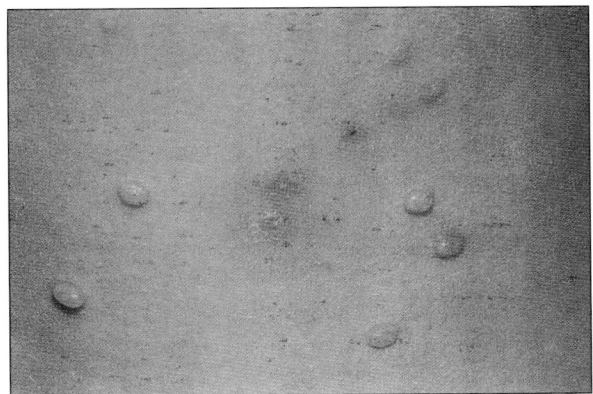

Fig 2-123 Circular rings and a central caseous plug are typical features of molluscum contagiosum.

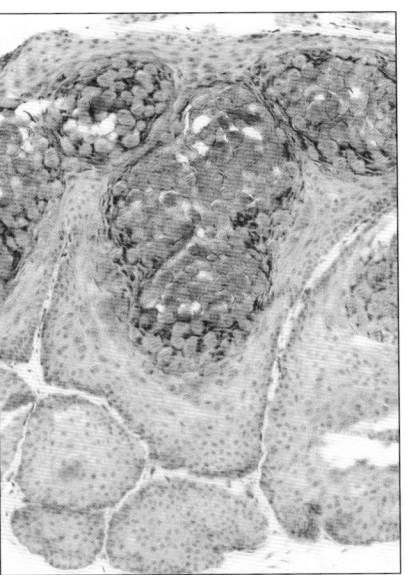

Fig 2-124a Low-power view showing the architecture of molluscum contagiosum.

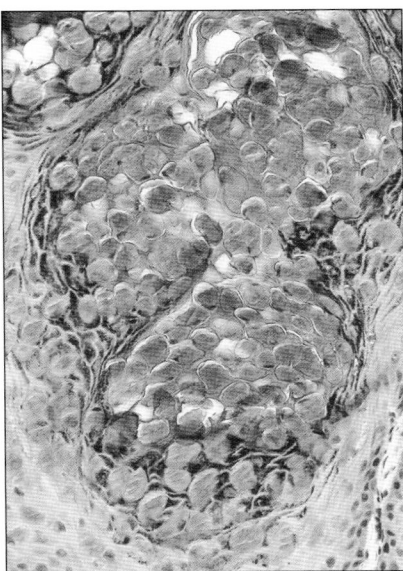

Fig 2-124b High-power view of Fig 2-124a showing the large inclusions that compress the nuclei peripherally.

Immunocompromised individuals, particularly those with HIV infection, have a high incidence of molluscum contagiosum. Some will present with numerous lesions, particularly on their facial skin and genitals. Because these individuals are immunocompromised, the natural course of the disease— spontaneous resolution and healing—does not occur. Instead, the lesions persist as chronic ulcers.

Molluscum contagiosum is caused by an unclassified pox virus. It is transmitted by direct contact with others, then spread by hand-face, hand-genitals, or hand-abdomen autoinoculation. The site of inoculation is the site of the lesion, but the incubation time is long (2 to 3 months).

DIFFERENTIAL DIAGNOSIS ▶ Individually, the skin lesions bear a resemblance to *cystic acne*. They may also mimic the course of a *keratoacanthoma*. Multiple lesions may even suggest *Torre syndrome,* one component of which is multiple keratoacanthomas. In addition, multiple keratoacanthomas are found in children (*Ferguson-Smith type*) and in adults (*Grybowski type*). Similarly, the individual lesions can appear like a *skin squamous cell carcinoma* or a *basal cell carcinoma*. Multiple lesions may even suggest *basal cell nevus syndrome*.

DIAGNOSTIC WORK-UP ▶ Diagnosis is made by microscopic examination of a single lesion or a representative lesion among many.

HISTOPATHOLOGY ▶ Low-power views show a crateriform or cup-shaped lesion in which the folded, acanthotic epithelium is pushed down into the underlying connective tissue (Fig 2-124a). In addition to this striking architecture, the cellular component is remarkable in that viral intracytoplasmic inclusions are present. These inclusions develop in the lower prickle cell layer as small ovoid eosinophilic structures. As they progress through the epithelium, they enlarge. When they reach the keratinized layer, they may measure as much as 35 μm in diameter. At this level, the eosinophilic inclusion is more basophilic, and the nucleus is compressed at the periphery of the cell (Fig 2-124b). These cells, or molluscum bodies, are released, resulting in the formation of a crater. The connective tissue shows little inflammation. If the lesion ruptures and extrudes into the connective tissue, a marked inflammatory reaction will result. Regression is accompanied by mononuclear infiltration, suggesting a cell-mediated immunologic reaction.

TREATMENT ▶ Lesions will be self-healing except in the immunocompromised host. However, treatment to more quickly eradicate the lesion and prevent further spread by autoinoculation is common. Curettage of the central core will theoretically shorten the course and may be the preferred therapy if numerous lesions

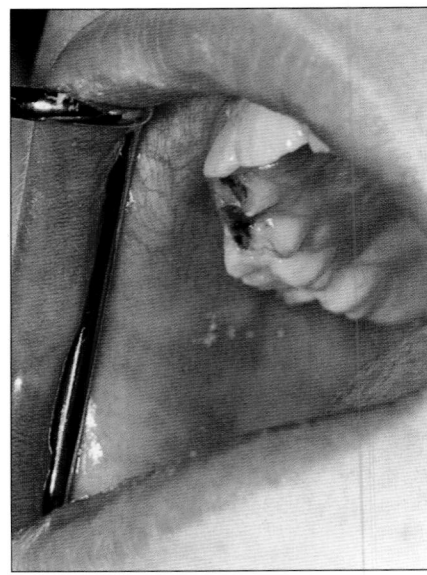

Fig 2-125 Koplik spots in the prodromal stage of measles (rubeola). (Reprinted from Bork K et al, *Diseases of the Oral Mucosa and the Lips*, with permission from WB Saunders Co.)

are present. If a single or small number is present, excision is preferred. As alternatives, liquid nitrogen freezing, electrodessication, and topical corrosive chemicals such as 25% podophyllum, applied once weekly for 3 weeks, may be used. More recently, imiquimod (Aldara, 3M), an inducer of local interleukin-2 production, has been used. It is applied 3 to 7 times weekly for 4 to 8 weeks.

PROGNOSIS ▶

Self-healing or treatment results in resolution without recurrence over 2 months. In the HIV-infected individual, immune restoration with proteinase inhibitors or other therapies will stimulate a spontaneous regression of the molluscum contagiosum.

Measles (Rubeola)

CLINICAL PRESENTATION AND PATHOGENESIS ▶

The most typical presentation of measles is a child who abruptly develops high fever (in the range of 104°F to 105°F) with nasal stuffiness, sneezing, and sore throat (called *coryza*). The child usually has a nonproductive cough, photophobia due to conjunctivitis, and often a discharge or crusting around the eyes. This set of signs and symptoms is often called the *prodrome* because it precedes any skin rash. Oral lesions called *Koplik spots* also appear during this prodrome and are pathognomonic of the disease. Koplik spots appear as flat, erythematous macules with tiny white "salt crystal" centers (Fig 2-125). They will characteristically precede the skin rash by 1 or 2 days. Koplik spots may also be seen on the conjunctiva.

The child generally will appear ill and irritable. There is usually a diffuse pharyngitis and bilateral cervical lymphadenitis. The rash will appear on the facial skin and behind the ears before spreading to the chest and trunk and then to all extremities. The skin rash will begin as pinhead-sized papules and then spread to form irregular red blotches, which may further coalesce to a more uniform erythema over a large area.

The measles virus is a DNA paramyxovirus transmitted by air–water-droplet vectors. The clinical prodrome occurs about 10 to 14 days after exposure. The infected individual is contagious from just before the prodromal stage until 4 days after the appearance of the rash. One clinical infection confers permanent immunity.

The incidence of measles in the United States took a dramatic downturn in 1963 with the federal funding of the measles, mumps, and rubella (MMR) vaccine. In 1963, about 800,000 cases were reported compared to only 1,500 cases in 1983. However, since then, the incidence has risen: More than 17,000 cases of measles were reported in 1989. This was attributable to unvaccinated children (primarily the inner-city poor) and a previously vaccinated teenage group. The first group indicates the need for inner-city children to have access to the vaccinations and the second group indicates the need for a booster vaccination in the junior high school age group. Today it is recommended that children receive their first dose at 12 to 15 months of age and a second dose at 4 to 6 years of age. Any doubt about serologic immunity can be resolved with assessment of antibody titers. When a nonimmunized individual is exposed to measles, the live virus vaccine can prevent the disease if given within 5 days of exposure. Pregnant women and immunosuppressed individuals should not receive the live virus vaccine except in rare individual circumstances.

DIFFERENTIAL DIAGNOSIS ▶

The clinical picture of an acutely ill child who develops oral lesions followed by a skin rash suggests *varicella* (*chickenpox*) and the *Stevens-Johnson syndrome variant of erythema multiforme*. If the oral lesions were overlooked, the clinical picture would resemble that of *rubella* (*German measles*) and possibly *scarlet fever*, both of which have an oral and pharyngeal erythema but no true Koplik spots.

DIAGNOSTIC WORK-UP ▶

The diagnosis is made from the history and presenting clinical characteristics. Laboratory confirmation can be gained by identifying a rise in antibody titers over several specimens taken 2 days apart. The most commonly used tests are immunofluorescent antibody and complement fixation tests. A one-time serum test that tests for measles-specific IgM antibodies is now available.

HISTOPATHOLOGY ▶

In the eruption of skin and mucosa, which represents a reaction to the development of antibody, infected epithelial cells show intracellular vacuolization, hyperkeratosis, and ultimately necrosis. The connective tissue is hyperemic and edematous, with perivascular lymphocytes and macrophages. Koplik spots show more epithelial necrosis and infiltration by neutrophils. The characteristic multinucleated giant cells of Warthin-Finkeldey are seen in hyperplastic lymphoid tissues, including tonsils and adenoids. They are usually present in the prodromal phase and disappear as antibody titers rise. These large cells have eosinophilic cytoplasm and centrally placed clusters of darkly stained nuclei.

TREATMENT ▶

Measles is self-limiting and runs a 2-week clinical course. However, the child needs to be isolated as the disease is highly transmissible to all who do not have either natural or vaccine-acquired immunity. Supportive care consisting of rest, hydration, analgesics, and antipyretics is important. Vitamin A, 400,000 U orally each day during the illness, has been shown to reduce complications. If secondary bacterial infections, such as otitis media, cervical lymphadenitis, or pneumonia, develop (15% of cases), appropriate antibiotic administration is required.

PROGNOSIS ▶

Measles is well-known to result in postdisease complications, some of which can be debilitating and life threatening. Encephalitis develops in 1:1,000 to 1:2,000 cases, with 10% to 20% of these cases eventuating in death and another 50% of these cases in mental retardation. Pneumonia occurs in 1% to 7% of patients, and other bacterial infections occur in 15% of patients. Measles during pregnancy can result in premature labor, spontaneous abortion, and low birth weight. Unlike rubella (German measles), rubeola does not have a high incidence of birth defects.

Rubella (German Measles)

CLINICAL PRESENTATION AND PATHOGENESIS ▶

The individual presenting with rubella (German measles) is usually a child or young adult who presents with fever, mild malaise, and cervical lymphadenitis. The general intensity of symptoms in rubella is less than that in rubeola (measles). The posterior lymphatic chains are usually more involved than are the anterior chains. In fact, suboccipital lymphadenopathy is common.

The face will develop a fine reddish maculopapular rash, and the palate and throat will develop an erythema. However, there will be no true Koplik spots as is seen in rubeola. The rash begins on the face, progressing down the trunk and upper extremities in 1 or 2 days. Characteristically, the rash will disappear behind its advancing front. It will fade from each area after 24 to 36 hours.

The disease, caused by a togavirus, is transmitted by air-water droplets. The virus stimulates humoral immunity of the IgM class and the IgG class, which confers postinfection permanent immunity. The MMR vaccine also confers permanent immunity. Because live attenuated rubella virus is used, it is not given to pregnant women, and birth control must be practiced for at least 3 months after vaccination.

DIFFERENTIAL DIAGNOSIS ▶

The facial rash and palatal erythema will suggest *rubeola* (*measles*). The clinician must examine the oral lesions carefully to assess the presence or absence of true Koplik spots. In addition, *scarlet fever, infectious mononucleosis*, and *adenovirus pharyngitis* will present with a similar general picture.

DIAGNOSTIC WORK-UP ▶

Rubella is one of the most worrisome diseases because of the high incidence of congenital rubella (85% in women infected during their first trimester) and the high probability that the baby will have some type of malformation. Therefore, confirmation of suspected rubella is essential. A definitive diagnosis of rubella is made with a fourfold rise in antirubella antibody levels. The rubella virus fluorescent antibody test is most often used.

HISTOPATHOLOGY ▶

Rubella is a mild, transient disease in which histology does not have a diagnostic role.

TREATMENT ▶

The patient requires no specific therapy. Rubella is a short-duration, self-limiting viral disease. Supportive care consisting of hydration, antipyretics, analgesics, and rest is recommended. It is important to isolate those infected from nonimmunized women of child-bearing age for 1 week after the rash has dissipated and to recognize that transmission may have occurred in the 1 week before the appearance of the rash.

PROGNOSIS ▶

The individual's prognosis is excellent, but transmission to a first-trimester embryo can be devastating. Such infection has been associated with congenital heart defects, cataracts, deafness, and growth retardation among other outcomes.

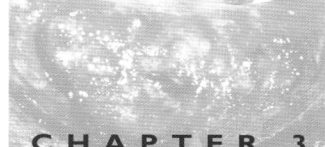

Immune-Based Diseases

► "The art of medicine is to amuse the patient while nature cures the disease."
—*Voltaire*

CHAPTER 3

Inflammatory processes, which were discussed in the last chapter, are precipitated by external factors such as microorganisms, to which, in many cases, immunologic reactions occur in response. This chapter discusses diseases precipitated by an actual disturbance in immune function, which in turn usually provokes an inflammatory response. Current knowledge suggests that these are caused by internal factors such as are seen in systemic lupus erythematosis, where autoantibodies develop against the body's own DNA. However, the possibility that immune-based diseases may sometimes be initiated by external factors, such as viruses, would mean a blurring of these seemingly distinct categories.

The mechanisms of the inflammatory diseases examined in Chapter 2 are not all clearly separated from the mechanisms of some of the immune-based diseases in this chapter. In many instances (eg, in leprosy and tuberculosis), chronic inflammation triggers an excessive immune response that damages tissue and is critical in the clinical manifestation of the disease. Immunologic responses that damage tissue and are significant in a disease process are termed *hypersensitivity reactions* in contradistinction to immune processes, which are usually protective. The immunologic protection-destruction imbalance is exemplified in tuberculosis. The variety of mechanisms involved in hypersensitivity reactions have been classified by Gell and Coombs. In the clinical situation, one type of the hypersensitivity reactions described below may trigger another. An understanding of the fundamentals of hypersensitivity reactions is helpful in appreciating the clinical and histologic changes seen in many of the diseases described in this chapter.

Hypersensitivity Reactions

Type I. Immediate or Anaphylactic Hypersensitivity

Inmmediate or anaphylactic hypersensitivity is mediated by IgE antibodies, which are bound to mast cells and basophils. When the allergen reacts with them, mediators, which are preformed and stored within the cell's granules, are released (degranulation). The reaction is immediate; the clinical effect is usually severe and dependent on the site of exposure to the antigen. Of the released inflammatory mediators, the most significant is histamine, which causes smooth muscle contraction and vascular permeability, and this in turn produces bronchoconstriction and edema. In addition, heparin, proteolytic enzymes, and neutrophil and eosinophil chemotactic factors are liberated. Mast cells also initiate formation of inflammatory mediators such as prostaglandins and leukotrienes (including slow-reacting substance of anaphylaxis). These contribute to reactions that develop several hours after exposure. Therefore, hypotension and even cardiovascular or respiratory arrest may occur.

Type II. Antibody–Cell Surface Reaction or Cytotoxic Hypersensitivity

In this type of hypersensitivity, cells are killed by the direct action of antibody against antigen on cell surfaces or in extracellular matrix, such as basement membrane. The suprabasilar split and acantholytic (degenerating) cells in pemphigus and the infrabasilar split of a partially lysed basement membrane in the pemphigoids are examples of this. The antibody may also activate complement, which leads to destruction of target cells by direct lysis (as of red blood cells in transfusion reactions) or indirectly by opsonization, as seen in some drug reactions. Other reactions are independent of complement, and the antibody that binds to the target cells may produce changes other than cell death within the cells. This can be seen in autoimmune-mediated hyperthyroidism (Grave disease), where autoantibodies bind to thyroid-stimulating hormone (TSH) receptor sites within the gland. The autoantibodies then simulate the effect of TSH itself on the thyroid and cause an excess secretion of thyroid hormone.

Type III. Immune Complex Disease

In this type of reaction, tissue damage results from antigen-antibody complexes. Antibodies are formed against circulating or tissue-derived antigen. The resultant antigen-antibody complexes may be deposited in tissue, where they inflict damage by activating complement with a resultant influx of neutrophils and macrophages, which in turn release proteases and oxygen radicals. Deposits tend to occur in areas of high pressure and filtration, such as the kidney, and in diseases in which there is abundant antigen, such as infection and autoimmune disease. These include leprosy, bacterial endocarditis, systemic lupus erythematosus, rheumatoid arthritis, dermatomyositis, and various forms of vasculitis.

Type IV. Cell-Mediated (Delayed) Hypersensitivity

Antigen-reactive cells, not antibody, are involved in cell-mediated hypersensitivities. Antigen is processed by macrophages or Langerhans cells and presented to antigen-specific T lymphocytes. The activated T cells release lymphokines, which recruit and activate lymphocytes, macrophages, and fibroblasts. Injury is induced by T cells and/or macrophages. These reactions are seen in tuberculin hypersensitivity and in granulomatous diseases, such as sarcoidosis and tuberculosis. Other examples of cell-mediated hypersensitivity include lichen planus and contact hypersensitivity, in which the Langerhans cells within the epithelium play a significant role.

Pemphigus Vulgaris

Pemphigus vulgaris is a B cell–mediated autoimmune disease in which autoantibodies develop to antigens within the desmosome-tonofilament junction of the intercellular bridges. Such autoantibodies fix complement and initiate inflammation, which causes a suprabasilar split (intraepithelial blister) as the primary pathogenesis.

CLINICAL PRESENTATION AND PATHOGENESIS ▶

Pemphigus vulgaris usually presents with painful skin and/or oral ulcers (Fig 3-1a). The lesions actually begin as short-lived vesicles that rapidly rupture because of their suprabasilar position. Skin lesions will more likely show vesicles or even bullae because of the increased thickness of skin epithelium and a greater keratin layer as compared with mucosa (Fig 3-1b). Many physicians without dental or oral and maxillofacial experience believe that pemphigus vulgaris is primarily a skin disease in which oral lesions precede skin lesions in 60% of cases. While this is correct, many patients will develop oral pemphigus lesions and no skin lesions. Such "oral pemphigus" represents a distinctive clinical form of pemphigus vulgaris. In this form, blacks are affected more frequently than are other races.

With either clinical presentation, the oral lesions are particularly painful. They form on all oral mucosal sites and may exhibit a Nikolsky sign, which is not pathognomonic of pemphigus as it can be elicited

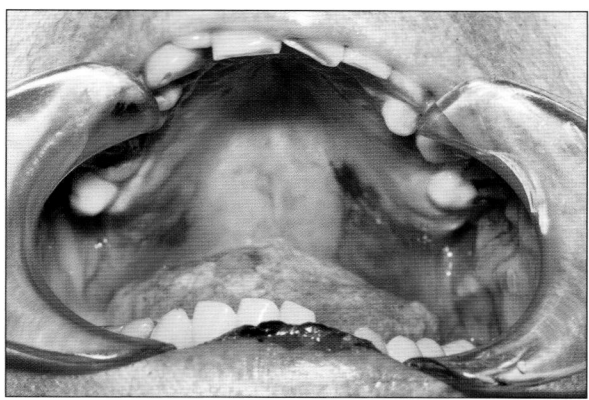

Fig 3-1a Bilateral small vesicles and larger ulcers of the oral mucosa in a case of pemphigus vulgaris.

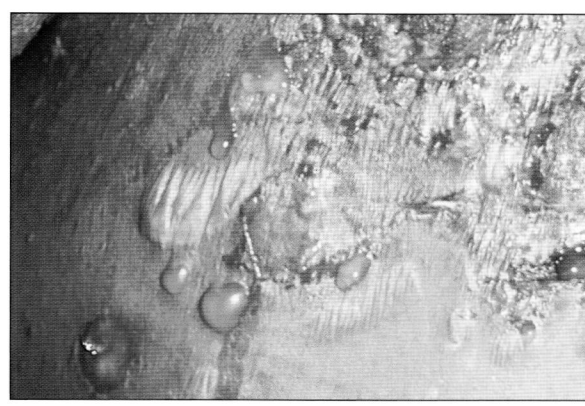

Fig 3-1b Pemphigus vulgaris of skin will show more unruptured vesicles because of the increased hyalinization and thickness of skin as compared with mucosa.

in other mucocutaneous diseases such as erythema multiforme and bullous lichen planus. Nikolsky sign identifies a loss of mucosal cohesiveness.

The individual will often present with irritability from the pain, fever from secondary infection and dehydration, and cervical lymphadenitis from secondary infections of numerous oral ulcers. The individual may not be eating because of the pain and may appear listless from dehydration, hypoglycemia, and analgesic use.

Pemphigus vulgaris is the type associated with oral mucosal lesions. *Pemphigus foliaceus* and its variant *pemphigus erythematosus* occur only on skin and have no oral mucosal involvement. The specific antigen in pemphigus vulgaris is a glycoprotein found in the desmosomes of intercellular bridges. The specific antigen in pemphigus foliaceus is a complex of several desmosomal proteins called desmoglein I, which is more common in skin epithelium, hence the limitation of this form of pemphigus to skin.

The autoantibodies (IgG type) in pemphigus vulgaris (desmoglein III) degrade the desmosome by initiating the release of intracellular lysosomes and proteolytic enzymes, causing the squamous cells to separate from each other (acantholysis). As individual squamous cells lose their intercellular bridge connections to adjacent cells, they retract into rounded cells called *acantholytic cells*. This occurs mostly at the level just superficial to the basal cells. Once the vesicle forms, its superficial nature lends itself to rapid rupture, exposing the basal cell layer where the close proximity of free nerve endings and the fixation of complement initiate inflammation and pain.

Initially, pemphigus vulgaris was described as a disease limited to people of Jewish descent. It actually occurs in nearly all ethnic and racial groups, but does have a higher incidence in people of Ashkenazic Jewish descent and in blacks. It is also associated with certain human lymphocyte antigens, specifically HLA-DR4, HLA-DQW3, HLA-DRW6, and HLA-DQWl, suggesting a genetic vulnerability in some individuals.

DIFFERENTIAL DIAGNOSIS ▶ The oral-only pemphigus presentation will include a subset of diseases that can produce painful oral lesions without concomitant skin lesions. The most common similar presentation is *erosive lichen planus*, which may be further confused with pemphigus vulgaris by its own tendency to form mucosal vesicles. However, lichen planus targets the dorsum of the tongue, buccal mucosa, and attached gingiva. Mild forms of pemphigus vulgaris may closely resemble *pemphigoid*. However, pemphigus does not usually produce a conjunctivitis, which is frequently present in pemphigoid cases, and pemphigus is much more painful than pemphigoid. A set of painful oral lesions with some vesicles is also consistent with the general picture of *primary herpetic gingivostomatitis*. *Erythema multiforme* does not usually manifest oral lesions without concomitant skin lesions and, therefore, is not as serious a consideration for this clinical picture.

The presentation of pemphigus vulgaris that expresses vesicular skin lesions in addition to painful oral lesions includes a subset of diseases that present in both areas, including *erythema multiforme*. If the skin lesions show larger vesicles suggesting bullae (greater than 2 cm in diameter), a diagnosis of *bullous pemphigoid* should be considered. If the oral lesions are not especially painful and more prominent than the skin lesions, and if the individual is older than 50 years, *pemphigoid* becomes a realistic consideration. *Bullous-erosive lichen planus* is another possibility, but lichen planus lesions of skin associated with bullous-erosive lichen planus are rare and more pruritic than painful. They are also violet-red, not the pale gray vesicles seen in pemphigus vulgaris.

DIAGNOSTIC WORK-UP ▶

The diagnosis of pemphigus vulgaris is made from a mucosal or skin biopsy that includes tissue that appears clinically normal. The oral mucosa is the preferred biopsy site. The identifiable suprabasilar separation and acantholysis is seen best in such tissues. Biopsy in an ulcerated area may be misleading because it may not show the roof of a vesicle or it may be obscured by secondary inflammation and necrosis. Obtaining two biopsy specimens or one specimen separated into two equally representative pieces is ideal. One is placed into 10% neutral-buffered formalin for hematoxylin & eosin (H&E) staining, and the other in Michel's medium for possible direct immunofluorescence studies. Direct immunofluorescence is not required in unequivocal cases but will confirm or rule out the diagnosis when there is doubt. Alternatives to Michel's medium are freezing of the specimen with liquid nitrogen or direct immunofluorescence of the fresh specimen within 4 hours. Once a tissue specimen has been placed into formalin, direct immunofluorescence studies cannot be performed on that specimen.

Indirect immunofluorescence may be performed to assess the titer of circulating autoantibodies and is thought to be an index of disease severity against which to adjust treatment dosage. However, assessing the titer of circulating antibodies is costly and is not as accurate as the patient's observed clinical disease severity.

HISTOPATHOLOGY ▶

The histopathologic features of pemphigus vulgaris reflect the action of the circulating antibody on the cell surface of the prickle cells and the consequent destruction of the desmosomes, which are responsible for maintaining the adhesion of these cells. Basal cells are attached to each other by desmosomes and can thus separate from each other. However, because they are attached to the basement membrane by hemidesmosomes, they are not affected in this area (Fig 3-2a), and the basal cells do not separate from the basement membrane. With loss of epithelial adhesion, a bulla is formed. This is seen in a predominantly suprabasilar location because this is the area of greatest cellular activity (Fig 3-2b). Within the bulla, acantholytic cells are seen. These are the detached prickle cells that have lost their polyhedral shape and become rounded. The nucleus is typically larger and hyperchromatic (Fig 3-2c). Acantholytic cells are crucial to the diagnosis. They can also be demonstrated by taking a cytologic smear of the contents of an unroofed bulla, a procedure for which Giemsa stain is usually used.

A feature that is often helpful diagnostically is the villous projections that may develop at the base of a bulla. When the surface epithelium ultimately separates, the mucosa will appear to have a surface of papillary projections lined by basal cells with some acantholytic cells (Figs 3-2d and 3-2e). Once the bulla has ruptured, the underlying connective tissue becomes densely inflamed. The eosinophilic infiltrate often seen in the skin occurs infrequently in oral mucosa. Study of perilesional tissue by direct immunofluorescence demonstrates the presence of IgG antibodies intercellularly in almost all cases (Fig 3-3). Direct immunofluorescence may remain positive even when the patient is in prolonged remission. The antigen is a 165kD protein (desmoglein), which is present within the desmosomal plaques and cell-cell adhesion junctions. Indirect immunofluorescence can also be useful. Most patients will demonstrate circulating autoantibodies, and in this disease the antibody titer loosely correlates with disease severity.

In some cases of pemphigus vulgaris, the histologic picture is primarily one of an epithelial hyperplasia that often has a verrucous surface. This develops on the villous formations described above, and the acanthotic epithelium appears to form a network (Fig 3-4). Clusters of eosinophils (abscesses) are found within the epithelium (Fig 3-5). Immunofluorescence studies yield the findings previously noted.

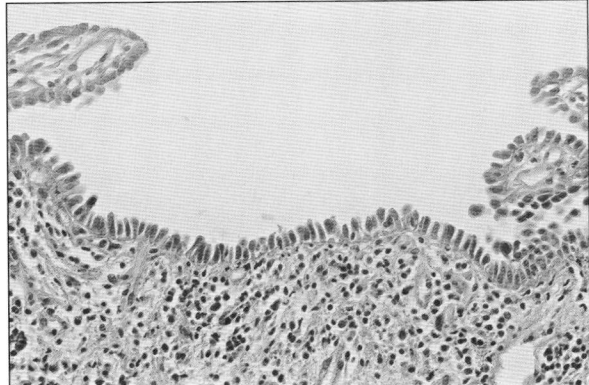

Fig 3-2a A case of pemphigus vulgaris in which the epithelium has separated suprabasilarly. The basal cells are attached to the basement membrane zone by means of hemidesmosomes. The desmosomal attachment of the basal cells to each other and to the prickle cells above have been lost. Consequently, the epithelium sloughs off and the basal cells remain attached to the basement membrane zone but separated from each other.

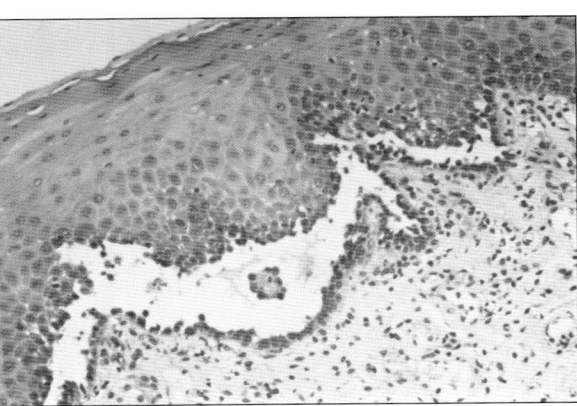

Fig 3-2b The typical suprabasilar separation seen in pemphigus vulgaris with some acantholytic cells in the vesicular fluid.

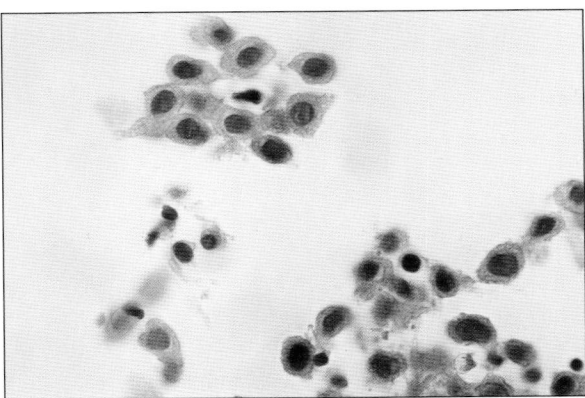

Fig 3-2c Cells from within a bulla in a case of pemphigus vulgaris. Some cells remain attached to each other and preserve their polygonal shape. Those that have separated are rounded.

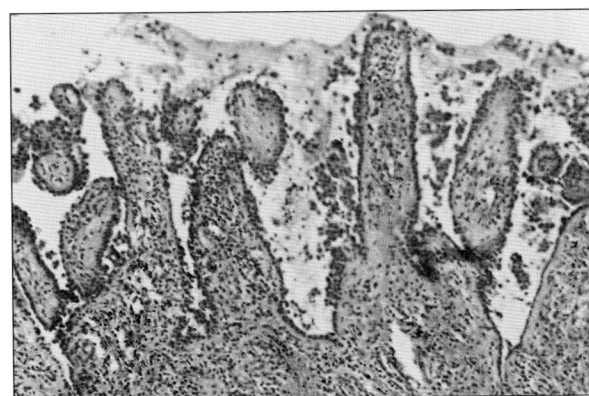

Fig 3-2d Villous projections are frequently seen in oral mucosal lesions of pemphigus vulgaris. The projections are lined by basal epithelial cells, and separated acantholytic cells are present.

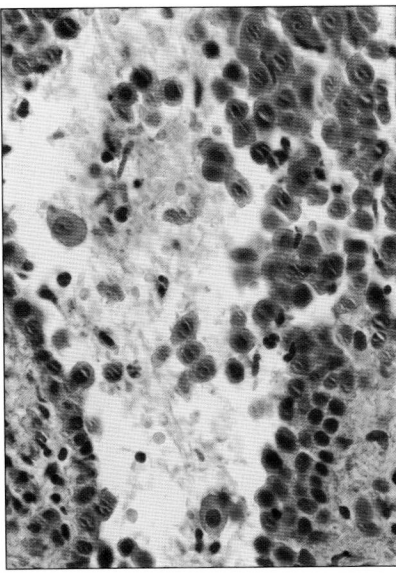

Fig 3-2e A higher-power view of Fig 3-2d shows acantholytic cells that are rounded and have dark-staining nuclei.

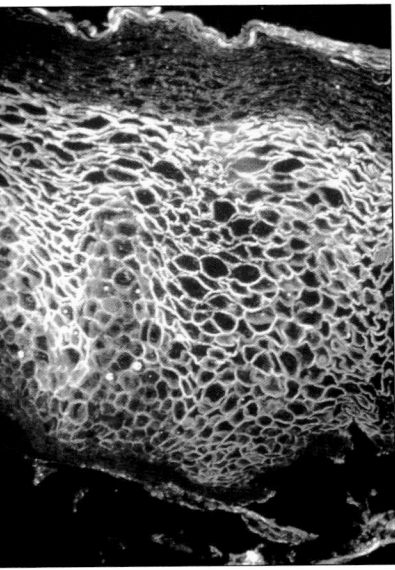

Fig 3-3 Direct immunofluorescence of a portion of mucosa from a patient with pemphigus vulgaris shows the intercellular deposition of IgG.

TREATMENT "Oral-only pemphigus vulgaris" responds well to systemic corticosteroid regimen I (see page 205). Approximately 70% of pemphigus vulgaris with both oral and skin lesions also respond to systemic corticosteroid regimen I (Figs 3-6a and 3-6b). The remaining 30% of cases of this type of pemphigus vulgaris respond incompletely to prednisone and require the addition of either cyclophosphamide (Cytoxan, Mead Johnson), 50 to 100 mg by mouth twice daily, or azathioprine (Imuran, Glaxo Wellcome), 50 to 100 mg by mouth twice daily, as in systemic corticosteroid regimen IIIB (see pages 205 to 206). In cases that remain refractory to this regimen, methotrexate, 25 mg per week, may be substituted for azathioprine, or plasmapheresis combined with azathioprine may be used as a method for reducing the corticosteroid dosage. In resistant or progressive cases or in cases in which the effects of long-term corticosteroids accumulate, dapsone, 100 mg per day, combined with either gold sodium thiomalate as used for rheumatoid arthritis or azathioprine or plasmapheresis, has also been used as a corticosteroid-sparing regimen.

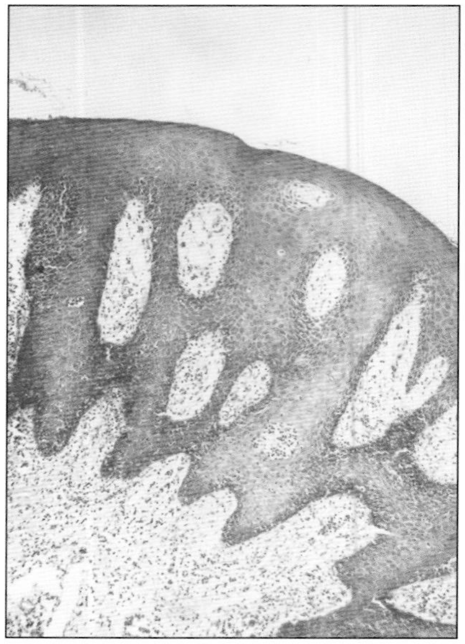

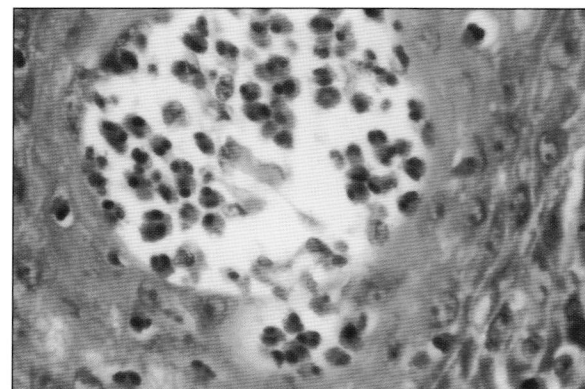

Fig 3-4 Pemphigus in which there is an epithelial hyperplasia that forms a net-like pattern.

Fig 3-5 High-power view of Fig 3-4 showing aggregates of eosinophils.

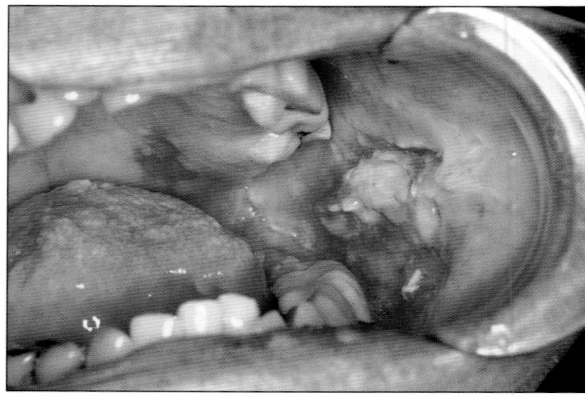

Fig 3-6a Large painful ulcers of the oral mucosa—only type of pemphigus vulgaris.

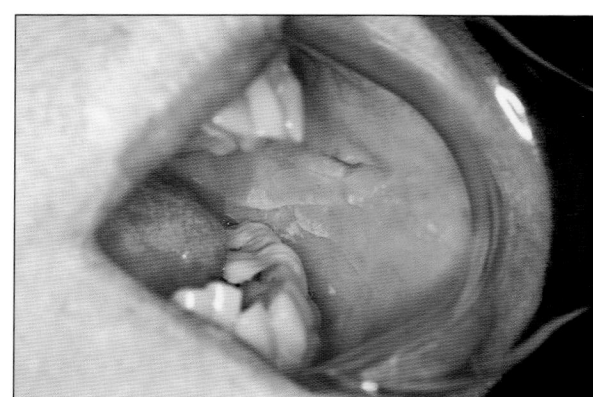

Fig 3-6b Healing and painless ulcers (shown in Fig 3-6a) after 3 weeks of treatment with corticosteroid regimen I.

Because patients will present with a recent history of a decreased oral intake and frequently secondary infection, it is often necessary first to provide hydration with intravenous fluids and to begin antibiotic therapy and pain control measures while the biopsy specimen is being processed. The clinician must resist the temptation to begin prednisone therapy before the diagnosis is confirmed. If corticosteroid therapy is initiated and the biopsy specimen is nondiagnostic, a second biopsy will have an altered tissue response, obscuring diagnosis and complicating treatment.

PROGNOSIS ▶ Untreated pemphigus vulgaris is usually fatal in 2 to 5 years. Treatment results in a residual 10% to 15% mortality rate at 15 years because of complications of long-term prednisone therapy and other immunosuppressive drugs. The most common cause of death is *Staphylococcus aureus* septicemia, which is often difficult to detect because of the immune suppression caused by concomitant corticosteroid therapy.

Oral-only pemphigus vulgaris is more responsive to therapy and has a much greater remission rate in patients either on maintenance therapy or in a drug-free state. It also has a reduced mortality rate due to a more complete response to corticosteroid therapy and hence fewer complications.

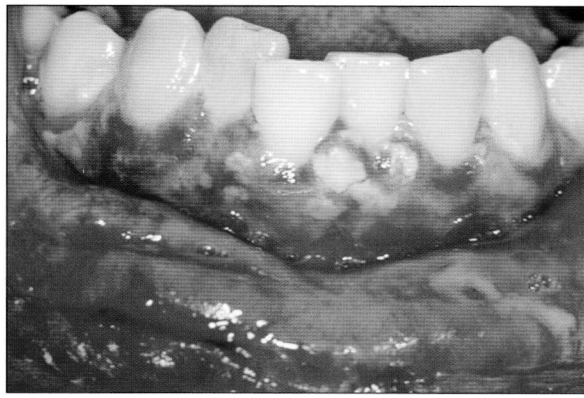

Fig 3-7a Oral lesions in paraneoplastic pemphigus are typically vesiculobullous and very painful. Mucosal involvement is extensive. Skin lesions also may be vesiculobullous, but may also resemble lichen planus. (Courtesy of Dr L. R. Eversole.)

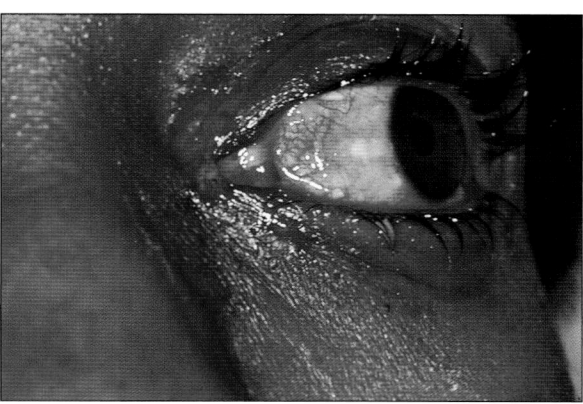

Fig 3-7b Paraneoplastic pemphigus frequently involves the conjunctiva. Scarring may occur as in ocular pemphigoid. (Courtesy of Dr L. R. Eversole.)

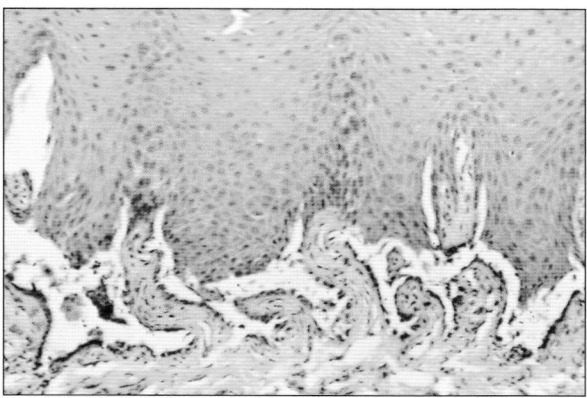

Fig 3-7c A suprabasilar separation in a case of paraneoplastic pemphigus. (Courtesy of Dr L. R. Eversole.)

Paraneoplastic Pemphigus

CLINICAL PRESENTATION AND PATHOGENESIS ▶

The clinician should be aware that a severe clinical picture of pemphigus vulgaris can occasionally represent a complication of a malignancy. When this happens, the malignancy is usually a Hodgkin lymphoma, a non-Hodgkin lymphoma, or a leukemia, but it can be associated with literally any malignancy and rarely a benign neoplasm. In such cases, numerous painful lesions develop on both the oral mucosa and the skin and are often evidence of an uncontrolled malignancy (Figs 3-7a and 3-7b). The course is usually rapid and fatal despite steroid and/or immunosuppressive therapy.

The mechanism of paraneoplastic pemphigus is thought to be a result of the neoplasm's ability to structurally alter normal epidermal proteins into antigenicity or to systemically secrete an antigenically similar protein to which autoantibodies develop and cross react with epidermal proteins. In either case, autoantibodies against epidermal desmoplakin I and II proteins are detected on skin biopsies by direct immunofluorescence and circulating in the serum by indirect immunofluorescence.

HISTOPATHOLOGY ▶

The histologic findings of paraneoplastic pemphigus are frequently a combination of pemphigus vulgaris and lichen planus. Suprabasilar separation of the epithelium with acantholysis can be seen in conjunction with vacuolization of basal cells, individual cell necrosis within the prickle cell layer, and a lymphoid infiltrate at the epithelial-connective tissue interface. In some cases, only one of these patterns will occur (Fig 3-7c).

Direct immunofluorescence shows intercellular deposition of IgG and complement, but, in addition, a granular deposition of complement occurs at the basement membrane zone. Indirect immunofluorescence testing using rat bladder transitional epithelium is highly specific for this disease. The antibodies react with 250-kD (desmoplakin I), 230-kD (BPAgI), 210-kD (desmoplakin II), and 190-kD proteins.

The Pemphigoid Group and Other Basement Membrane Autoimmune Diseases

The pemphigoids are a group of B cell–mediated autoimmune diseases that characteristically form vesicles and bullae. In overlapping clinical presentations, they may present with skin, oral mucosa, ocular mucosa, and other mucous membrane involvement. Traditionally, this group of diseases has been classified

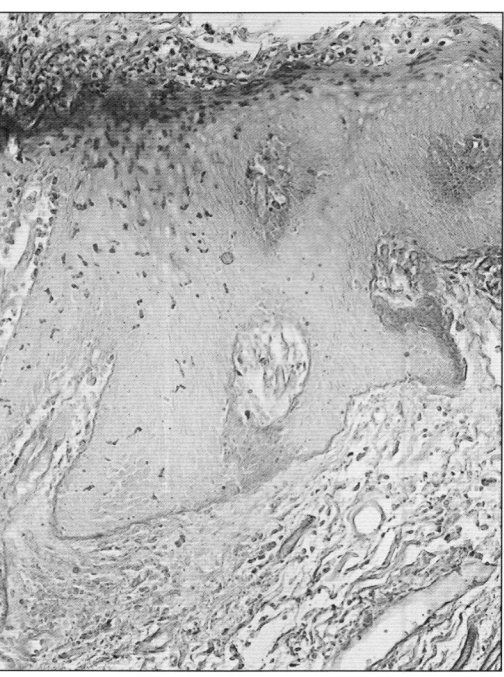

Fig 3-8 Periodic acid–Schiff (PAS) stain demonstrating the basement membrane as a thin line.

into two main clinical subgroups: bullous pemphigoid, which usually involves skin but 30% of the time involves oral mucous membranes as well; and cicatricial pemphigoid (mucous membrane pemphigoid), which involves mucous membranes (usually oral and/or conjunctival) and skin to a lesser extent (20%) and with less severity. Today, this group of diseases is categorized into two main clinical groups: cutaneous pemphigoid and mucosal pemphigoid. The mucosal pemphigoids are subclassified into three subgroups as follows:

• Cicatricial pemphigoid
• Oral mucous membrane pemphigoid
• Ocular pemphigoid

With specific direct immunofluorescent markers, it has been discovered that the related but different clinical presentations of cutaneous pemphigoid and mucosal pemphigoid are caused by autoantibodies to different molecules within the basement membrane zone. Moreover, what had been grouped together under "cicatricial pemphigoid" has been found to represent autoantibody formation to at least three different basement membrane zone proteins. Therefore, the spectrum of pemphigoid diseases today includes clinical presentations that may concentrate on skin, on oral mucosa, or on ocular mucosa. Numerous different basement membrane antigens are implicated. Both the clinical presentations and the antigenic proteins may overlap. In addition, two other diseases have autoantibody formation to basement membrane zone proteins and produce a similar light microscopic histopathology and clinical disease. Linear IgA disease and epidermolysis bullosa acquisita are such diseases but are not usually considered pemphigoids. To understand their similarities, their differences, and their overlapping clinical presentations, a study of the specific components of the basal cell–basement membrane junction is necessary.

All epithelia are separated from adjacent stroma by a continuous basement membrane. Most endothelial cells have basement membranes, as do some other cells such as those composing skeletal muscle and Schwann cells. The basement membrane is not stained by H&E but is well demonstrated by periodic acid–Schiff (PAS) as a homogeneous band 0.5 to 1.0 µm thick (Fig 3-8). It is, however, a complex structure best appreciated at an ultrastructural level (Figs 3-9a and 3-9b).

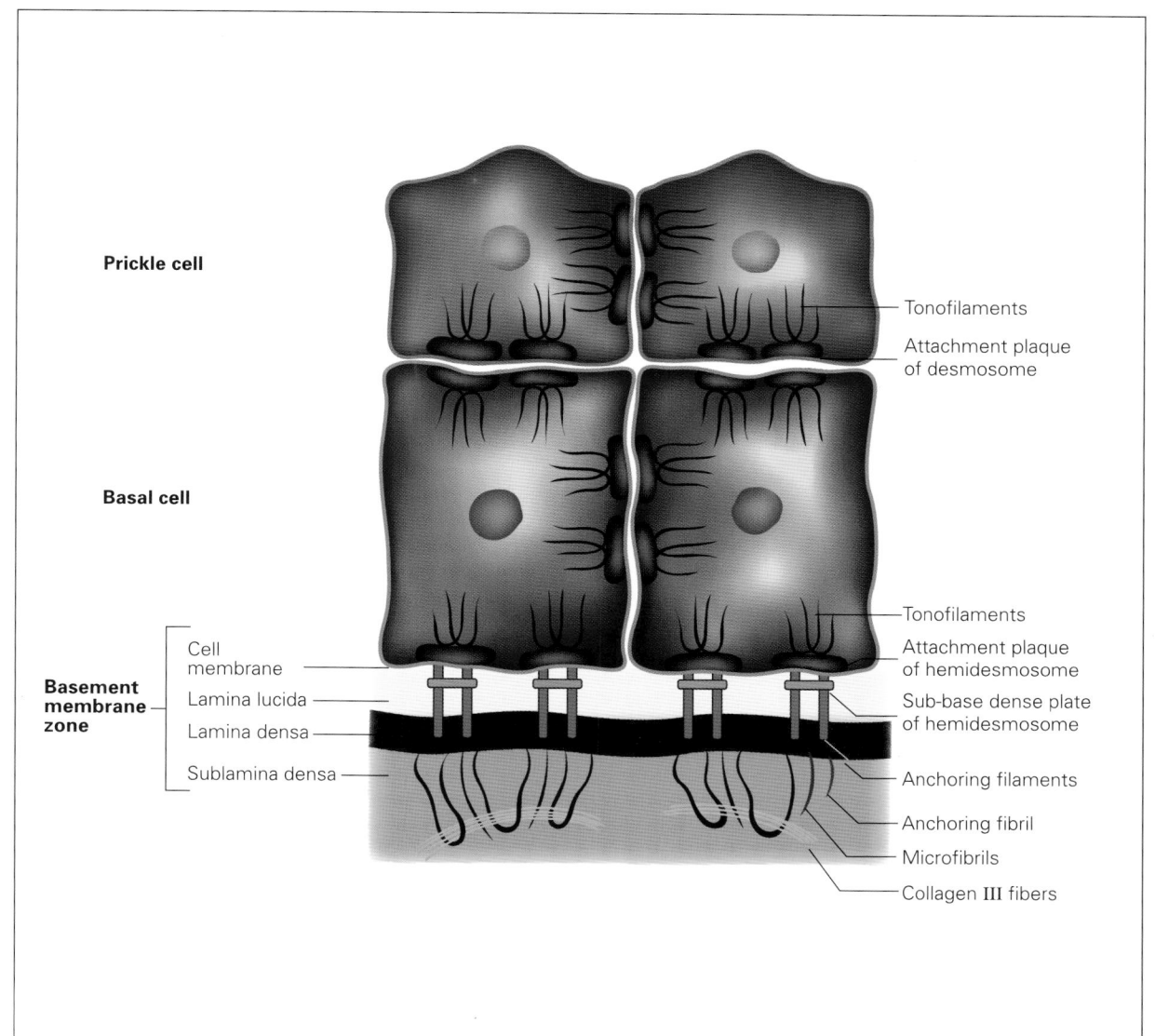

Fig 3-9a Stratified squamous epithelium and the basement membrane zone.

The components of the basement membrane are elaborated by the epithelium with the exception of the anchoring collagen fibrils and the elastic microfibrils. Numerous proteins exist in the basement membrane zone. The hemidesmosomes consist of an intracellular component of plectin and BPAgl (a 230-kD protein). BPAg2 (a 180-kD protein), and alpha-6-beta-4 integrin are transmembrane proteins combined with type XVII collagen, and their extracellular domains are within the lamina lucida. Anchoring filaments contain laminin 5 (epiligrin, kalinin, nicein), laminin 6, and uncein. These filaments extend from the hemidesmosomes into the lamina densa. Anchoring fibrils are composed of type VII collagen. Damage to this wide range of proteins can result in loss of attachment of the epithelium to the basement membrane zone with the clinical presentation of a pemphigoid phenotype. The initial damage may be caused by a variety of factors, including autoimmunity and gene mutation.

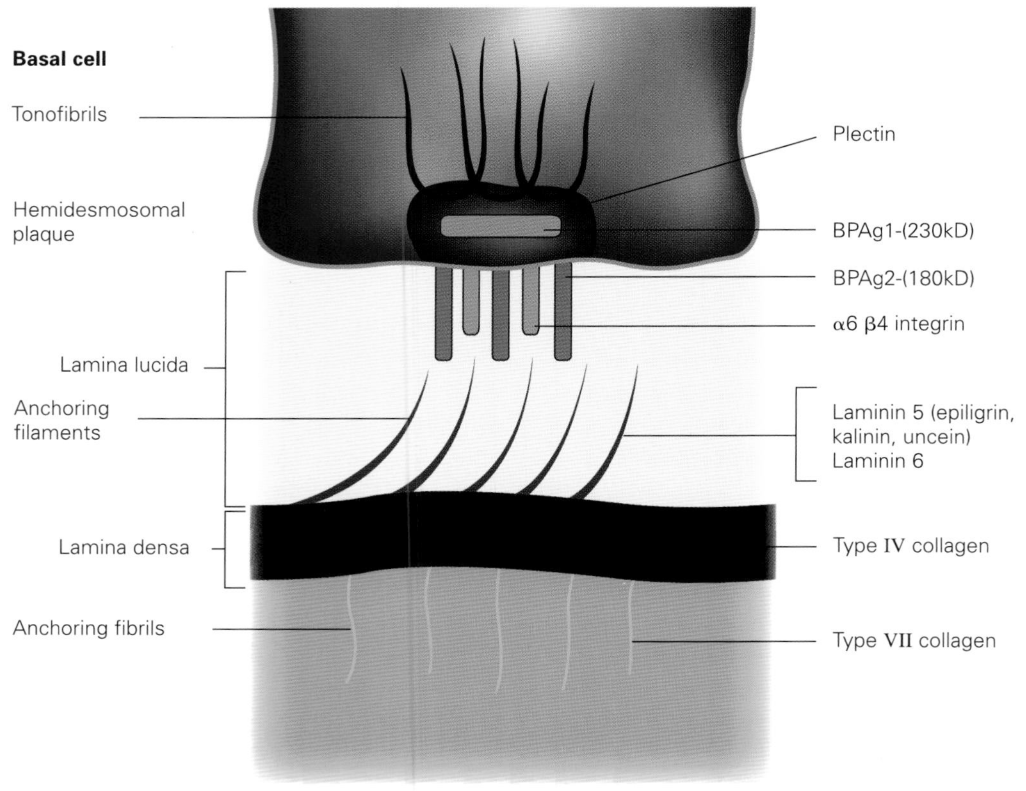

Fig 3-9b The hemidesmosome and the basement membrane zone.

Cutaneous Pemphigoid (Bullous Pemphigoid)

Cutaneous pemphigoid is a B cell–mediated autoimmune disease producing autoantibodies that target two proteins of the basal cell–basement membrane zone junction and the basement membrane proper. More than 80% of patients demonstrate autoantibody formation (usually IgG) to the BPAG-1 protein in the basal cell–upper lamina lucida area. This protein is a 230-kD protein that comprises part of the hemidesmosome in the basal cell and is involved in anchoring the basal cell to the lamina lucida of the basement membrane by interacting with the cytoplasmic portion of transmembrane integrins. About 50% of individuals with cutaneous pemphigoid have BPAG-2–directed autoantibodies in place of or in addition to BPAG-1–directed autoantibodies. The BPAG-2–directed autoantibody corresponds to a 180-kD antigen that is a transmembrane protein connecting the basal cell to the lamina lucida of the basement membrane. Both proteins are, therefore, found in the upper portion of the basement membrane zone with a resultant separation within the basement membrane.

Cutaneous pemphigoid is primarily a skin disease, forming oral lesions in only 30% of cases. The skin lesions are characteristically large bullae (3 to 15 cm in diameter), tense, and erythematous. They have a site preference for flexural creases of the trunk and extremities. The bullae and surrounding erythematous skin are characteristically pruritic (Fig 3-10a).

CLINICAL PRESENTATION AND PATHOGENESIS ▶

Cutaneous pemphigoid affects both sexes equally, unlike mucosal pemphigoid, which has a female predilection; however, like the mucosal pemphigoid groups, it occurs mostly in elderly individuals. Patient history may include intermittent episodes of exacerbations and spontaneous remissions. Most individuals will relate such a history over 2 to 3 years. After 5 or 6 years, the disease usually subsides into remission or only mild symptomatology.

The pathogenesis of cutaneous pemphigoid involves circulating IgG-type antibodies, which attack the BPAG-1 and BPAG-2 protein antigens within the basement membrane basal cell–lamina lucida layer. The antigen-antibody complexes fix complement (C3 in particular is found at the basement membrane zone by direct immunofluorescence), which initiates the series of steps that lead to inflammation. Inflammatory cells such as neutrophils, eosinophils, and macrophages release proteases such as lysozyme, which degrade the basement membrane at the lamina lucida level and generate pain by the formation of bradykinin, kallikrein, and slow-reacting substance P. Thus, the lesions are cutaneous in nature, somewhat painful, and clinically erythematous.

DIFFERENTIAL DIAGNOSIS ▶

Cutaneous pemphigoid must be distinguished from *pemphigus vulgaris*, which may also present with skin vesicles or bullae and oral lesions. However, the bullae of pemphigus are smaller and not as pruritic and will not have the marked erythema associated with cutaneous pemphigoid. The oral vesicles or ulcers of pemphigus vulgaris are also more painful. Although the *mucosal pemphigoids* have a similar pathogenesis, their skin lesions are not as prominent and occur in only 20% of cases. In addition, many of them will have a concomitant conjunctivitis, which cutaneous pemphigoid does not have. *Cutaneous-erosive lichen planus* remains a serious consideration because of its violaceous pruritic skin lesions, which may have corresponding oral lesions.

DIAGNOSTIC WORK-UP ▶

The diagnosis of cutaneous pemphigoid is made by biopsy of either oral mucosal or skin lesions in which a vesicle's edge or normal-appearing tissue adjacent to a lesion is sampled. Two biopsy specimens or one biopsy specimen separated into two equally representative halves should be taken. One specimen is submitted in 10% neutral-buffered formalin for routine H&E histopathologic studies, and the other specimen is placed in Michel's medium for direct immunofluorescence. Alternatives to Michel's medium include liquid nitrogen freezing or direct immunofluorescence processing of the fresh specimen within 4 hours. Most cases can be diagnosed with H&E histopathology correlated with a distinctive clinical presentation. Direct immunofluorescence is used to confirm the diagnosis by identifying specific anti–basement membrane zone autoantibodies to BPAG-1 and/or BPAG-2.

HISTOPATHOLOGY ▶

The histologic features of cutaneous pemphigoid are similar to those of mucosal pemphigoid. Eosinophils and neutrophils may be more prominent (Fig 3-10b). As in mucosal pemphigoid, separation occurs within the lamina lucida, but at a higher level. Antibodies bind to two antigens, BPAg1, a 230-kD protein, and BPAg2, a 180-kD protein. The proposed sequence of events that follows includes activation of the complement cascade, mast cell degranulation, eosinophil degranulation, and release of proteolytic enzymes. Direct immunofluorescence will show a homogeneous band of IgG in the basement membrane zone in almost 100% of cases as well as C3. Unlike in mucosal pemphigoid, circulating IgG antibodies to basement membrane will be seen in as much as 80% of cases. There is no correlation between titers and the clinical picture.

TREATMENT ▶

The treatment of choice is systemic corticosteroids. Systemic corticosteroid regimen I is preferred, but refractory cases may require regimen IIIB (see pages 205 to 206). For those who cannot take corticosteroids, a regimen of tetracycline or erythromycin, 500 mg twice daily, combined with nicotinamide (*not* nicotinic acid), 500 mg twice daily, will gradually but slowly decrease the disease activity.

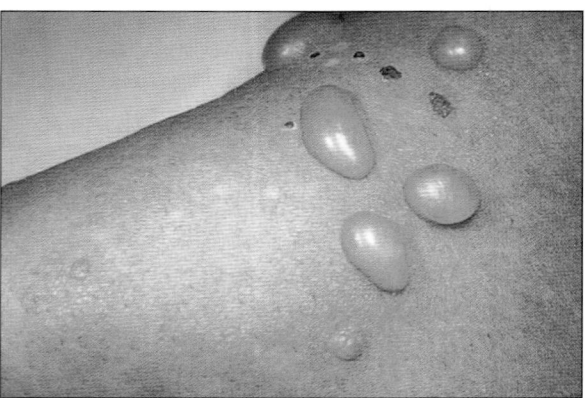

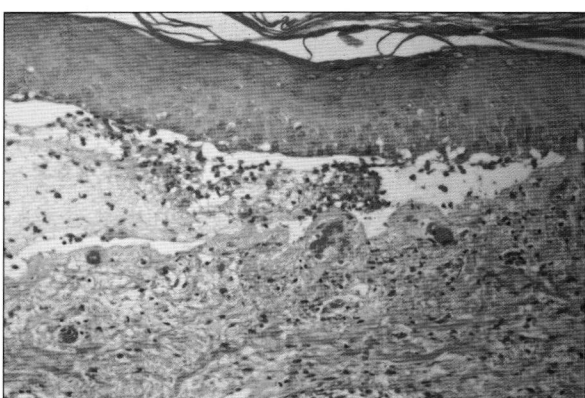

Fig 3-10a Bullae of cutaneous pemphigoid are characteristically large and have a red base. They are mostly pruritic and/or painful and more common in the flexure surfaces of skin. (Reprinted from Callen JP et al, *Color Atlas of Dermatology*, with permission from WB Saunders Co.)

Fig 3-10b Cutaneous pemphigoid showing essentially the same picture as mucous membrane pemphigoid with a separation of the epithelium from the underlying connective tissue. Eosinophils are present in this infiltrate.

PROGNOSIS ▶

Unlike pemphigus vulgaris, cutaneous pemphigoid is not fatal if untreated. Instead, spontaneous remissions are likely to occur in 5 to 6 years. Treatment often involves a drug-induced remission to reduce symptoms and alleviate the large bullae formation; it may hasten a complete remission.

The Mucosal Pemphigoids

Cicatricial Pemphigoid

Cicatricial pemphigoid is a B cell–mediated autoimmune disease of the mucosal pemphigoid group in which autoantibodies of the IgG and IgA class are directed against either the same BPAG-1 and BPAG-2 antigens as noted in cutaneous pemphigoid or other protein antigens of the basement membrane zone. Epiligrin (laminin-5), an anchoring filament connecting the lamina lucida to the lamina densa, and beta 4-integrin, a transmembrane protein into which anchoring filaments are attached to the basal cell surface, have also been implicated as the antigens. These antigens are variably seen in oral mucous membrane pemphigoid and ocular pemphigoid as well. Therefore, some overlap of clinical presentation is to be expected because each disease produces autoantibodies that attack the general basement membrane zone to cause a separation of epithelium from the underlying connective tissue. Cicatricial pemphigoid targets mucous membranes more than skin; oral and conjunctival mucous membranes are those most commonly involved. Involvement of more than one type of mucous membrane is characteristic of cicatricial pemphigoid.

CLINICAL PRESENTATION AND PATHOGENESIS ▶

Patients are generally older than 45 years; the average patient age is around 60 years. Women are affected more often than men. Cicatricial pemphigoid may present with one of two oral clinical pictures coupled with other mucous membrane involvement, most often ocular. The first symptom may be a reddened, burning attached gingiva, a presentation often referred to in the past as *desquamative gingivitis* or *postmenopausal gingivitis* (Fig 3-11a). The second is a diffuse series of vesicles, ulcers, and erythematous territories involving palatal mucosa, buccal mucosa, or labial mucosa (Fig 3-11b). The most common other mucous membrane involvement is ocular (Fig 3-11c), but nasal, pharyngeal, laryngeal, anal, and genital mucous membranes may become involved. Skin lesions, occurring in 20% of cases, appear as vesicles on an erythematous base that rupture, then crust (Fig 3-11d). They may be seen in either of the presentations, but are most often noted in the more intense and widespread presentations.

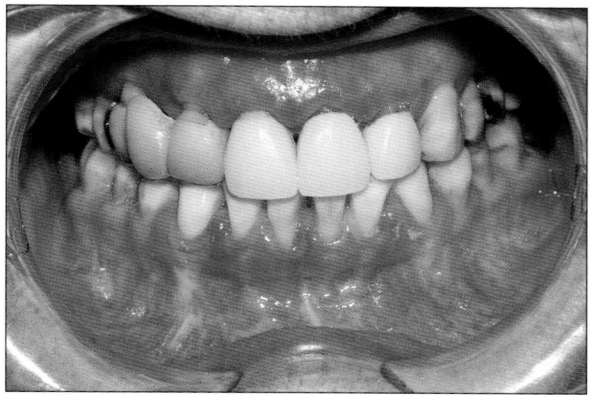

Fig 3-11a The mucosal pemphigoid group may present with a burning, red attached gingiva. A Nikolsky sign is usually present.

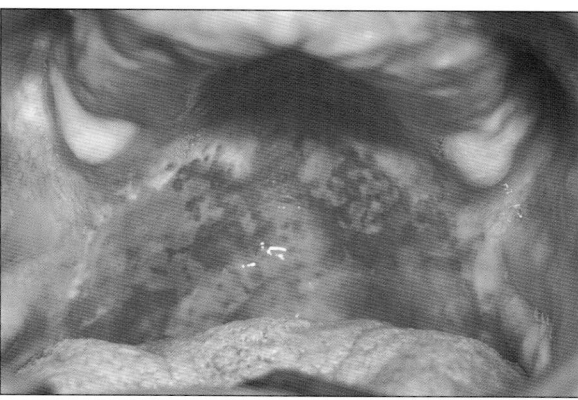

Fig 3-11b Mucosal pemphigoid with two vesicles and a diffuse area of inflammation and mild pain.

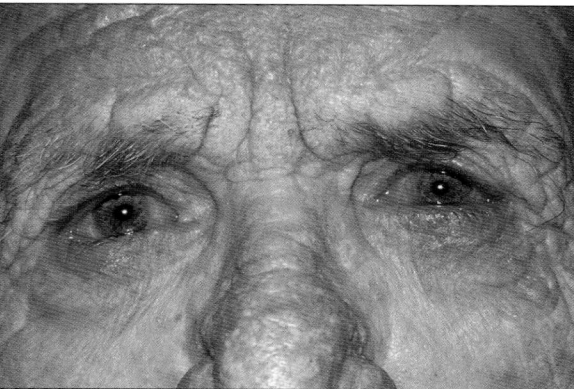

Fig 3-11c Mucosal pemphigoid will often have an ocular component, or an ocular pemphigoid may occur independently. Here a nonsuppurative conjunctivitis is present as an ocular component in mucosal pemphigoid.

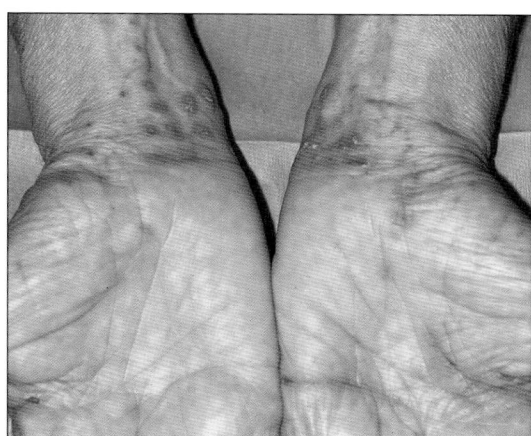

Fig 3-11d Mucosal pemphigoid will have skin vesicles and ulcers present in 20% of cases. Here the volar aspects of the forearms have multiple, minimally painful vesicles.

The conjunctival involvement is a nonsuppurative conjunctivitis. Occasional secondary infections may confuse the picture with pus formation. The conjunctiva will be reddened but will produce minimal symptoms. Scarring, particularly of the conjunctiva, is the mechanism of debilitation associated with cicatricial pemphigoid (hence its name). As the disease continues, scar bands form between the bulbar conjunctiva (the conjunctiva over the globe) and the palpebral conjunctiva (the conjunctiva over the inner eyelids), called *symblepharon* (Fig 3-12). This scar band in particular contracts to invert usually the lower lid eyelashes toward the cornea in a condition called *trichiasis*. This, in turn, abrades the cornea, causing ulceration, which leads to opacifications and even blindness in 15% of cases. In severe cases, scar bands will connect the upper and lower palpebral conjunctiva to partially close the eye, a condition called *ankyloblepharon*.

Cicatricial pemphigoid is similar to cutaneous pemphigoid. These diseases share similar immunopathologic and histopathologic characteristics, but differ in their spectrum of specific antigens and in the intensity of the autoimmune response and, therefore, their clinical presentation. Cutaneous pemphigoid targets skin with large bullae and has a lesser propensity for oral mucosa (30% of cases). Cicatricial pemphigoid targets mucous membranes with erythematous inflammation and small vesicles and has a lesser propensity for skin (20% of cases).

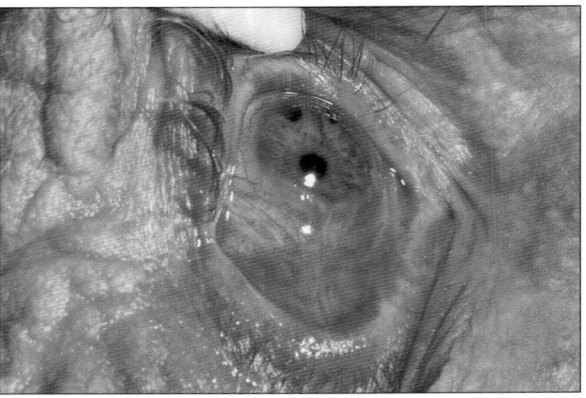

Fig 3-12 Ocular involvement of pemphigoid will produce scarring. Here a scar band is seen between the bulbar conjunctiva and the palpebral conjunctiva (symblepharon).

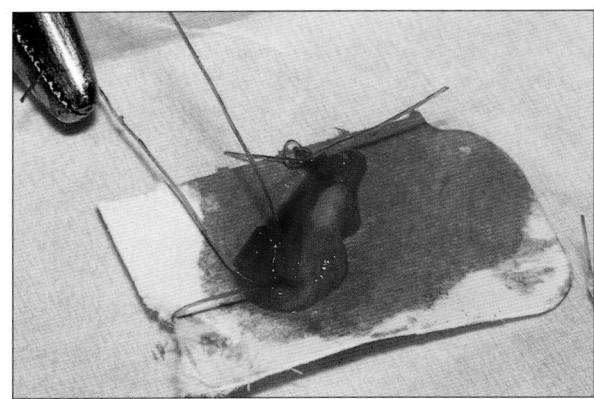

Fig 3-13 Suturing a thin mucosal biopsy specimen to the suture pack cardboard will assist the pathologist in determining the surface orientation of the specimen.

The diseases share some specific antigens. As circulating autoantibodies attach to these antigens, they fix complement and thus initiate the cascade of inflammation including neutrophil chemotaxis, phagocyte stimulation, and release of bradykinin and kallikrein, which mediate the mild pain and discomfort these patients perceive. Neutrophils and other phagocytes release lysosomes and proteases, which digest the basement membrane zone specifically at the lamina lucida area. Therefore, the epithelium can separate from the connective tissue in the classic infrabasilar split.

DIFFERENTIAL DIAGNOSIS ▶ The most important disease from which to distinguish cicatricial pemphigoid is the *cutaneous/erosive form of lichen planus*. Although erosive lichen planus is usually more painful, a milder presentation exists that bears close resemblance to cicatricial pemphigoid. In particular, lichen planus often has the reddened "desquamative gingivitis" presentation and thus resembles one of the clinical types of cicatricial pemphigoid. If there are clinical lesions on the dorsum of the tongue, lichen planus is strongly suggested, since cicatricial pemphigoid rarely involves that area. *Pemphigus vulgaris* is another vesiculocutaneous disease with oral lesions that may resemble those of cicatricial pemphigoid. Pemphigus vulgaris, however, occurs more often in younger patients than does cicatricial pemphigoid and is usually more symptomatic. The mild symptomatology of cicatricial pemphigoid and the diffuse erythematous territories are features seen in medication-related and contact hypersensitivities called *lichenoid drug reactions*. A presentation of cicatricial pemphigoid skin lesions together with oral lesions and conjunctival lesions may suggest *erythema multiforme,* which, however, affects skin more than mucous membranes and is very painful and debilitating.

DIAGNOSTIC WORK-UP ▶ Biopsy confirmation is required to diagnose cicatricial pemphigoid. Two biopsies or one biopsy that can be separated into two specimens, one for routine H&E sections and the other for direct immunofluorescence, are recommended. The biopsy should include a significant area of clinically normal-appearing tissue. If ulcerations are taken for biopsy, secondary inflammation will often obscure the diagnostic immunopathologic pattern required for diagnosis.

When performing mucosal biopsies where the tissue is only a few millimeters thick, it is useful to suture the specimen flat onto the cardboard of the suture pack to keep the specimen from curling in the fixative (Fig 3-13). This is especially important in the diagnosis of vesiculocutaneous and/or immune-based diseases, in which the relationships of the prickle cell layer, the basement membrane, the lamina propria, and the submucosa need to be seen without distortion.

One of the two specimens can be fixed in 10% neutral-buffered formalin; the second specimen should be fixed in Michel's medium for direct immunofluorescence. If the diagnosis is evident by clinical features and H&E histopathologic features, the direct immunofluorescence specimen may not be needed. However, a Michel's medium–fixed specimen becomes useful in equivocal situations in which confirma-

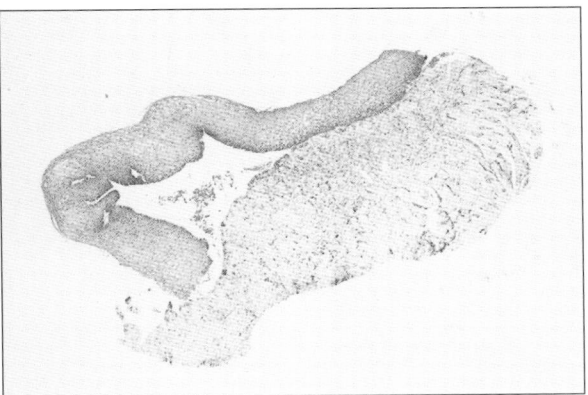

Fig 3-14a Mucosal pemphigoid showing the separation of the entire epithelium from underlying chronically inflamed fibrous tissue.

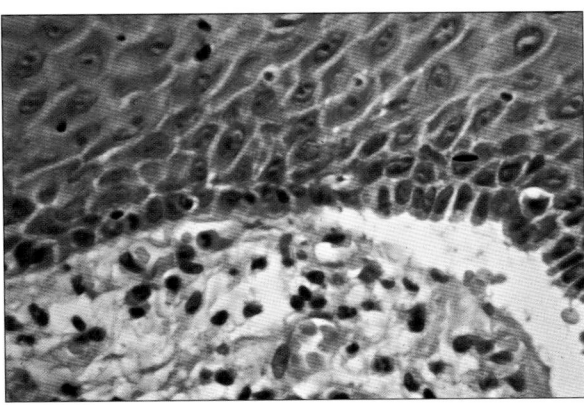

Fig 3-14b Mucosal pemphigoid with a well-defined separation of the epithelium showing the intact basal cells and inflammatory cells within the fibrovascular tissue.

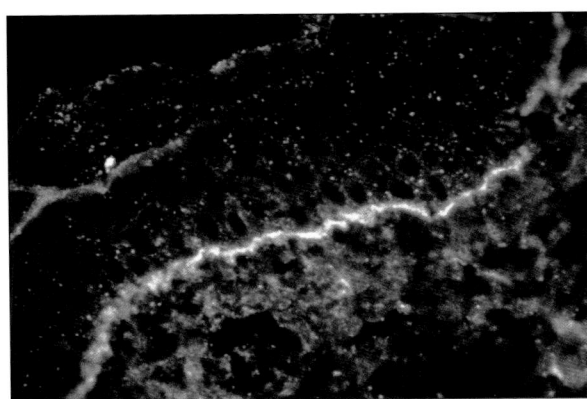

Fig 3-14c The smooth linear deposition of IgG along the basement membrane zone as seen in mucosal pemphigoid by direct immunofluorescence.

HISTOPATHOLOGY

tion is needed. As an alternative to Michel's medium, the tissue can be processed fresh (within 4 hours) or frozen in liquid nitrogen.

In cicatricial pemphigoid, bulla formation occurs subepithelially. The epithelium separates very cleanly from the underlying connective tissue so that an intact basal cell layer is present (Figs 3-14a and 3-14b). The epithelium shows no significant change other than degeneration following extended separation from the connective tissue. The lamina propria usually contains a lymphocytic infiltrate that may also include plasma cells and, less frequently, neutrophils. Initial changes have been described as extracellular edema with vacuolation in the basement membrane zone, followed by an influx of neutrophils into the vesicle and a perivascular distribution of lymphocytes and macrophages. On an ultrastructural level, separation of the epithelium occurs within the lamina lucida, but at a deeper level than in cutaneous pemphigoid.

Direct immunofluorescence studies, which should be performed on perilesional tissue, will show a homogeneous linear pattern of IgG at the basement membrane zone in 80% to 95% of patients (Fig 3-14c). The same distribution of C3 will be seen, and IgM and IgA may also be found. About 20% of patients will have circulating IgG antibodies, usually in low titers. There is no correlation between severity of disease and circulating antibody level. Targeted antigens include 180 kD (BPAg2), 230 kD (BPAg1), laminin-5 and -6, uncein, 200 kD, 168 kD, and 45 kD.

TREATMENT

Mild cases may require no specific treatment, only reassurance. Many patients with cicatricial pemphigoid are concerned that the oral lesions represent malignancies or premalignant conditions. Many mild cases can be managed with topical corticosteroids. The drug of choice for oral lesions is 0.05% fluocinonide gel (Lidex gel, Medicis Dermatologics). The patient is instructed to dry the affected mucosa, apply the gel, and massage it into the tissues four times daily. The patient should be cautioned not to eat or drink for an hour afterward and advised that application before sleep is advantageous.

The most predictable therapy for the oral lesions coupled with other mucous membrane lesions or the rare skin lesions is systemic corticosteroids. Patients with cicatricial pemphigoid respond well to systemic corticosteroid regimen I or II (see page 205) (Figs 3-15a and 3-15b). Because most cicatricial pemphigoid patients are older than 60 years, assessment for osteoporosis and cataracts is especially important. As a supplement to corticosteroid therapy or even for reassurance, excision of affected areas and replacement with a split-thickness skin graft is effective. In selected patients and at selected sites, such as the vestibule or floor of the mouth, replacement of affected mucosa with skin, which has a much lower propensity for this disease, often eliminates the restriction of scar contractions in addition to replacing the surface area of involved mucosa (Figs 3-15c and 3-15d). This approach is not recommended on the buccal mucosa because the tongue fixates on the rough texture of the skin, causing tongue abrasions.

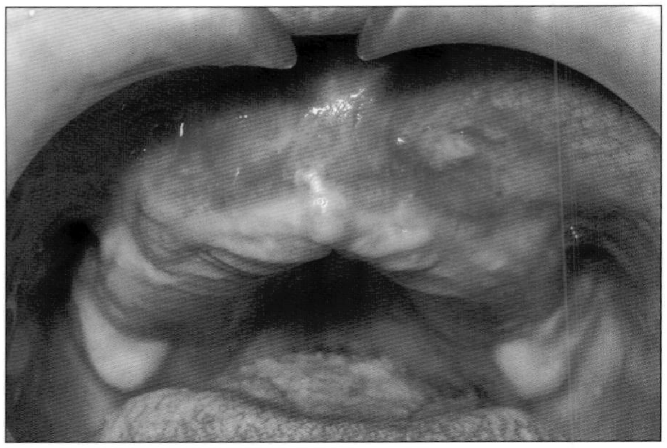

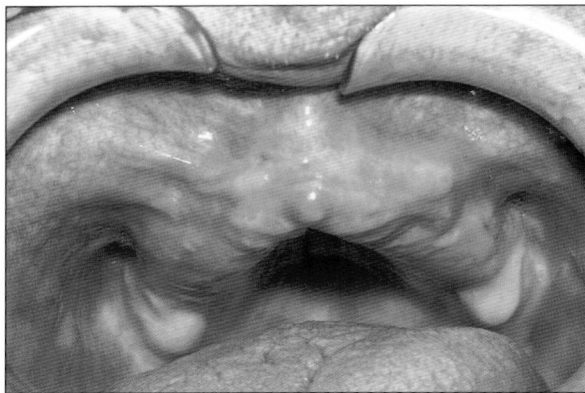

Fig 3-15a Oral mucosal pemphigoid lesions before treatment.

Fig 3-15b Oral mucosal pemphigoid shown in Fig 3-15a in a drug-free remission after corticosteroid regimen I.

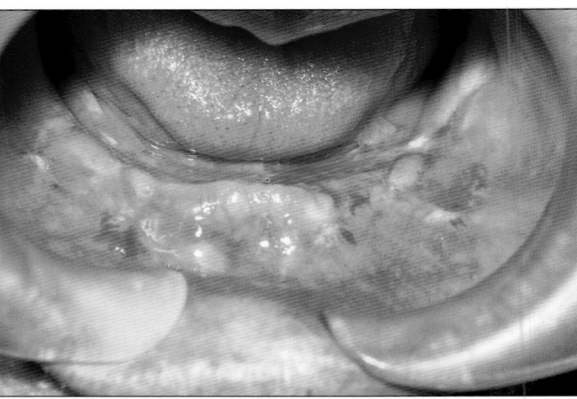

Fig 3-15c Scar tissue and active vesicles in the buccal vestibule in a patient with oral cicatricial pemphigoid before treatment.

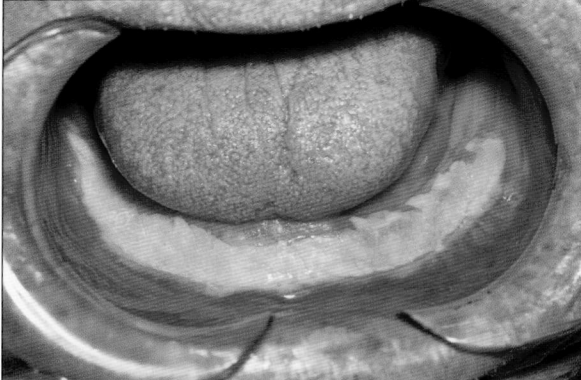

Fig 3-15d Replacement of scar and affected mucosa shown in Fig 3-15c with a split-thickness skin graft, which also provided a better ridge form and vestibule for the denture.

The conjunctivitis component in any case of cicatricial pemphigoid requires treatment. Complications and debility associated with cicatricial pemphigoid center on the symblepharon and trichiasis complications. Cortisporin ophthalmic drops (GlaxoSmithKline) or their equivalent are most commonly used in a regimen of two drops in each eye three times daily. In all cases of cicatricial pemphigoid, an ophthalmology consultation and follow-up are recommended.

PROGNOSIS ▶ Most cases of cicatricial pemphigoid can be controlled with systemic corticosteroids. Remissions can be maintained in either a drug-free state or an every-other-day maintenance dose. Exacerbations are uncommon and usually can be managed by reinitiating systemic corticosteroids. Poorly controlled disease will lead to continued inflammation and scarring. In the oral cavity, these conditions are seen most often as periodontal loss of tooth support or scar obliteration of the edentulous vestibules. In the eyes, poorly controlled disease will lead to vision loss from corneal opacification. More rarely, scar bands will affect pharyngeal or laryngeal function.

Oral Mucous Membrane Pemphigoid

When pemphigoid is limited to the oral cavity over several years and no ocular or other mucous membrane involvement develops, it is said to represent *oral mucous membrane pemphigoid* (OMMP). This may

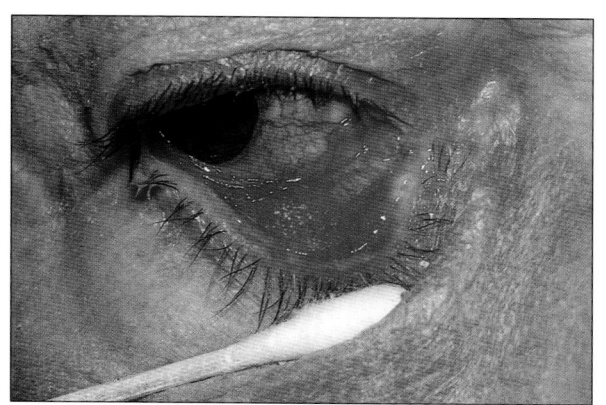

Fig 3-16 Severe conjunctivitis with secondary staphylococcus aureus infection as indicated by yellow flecks in a patient with ocular pemphigoid.

be a distinctive subgroup because of different autoantibody development to different basement membrane proteins.

Clinically, OMMP may present in the same two general oral presentations of cicatricial pemphigoid but without the presence or future development of ocular or other mucous membrane involvement. Therefore, OMMP may present with a reddened, boggy attached gingiva and a complaint of tenderness or burning pain (see Fig 3-11a). It may also present with diffuse vesicles, ulcers, and erythematous areas of the buccal, palatal, or labial mucosa. The same differential diagnostic considerations, work-up, and treatment options as discussed for cicatricial pemphigoid pertain to OMMP. The prognosis is usually better for OMMP than it is for cicatricial pemphigoid because of its more limited area of involvement and its less intensive activity.

Suggested basement membrane antigens seen in OMMP that differ from those seen in cicatricial pemphigoid are alpha-6 integrin, which is a transmembrane protein of the basal cell–lamina lucida junction, and laminin-6, which is an anchoring filament that connects the extracytoplasmic portions of these transmembrane proteins to the lamina densa. However, OMMP may also be a limited clinical expression of cicatricial pemphigoid, to which it has several identical antigens, such as BPAg2 and epiligrin (laminin-5). The difference may be one only of the degree of immune stimulation and disease intensity.

Ocular Pemphigoid

Ocular pemphigoid is a subgroup of mucosal pemphigoid in which only the conjunctiva is involved. This may also be a distinctive disease because specific antigens different from those of cicatricial pemphigoid and oral mucous membrane are seen, or it may be a variant with only a difference in disease activity and intensity. The specific antigens responsible for ocular pemphigoid seem to be the same beta-4 integrin protein and epiligrin (laminin-5) seen in cicatricial pemphigoid. However, ocular pemphigoid lacks the BPAg2 antigen seen in cicatricial pemphigoid. This suggests that each of the diseases in the pemphigoid group may have more than one antigenic focus within the basement membrane zone and that differences in clinical presentation may arise from the various combinations that are possible. Ocular pemphigoid may be limited to the conjunctiva because its BPAg2 protein is normal but the beta 4-integrin and epiligrin are antigenic.

Histologic changes in the conjunctiva in ocular pemphigoid include squamous metaplasia of the epithelium often with loss of goblet cells, which reverse after disease control. The underlying tissue contains a chronic inflammatory infiltrate and will show fibrosis.

Nevertheless, ocular pemphigoid remains a serious disease with a potential for blindness and will present like the ocular component in cicatricial pemphigoid (Fig 3-16); an ophthalmology consultation is required as it is for cicatricial pemphigoid. The scar potential of ocular pemphigoid is also the same. Therefore, concerns about symblepharon, trichiasis, corneal abrasions, and blindness also are the same.

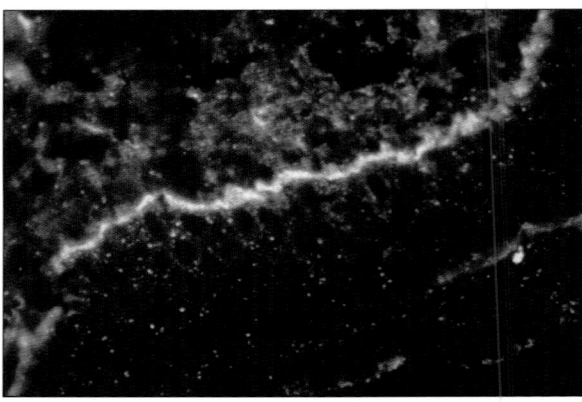

Fig 3-17 Deposition of IgA along the basement membrane zone seen by direct immunofluorescence, confirming the diagnosis of linear IgA disease.

Linear IgA Disease

Linear IgA disease is a rare autoimmune disease involving skin and oral mucosa. It is not considered part of the pemphigoid group but is a similar disease in which autoantibodies attack basement membrane proteins. The specific basement membrane antigens are not as well-known for linear IgA disease as they are for the pemphigoid group. The distinction of linear IgA disease is that the autoantibody is in the IgA class of immunoglobulins, whereas in the pemphigoid group it is primarily IgG.

CLINICAL PRESENTATION ▶   Like the pemphigoid group of diseases, linear IgA disease is a chronic disease found in adults. It will most often produce skin, oral mucosal, and ocular lesions simultaneously. Both the skin and oral lesions are bullous or vesicular, but may have ruptured into ulcers. Early vesicles will present as an erythema. The ocular lesions will present as the same conjunctivitis as is seen in cicatricial pemphigoid or ocular pemphigoid. If discomfort is experienced, it is mild.

DIFFERENTIAL DIAGNOSIS ▶   Linear IgA disease is sufficiently rare that it is not likely to be the expected diagnosis. Because the presentation is almost identical to that of *cutaneous pemphigoid* and *cicatricial pemphigoid*, these diseases are the two most important considerations. In addition, some clinical presentations of *lichen planus* and mild cases of *pemphigus vulgaris* may also present with oral and skin vesicles.

DIAGNOSTIC WORK-UP ▶   As in the pemphigoid group, the presentations described require a mucosal or skin biopsy. Specimens should be processed for both routine H&E–stained sections as well as placed in Michel's medium or frozen for direct immunofluorescence studies. It is important that the pathology laboratory use antisera to detect IgA autoantibodies. Although IgA autoantibody testing is usually part of the direct immunofluorescence battery, the clinician should request that it be included to ensure that this rare disease is not overlooked.

HISTOPATHOLOGY ▶   The distinguishing feature of linear IgA disease is the presence of IgA in a homogeneous, linear pattern at the basement membrane zone in lesional and perilesional tissue (Fig 3-17). Thus, direct immunofluorescence is necessary for the diagnosis. The vesicles are subepithelial and occur within the lamina lucida or below the basal lamina. Other findings are variable. In about half the cases, neutrophilic microabscesses at the tips of the connective tissue may be seen with or without eosinophils, as in dermatitis herpetiformis. In other cases, lymphocytes are seen at the dermal-epidermal tissue interface. Circulating antibodies are uncommon and when present are in low titers. Their presence does not correlate with disease activity. The antibodies react with 97-kD and 120-kD antigens, which seem to be fragments of the extracellular domain of type XVII collagen.

TREATMENT ▶   Mild cases may require no specific treatment or may be managed well with typical corticosteroid medications such as 0.05% fluocinonide gel for oral mucosa (Lidex gel, Medicis Dermatologics) or cream

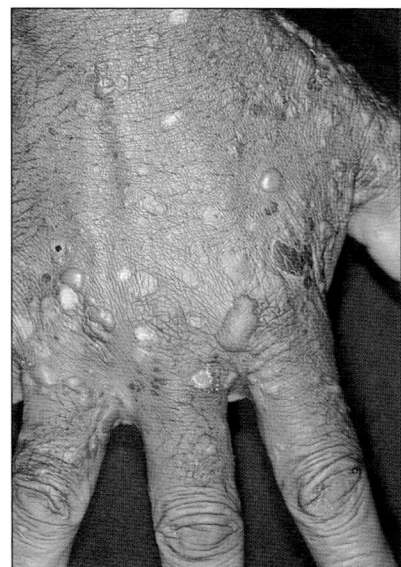

Fig 3-18 Epidermolysis bullosa acquisita will be remarkable for fragile hemorrhagic skin in addition to vesicles and bullae. (Reprinted from Callen JP et al, *Color Atlas of Dermatology*, with permission from WB Saunders Co.)

for skin (Lidex cream, Medicis Dermatologics). Ocular lesions may require cortisone ophthalmic drops (Cortisporin, GlaxoSmithKline). If ocular lesions are present, however, an ophthalmology consultation is indicated.

PROGNOSIS ▶

The prognosis for linear IgA disease seems good from the few known cases. It is usually not severe or debilitating and is controlled well with either topical or systemic corticosteroid management.

Epidermolysis Bullosa Acquisita

CLINICAL PRESENTATION AND PATHOGENESIS ▶

Epidermolysis bullosa acquisita is another B cell–mediated autoimmune disease that affects the basement membrane zone. The antigen, however, seems to be type VII collagen, the main protein of the lamina densa, which is in the lower portion of the basement membrane. Epidermolysis bullosa acquisita is the acquired or nonhereditary type of epidermolysis bullosa and should not be confused with the several hereditary types seen in children and caused by genetic defects in the basement membrane zone. Instead, epidermolysis bullosa acquisita is an IgG-mediated autoantibody disease that begins in mature to elderly adults.

Epidermolysis bullosa acquisita will present mostly with skin bullae and vesicles and only rarely with oral vesicles. The skin bullae will be larger and more dominant. The bullae and vesicles are well-known to emerge after minor trauma or simple skin contact. Patients will note a skin fragility. The oral mucosa is equally fragile and, when involved, will form large hemorrhagic bullae, usually seen on the buccal mucosa (Fig 3-18). Both the skin and oral lesions will heal with scar formation. Ocular lesions have not been reported.

DIFFERENTIAL DIAGNOSIS ▶

Epidermolysis bullosa acquisita should not be confused with its hereditary counterpart, *epidermolysis bullosa*, because the former occurs exclusively in older adults, whereas the latter is seen in early childhood. However, *cutaneous pemphigoid* and *cicatricial pemphigoid* with some skin lesions will appear similar. In addition, *pemphigus vulgaris* may also form large skin bullae and oral vesicles. Because of the advanced age of most affected patients, a *paraneoplastic pemphigus* also bears some consideration.

DIAGNOSTIC WORK-UP ▶

The disease may be anticipated by the age of the patient and the extreme fragility of both skin and mucosa; however, a biopsy either of mucosa or of skin is required to establish the diagnosis. The biopsy may include part of a vesicle, but it should also include adjacent normal-appearing tissue. Routine formalin-fixed H&E specimens and Michel's medium or frozen-fixed direct immunofluorescence specimens are required for diagnosis.

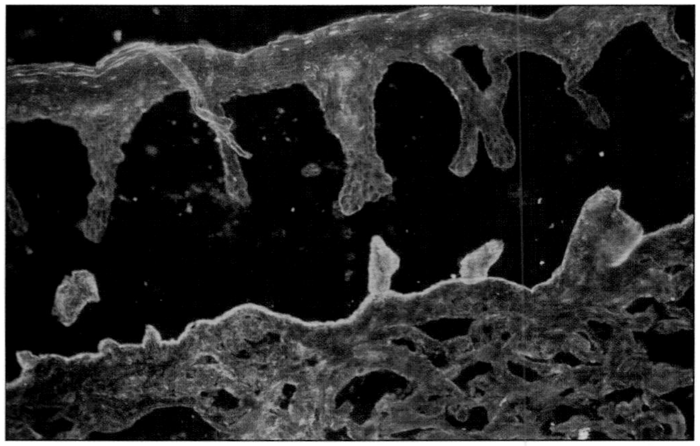

Fig 3-19 In this section of salt-split skin, antibodies (IgG) are present at the base in epidermolysis bullosa acquisita (dermal side). In pemphigoid, antibodies are found at the roof (epidermal side). (Courtesy of Dr Ellen Eisenberg.)

HISTOPATHOLOGY ▶

Bullae form below the basal lamina. Some forms are noninflammatory, but more frequent is a lymphocytic and neutrophilic infiltrate that is perivascular and infiltrates the dermal papillae. Eosinophils may be present. By direct immunofluorescence, perilesional tissue will show linear deposits of IgG and complement at the basement membrane zone. Circulating IgG antibodies are seen in about 50% of cases. In this disease, antibody is directed to type VII collagen so that the anchoring fibrils are affected. Separation occurs in the upper lamina densa, so that the lamina densa is seen on the roof of the blister. While electron microscopy will be diagnostic, the use of saltsplit skin (skin biopsy treated with salt to effect a split within the basement membrane zone) for diagnosis is most helpful and distinguishes this condition from cutaneous pemphigoid (Fig 3-19). In epidermolysis bullosa acquisita, IgG is seen on the floor of the vesicle, whereas in cutaneous pemphigoid it is on the roof.

TREATMENT AND PROGNOSIS ▶

Treatment responses are minimal. Although systemic corticosteroids with and without immunosuppressive drugs, as in the systemic corticosteroid regimens IIIA and IIIB (see pages 205 to 206), have been used, as have various chemotherapeutic agents often reserved for malignancies, the response is inconsistent and incomplete. Patients are, therefore, treated with adjusted doses of prednisone, dapsone, retinoids (such as Accutane, Roche), or beta carotene and further supported with protective clothing and an effort to avoid skin and mucosal friction or trauma.

Lichen Planus

CLINICAL PRESENTATION AND PATHOGENESIS ▶

Lichen planus is a T-cell–mediated autoimmune interface disease in which the basal cell layer of mucosa and/or skin is attacked.

Lichen planus presents in one of three different clinical forms that rarely transform from one to another. All forms are seen mostly in patients older than 40 years and in men and women equally; in addition, all have a predilection for the buccal mucosa, the tongue, and the attached gingiva, particularly the buccal regions. The three forms, in order of advancing severity and symptomatology, are reticular, plaque, and erosive.

Reticular Form

The reticular form is characterized by so-called Wickham striae of lacy, white interlacing lines found mostly on the characteristic sites of the buccal mucosa, attached gingiva, and tongue (Fig 3-20). These striae are usually asymptomatic, reach a certain area of involvement, and then cease to extend. This form requires no specific diagnostic measure or treatment.

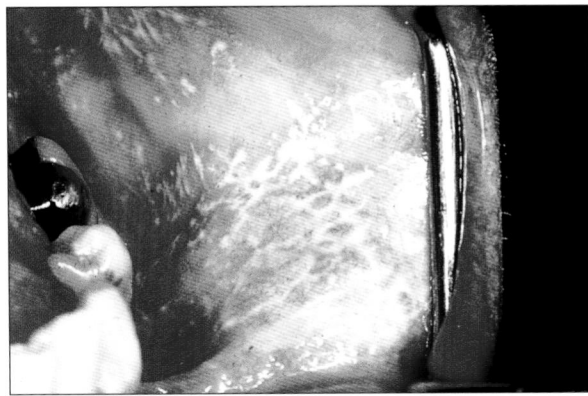

Fig 3-20 White striae and annular pattern with small white papules, which are characteristic of reticular lichen planus.

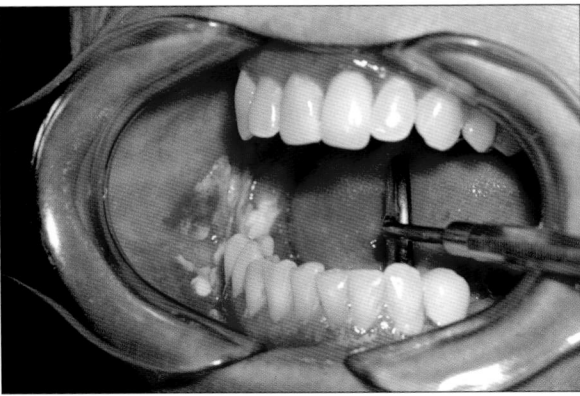

Fig 3-21 The plaque form of lichen planus is often found on the buccal mucosa and/or tongue. It will be slightly elevated and irregular.

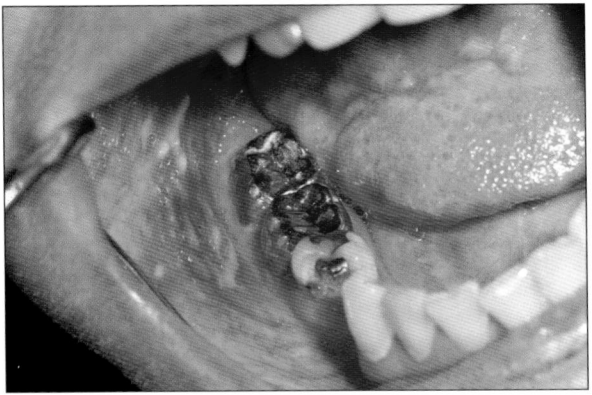

Fig 3-22a The most common location for erosive lichen planus is the buccal mucosa, where red, fibrinous, painful ulcerations will be seen.

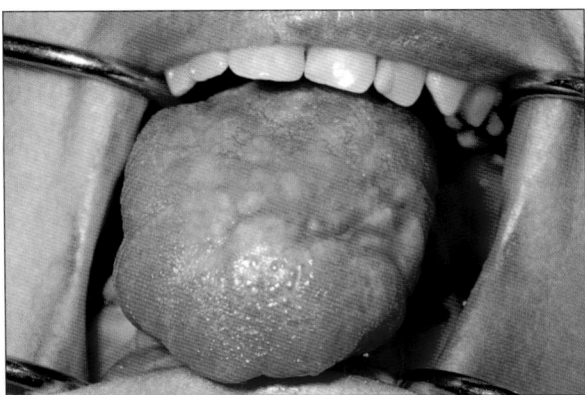

Fig 3-22b The second most common location for erosive lichen planus is the dorsum of the tongue. Here, white patches, red patches, and fibrinous ulcers are seen together.

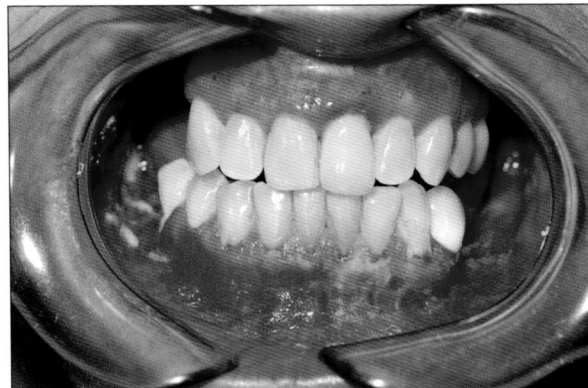

Fig 3-22c The third most common site of erosive lichen planus is the attached gingiva, which will be friable and painful with a reddened base in which some white patches may appear.

Plaque Form

The plaque form is characterized by a white patch or leukoplakia appearance. In this form, slightly elevated, irregular hyperkeratotic plaques develop at the characteristic sites (Fig 3-21). These patches are usually asymptomatic but may be associated with some discomfort. Biopsy is required to differentiate this form from premalignant or malignant mucosal changes.

Erosive Form

The erosive form is characterized by intense pain and erythematous mucosal inflammation. When it involves the buccal mucosa or the tongue, it will produce fibrinous-based ulcers against a background of erythema and sometimes white hyperkeratotic foci (Figs 3-22a and 3-22b). When it involves the attached gingiva, it will produce a boggy, red, friable tissue that bleeds easily (Fig 3-22c). Because the inflammatory destruction is focused on the basal cells, some presentations will demonstrate vesicle formation, and a Nikolsky sign may even be elicited. Some label this finding a separate form, *bullous lichen planus*, but it merely represents a part of the erosive lichen planus spectrum. Similarly, the attached gingiva presentation of erosive lichen planus closely resembles what many in the past referred to as *desquamative gin-*

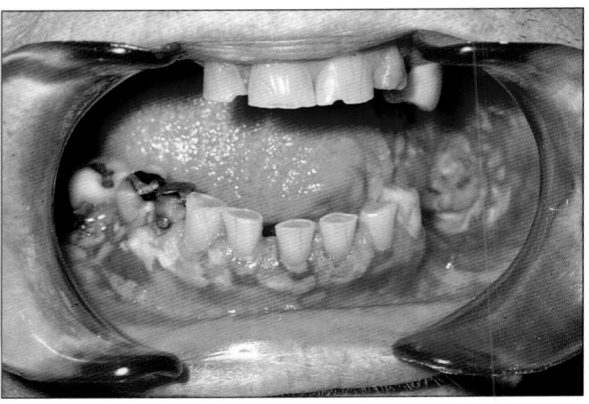

Fig 3-23a This field dysplasia presented with pain and a clinical picture indistinguishable from erosive lichen planus. Dysplasia and squamous cell carcinoma should always be considered along with lichen planus on a differential diagnosis.

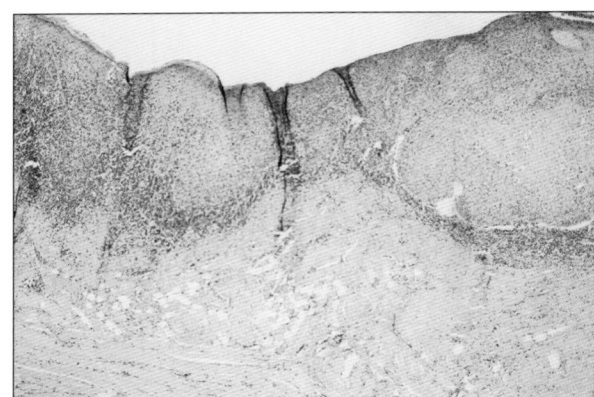

Fig 3-23b Here, epithelial dysplasia mimics erosive lichen planus with acanthosis, a disrupted basement membrane, and a band-like inflammatory infiltrate. However, cytologic atypia of the epithelial cells identify this as a premalignant condition.

givitis, and what some today refer to as an *atrophic form*, but this represents an unnecessary splitting of terminology as this is again merely part of the erosive lichen planus spectrum.

The postulated pathogenic mechanism for lichen planus is that native proteins are falsely identified as foreign antigens. This may result from basal cells expressing surface proteins that bear a close structural resemblance to a foreign protein, thus stimulating a delayed cell-mediated hyperimmune response. It may also result from the exposure of basal cell proteins, which are normally hidden from lymphocytes, to lymphocytes or macrophages, which can then process them as antigens. Basal cells that do not normally express class II histocompatibility antigens are induced to do so by injury, drugs, nonspecific activated lymphocytes secreting gamma-interferon, or other factors. They then express human lymphocyte antigen HLA-DR, which is also expressed by lymphocytes and antigen-processing macrophages called Langerhans cells. If both basal cells and lymphocytes carry HLA-DR surface antigens, they can come into contact and transfer antigenic information, as is common to Langerhans cell–lymphocyte interactions, which confer normal cell-mediated immunity. In this sense, basal cell antigen may become transferred to these lymphocytes and initiate the cell-mediated autoimmunity that is known to be the mechanism of lichen planus.

DIFFERENTIAL DIAGNOSIS ▶

The reticular form of lichen planus is clinically distinct. The plaque form of lichen planus could be described as "clinical leukoplakia." Such "clinical leukoplakia" carries with it a subset of different lesions that, like lichen planus, can produce a white leukoplakic patch. These include the nonspecific *benign hyperkeratoses*, a spectrum of *epithelial dysplasias*, *verrucous hyperplasia*, *verrucous carcinoma*, and *invasive squamous cell carcinoma*. In addition, *hypertrophic candidiasis* is also known to produce a white patch that will not rub off as do other forms of candidiasis.

The erosive form of lichen planus can be particularly treacherous because its clinical presentation may be identical to that of *dysplasia* (Fig 3-23a). The similarity of clinical and even histopathologic appearance has stirred a controversy in which lichen planus is considered a premalignant disease by some (Fig 3-23b). The term *lichenoid dysplasia* correctly describes the histopathologic similarities of the two entities but is confusing because atypical cells are part of dysplasia from its onset but are not part of uncomplicated lichen planus. Therefore, a field dysplasia exists separate from lichen planus and should be included in the differential diagnosis. However, recent documentation of lichen planus transforming into squamous cell carcinoma has identified erosive lichen planus to indeed have this premalignant potential.

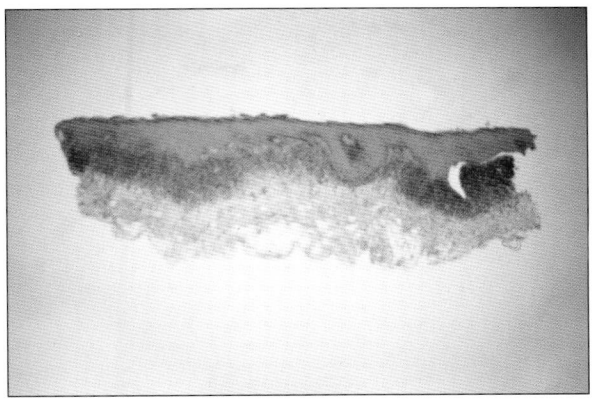

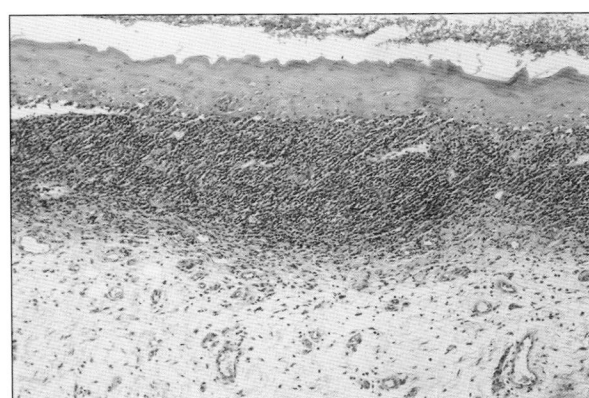

Fig 3-24a A low-power view of a case of lichen planus shows the typical band-like infiltrate of lymphocytes that is well demarcated and just below the basement membrane.

Fig 3-24b A higher-power view of Fig 3-24a shows that the lymphocytic band is well delimited at its inferior border and that it hugs the epithelium. A so-called Max-Jacob space, an artifactual separation of the epithelium, is also seen, a finding often noted in lichen planus.

Although its transformation incidence is about 1% to 3%, erosive lichen planus transitioning into an invasive squamous cell carcinoma is a realistic inclusion in the differential diagnosis.

The presentation of painful, red attached gingiva in particular will closely resemble *pemphigoid*, and the generally painful oral lesions, usually without skin lesions, will strongly suggest *pemphigus vulgaris* at times. *Chronic ulcerative stomatitis* may present with ulceration and desquamation of the gingiva.

DIAGNOSTIC WORK-UP ▶ The diagnosis is made from a mucosal biopsy; skin biopsies are also diagnostic if skin lesions are present. The critical guideline to obtaining a diagnostic tissue specimen is to avoid biopsy of an ulcerated area. Ulcerated areas will be distorted by epithelial loss and secondary nonspecific inflammation. It is best to biopsy a red or white area and include some surrounding normal-appearing tissue. The use of direct immunofluorescence is not specifically required to diagnose lichen planus because it is a T-cell–mediated disease in which there are no autoantibodies or other specific markers to identify. However, biopsies also submitted in Michel's medium for direct immunofluorescence may be required to rule out other immune-based diseases such as pemphigus vulgaris and pemphigoid, which have a definitive direct immunofluorescence marker.

HISTOPATHOLOGY ▶ Lichen planus involves a cell-mediated immune reaction that damages epithelial basal cells. Langerhans cells are increased in number in lichen planus. These are the antigen-presenting cells to which T cells respond and are consequently drawn into the area, forming a banded infiltrate subjacent to the epithelium (Figs 3-24a and 3-24b). The infiltrate is typically well demarcated inferiorly, but it invades the epithelium, effacing the epithelial–connective tissue junction (Fig 3-25a). The T cells are cytotoxic to the basal cells, which undergo vacuolation and destruction (liquefaction degeneration) (Fig 3-25b). Secondary to the loss of basal cells, melanin may be released into the connective tissue, where it is picked up by macrophages which then are termed melanophages. Known as melanin incontinence, this process is responsible for the frequent violaceous color that may be associated with lichen planus (Fig 3-25c). The rete ridges lose their well-defined architecture and often appear to "melt" into the fibrous tissue (Fig 3-25d). The epithelium also reacts to the assault, possibly through lymphocyte mediation, so that hyperkeratosis and/or hyperparakeratosis is seen with varying degrees of acanthosis and/or atrophy. Round to oval eosinophilic cells are frequently found in the lower epithelium or lamina propria. These represent necrotic epithelial cells and have been called *Civatte bodies, colloid bodies,* or *apoptotic cells* (Fig 3-25e).

The histologic features of lichen planus vary according to the age of the lesion. Following regeneration of the basal layer, a discrete eosinophilic band that separates the epithelium from the underlying lymphocytic infiltrate is often seen (Fig 3-25f). Secondary to the destruction of basal cells, desquamation of

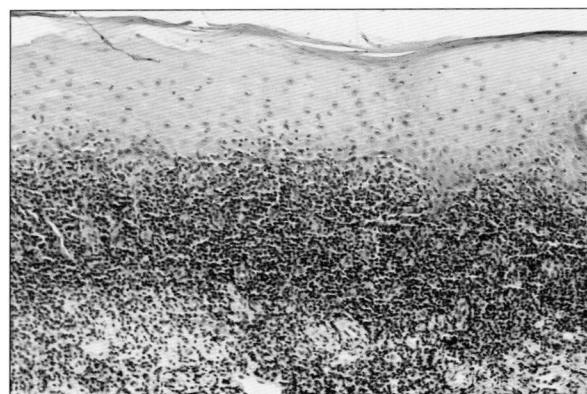

Fig 3-25a A lesion of lichen planus from the buccal mucosa shows some hyperparakeratosis and the typical masking of the epithelial–connective tissue junction by the lymphocytes (interface mucositis).

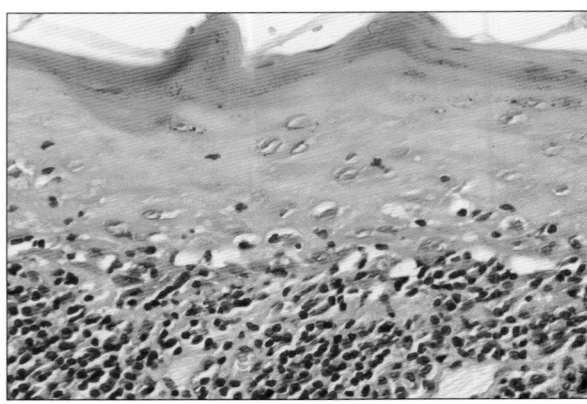

Fig 3-25b The vacuolation of basal cells (liquefaction degeneration) can be seen.

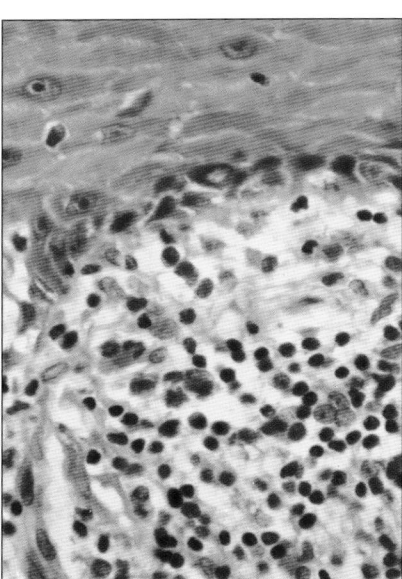

Fig 3-25c Within the lymphocytic infiltrate, melanophages can be seen.

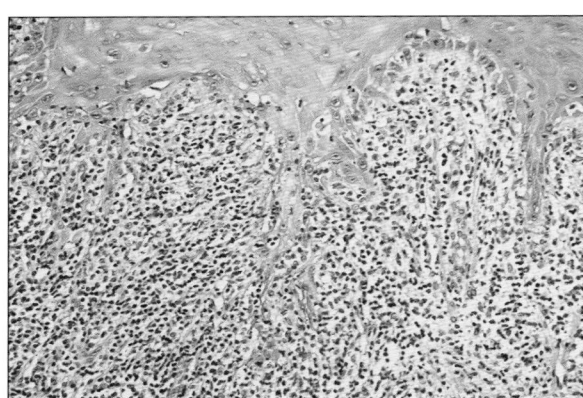

Fig 3-25d The "melting" or fading of the rete ridge into the inflamed connective tissue can be seen. This finding, which is caused by the epithelial destruction that has occurred, should not be misconstrued as an invasive process.

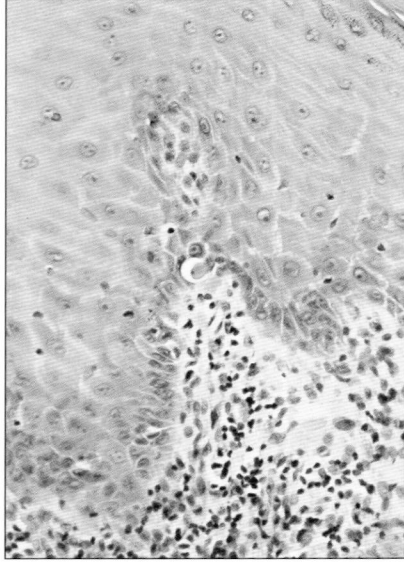

Fig 3-25e Immediately below the epithelium, in the center of the field, an apoptotic cell can be seen.

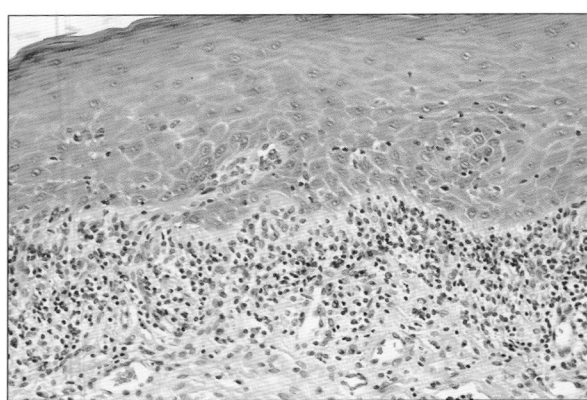

Fig 3-25f In this area, a thin eosinophilic band separates the epithelium from the underlying lymphocytic infiltrate.

the epithelium may occur (as in desquamative gingivitis) or a bulla may develop (as in bullous lichen planus). These bullae may be distinguished by the lack of basal cells and the fact that the base of the lesion is formed by connective tissue while the roof consists of prickle cells (Fig 3-26). In erosive lichen planus, the inflammatory infiltrate is extremely dense and, because of the ulceration, more pleomorphic.

Lichen planus does not produce a single definitive histologic picture and, depending on the stage, the changes may be nonspecific. It is significant, however, that dysplastic changes within the epithelium rule out the diagnosis of lichen planus. Dysplastic disease can also be associated with banded lymphocytic in-

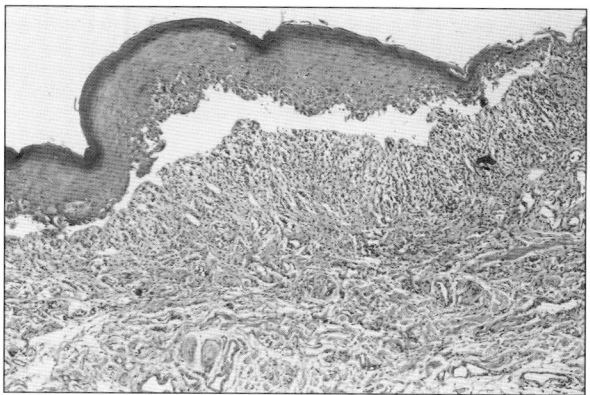

Fig 3-26 A case of bullous lichen planus shows the separation of the epithelium. The base of the bulla consists of connective tissue, and the roof is composed of prickle cells, the basal cells having undergone vacuolation.

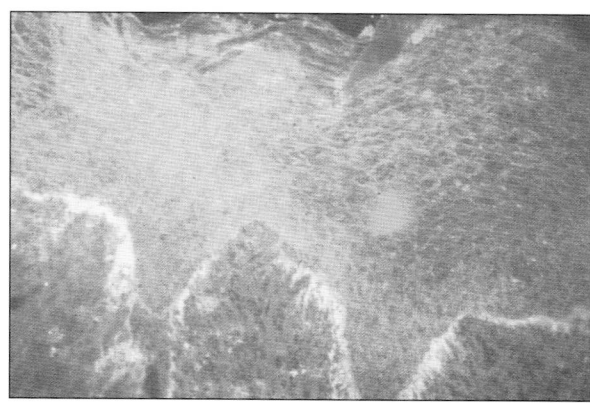

Fig 3-27 Direct immunofluorescence in lichen planus shows positivity only for fibrin, which forms a shaggy pattern below the epithelium.

filtrates, which should not be construed as representing lichen planus. By means of direct immunofluorescence, fibrinogen may be demonstrated in the basement membrane zone, extending in little tags into the connective tissue (Fig 3-27). This is nonspecific and may be seen in other inflammatory conditions. The colloid apoptotic cells can also be demonstrated by direct immunofluorescence. They typically stain for IgM, but IgG, IgA, C3, and fibrin may also be seen. Although not unique to lichen planus, when seen in large numbers they are strongly suggestive of this disease.

Chronic ulcerative stomatitis is a condition that mimics lichen planus histologically. However, the immunopathologic picture is different. It is characterized by anti-nuclear antibodies directed against the stratified squamous epithelium. This can be demonstrated by both direct and indirect immunofluorescence. Significantly, this disease is not as responsive as lichen planus to corticosteroids but will respond to hydroxychlorquine (Plaquenil, Sanofi Winthrop).

TREATMENT ▶ Reticular and plaque forms usually do not require treatment other than reassurance and follow-up. The milder cases of erosive lichen planus and some symptomatic cases of the other forms often can be managed with topical corticosteroids, usually 0.05% fluocinonide gel (Lidex gel, Medicis Dermatologics), four times daily, or combined with the antifungal agent griseofulvin (Fulvicin, Schering), 250 mg of the micronized form twice daily. The efficacy of this agent seems to be related to its side effect of promoting epithelial cell differentiation and maturity. Intralesional triamcinolone (Kenalog 0.5%), injected in 1-mL increments, may also be used for focal symptomatic areas.

Most erosive lichen planus requires systemic corticosteroid regimen I or II and only rarely IIIA or IIIB (see pages 205 to 206) (Figs 3-28 and 3-29). Griseofulvin or topical fluocinonide can be added to either regimen to reduce the prednisone requirements or help maintain a remission.

Recently, some authors have suggested topical retinoids (isotretinoin), a vitamin A analog, for reticular lichen planus. However, almost all reticular lichen planus is asymptomatic and nonprogressive. In addition, the striae return if the drug is discontinued. Systemic retinoids have also been attempted, but their value is questionable owing to their minimal effect on the disease and significant side effects, such as increase of liver enzyme levels, hypercholesterolemia, hypertriglyceridemia, mucositis, mood changes, and possible teratogenicity.

Dapsone (diaminodiphenylsulfone) has been effective for mild cases of lichen planus involving skin. If used, the patient's serum should be tested for the presence of glucose-6-phosphate dehydrogenase (G6PD) because dapsone may precipitate a G6PD-deficiency hemolytic episode. Dapsone is given in a dose of 50 mg per day and may be continued for several weeks.

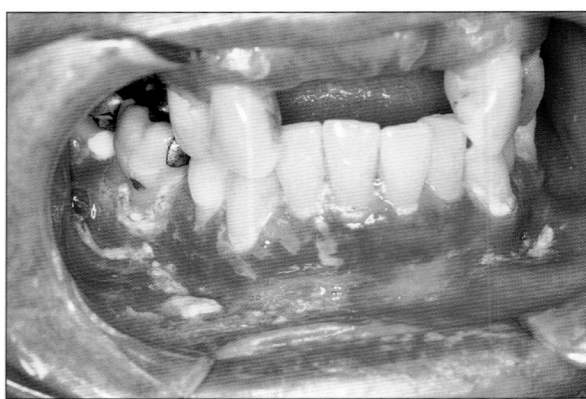 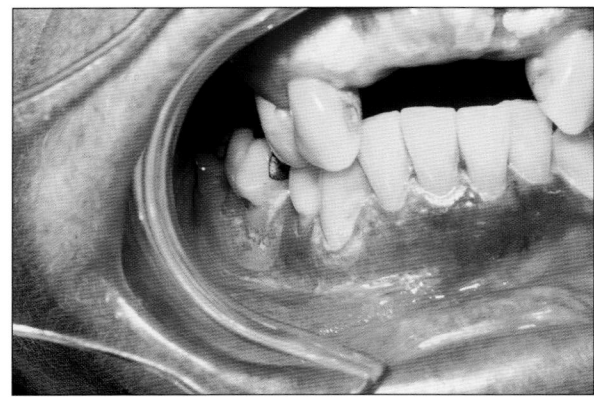

Fig 3-28 Erosive lichen planus before treatment with corticosteroid regimen I and griseofulvin.

Fig 3-29 Within 2 months, a marked improvement of 80% is noted with some residual erythema and no ulcerations, white patches, or pain.

PROGNOSIS

Erosive lichen planus responds well to systemic corticosteroids but not as completely as does pemphigus vulgaris or the various pemphigoids. A milder, residual clinical disease often persists and consequently a drug-free remission is less common than a maintenance-control remission. Often the disease can be suppressed with prednisone to a point at which topical fluocinonide and/or griseofulvin can maintain the remission without continued prednisone or with only a low, every-other-day prednisone schedule.

The premalignant potential of erosive lichen planus is now proven. Certainly there is a higher incidence of oral mucosal squamous cell carcinoma in patients with a history or a diagnosis of erosive lichen planus than in the general population. The transformation is uncommon (1% to 3%) and usually takes 15 years or more. Therefore, any erosive lichen planus that does not respond to therapy, especially prednisone, should be viewed with suspicion. These patients should undergo another biopsy. The original histopathology slides should be reviewed for subtle evidence of cellular atypia and the features of true lichen planus and then compared to the new slides.

Erythema Multiforme

Erythema multiforme historically has been a confusing disease for most clinicians for two reasons. First, the diagnosis of "erythema multiforme" has been attached to many disease states associated with oral lesions for which no other specific diagnostic name could be applied. Second, a spectrum of clinical signs and symptoms may be seen; this is related to the great variability in disease severity. Therefore, diagnosis of true erythema multiforme must fulfill specific criteria, and a division into erythema multiforme minor and major is appropriate.

Erythema Multiforme Minor

CLINICAL PRESENTATION AND PATHOGENESIS

Most afflicted individuals are young adults who develop both skin lesions and oral lesions after an infection or other physiologic stress (Fig 3-30). Many of these cases follow a mycoplasma pneumonia or herpes simplex infection. The skin lesions are more prominent than the oral lesions, and they are often described as classic "target" or "iris" lesions because they appear to have a background erythematous center with concentric rings of more intense erythema at the periphery (Fig 3-31). The palms of the hands will show target-like lesions more than any other skin surface. However, early lesions will often be merely macular erythematous areas, and some will crust over or develop vesicles without demonstrat-

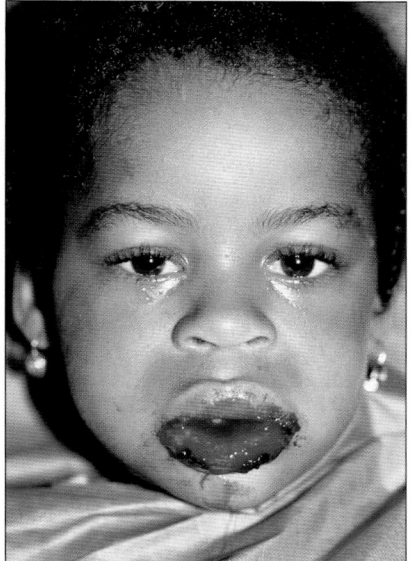

Fig 3-30 Erythema multiforme minor has severe pain and a fast onset. Here a 5-year-old developed three target skin lesions and a painful lower lip lesion within 18 hours after taking the antibiotic cefaclor.

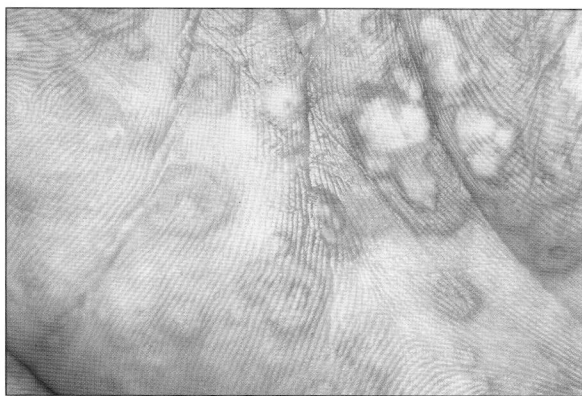

Fig 3-31 "Classic" erythema multiforme skin lesions will appear target-like and are best seen on the palms of the hands.

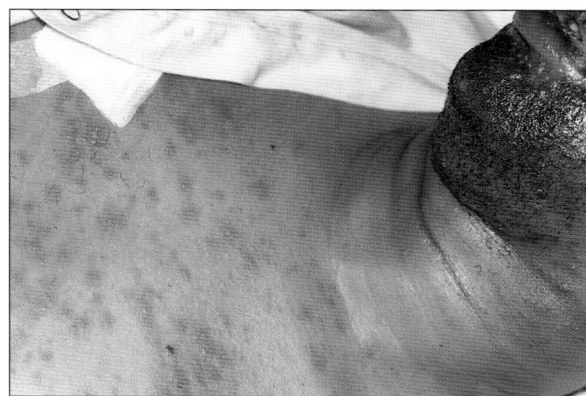

Fig 3-32 Early erythema multiforme skin lesions will not be target-like and will be more prominent on the trunk and extremities.

CLINICAL PRESENTATION AND PATHOGENESIS ▶

ing a target pattern. The skin lesions will be symmetric, and distribution will occur more prominently on the extremities and trunk (Fig 3-32).

Oral lesions tend to be hemorrhagic ulcers that crust and may be seen on any portion of the oral mucosa. However, the lip vermilion is the site of predilection (see Fig 3-30). Oral lesions will occur in only 50% of cases with skin lesions and will emerge concurrently. Oral lesions suggestive of erythema multiforme without concomitant skin lesions probably do not represent true erythema multiforme. Such cases often represent a lichenoid drug eruption or an immune-based disease not documented by a biopsy.

The skin lesions and oral lesions produce pain, but it will not be nearly as severe and debilitating as that associated with erythema multiforme major. The pain will decrease over the first week and nearly disappear for the remaining 2 to 4 weeks of the lesions' duration.

Erythema Multiforme Major (Stevens-Johnson Syndrome)

This variant of erythema multiforme represents a life-threatening and debilitating hypersensitivity. It is most often seen in children younger than 15 years, but it also occurs in adults. The clinical symptoms arise quickly and progress rapidly in what is often called an "explosive onset," mostly after ingestion of a therapeutic drug (Figs 3-33a and 3-33b). Skin lesions will begin as erythematous macules but rapidly progress to so-called target lesions and vesicles. These progress to skin necrosis, producing large denuded areas with loss of electrolytes and tissue proteins, as well as frequent secondary infections resembling a burn. In the past, patients were described as having "ocular-genital lesions." Skin lesions involve necrosis of scrotal skin (Fig 3-34), penile skin, or vulval and labial surfaces. The ocular component is epithelial necrosis of the cornea and conjunctiva, which is analogous to the skin lesions. The conjunctiva and cornea develop prominent ulceration and necrosis, often leading to blindness directly or to visual loss caused by secondary infection (Fig 3-35).

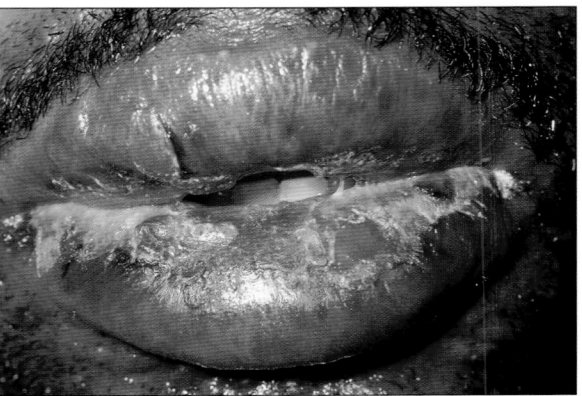

Fig 3-33a Early onset of erythema multiforme major with beginning erosive surface lesions of the vermilion.

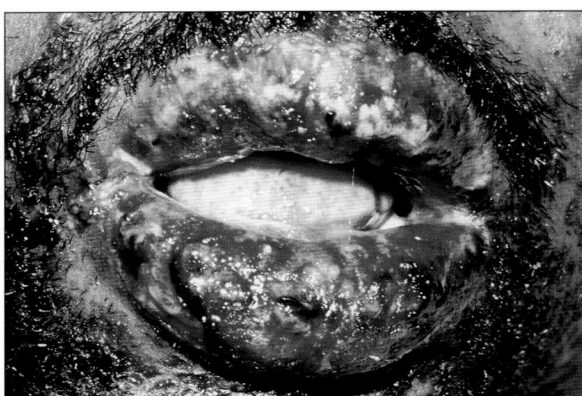

Fig 3-33b Within 24 hours, the beginning erosions have necrosed the entire vermilion surface to create a painful hemorrhagic crusting lip.

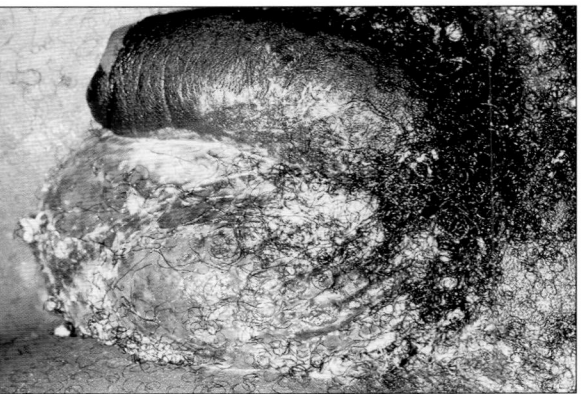

Fig 3-34 The genital lesions of erythema multiforme major are skin necroses of the scrotum and penis. One-percent silver sulfadiazine is used here as an antimicrobial cream similar to burn wound management.

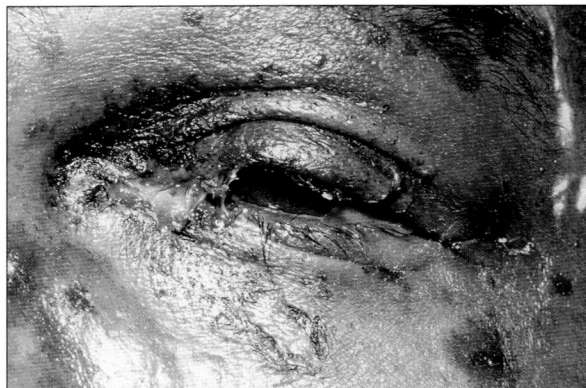

Fig 3-35 The ocular lesions of erythema multiforme major are corneal and conjunctival necrosis along with some skin necrosis. This eye lost vision within 36 hours because of corneal loss.

Oral lesions are large, hemorrhagic, crusting ulcers, particularly of the lips and labial mucosa. Mucosal and vermilion necrosis is common. The oral lesions as well as the skin lesions are severely painful. The oral lesions will secondarily produce drooling, which exacerbates fluid and electrolyte loss and frequently leads to secondary infection, ultimately resulting in cervical lymphadenitis. The pain prevents oral intake of fluids or solids. The progression from the initial emergence of lesions to a full debilitating clinical picture with skin and mucous membrane necrosis often occurs within 24 hours.

The pathogenesis of erythema multiforme is that of an intense vasculitis. It represents an antibody-based hypersensitivity in which a range of inflammatory intensities from mild to fulminant are possible. The end products are initiation of epithelial cell necrosis by the secretory enzymes of inflammatory cells directly on the epithelium and on the nutrient vessels in the subjacent connective tissue.

Erythema multiforme is thought to represent a combined type III and IV immune reaction. The more deeply located lymphocytes are primarily CD4 cells, while those associated with the epithelium and located closer to the basement membrane are CD8 cells. With direct immunofluorescence, the superficial vessels of the connective tissue are seen to contain IgM and C3 in their walls. At the dermal-epidermal junction, granular deposits of IgM, fibrinogen, and C3 may be seen. Circulating immune complexes have also been found.

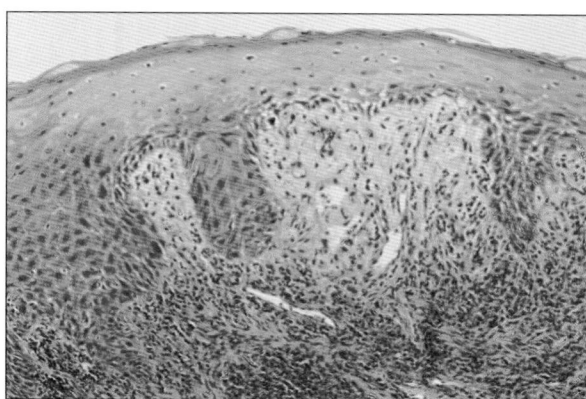

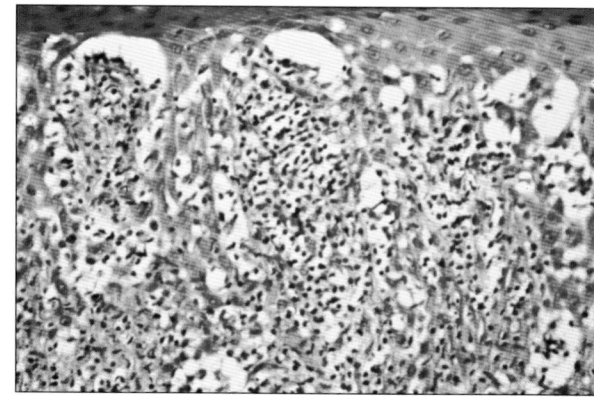

Fig 3-36a Erythema multiforme with edema, inflammation, and vascular proliferation in the connective tissue and some intercellular and intracellular edema in the basal area of the epithelium.

Fig 3-36b Vesicle formation is seen in the basement membrane zone accompanied by a marked inflammatory response in a case of erythema multiforme.

DIFFERENTIAL DIAGNOSIS ▶

Erythema multiforme minor can resemble several other diseases that have painful skin and oral lesions, specifically *lichenoid drug eruptions*, *lichen planus*, and *pemphigus vulgaris*. Because this type of erythema multiforme may follow a herpes simplex infection, an extension or exacerbation of a *herpes infection* must be considered. The general picture of oral, skin, and ocular lesions may cause some to consider *pemphigoid*, *Behçet syndrome*, or the mucosal component of *reactive arthritis*. However, pemphigoid is found in a much older group and manifests much less skin involvement. Behçet syndrome skin lesions are more discrete and less widespread, and its ocular lesions do not involve the conjunctiva or cornea; instead, an iritis that frequently produces pus in the anterior chamber (hypopyon) is found. Reactive arthritis produces painless oral lesions, and the eye involvement is limited to conjunctivitis.

Erythema multiforme major is such a dramatic and distinctive clinical-symptom complex that few other diseases are confused with it. The main differential lesion is *toxic epidermal necrolysis*, which some believe is merely another name for the same disease process. Severe cases of *pemphigus* or *cutaneous pemphigoid* may also mimic erythema multiforme major, but the progression of signs and symptoms is not nearly as rapid.

DIAGNOSTIC WORK-UP ▶

Both types of erythema multiforme are clinical diagnoses. Nevertheless, a mucosa or skin biopsy is recommended to rule out identifiable immune-based and viral diseases. The histopathologic features are not pathognomonic unless a fresh, early lesion is sampled.

HISTOPATHOLOGY ▶

The histologic appearance of erythema multiforme depends in part on the stage of the lesion and the area of the biopsy (Figs 3-36a and 3-36b). Initially, there is vacuolation of basal cells and some exocytosis. Lymphocytes may be seen along the dermal-epidermal junction as well as perivascularly. Necrosis of prickle cells is a significant finding. There may be considerable edema, particularly within the connective tissue papillae.

Some differences have been noted between lesions that are associated with herpes simplex and those that are drug induced. In the former, there is more connective tissue edema, spongiosis, exocytosis, and liquefaction degeneration of basal cells. Drug-induced lesions manifest more epithelial necrosis. Epithelial necrosis is also very prominent within the center of "iris" lesions. Ultrastructural examination of the bullae of erythema multiforme shows that the basal lamina may be on either the roof or the floor.

TREATMENT ▶

Erythema multiforme minor usually requires no treatment. It is self-limiting, will improve after 5 to 8 days, and will completely resolve within 2 to 4 weeks. In some cases, antibiotics are required to treat secondary skin or oral infections. Skin infections are treated with antibiotics that are effective against *Staphylococcus* species; oral infections are treated with antibiotics that are effective against *Streptococcus* species. Drugs effective against both species include amoxicillin with clavulanate (Augmentin, SK Beecham), dicloxacillin, and erythromycin. One should resist the temptation to treat erythema multiforme minor with systemic corticosteroids. In these cases, such therapy neither shortens the disease course nor reduces symptoms and actually predisposes the patient to secondary infections.

Erythema multiforme major (Stevens-Johnson syndrome), however, requires systemic corticosteroids. Initially, high doses of prednisone, 100 to 160 mg per day, are used for about 2 weeks as in systemic corticosteroid regimen II (see page 205). Because most of these patients cannot swallow well, intravenous methylprednisolone (Solu-Medrol, Pharmacia and Upjohn), 500 to 750 mg, is given until swallowing improves. Hydration with intravenous fluids and antibiotics such as vancomycin, ampicillin with sulbactam (Unasyn, Pfizer US), or erythromycin are given concomitantly. The necrosed skin is treated as a burn with topical antimicrobial creams (1% silver sulfadiazine; Silvadene, Aventis), and the eyes are irrigated and patched.

Once the intensity of the disease resolves and no new skin lesions are developing, corticosteroids are discontinued. The use of corticosteroids in this form of erythema multiforme does not fit a specific regimen; the goal is to reduce the inflammation-mediated tissue destruction and then discontinue the drug to prevent secondary infections of the many denuded skin areas.

PROGNOSIS ▶ Erythema multiforme minor is self-limiting, lasts 2 to 4 weeks, and may recur. It has frequently been noted to recur seasonally, in the spring and the fall. Erythema multiforme major is also self-limiting and lasts 2 to 4 weeks; however, it usually does not recur and is associated with some mortality because of fluid and electrolyte loss and in some cases skin infections unresponsive to antibiotics. In addition, blindness, impotence, and disfiguring scar formation may be seen and may result in lifelong disability.

Systemic Drug Reactions

Reactions to systemically administered drugs are more common than realized. The target organ is the skin in most cases, but it may be the oral mucosa in others. Some drug reactions produce a specific clinical presentation and, therefore, may be distinguished as a distinct entity or given a specific name. The 50% or more of cases of erythema multiforme that are triggered by a drug, including the major form called Stevens-Johnson syndrome (erythema multiforme major), are examples of systemic drug reactions. The entity that produces erythematous and erosive lesions limited to the oral mucosa and resembles erosive lichen planus is distinguished by some and called *lichenoid drug reactions*.

CLINICAL PRESENTATION ▶ The clinical presentation of the drug reaction depends on many factors. The most significant factors are the type of immune mechanisms; the susceptibility of the individual (those with a history of multiple, frequent reactions and allergies are referred to as *atopic*); and the triggering drug.

There are four general drug-reaction mechanisms, each of which produces a somewhat different general clinical picture. They are histamine release, IgE-mediated reactions, antigen-antibody complexes, and cytotoxic drug reactions.

Histamine Release

This is the only nonimmune-based mechanism. Certain drugs directly stimulate degranulation of fixed tissue mast cells. The histamine they release causes a vasodilation and a discharge of action potentials at free nerve endings, which results in an erythema and itching characteristic of histamine release. Common offending drugs of this type include the narcotics morphine, meperidine hydrochloride (Demerol), and codeine, and many antimicrobials such as vancomycin and amphotericin B.

IgE-Mediated Reactions

Other drugs indirectly cause varying degrees of histamine release and the release of other vasoactive/inflammation-initiating chemicals. This occurs when the drug contains an antigenic site that causes it to be

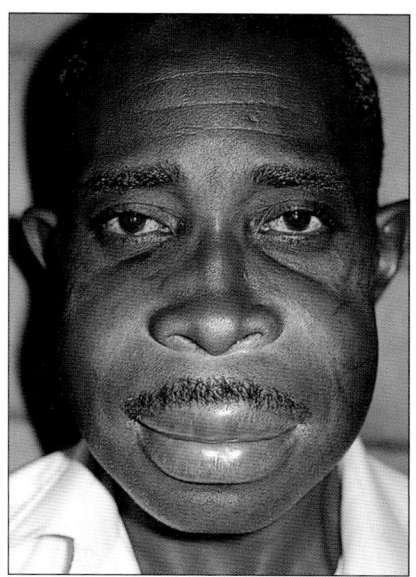

Fig 3-37 Angioedema often involves the soft tissue of one or both lips, usually in a painless manner.

bound to IgE fixed to the cell membranes of mast cells. The IgE previously became fixed to mast cells and was produced with a specific antigenic site by previous sensitization often believed to be topical sensitization. Clinically, this mechanism may produce a simple skin rash or a series of more severe reactions up to anaphylaxis. This is the mechanism responsible for most food allergies, particularly milk and shellfish reactions and acquired angioedema. Acquired angioedema will appear as a soft, diffuse, but usually large painless swelling of the lips and facial skin (Fig 3-37). Unlike most other drug reactions, angioedema does not cause an erythema. It seems to affect vascular permeability without a prominent release of the initiators of inflammation and, therefore, inflammatory cells. Such angioedema is, however, self-limiting and lasts only 3 to 5 days. This type of angioedema should be distinguished from hereditary angioedema, which creates an identical clinical presentation but is caused by an autosomal-dominant trait in which there is a deficiency of the inhibitor of CI esterase, the first component of the complement cascade. Therefore, the complement cascade can be triggered and expressed without modulation.

Antigen-Antibody Complexes

If a drug is taken over a long period, circulating antibodies to it may slowly develop. Over time, antibody titers may rise so that further drug administration creates sufficient numbers of new circulating antigen-antibody complexes that may lodge in the skin or any organ to initiate inflammation. This mechanism is involved when patients claim to have developed a sudden allergy to a medication they have taken before or have been taking for some time. This mechanism is referred to as *serum sickness* and is responsible for many internal-organ drug reactions, such as nephritis and arthritis.

Cytotoxic Drug Reactions

Some drugs become bound to cell membranes in one or many organs as part of their mechanism of action or their elimination. If, through sensitization, the drug has stimulated antibody production by the coupling of antibody to the antigen fixed to the cell membrane, the drug in question may cause cell lysis. This type of reaction, which may be very severe and cause extensive tissue destruction, is thought to be the mechanism responsible for erythema multiforme and, although less severe, so-called lichenoid drug reaction (Fig 3-38a). It has been known to produce a hemolytic anemia when the drug is fixed to red blood cell membranes.

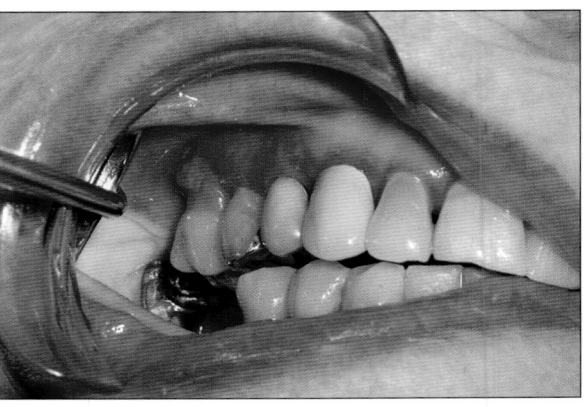

Fig 3-38a This diffuse and modestly painful erythema was due to the yellow dye tartrazine in the patient's Synthroid (levothyroxine) tablets.

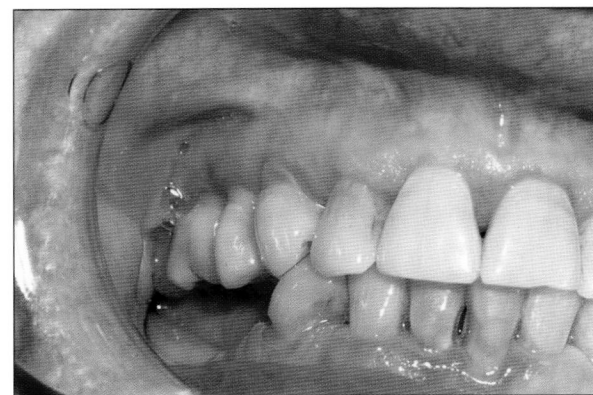

Fig 3-38b After the Synthroid tablets were changed to another color, the systemic drug reaction resolved.

Offending Drugs

While any drug can cause a systemic drug reaction, some drugs historically have produced a higher incidence than others. The following substances have the highest incidence of these reactions: (1) levothyroxine sodium (Synthroid); (2) FD&C yellow no. 5 (tartrazine), a dye used in many yellow-colored tablets. (Its use in the Synthroid 100-µg tablet is associated with a higher-than-usual incidence of so-called lichenoid drug reactions in particular); (3) gold salts; (4) allopurinol; (5) colchicine; (6) methyldopa; (7) nifedipine (Procardia); (8) penicillin (particularly ampicillin); (9) codeine; (10) propranolol.

HISTOPATHOLOGY ▶ Tissue changes secondary to drug reactions are essentially inflammatory but can present a varied picture. Some have a lichenoid appearance with a mononuclear subepithelial banded infiltrate. Others resemble lupus erythematosus and demonstrate perivascular mononuclear infiltrates. Still others produce a pemphigus-type reaction. For all of these, the histologic and immunologic features are the same as those in the nondrug-related cases. Erythema multiforme is often secondary to drug reactions.

TREATMENT ▶ The obvious treatment for drug reactions is to identify the offending drug and discontinue its use. This may be easy if the offending drug is a new drug just introduced, or it may be difficult if it occurs in a situation of multiple, long-term drug usage.

If the reaction is anaphylaxis, full cardiopulmonary resuscitation and cardiac life support may be needed. If the reaction is known to be drug precipitated, 0.3 mL of 1:1,000 epinephrine solution subcutaneously should be part of the resuscitation.

If the reaction is clinically obvious angioedema, no specific treatment may be necessary other than airway observation. For histamine-releasing reactions, diphenhydramine hydrochloride (Benadryl, Warner Lambert), 50 mg intravenously, remains one of the best H1 antihistamines for quick reversal of symptoms. To prevent symptoms in an anticipated reaction or to treat recurrent histamine release, diphenhydramine hydrochloride, 50 mg twice daily by mouth, or terfenadine (Seldane), 60 mg orally twice daily, may be needed. Terfenadine is associated with little drowsiness and sedation compared to other antihistamines and may be the drug of choice if the symptomatic response is good.

If the offending drug is the tartrazine yellow dye of Synthroid (levothyroxine) 100-µg tablets, a change to two 50-µg Synthroid tablets, which does not have the tartrazine yellow dye, often solves the problem. If the offending drug is the Synthroid itself, the clinician should consult the endocrinologist about other thyroid replacements. If the offending drug cannot be discontinued, prednisone is a reasonable therapeutic choice, but in the lowest dose possible to maintain control of the reaction (Figs 3-38a and 3-38b).

When an offending drug that has been a long-standing part of a patient's medications is discontinued, the drug reaction will be slow to respond. The clinician should warn the patient that it may take up to 3 months to see clinical improvement.

Contact Drug Reactions

CLINICAL PRESENTATION ▶

Contact drug reactions are of three types. The first type is a direct drug toxicity, whereby the pH or an active chemical site produces a physical injury to the tissue. "Aspirin burn" caused by the acidic pH of aspirin and the chemical burn of capsiscum in sharp peppers are examples of direct drug toxicity. Such reactions are direct physical injuries, not actual immune-based reactions. The lesions are usually a localized, white painful area with a fibrinous base or slough surrounded by a small zone of erythema.

The second and most predominant type is a T-cell–mediated immune reaction. Initially the offending drug is topically absorbed through intact skin or mucosa. During absorption, the drug contacts the Langerhans cells, which exist in the middle zone of the prickle cell layer in both skin and mucosa. The Langerhans cell, which seems to be a type of histiocyte, processes the drug as an antigen. It will present the drug on its cell membrane to T lymphocytes, creating antigen-sensitized T lymphocytes. When the drug is topically absorbed a second time, the sensitized T lymphocytes will react by secreting an array of lymphokines that produce inflammation and tissue injury characteristic of contact reaction "allergies." This may affect skin (contact dermatitis) or oral mucosa (contact stomatitis) (Fig 3-39). Such reactions will mostly be areas of boggy erythema corresponding to the drug contact and the pattern dispersal by tongue, lip, and swallowing movements. If the reaction is more severe, actual vesicles or ulcers may form. The prime offending agents have been cosmetics, including lipsticks and lip balm, and dental preparations, such as toothpaste and some of its ingredients. In particular, mint and cinnamon flavorings have been implicated in oral-contact stomatitis. Cosmetic and skin care preparations have been such prominent offenders that complete lines of hypoallergenic products have been developed. Included in this group is hypoallergenic surgeon gloves, which were developed because the powdered starch in many gloves induced a typical contact dermatitis. One supposed cause of contact stomatitis that has been grossly overstated for years is that related to denture acrylic. There is little if any direct evidence to support a true "denture contact stomatitis." Most so-called denture reactions represent other diseases, such as candidiasis, pemphigoid, lichen planus, or mere chronic injury from an ill-fitting denture.

The third type of contact drug reaction is a B-cell–mediated immune reaction whereby antibodies are produced. In a fashion similar to the mechanism noted for T-cell–mediated immune reaction, Langerhans cells may present processed antigen to B lymphocytes, which in turn manufacture specific antibody to the absorbed drug. On a subsequent absorption, antibodies attack the antigen at the epithelial or subepithelial level to produce inflammation and tissue injury. In plasma cell gingivitis, for example, the plasma cells are prominent because they produce specific antibody in the area of antigen (the contact drug) absorption. Plasma cell gingivitis was common in the late 1960s and early 1970s but is rare today. It is believed that the peak of incidence was related to formula changes and ingredients in several dental preparations, which have since been eliminated by the manufacturers.

Clinically, contact drug reactions produce a soft, spongy, red attached gingiva. They may also affect to a lesser degree the labial mucosa, tongue, and commissures. The gingiva and tongue are reported to have a dull, burning sensation (Fig 3-40).

DIFFERENTIAL DIAGNOSIS ▶

The clinical picture of diffuse, red, burning lesions on the oral mucosa without concomitant skin lesions is the classic "burning mouth syndrome" that frequently confronts practitioners. Indeed, many of these represent some type of contact drug reaction that should be meticulously sought out from the patient's history. However, *systemic drug reactions*, *candidiasis*, *recurrent herpes*, *pemphigoid*, *pemphigus*, and *erosive lichen planus* also produce a complaint of burning mouth.

DIAGNOSTIC WORK-UP ▶

If the offending drug is apparent, no further work-up is required. If not, a biopsy including PAS staining to assess for invasive candidiasis, routine H&E staining, and possibly direct immunofluorescence studies to rule out pemphigus and pemphigoid may be required.

HISTOPATHOLOGY ▶

The histologic picture is variable. Some will be indistinguishable from lesions of lichen planus, although lymphoid aggregates are often found in deeper areas of connective tissue in addition to the interface pattern. Plasma cells also may be more prominent, and eosinophils may be present. Plasma cell gingivitis, in

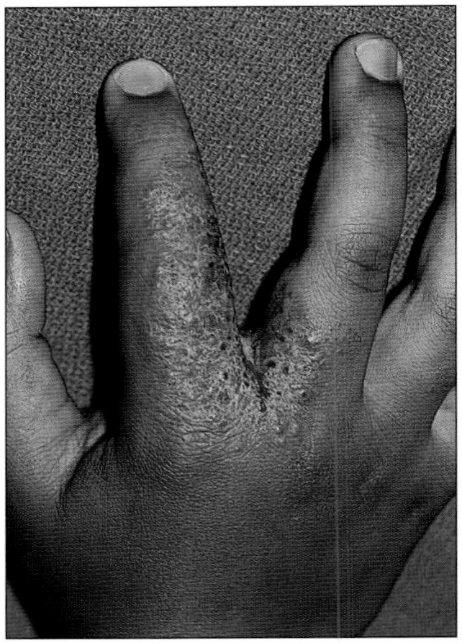

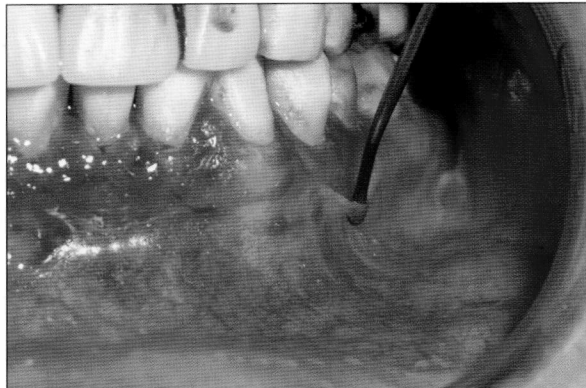

Fig 3-39 Contact dermatitis caused by a topical medicament used as a lubricant to remove a ring.

Fig 3-40 A contact drug reaction from a topical antibiotic produced painful gingival inflammation, erosive ulcers, and even a Nikolsky sign.

addition to a dense plasmacytic infiltrate in the connective tissue, shows spongiosis of the epithelium, often with a neutrophilic infiltrate. Langerhans cells are increased in number.

TREATMENT ▶ Discontinuation of the offending drug is the obvious treatment of choice. However, the patient should be cautioned that improvement may be slow and may take up to 3 months. The delay seems to be caused by the fixation of antigen (drug) to cell membranes, slowing the clearance of the drug. Topical corticosteroids, 0.05% fluocinonide cream for skin (Lidex cream, Medicis Dermatologics) or 0.05% fluocinonide gel (Lidex gel) for mucosa will reduce the symptoms and erythema during the course of antigen clearance.

Discoid Lupus Erythematosus

CLINICAL PRESENTATION AND PATHOGENESIS ▶ Discoid lupus erythematosus (DLE) is an inflammatory disease that targets primarily skin and, to a lesser degree, mucosa. Unlike systemic lupus erythematosus (SLE), DLE has no sex predilection and usually presents with no symptoms. Individuals will seek attention because of the development of dusky red localized skin plaques, 5 to 20 mm in diameter, on the face (Fig 3-41). These plaques will have a predilection for the hairline and sun-exposed areas. A butterfly malar rash develops in DLE, just as it does in SLE. The skin lesions are often referred to as "grass fire" lesions because, as they mature, they develop a broad atrophic white area with a perimeter of red resembling the pattern of a grass fire (Fig 3-42). The scar within this white area will be devoid of hair follicles, leaving patchy bald areas in men's beards or a patchy alopecia on the scalp. In darker-skinned individuals, these lesions leave multiple depigmented regions. Some skin lesions will become scaly, resembling psoriasis.

The oral lesions appear similar to the oral lesions seen in SLE. They are shallow red ulcers that produce minimal symptoms (Fig 3-43) and are most commonly noted on the hard palate mucosa and around the marginal gingiva.

DLE represents an autoimmune inflammatory disease without identifiable autoantibodies. If identifiable autoantibodies exist, the diagnosis is SLE. The autoimmune stimulus is unknown, but it seems to spare B cell involvement and produces a local inflammatory response.

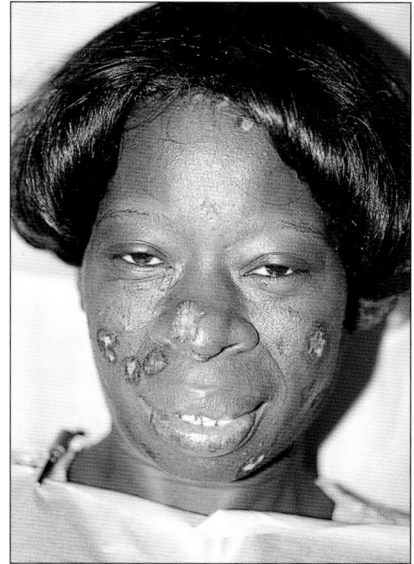

Fig 3-41 Dusky red disfiguring skin lesions are characteristic of discoid lupus erythematosis.

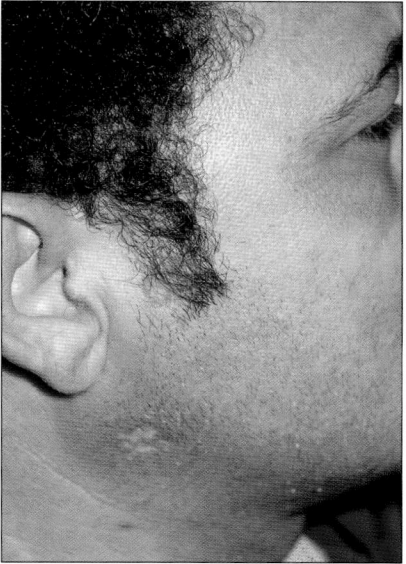

Fig 3-42 Discoid lupus erythematosus lesions may be subtle but will appear like scars and be clustered around hairlines and in sun-exposed areas.

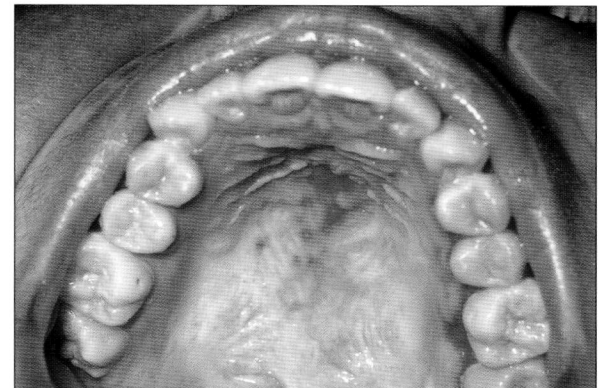

Fig 3-43 Oral lesions in discoid lupus erythematosus often appear on the palate or the marginal gingiva as shallow painless ulcers.

DIFFERENTIAL DIAGNOSIS ▶

Cases that present with prominent skin ulcers, plaques, and perhaps oral lesions and a malar butterfly rash need to be distinguished from *systemic lupus erythematosus*. As an abbreviated screening test to rule out SLE, a battery of tests that include antinuclear antibodies (ANA), anti–double-stranded (native) DNA antibodies, and serum complement level is effective. All are negative or normal in DLE, whereas SLE yields at least one positive or abnormal finding. In particular, 95% of SLE patients will show hypocomplementemia because the systemic antigen-antibody complexes of that disease will consume complement nearly to the point of depletion.

The skin lesions also look like those of *psoriasis*, particularly if they are scaly and plaque-like; *skin tuberculosis* (lupus vulgaris); *sarcoidosis*; or even an early *lepromatous leprosy* if similar multiple facial lesions are visible. Individual lesions may not be distinguishable from those of a *sclerosing morphea type of basal cell carcinoma* or *seborrheic dermatitis*.

DIAGNOSTIC WORK-UP ▶

A topographic and oral-clinical examination is the most important part of a DLE work-up. Screening laboratory tests of an ANA, anti–double-stranded DNA antibodies, and serum complement levels should be accomplished to rule out SLE. Biopsy of one of the skin or mucosal lesions is useful to rule out the other considerations on the differential diagnosis and to establish a firm diagnosis of DLE.

HISTOPATHOLOGY ▶

The microscopic changes associated with DLE include hyperkeratosis and/or hyperparakeratosis, sometimes with keratin plugging, varying areas of acanthosis and atrophy, hydropic degeneration of basal cells, and edema of the lamina propria and inflammatory infiltrates (Figs 3-44a and 3-44b). The inflammatory component is essentially lymphocytic and may be diffuse or perivascular in distribution. It often lies subjacent to the epithelium with cells migrating into the epithelium, known as an *interface reaction* (Fig 3-45a), or it may be seen more deeply within the connective tissue in a perivascular arrangement (Fig 3-45b). Most cases will demonstrate a granular pattern of IgG, IgM, IgA, C3, and fibrinogen in the basement membrane zone on direct immunofluorescence of involved mucosa or skin (Fig 3-46). The histologic features of DLE bear a close resemblance to those of lichen planus because both demonstrate an interface process with reactive epithelial changes. The features that are more suggestive of lupus, and thus should be stressed, are the keratin plugs, the varied atrophy and acanthosis, connective tissue

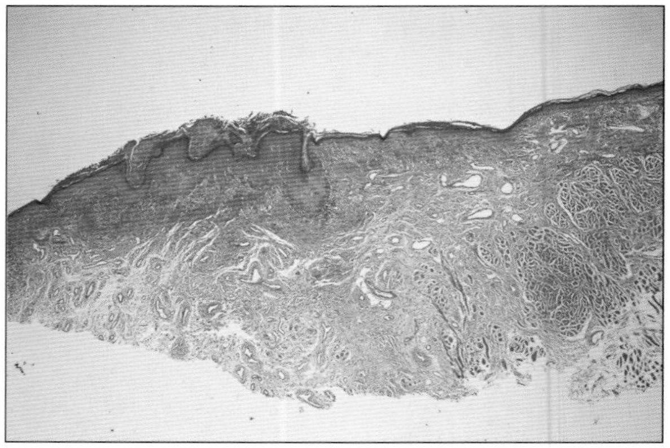

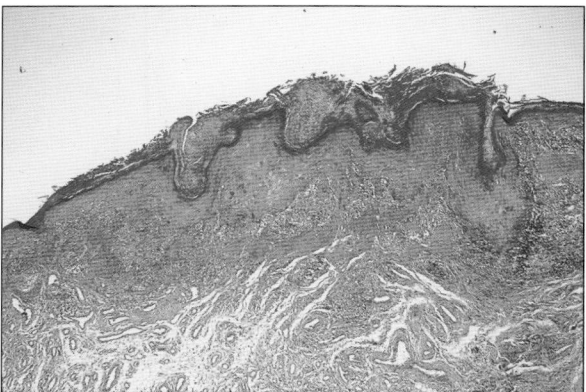

Fig 3-44a Chronic discoid lupus erythematosus of the lower lip. Atrophic and hyperplastic areas are continuous.

Fig 3-44b Higher-power view of Fig 3-44a shows keratin plugging, hyperkeratosis, and hypergranulosis with a subepithelial lymphocytic infiltrate.

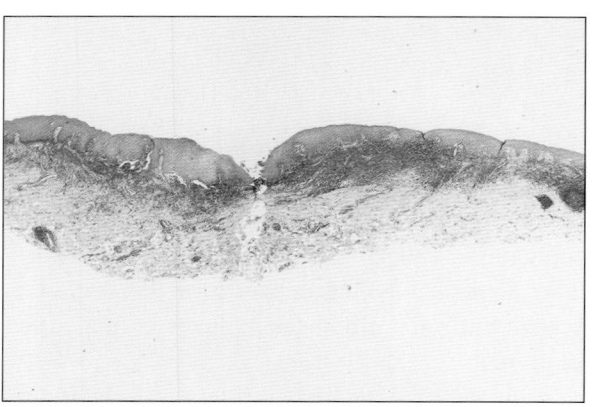

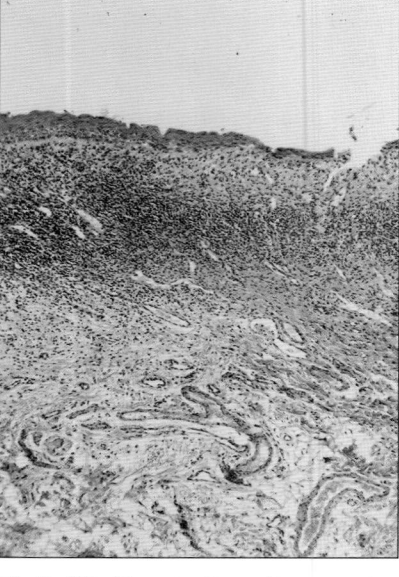

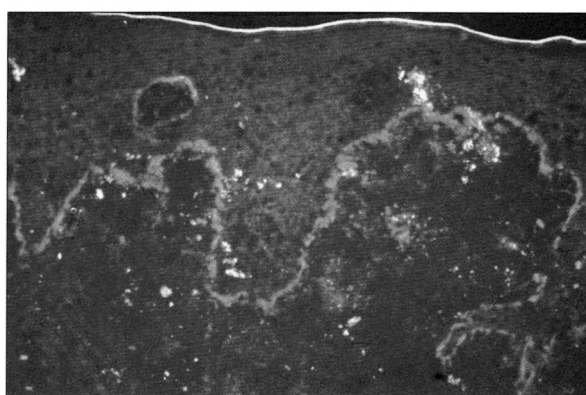

Fig 3-45a Chronic discoid lupus of oral mucosa showing a banded lymphocytic infiltrate as may be seen in lichen planus.

Fig 3-45b Chronic discoid lupus with a midzonal banded lymphocytic infiltrate.

Fig 3-46 Direct immunofluorescence showing a granular deposition of IgG in the basement membrane zone. Systemic lupus produces the same finding.

edema, the deeper perivascular infiltrate, and the less compact band of lymphocytes at the interface. In addition, immunoglobulins are identified in the basement membrane zone only in lupus.

TREATMENT ▶ The oral lesions usually require no treatment. Skin lesions may be treated, and some prevention may be helpful. Prevention takes the form of avoiding sun exposure and photosensitizing drugs such as tetracyclines, thiazole diuretics, and piroxicam. Topical corticosteroids such as 1% hydrocortisone cream (Topicort 1%, Aventis) or 0.05% fluocinonide (Lidex cream, Medicis Dermatologics) are somewhat effective, as are intralesional corticosteroids such as triamcinolone (Aristocort, Fujisawa), 5 mg/mL once a month. In severe cases, prednisone is used as directed in systemic corticosteroid regimen I or II (see page 205).

PROGNOSIS ▶ DLE is persistent and long term. It is not life threatening, nor is it usually debilitating, but it is often disfiguring because of alopecia and hypopigmentation. Only rarely is DLE reported to transform into SLE, and these cases may not have been DLE but a mild early SLE that had not yet developed significant autoantibody production.

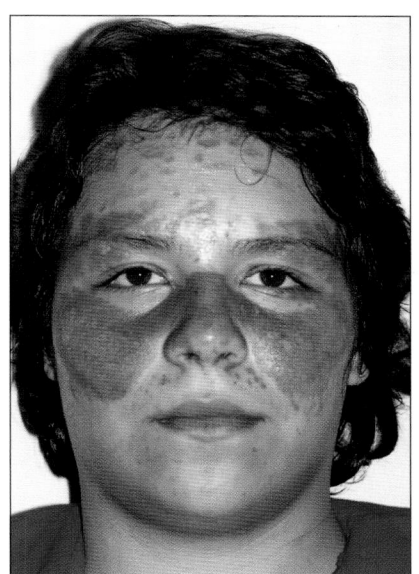

Fig 3-47 Systemic lupus erythematosus will often show the classic malar butterfly rash, which spares the nasolabial crease. Note the hairline cluster of other lesions around the eyebrows and forehead.

Systemic Lupus Erythematosus

CLINICAL PRESENTATION AND PATHOGENESIS ▶

Systemic lupus erythematosus is an autoimmune disorder in which antigen-antibody complexes become entrapped in the capillaries of most organs. These complexes initiate the complement cascade and inflammation. The clinical presentation, therefore, may show evidence of single-organ disease or widespread multiorgan disease. It may also present in a mild episodic form or a rapidly progressive form leading to death, depending on the organs involved and the degree of autoimmune abnormality.

The classic presentation is a young woman of so-called child-bearing age. Eighty-five percent of patients are women, and indeed the peak incidence is between the ages of 20 and 40 years. There is a higher incidence in blacks than in any other race, although it is not found in Africa. The most notorious feature of SLE is the malar butterfly rash (Fig 3-47). However, the clinician should remember that other diseases, such as DLE, pemphigus, and drug-induced conditions, can produce a similar rash and that the rash alone does not establish a diagnosis of SLE. In fact, the malar butterfly rash is only 1 of a possible 11 clinical-laboratory findings that may be present (Table 3-1). The American Rheumatism Association (ARA) requires that at least 4 of these 11 criteria be present, together with a positive serum ANA, before a definitive diagnosis of SLE can be made. Familiarity with these criteria helps the clinician know what to look for and which diagnostic tests to pursue.

In addition to the malar rash, which will usually spare the nasolabial crease, there may be other skin lesions, known as a *discoid rash* (Fig 3-48). These lesions are seen clustered around hairline areas and are exacerbated by exposure to sunlight (photosensitivity). The oral ulcers (Fig 3-49) are red, shallow ulcers most commonly found on the palate and the marginal gingiva. At times, the oral lesions will take the form of a nonulcerated inflammatory area or a line of inflammation. They may mimic a marginal gingivitis.

Joint symptoms (painful joints, mild swelling) occur frequently (90% of patients) and are often an early sign. This "arthritis" is not a deforming type of arthritis and will not show radiographic changes. Individuals with systemic lupus erythematosus also frequently exhibit Raynaud phenomenon. This phenomenon relates to color changes of the fingers in response to exposure to cold. It can be elicited by placing the patient's hand in ice water, which will produce vasoconstrictions and vasodilations, creating the so-called patriotic sign, that is, red, white, and/or blue changes in the skin color. Ocular manifestations may include blurred vision, transient blindness, conjunctivitis, and photophobia. A slit-lamp or ophthalmoscopic examination may show fluffy cotton-wool spots, called *cytoid bodies*, on the retina.

Table 3-1 American Rheumatism Association 11 criteria for systemic lupus erythematosus*

System or Criterion	Description
1. Malar rash	Red rash over cheeks and bridge of the nose
2. Discoid rash	Red, scaly rash on the face, scalp, ears, arms, or chest
3. Photosensitivity	Unusual reaction to the sun
4. Oral ulcers	Small sores on the moist lining of the nose or mouth
5. Arthritis	Pain in the joints of the hands, arms, shoulders, feet, legs, hips, or jaws that may move from joint to joint and be accompanied by heat, redness, and swelling
6. Serositis	Pleurisy—chest pain or abnormal sounds heard by physician Inflammation of the lining of the heart. Documented by ECG or heard by physician
7. Renal (kidney)	Excess protein and/or cellular casts in the urine
8. Neurologic	Seizures and/or psychosis
9. Hematologic (blood)	Disorder that can include a decrease in the number of red and white blood cells or platelets
10. Immunologic	Immunologic positive anti-DNA test
11. Antinuclear antibody	Antinuclear antibody (ANA) positive

*A patient who has four or more of these symptoms over a period of time may have systemic lupus.

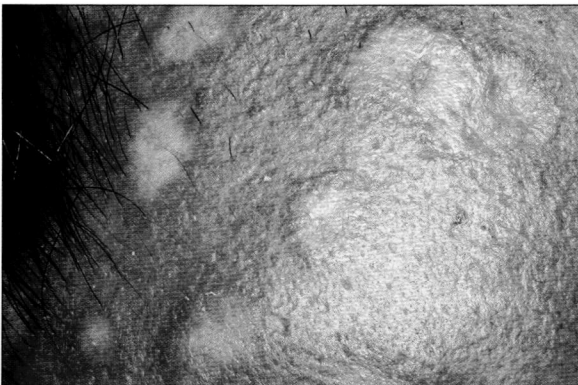

Fig 3-48 The skin lesions of SLE will be like those of DLE and are called a *discoid rash*. In both, they will form around hairlines and have the "grass fire" appearance.

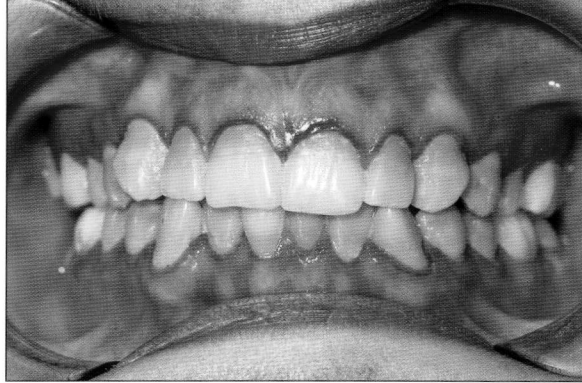

Fig 3-49 Oral lesions of systemic lupus erythematosus are often located on the marginal gingiva and palate as shallow painless ulcers.

Lung involvement will take the form of pleuritis with effusion, and there is also frequently a pneumonia and restrictive lung disease. The heart often develops pericarditis "serositis" and a verrucous nonbacterial endocarditis called *Libman-Sacks endocarditis* that is known to produce a mitral valve regurgitation.

The "renal disease" takes the form of glomerulonephritis, mostly where glomerular thickening produces a "wire loop" nephritis also called *lupus nephritis*. Interstitial nephritis is also seen. The "neurologic disease" is often manifested as seizure activity and psychosis, particularly depression.

The pathogenesis of SLE centers around the development of autoantibody against native double-stranded DNA or other ribonuclear proteins (Table 3-2). SLE seems to have a familial predisposition; it has been reported in identical twins on several occasions, and aggregations of abnormal serologic characteristics (ANA, hyperglobulinemia, anti-DNA antibodies) are seen in asymptomatic family members. Nevertheless, clinical disease is initiated when sufficient numbers of autoantibody complexes accumulate in tissues to initiate inflammatory destruction of the host tissue. In the process, they fix and consume complement. The inflammatory process is destructive but normal. It is unceasing because of ongoing antigen-antibody complex reinitiation of inflammation.

Table 3-2 Frequency (%) of autoantibodies in rheumatic diseases

Disease	ANA*	Anti-native DNA	Rheumatoid factor	Anti-Sm	Anti-SS-A	Anti-SS-B	Anti-SCL-70	Anti-centromere	Anti-Jo-1	ANCA†
Rheumatoid arthritis	30–60	0–5	72–85	0	0–5	0–2	0	0	0	0
Systemic lupus erythematosus	95–100	60	20	10–25	15–20	5–20	0	0	0	0–1
Sjögren syndrome	95	0	75	0	60–70	60–70	0	0	0	0
Diffuse scleroderma	80–95	0	25-33	0	0	0	1	1	0	0
Limited scleroderma (CREST syndrome)	80–95	0	25–33	0	0	0	50	50	0	0
Polymyositis/dermatomyositis	80–95	0	33	0	0	0	0	0	20–30	0
Wegener granulomatosis	0–15	0	50	0	0	0	0	0	0	93–96‡

*ANA—Antinuclear antibodies.
†ANCA—Antineutrophil cytoplasmic antibody.
‡Frequency for generalized, active disease.

DIFFERENTIAL DIAGNOSIS ▶

The most important differentiation to make when pursuing a suspected case of SLE is to distinguish it from a *drug-induced lupus syndrome*. In particular, methyldopa, hydralazine, chlorpromazine, procainamide, isoniazid (INH), and quinidine have a strong association with the production of a lupus-like syndrome. To distinguish this clinically similar entity, the clinician must strictly adhere to the 11 ARA criteria and consider the following facts concerning a drug-induced lupus syndrome:

1. Males are affected equally.
2. There are no neurologic or renal components.
3. Anti–native DNA antibodies are not present.
4. The clinical picture improves if the suspicious drug is withdrawn.

Other diseases that may present with an initial picture similar to that of SLE include *discoid lupus erythematosus*, *erythema multiforme*, and *rheumatoid arthritis*.

DIAGNOSTIC WORK-UP ▶

The physical examination and radiographic and laboratory studies are guided by the ARA criteria and are straightforward. Included should be a routine urinalysis and a 24-hour urine collection specimen to assess for proteinuria and cellular casts indicative of glomerular damage. In addition, a routine chest auscultation, chest radiograph, and pulmonary function tests particularly assessing for pleural effusions, restrictive lung disease, and mitral valvular incompetence should be included.

The blood abnormalities in lupus are mainly cytopenia from marrow depression caused by immune effects. Therefore, a routine complete blood count should identify either anemia, leukopenia (particularly lymphopenia), or thrombocytopenia. In addition, hypocomplementemia is commonly found in SLE (95% of cases) because the antigen-antibody complexes continually fix complement, thereby depleting their serum values. An ANA is required and is positive but is not specific for SLE. Other serum immunologic studies should include anti-DNA antibody, anti-Sm (Smith), which is a specific antiribonuclear protein, and a VDRL (Venereal Disease Research Laboratory) (the positive VDRL is often false positive in SLE). The anti–native DNA antibody is reasonably specific for SLE, and when first introduced, was hoped to be a single diagnostic test for SLE, but its sensitivity is low. Only 30% to 40% of SLE patients test positive for anti-DNA antibody.

HISTOPATHOLOGY ▶

The histologic changes of systemic lupus as observed in the oral mucosa do not differ appreciably from those in discoid lupus, and it has been observed that even the ulcerative lesions of SLE evolve from the same basic mechanism of destruction secondary to the interface reaction. In general, how-

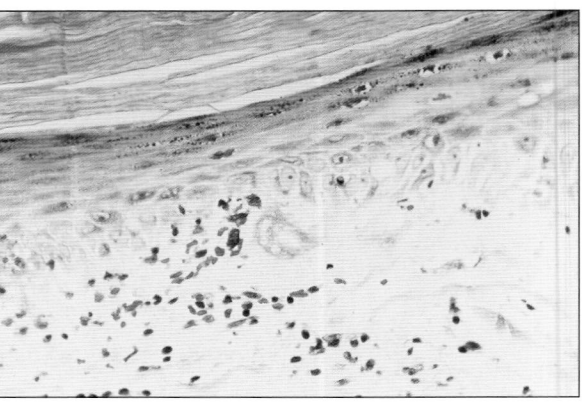

Fig 3-50 Systemic lupus erythematosus involving the skin, showing marked edema, scant inflammatory cells, extravasated erythrocytes, and some fibrin.

ever, particularly in the early skin lesions of SLE, the changes vary in degree. In these cases, connective tissue edema is more pronounced, as is hydropic degeneration of basal cells, and the inflammatory component and hyperkeratosis are diminished. Extravasation of erythrocytes is more pronounced, and colloid bodies are more likely to be seen. Deposits of fibrin are more prominent. This occurs within the connective tissue, causing thickening of collagen bundles, as well as within vessel walls and basement membrane zone (Fig 3-50). These deposits are strongly PAS positive. Subcutaneous fat may also show involvement with mucoid degeneration and lymphocytic infiltrates. In virtually all cases of SLE, the granular deposits of immunoglobulin are seen on direct immunofluorescence, a phenomenon that may also occur in cases of DLE.

TREATMENT ▶ Many people have a mild form of SLE that runs an unprogressive course and requires only supportive care. Nonsteroidal anti-inflammatory drugs or, for mild flare-ups, antimalarial drugs such as hydroxychloroquine (Plaquenil, Sanofi Winthrop), 400 mg by mouth every day, can be used to alleviate symptoms.

Most patients with SLE, particularly those with multiorgan involvement and/or progressive disease, require systemic prednisone (systemic corticosteroid regimens IIIa and IIIb; see pages 205 to 206). These patients usually require such therapy at adjusted dosages throughout their lives.

PROGNOSIS ▶ The prognosis of patients with SLE improved in the 1980s. Currently, 10-year survival rates are at 85%. Most patients have a mild form of the disease requiring intermittent courses of prednisone. As the patient ages, the exacerbations become fewer and less intense, with longer disease-free remissions in between. After 5 years, the elevated erythrocyte sedimentation rate (ESR), ANA, and anti-DNA antibody titers are reduced and may even be normal. Because more SLE patients now survive for many years, long-term corticosteroid complications, especially avascular necrosis of the hip and cataracts, develop in most. A small number die from opportunistic infectious agents causing pneumonia.

If a patient has a virulent progressive course of SLE, it is evident from the onset. Those who survive the first 4 years generally have long-term survival. The rapidly progressive form of SLE causes severe kidney damage, heart damage, or lung damage leading to death mostly from renal failure or pneumonia.

Antiphospholipid Antibody Disease

Antiphospholipid antibody disease may be part of the SLE picture or exist as a separate primary antiphospholipid antibody syndrome. Antiphospholipid antibodies compose 32% of the autoantibodies found in SLE, and three different types are found. The first causes the biologic false-positive VDRL for syphilis and is found in 25% of SLE patients. The second is the lupus anticoagulant antibody, which, despite its name, causes both venous and arterial thrombosis, which in turn cause miscarriages. It is most commonly identified by an elevated partial thromboplastin time (PTT) and is found in 7% of SLE patients.

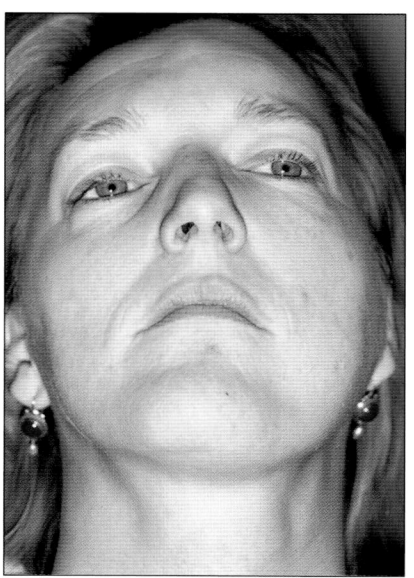

Fig 3-51 The coup de sabre deformity, a depressed ridge in the midline or paramidline of the forehead, is seen in progressive systemic sclerosis and in several other conditions.

The third type is an anticardiolipin antibody and has been associated with fetal death in pregnant women with SLE. It is found in 25% of SLE patients.

A primary antiphospholipid antibody syndrome unassociated with SLE also exists. Its main presentation is one of recurrent arterial and venous occlusions without any other features of SLE. Repeated venous or arterial occlusions in women and repeated unexplained miscarriages require a work-up for SLE as well as antiphospholipid antibody determinations.

Progressive Systemic Sclerosis (Scleroderma) and the CREST Syndrome

CLINICAL PRESENTATION AND PATHOGENESIS ▶

Progressive systemic sclerosis (PSS) is an autoimmune disease that produces systemic cellular damage focused on connective tissues that leads to fibrosis in the dermis of the skin and in internal organs (see Table 3-2). Like any autoimmune disease, it results from a cellular component that becomes antigenic. In the case of scleroderma, one or several ribonucleic proteins, most commonly (55%) the SCL-70 protein, is the antigenic focus. In a milder PSS variant of scleroderma known as the CREST (calcinosis, Raynaud phenomenon, esophageal hypomotility, sclerodactyly, and telangiectasias) syndrome, the cytoplasmic organelle, the centromere, is the antigen. Because several different antigenic nuclear proteins may be involved, some of which may stimulate a more intense antibody response than others, a spectrum of severity ranging from localized sclerosis to CREST syndrome to widespread systemic sclerosis to a rapidly progressive and fatal systemic sclerosis is to be expected.

Localized Systemic Sclerosis

This milder variant is limited to the skin and will involve one side more than the other. Women are affected more than men (4:1). Although this variant does not include all of the components of the CREST variant, Raynaud phenomenon is an early finding or one that may precede skin involvement. The skin involvement will be in either plaque or linear form. When the linear form occurs vertically across the forehead it is termed the *coup de sabre deformity* (Fig 3-51) to highlight its resemblance to the gash of a sword.

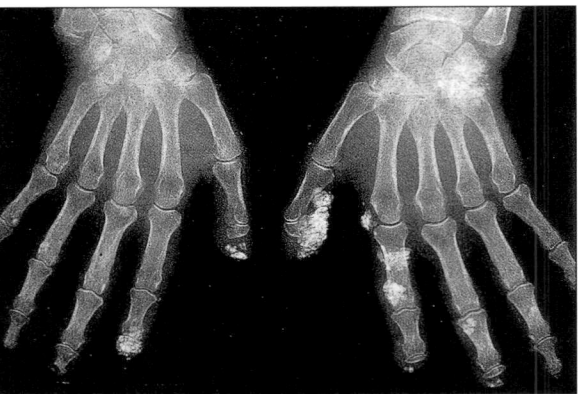

Fig 3-52a The *C* in the CREST syndrome refers to calcinosis, which is most frequently seen in the tendon sheaths of the fingers and within the finger pads.

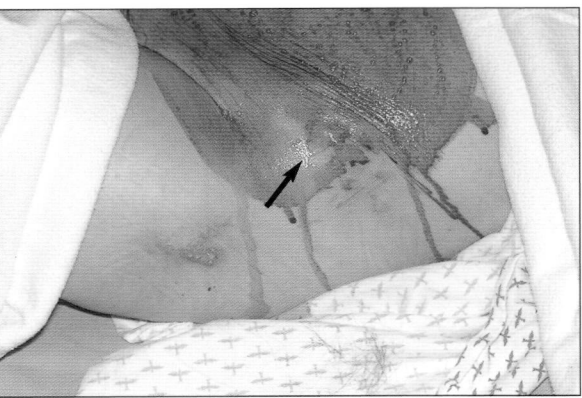

Fig 3-52b Calcinosis in the CREST syndrome is also frequently observed over bony prominences. Here, calcinosis is seen over the prominence of the greater trochanter of the femur (*arrow*).

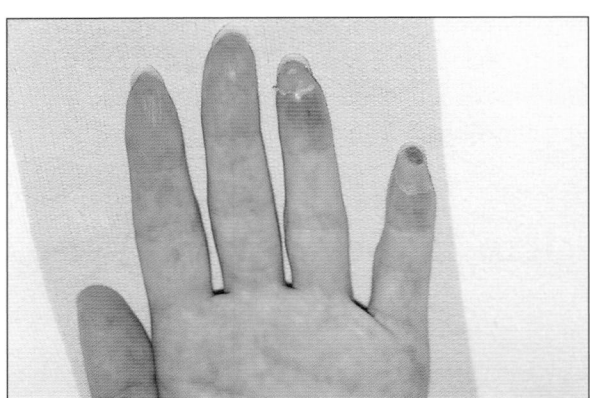

Fig 3-52c The *R* in the CREST syndrome refers to Raynaud phenomenon, a vasospastic response to cold that produces red, white, and blue features in the hands and fingers (often referred to as the "patriotic sign").

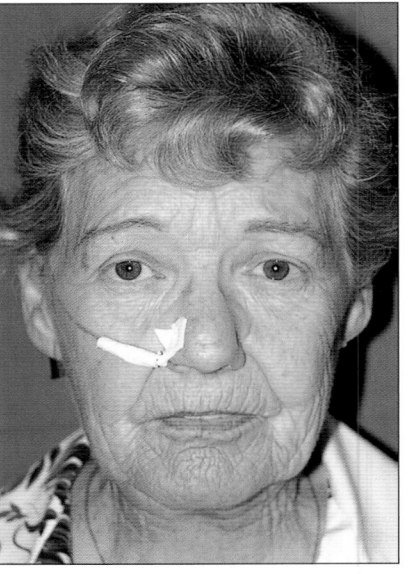

Fig 3-52d The *E* in the CREST syndrome refers to esophageal hypomotility, which may require a nasogastric feeding tube or a gastrostomy.

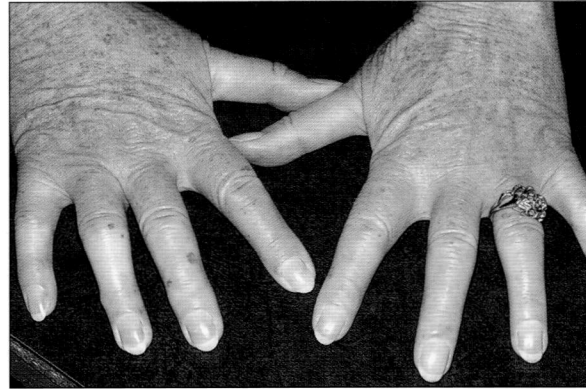

Fig 3-52e The *S* in the CREST syndrome refers to sclerodactyly, which is characterized by thin pointed fingers with circumferentially tight skin.

CREST Syndrome

The CREST syndrome is a less progressive, lifelong, chronic form of PSS. Individuals with the CREST variant may show radiographically apparent calcification (calcinosis) at the finger tips (Fig 3-52a) or in the subcutaneous tissues over the bony prominences of the femur, the iliac crest (Fig 3-52b), the elbows, or the knees. Raynaud phenomenon is present in almost all forms of PSS, and the CREST variant is no exception.

Raynaud phenomenon is a vasospastic response brought on by cold. It is the initial clinical manifestation of all forms of PSS in 50% of cases. It can be brought about by immersing the individual's hands in cold water. Raynaud phenomenon occurs in three stages: the first is pallor (white), which is due to vasospasms that are painful and paresthetic; the second is cyanosis (blue), which heralds relaxation of the vasospasm and is caused by pooling of venous blood; and the third is hyperemia (red), in which the re-

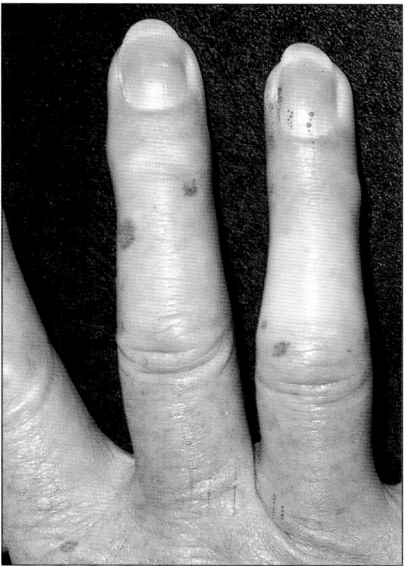 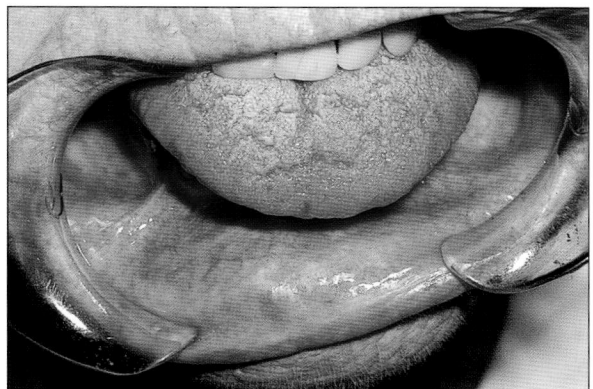

Fig 3-52f The *T* in CREST syndrome refers to telangiectasias, which are most commonly seen on the tight skin of the fingers.

Fig 3-52g Oral telangiectasias on the lips and tongue may also be seen in CREST syndrome.

laxation of the vasospasm creates a reactive hyperemia that actually represents a mild reperfusion injury. Because the red, white, and blue are often seen together, Raynaud phenomenon is known as the "patriotic sign" (Fig 3-52c).

Esophageal hypomotility is caused by fibrosis and atrophy of the smooth muscles of the entire gastrointestinal tract. The esophageal involvement is most easily recognized, however, and often requires nasogastric or gastrostomy tube feedings (Fig 3-52d).

Sclerodactyly is the dermal fibrosis involving the skin around each finger, causing the finger to appear narrow and pointed. The fingertips may be narrowed with ulcerations or loss of the nail. The skin will be noticeably tight and telangiectasias on the skin of the fingers are common (Fig 3-52e).

Telangiectasias in the CREST variant have a unique morphology. They are flat and mat-like with irregular edges. They are most commonly seen on the skin of the hands, fingers, face, and back and on the mucosa of the tongue and lips (Figs 3-52f and 3-52g). Like all true telangiectasias, they do not blanch.

Diffuse Progressive Systemic Sclerosis

The diffuse type of PSS is the form previously referred to as *scleroderma*. This type is diagnosed by the clinical identification of either one major criteria or two or more minor criteria as defined by the American Rheumatism Association (Table 3-3). The single major criterion, proximal sclerosis, is sclerosis proximal to the knees and elbows. Minor criteria include sclerodactyly, loss of finger pads or pitting of the fingertips, and pulmonary fibrosis.

Diffuse PSS will initially present with either Raynaud phenomenon or a thickening of the skin on the hands and fingers. Nonspecific joint pains, weakness, weight loss, and muscle aches may also be seen. As the disease progresses, more obvious signs develop. The skin becomes overtly firm and bound down and possibly hyperpigmented. In addition, hair loss and dryness of the skin will develop because of fibrosis around skin appendages. The fingers and wrists may eventually undergo a flexion deformity resulting from a greater quantity of muscle and tendon in the flexors versus the extensors (Fig 3-53a). The oral and maxillofacial specialist may observe a somewhat limited mouth opening due to tightness at the commis-

Table 3-3 American Rheumatism Association diagnostic criteria for progressive systemic sclerosis

Major criteria
Proximal sclerosis (91% sensitivity and greater than 99% specificity)

Minor criteria
Sclerodactyly
Digital pitting scars of fingertips or loss of substance of the finger pad
Pulmonary fibrosis—bibasilar

One major or two minor criteria were found in 97% of patients with definite systemic sclerosis.

sures (Fig 3-53b) and a stiff, thin lip quality. Radiographs may show a symmetric widening of the periodontal membrane space (Fig 3-53c) or bony resorption at the angle and posterior ramus. This resorptive pattern has been termed the "tail of the whale" deformity because the thinned ramus resembles the base of a whale's tail and the condyle and coronoid process resemble the flutes of the tail (Fig 3-53d). In addition, fibrosis often produces a retrognathia of the mandible and an absolute transverse deficiency in the maxilla. The overall appearance will usually be that of a skeletal Class II with a high arched palate.

DIFFERENTIAL DIAGNOSIS ▶ Progressive systemic sclerosis and its variants are difficult to diagnose in their early stages but become more apparent as the disease develops. If Raynaud phenomenon is the first manifestation, similar autoimmune diseases such as *systemic lupus erythematosus, Sjögren syndrome*, and *mixed connective tissue disease* would be considered. If nonspecific arthralgias, muscles aches, and thickening of the skin are the first signs, *Hashimoto thyroiditis, eosinophilic fasciitis, dermatomyositis*, and *chemical-induced scleroderma-like conditions* would be the considerations. Agents such as bleomycin, pentazocine, and vinyl chloride produce significant fibrosis, which may mimic scleroderma. In the CREST variant, the telangiectasias may initially mimic *hereditary hemorrhagic telangiectasia*, and the esophageal hypomotility may mimic *Plummer-Vinson syndrome*.

DIAGNOSTIC WORK-UP ▶ The work-up should include a physical examination guided by knowledge of the manifestations of PSS. Once all positive physical findings are noted, a panoramic radiograph, a chest radiograph, a barium swallow, an arterial blood gas, pulmonary function tests, a serum creatinine, and antibody tests for the general antinuclear antibody (ANA) as well as the more specific SCL-70 and anti-centromere antibody are recommended. A panoramic radiograph may identify widened periodontal membrane spaces and angle resorption. The chest radiograph is needed to assess for pulmonary fibrosis, which will be confirmed by the arterial blood gas and pulmonary function tests. In PSS, the vital capacity is often < 50% of predicted and the PaO_2 < 70 mm Hg. The barium swallow will identify esophageal hypomotility. The creatinine will assess for possible renal fibrosis. The ANA is positive in 96% of PSS cases and the anti-centromere antibody test is positive in 96% of the CREST variants. The SCL-70 antibody is positive in 55% of PSS cases.

HISTOPATHOLOGY ▶ Within the skin, there is initial edema, which is followed by induration due to an increase in collagen deposition within the reticular dermis. This is accompanied by a thinning of the epidermis with loss of rete ridges and atrophy of dermal appendages (Fig 3-53e). Mild mononuclear T-cell infiltrates occur within the subcutaneous tissue and around vessels. Hyalinization and obliteration of arterioles may be seen. Within the collagen, calcific deposits may form. Similar changes can be seen in other organ systems. Vascular changes are prominent in the kidney with luminal narrowing and fibrosis. The lungs show diffuse interstitial fibrosis, and the esophagus may undergo atrophy of smooth muscle with fibrosis. Interstitial fibrosis and acinar atrophy may also affect salivary glands.

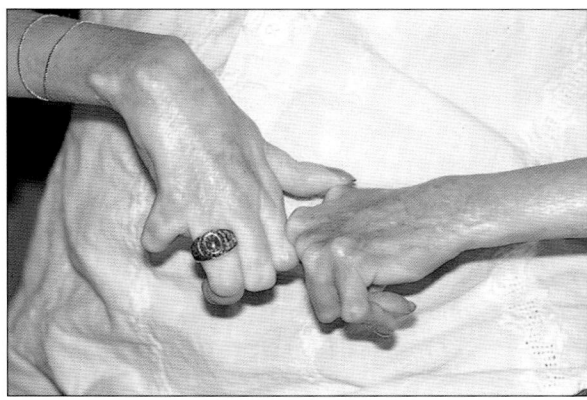

Fig 3-53a Severe flexion deformity of the hands related to PSS.

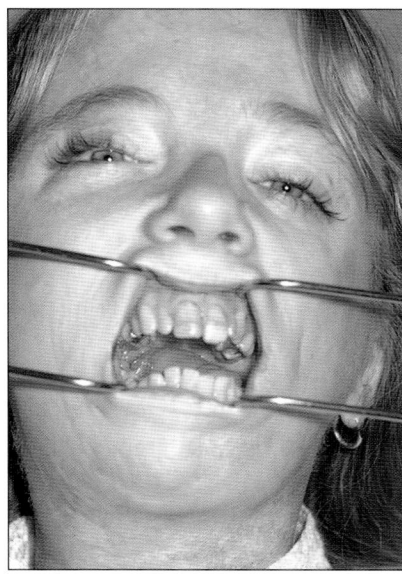

Fig 3-53b Limited mouth opening in PSS is due in part to fibrosis at the commissures and within the cheek and in part to fibrosis in the muscles of mastication.

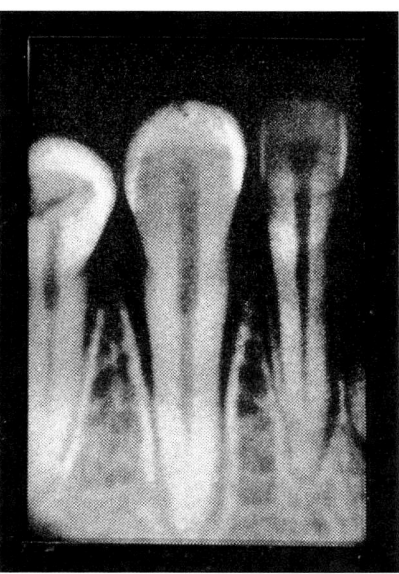

Fig 3-53c A symmetric widening of the periodontal membrane space is also noted in many cases of PSS.

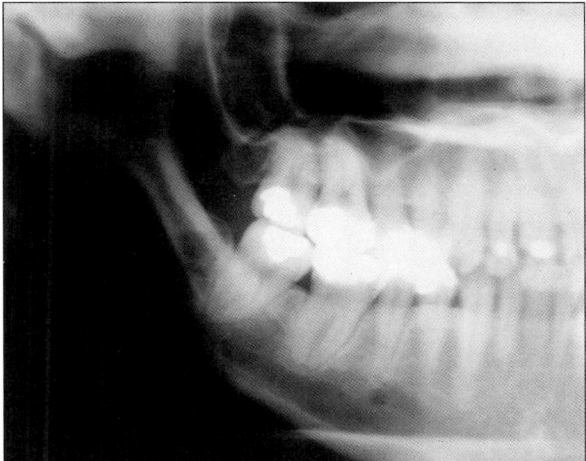

Fig 3-53d A resorption of angle and posterior ramus border in PSS creates a "tail of the whale" appearance on a panoramic radiograph.

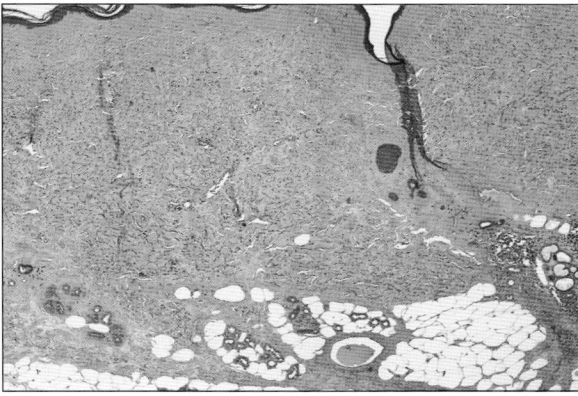

Fig 3-53e Systemic sclerosis showing excessive deposition of collagen extending into the fat. The overlying epithelium and skin appendages are atrophic.

TREATMENT AND PROGNOSIS ▶

There are few effective therapies to reverse or even significantly slow the progress of PSS. Like most autoimmune diseases, PSS will progress at a predetermined rate. Those with early and progressive internal organ involvement of the lungs, heart, or kidneys succumb to the disease often in their 30s or 40s. Most individuals with more slowly progressive PSS live into their 60s and 70s. In the past, attempts to halt the progression with steroids, azathioprine, chlorambucil, cyclophosphamide, and colchicine have proven ineffective. However, penicillamine, which blocks the cross-linking in collagen synthesis in dosages of 500 to 1500 mg per day, has some therapeutic benefit. It reduces skin thickness and slows the progression of internal fibrosis. As part of the overall management of PSS, physical therapy to maintain joint

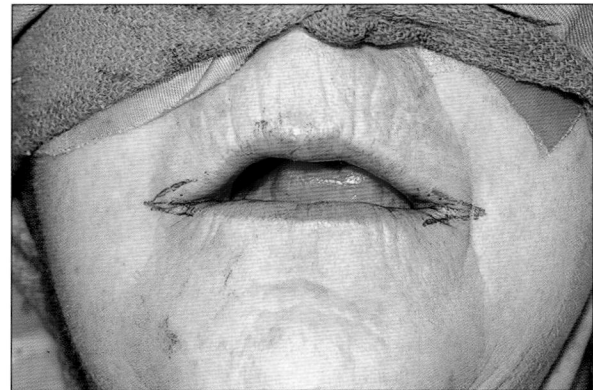

Fig 3-54a A bilateral commissurotomy may be necessary to allow for insertion of appliances and to gain access for dental care. Excision of some fibrosis is usually necessary in PSS patients.

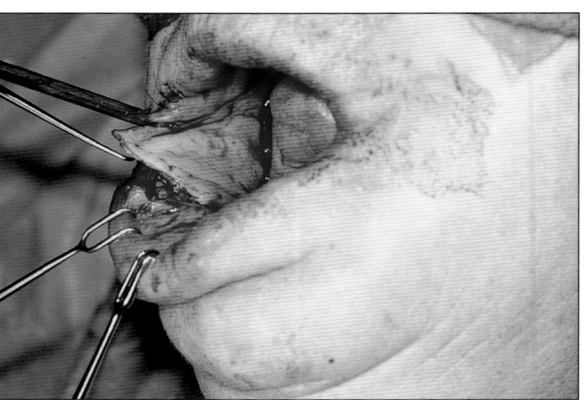

Fig 3-54b An advancement flap of buccal mucosa is often required to reline the surface of the commissures.

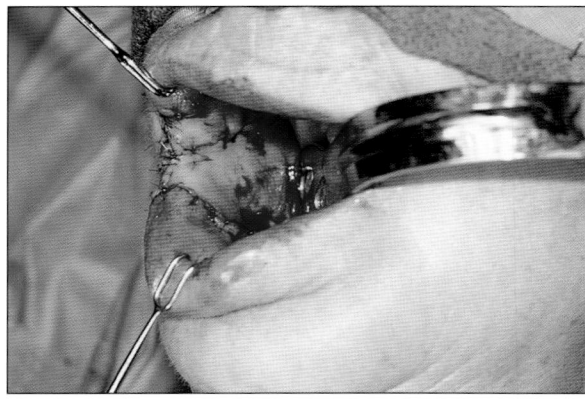

Fig 3-54c The advancement of buccal mucosa should overlap a portion of both the upper and lower vermilions.

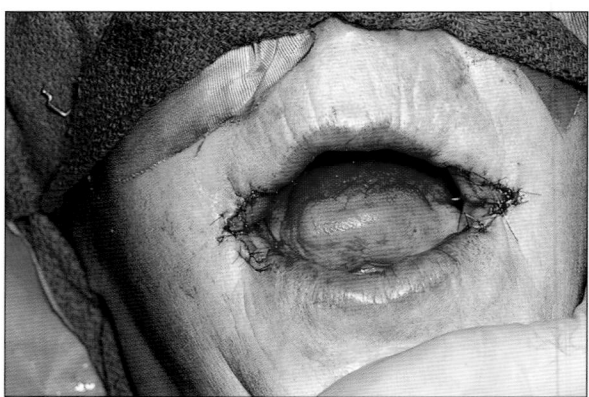

Fig 3-54d The commissurotomies should be symmetrical and create an internal fold to accommodate mouth closures without tissue redundancy.

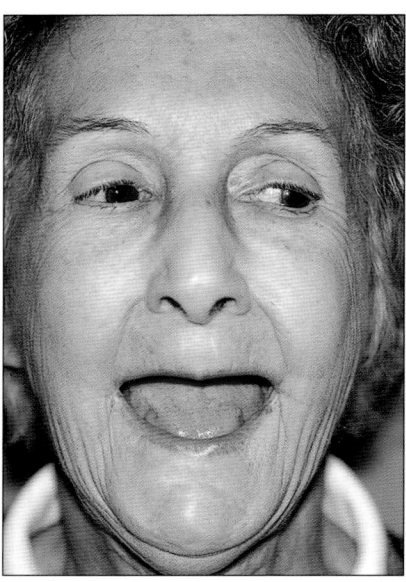

Fig 3-54e A successful commissurotomy surgery in a PSS patient will not necessarily increase the vertical opening. It will, however, increase the stoma, allowing access for dental care, oral hygiene, and the insertion of appliances.

motion and mouth opening is recommended. The oral and maxillofacial specialist should not hesitate to prescribe such physical therapy as well devices such as the Therabite (Therabite) to resist further limitation of jaw opening.

The oral and maxillofacial surgeon also may be called upon to accomplish a bilateral commissurotomy to improve jaw opening. Such surgery can be accomplished without wound-healing complications and the need for hyperbaric oxygen, although it will not increase the absolute interincisal opening. This is due to the fibrosis, which is not only within the commissures but also within the buccinator, cheek, and pterygomasseteric sling. Nevertheless, the commissurotomy surgery will benefit the individual by increasing the lateral slit opening of the mouth to allow for insertion of appliances, improved access for dental care and oral hygiene, and an improved eating ability (Figs 3-54a to 3-54e).

Kawasaki Disease (Mucocutaneous Lymph Node Syndrome)

Kawasaki disease fits the very definition of a syndrome; that is, a complex of clinical signs and symptoms. In this syndrome, mucocutaneous lesions and cervical lymphadenopathy are the two central findings and are often responsible for bringing it to the attention of the oral and maxillofacial specialist.

Although the syndrome suggests a bacterial etiology, none has been found. Its mechanism is thought to be related to a subtle staphylococcal infection or colonization. This produces an exotoxin, which in turn acts as a potent antigen. This toxin-antigen subsequently stimulates a profound T-cell response that produces the observed signs and symptoms of the syndrome. An overstimulated immune response causing tissue injury and clinical signs is a common finding in several infection-based–immune-based diseases of which tuberculosis, leprosy, and rheumatic fever are other good examples.

CLINICAL PRESENTATION ▶

Kawasaki syndrome is most often seen in children younger than 10 years and of Asian heritage. Occasionally adults and rarely non-Asian children are seen with Kawasaki syndrome. Outbreaks among several individuals may develop in an epidemic pattern. Fever is the most common finding combined with a variable mucous membrane presentation of inflamed tongue (the so-called strawberry tongue), pharyngitis, cracked and fissured lips, and bilateral nonsuppurative conjunctivitis. The cervical lymphadenopathy is mildly tender with multiple palpable lymph nodes of about 1.5 cm. These findings are coupled with extremity signs consisting of either edema, erythema, and/or a desquamation of skin.

The most serious complication of Kawasaki syndrome is coronary arteritis, which occurs in 25% of untreated cases. This has caused coronary artery aneurysms and even myocardial infarction in children, making Kawasaki syndrome one of the more common causes of acquired pediatric heart disease in the United States.

DIFFERENTIAL DIAGNOSIS ▶

The presentation of oral mucosal infections, fever, pharyngitis, and cervical lymphadenitis is suggestive of several specific diseases such as *streptococcal pharyngitis*, *diphtheria*, and *infectious mononucleosis*. In addition, *HIV-related lymphadenopathy* and *tuberculosis lymphadenitis* in an HIV-positive child are considerations in certain individuals. Once extremity signs or symptoms related to coronary arteritis such as chest pain and tachycardia develop, a serious consideration for *rheumatic fever* is warranted. Mild cases will mimic nonspecific *viral influenza*, particularly when associated with other cases in an epidemic pattern.

DIAGNOSTIC WORK-UP ▶

The diagnosis of Kawasaki syndrome is made by the clinical correlation of signs and symptoms and only after rheumatic fever and streptococcal pharyngitis have been ruled out. Therefore, throat cultures are recommended with a specific attention to group-D hemolytic streptococci. Otherwise, a complete blood count with a differential white blood cell count and c-reactive protein are recommended. Kawasaki syndrome usually will be associated with leukocytosis and an elevated c-reactive protein. In cases where extremity involvement is significant or oral/pharyngeal lesions are severe, a cerebrospinal fluid tap will reveal a leukocytosis. The value of this diagnostic test toward the diagnosis must be weighed against its morbidity and possible complications.

Lymph node biopsy is not indicated unless other disease considerations in the differential diagnosis require it: Cultures of the oral or pharyngeal lesions are usually nonspecific.

HISTOPATHOLOGY ▶

Mucocutaneous lesions show only a nonspecific perivascular infiltration of lymphocytes and histiocytes.

The cutaneous lesions show changes similar to those found in polyarteritis nodosa, including a panarteritis and perivascular infiltrates of neutrophils. The lymph nodes may show localized necrosis, small thrombi, and inflammation of small vessels with a proliferation of immunoblast-like cells around postcapillary venules.

TREATMENT ▶

Although the association with a staphylococcal infection or colonization is suspected, there is no clear-cut indication for antibiotics. However, because of this suspicion and the concern of secondary infections, antibiotics with staphylococcal coverage have sometimes been used.

The management of Kawasaki syndrome has focused on reducing the fever and the inflammation. This is usually accomplished with aspirin, 80 to 100 mg/kg per day in divided doses, coupled with intravenous immune globulin in high doses. In refractory cases, plasmapheresis is used. Corticosteroids are not recommended to treat Kawasaki syndrome because of the fear of further weakening coronary artery walls and thus increasing the likelihood for coronary artery aneurysms or worsening those already present. In rare cases where coronary artery aneurysms obtain a size of 6.5 mm or larger, anticoagulation with Coumadin (DuPont) is recommended.

PROGNOSIS ▶

Prompt recognition and treatment leads to recovery without sequelae. However, uncommon refractory cases or those left untreated can lead to severe cardiac disabilities and even death.

Dermatitis Herpetiformis

CLINICAL PRESENTATION AND PATHOGENESIS ▶

Dermatitis herpetiformis is a papulovesicular disease associated with gluten hypersensitivity. Eighty-five percent of affected individuals have a gluten-sensitive enteropathy associated with very pruritic skin lesions. The skin lesions are broad areas seen most commonly on the knees, elbows, buttocks, posterior neck, and scalp. The disease has only rare oral involvement. When it does, the lesions appear as discrete vesicles on the palate or buccal mucosa (Fig 3-55).

The disease process is not herpes-related; it derives its name from the appearance of the skin lesions, which resemble those seen in herpes zoster (Fig 3-56). The pathogenesis relates to IgA antibody production, which collects at and apparently produces inflammation around the dermal papillae. The collections of IgA are granular-focal as opposed to the linear IgA disease or those seen at the basement membrane zone in the spectrum of pemphigoid diseases. The role of gluten may involve the inducement of antigluten antibodies, which become fixed to gluten attached to gut mucosa and the dermal papillae, or perhaps gluten-altered intestinal permeability, which allows other dietary products to enter the circulation as larger molecules and therefore become antigenic.

DIFFERENTIAL DIAGNOSIS ▶

Skin lesions closely resemble *psoriasis* and *skin lichen planus* because of their broad crusty papules and pruritus. Their raised nature and distinctive rolled borders may also suggest *sarcoidosis* (particularly in Scandinavians, who have a higher incidence of both diseases). Because of the pruritus and redness of the lesions, the erythrodermic stage of the cutaneous lymphoma *mycosis fungoides* is a concern. Early cases may seem to arise over a single dermatome. Because the clinical lesion resembles a herpes skin eruption (hence its name), *herpes zoster* becomes a consideration.

DIAGNOSTIC WORK-UP ▶

Dermatitis herpetiformis can be distinguished from all of the other entities on the differential diagnosis by a direct immunofluorescence biopsy. A representative biopsy specimen of the lesion's edge, along with clinically normal-appearing skin, is diagnostic. Unlike several other immune-based diseases, such as pemphigus vulgaris and cicatricial pemphigoid, in which direct immunofluorescence is optional and required only in equivocal cases, direct immunofluorescence is required in all cases suggestive of dermatitis herpetiformis. Therefore, biopsy specimens should be sent both in 10% neutral-buffered formalin for routine H&E slides and in Michel's medium for direct immunofluorescence. As an alternative to Michel's medium, the tissue specimen can be frozen with liquid nitrogen or sent fresh within 4 hours. Because circulating anti-endomysium antibodies can be detected in all cases of dermatitis herpetiformis, this should be tested if the laboratory has that capability.

HISTOPATHOLOGY ▶

The early erythematous lesions of dermatitis herpetiformis show an infiltrate of neutrophils in the tips of connective tissue papillae. These develop into microabscesses, and an influx of eosinophils ensues. Vesicles form as separation occurs over the tips of the papillae (Fig 3-57). Initially multilocular, the lesion becomes unilocular as the separation widens. The deeper tissue contains perivascular infiltrates of mononuclear cells. Early lesions show that separation occurs above the lamina lucida, but that in more advanced lesions there is destruction of the lamina densa. By means of direct immunofluorescence, IgA may be demonstrated in the basement membrane zone, usually in a granular pattern over the tips of the papillae, although deposits may occur throughout the papilla. This may be seen in both lesional and nonlesional tissue. Circulating IgA antibodies may be present.

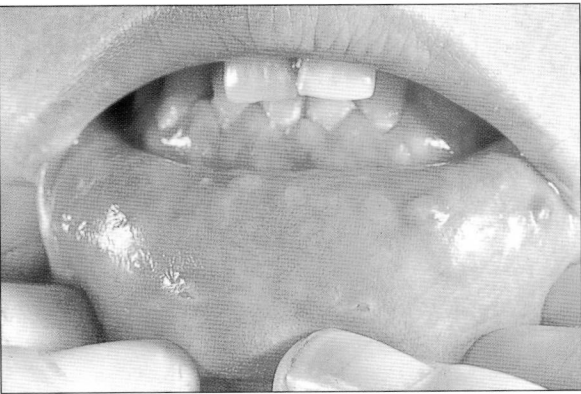

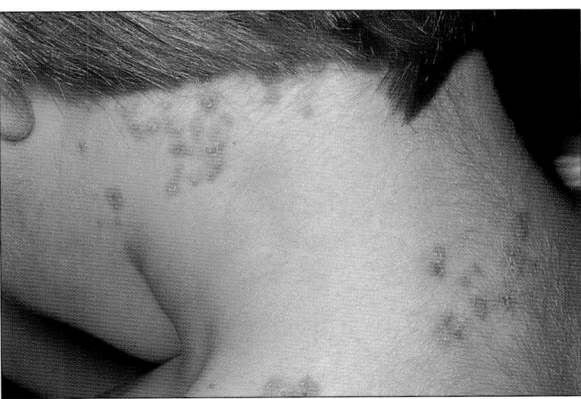

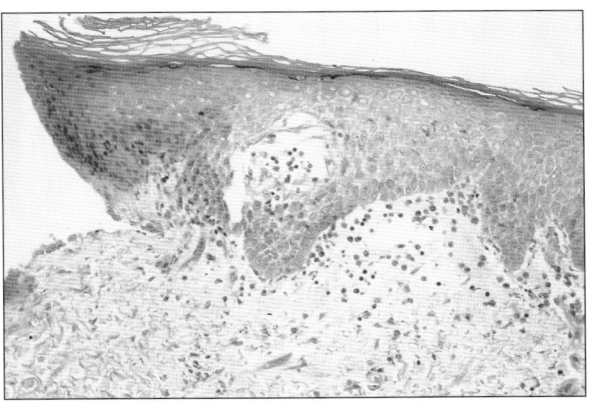

Fig 3-55 The rare oral lesions of dermatitis herpetiformis will be clinically nonspecific but may show small vesicles on an erythematous base similar to those found in pemphigus or oral pemphigoid. (Reprinted from Strassburg M and Knolle G, *Diseases of the Oral Mucosa*, with permission from Quintessence Publishing Co.)

Fig 3-56 Dermatitis herpetiformis is not related to the herpes virus. The skin lesions will be vesicles and bullae often in a linear arrangement mimicking herpes zoster. However, dermatitis herpetiformis is more pruritic and herpes zoster is more painful. (Courtesy of Dr Drore Eisen.)

Fig 3-57 Dermatitis herpetiformis showing edema and an infiltrate of neutrophils and eosinophils in the papillae. Initially this produces a multilocular pattern, but these areas subsequently become confluent.

The enteric component involves the jejunum with atrophy of villi and lymphocytic infiltration of the epithelium.

TREATMENT ▶

Both the enteropathy and the skin lesions resolve when a gluten-free diet has been followed for 4 to 36 months and will recur if gluten is reintroduced. The skin lesions respond well to drug therapy, but the enteropathy does not. The drug of choice is either dapsone, 100 mg per day (range, 50 to 400 mg per day), or sulfadiazine, 500 mg twice per day (range, 500 to 1,000 mg per day). With the use of either of these, most if not all of the skin lesions will resolve. Dapsone is the treatment of choice if the patient can tolerate it. In the 22% who develop side effects, or in the elderly patients who develop dapsone-induced hemolysis, sulfamethoxypyridazine is the drug of choice.

PROGNOSIS ▶

Disease control with diet alone and/or diet and drugs is excellent. Diet control is ideal because it is the only known means of controlling the small bowel changes. However, because an absolutely gluten-free diet is difficult to maintain, most patients require intermittent drug therapy.

Dermatomyositis

CLINICAL PRESENTATION AND PATHOGENESIS ▶

Dermatomyositis is a disease of unknown etiology, but probably represents an autoimmune disease of striated muscle. It produces inflammation followed by degenerative changes in the larger (proximal) muscles first, followed by weakness in all muscle groups. Women are affected twice as commonly as men, and it is found in individuals of all ages. Initial symptoms are weakness at the pelvis or shoulder girdle areas. Patients may not be able to rise from a sitting position or lift their arms above their head. Pain is usually not a significant part of the presentation although mild discomfort does occur.

A skin rash that is characteristically dusky red may mimic the butterfly rash more commonly associated with either type of lupus erythematosus. A periorbital (Fig 3-58) purplish edema over the upper eyelids is characteristic, as are scaly patches, called *Gottron sign*, over the dorsum of the proximal interphalangeal and metacarpophalangeal joints. The skin rash usually precedes the development of muscle weakness (Fig 3-59).

In the oral and maxillofacial area, the flexor muscles of the neck are especially weakened, leading to an upward facial gaze. Involvement of the pharyngeal and esophageal musculature often leads to dysphagia and silent regurgitation. Laryngeal muscle weakness will produce a coarse or raspy voice.

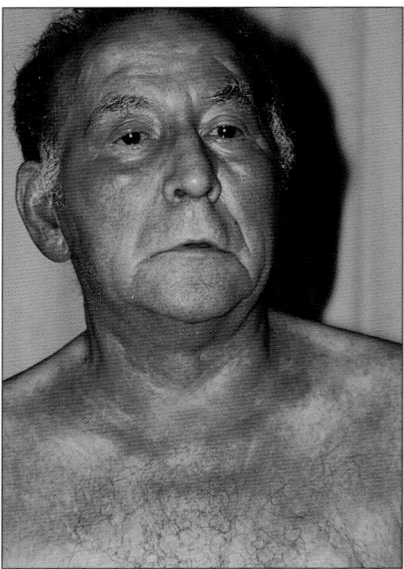

Fig 3-58 A periorbital purple edema is characteristic of dermatomyositis. The discoloration also involves the cheeks, neck, and upper chest. This patient had a carcinoma of the rectum.

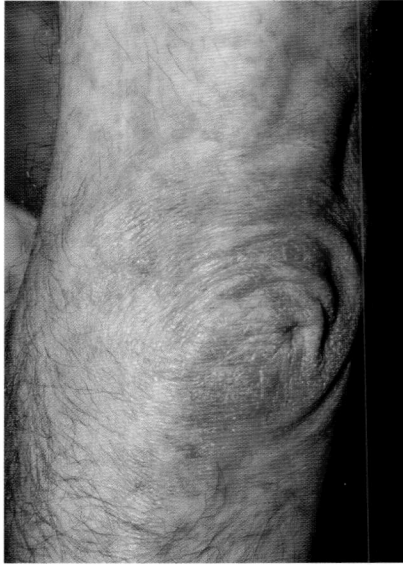

Fig 3-59 A skin rash of dermatomyositis along with redundant skin folds resulting from muscle weakness and atrophy.

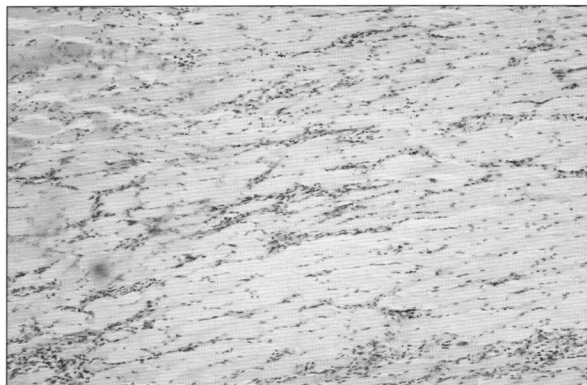

Fig 3-60 Mononuclear cell infiltrates within skeletal muscle in a patient with dermatomyositis.

Dermatomyositis is a combined cell-mediated and humoral immune-based disease. The specific antigen or stimulus remains unknown. There is a noted association with malignancy and it tends to precede infection, which implies either that it may offer the immune system an antigen similar to a muscle component or that it may alter a normal muscle component to make it antigenic. In either case, the full array of inflammatory cells proceed to degrade muscle fibers, producing clinical fatigue and decreased strength. If and when cardiac muscle is attacked, the prognosis dramatically worsens because arrhythmias and heart blocks develop.

DIFFERENTIAL DIAGNOSIS ▶ Like dermatomyositis, both *hypothyroidism* and *hyperthyroidism* are noted for muscle weakness together with elevated levels of creatinine phosphate kinase (CPK). Careful examination of the type, distribution, and character of the skin rash will, however, distinguish dermatomyositis from either of the two. *Multiple sclerosis* and *myasthenia gravis* are also known for muscle weakness but will have a distinctly different electromyographic pattern from that of dermatomyositis. Additionally, many drugs, including alcohol, glucocorticoids, and penicillamine, can produce a *drug-induced polymyositis*. In particular, HIV-infected individuals on zidovudine (AZT) frequently develop a polymyositis.

DIAGNOSTIC WORK-UP ▶ Four components should be included in a work-up to rule out dermatomyositis. The first is measurement of serum CPK, which is indicative of muscle degeneration. The second is an ANA test, which is a nonspecific screening test for autoimmune disease; over 70% of dermatomyositis patients have positive results. It is also recommended that anti-Jo-1 autoantibodies be assessed because they are found in a small subset of dermatomyositis patients who have interstitial fibrosis as part of their disease. The third component is electromyographic testing, which can help distinguish dermatomyositis from other diseases that cause muscle weakness. Characteristically, dermatomyositis will show high-frequency action potentials in a pattern of polyphasic potentials and fibrillation. The fourth is a muscle biopsy of a clinically involved muscle. Often the muscle biopsy is from the hip or shoulder girdle, but if the flexors of the neck are involved, the sternocleidomastoid muscles serve as readily accessible muscle biopsy sites. If jaw closure reveals clinical weakness, the anterior border of the masseter muscle can be accessed from a transoral approach.

Dermatomyositis is associated with a general increased risk for malignancy. The general physical examination should specifically look for and include diagnostic tests for malignancy common to the age, sex, and other risk factors of the individual.

HISTOPATHOLOGY ▶

Skin lesions may show a nonspecific inflammatory infiltrate, but very often the changes are akin to those of SLE. They show perivascular lymphoid infiltrates, connective tissue edema, liquefaction degeneration of epithelial basal cells, and PAS-positive deposits in the basement membrane zone and around capillaries. However, there is no deposition of immunoglobulins at the epidermal-dermal junction. The changes within muscle consist of scattered degeneration and regeneration of muscle fibers. These areas, as well as blood vessels, may be surrounded by mononuclear infiltrates (Fig 3-60). Because these inflammatory components are focal, they may be missed on biopsy. A typical degenerative-regenerative reaction may be seen at the periphery of muscle fascicles. In older lesions, muscle fibers may be replaced by fibrotic tissue. The mononuclear infiltrates are predominantly activated T cells that show sensitization to muscle antigens and natural killer cells, which are cytotoxic to muscle fibers.

TREATMENT ▶

Most patients respond to prednisone. Systemic corticosteroid regimen I or IIIA is used most often. Systemic corticosteroid regimen IIIB is used rarely and only in refractory cases (see pages 205 to 206).

PROGNOSIS ▶

Long-term use of prednisone is often needed, and exacerbations after discontinuation are common. CPK serum levels are indicative of disease activity and are a part of the follow-up assessment. Patients with an associated malignancy do not respond as well to treatment and have a poorer prognosis. However, treatment of the malignancy alleviates the dermatomyositis. Children respond much better than do adults, and many achieve permanent drug-free remissions.

Aphthous Stomatitis

CLINICAL PRESENTATION AND PATHOGENESIS ▶

Aphthous ulcers, well-known to healthcare providers, are known as "canker sores" to the layperson. Aphthous ulcers are divided into two types: minor and major. Minor aphthous ulcers appear as single discrete ulcers or in groups of two or more (Figs 3-61a and 3-61b). They are characteristically found on the free movable oral mucosa rather than the attached mucosa. The formed ulcers are discrete with a white-yellow base, which is a fibrinous slough, and a distinct irregular border with a red halo. The lesions emerge in four stages. In the first or prodromal stage, the individual will experience a tingling or burning pain in a clinically normal-appearing site; during the second or preulcerative stage, red oval papules appear and the pain intensifies; in the third or ulcerative stage, the classic ulcer appears; it will measure between 3 and 10 mm and may last 7 to 14 days. The fourth stage is the healing stage in which granulation tissue followed by epithelial migration incurs healing without scar.

Major aphthous ulcers are identical in their developmental stages and their general appearance except that they are larger (exceeding 10 mm), deeper (extending into the deep layers of the submucosa and into underlying muscle at times), and longer lasting (up to 6 weeks) (Fig 3-62). Most individuals with major aphthous ulcers (formerly called *Sutton major aphthae* and before that incorrectly called *periadenitis mucosa necrotica recurrens*) harbor at least one or two lesions at all times.

The pathogenesis of aphthous stomatitis remains unknown. The theories are even more numerous than its suggested treatment schedules. The most plausible theory explaining most clinical observations is that of an immune-based leukocytoclastic vasculitis. In this theory, either autoantibodies to oral mucous membrane epithelium or circulating antibodies to the microorganism *Streptococcus sanguis* form antigen-antibody complexes within local vessel walls. These immune complexes together with complement initiate an intense cascade of inflammation mediated mostly by neutrophils. The secretion of cytopathic enzymes by neutrophils and other leukocytes causes the tissue destruction and necrosis of epithelium recognized as an aphthous ulcer.

DIFFERENTIAL DIAGNOSIS ▶

Aphthous stomatitis is somewhat distinctive. However, minor aphthae will often be confused with recurrent *herpes lesions*. This similarity is sufficient to compel some authors to distinguish yet another type

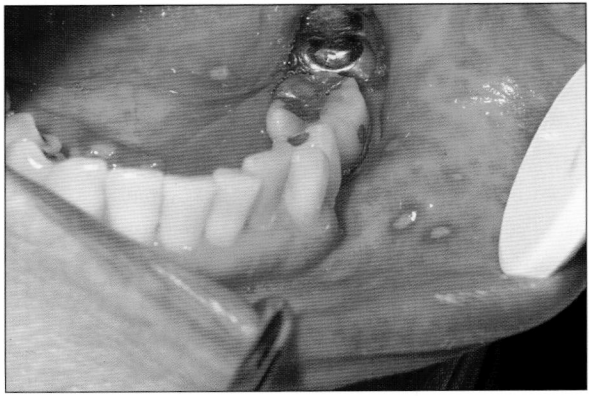

Fig 3-61a Minor aphthous ulcers are single or in small clusters. Each will be painful with a white-yellow fibrinous center and a peripheral "halo" of erythema.

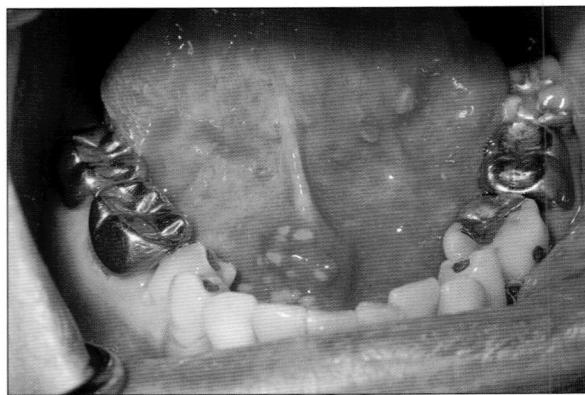

Fig 3-61b A cluster of minor aphthous ulcers located on the free mucosa of the floor of the mouth.

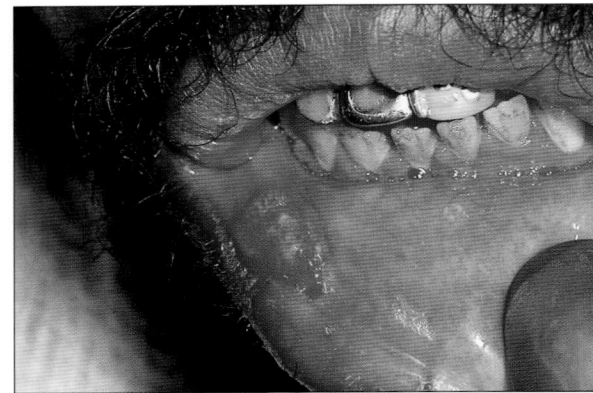

Fig 3-62 Major aphthous ulcers are larger (here 11 mm × 18 mm), deeper, and longer-lasting.

of aphthous ulcer, the so-called herpetiform aphthous ulcer; however, there is no real distinction. The lesions of *Behçet syndrome* will look very much like those of major aphthous stomatitis and will require that the clinician examine for iritis-hypopyon and similar-appearing genital skin lesions characteristic of Behçet syndrome. The oral lesions of *hand-foot-and-mouth disease* will also resemble aphthae. However, a close examination of fingers, toes, and palms will confirm or rule out this entity.

DIAGNOSTIC WORK-UP ▶ No specific work-up is required. Aphthous stomatitis is a clinical-recognition diagnosis.

HISTOPATHOLOGY ▶ Histologic examination is not usually indicated for aphthous ulcers, although it is sometimes helpful for difficult clinical cases. The findings are rather nonspecific. The ulcer often appears punched out (Fig 3-63a), and the epithelial margins show no significant change, although occasionally edema may cause a slight separation of the epithelium from the underlying connective tissue (Fig 3-63b). There may be some spongiosis, and there is usually an intense inflammatory infiltrate at the base. While neutrophils are typically seen on the surface of the ulcer, lymphocytes and macrophages are the major component. Major aphthae show changes identical to those in the minor form, but the inflammatory infiltrate extends more deeply (Fig 3-63c). Because this often involves underlying mucous glands, it is understandable that at one time major aphthae were thought to be associated with salivary glands, hence the term *periadenitis mucosa necrotica recurrens*. The depth of the involvement is also responsible for the chronicity and scarring of these ulcers. Studies have indicated that aphthae may be the consequence of an immune complex vasculitis. This is supported by the fact that foci of extravasated erythrocytes are seen and that perivascular aggregates of neutrophils are found. The development of the lesion may relate to a lymphocytotoxic process because early lesions contain predominantly T4 lymphocytes before ulceration. In the ulcerative phase, most are T8 lymphocytes, while during healing the T4 cells again dominate.

TREATMENT ▶ Because there is no known single effective treatment for aphthous stomatitis, there is a plethora of published and unpublished treatment schedules and drugs. They include antibiotics; vitamins; zinc; levamisole as an immune stimulant; and either topical, intralesional, or systemic corticosteroids. In addition, chlorhexidine gluconate 0.12%, sulfones, and iron therapy, among other treatments, have been recommended, confusing the situation.

A rational approach to aphthous stomatitis requires an understanding that minor aphthous ulcers are few and of short duration. No specific therapy is ideal. It is reasonable to simply reassure the patient and provide no specific treatment. Most individuals can endure the minor level of discomfort, which is preferable to risking therapy with agents of unfounded efficacy and potential side effects. Single or small groups of ulcers that are uncomfortable may be directly cauterized with silver nitrate ($AgNO_3$) or phenol, thereby avoiding systemic side effects.

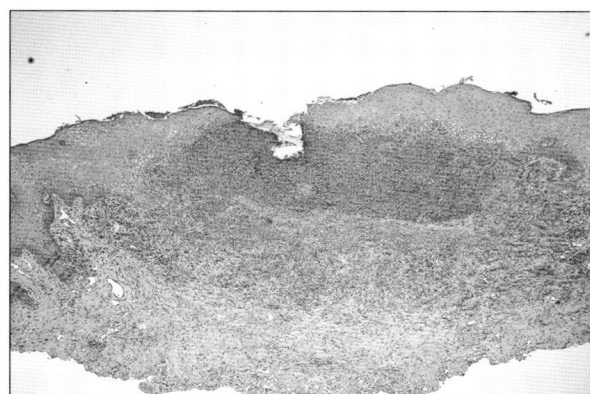

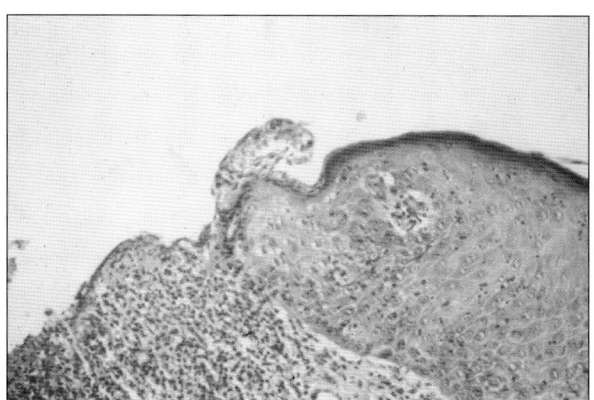

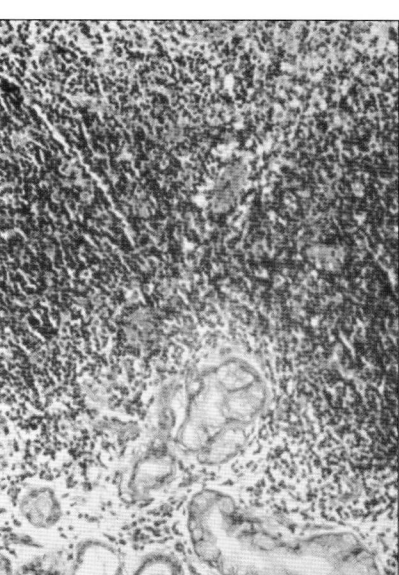

Fig 3-63a A punched-out ulceration with an intense inflammatory reaction is a typical finding in aphthous stomatitis.

Fig 3-63b Other than some edema below the epithelium, the margin of the aphthous ulcer shows no changes in the epithelium. This finding can help distinguish these lesions from herpetic ulcers in which the viral infection produces significant epithelial changes.

Fig 3-63c In major aphthae, the inflammatory reaction tends to extend deeply into the connective tissue. Seen here is obvious involvement of mucous glands.

For aphthous ulcers that are numerous and frequent enough to debilitate patients, a trial with antibiotics is useful before resorting to systemic corticosteroids. The three most effective antibiotic regimens are: (*1*) erythromycin, 250 mg by mouth four times daily; (*2*) tetracycline (Achromycin, Lederle), 250 mg by mouth four times daily; and (*3*) a mixture often called "tetranydril elixir," which consists of 250 mg tetracycline and 12.5 mg diphenhydramine hydrochloride (Benadryl, Warner Lambert) per 5 mL of Kaopectate (Pharmacia and Upjohn). The patient is instructed to use 1 tsp at a time and swish, hold the solution in their mouth as long as possible, and swallow, three times daily. These regimens have been variably useful in controlling the number, frequency, and duration of lesions. Patients will have "breakthrough" lesions, but they are few and much more tolerable. Any of these regimens can be continued for extended periods (2 to 6 months) before withdrawal to attempt continued control in a drug-free stage.

If these antibiotic regimens fail, systemic corticosteroids are the treatment of choice. Topical corticosteroids have little effect on major lesions. Most lesions that seem to benefit from topical treatment may not warrant any treatment. The corticosteroid of choice is prednisone and should follow the systemic corticosteroid regimen I or II (see page 205) in an attempt to gain a corticosteroid-induced remission and maintain the remission in a drug-free state.

PROGNOSIS ▶

Aphthous stomatitis is most active in young adulthood. There may be a period of 10 to 15 years in which intermittent flare-ups occur where lesions appear more frequently and are more intense. The treatment schedules described attenuate and control the lesions and will likely alleviate their symptoms. With time and advancing age, the condition becomes less intense and usually remits altogether.

Behçet Syndrome

CLINICAL PRESENTATION AND PATHOGENESIS ▶

Behçet syndrome most often presents in young men with oral lesions identical to large aphthous ulcers (Fig 3-64a). The syndrome is said to include ocular and genital lesions, so that, in addition to recurrent oral lesions, recurrent aphthous-looking lesions also appear on the skin around the penis and scrotum

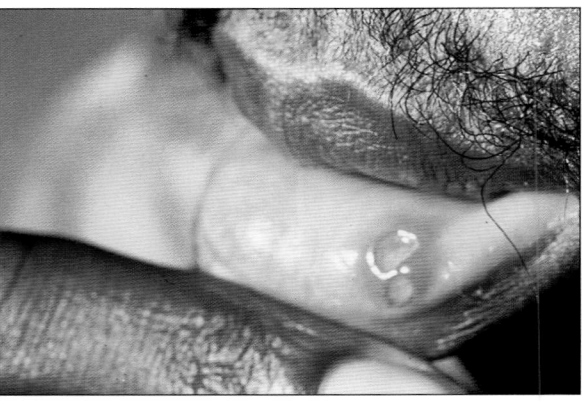

Fig 3-64a Behçet syndrome ulcers will be painful and resemble major aphthous ulcers.

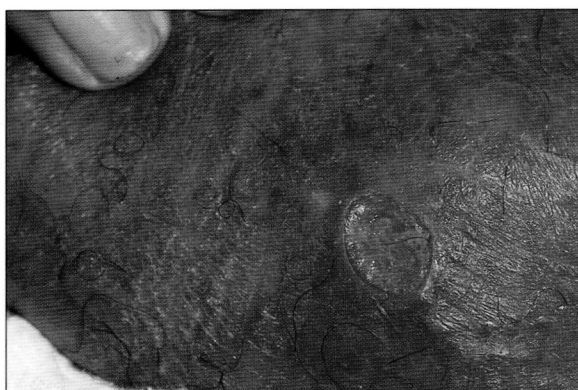

Fig 3-64b The genital lesions of Behçet syndrome in men are aphthous-like ulcers located on the skin of the scrotum, as seen here, or on the penis. The rare cases in women will have the ulcers on the labia or vulva.

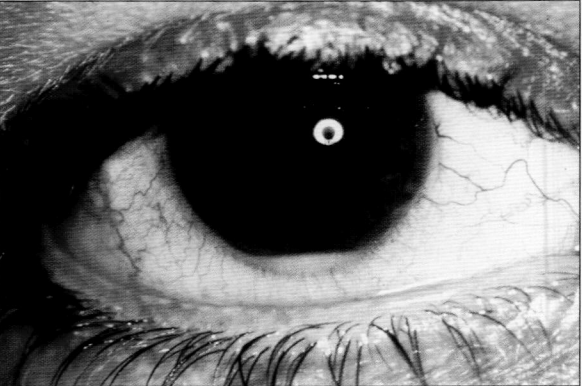

Fig 3-64c The ocular lesions in Behçet syndrome result from inflammation in the iris (iritis) and/or uveal tracts (uveitis), which often produces pus in the anterior chambers (hypopyon) as seen here.

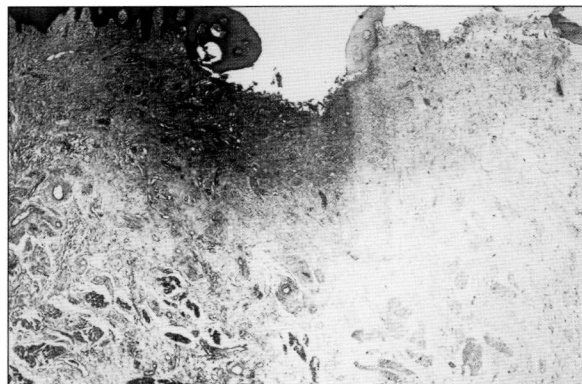

Fig 3-64d The histologic appearance of a lesion from a patient with Behçet syndrome who had painful oral ulcers. The punched-out appearance with the intense inflammatory reaction is similar to that seen in the aphthous ulcer shown in Fig 3-63a.

(Fig 3-64b). In women, lesions occur on the labia and vulva. Specifically, the ocular lesions comprise inflammation of the iris and uveal tracts (iritis and uveitis), which will produce a level of pus in the anterior chamber (hypopyon) (Fig 3-64c). Because the basis of this disease seems to be a vasculitis, red-nodular skin lesions (erythema nodosum) and a nonrheumatoid (seronegative) arthritis appear in two thirds of patients (localized to the knees and ankles). In one variant of Behçet syndrome, termed MAGIC (mouth and genital ulcers with inflamed cartilage) syndrome, auricular and nasal cartilage is targeted along with the other manifestations. In rare severe cases, the vasculitis may cause vascular thrombosis, cranial nerve palsies, and encephalitis.

The oral lesions are usually the feature that brings the individual to seek medical attention. The lesions are painful and are usually 2 to 10 in number. They often precede the iritis, or the iritis is present but subclinical at the time of presentation.

The cause of Behçet syndrome is still unknown. It is currently believed to represent an autoimmune vasculitis in susceptible individuals related to HLA-B51 as a part of a recently recognized class of diseases referred to as *leukocytoclastic diseases*.

DIFFERENTIAL DIAGNOSIS ▶ Behçet syndrome initially resembles an *aphthous stomatitis*, making it incumbent on the clinician to search for other features of this syndrome. Conversely, *reactive arthritis* may present with arthritis and a conjunctivitis resembling Behçet syndrome, but the oral lesions are not aphthous-like and are nonpainful. If skin lesions are prominent and include skin outside the genital area, *erythema multiforme* also must be considered.

Behçet syndrome requires only a recognition of its clinical symptom complex. However, a complete ophthalmologic examination is indicated to assess the degree of uveitis.

Behçet syndrome may show the same histologic features as noted for aphthous stomatitis (Fig 3-64d). Although the lesions may show only diffuse infiltration of neutrophils or mononuclear cells, there is often a vasculitis that may be lymphocytic or leukocytoclastic and in which fibrin is deposited in the wall of small blood vessels.

Prednisone is the treatment standard for Behçet syndrome. Systemic corticosteroid regimen I or III is most commonly used (see pages 205 to 206).

Behçet syndrome is difficult to control even with systemic corticosteroids. Cytotoxic drugs such as cyclophosphamide (Cytoxan, Mead Johnson), 50 mg twice daily, or azathioprine (Imuran, GlaxoSmith-Kline), 50 mg twice daily, as in systemic corticosteroid regimen III, are frequently required or, alternatively, chlorambucil may be used. The disease course is most active in youth, and exacerbations are frequent. As the patient ages, the disease becomes more controllable and often goes into permanent remission.

Reactive Arthritis (Formerly Reiter Syndrome)

Reactive arthritis is said to be a postinfection syndrome with a tetrad of findings consisting of urethritis, conjunctivitis, arthritis, and painless oral-skin lesions (mucocutaneous lesions). Originally named for Hans Reiter, who described a postdysenteric collection of findings in a World War I German military officer in 1916, the syndrome occurs primarily in young adult men. Those afflicted seek attention because of either arthritis or concern about penile lesions that usually develop a few weeks after a gastrointestinal infection, or, more rarely, a venereal infection. The oral lesions (50% of cases) are characteristically painless red papules that are seen on the palate, buccal mucosa, tongue, and gingiva (Fig 3-65a). The skin lesions are very distinctive and consist of two types: *(1)* painless lesions of the penis tip and scrotum, called *balanitis circinata,* which represent shallow erosions and striated erosions (Fig 3-65b), and *(2)* pustular hyperkeratotic plaques and vesicles, called *keratoderma blennorrhagicum,* which appear on the weight-bearing portions of the soles and on the palms (Fig 3-65c).

The arthritis characteristically focuses on the joints of the hips, knees, ankles, and metatarsals. The local tendon insertions are also inflamed, and painful Achilles tendinitis and plantar fasciitis are very common. The ocular lesions are most commonly a mild, culture-negative but purulent conjunctivitis. They will produce some pain, photophobia, and conjunctival erythema ("red eye"). Less commonly, uveitis and iritis may be present. The urethritis is usually manifested as mild dysuria. It is often referred to as *nongonococcal urethritis* because gonorrhea is the cause of most cases of urethritis. Occasionally, prostatitis and epididymitis develop in men. In the uncommon cases in women, vaginitis and cervicitis may develop.

Reactive arthritis is a reactive disease occurring in susceptible individuals—those with human leukocyte antigen HLA-B27 positivity—caused by an unknown immune stimulation resulting from dysenteric or venereal infection. It is a disease primarily of young men; the male to female ratio is 9:1 when it arises after a dysenteric infection and 99:1 when it arises from a venereal infection. The most common infective agents include *Chlamydia, Campylobacter, Shigella,* and *Salmonella* species. Today, there is a strong association of reactive arthritis with the later stages of HIV infection and AIDS. One study noted reactive arthritis in 5% of HIV-infected patients. In such patients, the arthritis is much more destructive and the oral-skin lesions more persistent. The onset of reactive arthritis appears 1 to 4 weeks after the infectious stimulation.

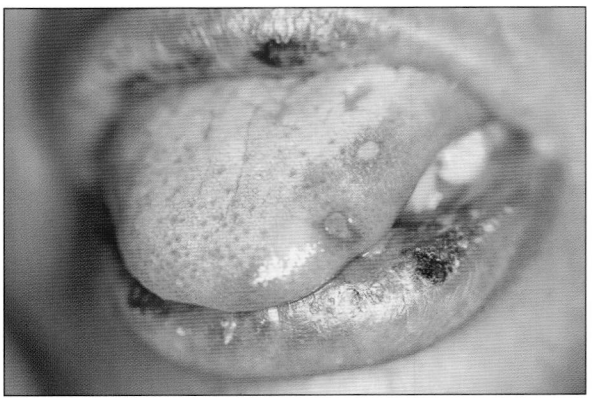

Fig 3-65a The oral manifestations of reactive arthritis may appear to be painful, but they actually represent painless eruptions.

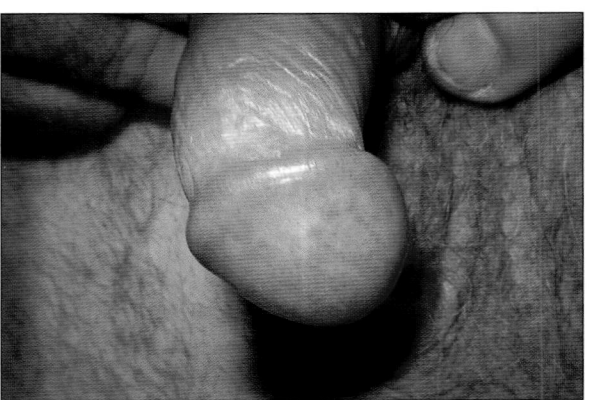

Fig 3-65b The genital lesions in reactive arthritis, called *balanitis circinata,* will also be painless and usually involve the tip of the penis and scrotum.

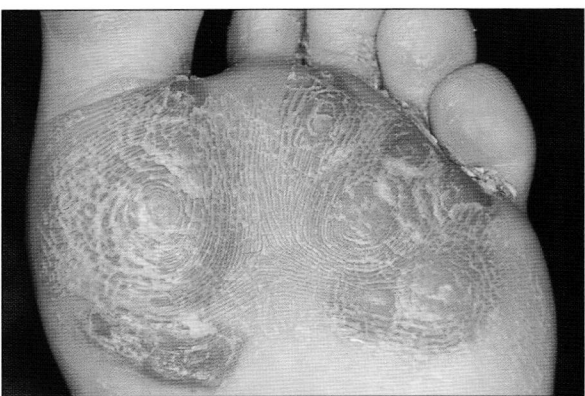

Fig 3-65c Reactive arthritis also will often develop hyperkeratotic plaques, termed *keratoderma blennorrhagicum,* on the palms of the hands or sole of the feet.

DIFFERENTIAL DIAGNOSIS ▶

The most important differential feature of reactive arthritis is the painless quality of the oral and skin lesions. Otherwise, several diseases that may present with concomitant oral and skin lesions, such as *erythema multiforme, Behçet syndrome,* and *lichen planus,* must be considered. The dysuria and skin lesions may also suggest *primary syphilis, secondary syphilis,* or *gonorrhea.*

DIAGNOSTIC WORK-UP ▶

Reactive arthritis appears to be more common in patients infected with HIV and may precede or occur during AIDS. It is reasonable to gain the patient's consent for HIV testing. A urinalysis for Gram staining and culture to rule out gonorrhea is also appropriate. An ANA and a rheumatoid factor (RF) analysis are frequently accomplished to rule out rheumatoid disease as the cause of the arthritis. A routine complete blood count (CBC) will often show a normochromic, normocytic anemia and a leukocytosis with a neutrophilia. Because HLA-B27 positivity is highly associated with reactive arthritis (60% to 90%), testing for this may be performed.

HISTOPATHOLOGY ▶

The lesions of reactive arthritis, whether on oral mucosa, skin, or genitalia, have a psoriasiform appearance. Pindborg et al described them as showing parakeratosis and acanthosis with elongation of rete ridges. Neutrophils infiltrate the epithelium and form microabscesses. The underlying connective tissue contains lymphocytes with some plasma cells and leukocytes.

TREATMENT ▶

Reactive arthritis is self-limiting in most cases. Reassurance and supportive management of the tetrad of involved areas are indicated. The mild conjunctivitis is not treated, but an anterior uveitis/iritis may be treated with atropine and topical corticosteroids. The urethritis is treated with a 7- to 14-day course of doxycycline (Vibramycin, Pfizer), 100 mg twice daily, or erythromycin, 500 mg four times daily, to treat chlamydia if present. If dysentery was the stimulus for reactive arthritis, administration of one of the quinolones or chloramphenicol is recommended. The arthritis is treated with nonsteroidal anti-inflammatory agents such as ibuprofen (Advil, McNeill), 400 mg three times daily, or with Cox-2 inhibitors such as rofecoxib (Vioxx, Merck), 50 mg by mouth per day, which is very effective in reducing symptoms. The oral-skin lesions usually require no specific therapy, only time for resolution. However, they will respond very rapidly to methotrexate, 25 to 50 mg by mouth every day, or azathioprine (Imuran, GlaxoSmithKline), 50 mg twice daily.

PROGNOSIS ▶

While most cases resolve completely over a 2-month period after treatment, about 40% develop periodic relapses and another 10% to 25% suffer severe disability.

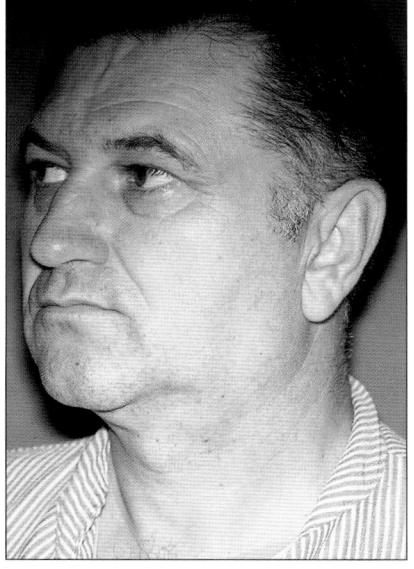

Fig 3-66a This limited neck rotation and neck pain were due to ossification of the stylohyoid ligaments and ossification of the intervertebral ligaments.

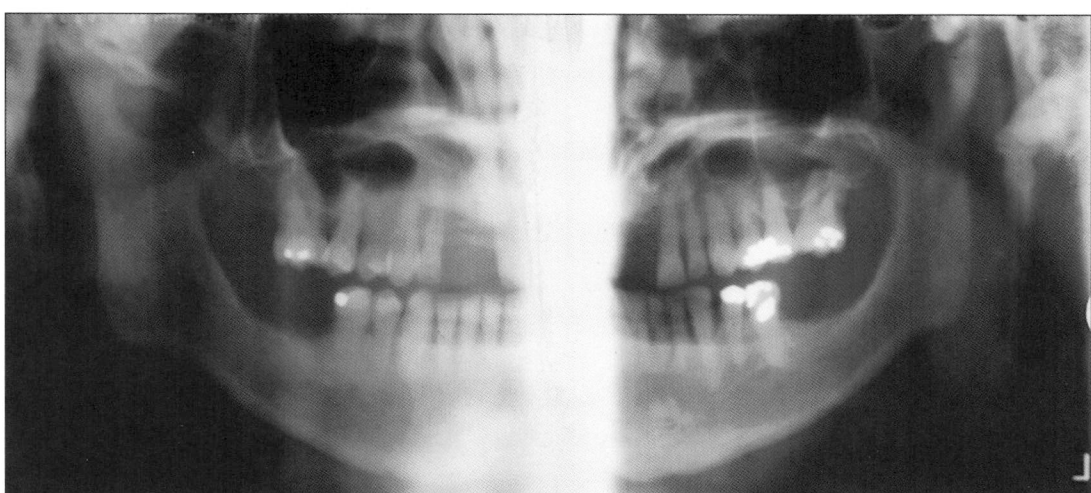

Fig 3-66b Panoramic radiograph showing ossification of the stylohyoid ligaments.

Diffuse Interosseous Skeletal Hypertrophy (DISH) Syndrome

CLINICAL PRESENTATION AND PATHOGENESIS ▶

Diffuse interosseous skeletal hypertrophy (DISH) syndrome is often mistaken for Eagle syndrome by many oral and maxillofacial specialists. Individuals with DISH present with ossification of their interosseous ligaments that restricts neck motion and induces pain (Fig 3-66a). Ossification of intervertebral ligaments produces cervical pain during neck rotation and extensions, and the stylohyoid ligament ossifies to produce pain on swallowing. The latter is readily apparent on a panoramic radiograph (Fig 3-66b). In contrast, so-called Eagle syndrome causes neck and swallowing pain related to tonsillar infections and complicated tonsillectomies. The mechanism for this pain was suggested to be scarring of the stylohyoid ligament and other pharyngeal muscles of the mucosa in the tonsillar fossa. When panoramic radiographs became commonplace in the 1960s, the frequent finding of elongated stylohyoid processes (most of which were within normal range) prompted the addition of an elongated or "calcified" stylohyoid ligament to the syndrome. Consequently, many patients with neck pain or dysphagia arising from other sources who radiographically demonstrated longer-than-average stylohyoid ligaments were said to have Eagle syndrome. Included in this group were some individuals with true DISH syndrome in whom the more important cervical and even thoracolumbar involvement remained unrecognized.

Patients with DISH syndrome will indeed present with variable complaints relating to dysphagia and pain during neck motion. Upon questioning, many will also relate pain and/or paresthesias radiating to one or both arms and even to their fingertips. This is indicative of cervical nerve root compression (radiculopathy). Most will be between 40 and 60 years of age and will not identify a complicated tonsillectomy in their history. There is an equal distribution between men and women.

DIFFERENTIAL DIAGNOSIS ▶

Neck pain and dysphagia is always a worrisome finding. The clinician should consider malignancies such as *squamous cell carcinoma* or *lymphoepithelioma* in this area, as well as *salivary gland malignancies*. If the patient is a fair-skinned woman, the *Plummer-Vinson (Paterson-Kelly) syndrome* of iron-deficiency anemia with dysphagia due to esophageal webs, which carries a high risk for pharyngeal carcinoma, becomes a consideration. In any individual with a history of whiplash trauma, *ligamental injuries* with inflammation

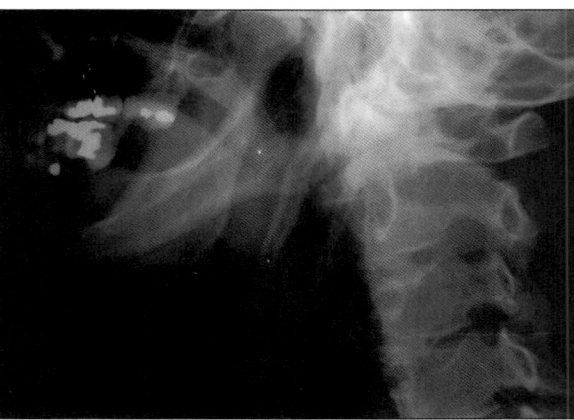

Fig 3-66c Oblique radiograph of the mandible and upper cervical spine showing significant ossification of the intervertebral ligaments and the stylohyoid ligaments.

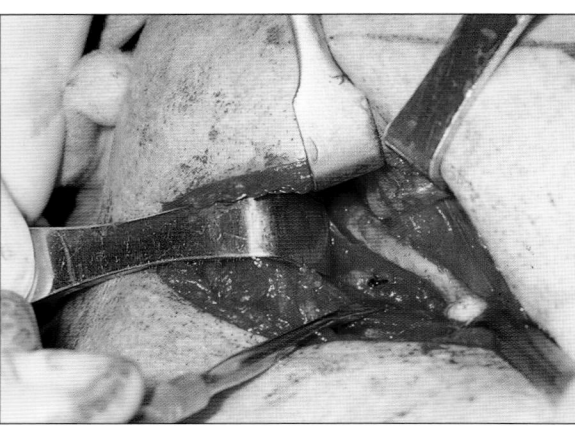

Fig 3-66d Complete ossification of the stylohyoid ligament may fix the hyoid to the base of the skull by means of a continuous bony connection.

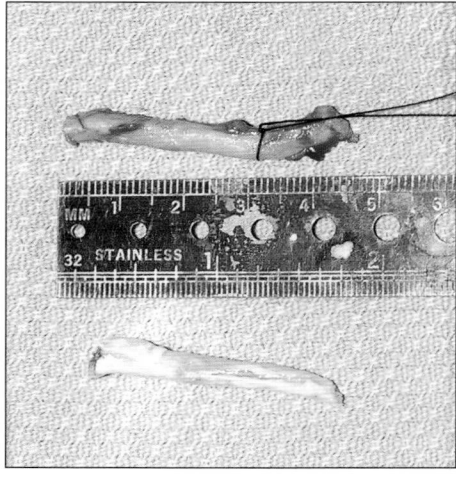

Fig 3-66e Resection specimens of bilateral ossified stylohyoid ligaments in an individual with DISH syndrome.

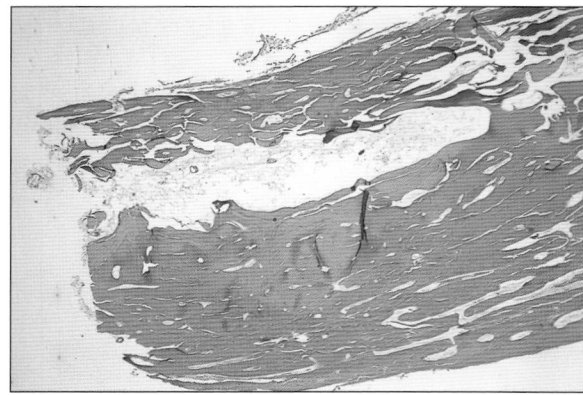

Fig 3-66f Histology of the stylohyoid ligament from a DISH patient will document that the ligament is ossified rather than merely calcified.

is possible, and of course *rheumatoid arthritis, juvenile rheumatoid arthritis*, and age-related *degenerative joint disease* (DJD) must also be considered.

DIAGNOSTIC WORK-UP ▶ Individuals with DISH syndrome will exhibit radiographically identifiable ossifications of their intervertebral ligaments. Many of these can be seen on a routine panoramic radiograph that includes the cervical spine in the field. Otherwise, oblique plain neck radiographs (Fig 3-66c) or tomographs will show them well and a CT scan will provide the most obvious and detailed picture. A CT scan is recommended in all cases, not only to identify the intervertebral ossifications but to rule out subtle masses suggestive of malignancy or signs of actual joint-related arthritis. If the Plummer-Vinson (Paterson-Kelly) syndrome is considered, a barium swallow study may be useful as well as a complete blood count with Wintrobe indices. If rheumatoid arthritis is a serious consideration, a serum antinuclear antibody (ANA) and a rheumatoid factor (RF) test may be useful.

TREATMENT AND PROGNOSIS ▶ The identification of symptomatic "elongated" or "calcified" (they are actually ossified) stylohyoid ligaments that are proven to be DISH by vertebral radiographs should be co-managed with a rheumatologist. While it is reasonable to consider excision of the ossified stylohyoid ligaments, this should be accomplished within the context of a more comprehensive management. DISH is incurable and slowly progressive. The goal of therapy is to relieve pain and maintain motion and activity. Cervical collars, neck or back braces, and physical therapy are usually needed for the vertebral involvements. Patients also benefit from nonsteroidal anti-inflammatory drugs (NSAIDs), particularly the Cox-2 inhibitors such as rofecoxib (Vioxx, Merck), 25 mg daily, and celecoxib (Celebrex, Searle), 200 mg daily for a prescribed length of time.

Since nearly every vertebrae will have some ossifying of its respective intervertebral ligaments, cervical surgery is not helpful and therefore not indicated. However, excising the ossified stylohyoid ligaments can reduce pain, particularly the pain on swallowing. The patient should be informed that such surgery will not relieve all and perhaps not even the majority of the pain because of the numerous vertebrae affected.

The surgical approach is via a horizontal incision within a skin fold of the neck paralleling the inferior border of the mandible. The incision should be located over the lower portion of the submandibular gland in the area of the intermediate tendon. The dissection should proceed through the platysma and superficial layer of the deep cervical fascia to identify the intermediate tendon between the anterior and posterior digastric muscles. The intermediate tendon is then followed inferiorly for about 1 cm to identify the stylohyoid muscle, which lies superficial to the posterior digastric muscle, and to identify the lesser horn of the hyoid bone. In some cases the entire length of the stylohyoid ligament will have ossified, thereby fixing the hyoid in position via one solid cord of bone from the stylomastoid foramen area to the lesser horn of the hyoid (Fig 3-66d). The ossified stylohyoid ligament is then followed superiorly from the lesser horn of the hyoid. The ligament will be just deep to the stylohyoid muscle. The soft tissues are separated from the ossified stylohyoid ligament before it is separated from the styloid process proper. This includes ligating the facial artery, which courses deep to the stylohyoid ligament to enter the submandibular triangle. Removal of the ossified stylohyoid ligament can be accomplished with a rongeur or an osteotome and is straightforward since the ossified stylohyoid ligament is usually connected to the native styloid process by a fibrous band in a pseudojoint fashion. The residual styloid process is rounded off before closing in layers.

Since the stylohyoid ligament is ossified (Figs 3-66e and 3-66f) to or nearly to the hyoid bone and since the facial artery and retromandibular vein are in close approximation, a transoral approach is not recommended. Transoral approaches have not been able to completely remove the diseased ligament, and significant bleeding with limited access to control it has been encountered.

FOLLOW-UP ▶

Excision of the ossified stylohyoid process provides some pain relief and may improve swallowing. Patients should be informed of the slowly progressive nature of DISH and followed lifelong. They also must be made aware that continuing physical therapy and medications will be necessary.

Juvenile Periodontitis

CLINICAL PRESENTATION AND PATHOGENESIS ▶

Juvenile periodontitis is composed of three disease presentations—prepubertal periodontitis, juvenile periodontitis, and rapidly progressing periodontitis—all of which share the common pathogenesis of a genetic leukocyte adhesion deficiency (LAD) and a loose association with specific microorganisms, most commonly *Actinobacillus actinomycetemcomitans* and sometimes different *Capnocytophaga* species.

Prepubertal periodontitis is broken down further into a localized form and a generalized form. The localized form shows minimal inflammation but deep periodontal pockets localized to the primary molars first, followed soon thereafter by the primary incisors. The generalized form shows severe proliferative gingival inflammation in addition to deep intrabony pockets and affects all primary teeth. The LAD underlies both forms and seems to be a matter of degree. The children with the localized form of prepubertal periodontitis are otherwise healthy, but the children with the generalized form frequently have histories of repeated infections, pneumonias, delayed wound healings, and a peripheral blood leukocytosis.

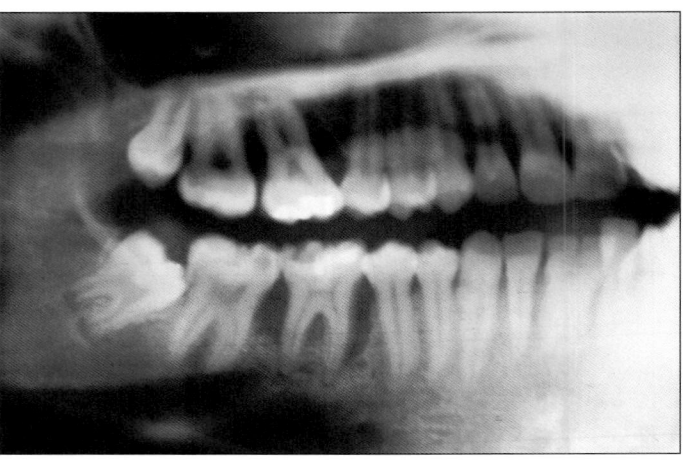

Fig 3-67 This localized form of juvenile periodontitis in a 17-year-old had extensive bone loss limited to all first molars and around the mesial aspect of the second molars.

Juvenile periodontitis affects the first permanent molars and then the incisors in otherwise healthy preteens and teenagers (Fig 3-67). Inflammation, periodontal pockets, and alveolar bone loss are seen with tooth mobility. The bone destruction progresses rapidly, but periods of quiescence also occur.

Rapidly progressive periodontitis, which has a similar clinical presentation, occurs in adults younger than 35 years. It tends to be more generalized and mimics the more common chronic periodontitis, but is quick in onset and destruction and is more severe around molars and incisors. The picture of bone loss and tooth mobility is more advanced than would be consistent with the individual's plaque control.

LAD is an autosomal-recessive trait. Most patients with clinical disease are homozygous. The defective or absent glycoproteins on the cell surface of neutrophils and macrophages prevent adhesion to each other or to the wound so that they do not concentrate at a site of inflammation. Therefore, a specific pathogen or other pathogenic microorganisms can be more destructive and proceed unchecked. In all of the juvenile periodontitis forms, *A actinomycetemcomitans* is thought to specifically contribute to the progression of this disease because it produces a neutrophil chemotaxis inhibiting factor, a lymphocyte suppressing factor, bone-resorbing toxin, collagenase, and fibroblast-inhibiting factors.

DIFFERENTIAL DIAGNOSIS ▶ Unexpected bone loss in a child or young adult, which will sometimes create the radiographic appearance of a tooth (usually a molar) floating in the alveolus, is a classic feature of several serious diseases, in particular *Langerhans cell histiocytosis*, *Papillon-Lefèvre syndrome*, *acute lymphocytic leukemia* in children and preteens, and *acute myelogenous leukemia* in late teens and early adults. In addition, systemic diseases that suppress leukocyte function or cause immune suppression will predispose patients to a more rapid progress of chronic periodontitis, which may resemble one of the forms of juvenile periodontitis. Therefore, *diabetes-*, *HIV-*, *AIDS-,* and *neutropenia-related periodontitis,* among others, are also considerations.

DIAGNOSTIC WORK-UP ▶ The index of suspicion for either form of this disease directs the collection of clinical and radiographic data. If the index of suspicion is high, tissue biopsies to rule out other diseases are required, as are blood tests to assess the LAD. In addition to a routine complete red cell and white cell count with a differential (particularly to assess for neutrophilia), in vitro testing of the following is suggested: neutrophil and monocyte adherence, random and directed migration assessment of neutrophils and monocytes, intracellular microbicidal activity, and oxygen consumption during organism digestion.

Testing of neutrophil and monocyte cell surface glycoproteins also may be necessary because these are the actual deficiencies that result in absence of leukocyte adhesion and, consequently, in their failure to aggregate and perform their usual functions at a site of inflammation. They are MAC-1 (complement receptor type 3), LFA-1 (lymphocyte function–associated antigen), p150, and p95 cell surface glycoproteins. The assessment of each requires a sophisticated laboratory capable of immunofluorescence flow cytometry, gel electrophoresis, and immunoprecipitation. It is, therefore, advisable to discuss the specimens, their quantity, their handling, and their transport with the laboratory before the specimens are released.

Because there remains an association with *A actinomycetemcomitans* and *Capnocytophaga* species, tissue specimens should also be submitted for culture identification of each.

HISTOPATHOLOGY ▶ The epithelium shows widening of intercellular spaces and migration of the junctional epithelium apical to the cementoenamel junction. This epithelium forms numerous rete ridges and is infiltrated by inflammatory cells, as is the subjacent connective tissue. Plasma cells are prominent. This is a nonspecific picture identical to the common form of chronic periodontitis.

TREATMENT ▶ The goal in treatment is to remove hopeless teeth and salvage as much of the remaining dentition as possible. The treatment, therefore, takes the form of tooth extraction and an individualized periodontal surgery plan. In addition, tetracycline, 250 mg four times daily, started 2 days before definitive surgery and extending for 21 to 28 days, is recommended.

In patients with histories of recurrent systemic infections, of multiple local infections that do not produce pus, or of delayed wound healing, the genetic expression of LAD is higher and makes them more prone to continued infection and surgical complications. These patients need to be made aware of their general health risks as well as their dental disease. These patients are more susceptible to a wide range of infections at multiple sites, such as mastoiditis, otitis, pneumonia, and skin infections. In very severe deficiencies, bone marrow transplantation to restore normal leukocyte function may be necessary.

PROGNOSIS ▶ Plaque control, antimicrobial therapy, and periodontal surgery have been successful in maintaining salvageable teeth in all but the most severe expressions.

Papillon-Lefèvre Syndrome

CLINICAL PRESENTATION AND PATHOGENESIS ▶ Papillon-Lefèvre syndrome is an autosomal-recessive trait associated with an LAD similar to those seen in the three forms of juvenile active periodontitis (Fig 3-68a). In fact, Papillon-Lefèvre syndrome combines the severe generalized prepubertal form of juvenile periodontitis with palmoplantar keratoderma and at times other less frequent manifestations.

Primary teeth erupt normally, but between the ages of 2 and 4 years patients simultaneously develop severe periodontal inflammation, bone loss (Fig 3-68b), and tooth mobility together with a red, scaly palmoplantar keratoderma. As the hyperkeratosis matures, the afflicted area may appear furry and brown or even have black areas (Fig 3-68c) caused by keratin layers. The hyperkeratotic areas are well demarcated and characteristically approach the edges of the thenar eminence and spread up onto the skin over the Achilles tendon.

The periodontal bone loss usually starts when the second primary molar erupts, and it causes almost all of the primary teeth to be lost by the age of 4 or 5. When the permanent teeth erupt, the process begins again, starting with the teeth that erupt first, ie, the first molars and the incisors. As the children progress through their preteen and teen years, the permanent dentition, with the exception of the third molars, is lost as is the alveolar bone, creating an atrophic mandible.

DIFFERENTIAL DIAGNOSIS ▶ The palmoplantar keratoderma should distinguish Papillon-Lefèvre syndrome from other entities and is a required finding for diagnosis. However, severe alveolar bone loss in a child is worrisome. Certainly *juvenile periodontitis, Langerhans cell histiocytosis, acute lymphocytic leukemia, neutropenia*, and *Chédiak-Higashi syndrome*, which also has a neutrophil dysfunction component, are other considerations.

DIAGNOSTIC WORK-UP ▶ Because this syndrome contains a component of juvenile periodontitis, the work-up should assess neutrophil function and test for neutrophil and macrophage surface glycoproteins MAC-1, LFA-1, p150, and p95 as in juvenile periodontitis. In addition, a complete battery of lymphocyte transformation tests and skin antigen tests for cell-mediated immune responses is recommended.

HISTOPATHOLOGY ▶ The palmoplantar keratoderma shows a nonspecific picture of hyperkeratosis, hypergranulosis, and acanthosis. The upper dermis contains a mild chronic inflammatory infiltrate. Periodontal lesions are

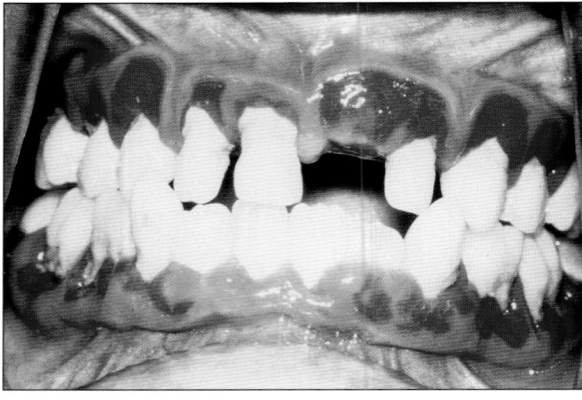

Fig 3-68a Severe inflammation, gingival recession, and underlying periodontal bone loss in a teenager with Papillon-Lefèvre syndrome.

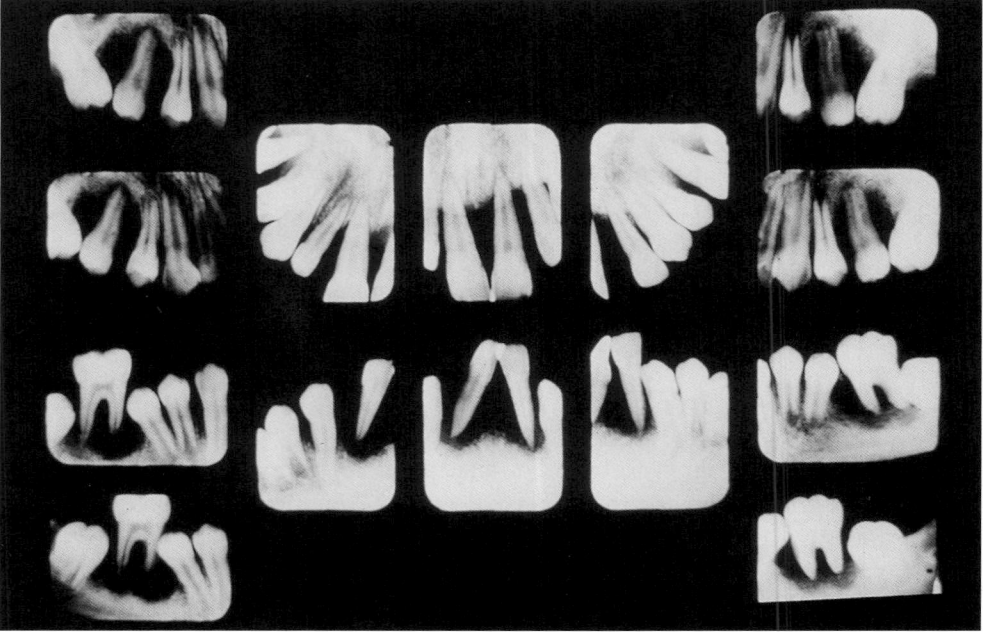

Fig 3-68b The pattern of bone loss in Papillon-Lefèvre syndrome is generalized but begins and is most severe around first molars and incisors, similar to that seen in juvenile periodontitis.

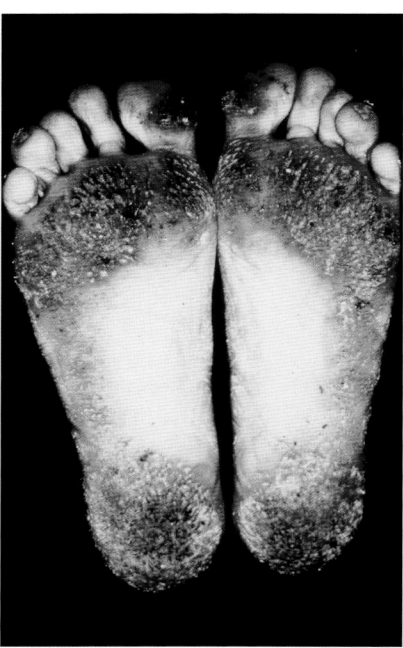

Fig 3-68c Plantar hyperkeratosis as seen here may be overt and is most prominent on the weight-bearing areas.

identical to those described in juvenile periodontitis. As in all LADs, neutrophils are markedly decreased or absent from inflammatory infiltrates.

TREATMENT ► In the past, Papillon-Lefèvre syndrome has been treated with removal of hopeless teeth only. Although this remains a component of necessary care, retention of teeth for a longer period often can be accomplished with intense periodontal care and a tetracycline, given four times daily, in doses adjusted for body weight. Because third molars often are not involved in this syndrome, their prophylactic removal is not indicated, and their retention is often useful in later prosthetic rehabilitation.

PROGNOSIS ► The prognosis of the dentition remains poor. Most patients become edentulous (except for the third molars) and have a small mandible and maxilla, which presents problems for obtaining prosthetic stability and retention. To date, osseointegrated fixtures have not been researched in this disease. While their success in edentulous states with normal immune function is excellent, their success in patients with host defense cell deficiencies is likely to be diminished. They are, therefore, not recommended at this time as a treatment except in the case of a special informed-consent research study.

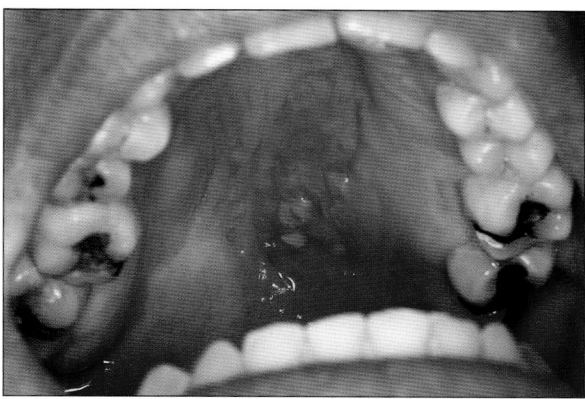

Fig 3-69a Wegener granulomatosis with a cobblestone appearance and painful ulcers.

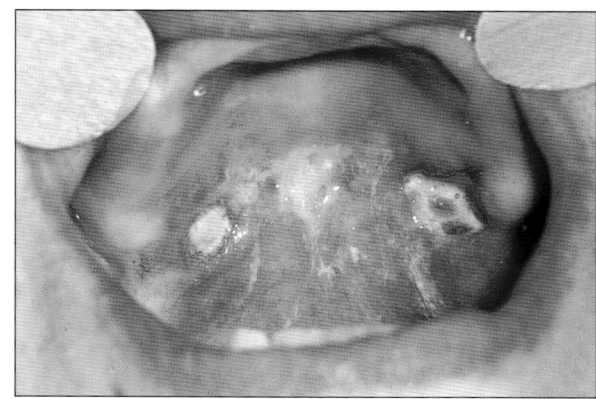

Fig 3-69b Bilateral necrotic ulcers of the palate were the presenting signs in this patient with Wegener granulomatosis.

Wegener Granulomatosis

CLINICAL PRESENTATION AND PATHOGENESIS ▶

Wegener granulomatosis is a rare idiopathic vasculitis of small arterioles and capillaries. Consequently, it attacks the lungs, kidneys, and oral regions, all of which have numerous small arterioles and capillaries.

Wegener granulomatosis usually presents with a 4- to 12-month onset of upper respiratory tract symptoms in an adult between 30 and 50 years of age. These may include nasal congestion, sinusitis, otitis media, cough, dyspnea, or hemoptysis. Oral symptoms and signs may include a painful cobblestone (Fig 3-69a) or ulcerative (Fig 3-69b) appearance of the palatal mucosa or the gingiva. Fever, weight loss, and fatigue are common. Palatal bony erosion has been overstated; even severe cases, in which much of the palatal mucosa is lysed, rarely if ever exhibit perforation of the palate into the nasal cavity.

Wegener granulomatosis is an immune-based disease. Antibodies develop to cytoplasmic components in the neutrophil; these are known as cANCA, which stands for *c*ytoplasmic pattern *an*tineutrophil *c*ytoplasmic *a*ntibodies. pANCA, which stands for *p*erinuclear *an*tineutrophil *c*ytoplasmic *a*ntibodies, relates to antibodies that develop to the myeloperoxidase granules, and are located in the cytoplasm of neutrophils in a perinuclear pattern. Wegener granulomatosis has a 70% positivity for cANCA and a 20% positivity for pANCA. In either, the antibody is thought to lyse the neutrophil, releasing its multiple enzymes and proteases, which induce further inflammation and directly necrose local tissues.

DIFFERENTIAL DIAGNOSIS ▶

The picture of a chronically ill or anemic individual with respiratory tract symptoms and the more common presentation of palatal granulation tissue and ulcers is also suggestive of systemic fungal diseases such as *histoplasmosis, coccidioidomycosis,* and *blastomycosis,* as well as local fungal diseases such as *mucormycosis* and an *Aspergillus infection.* Mucormycosis and aspergillosis are usually associated with a significant immune compromise, such as uncontrolled diabetes, HIV infection, or immunosuppressive therapy. Mucormycosis will cause bone necrosis, whereas Wegener granulomatosis should not. Both fungal diseases render tissue black, mucormycosis by avascular necrosis of bone and aspergillosis by virtue of the black appearance of its organismal colonies. *Histoplasma, Coccidioides,* and *Blastomyces* species will appear in the biopsy specimen, as will *Mucor* and *Aspergillus* species. A PAS or methenamine silver stain is useful in identifying these organisms in tissue.

In addition to these infectious diseases, the more common *oral squamous cell carcinoma* should be considered in the presence of a palatal ulceration. If the granulation tissue and inflammation are submucosal with an intact surface, a *non-Hodgkin lymphoma* of the mucosal type bears consideration, as might the more rare *angiocentric T cell* and *natural killer cell lymphoma* formerly termed *midline lethal granuloma.*

DIAGNOSTIC WORK-UP ▶

Because Wegener granulomatosis produces a normochromic, normocytic anemia, leukocytosis, and thrombocytosis, a complete blood count is recommended. A chest CT scan is preferred over a plain ra-

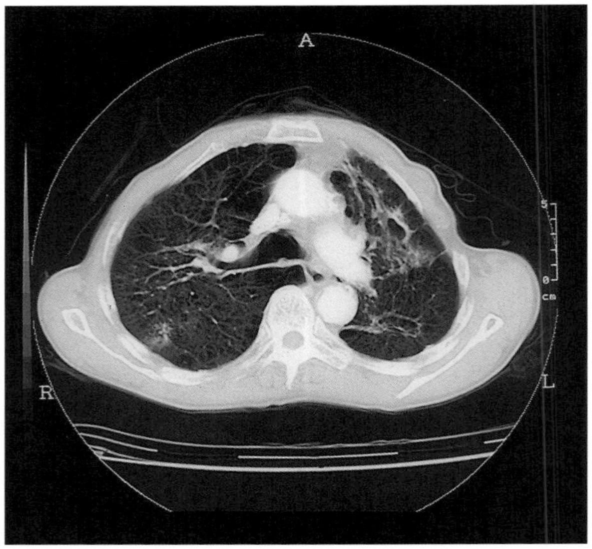

Fig 3-70 CT scan of the lungs in an individual with Wegener granulomatosis. Areas of cavitation, alveolar thickening, and fibrosis, as well as nodules, can be noted.

diograph because of the multiple patterns that may be seen, ranging from infiltrates to nodules to thickening of alveoli to large cavities (Fig 3-70). Because of the possibility of renal disease, a urinalysis and serum renal function test are indicated. The oral and maxillofacial area is also best studied with a CT scan to asses sinus, nasal, mastoid, and middle ear involvement.

A definitive diagnosis requires a biopsy, which should show an intense necrotizing vasculitis of small vessels and a positive serum ANCA determination. It is recommended to test for both cANCA and pANCA, although a positive cANCA is more closely associated with Wegener granulomatosis.

The oral biopsy offers a straightforward opportunity to make an important diagnosis. It should sample a large portion of the clinically apparent lesion. Because several fungal diseases are part of the differential diagnosis, this tissue will require cultures in Sabouraud medium for fungi, as well as both aerobic and anaerobic cultures. It is advisable to include areas that are not necrotic since the preponderance of organisms will be found at the edge of viable and necrotic tissue.

HISTOPATHOLOGY ▶

The characteristic change is a necrotizing vasculitis of small vessels, in which there is an infiltration of neutrophils, and fibrinoid necrosis (Figs 3-71a and 3-71b). This type of necrosis appears as an eosinophilic, structureless mass that stains positive for fibrin. There may be thrombosis of vessels with ulceration. The second major histologic finding is formation of necrotizing granulomas, which tend to have necrotic centers surrounded by neutrophils, lymphocytes, and plasma cells. Epithelioid cells are uncommon, but multinucleated giant cells of Langerhans and/or foreign-body type are usually prominent. These may be seen within, adjacent to, or at some distance from vessel walls (Fig 3-71c). Gingival lesions do not usually demonstrate necrotizing vasculitis, although vessel damage probably results in the inflammatory infiltrate and hemorrhages that are seen. The gingiva will often show a reactive epithelial hyperplasia, and the epithelium may be infiltrated by neutrophils. The connective tissue usually contains infiltrates of neutrophils and eosinophils with formation of microabscesses. Plasma cells and lymphocytes may also be present, and multinucleated giant cells are seen. Sometimes, however, the clinical changes are accompanied by a nonspecific inflammatory reaction.

TREATMENT AND PROGNOSIS ▶

Without treatment, Wegener granulomatosis is fatal in less than 1 year. Prompt treatment is essential to prevent involvement of the kidneys or to reverse kidney involvement to avoid renal failure, which is the most common cause of death.

The treatment of choice is cyclophosphamide (Cytoxan, Mead Johnson), 50 mg orally twice daily, combined with prednisone, 20 to 60 mg per day orally. The dosages of each are then adjusted to prevent recurrence at the lowest dose. Once the disease is under control, oral methotrexate, 25 mg per week,

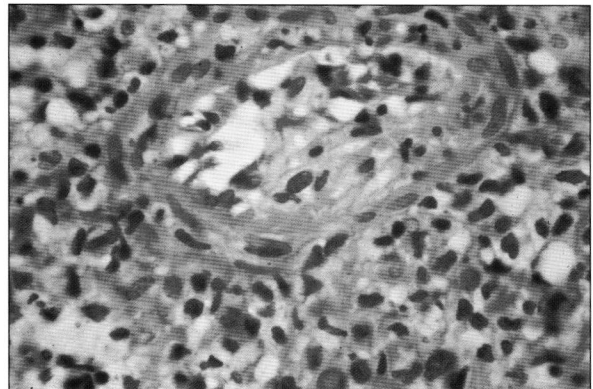

Fig 3-71a Wegener granulomatosis of the palate showing a necrotizing vasculitis with a fibrinous thickening and inflammation.

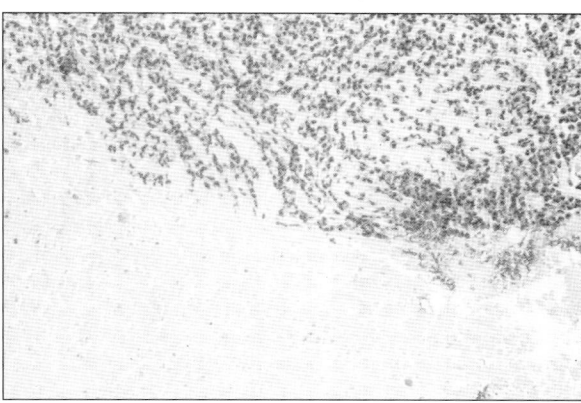

Fig 3-71b The lesion produced extensive fibrinoid necrosis.

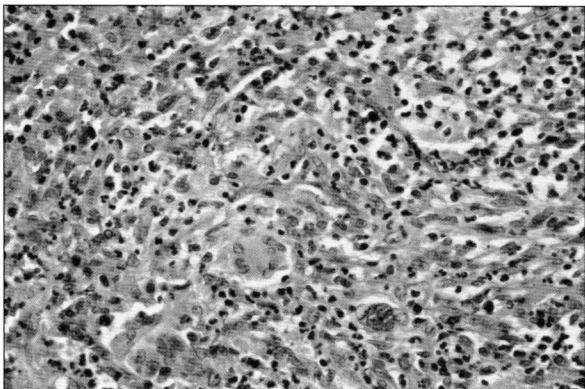

Fig 3-71c A granulomatous response with some multinucleated giant cells.

is a reasonable substitute for cyclophosphamide to maintain a remission. In addition, the antibiotic trimethoprim sulfamethoxazole (Bactrim, Roche) can also maintain a remission and allow for a discontinuance of cyclophosphamide and prednisone. Methotrexate and trimethoprim sulfamethoxazole are both folate antagonists, which may explain their effectiveness and should alert the clinician to avoid folate dietary supplementation as well as to watch for signs of marrow suppression and anemia.

The prognosis is good with treatment. However, delayed treatment or severe disease may result in death. Most patients experience long-term remissions. Some require repeated treatments or ongoing maintenance therapy. The cANCA levels do not correlate well with disease activity and are not recommended for planning changes in treatment.

Giant Cell Arteritis

Giant cell arteritis is a serious inflammatory disease of medium- and large-sized arteries. It occurs in nearly all vessels of that caliber but is most frequent in the branches of the external carotid system. In fact, the disease was once called *temporal arteritis* because it was most readily visible in the temporal artery and seemed to explain the frequent complaint of headache (Fig 3-72). About 50% of patients with giant cell arteritis also have polymyalgia rheumatica, which causes inflammatory-based pain in the shoulder and pelvic regions. These diseases share predisposed HLA antigens and a similar age range of 50 years and older, and they frequently coexist. However, giant cell arteritis either alone or with polymyalgia rheumatica is a more serious condition because of its high risk for blindness.

CLINICAL PRESENTATION ▶ The individual will be older than 50 years and may complain of headache, scalp tenderness, twitching of the masseter reported as "jaw spasms," and throat pain. A few may complain of visual disturbances, which should be treated as a serious sign and a prelude to possible ischemic optic neuropathy and blindness. Although the temporal artery may be tender and even nodular, it may also be normal. Fever is a frequent presenting sign. In fact, giant cell arteritis reportedly accounts for 15% of fevers of unknown origin in people older than 65 years. More advanced cases may have asymmetry of their radial pulses, a murmur indicating aortic regurgitation, and subclavian artery bruits caused by stenosis in that vessel.

DIFFERENTIAL DIAGNOSIS ▶ Giant cell arteritis, the symptoms of which may be subtle, may mimic *myofascial pain dysfunction* from occlusal abnormalities or bruxism. If scalp tenderness and muscle pain are prominent, *polymyositis* may be suggested. If fever and anemia are present, a *non-Hodgkin lymphoma* or *multiple myeloma*, or even a *septicemia from bacterial endocarditis*, are possibilities.

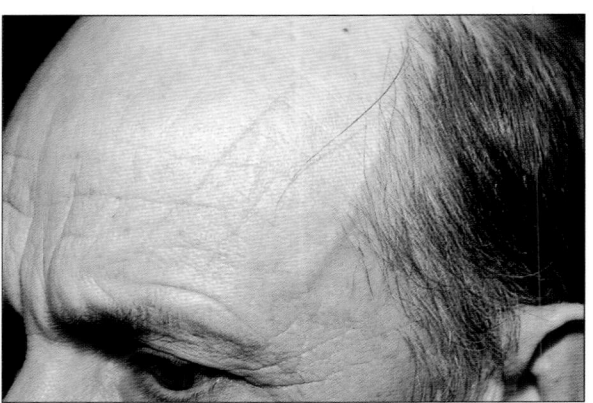

Fig 3-72 The temporal arteries are readily visible and prominent in an individual with giant cell arteritis. They are also tender or even painful to palpation.

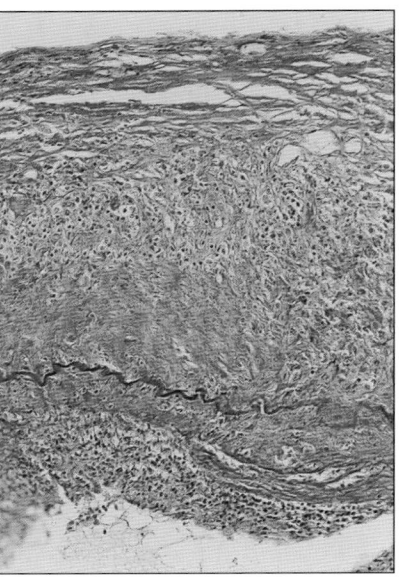

Fig 3-73 Giant cell arteritis shows degeneration of the internal elastic membrane with an inflammatory infiltrate and giant cells.

DIAGNOSTIC WORK-UP ▶ Although the diagnosis may be established with a temporal artery biopsy, this procedure is generally unnecessary and will eliminate an important physical diagnostic sign, which correlates with treatment response. Once diagnosed, the pain and edema of the temporal arteries will diminish with effective treatment. When a unilateral temporal artery biopsy is taken, it is positive in 80% to 85% of cases. However, the biopsy must include a 4- to 5-cm length of the temporal artery for an assured diagnosis. Because giant cell arteritis is segmental along the course of each vessel, a small portion of the artery may be nondiagnostic.

Consistent with the diagnosis of giant cell arteritis is a high erythrocyte sedimentation rate (ESR). Whether fever is present or not, the white blood cell count is normal. This will distinguish giant cell arteritis from some infectious diseases. A normochromic, normocytic anemia is almost always present. The findings of anemia and an elevated ESR coupled with the clinical findings of an enlarged and tender superficial temporal artery establish the diagnosis.

HISTOPATHOLOGY ▶ The involved artery shows a nodular thickening. The lumen is compromised and may be thrombosed. Essentially, there is a granulomatous inflammation of the media and intima, consisting of macrophages, lymphocytes, and plasma cells. Eosinophils and neutrophils are variably present and concentrate in the area of the internal elastic lamina, which undergoes degeneration with swelling and fragmentation (Fig 3-73). Portions of the elastic lamina may be found within giant cells. Subsequently, there is intimal thickening and fibrosis of the media. Distribution of these lesions is patchy within the artery so that it is not uncommon for biopsies to be nondiagnostic.

TREATMENT AND PROGNOSIS ▶ Prevention of blindness, which is irreversible, is the goal of treatment. Blindness does not result from the temporal artery disease, but from occlusion of the posterior ciliary branch of the ophthalmic artery, underscoring the involvement of all medium to large arteries, even those branches of the internal carotid system.

The treatment is oral prednisone, 60 mg per day. Prednisone therapy is recommended in almost all cases, and the prompt use of it may prevent blindness. In addition, a reduction in symptoms within 72 hours strongly supports the diagnosis of a giant cell arteritis.

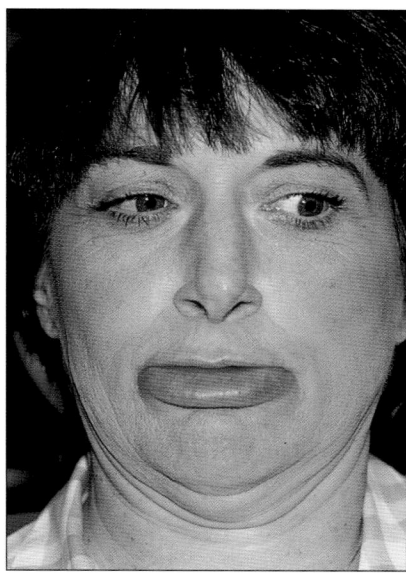

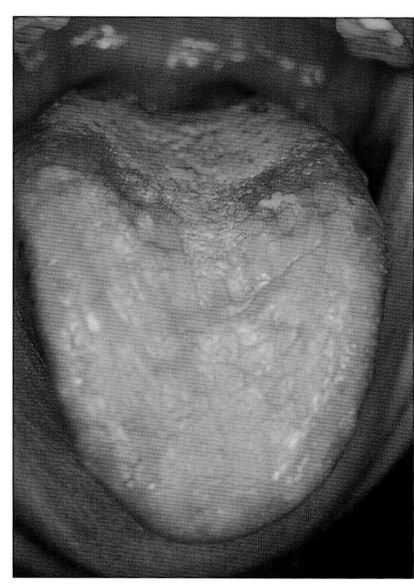

Fig 3-74a Melkersson-Rosenthal syndrome with lip edema and left facial nerve paresis.

Fig 3-74b Prominently fissured tongue associated with Melkersson-Rosenthal syndrome in the patient shown in Fig 3-74a.

Prednisone should be continued at 60 mg per day for 1 to 2 months before tapering. The clinical symptoms are more reliable than the ESR in the decision to start tapering the prednisone, although the ESR does decrease with therapy. Recurrence can occur, necessitating reinstitution of prednisone at the same dose as used initially. In such cases, a more gradual tapering schedule is recommended. Some refractory cases may be active for several years and require prednisone at adjusted dosages throughout that time.

Melkersson-Rosenthal Syndrome

CLINICAL PRESENTATION AND
PATHOGENESIS ▶

Melkersson-Rosenthal syndrome is a clinical symptom complex consisting of chronic lip and facial edema (Fig 3-74a), fissured tongue (Fig 3-74b), and intermittent unilateral or bilateral facial nerve palsy. Its etiology remains completely unknown. Although some cases have revealed an inheritance pattern, most have no identifiable inheritance. This author (REM) has seen two cases that have responded to a gluten-free diet, implying a hypersensitivity reaction, yet such a cause remains unproven.

The syndrome usually presents with only one or two of the three components of the classic triad. In one study, 39% had all three components, 57% had two of the three, and 4% had only one component.

The onset of the lip and facial edema is sudden and usually precedes the facial paralysis. The facial paralysis may occur simultaneously with the lip edema, or it may follow weeks to months later or not occur at all. The syndrome usually begins in childhood, the teenage years, or the early 20s. The lip edema can be extreme and may increase the lip to three to four times its normal size. The lip edema is expected to be permanent.

Facial palsy, which develops in only about 20% of cases, may be complete or incomplete and may be unilateral or bilateral. It may also resolve slowly only to recur again. When it does occur, this component slowly recovers and returns to normal.

The fissured, or *scrotal* tongue is characterized by deep furrows that do not interfere with function and cause only a slight alteration of taste in some of those affected. About 40% of patients develop this component, which is also present in 1% to 3% of the normal population. Sometimes the buccal mucosa also is fissured with deep furrows separated by smooth rounded margins, giving it the appearance of palatal rugae. The fissured tongue is expected to be permanent.

DIFFERENTIAL DIAGNOSIS ▶

The differential diagnosis will vary depending on which and how many of the three components are present at the time of presentation and to what degree. In the rare instance when a facial paralysis is not accompanied by any other component of the syndrome, a *viral Bell's palsy* or an early case of *Ramsay Hunt syndrome* may be expected. In the more usual presentation of a lip edema accompanied by some facial edema, *angioneurotic edema* might be suspected, as would *cheilitis granulomatosis, multiple endocrine neoplasia syndrome type III*, or *Hughes syndrome*, which is an autosomal dominant trait that produces features of acromegaly but begins with prominent thickening of the lips.

DIAGNOSTIC WORK-UP ▶

Like many other syndromes, Melkersson-Rosenthal syndrome is diagnosed mainly on the basis of clinical recognition. A biopsy of the lip edema is often useful, however, if it includes some of the minor salivary glands in the lip. The salivary glands are expected to show sarcoid-like granulomas and thus may suggest cheilitis granulomatosa unless one other component of the syndrome is present.

HISTOPATHOLOGY ▶

The lamina propria is edematous with dilation of lymphatics and a lymphocytic infiltrate. Noncaseating granulomas similar to those seen in Crohn disease and sarcoidosis may be present. As in Crohn disease, the epithelioid cells, multinucleated giant cells, and lymphocytes may not be compactly arranged.

TREATMENT AND PROGNOSIS ▶

The facial palsy component spontaneously resolves, while the fissured tongue and lip edema are usually permanent. However, a strict gluten-free diet is a worthwhile recommendation, particularly since no other therapy has been known to improve this syndrome. Gluten is a storage protein that is present in wheat, barley, oats, and rye, but not in corn or rice. In the susceptible host, gluten is known to incite humoral and cellular immune responses, known as *sprue*, in the gastrointestinal mucosa.

The lips may be separately treated with either intralesional steroids using a 10 mg/mL concentration of triamcinolone in 1% xylocaine and injecting 2 to 5 mL in each lip every month, or by systemic prednisone using systemic corticosteroid regimen 1 (see page 205), or by cheiloplasty surgery. The surgery would excise a portion of the lower lip labial mucosa from one commissure to the other and some of the contents of the submucosal compartment and is reserved for severe cases. Recurrence after either type of steroid therapy or surgery is common.

Systemic Corticosteroid Therapy

Systemic corticosteroids are the most predictable medications used to control autoimmune diseases and certain immune-based inflammatory diseases. Most of these diseases are incurable; the goal of therapy is a drug-induced remission, a point the clinician is well advised to discuss with each patient. It is hoped that a drug-induced remission can be long term and in some cases permanent in a drug-free state.

The drug of choice is prednisone, an anti-inflammatory glucocorticoid that affects mostly the cellular phase of inflammation, lymphocytes in particular. (This is one of the reasons prednisone is part of nearly every chemotherapy protocol for lymphoma.) Dexamethasone (Decadron, Merck), while more potent, affects mostly the exudative phase of inflammation by stabilizing cell membranes. It, therefore, remains an excellent drug for reducing surgical inflammation (mostly edema fluid) but is limited in reducing T-lymphocyte elaboration of lymphokines or B-lymphocyte production of antibodies, which mediate most immune-based diseases. Therefore, prednisone remains the corticosteroid drug of choice for immune-based diseases.

There are three clinically effective prednisone regimens. The choice of prednisone regimen is the clinician's decision to make and should be based on the specific diagnosis, the intensity of the disease, and the organ systems involved.

Systemic Corticosteroid Regimen I

This regimen begins with prednisone, 100 to 120 mg per day by mouth (1.5 mg/kg per day) for 2 weeks. A tapering schedule reduces prednisone by 20 mg per day each week over several weeks until a dose of 20 mg per day is reached. This dose is continued for 1 month, followed by 10 mg per day for 3 months. The dose is then reduced to 10 mg every other day for another 3 months, followed by 5 mg every other day for 6 months. After 6 months of a 5-mg dose of prednisone every other day, the drug may be discontinued with a high possibility of an extended remission in a drug-free state.

The rationale for this approach is to gain a rapid suppression of disease activity with a high loading dose and to taper this dose rapidly enough to avoid most of the more serious side effects of high-dose prednisone. The 20-mg-per-day dose is significant because at that dose or below, side effects are significantly reduced. The tapered dose is extended in length with each decrease in dose to prevent an exacerbation at the time of dose reduction or after drug discontinuation. The every-other-day dose is designed to permit the hypophyseal-adrenal cortical axis to regain its function. The 5-mg, every-other-day dose is called a "maintenance dose" because 5-mg of prednisone equals the daily 20 mg of cortisol the adrenal cortex produces in an unstressed individual, and the every-other-day use continues to allow the adrenal cortex to regain activity.

This regimen is the preferred regimen because it facilitates a long-term remission and has reduced side effects. It is indicated for most oral lesions associated with pemphigus vulgaris, erosive lichen planus, and severe nonocular pemphigoid. It is very effective but requires close attention by the clinician and absolute compliance by the patient.

Systemic Corticosteroid Regimen II

This regimen begins with prednisone, 100 to 120 mg per day by mouth (1.5 mg/kg per day), for a period of 2 weeks, at which time the drug is abruptly discontinued. The rationale for this approach is to gain rapid suppression of disease activity and then discontinue the drug before side effects develop or significant adrenal suppression occurs. This approach is effective and much more straightforward than systemic corticosteroid regimen I. Its drawback is that exacerbations are more frequent, and the disease process is less controlled.

This regimen also is indicated in pemphigus vulgaris, erosive lichen planus, and severe nonocular pemphigoid. It is the preferred regimen in the Stevens-Johnson form of erythema multiforme.

Systemic Corticosteroid Regimen IIIA

This regimen begins with prednisone, 100 to 120 mg per day by mouth for 2 weeks. A tapering schedule reduces prednisone by 20 mg per day each week until the lowest possible prednisone level is reached without exacerbating the disease. Many individuals remain on 20 mg per day or even higher doses for long periods because lesser dosages are associated with disease exacerbations.

This approach is suited to those cases with disease intensity and organ involvement that lower doses of prednisone cannot control. It is usually applied to resistant pemphigus cases and selected cases of systemic lupus erythematosus or sarcoidosis. These patients require lifelong dosage adjustments and follow-up. They also develop many of the late complications of ongoing corticosteroid therapy (Table 3-4).

Systemic Corticosteroid Regimen IIIB

This regimen begins with prednisone, 100 to 120 mg per day by mouth for 2 weeks. A tapering schedule reduces prednisone by 20 mg per day each week until a prednisone level is reached at which the disease is exacerbated. This level and slightly higher levels of prednisone may still be associated with dis-

Table 3-4 Short-term and long-term side effects of systemic corticosteroid therapy

Short-term effects	Long-term effects
Sodium and water retention	Muscle wasting/fat deposits
Hypertension	Delayed wound healing
Hypernatremia/hypokalemia	Osteoporosis
Hyperglycemia	Cataracts
Infections (candidiasis, *Pneumocystis carinii* infection)	
Mood changes	
Increased risk for peptic ulcer disease	

ease activity. Cyclophosphamide (Cytoxan, Mead Johnson), 50 to 100 mg twice daily by mouth; azathioprine (Imuran, GlaxoSmithKline), 50 to 100 mg twice daily by mouth; and methotrexate, 25 to 50 mg per week, individually or in combinations, is then added to the prednisone therapy.

The rationale for this approach is to affect the disease with double-drug therapy so that the dosage and, therefore, the side effects of each can be reduced. This approach is reserved for refractory cases and for patients in whom corticosteroid complications pose a greater risk, such as those with diabetes, a history of tuberculosis, peptic ulcer disease, osteoporosis (in women), and cataracts. It is also strongly recommended as a regimen for ocular pemphigoid.

Corticosteroid Side Effects and Complications

Systemic corticosteroids have short-term and long-term side effects. Both are related to the basic physiologic effect of mixed glucocorticoid mineralocorticoid drugs, which also include membrane effects, the end result of which is sodium retention and potassium loss. With the sodium retention comes water gain and, consequently, weight gain. In addition, the effect of the sodium depletion on the brain may affect mood: Swings in mood from euphoria to depression are the types of mood changes observed. The glucocorticoid portion causes gluconeogenesis at the expense of protein synthesis and fat stores. Therefore, in the short term, hyperglycemia is noted and in the longer term defective wound healing, muscle wasting, osteoporosis, and cataract formation are seen.

The classic fat deposits and "buffalo hump" seen in long-term corticosteroid use and in hyperadrenocorticism (Cushing disease) are also related to gluconeogenesis. The complex mechanism is one in which the breakdown and re-formation of triglycerides in fat stores is dependent on fresh glycerol derived from glucose. The reuse of glycerol from the breakdown of triglycerides is not possible. Therefore, the availability of glycerol from abundant glucose via gluconeogenesis will drive the equilibrium toward triglyceride re-formation, causing the development of fat deposits. The short-term anti-inflammatory effects inhibit leukocyte chemotaxis and migration as well as the ability of leukocytes to phagocytose and digest organisms. Therefore, colonization of *Candida* species becomes common and frequently leads to a true invasive candidiasis. Other, longer-term opportunistic infections may be seen, particularly *Pneumocystis carinii*. The long-term anti-inflammatory effects will cause involution of lymph nodes and reductions in lymphocytes, which is part of the goal of autoimmune disease control, but in general predisposes the patient to a variety of other infectious disease states. Their inhibitory effects on prostaglandin synthesis also predispose the gastric mucosa to injury, thereby increasing slightly the risk for peptic ulcer disease.

Conditions of Developmental Disturbances

CHAPTER 4

▶ "Disease is life under abnormal conditions."
—*Perez Tamayo*

Persistent Lingual Thyroid Gland

CLINICAL PRESENTATION ▶

A persistent lingual thyroid gland is usually an incidental finding in a child younger than 10 years of age. Occasionally, it may be brought to the attention of parents or the child by persistent gagging due to its size or to bleeding. The persistent lingual thyroid will be located at or posterior to the foramen cecum in the midline or paramidline of the tongue. The tongue will require anterior traction for ideal visualization of a lingual thyroid, which will appear as a soft, fleshy, painless mass with a thin but usually intact mucosa (Fig 4-1a).

DIFFERENTIAL DIAGNOSIS ▶

A mass in the posterior one third of the tongue in a child or young adult should include a persistent lingual thyroid in the differential because when this rare entity is confirmed, it is almost always the only thyroid tissue the child has. Other entities that can produce a soft, fleshy mass in this location of the tongue are *hemangioma, lymphangioma*, and *a mucous retention phenomenon* from the glands of von Ebner around the base of the circumvallate papillae. In addition, the clinician should also be concerned about a *rhabdomyosarcoma* in this location in a child. Rarely, a *thyroglossal tract cyst* rather than an entire persistent gland will occur in the tongue rather than the neck, but these generally occur later in life.

DIAGNOSTIC WORK-UP ▶

Biopsy should not be performed until a persistent lingual thyroid is ruled out. Removal of even a seemingly small portion of a persistent lingual thyroid could result in hypothyroidism. An ^{131}I radionucleotide scan is the diagnostic test of choice. The radioactive iodine will be selectively taken up by thyroid tissue and will reveal whether the lingual mass is indeed thyroid and if other thyroid tissue is present at the laryngeal level (Fig 4-1b).

HISTOPATHOLOGY ▶

Persistent lingual thyroid glands typically consist of normal thyroid tissue, that is, follicles lined by cuboidal to squamous epithelium with eosinophilic colloid in the lumen (Fig 4-2). This tissue also has the potential to undergo pathologic change (eg, goiter, adenomas, or adenocarcinomas), which, however, is very uncommon.

TREATMENT ▶

Most persistent lingual thyroid glands do not require specific treatment. They do require a discussion with and education of the parents as well as thyroid function tests to determine the functional status of the persistent gland. Parents must be informed that the thyroid is related to the growth and development of the child. They should be alerted to the fact that the persistent lingual thyroid may hypertrophy and produce some gagging and may even bleed at times. They should be cautioned not to have it removed or cauterized if some bleeding does occur. In cases where the gland produces recurrent bleeding or significant gagging or even obstructs the airway, it may be transplanted into the neck or within a muscle anywhere in the body. Because the thyroid is an endocrine gland, which, by definition, secretes hormone directly into the bloodstream, it can be transplanted to a vascular site with every expectation of full function.

PROGNOSIS ▶

Persistent lingual thyroid glands remain permanently functional as a rule. In rare cases of a hypothyroid state, replacement therapy with sodium levothyroxine (Synthroid, Knoll) at sufficient doses to

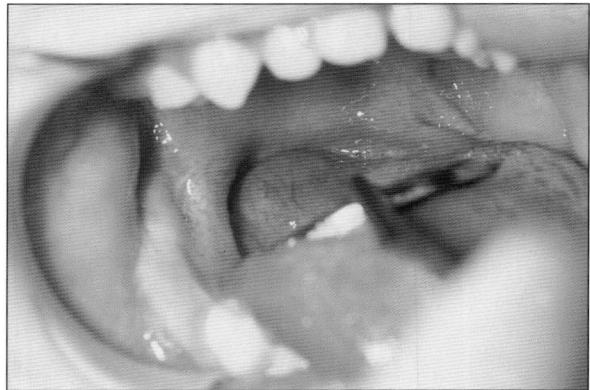

Fig 4-1a Persistent lingual thyroid mass at midline of posterior tongue in a 5-year-old. Note thin intact mucosa and vascularity.

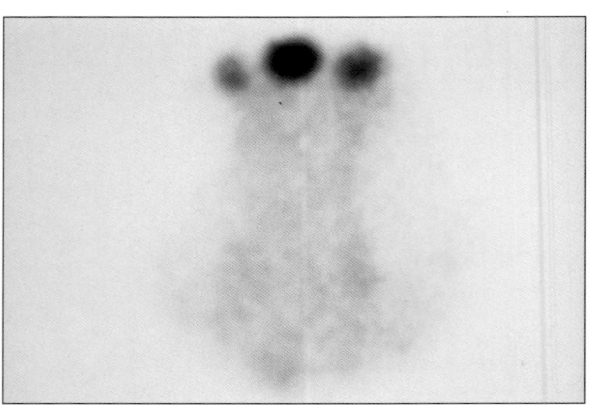

Fig 4-1b ^{131}I radionucleotide scan showing mass of persistent lingual thyroid in midline and no uptake in neck (absent thyroid).

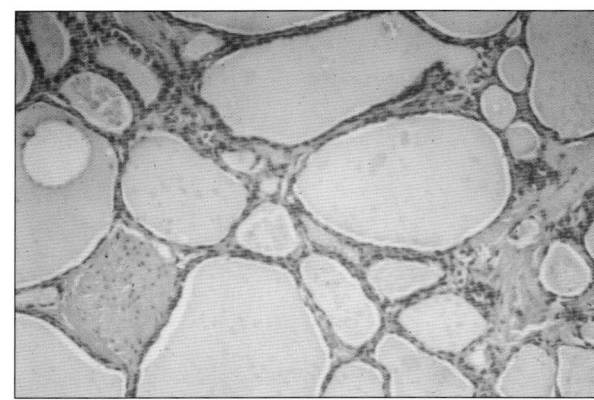

Fig 4-2 Tissue from a lingual thyroid showing follicles containing colloid and lined by normal-appearing thyroid glandular epithelium.

gain a euthyroid state is required. In all cases, annual follow-up, including thyroid function tests, is advised. Because the thyroid arises from the third branchial pouch and the parathyroid glands from the fourth branchial pouch, the parathyroids are not in this condition.

Osteoporotic Bone Marrow Defects

CLINICAL PRESENTATION AND PATHOGENESIS ▶

An osteoporotic bone marrow defect is, paradoxically, both an uncommon and a common entity in that it is common but rarely of sufficient size to be seen on the usual dental periapical or panoramic radiograph and therefore is uncommonly diagnosed. Since the marrow compartment does not normally contribute significantly to the radiographic density of a mandible or maxilla, a marrow defect within it is not expected to be noticed. However, most postmenopausal women and many men of advanced age have some degree of osteoporosis. Such defects, though not easily seen on a plain radiograph, today can be seen on a computed tomography (CT) scan and are now more frequently noted.

Nearly all studies concerning osteoporotic bone marrow defects report at least a 70% predilection in postmenopausal women, underscoring the fact that this entity is an asymptomatic hormonal and age-related systemic effect on bone that is recognized in the jaws. The reader should note that the unfortunate term used to describe a condition referred to as neuralgia-inducing cavitational osteonecrosis (NICO) is actually an osteoporotic bone marrow defect in someone who reports pain from an unrelated etiology, usually a deafferentation neuropathy from local nerve damage. This purported but nonexistent entity (see Chapter 20) also has its highest incidence (over 80%) in postmenopausal women.

RADIOGRAPHIC PRESENTATION ▶

On plain radiographs, an osteoporotic bone marrow defect will appear as a faint or more obvious radiolucency usually with an indistinct margin (Fig 4-3). While it is most commonly seen in the posterior body region of the mandible, it can affect any location within the mandible or maxilla, including the ramus and condyle. On a CT scan it will appear as an absence of trabecular bone in the marrow space. It will lack expansion and may exhibit a slight thinning or resorptive remodeling of the medullary surface of the cortex. When this occurs it is likely to be seen on plain radiographs as well.

DIFFERENTIAL DIAGNOSIS ▶

A nonexpansile radiolucency in the mandible may appear to be a *dental abscess* or a *radicular cyst*. Since the patient is most likely to be older than 40 years, an idiopathic bone cavity would not be a serious consideration, but a *metastatic malignancy* or a *primary malignancy* in the jaws would. In addition, numerous other radiolucent lesions may be considered depending on the size, shape, location, and association with tooth structures. Some of the more likely ones would be an *osteomyelitis*, some *odontogenic tumors*, and an *odontogenic keratocyst*.

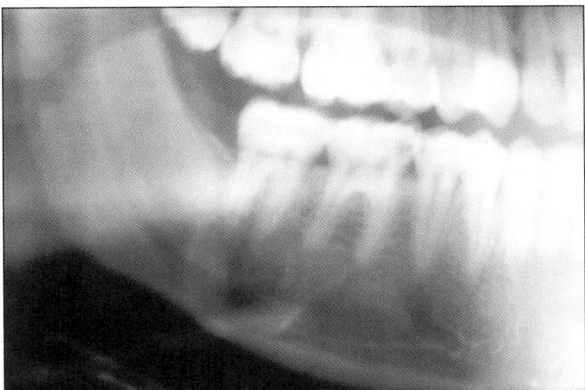

Fig 4-3 Unilocular radiolucency in the posterior mandible, which, when explored, revealed an asymptomatic cavity containing fibrofatty marrow.

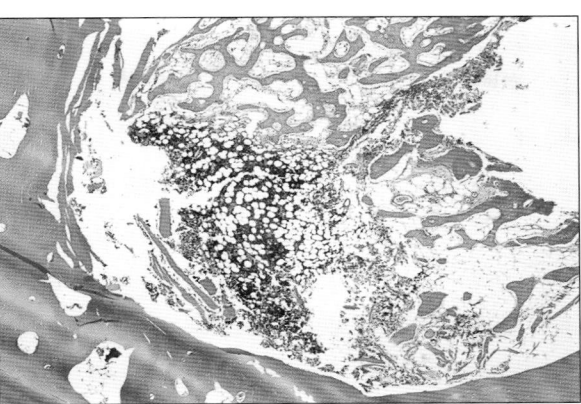

Fig 4-4a Asymptomatic osteoporotic bone marrow defect. Normal marrow cells and reactive new bone formation is evident.

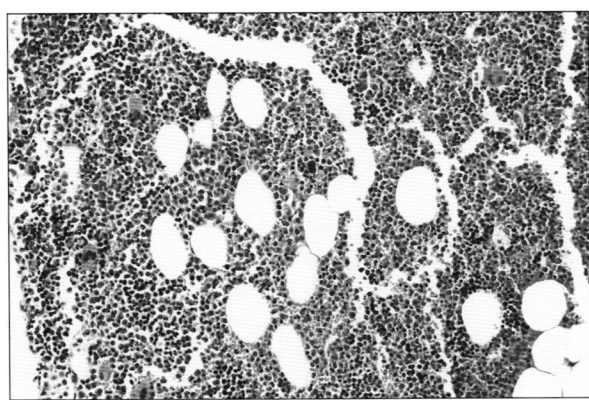

Fig 4-4b High-power view of an osteoporotic bone marrow defect showing megakaryocytes and normal red blood cell and white blood cell precursors.

HISTOPATHOLOGY ▶

Osteoporotic bone marrow defects will appear as empty spaces in bone that may actually contain clusters of identifiable bone marrow cells such as thrombocytes, promyelocytes, normoblasts, metamyelocytes, or other red blood cell and white blood cell precursors (Figs 4-4a and 4-4b), or it may contain fatty marrow. The older the patient, the more likely the defect will contain a preponderance of fibrofatty tissue.

TREATMENT AND PROGNOSIS ▶

No treatment is required. However, for those defects initially identified on a panoramic radiograph, a CT scan is recommended to rule out primary or metastatic malignancies as well as the other possibilities noted on the differential diagnosis. For those cases in which a CT scan cannot be accomplished or where uncertainty remains, these significant differential diagnostic considerations indicate the need for an exploration and biopsy.

Lingual Salivary Gland Depressions

CLINICAL PRESENTATION ▶

Lingual salivary gland depressions may be located in either the submandibular or the sublingual gland area. They have no real clinical presentation other than a radiographic presence. They are innocuous convexities in the lingual cortex of the mandible that would be of no consequence if they did not produce a radiolucency in jaw radiographs that may be difficult to distinguish from more serious conditions, such as cysts and benign or even malignant tumors. Radiographic diagnoses of tumors or cysts have been made, resulting in unnecessary surgery and removal of bone.

RADIOGRAPHIC FINDINGS ▶

Depressions of the submandibular gland will usually create a well-demarcated radiolucency in the posterior mandibular body below the mandibular canal outline (Fig 4-5). Such radiographic pictures in the past have been termed *Staphne's bone cysts*, an obvious misnomer and misleading term. However, not all submandibular salivary gland depressions will be well demarcated with a seemingly sclerotic border. Rare depressions will be more irregular in their borders and truly suggest a neoplastic process.

Depressions of the sublingual gland will appear ovoid (longest dimension in the horizontal plane) or round radiolucencies that are well demarcated but do not have a sclerotic border (Fig 4-6). These are more diagnostically troublesome than the submandibular gland depressions because they are less common and, therefore, more often overlooked. Additionally, the radiolucencies are superimposed over the root apices of the anterior teeth and, therefore, strongly mimic a periapical granuloma or a radicular cyst.

DIFFERENTIAL DIAGNOSIS ▶

Depressions producing a radiolucency in the posterior mandibular body may suggest an *odontogenic keratocyst*; an odontogenic tumor such as an *ameloblastoma* or a *myxoma*; an *idiopathic bone cavity*; *metastases from breast or lung*; or *multiple myeloma*.

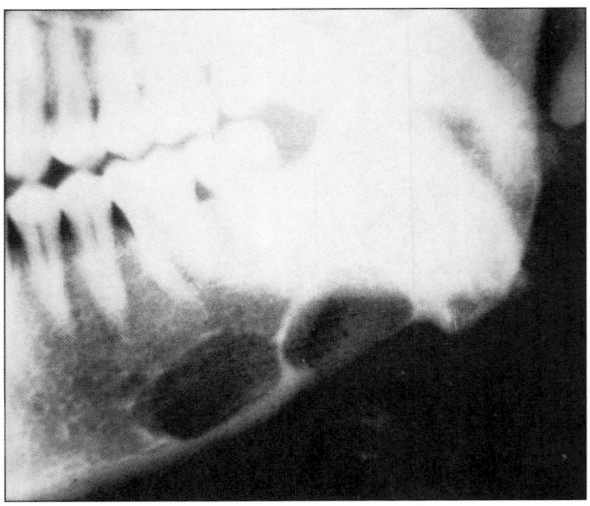

Fig 4-5 Lingual salivary gland depressions from the submandibular gland. Note well-demarcated borders and even resorption of the inferior border.

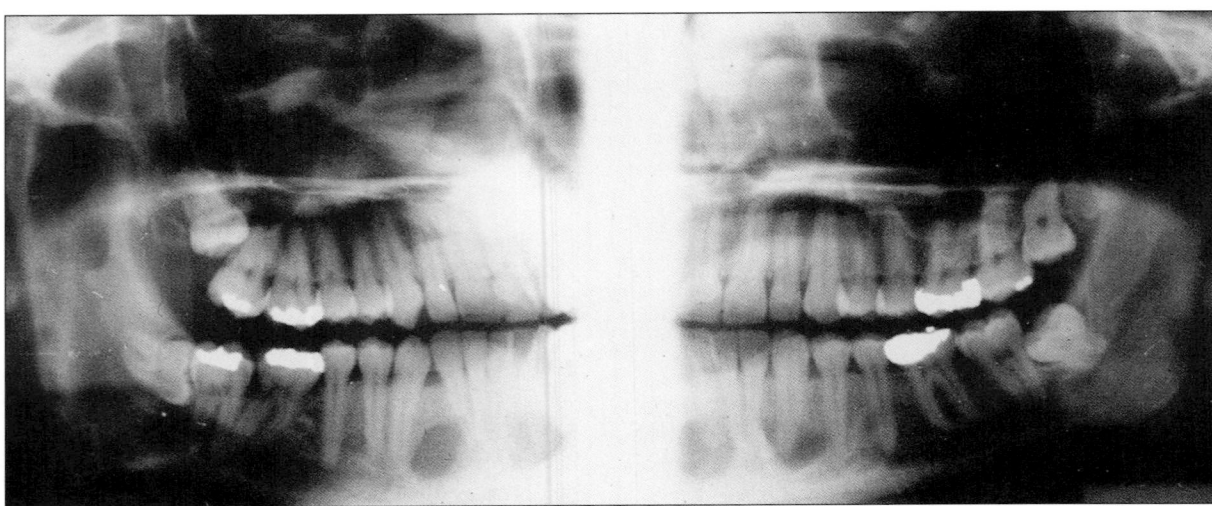

Fig 4-6 Bilateral sublingual gland depressions mimicking several different odontogenic pathologies.

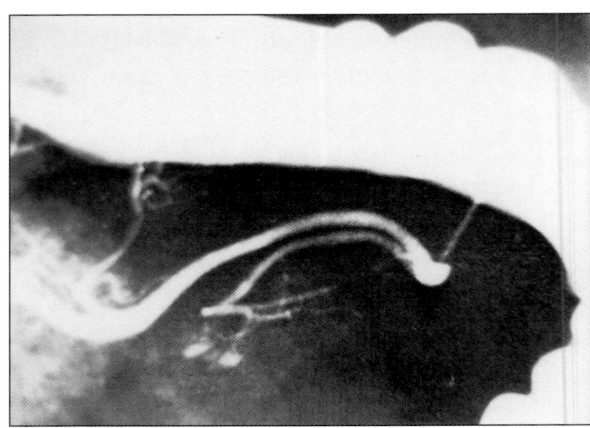

Fig 4-7 Occlusal sialogram showing ducts to both a submandibular and a sublingual gland depression.

Depressions arising from the sublingual gland and thus appearing in the anterior mandible are less likely to be suggestive of metastasis but may suggest a *keratocyst,* an *odontogenic tumor,* or an *idiopathic bone cavity*. If superimposed over a tooth root, a *periapical granuloma* and/or a *radicular cyst* are the most serious considerations.

DIAGNOSTIC WORK-UP ▶ Lingual salivary gland depressions that produce a characteristic radiographic pattern and show no signs or symptoms of other pathology may be diagnosed by evaluation of the discovering radiograph. Pulp testing should be performed to rule out inflammatory dental disease, and a right-angled (eg, occlusal) radiograph should be taken to rule out expansion.

The most direct way to confirm a lingual salivary gland depression is with CT scan sialography or plain CT scan with contrast. A CT scan sialography is accomplished by injecting 0.5 mL of a water-soluble radiographic dye into the submandibular duct followed by CT scanning using 1-mm cuts. If the dye cannula is introduced only 2 to 3 mm into the submandibular duct, it will often fill accessory ducts (Bartholin ducts) adjoining it to the sublingual gland, thereby filling the sublingual gland as well (Fig 4-7). The position of the glands in relation to the lingual cortex can then be examined. If a CT sialography cannot be accomplished, a venous injection CT scan with contrast will usually show the relationship of both glands to the lingual cortex and thus confirm the diagnosis.

HISTOPATHOLOGY ▶ No histopathology should be required.

TREATMENT ▶ No treatment is indicated.

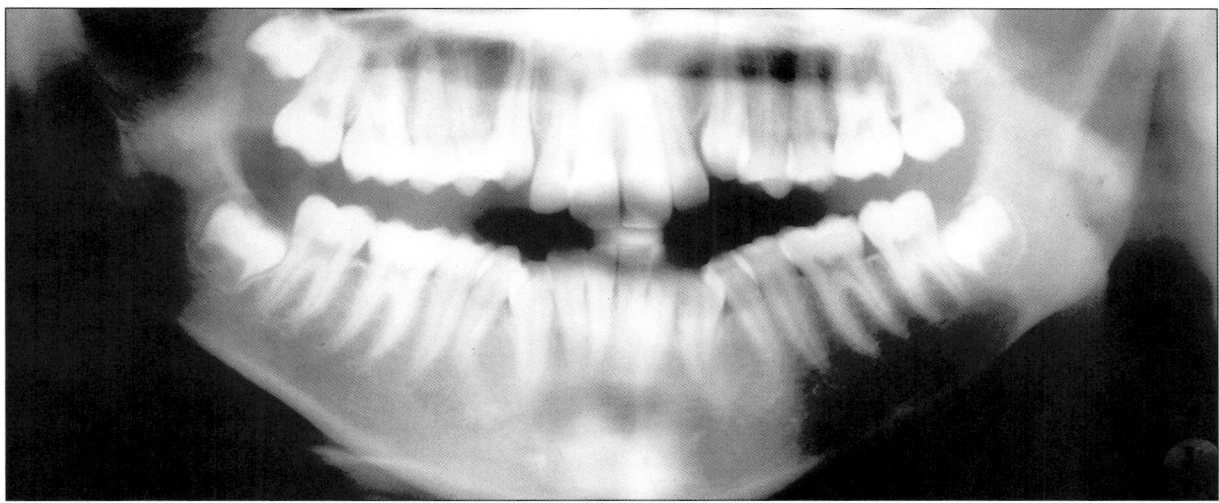

Fig 4-8a The most common radiographic appearance of an idiopathic bone cavity is a radiolucency in the body region of the mandible that scallops between teeth and thins the inferior border but does not displace tooth roots or the mandibular canal.

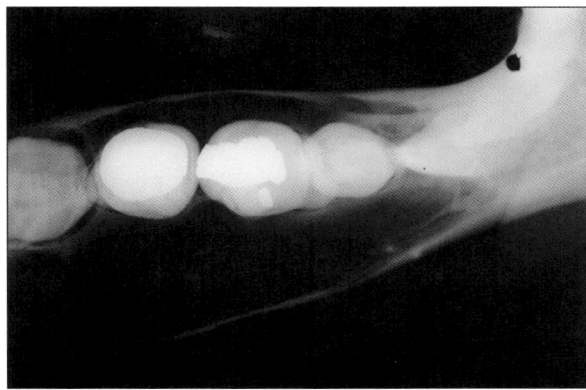

Fig 4-8b Idiopathic bone cavity with slight expansion and thinned buccal cortex.

Idiopathic Bone Cavities

CLINICAL PRESENTATION AND PATHOGENESIS ▶

Idiopathic bone cavities are empty cavities in bone that have an unknown cause. They have erroneously been called "traumatic bone cysts" for many years. However, they lack an epithelial lining required of a cyst and are not specifically related to trauma (see Chapter 20). Most idiopathic bone cavities in the jaws occur in the mandible; only a very few have occurred in the maxilla. Long bones, especially the humerus, also have some incidence of idiopathic bone cavities. Most are discovered as an incidental finding on radiographs in individuals who are usually in their late teens or early 20s. Few if any idiopathic bone cavities occur in individuals older than 40 years.

The most common location in the jaws is in the body of the mandible, although some have occurred in the symphysis, ramus, and even the condyle. There is often mild expansion, and the cortices are thinned but not perforated (Fig 4-8a). Associated teeth are vital, and no change in sensory nerve function is noted. Rare cases have occurred bilaterally.

The pathogenic mechanism of idiopathic bone cavities is truly unknown. The previous belief in a traumatic etiology has no scientific basis. Individuals in high-trauma professions, such as boxers and martial arts instructors, do not have a higher incidence of idiopathic bone cavities, and none has been produced in laboratory animals after trauma. Indeed, trauma centers do not see idiopathic bone cavities after facial trauma with or without mandibular fractures in any greater frequency than that in the general population. Those studies that have suggested an association with trauma are invalid because of inadequate controls (nearly all young adults will identify some type of minor trauma to their jaws). It seems more likely that idiopathic bone cavities represent a disturbance in the remodeling of trabecular bone related to biochemical or hormonal changes during the peak incidence of the teen years.

RADIOGRAPHIC FINDINGS ▶

The classic description of an idiopathic bone cavity in the jaws is a radiolucent lesion that scallops between teeth into the interradicular bone (see Fig 4-8a). Because the cavity does not expand from a central point in the jaws but instead resorbs bone without prominent expansion, tooth roots, teeth, and the mandibular canal are not displaced. A panoramic radiograph at a reduced kilovoltage may be used to highlight the bony walls of the mandibular canal. In an idiopathic bone cavity, the canal outline is seen to course through the radiolucency instead of being displaced by it.

Right-angle radiographs, such as occlusal radiographs and axial CT scans, will show the thinned but unperforated cortices (Fig 4-8b). Because idiopathic bone cavities are not static and may be radiographed

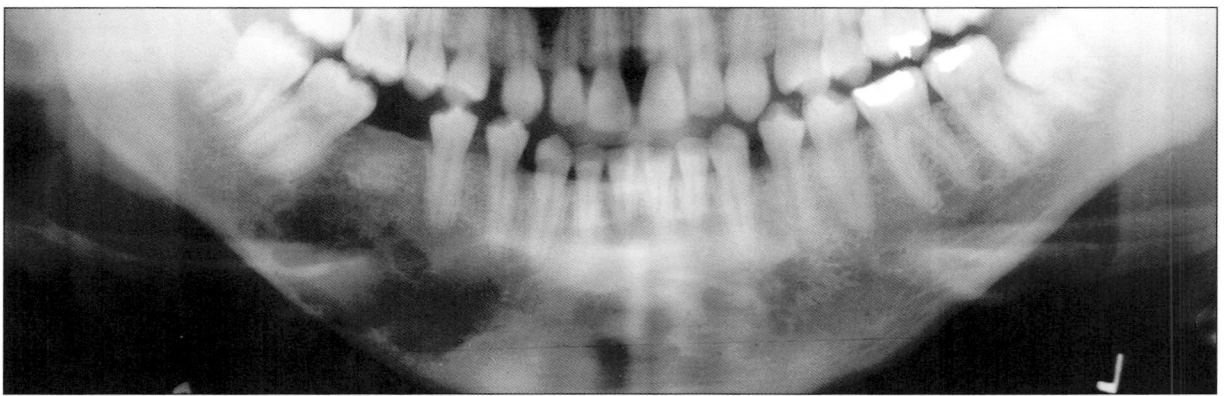

Fig 4-9 Idiopathic bone cavities sometimes partially fill in or appear irregular, mimicking an osteomyelitis or a malignancy.

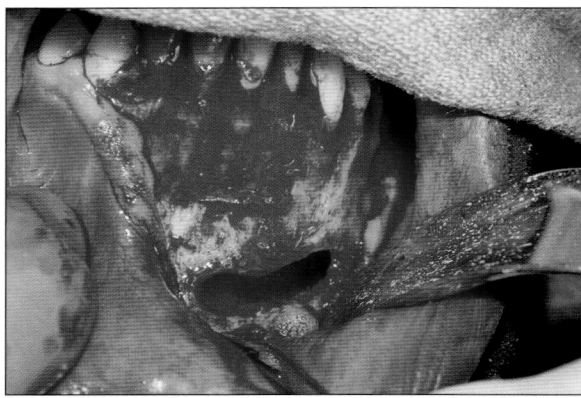

Fig 4-10 Exploration of an idiopathic bone cavity requires the removal of a cortical window and curettage of the cavity. Sometimes a small fibrin mass is found in what usually is a completely empty cavity within bone.

DIFFERENTIAL DIAGNOSIS ▶

DIAGNOSTIC WORK-UP AND TREATMENT ▶

HISTOPATHOLOGY ▶

in an ascending or involutional stage, not all radiographs will show the classic appearance. Some idiopathic bone cavities will show an irregular radiolucency (Fig 4-9). Others may show a partial fill with bone that will not scallop between teeth and therefore may resemble odontogenic cysts or tumors.

An idiopathic bone cavity is not a worrisome lesion. However, because it produces a dramatic radiolucent lesion of significant size in bone, it must be explored to rule out the more common and more significant odontogenic cysts, tumors, and fibro-osseous lesions that can produce similar radiolucencies. In particular, *odontogenic keratocysts, central giant cell tumors, central hemangiomas of bone,* and *ameloblastomas* or *odontogenic myxomas* are the more serious considerations.

Idiopathic bone cavities are diagnosed by observation during exploration. Because these lesions are almost never seen in patients older than 40 years and because many have been observed to remodel with normal bone over time without exploration, they could probably be left to observation if the diagnosis were known and the more serious diseases on the differential list did not need to be ruled out. Therefore, all idiopathic bone cavities are best diagnosed and treated by aspiration followed by exploration.

Aspiration of an idiopathic bone cavity will often return blood (see Fig 1-10). It does so not because it is a blood-filled lesion, but because a tight needle fit through the cortex will cause an excessive negative pressure in the marrow space, which disrupts capillaries and causes a return of blood. To distinguish this phenomenon from the return of blood associated with an arteriovenous malformation or a cavernous hemangioma, 1 mL of saline should be placed in the syringe before aspiration and the first part of the return observed carefully. An idiopathic bone cavity will return a few air bubbles or a small amount of straw-colored fluid into the syringe before blood appears. The syringe should be disconnected from the needle after a syringe of blood is obtained, keeping the needle in place. If an idiopathic bone cavity is present, the oozing of blood from the needle will cease, whereas more prominent vascular lesions will show a continued brisk oozing or even a spurting.

After aspiration, a cortical window is removed and the bony walls are curetted. Occasionally, a small fibrin mass is found in the cavity (Fig 4-10). During exploration, it is important to visually inspect the bony walls to ensure that there is no soft tissue lining. Odontogenic keratocysts have a very thin lining, which may be removed with the cortical window and, therefore, may be overlooked.

Submitted specimens from these lesions usually consist of portions of bone that may have no discernible lining or may be lined by delicate fibrous tissue containing capillaries. There is no epithelial component (Fig 4-11). The lumen may contain serosanguinous material. The osseous wall frequently appears inactive. However, because these lesions are not static, it is not surprising that reactive bone and osteoclastic activity have been reported in these areas.

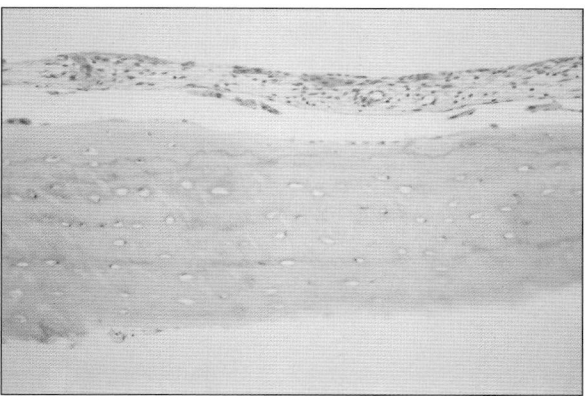

Fig 4-11 The wall of an idiopathic bone cavity shows only normal bone and a thin fibrous connective tissue lining.

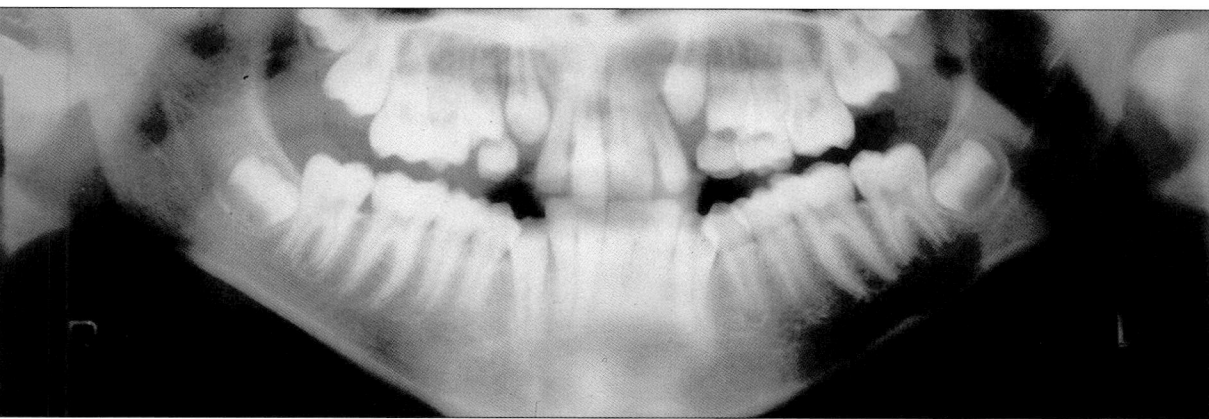

Fig 4-12a Idiopathic bone cavity 1 year prior to the view shown in Fig 4-8a.

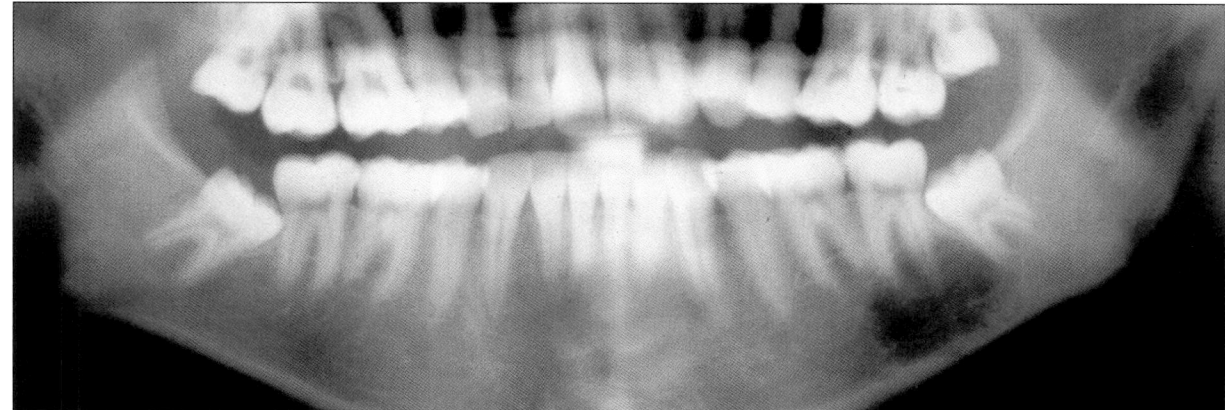

Fig 4-12b Idiopathic bone cavity in state of spontaneous involution 3 years after the view shown in Fig 4-12a and 2 years after the view shown in Fig 4-8a.

PROGNOSIS ▶

The exploration itself stimulates bony fill and remodeling within the bone cavity in 95% of lesions. Rarely, one will recur and may even progress to cause severe resorption. Such recurrent and more aggressive lesions require a wider exploration and a more complete curettage of the bony walls. There is no indication for bone grafting of these cavities except perhaps for the recurrent, progressive few. Bony remodeling is predictable and is usually complete (Figs 4-12a and 4-12b). It is especially advisable to avoid placement of foreign materials, such as hydroxyapatite preparations, because the material will occupy space into which bone should regenerate. Such foreign materials will also obscure the radiographic appearance used to follow the patient's progress.

White Sponge Nevus

CLINICAL PRESENTATION ▶

White sponge nevus is an autosomal-dominant disease producing a soft, spongy type of clinical leukoplakia. These white, asymptomatic, folded lesions usually develop in the preteen years and reach a plateau in early adulthood. White folded areas are most prominent on the buccal mucosa and the lateral border of the tongue (Fig 4-13). Characteristically, the oral mucosa is the only mucosa involved with the exception of isolated cases with lesser involvement of the anal, vaginal, or pharyngeal mucosa. The conjunctiva and cornea are not involved.

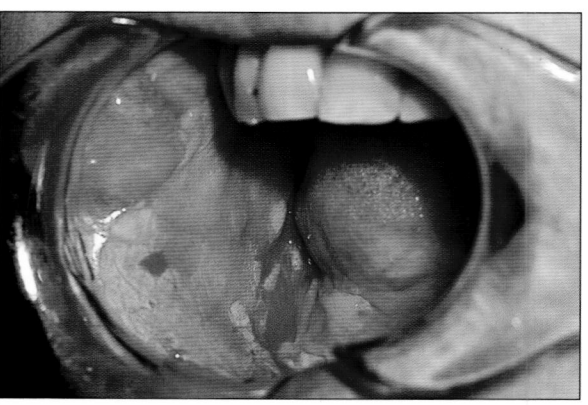

Fig 4-13 White sponge nevus will present as a clinical leukoplakia that is rolled and folded.

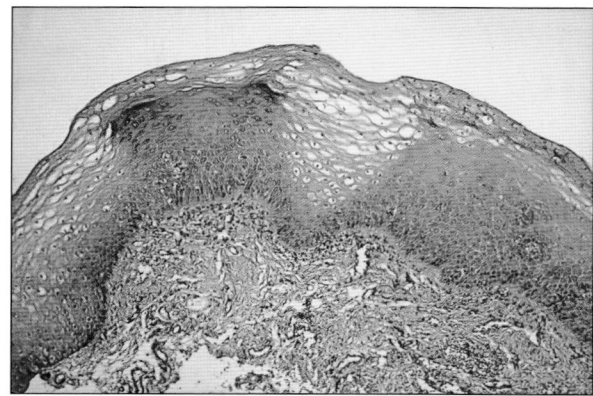

Fig 4-14 The white sponge nevus showing a basket-weave pattern within the epithelium. Basal cells appear normal. (Reprinted from McCarthy PL, *Diseases of the Oral Mucosa*, Philadelphia: Lea & Febiger, 1980, with permission from Lippincott Williams & Wilkins.)

DIFFERENTIAL DIAGNOSIS ▶

White sponge nevus is essentially a leukoplakia, that is, a white patch. Its main differential lesions are a *benign hyperkeratosis* and a *dysplastic* or *premalignant lesion,* which may also present as clinical leukoplakia. In addition, *hereditary benign intraepithelial dyskeratosis,* which is another autosomal-dominant trait, causes identical white oral lesions but has concomitant conjunctival plaques with hyperemia. *Lichen planus* is a more common disease that produces white oral lesions, particularly on the buccal mucosa and tongue; however, lichen planus is a disease of adults and is not usually seen in the preteen and teen years. *Candida* of the hypertrophic type, which will not come off on scraping, is also a consideration. Lastly, the two pachyonychia congenita syndromes, *Jadassohn-Lewandowsky syndrome* and *Jackson-Lawler syndrome,* produce similar white oral patches; however, each also shows palmar and plantar hyperkeratosis and nail bed elevations, which distinguish them from white sponge nevus.

DIAGNOSTIC WORK-UP ▶

A mucosal biopsy is indicated to confirm the diagnosis and distinguish this condition from the other more serious diseases in the differential diagnosis.

HISTOPATHOLOGY ▶

There is a thickening of the epithelium due to hyperparakeratosis, acanthosis, and intracellular edema of prickle cells. The change in the prickle cells may affect all layers, and the nuclei are also pyknotic. The basal cells are unaffected. Parakeratotic plugs may extend into the prickle cells, giving a so-called basket weave appearance to the epithelium. The underlying connective tissue is unremarkable (Fig 4-14).

TREATMENT ▶

No specific treatment is necessary. Reassurance should be given to the patients and their families that the lesions do not represent a premalignant condition and that transformation to a malignancy does not occur.

Hereditary Benign Intraepithelial Dyskeratosis

CLINICAL PRESENTATION AND PATHOGENESIS ▶

Hereditary benign intraepithelial dyskeratosis (HBID) is a rare autosomal-dominant trait, most cases of which have been traced to a single ancestor. It was first noted in an isolated population of individuals in Halifax County, North Carolina, whose ancestors were a mix of African-heritage blacks, Native Americans, and Caucasian whites. The 75 individuals initially described with HBID were traced back to a common female ancestor who lived 130 years earlier.

The signs of HBID are usually apparent within a few months after birth but may go unnoticed. The syndrome primarily affects oral and conjunctival mucosa. The oral mucosa is affected throughout, with the exception of the dorsum of the tongue, and develops wide areas of soft, spongy white lesions resembling clinical leukoplakia (Fig 4-15a). The buccal mucosal lesions are the most prominent and will

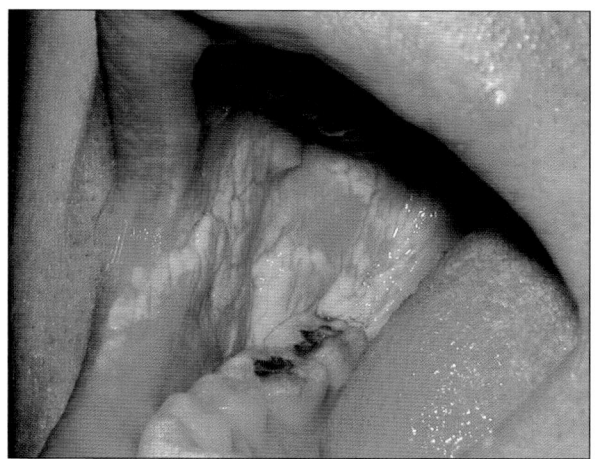

Fig 4-15a HBID will present as a clinical leukoplakia that is thin, soft, and spongy.

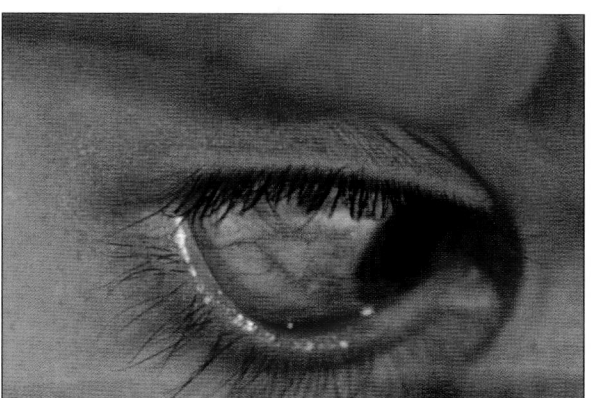

Fig 4-15b Foamy gelatinous plaques on the bulbar conjunctiva also are formed in HBID. (Reprinted with Tiecke RW [ed], *Oral Pathology*, with permission from McGraw-Hill Co.)

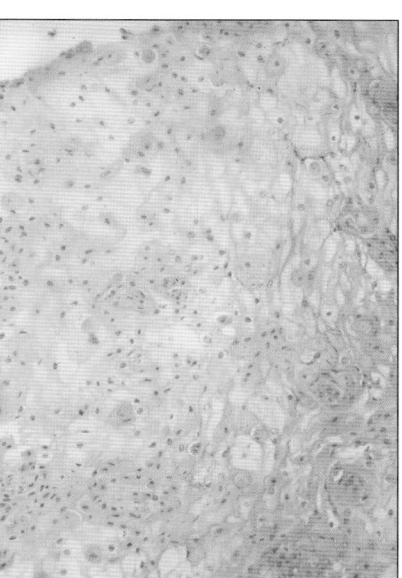

Fig 4-16 Acanthotic epithelium with pale cells and some darker cells with eosinophilic cytoplasm, representing the dyskeratotic cells in hereditary benign intraepithelial dyskeratosis.

often extend onto the commissure. As the individual matures, the lesions increase in area and often become folded and variegated in appearance between white and a translucent mucosal color.

The conjunctival lesions are superficial, foamy, gelatinous plaques of the bulbar conjunctiva (ie, the conjunctiva covering the globe) that form just outward from the limbus (the junction of the cornea and bulbar conjunctiva) (Fig 4-15b). These plaques are associated with a conjunctival hyperemia, as noted by an increased number and size of vessels, but not a true conjunctivitis, as has been reported. There is no true inflammation. Some patients will develop photophobia. In rare cases, these plaques can cover the cornea and cause blindness as the plaques exfoliate and scar the cornea.

DIFFERENTIAL DIAGNOSIS ►

The oral lesions are very similar to those seen in *white sponge nevus, lichen planus,* and the oral component of the two pachyonychia congenita variants, *Jadassohn-Lewandowsky syndrome* and *Jackson-Lawler syndrome.* However, neither white sponge nevus nor lichen planus produces conjunctival plaques as are seen in HBID. Lichen planus can produce a diffuse conjunctivitis at times, but not plaques. The pachyonychia congenita syndromes can be distinguished by their palmar and plantar hyperkeratosis as well as their prominent elevations of the toenails and fingernails. *Benign nonspecific hyperkeratosis* and even *dysplastic* or *premalignant erythroleukoplakia* may be considered in adult cases with mature HBID lesions. These lesions require a biopsy to distinguish them.

DIAGNOSTIC WORK-UP ►
HISTOPATHOLOGY ►

An oral biopsy to obtain tissue confirmation of the diagnosis is recommended.

The epithelium is thickened by acanthosis and intracellular edema. The dyskeratotic cells are large, waxy-appearing eosinophilic cells in the upper portions of the epithelium. Basal cells and deep prickle cells are normal, as is the underlying connective tissue (Fig 4-16).

Ultrastructurally, the eosinophilic cells contain large numbers of tonofilaments and degenerated nuclei, and there is a loss of desmosomes.

TREATMENT ►

No specific treatment is necessary. On rare occasions, conjunctival plaques that threaten the cornea may need to be removed. Reassurance to family and individuals that the lesions are not premalignant and will not transform into a malignancy is recommended.

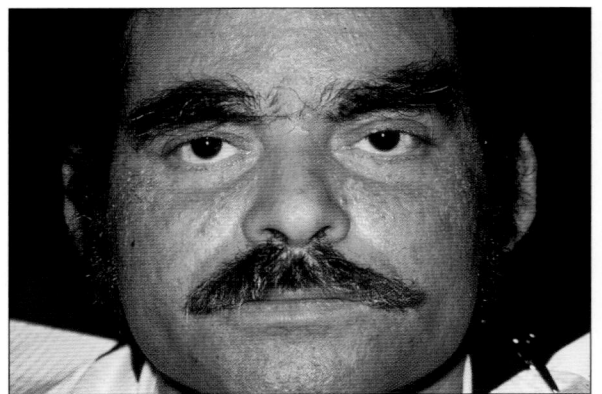

Fig 4-17a Darier disease with multiple small papules of hyperkeratosis on the face that will worsen with age.

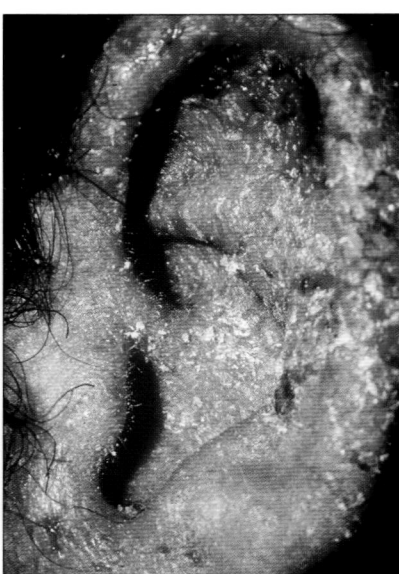

Fig 4-17b Coalesced papules develop a cobblestone appearance, shed keratin, and become brown or black because of keratin accumulation. (Reprinted from Prindiville DE, Stern D, J Oral Surg 1976;11:1001–1006, with permission from WB Saunders Co.)

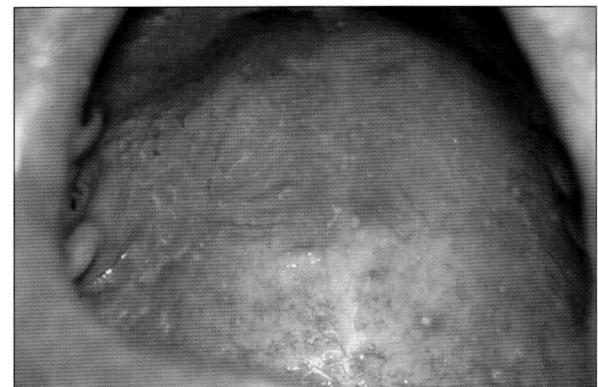

Fig 4-17c Oral lesions are similar to those on skin and represent papules of hyperkeratosis. The palate, which here has a cobblestone appearance, is a common location for oral lesions. (Reprinted from Prindiville DE, Stern D, J Oral Surg 1976;11:1001–1006, with permission from WB Saunders Co.)

Darier Disease

CLINICAL PRESENTATION AND PATHOGENESIS ▶

Darier disease is an autosomal-dominant trait that causes a defect in the maturation and keratin production of epithelial cells in the skin and, to a lesser extent, in the oral mucosa. The disease begins in late childhood or early adolescence and progresses into a more overt form in adulthood (Fig 4-17a).

Beyond the genetic inheritance, little is understood about the pathogenesis of Darier disease. There seems to be a defect in the desmosome-tonofilament complex of intercellular bridges, which explains the epithelial clefting and the histopathologic findings of corps ronds and grains. There may also be a defect in the formation or regulation of keratin production and vitamin A utilization, resulting in the overproduction of keratin.

Early cases will present with small, symmetrically located papules over the face, chest, and back. After a few years, the papules coalesce and the area of involvement develops a shiny yellow-brown to black color (Fig 4-17b) indicative of heightened keratin production. Adults will present with a dramatic and unmistakable odor generated by the keratin and colonizations of organisms within it. Adults will have such a coalescence of papules that fields of pebbly verrucous vegetations will occur. They also begin to develop keratin-producing vegetations on their soles and palms as well as the dorsum of the hands. In some cases, noticeable changes in the fingernails will be present. Pitting, splintering, and subungual keratosis has been noted.

Oral lesions do not occur without skin lesions and are found in only about 50% of cases. The oral lesions are usually small papules (Fig 4-17c) that may coalesce to give a cobblestone appearance. This tends to be most prominent on the naturally keratinized mucosa of the palate and attached gingiva. In adults, the oral lesions become more prominent and may extend to the pharynx.

DIFFERENTIAL DIAGNOSIS ▶

The distinctive odor and greasy brown to black keratotic plugs are somewhat pathognomonic. However, less advanced cases will bear a clinical resemblance to the two pachyonychia congenita syndromes, *Jadassohn-Lewandowsky syndrome* and *Jackson-Lawler syndrome,* both of which have a component of hyperkeratosis particularly involving palms, soles, and nail beds. However, the degree of hyperkerato-

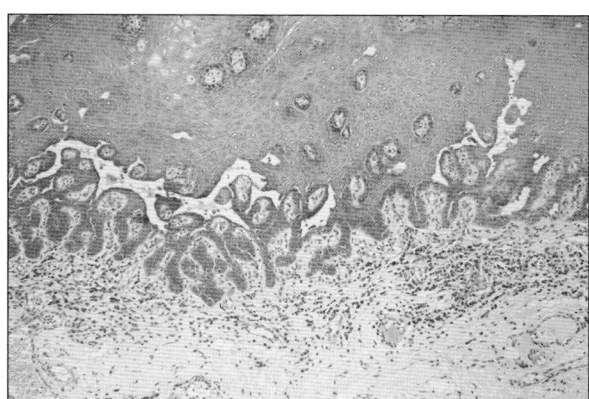

Fig 4-18a Low-power view of Darier disease showing small horizontal suprabasilar separations called *lacunae*, as well as some vertical clefts. A chronic inflammatory infiltrate is apparent.

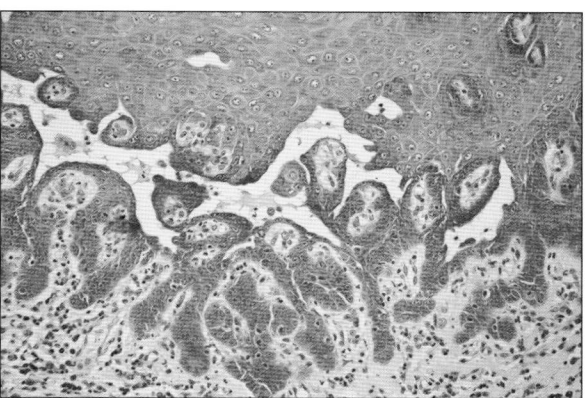

Fig 4-18b Higher-power view of Fig 4-18a in which some acantholytic cells are visible. Basilar epithelium proliferates in cords into the connective tissue.

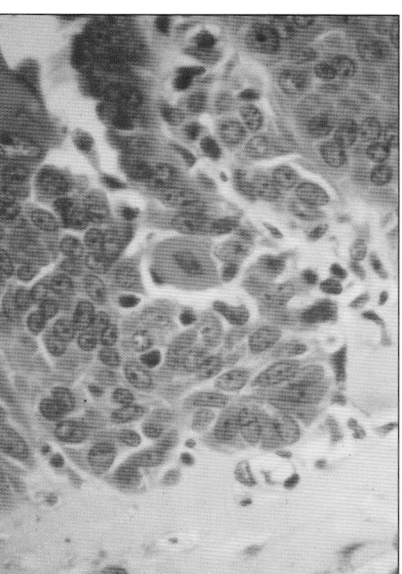

Fig 4-18c Acantholytic cells are seen, together with a corps ronds in the center of the field.

sis never becomes as prominent as in Darier disease, and these two syndromes begin or are noticed just after birth. Similarly, the thickened and darkly hyperpigmented skin associated with palmar and plantar hyperkeratosis in the malignant form of *acanthosis nigricans* may resemble Darier disease; however, the axillary, genital, and neck distribution in acanthosis nigricans as well as the lack of odor should distinguish the two. *Papillon-Lefèvre syndrome* is also associated at times with dramatic palmar and plantar hyperkeratosis but lacks skin lesions elsewhere and is associated with alveolar bone loss and tooth mobility.

HISTOPATHOLOGY ▶

The histologic picture of Darier disease includes hyperkeratosis/hyperparakeratosis and acanthosis, sometimes with papillomatosis. One of the characteristic features, however, is suprabasal acantholysis, which results in the formation of suprabasalar separations or *lacunae* (Figs 4-18a and 4-18b). At the lacunar base, villus projections may develop into the space, and the basal cells can proliferate as narrow cords into the connective tissue. In addition to these horizontal separations, vertical clefts may be seen extending to the surface of the epithelium (see Fig 4-18a). The underlying connective tissue usually will show varying amounts of chronic inflammation.

Two types of benign dyskeratotic cells can be seen in Darier disease. Corps ronds (ie, round bodies) are rounded epithelial cells with a homogeneous, pyknotic, basophilic nucleus surrounded by a clear halo, which is sometimes partly replaced by eosinophilic material (Fig 4-18c). The periphery of the cell consists of basophilic dyskeratotic material. These cells are usually seen in the upper layers of the epithelium. Grains are epithelial cells with elongated nuclei and basophilic or eosinophilic cytoplasm that are seen in the keratin layers or within lacunae.

Ultrastructurally, the corps ronds show extensive vacuolation of the cytoplasm with bundles of tonofilaments at the periphery. Grains show nuclear remnants, compression of vacuoles, and bundles of tonofilaments throughout the cytoplasm. The tonofilaments separate from the desmosomes and proliferate, creating the dyskeratotic process. Corps ronds and grains, while characteristic of the disease, are not pathognomonic, and they are not usually present in oral mucosal lesions.

TREATMENT ▶

The treatment of choice is systemic isotretinoin (Accutane, Roche), 0.5 to 2.0 mg/kg per day given in two doses each day (usually 40 mg twice daily). Although the treatment is not curative, it effectively reduces the number of papules and the overproduction of keratin. With 6% salicylic acid and warm water soaks, control can be maintained.

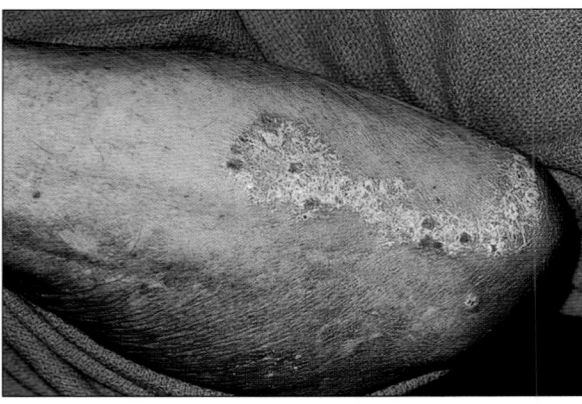

Fig 4-19 White scaly plaques on a reddened base are typical of psoriasis. Location of lesions on exterior surfaces of extremities also is common.

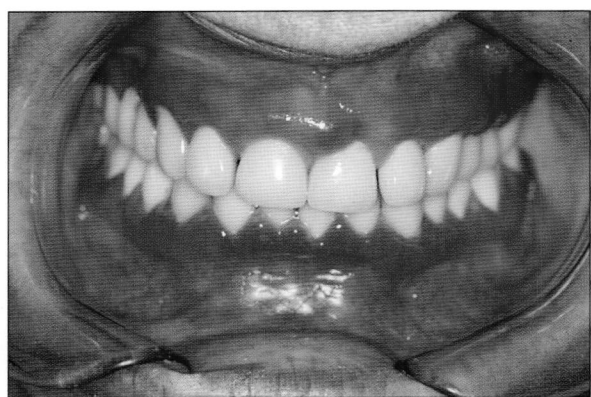

Fig 4-20 Patient with active psoriasis. The histologic changes in the gingiva also were consistent with psoriasis.

PROGNOSIS ▶

Darier disease is an incurable, progressive disease. The limitation of control is the frequent side effects of systemic isotretinoin. Most patients develop mucositis and dry skin; less frequently, mood alterations or elevation of liver enzymes is observed. Many patients require either downward adjustments in dose or periodic discontinuation. Exacerbation of the disease within weeks to months usually follows discontinuation of isotretinoin.

Psoriasis

CLINICAL PRESENTATION AND PATHOGENESIS ▶

Psoriasis is a common (1% of the United States population) acute or chronic inflammatory skin disease that is dependent on an individual's genetic susceptibility. It is usually triggered by an infection, trauma, drugs, or psychologic stress. Bright-red plaques with central silver scales are typical lesions of psoriasis. They are mostly seen on the elbows, knees, and scalp (Fig 4-19). A subtle stippling of the fingernails, a type of pitting, is an early sign and is very suggestive of psoriasis. The lesions are usually asymptomatic, but some may be mildly pruritic, and a few are severely pruritic. Severely pruritic forms are often termed *eruptive psoriasis*. The forms with central pustules rather than silvery scales are termed *pustular psoriasis*.

A thorough skin examination will frequently identify a red line in the gluteal folds and psoriatic-appearing lesions on the soles of the feet. If normal skin is traumatized, a psoriatic lesion, called *Koebner phenomenon,* will often appear at that site within 1 to 3 days. If a silvery scale is removed, a pinpoint bleeding site is often seen, which represents thinned epithelium over a hypervascular dermal papilla. This test or observation is called *Auspitz sign*.

Oral lesions in psoriasis are overstated. Rarely, they can occur concomitantly with skin psoriasis but, contrary to some beliefs, oral lesions are not an early sign of psoriasis and probably do not occur in a limited oral form (Fig 4-20). When they do occur with skin psoriasis, they are usually gingival or mucosal white or red-white thickenings. Much of the dermatology literature has associated a high incidence of the so-called geographic tongue with psoriasis, but geographic tongue probably represents only a coincidental finding.

The pathogenesis of psoriasis is unknown, but there are obvious links to a genetic predisposition related to several HLA antigens. Recent investigations have shown beneficial responses to cyclosporine, which strongly suggests an immune basis, but this has not been confirmed.

DIFFERENTIAL DIAGNOSIS ▶

Psoriasis in the oral and maxillofacial area manifests with scaly skin and scalp lesions that may itch. If the scalp lesions are more prominent, *seborrheic dermatitis* is a consideration. Seborrheic dermatitis is

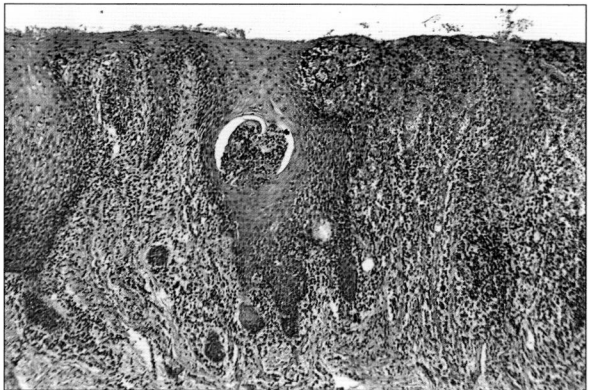

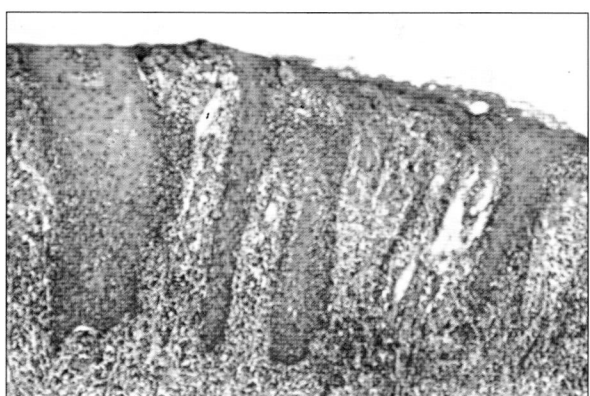

Fig 4-21 Low-power view of psoriasis in which a micro-abscess can be seen within the epithelium.

Fig 4-22 Low-power view of psoriasis with elongated test tube–shaped rete ridges and thinned epithelium overlying the connective tissue papillae, which contain dilated capillaries and neutrophils.

usually more diffuse whereas psoriasis has more well-demarcated lesions. In addition, skin lesions with prominent pruritis are suggestive of *skin lichen planus* and the cutaneous lymphoma, *mycosis fungoides*. However, lichen planus should be more purple in color; mycosis fungoides should be more diffuse and will appear more on surfaces other than knees and elbows. *Cutaneous candidiasis* as well as other skin fungal diseases may also produce this type of clinical presentation. In such cases, an immune deficiency should be suspected.

DIAGNOSTIC WORK-UP ▶

The combination of red plaques with silvery scales on elbows and knees, with scaliness in the scalp or nail findings, is diagnostic. The identification of an Auspitz sign or the Koebner phenomenon is helpful. No laboratory tests facilitate diagnosis, and the histopathology is suggestive but not pathognomonic.

HISTOPATHOLOGY ▶

The histologic picture of psoriasis changes with time. Initially, there is dilation of capillaries in the connective tissue papillae with perivascular collections of mononuclear cells, which then infiltrate the deeper layers of the epithelium. Focal vacuolation and loss of granular cells occur, followed by parakeratinization. The characteristic "squirting papilla" as described by Pinkus and Mehrigan becomes manifest with the intermittent migration of neutrophils from the connective tissue papillae. The neutrophils ascend rapidly to the areas of parakeratosis, where they aggregate to form microabscesses of Munro (Fig 4-21). Ultrastructurally, neutrophils are seen to enter epithelial cells, and as these aggregate within and between damaged epithelial cells overlying the papilla, they form spongiform pustules of Kogoj. As the lesion ages, the inflammatory component diminishes and the abscesses and pustules recede.

The rate of replication of epithelial cells is markedly increased in psoriasis, which is reflected in the high incidence of mitoses. There is also acanthosis with elongation of rete ridges to an equal length. The rete ridges are relatively narrow and test-tube shaped but may thicken toward their base, presenting a club-like appearance. There is also thinning of the epithelium over the connective tissue papillae, which contain dilated and tortuous capillaries (Fig 4-22). The scale is a lamellar structure that contains areas of hyperparakeratosis alternating with areas of hyperkeratosis. The connective tissue often contains a mononuclear cell infiltrate.

Ultrastructurally, tonofilaments and keratohyaline granules are reduced in number and are malformed. There is widening of intercellular spaces due to deficiency in the glycoprotein cement substance.

TREATMENT ▶

Psoriasis therapy is complex and requires ongoing follow-up. It often requires trials of treatments to assess the individual's response and relapse rate. For limited psoriasis, which involves less than 30% of the skin surface, topical corticosteroid creams such as 0.05% fluocinonide (Lidex, Medicis Dermatologics) or 0.1% triamcinolone cream (Kenalog) are used alone or mixed with a coal tar. Coal tar preparations such as Polytar (Stiefel Labs) or Tegrin (GlaxoSmithKline), liquid carbonic detergents

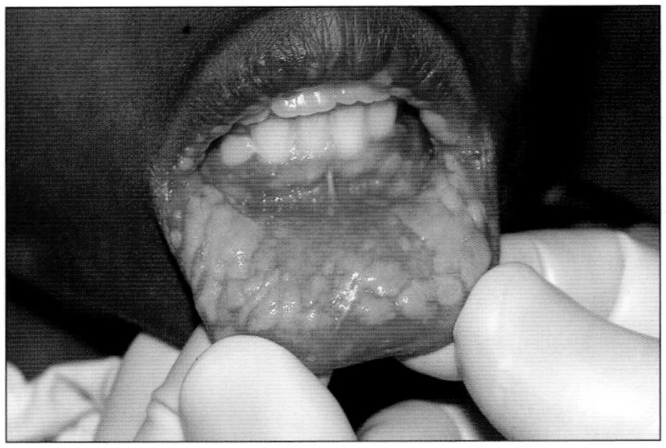

Fig 4-23 Focal epithelial hyperplasia presents with slightly raised white mucosal patches. The whiteness is due to the increased thickness of the prickle cell layer.

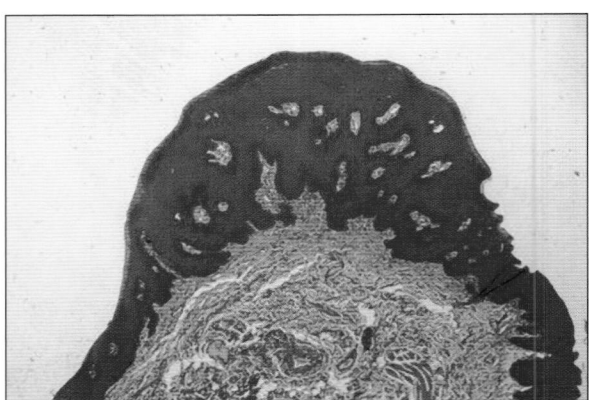

Fig 4-24 Low-power view showing epithelial hyperplasia (acanthosis) with broad, elongated rete ridges.

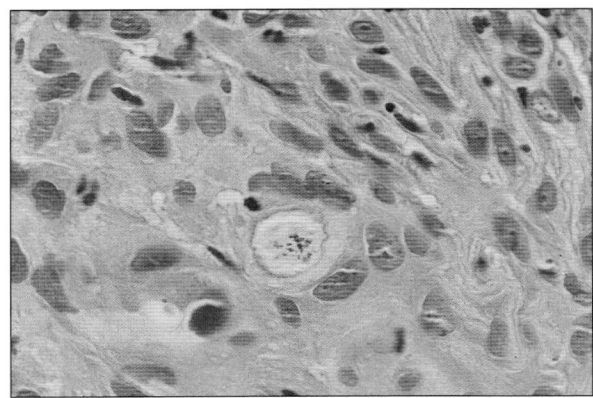

Fig 4-25 High-power view of a "mitosoid" cell in focal epithelial hyperplasia. This is the result of virally induced changes that resemble atypical mitoses.

(LCD, coal tar), and LCD 10% in Nutraderm lotion are best when mixed with a corticosteroid cream. Tar gels such as Estargel or Psorigel are also more effective mixed with a corticosteroid cream. Response becomes apparent in 1 to 2 weeks, but relapses are common. Some clinicians prefer to use coal tar preparations without topical corticosteroids because of the skin atrophy associated with chronic corticosteroid use and exacerbations that are less responsive to other treatments.

For scalp psoriasis, the Polytar or Tegrin shampoo preparations are useful. In addition, the same topical corticosteroid creams as described above applied to the scalp are also reasonably effective.

For more severe and generalized psoriasis that involves more than 30% of the skin surface area, the treatment of choice is ultraviolet (UV) B light exposure three times weekly. UVB light therapy can be performed on an outpatient basis with lesions clearing in about 2 months, but maintenance retreatments are usually necessary because of relapses. Very severe psoriasis is often treated with what is called *Goeckerman therapy*, which involves long hours of exposure to crude coal tar and UVB light. This treatment is time-consuming but provides prolonged remissions with fewer relapses.

PUVA (psoralen plus ultraviolet A light, which is in the 320- to 400-nm wavelength range ["black light"]) is a popular long-term therapy. Relapse rates are at 63% in 6 months, but retreatment and maintenance treatments can achieve longer remissions. However, skin atrophy and skin cancers remain a concern because of the cumulative damage of UV light therapy and the fact that the total safe dosage remains unknown.

PROGNOSIS ▶ Psoriasis is a chronic, incurable disease that usually requires lifelong management.

Focal Epithelial Hyperplasia (Heck Disease)

CLINICAL PRESENTATION AND PATHOGENESIS ▶ Focal epithelial hyperplasia presents with white, sessile, raised mucosal patches and nodules between 1.0 and 1.5 cm in diameter. Lesions are most commonly seen on the labial mucosa, buccal mucosa, and tongue (Fig 4-23). They are painless and do not blanch, and the surrounding mucosa is normal in appearance and texture.

Historically, this disease was believed to occur only within racial isolates of Native Americans, Brazilians, and Eskimos. It has now been described among all ethnic and racial groups. It occurs at any age, but seems to have one peak incidence in preteen children and another around age 50 years.

There has been an association with human papillomavirus (HPV-13). However, the pathogenesis of this disease remains uncertain.

DIFFERENTIAL DIAGNOSIS ▶

The clinical appearance of focal epithelial hyperplasia resembles clusters of papillomas. It is, therefore, often confused with *multiple squamous papillomas* or *condyloma accuminatum*. A confluence or tightly grouped cluster will resemble a *verrucous carcinoma* or even a *squamous cell carcinoma* at times. Lesions that are more widespread and nodular may resemble the oral submucosal granulomas seen in *Crohn disease*.

DIAGNOSTIC WORK-UP ▶

Lesions suspected of focal epithelial hyperplasia are biopsied to include an edge of the surrounding normal-appearing mucosa, which will best show the contrast in epithelial thickness and the degree of hyperkeratosis (Fig 4-24).

HISTOPATHOLOGY ▶

The epithelial hyperplasia consists of acanthosis with broadening and elongation of rete ridges, which tend to anastomose.

Viruses have been found within the nuclei and cytoplasm of the epithelium in some cases. Changes suggestive of viral etiology may sometimes be seen in the form of koilocytotic cells with clear perinuclear halos, or as nuclear changes that resemble atypical mitotic figures (mitosoid figures) (Fig 4-25). The connective tissue is vascular and may contain a mild chronic inflammatory infiltrate.

TREATMENT ▶

No treatment is indicated. Spontaneous involution over 3 years is the most common outcome, especially in children. However, longer periods of time up to 30 years have also been reported. If the lesions are a concern to the patient, accessible, and few in number, excision is reasonable.

PROGNOSIS ▶

When lesions spontaneously involute or are excised, recurrence is rare. In most cases, clinical lesions develop slowly, reach a peak in number and area of involvement, and then remain static before showing partial or complete involution.

Hereditary Gingival Fibromatosis

CLINICAL PRESENTATION AND PATHOGENESIS ▶

Hereditary gingival fibromatosis is the most common of several syndromes of gingival fibromatosis. Inherited as an autosomal-dominant trait, it has as its primary feature a firm, fibrous enlargement of the attached gingiva. Cases will express varying degrees of gingival enlargement dependent on the genetic penetrance and expressivity of the genotype. Mild cases will present with firm enlargements of the interdental papillae and attached gingiva of both jaws (Fig 4-26). More severe cases will manifest larger gingival masses, which frequently cover the teeth (Fig 4-27). Occasionally, one will encounter dramatic presentations of large gingival masses leading to lip protrusion and prevention of lip closure (Fig 4-28).

The gingival enlargement is hereditary but not congenital. The gingiva is usually normal until age 3 or 4 years, and some patients will not develop gingival enlargement until their early teen years. The full syndrome is said to include hypertrichosis (excessive hair and hair growth in usually non–hair-bearing skin), mental retardation, and epilepsy. These three components are less frequent and quite variable. Most cases present with fibrous gingival enlargement only.

DIFFERENTIAL DIAGNOSIS ▶

Drug-induced gingival enlargement is a well-known phenomenon. Phenytoin is particularly well-known to cause such a reaction in up to 50% of patients receiving the drug. However, the immunosuppressant cyclosporine and the calcium channel blockers, such as nifedipine and verapamil also cause gingival enlargement. Such drug-induced gingival enlargements can be elicited by history, and they are generally not so severe as to cover teeth as do many of the more severe cases of hereditary gingival fibromatosis. *Leukemic gingival infiltrates* are rare but do occur. However, leukemic infiltrates are soft and friable unlike the lesions of hereditary gingival fibromatosis, which are firm and resistant. Several other syndromes also produce a firm gingival enlargement, particularly *hereditary neurofibromatosis*. These must be distinguished from hereditary gingival fibromatosis by their other components:

1. *Murray-Puretic-Drescher syndrome*: Gingival fibromatosis with multiple hyaline fibromas of the skin and scalp
2. *Laband syndrome*: Gingival fibromatosis with formative defects of the ear, nose, nails, and bone and hepatosplenomegaly

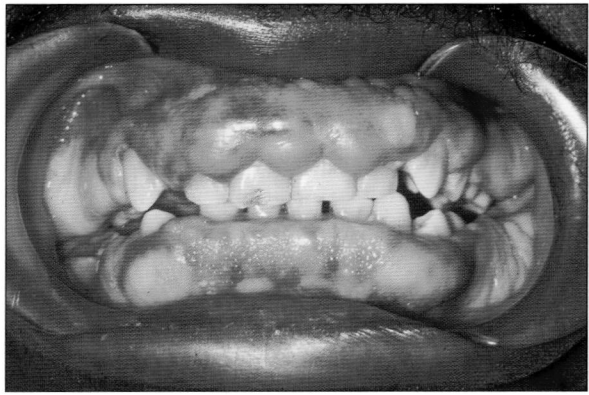

Fig 4-26 Mild to moderate expression of hereditary gingival fibromatosis enveloping one third of the tooth crown. Typically, the attached gingiva of both jaws is involved and pseudoperiodontal pockets are formed.

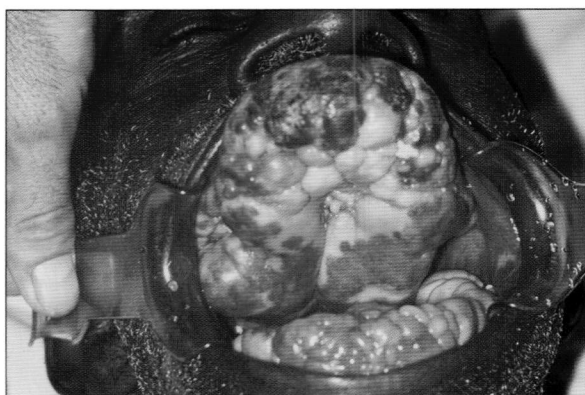

Fig 4-27 Severe expressions of hereditary gingival fibromatosis completely cover teeth and may be massive enough to prevent lip or jaw closure.

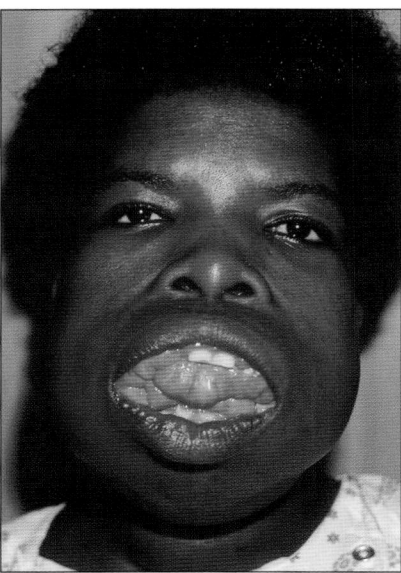

Fig 4-28 Severe expressions produce large masses as early as the teenage years. The size of the fibromatous masses is a function more of the degree of the genetic expression than of the duration of the masses.

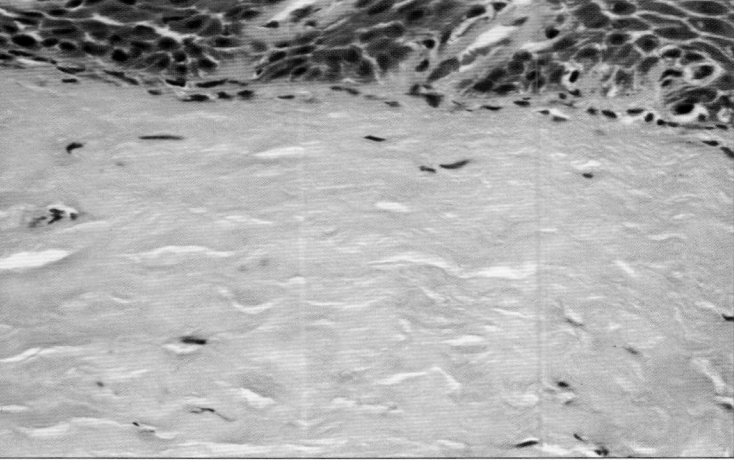

Fig 4-29 Histologically, hereditary gingival fibromatosis appears similar to a keloid with dense collagen bands and very few fibroblasts.

3. *Rutherfurd syndrome*: Gingival fibromatosis and corneal opacities
4. *Cross syndrome*: Gingival fibromatosis with microphthalmia, skin hypopigmentation, mental retardation, and corneal opacities

In each of the above syndromes, the gingival fibromatosis is usually less severe than it is in hereditary gingival fibromatosis.

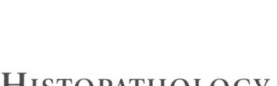

HISTOPATHOLOGY ► There is proliferation of densely collagenized fibrous tissue, which is sparsely cellular (Fig 4-29). There is no sigificant inflammatory component. The overlying epithelium is often acanthotic.

TREATMENT ► Most patients function very well either with their natural dentition or by occluding on their tough, fibrous ridges. Excision of the fibromatosis can expose greater tooth surface, but regrowth within 1 year to 18 months is common. If the teeth are only partially covered, ongoing plaque control and prophylaxis to manage plaque buildup in the pseudoperiodontal pockets will reduce caries and periodontal bone loss. In edentulous areas, the fibromatosis involutes incompletely to a bulbous and fibrous ridge.

Most cases require very little if any surgery. When surgery is performed on these tissues, a dense, white, avascular connective tissue resembling a mature scar is encountered.

PROGNOSIS ► Hereditary gingival fibromatosis is compatible with a normal life span. Frequently teeth are lost because of cervical caries and plaque-induced periodontal bone loss.

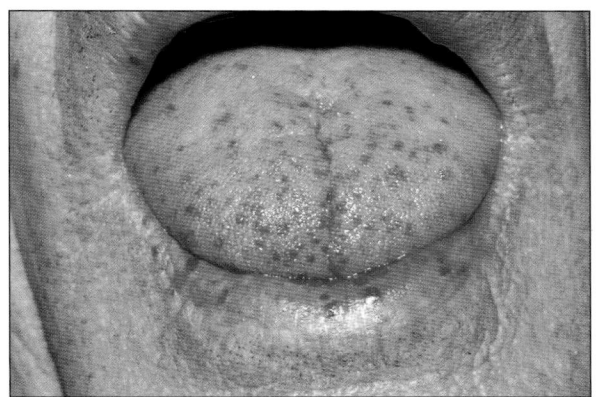

Fig 4-30a Multiple telangiectasias of the lip and tongue mucosa in a 51-year-old man with hereditary hemorrhagic telangiectasia.

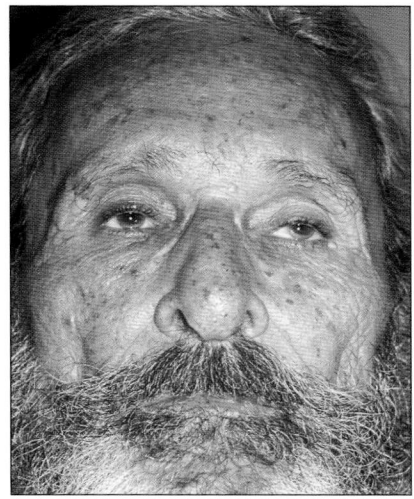

Fig 4-30b Telangiectasias are commonly found on the face as well as the oral mucosa. They increase in number with age.

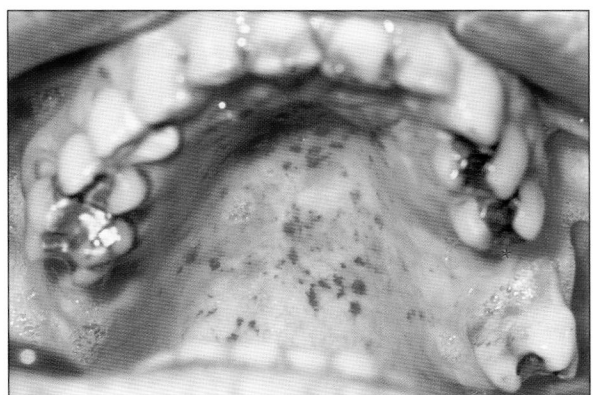

Fig 4-30c Telangiectasias in the oral cavity are most commonly found on the palate, lips, and tongue. They too will increase with age and periodically bleed.

Hereditary Hemorrhagic Telangiectasia (Rendu-Osler-Weber Syndrome)

CLINICAL PRESENTATION AND PATHOGENESIS ▶

Hereditary hemorrhagic telangiectasia is an autosomal-dominant trait of weakened capillaries in the skin and mucosa, seemingly due to defective endothelial interconnections. Clinically, patients develop telangiectatic capillary dilations within the superficial layers of skin and mucous membrane, which always blanch on compression (Fig 4-30a).

The genetic defect involves the endothelial cells, which are unable to produce overlapping cytoplasmic villi that normally interdigitate with an adjacent endothelial cell. The result is an ultrastructural gap between endothelial cells. Initially, they will appear as normal capillaries that are nevertheless weak. The capillaries spread and balloon into telangiectasias after years of systemic vascular pressure.

Telangiectasias characteristically do not become apparent until the individual reaches the upper 30s or the 40s. Rare exceptions manifest lesions earlier in life, even childhood. Once they appear, the lesions will extend in area and in number to provide symptoms of bleeding after seemingly trivial trauma or even spontaneously.

The incidence is about 1 or 2 per 100,000. Whites are affected much more frequently than blacks. Skin lesions are common on the facial skin and on the fingers and are usually quite apparent (Fig 4-30b; see also Fig 3-52f). Oral lesions are most notable on the lips, tongue, and palate (Fig 4-30c). The most troublesome and most frequent presenting symptom is epistaxis from lesions of the anterior septal mucosa within Kesselbach plexus. Oral hemorrhages also occur. Occasionally, persistent epistaxis of unknown cause will be a forerunner and early sign of hereditary hemorrhagic telangiectasia. Because gastric, visceral, and lung mucosa may also be involved, hematemesis, melena, or hemoptysis may be part of the presenting symptomology.

DIAGNOSTIC WORK-UP ▶

The most important differential of hereditary hemorrhagic telangiectasia is a variation of normal. Specifically, *cherry angiomas* (Campbell de Morgan spots) develop in about 90% of individuals older than 40 years. They are, however, more diffuse, less clustered, and do not increase their numbers as quickly with age. *Spider nevi* are seen as a developmental malformation even in children and continue unchanged into adult life. *Spider telangiectasias* are also a physical diagnostic sign of liver dysfunction and are seen in many alcoholics with cirrhosis.

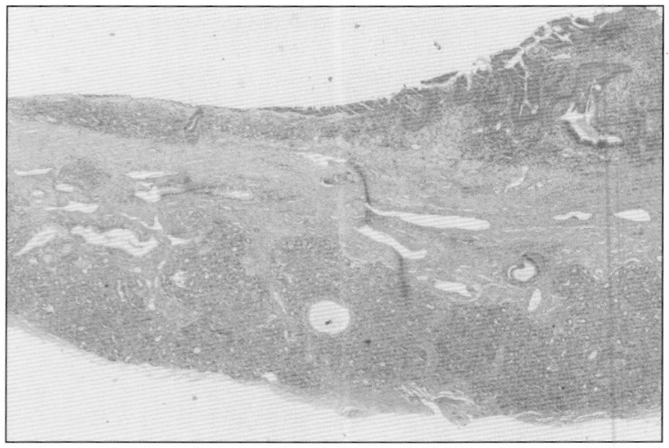

Fig 4-31 Dilation of capillaries is evident within the mucosa of a patient with hereditary hemorrhagic telangiectasia.

Several other syndromes also manifest telangiectasias. Notably, the glycosphingolipid metabolic defect of *Fabry syndrome* contains diffuse, full-body telangiectasias, which do not blanch like those in hereditary hemorrhagic telangiectasia but begin in childhood and increase in both number and area with age. *Maffucci syndrome* will show small tongue hemangiomas in addition to the enchondromas of the digits and phleboliths, but these are seen in childhood with the hands and feet becoming prominently distorted. The variant of progressive systemic sclerosis (scleroderma) known as *CREST syndrome* manifests oral, facial, and finger telangiectasias similar to those of hereditary hemorrhagic telangiectasia, and CREST develops in the 30- to 50-year age range. To distinguish CREST syndrome, the clinician must identify its other features: calcinosis within muscles or tendons, Raynaud phenomenon, esophageal hypomotility, sclerodactyly, as well as telangiectasias.

DIAGNOSTIC WORK-UP ▶ Persistent and recurrent bleeding episodes may produce an iron deficiency anemia requiring a complete blood count with assessment of Wintrobe indices, serum iron, and total iron binding capacity. If symptoms have suggested gastrointestinal bleeding, gastroscopy and colonoscopy may be needed.

HISTOPATHOLOGY ▶ Skin and mucosa show the same changes. The upper portions of the connective tissue contain irregularly dilated capillaries and venules lined by flattened endothelial cells (Fig 4-31). The walls are thinned.

Ultrastructurally, dilated capillaries lack pericytes, and endothelial cells of venules show gaps. In addition, perivascular supporting tissue is edematous and contains abnormally constructed fibrils. Thus, venules with a defective support structure are likely to hemorrhage.

TREATMENT ▶ No treatment is usually necessary other than local hemostatic measures during small bleeding episodes, such as silver-nitrate cautery, Surgicel dressings (Ethicon), etc. Corticosteroid nasal sprays such as beclomethasone (Vancenase, Schering), one spray four times daily, will reduce minor, recurrent nasal bleeds. For those nasal bleeds or oral bleeds that are persistent and frequent, superficial excision of a field, including the largest cluster of telangiectasias, combined with split-thickness skin grafting, is very effective.

PROGNOSIS ▶ Hereditary hemorrhagic telangiectasia is not curable but is manageable. Many patients do not require any intervention, and those who do usually do so because of epistaxis. Recurrent bleeding points should be treated early as they will characteristically become worse with time. Those that undergo skin grafting gain the best long-term reduction of bleeds.

Encephalotrigeminal Angiomatosis (Sturge-Weber Anomaly)

CLINICAL PRESENTATION AND PATHOGENESIS ▶ Encephalotrigeminal angiomatosis (ETA) is not a genetic inheritable defect but a disturbance of fetal development in utero, an anomaly that is present from birth. The most notable clinical manifestation (infant or adult) is an ipsilateral facial angioma that ends abruptly at the midline in most areas and thus seems

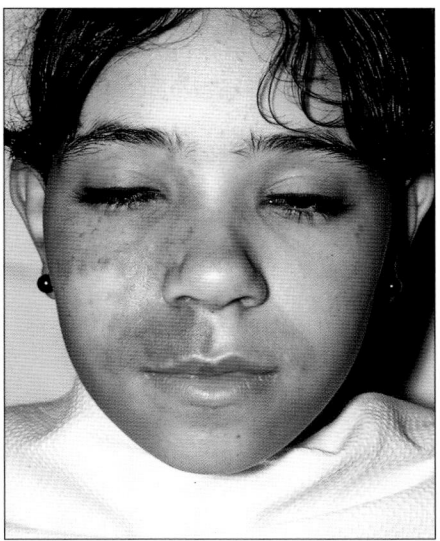

Fig 4-32a Dermal-level facial heman-giomas corresponding to the maxillary distributions of the trigeminal nerve represent the most common presentation of encephalotrigeminal angiomatosis.

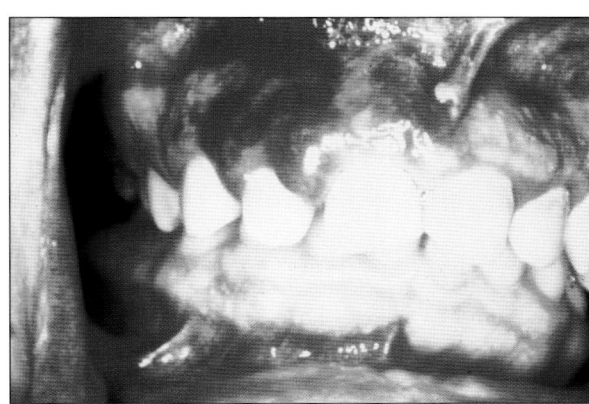

Fig 4-32b Submucosal-level oral angiomas corresponding to the facial distribution of angiomas.

to follow the distribution of the trigeminal nerve (Fig 4-32a). This and the other angiomas are the result of a persistent fetal vascular plexus that has failed to involute. By the sixth week of normal fetal development, a vascular plexus forms between the neural tube ectoderm destined to become brain and the skin ectoderm destined to become facial skin. This plexus normally involutes by the ninth week. In ETA, failure of involution results not only in a visible dermal-level angioma, but in angiomas of the meninges as well. The facial pattern of the angioma has nothing to do with the trigeminal nerve per se, except that it shares the same developmental and anatomic location.

Meningeal angiomas are venous in type with low-flow characteristics. They, therefore, frequently calcify, which makes them visible radiographically and produces a seizure disorder in 75% to 90% of individuals. If the meningeal angiomas hypertrophy or extensively calcify, mental deficiency states (30% of individuals) and in some cases overt retardation can arise. Occasionally, the meningeal angiomas affect a motor area and produce a hemiplegia. Commonly, the angiomas will extend into the choroid plexus of the eyes, where they are mostly an incidental finding but rarely have been reported to produce glaucoma.

Oral angiomas either in bone or in soft tissue correspond to the facial lesions and may be more troublesome. They frequently enlarge and become bulbous, causing bleeding episodes and interfering with the occlusion (Fig 4-32b). Characteristically, the bone size is increased (usually the maxilla) on the involved side, and tooth eruption is accelerated compared to the unaffected side, presumably because of the increased blood supply.

DIFFERENTIAL DIAGNOSIS ▶

Encephalotrigeminal angiomatosis must be distinguished from *congenital hemangiomas* and *vascular malformation* not associated with ETA. Each will show no midface midline demarcation or cerebral calcifications. Another syndrome, *Klippel-Trenaunay-Weber syndrome (angio-osteohypertrophy),* also manifests ETA-like facial and oral angiomas. It differs from ETA in that it lacks meningeal angiomas and calcifications and also has overt limb enlargement. In fact, because the angiomas of Klippel-Trenaunay-Weber syndrome involve the trunk and enlarged limbs and no genetic inheritance is known, it may very well represent an ETA-like anomaly in a different location. *Beckwith-Wiedemann syndrome* also has a facial vascular component, but it occurs symmetrically across the midline in the glabellar region and will disappear within the first year. Beckwith-Wiedemann syndrome will of course be identified by its other features such as prognathism, macroglossia, and omphalocele.

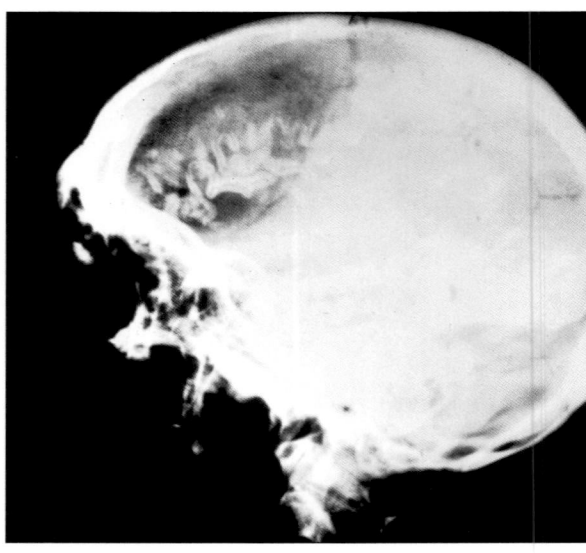

Fig 4-32c Calcification of meningeal angiomas appears in a wave-like pattern because the meninges tightly cover the brain and therefore outline the cerebral convolutions.

DIAGNOSTIC WORK-UP ▶

If ETA is suspected in the first 2 years of life, the meningeal angiomas can be mapped by internal carotid angiography. Beyond 2 years, cerebral calcification negates most of its diagnostic value (Fig 4-32c). Otherwise, plain skull radiographs and a panoramic radiograph are useful.

HISTOPATHOLOGY ▶

The angiomas (nevus flammeus) of this disorder show dilation of blood vessels, which increases with age. Endothelial proliferation is not present.

TREATMENT ▶

Most patients to date have not been treated for their facial angiomas because of the limited prognosis. Recently, subdermally focused laser ablation has shown promise in removing at least some of the angiomatous tissue without affecting the skin surface. Oral manifestations, which involve bulbous and inflamed gingival tissue due to plaque accumulation and bleeding episodes, may be treated by gingivectomy. Because the angiomatous tissue is venous and venous pressure is not great, bleeding is controllable.

Cleidocranial Dysplasia

CLINICAL PRESENTATION AND
PATHOGENESIS ▶

Cleidocranial dysplasia produces a pathognomonic facial and general physical appearance. Individuals will be short of stature (males, 5 feet average height; females, 4 feet 9 inches average height). They will appear to have a long neck with narrow, drooping shoulders due to absence of or hypoplastic clavicles. Their head will appear brachycephalic with obvious frontal and parietal bossing.

The cranium will be enlarged in the anteroposterior dimension and shortened in the superoinferior dimension, and the nasal bridge will appear flat and broad. There may be a groove in the midline of the forehead, and there may be palpable soft areas in the scalp due to open sutures. The supraorbital and infraorbital ridges are often prominent, and exorbitism may be seen because of a deficient orbital volume due to frontal bone thickening.

The absent clavicles have always been the focus of attention in cleidocranial dysplasia patients. The added motion of the shoulder girdle allows patients to touch their shoulders together in the midline. Many patients have residual hypoplastic clavicles rather than complete agenesis, with the residual portion articulating to the sternum. Some have only unilateral clavicular absence (more common on the right side).

An oral examination will be striking for a malocclusion with overretained primary teeth and missing permanent teeth. The maxilla will be hypoplastic with a deep, narrow palate that may harbor a submucosal cleft. The anteroposterior deficiency of the maxilla will create a pseudoprognathism. The nasolabial angle is usually excessively obtuse. Other skeletal abnormalities may also be variably present. These may

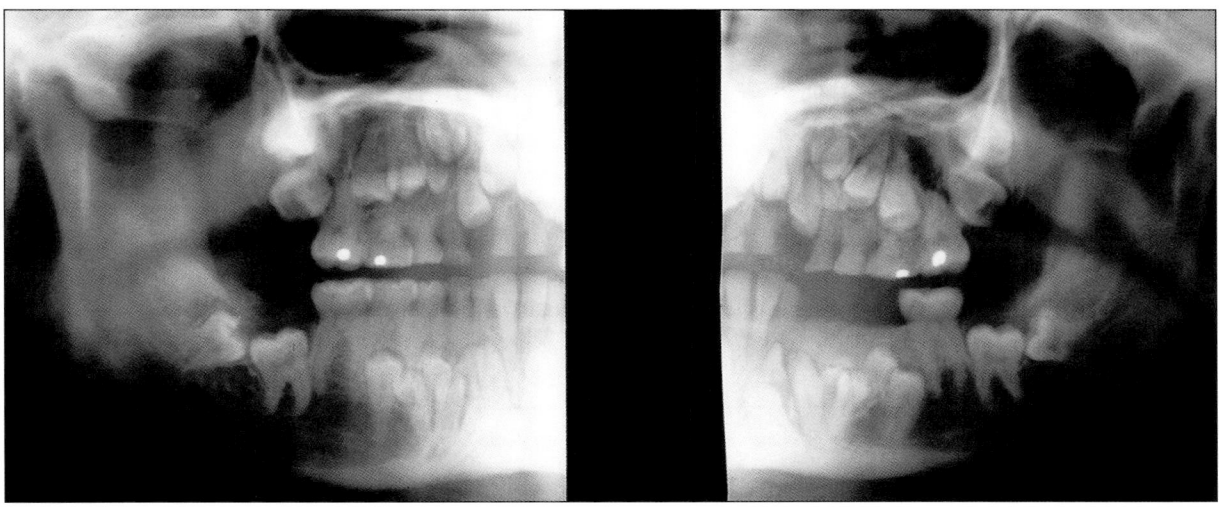

Fig 4-33a Panoramic radiograph of an individual with cleidocranial dysplasia showing numerous supernumerary premolar-shaped teeth as well as unerupted normal premolar teeth.

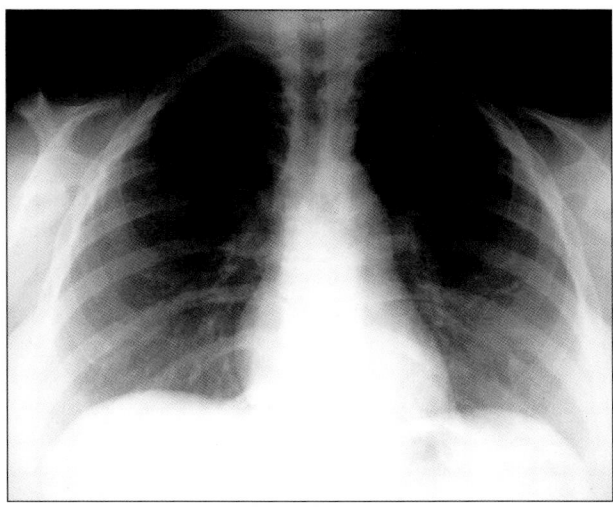

Fig 4-33b Chest radiograph of an individual with cleidocranial dysplasia showing absence of the left clavicle and only a small segment of the right clavicle in the sternoclavicular area.

include spina bifida, delayed closure of the pubic symphysis, and malformation of the metacarpals and phalanges, among others.

Cleidocranial dysplasia is an autosomal-dominant syndrome. The inheritance is not fully expressed, as one would expect in a dominant trait, but instead has a variable expressivity. About 35% of cases have no apparent inheritance and probably represent spontaneous mutations. The multiple unerupted teeth are believed to be due to absence of cellular cementum, and the delayed exfoliation of the primary dentition due to delayed root resorption. The multiple supernumerary teeth seem to be related to a delayed involution of the dental lamina, which becomes reactivated when the expected permanent tooth develops. Because the dental lamina arises from and forms the teeth from a lingual position, the supernumerary teeth lie lingual and occlusal to the permanent teeth.

RADIOGRAPHIC FINDINGS ▶ Skull radiographs will show areas of radiolucency corresponding to delayed cranial bone formation. They will also show radiopaque centers of secondary calcification and wormian bones in the sutures. The frontal and sphenoid sinuses will be small or absent, and the mastoid air cells will be missing. The maxillary and ethmoid sinuses will be absent or small. The orbital ridges will appear dense.

Panoramic radiographs will show, for those in the primary dentition stage (ages 2.5 to 6 years), normal eruption and formation of all 20 primary teeth. Those in the mixed-dentition stage and into adulthood will show numerous unerupted and supernumerary teeth (Fig 4-33a). The primary dentition will show delayed root resorption and physiologic exfoliation. As a general rule, there is one supernumerary tooth for every expected permanent tooth. This "double dentition" characteristically forms lingual and occlusal to the expected normal but unerupted permanent premolar teeth and prevents their eruption. The supernumerary teeth are premolar teeth morphologically even if they form in association with molars. In rare cases, there may be a radiolucent line in the mandibular symphysis indicating failure to unite in the midline.

Chest radiographs may reveal absent or incomplete clavicles. Hypoplastic clavicles often show a remnant at the sternoclavicular joint or medial and lateral segments with a central gap (Fig 4-33b).

DIFFERENTIAL DIAGNOSIS ▶ The clinical and radiographic appearance is distinctive and pathognomonic. The diagnosis is made by recognition of the components of this syndrome.

HISTOPATHOLOGY ▶ The few studies of teeth of these patients have shown almost complete lack of cellular cementum of both primary and secondary dentition.

Treatment is focused on reducing the dentofacial deformity and correcting the malocclusion. A coordinated treatment plan is required and generally involves removing some (but not necessarily all) supernumerary teeth. Those that seem to be forming dentigerous cysts or other pathologic entities or those that might interfere with orthodontic therapy and arch coordination are the ones indicated for removal. If a submucosal cleft exists, it can be corrected separately or at the time of orthognathic surgery, which is frequently required in these individuals. Follow-up orthodontic refinement and stabilization is necessary as is restorative and prosthetic dentistry for areas of carious or missing teeth. Uncovering of unerupted teeth with planned attempts to guide eruption by orthodontic means cannot be expected to be successful because of the lack of cellular cementum.

Osteogenesis Imperfecta

The osteogenesis imperfectas are an extremely varied and overlapping group with multi-organ and therefore heterogeneous clinical involvements that have the commonality of defective Type I collagen. Therefore, it would perhaps be better to collectively term these diseases *connective tissue imperfectas*. In the past, students have been taught to remember these diseases as a single entity through the phrase "brittle bones and blue scleras." While this is mostly true, some cases will be sufficiently subclinical as to lack brittle bones or fractures but have blue sclerae and several other features, and others will lack blue sclerae but will have multiple fractures that are more common at certain ages. This great variability relates to (*1*) different phenotypic expressions of the usually autosomal-dominant inheritance; (*2*) isolated cases of autosomal-recessive inheritance; (*3*) numerous cases of spontaneous mutations related to advanced parental age; (*4*) a wide subset of point mutations in different locations in procollagen synthesis; and (*5*) some cases resulting not from defective collagen synthesis but from faulty assembly of the triple helix conformation of the collagen molecule. The "brittle bones" result from normal mineralization of a defective Type I collagen, which does not have the elasticity of normal bone and is therefore prone to fracture following mild trauma. The blue sclerae are not due to an abnormal thinness of the sclera but rather to a decreased collagen fiber thickness and fiber diameter, allowing the retinal and uveal vessels and pigments to show through as blue (Fig 4-34a).

Since the osteogenesis imperfectas involve all collagen synthesis in the individual in addition to fractures (Fig 4-34b), they may also variably have aortic dilations, joint hypermobility, bowing of the long bones (Fig 4-34c), easy bruising, and various dentinogenesis imperfecta manifestations, among other organ involvements. Although various dentin abnormalities are associated with osteogenesis imperfectas, dentinogenesis imperfecta may occur as a single entity unassociated with osteogenesis imperfecta, and conversely, osteogenesis imperfecta may or may not have concomitant dentinogenesis imperfecta. In fact, this association has led to the classification of two subtypes of type I osteogenesis imperfecta.

In an attempt to develop a general categorization, the many clinical expressions of osteogenesis imperfecta have been divided into four major types as follows:

Type IA

Individuals with type IA will tend to have multiple bone fractures, although 10% will have no fractures. The number of fractures will range from 2 to more than 70 throughout the individual's lifetime. Such fractures will be more frequent in children and older individuals, and less frequent at puberty and for some years afterward. Fracture frequency thus increases with age and is particularly high among postmenopausal women. These individuals may also have varying degrees of kyphosis, scoliosis, bowing of long bones, and increased cranial size (macrocephaly).

Individuals with type IA will not have dentinogenesis imperfecta; the teeth are clinically and radiographically normal. However, 95% of those in this group over the age of 30 will develop some conduc-

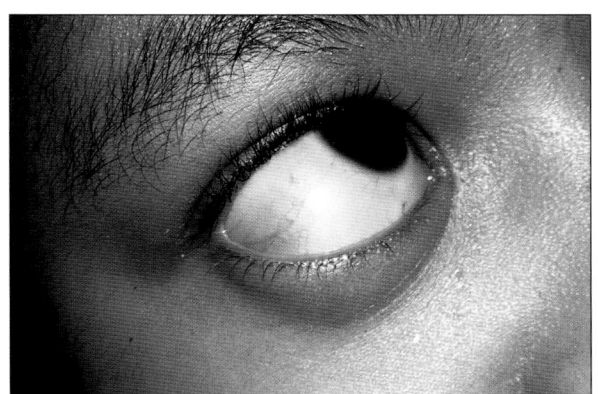

Fig 4-34a The blue sclerae seen in some types of osteogenesis imperfecta are due to the thinness and the defectiveness of the collagen fibers in the sclera.

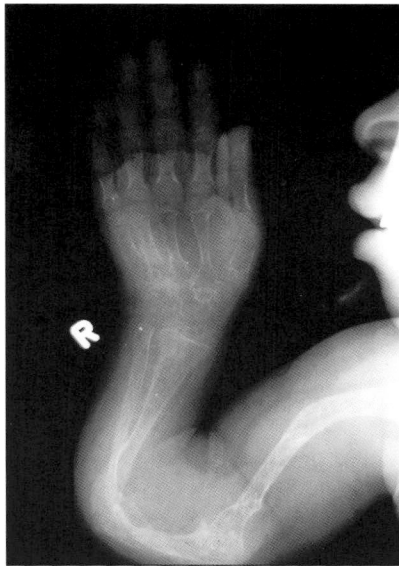

Fig 4-34b Because the main organic component of bone is collagen, the bone is bowed and brittle. Fractures are common.

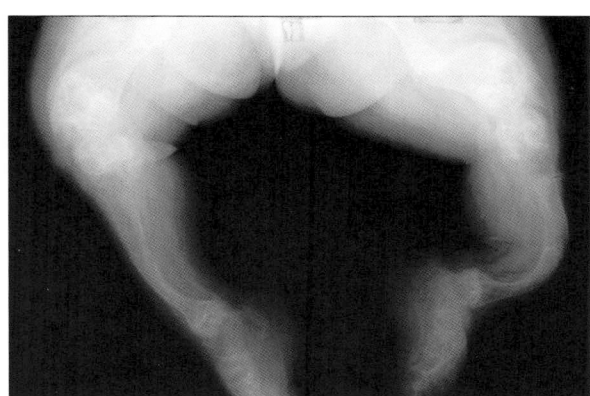

Fig 4-34c Long bones are more severely bowed than others and may be hypoplastic.

tive hearing loss due to immobility of the middle ear ossicles at the stapes footplate. This group may also have aortic dilations; however, only 24% of men and 4% of women have this involvement, and it is usually asymptomatic. Joint hypermobility may also be seen, but to a lesser degree than that seen in Ehlers-Danlos syndrome or Marfan syndrome, two other diseases of defective collagen synthesis or structure.

Type IB

Individuals with type IB may have any or all of the involvements of osteogenesis imperfecta in type IA, as well as various degrees of dentinogenesis imperfecta. Usually both the primary and secondary teeth erupt with opalescent dentin, which is the gray or blue-gray appearance of the teeth. Like the blue sclerae, the malformed collagen component of the dentin allows the pulp vascular network to reflect light through the teeth as blue (Fig 4-35a). A widened pulp chamber, resulting from incomplete and shortened dentinal tubules, may also contribute to this effect. The enamel is normal, but the dentinoenamel junction is usually flat. Therefore, the enamel rods wear off rapidly to expose the dentin, producing a brown discoloration soon after eruption that may resemble a restorative crown preparation. Significant secondary dentin is deposited so that the teeth will lose their blue-gray opalescence, and a radiograph will show obliterated pulp chambers (Fig 4-35b). Therefore, depending on the timing, the teeth may appear gray-blue, normal, or brown clinically and show enlarged, normal, or obliterated pulp chambers radiographically.

Types IIA, IIB, and IIC

The three subgroups of type II osteogenesis imperfecta are distinguished by the mode of inheritance. Type IIA is thought to be the result of new mutations, which are autosomal dominant. Type IIB is thought to be inherited from parents who are carriers and is an autosomal-dominant inheritance. Type IIC is very rare but is thought to represent autosomal-recessive inheritance.

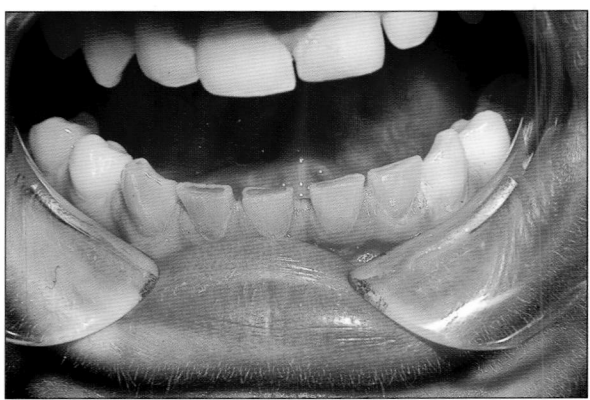

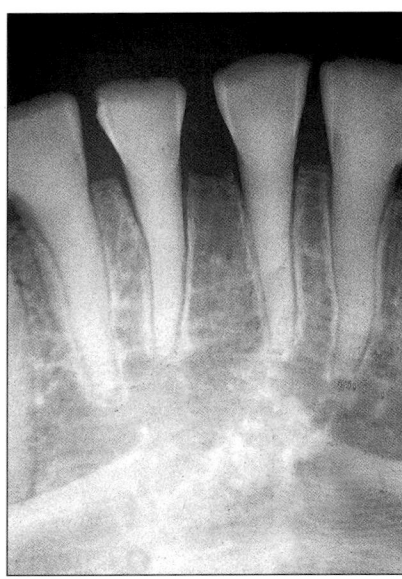

Fig 4-35a In osteogenesis imperfecta type IB, varying degrees of dentinogenesis imperfecta are present. The teeth may have a blue-gray appearance due to malformed dentin, which allows the pulp vasculature to show through. (Courtesy of Dr David E. Prindiville.)

Fig 4-35b Osteogenesis imperfecta type IB with dentinogenesis imperfecta will erupt with opalescent dentin but will progress to form significant secondary dentin, which will cause the teeth to lose their original blue-gray opalescence and develop obliterated pulp chambers. (Courtesy of Dr David E. Prindiville.)

In each of the subtypes, type II osteogenesis imperfecta is a severe expression characterized by extreme bone fragility and multiple early fractures, including fractures in utero and stillbirths or early infant deaths (14 hours to 4 weeks). In fact, much of the data available in this group have been derived from autopsies. Similar to type IB, type II has enlarged dental pulps with shortened and incomplete dentinal tubules, but no information is available concerning secondary dentin and eventual pulpal obliteration because of the short life spans. In this general type, radiographs show dramatically incomplete skeletal development with malformed ribs, wormian bones in the calvarium (island of bone), and absent ossifications of the distal segments in the extremities.

Type III

Type III osteogenesis imperfecta is also a more severe form than type I although not as severe as type II. This type progressively worsens so that about 38% survive long term, as do most type I individuals, but none dies in early infancy as do those with type II. Instead, this type is seen to have about a 25% mortality in the first year, another 25% mortality between the teen years and the early 20s, then another 20% mortality up to the age of 50 years. Most deaths result from complications of fractures or inadequate skeletal support of internal organs, leading to scoliosis, pulmonary hypertension, and cardiopulmonary failure.

This type will not have blue sclerae. The sclerae will appear normal clinically in adults, although children may have blue sclerae throughout their first year. The dentitions in this group have not been adequately reported; however, it seems that 50% will have some form of dentinogenesis imperfecta.

Type IV

Type IV osteogenesis imperfecta will have normal sclerae as does type III individuals. However, this type has more fractures at birth than type III and, also in contrast to type III, does not worsen over time but

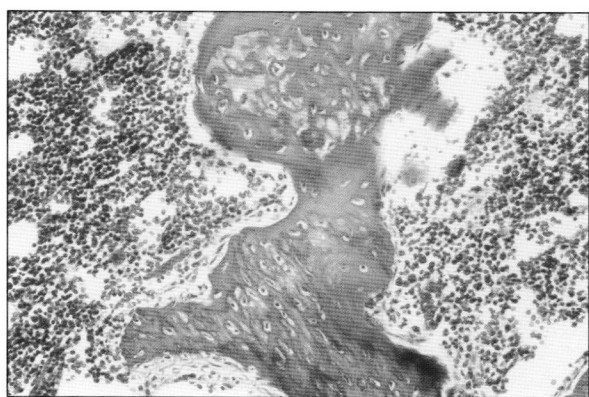

Fig 4-36 Osteogenesis imperfecta bone will be undermineralized and more cellular than is normal bone.

actually has fewer fractures after puberty. This type has a high incidence of concomitant dentinogenesis imperfecta similar to that of type IB. The specific degree of dentinogenesis imperfecta and its course are consistent within a family. They generally include a slight variation of opalescent teeth on eruption, enamel loss once in function, and obliterations of the pulp due to secondary dentin deposition.

DIFFERENTIAL DIAGNOSIS ▶

There are several rare syndromes that may produce bone radiolucency and fractures. These include *Cole-Carpenter syndrome, Campomelic syndrome,* and *Bruck syndrome.* If wormian bone in the calvarium is the prominent feature, *cleidocranial dysplasia, progeria, mandibuloacral dysplasia,* and *acroosteolysis* may be considered as well. If blue sclerae is the prominent feature, *Marfan syndrome* and *Ehlers-Danlos syndrome* may be included. If *dentinogenesis imperfecta* features predominate, it is well to remember that dentinogenesis imperfecta can exist independently and that *dentin dysplasia type I and type II* will produce dentin abnormalities similar to dentinogenesis imperfecta.

In a practical sense, a young child who presents with multiple fractures should be considered a potential "*battered child.*" This may be particularly difficult to distinguish from some of the osteogenesis imperfectas because of the easy bruising that may be a part of the collagen abnormality and the obvious bruising seen in a battered child. In such cases, the dental examination, the color of the sclerae, and the pattern of bony fractures become the important differential points.

DIAGNOSTIC WORK-UP ▶

A detailed complete-body physical examination, oral examination, jaw radiographs, and full skeletal radiographs are the baseline studies recommended. If these studies suggest a diagnosis of osteogenesis imperfecta, genetic testing of parents and patient may be accomplished as well as collagen mapping and DNA probe studies, which usually require biopsy material.

HISTOPATHOLOGY ▶

The ossification centers develop normally in cartilaginous bone, but no ossification occurs (Fig 4-36). Cortices are thin, and medullary trabeculae are few, fragile, and subject to microfractures. In the severely affected infant, the skull may be fibrous and in adults it may be composed of small wormian bones with irregular sutures.

TREATMENT ▶

There is no specific treatment for the disease itself. It will progress to its full expression as dictated by the degree of genetic mutation of the particular type, which in turn has dictated the degree and amount of "imperfect" collagen.

The oral and maxillofacial surgeon may be required to treat facial bone or jaw fractures in these individuals. In such cases, the rate and degree of bone regeneration is the same as for normal individuals. However, the bony callus and bony union will be of osteogenesis imperfecta–type bone. Therefore, standard fracture treatment approaches may be used with little modification. There is no compelling recommendation to use more rigid internal fixation plates in these individuals because the gain of rigidity is offset by the stress rizors that are more prominent in "brittle bones" when screw holes are drilled and the potential for new fractures adjacent to plates where the stress differential between plate and bone may be significant.

The dentinogenesis component is usually treated with onlay or full-crown coverage. In the anterior teeth, cosmetic full crowns or veneers may be used. Selective orthodontic therapy to correct the frequent malocclusions is feasible as these teeth will move through this type of bone, but the treatment risks are higher because of the increased mechanics required and the already shortened roots.

PROGNOSIS ▶ Prognosis is dependent on the type of osteogenesis imperfecta and the degree of genetic expression. As has been stated, this can vary greatly from intrauterine death to a full life span. In those with one of the milder expressions, cautious lifestyles and prompt medical and surgical management of disease-related complications can extend longevity.

Dentinogenesis Imperfecta

CLINICAL PRESENTATION AND PATHOGENESIS ▶ Dentinogenesis imperfecta (DI) is an autosomal-dominant trait that affects both the primary and permanent dentitions. It is, therefore, usually recognized early in life (ages 2 to 6 years) when teeth begin to appear brown or opalescent and the enamel seems to quickly wear off the crowns. When DI occurs as a component of osteogenesis imperfecta, it is classified as DI type I. When DI occurs as a separate isolated trait, it is classified as DI type II. Both type I and type II DI exhibit seemingly normal teeth at the time of early eruption. After several months, full eruption of the teeth will often disclose a bell-shaped crown and obvious discoloration in addition to enamel wear. Radiographs will indicate obliteration of the pulp chamber by dentin (Fig 4-37a). Because the primary dentition is more severely affected than the permanent dentition, children will be brought in by parents who seek consultation concerning "discolored teeth" (Fig 4-37b).

The opalescent color of some teeth is due not to the pulp showing through but to the collagen structural defect within the dentin, which may reflect either a bluish light through the enamel or a brown color. Also, the enamel does not actually "fall off" the dentinoenamel junction, as some believe; the dentinoenamel junction in DI seems to be structurally and functionally normal. Some enamel wears excessively because of hypoplastic and hypocalcified areas within the enamel rods. These are presumably due to the fact that amelogenesis is induced and initiated by the initial mantle dentin deposition in normal tooth formation. The abnormality in dentin formation results secondarily in enamel that is also microscopically somewhat defective.

The abnormal collagen is produced by abnormal odontoblasts. The preodontoblasts within the dental papilla seem to undergo normal cellular differentiation and form nearly normal mantle dentin. These odontoblasts die and are replaced by newly differentiated odontoblasts from the dental papillae that never mature into fully functional odontoblasts. These defective odontoblasts secrete an abnormal collagen, which is undermineralized and fails to form odontoblastic tubules. The result is the imperfect dentin that reflects light in the brown or blue spectrum but has formed a near normal dentinoenamel junction because of the less affected pre-odontoblasts and the mantle dentin they produce (Fig 4-38).

DI type III may represent a rare transitional link between dentinogenesis imperfecta and dentin dysplasia. DI type III also is an autosomal-dominant trait, but it is a specific dentin abnormality. It seems to be a specific defect only within the primary dentition, but it may produce secondary dystrophic dentin, which causes pulpal obliteration, or, paradoxically, it may underproduce such dystrophic dentin, creating an enlarged pulp cavity, resulting in shell-shaped teeth.

DIFFERENTIAL DIAGNOSIS ▶ The initial recognition of discolored and malformed teeth with excessive enamel wear may also suggest *amelogenesis imperfecta* or *fluorosis*. However, amelogenesis imperfecta can be recognized by its more clinically apparent enamel defect. Specifically, the enamel will be pitted and mottled in appearance, and globular enamel that produces a widening just apical to the incisal edges of lower incisor teeth is common. Moreover, both amelogenesis imperfecta and fluorosis are associated with normal pulp chambers, whereas DI produces obliterated pulp chambers. Dentinogenesis imperfecta must also be distinguished from *dentin dysplasia,* another autosomal-dominant trait that affects dentin in two types. These can be

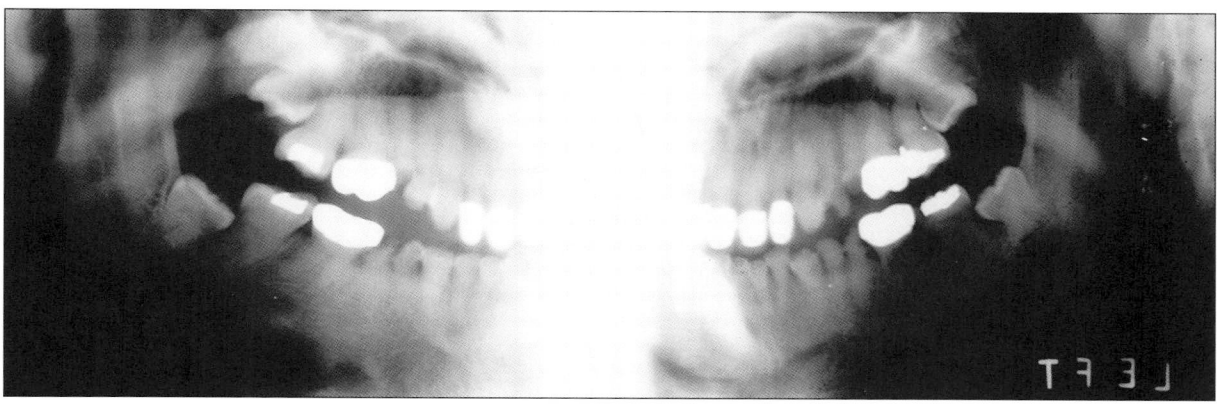

Fig 4-37a Panoramic radiograph of an individual with dentinogenesis imperfecta showing obliterated pulp chambers and normal root development without periapical radiolucencies. Here, crown coverage is an obvious part of treatment.

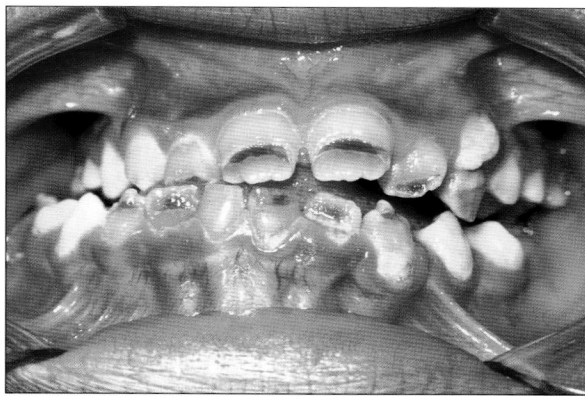

Fig 4-37b The effects of dentinogenesis imperfecta will not be apparent in newly erupted teeth (note the premolars). However, after eruption, enamel rods with internal defects become separated from the even more defective dentin as a result of function.

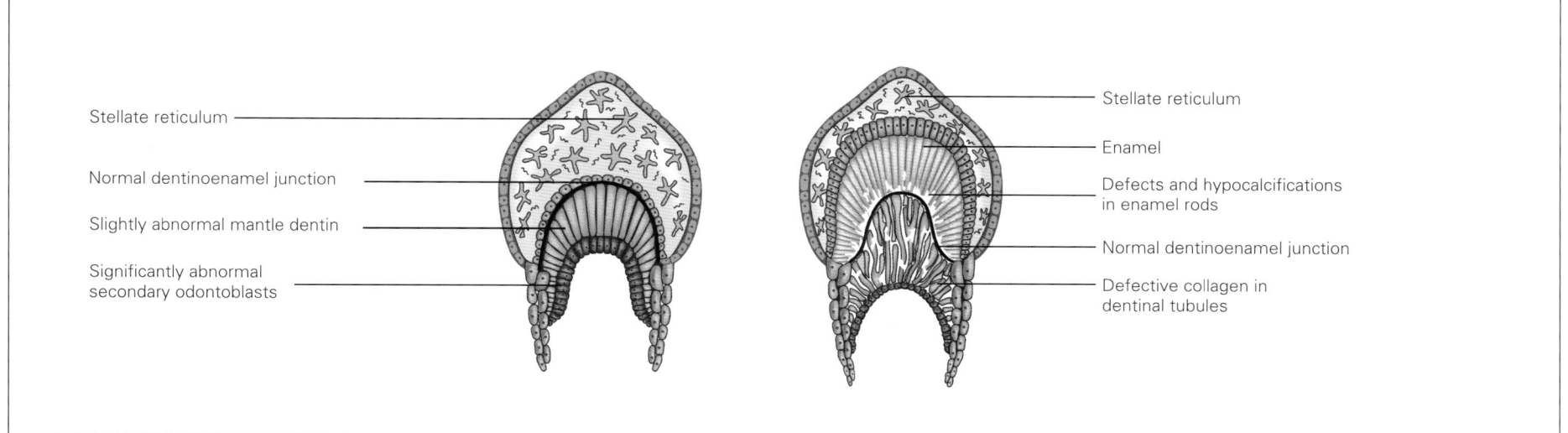

Stellate reticulum

Normal dentinoenamel junction

Slightly abnormal mantle dentin

Significantly abnormal secondary odontoblasts

Stellate reticulum

Enamel

Defects and hypocalcifications in enamel rods

Normal dentinoenamel junction

Defective collagen in dentinal tubules

Fig 4-38 Dentinogenesis imperfecta results in the formation of defective collagen deposition in the secondary dentin after initial mantle dentin deposition. Therefore, the dentinoenamel junction is normal, the mantle dentin is slightly abnormal, and the secondary dentin, which forms the dentinal tubules, is significantly abnormal. In addition, since enamel formation is induced by the deposition of mantle dentin, some voids and defects also occur within the lower portion of the enamel rods.

separated from true dentinogenesis imperfecta because one of its forms, *dentin dysplasia type I,* has normal coloration of both the primary and permanent dentition, although their pulps are almost completely obliterated. Unlike DI, it also manifests extremely short roots and periapical radiolucencies. The other form of dentin dysplasia, *dentin dysplasia type II,* does cause a discolored opalescent primary dentition with obliterated pulp chambers, but the permanent dentition is of normal color and the pulp chambers are enlarged.

DIAGNOSTIC WORK-UP ▶

Dentinogenesis imperfecta is a clinical-radiographic diagnosis best made from good-quality panoramic radiographs and full-mouth periapical series.

HISTOPATHOLOGY ▶

The enamel may appear to be normal; however, there are subtle hypocalcification defects in the enamel rods just above the dentinoenamel junction. The dentinoenamel junction appears flattened. The dentin is composed of broad, sparse, irregular tubules. Calcification is poor. Continued deposition of dentin may cause almost complete obliteration of the pulp chamber.

TREATMENT ▶

Treatment is aimed at protecting teeth from caries and wear. Most patients seek cosmetic dental improvement. Although the dentin is defective and the enamel is also secondarily abnormal, full crowns and veneer restorations are possible and will be very serviceable. Because the dentin is structurally somewhat brittle, excessive occlusal forces on a single tooth or teeth used as abutments for fixed partial dentures are not recommended because of risk for fracture.

PROGNOSIS ▶

If teeth are not protected with occlusal coverage, dysfunction and loss of teeth due to wear are likely.

Dentin Dysplasia

CLINICAL PRESENTATION AND PATHOGENESIS ▶

Dentin dysplasia is a rare autosomal-dominant trait that is associated with defective dentin formation but is separate from and unrelated to dentinogenesis imperfecta. Dentin dysplasia type I primarily affects the root, while type II primarily affects the crown.

In dentin dysplasia type I, the clinical crown appears normal in shape and color; however, the roots are short and will cause mobility and early tooth loss. The pulps will be obliterated in a manner similar to that found in dentinogenesis imperfecta, but they will be distinguished by their shortness, a conical shape, and an apical radiolucent notching.

In dentin dysplasia type II, the crowns of the primary dentition are opalescent because of large dentinal tubules ("thistle tube" dentin) and abnormal globules of dentin. However, the crowns of the secondary dentition are normal in color but radiographically will show enlarged pulp chambers due to the so-called thistle tube dentin. This normal crown coloring in the presence of an enlarged pulp chamber presumably is due to the thicker enamel and mantle dentin in permanent teeth.

Microscopically, both the enamel and the mantle dentin just below the dentinoenamel junction should be normal in both types of dentin dysplasia. It is the deeper dentinal tubules that are abnormal. These tubules are often just amorphous round nodules of dentin or disorganized interrupted tubules rather than actual tubules.

DIFFERENTIAL DIAGNOSIS ▶

Dentin dysplasia will most likely resemble either *amelogenesis imperfecta* or *dentinogenesis imperfecta as a component of osteogenesis imperfecta* or as an *isolated dentinogenesis imperfecta.* Amelogenesis imperfecta can be ruled out by the finding of clinically normal enamel in dentin dysplasia. Regardless of the color of the teeth (normal vs opalescent), in dentin dysplasia it will be smooth and complete without pits as is seen in amelogenesis imperfecta. Dentinogenesis imperfecta as part of osteogenesis imperfecta can be ruled out based on the absence of multiple old fractures, absence of blue sclerae (inconsistent), and the fact that the enamel in dentinogenesis imperfecta wears off the dentinoenamel junction because of induced defects in the lower portion of the enamel rods. In dentin dysplasia there is no exposed dentin since the enamel remains on the crown.

HISTOPATHOLOGY ▶

In dentin dysplasia type I, the enamel is normal, and a thin layer of normal dentin is found adjacent to the dentinoenamel junction. The deeper dentin is dysplastic, ranging from atubular to a few small tubules. Between these dysplastic masses are spaces presumed to have previously contained remnants of the dental papilla. The root dentin is entirely dysplastic. In type II, all dentin below the mantle layer is highly disorganized.

TREATMENT ▶

Teeth with reasonable root lengths may be treated with full crown coverage. Those with short roots often require removal and replacement with dental implant–retained fixed crowns or removable tissue-borne prostheses.

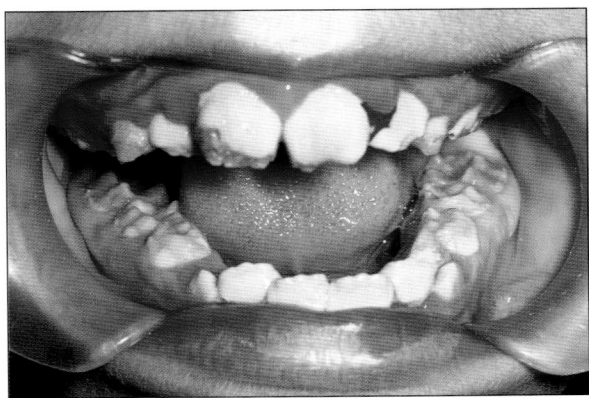

Fig 4-39a Pitted, grooved, and lost enamel resulting in yellow to brown exposed dentin in both the primary and permanent dentition in amelogenesis imperfecta. Note also the globular enamel on the mandibular incisors, which resembles calculus deposits.

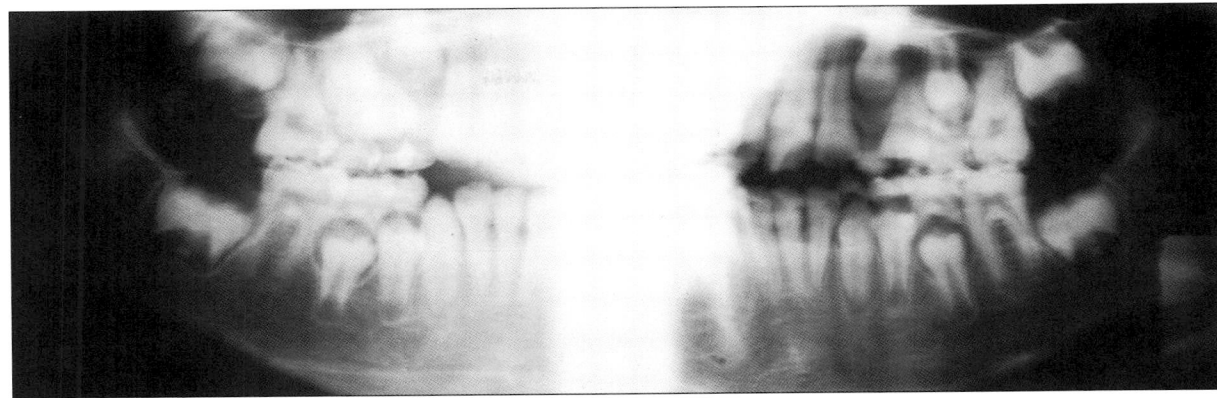

Fig 4-39b Panoramic radiograph showing normal pulp morphology, dentin, and root development in amelogenesis imperfecta.

Amelogenesis Imperfecta

CLINICAL PRESENTATION ▶

The term *amelogenesis imperfecta* encompasses a group of hereditary disorders that, alone or with other features such as epilepsy, taurodontism, and sclerotic bones, produces defective enamel. The enamel defects are of two major types: hypocalcified enamel rods and hypoplastic enamel rods. Various subtypes exist as do variable inheritance patterns, from X-linked recessive to X-linked dominant to autosomal dominant. Most occur as an autosomal-dominant trait unassociated with other abnormalities.

In the defect with hypoplastic malformed enamel rods, both primary and permanent teeth erupt with a thin enamel cover that may be absent on some surfaces. The incisal and cuspal thirds are the surfaces most often lacking enamel. The remaining part of the tooth surface may be pitted or grooved (Fig 4-39a). The disorder is apparent as soon as the teeth erupt.

In the defect with hypocalcified enamel rods, both the primary and permanent dentition appear normal at first. However, the enamel rods are soft, friable, and do not adhere to the dentinoenamel junction. The enamel layer is either lost at the dentinoenamel junction or split in the midenamel layer, leaving additional defective enamel on the dentin.

In both defects, the teeth become yellow and brown. In some cases, unerupted teeth are resorbed or partial agenesis occurs, leaving edentulous areas within a dentition that is otherwise affected by amelogenesis imperfecta.

RADIOGRAPHIC FINDINGS ▶

Radiographs will show a thinned and irregular enamel layer. Otherwise, the pulp chambers, dentinal layers, and root morphology are normal in all but the rarest of cases (Fig 4-39b).

DIFFERENTIAL DIAGNOSIS ▶

The eruption of teeth that are discolored or that soon become discolored suggests *fluorosis* or *dentinogenesis imperfecta*. Fluorosis may be clinically difficult to distinguish from amelogenesis imperfecta, but family history and testing of water sources can separate the two. In addition, teeth affected by amelogenesis imperfecta have soft enamel, whereas teeth affected by fluorosis have a hardened enamel. Amelogenesis imperfecta is best separated from dentinogenesis imperfecta by examination of the enamel, which will be pitted, globular at the incisors, and clinically soft. The radiographs will show normal pulp chambers in amelogenesis imperfecta, which in dentinogenesis imperfecta are usually obliterated. It is also well to remember that *high fevers, congenital syphilis,* and *rickets (avitaminosis D)* may also impair enamel formation (hypoplasia) or enamel calcification (hypocalcification). Of these, fevers will cause a line of affected enamel, and congenital syphilis will cause the typical mulberry-shaped first permanent molars and screwdriver-shaped permanent incisors without affecting the enamel of other teeth. Although rickets may affect the enamel of all teeth, its concomitant undermineralizing effect on bones will produce the stigmata of bowed legs, short stature, and bone pain, among other signs.

The hypoplastic type of amelogenesis imperfecta will show defects of the enamel matrix, which in some cases may be absent. The hypocalcified type shows abnormalities in the matrix and in calcification. Routine specimen processing that would require decalcification cannot be used to demonstrate these changes. Ground sections of undecalcified teeth are necessary.

Teeth affected by amelogenesis imperfecta are otherwise sound and are not more caries prone than normal teeth except for their exposed dentin. Cosmetic dentistry in the anterior dentition and occlusal coverage in the posterior dentition are indicated.

Hemifacial Hyperplasia

Hemifacial hyperplasia replaces the term *hemifacial hypertrophy*, which represented a double misnomer in that (*1*) the disease involves an increase in cell numbers (hyperplasia) and not an increase in cell size (hypertrophy), and (*2*) it usually occurs in a limited hemifacial form, but it may also occur in a hemibody form or variations in between. Thus the current term, *hemifacial hyperplasia*, is better but still somewhat misleading. The disease does not seem to show a definite hereditary pattern. Most cases are isolated and suspected to be the result of disturbances in fertilization or early embryologic development. The condition is present at birth (congenital) but becomes more obvious with growth in the succeeding years. The hemifacial hyperplasia includes enlargement of all soft and hard tissues.

Most patients present with prominent enlargement in the midcheek area, but lips, tongue, teeth, mandible, maxilla, and zygoma are also involved (Fig 4-40a). The enlargement is less noticeable above the level of the zygomatic arch and in the neck. The skin itself is thickened but soft and flabby. There may also be excessive hair (hypertrichosis) or sweating. The pinna is also overtly large.

Oral findings are of great importance in defining the condition and distinguishing it from other syndromes and diseases that present with unilateral hyperplasias and enlargements, none of which involves the teeth and few of which involve the oral soft tissues. In hemifacial hyperplasia, the tongue is unilaterally enlarged with a sharp midline demarcation and prominent, red, fungiform papillae. Occasional cases show a diffuse enlargement of the tongue. The dental arches are wide, and their overlying gingiva and mucosa are thickened. The palatal vault is strikingly thick on the affected side and is well demarcated at the midline or pushes the midline toward the unaffected side. The visible tooth crowns are increased in size by 25% to 45%. The roots are also proportionally enlarged. Both dentitions show this macrodontia, which in the primary dentition is limited to the second molar and canine and in the permanent dentition involves all teeth on the affected side but is most prominently seen in the first and second molars and the canines (Fig 4-40b). Tooth eruption is accelerated, with the primary dentition exfoliating by the age of 4 to 5 years. The difference in tooth size, tooth rotations, and eruption time often creates overt malocclusions, usually with an open bite on the unaffected side.

The two concerning features of this disorder are a 15% to 20% incidence of mental retardation due to unilateral enlargment of the cerebrum and malignancies of the adrenal cortex, liver, and kidney. Wilms tumor of the kidney, a tumor of embryonic origin, is the most common and is indicative of a relationship between hemihyperplasia and an oncogenic stimulation.

Hemifacial hyperplasia has a male to female predilection of 4:1. It occurs in approximately 1 in 86,000 live births. In males, the right side is more commonly affected; in females, both sides are affected equally. The cause is unknown, and many unproven theories exist. The lack of a genetic transmission and the variability in area of involvement from a single finger to hemifacial to hemibody implies some disturbance during fertilization or initial cleavage of the fertilized egg.

Unilateral facial enlargement is seen in conditions such as *craniofacial fibrous dysplasia* and *hereditary neurofibromatosis*. Neither will have definitive enlargement in tooth size. Although fibrous dysplasia may mimic hemifacial hyperplasia with expansion of the maxilla, it will not include the overlying soft tissue or the tongue and usually will not involve the mandible. Hereditary neurofibromatosis will cause soft tissue

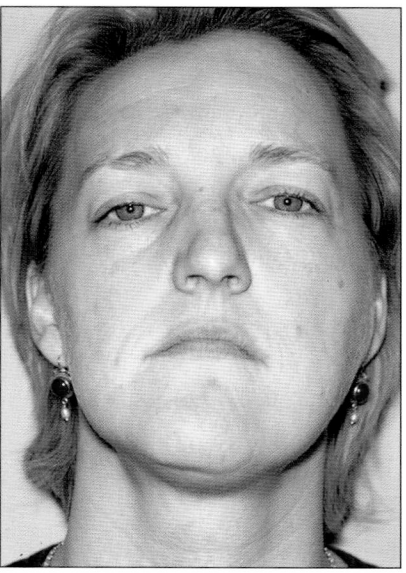

Fig 4-40a A generalized increase in the size of every facial unit is apparent on the left side of this individual with hemifacial hyperplasia. Note the abrupt demarcation at the midline.

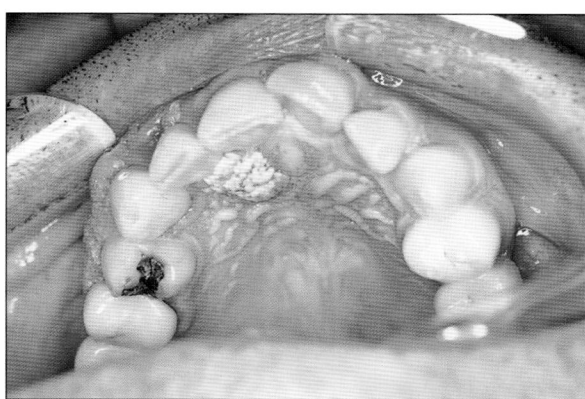

Fig 4-40b All structures on the involved side, including the teeth, will have a marked increase in size. In this case, the enlarged teeth also caused a unilateral crowding of the dentition.

enlargements including the hemitongue, but the bone is usually not involved or only one bone is involved and the teeth are of normal size. *Congenital lymphedema* and *vascular malformations* may also be considerations but are limited to soft tissue enlargements and will not necessarily be unilateral. *Klippel-Trenaunay-Weber syndrome* is a syndrome of angiomatous enlargements of several body areas, usually the extremities. It can also cause unilateral enlargement of the jaws. However, close inspection will show that this syndrome does not necessarily limit itself to one side, has a vascular component, and will not cause tooth enlargement.

DIAGNOSTIC WORK-UP ▶

During childhood, cognitive tests and IQ tests are recommended to assess for mental deficiencies. A complete physical examination and internal organ scanning are necessary to assess for the presence of internal malignancies.

It may be necessary to measure mesiodistal and buccolingual tooth widths on both sides. Plain radiographs or CT scans may be necessary to assess the size of affected bones and soft tissues if the diagnosis is unclear.

HISTOPATHOLOGY ▶

The limited number of histologic evaluations of this condition have indicated no significant change in the involved tissue other than overgrowth. The overgrowth is due to hyperplasia rather than hypertrophy.

TREATMENT ▶

In uncomplicated hemifacial hyperplasia, functional and cosmetic improvements may be achieved through orthodontic tooth alignment and serial staged surgeries. There are no wound-healing difficulties or bleeding tendencies in these patients. Corrective surgery requires a combination of mandibular and maxillary osteotomies along with bony contouring procedures. Soft tissue debulking of certain areas may also be necessary.

PROGNOSIS ▶

So few affected patients have undergone corrective surgery that surgical outcomes cannot be adequately assessed. Because the enlargement is related to all tissue levels, it is reasonable to assume that perfect symmetry cannot be obtained. Whether or not there is a tendency for redevelopment of tissue hyperplasia remains unknown.

Hemifacial Atrophy (Romberg Syndrome)

CLINICAL PRESENTATION AND PATHOGENESIS ▶

Hemifacial atrophy is a frightening and frustrating condition in which an otherwise normal-appearing pre-teen or teenage individual undergoes a 3-year period of progressive one-sided facial soft tissue and bone atrophy. The left side of the face is affected in more than 85% of cases. There is usually an accompanying Jacksonian type of sensory seizure disorder on the contralateral side. In about 10% of cases, the atrophy includes an entire half of the body. Most will also develop some skin hyperpigmentation, sparsity of hair, and an atypical trigeminal neuralgia in the affected area.

The first sign of this syndrome is a thinning over the body of the zygoma, which spreads from that point. The skin, subcutaneous tissues, muscle, and underlying bone decrease in size. The hair, including eyelashes and eyebrows, is also somewhat affected. The atrophic process sometimes spares the skin while the underlying fat, muscle, and bone atrophy. Orally, the upper lip and sometimes both lips and the hemitongue are involved. The maxilla is atrophic, and teeth may be incompletely erupted or unerupted. When the mandible is affected, all parts on the affected side are proportionally smaller. The teeth, however, seem to be of normal size.

The resultant facial appearance may progress to a retracted commissure and distortion of the nose, lips, and chin to the affected side (Fig 4-41a). A severe commissural and upper lip retraction produces an exposure of the maxillary teeth and may create a sardonic smile. The loss of orbital fat and the atrophy of the zygoma will produce enopthalmos and downward displacement of the lateral canthus. Less frequently, the eye will display lagopthalmos, ptosis, or a full Horner syndrome.

The contralateral sensory seizure activity begins when the facial atrophy is almost complete. However, the ipsilateral atypical trigeminal neuralgia may be an early sign.

After about a 3-year course, the atrophy stops and is not reactivated. The disease has an extremely wide range of severity from minor cheek thinning to a dramatic facial deformity.

The pathogenesis of hemifacial atrophy remains unsettled. Most theories today suggest a disturbance in the trophic sympathetic nervous system. In fact, one group of investigators was able to produce a similar condition in rats by performing a unilateral cervical sympathectomy.

DIFFERENTIAL DIAGNOSIS ▶

Hemifacial atrophy is quite distinctive clinically. The only two specific entities that remotely resemble it are *progressive systemic sclerosis* (scleroderma) and *hemifacial microsomia* (oculoauriculovertebral syndrome). The *coup de sabre* form of scleroderma is believed by some to represent a special type of progressive hemifacial atrophy. In this type of scleroderma, a facial hemisclerosis develops that often includes an atrophic indentation in the forehead above the lateral orbital area, which resembles the gash of a sword, hence the term *coup de sabre*. There is ongoing debate as to whether this entity is a form of hemifacial atrophy or a separate entity within the scleroderma spectrum. Hemifacial microsomia can be distinguished from hemifacial atrophy by virtue of its congenital nature, extrabulbar dermoids, and the fact that most have ear tags rather than an atrophic ear.

DIAGNOSTIC WORK-UP ▶

No diagnostic work-up will currently aid the diagnosis, which is one of clinical recognition. However, CT scans and magnetic resonance imaging (MRI) scans are useful in tracking the atrophy and planning treatment.

TREATMENT ▶

Attempts at reconstructive surgery during the active period of atrophy are not advised. During that time, atrophy or loss of transplanted tissue will occur, and such correction will not halt further atrophy. Reconstruction after a documented period of quiescence (6 months is recommended) may then be undertaken to deal with each unique defect.

In cases where the skin has been spared, a combination of onlay cranial bone grafts and soft tissue transplants, ranging from free nonvascularized dermal fat (Fig 4-41b) to a vascularized transfer of omental fat to a de-epithelialized radial forearm flap, are useful. In cases where the skin is atrophic, complete replacement with a skin-containing flap may be necessary. If available, trapezius or latissimus dorsi pedicled flaps can serve the purpose, as can vascularized free transfers of either the radial forearm or scapu-

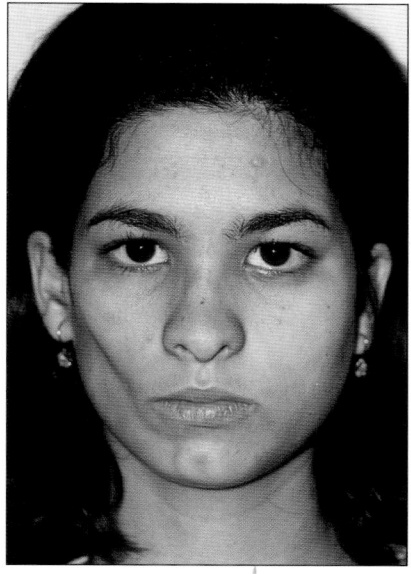
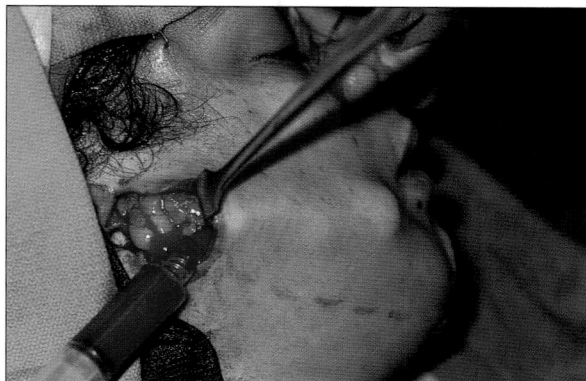
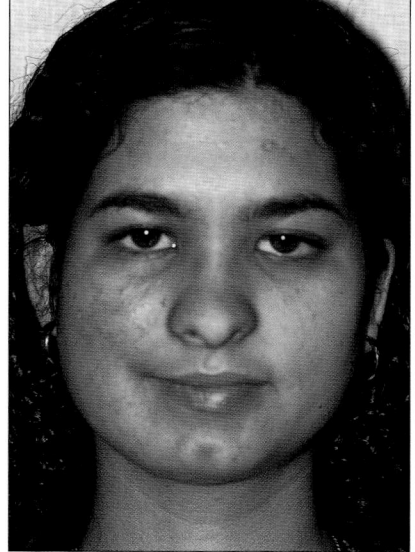

Fig 4-41a The 3-year period of facial atrophy will result in a generalized decrease in the size of all facial units on the involved side. Note the smaller lips, neck, and chin and the anterior temporal recess in addition to the more obvious cheek involvement.

Figs 4-41b and 4-41c A dermal fat graft supported with platelet-rich plasma growth factors and placed at the subcutaneous or SMAS level is a useful corrective surgery for hemifacial atrophy.

lar flap. A vascularized transfer of iliac bone with a skin subcutaneous composite based on the deep circumflex iliac artery can achieve simultaneous reconstruction of atrophied bone and soft tissue. Otherwise, second-stage cancellous bone grafts from the ilium or block calvarial bone grafts are placed after soft tissue reconstruction.

Orbital reconstruction may also be required and is best done after completion of the soft tissue phase. Orbital reconstruction is best accomplished with cranial bone grafts and soft tissue fat transfers into the orbital volume.

PROGNOSIS ▶

Hemifacial atrophy correction is an extremely difficult reconstruction. The multiple tissue types involved (skin, muscle, bone, fat) and the distortions they cause to key facial units such as the commissure, lip line, and orbital contours make it very difficult to achieve a close symmetry with the unaffected side. The syndrome does not return after its initial course, but reconstructions themselves can atrophy because of a hostile recipient-tissue bed; hence the preference for pedicled or vascularized reconstructions in the more severe patient involvements. Dermal fat grafts are the preferred and more straightforward reconstructions in patients with moderate involvements (Fig 4-41c).

Ehlers-Danlos Syndrome

CLINICAL PRESENTATION AND PATHOGENESIS ▶

There are now eight reported variants of Ehlers-Danlos syndrome related to faulty collagen metabolism. Four are autosomal dominant, including the rare periodontal form that results in rapid tooth mobility and loss by age 30, and one is X-linked. The remaining three autosomal-recessive forms tend to be more severe than the dominant forms, following the general rule for most syndromes. A spectrum of frequency of the severities has been suggested: severe, 30%; mild, 45%; benign hypermobile, 10%; ecchymotic, 5%; and X-linked, 10%.

The clinical features originate from incomplete and faulty collagen that lacks its usual unique strength and integrity. Consequently, tissues are friable and overly pliable. Even the fetal membranes are pliable so

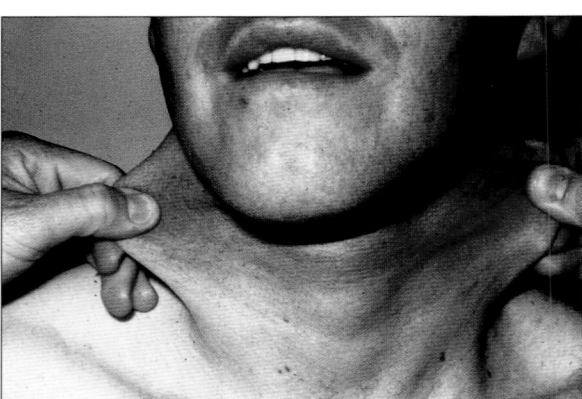

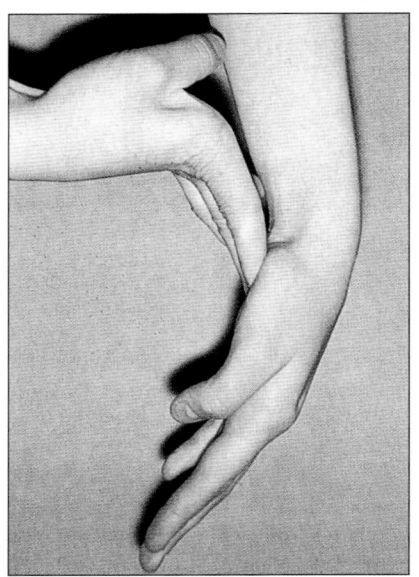

Fig 4-42a Hyperstretchable skin in an individual with Ehlers-Danlos syndrome.

Fig 4-42b Hyperextensible joints in an individual with Ehlers-Danlos syndrome.

that early membrane rupture and premature deliveries are common. In the ecchymotic form and the severe forms, cutaneous hemorrhages are common; even exsanguination has occurred. This is ostensibly due to fragile capillaries as well as to fragile large vessels.

Ehlers-Danlos syndrome is well recognized to cause hyperstretchable skin and hyperextensible joints (Figs 4-42a and 4-42b). This hyperstretchability of skin has spawned the term *Indian rubber man*, and the hyperextensibility of joints can be seen in the so-called human pretzel circus performances of those with the milder forms of this syndrome. The often-used term *hyperelastic* is a misnomer and thus should be avoided. Hyperelastic skin stretches excessively but returns to its normal position and contour, indicating normal elastic recoil and elastin fibers.

The skin of those affected is friable and will open into overt wounds on minor trauma. Wound healing is slow, and wound tissue has poor tensile strength. The scarring is often referred to as "cigarette paper scarring" because of its irregular surface and pitting. The skin is usually thin and in the ecchymotic form allows the subcutaneous vascular plexus to become visible. In addition, crumpled paper–like scars form over the major joints, and what are called *pseudotumors* of soft, disorganized collagen develop in the same locations.

The friability and stretchability of soft tissue contribute to an increased incidence of hernias and kyphoscoliosis. They also contribute to hiatal hernias, diverticulosis, aortic or other arterial ruptures, and in rare instances to bowel perforation. The more severe the disease, the greater the risk.

The hyperextensible joints permit a variety of voluntary contortions across all joints. The term *genu recurvatum* has been used to describe the opposite knee curvature seen in 25% of cases. The temporomandibular joint, along with other joints, has been reported to undergo and be at risk for dislocation.

Oral findings are not especially profound except in type VIII, the periodontal form, in which rapidly progressive periodontal disease causes a complete loss of teeth. Radiographically, the teeth are observed to contain pulp stones and a high percentage of deformed roots. The crowns will be heavily grooved and have deep fissures. More than half of all Ehlers-Danlos patients can touch their nose with the tip of their tongue as opposed to only 8% of the general population.

Epicanthal folds are seen in 25% of individuals, while blue sclerae are seen in only 10%. Eversion of the upper eyelids resulting in protrusion of the tarsal plates, called *metenier sign*, can occur.

The pathogenetic defect seems to be related to type III collagen. The primary sites of deformity—skin, vessels, joints, and tendons—are mainly composed of type III collagen. The collagen in Ehlers-Danlos syndrome does not seem to be crosslinked. Crosslinking of the left-sided triple helix of collagen is this protein's fundamental component of strength. It is postulated that enzyme deficiencies such as procollagen peptidase and lysine hydroxlyase fail to develop hydroxylysine crosslinking, and therefore fails to convert the extracellular soluble procollagen into insoluble mature collagen.

DIFFERENTIAL DIAGNOSIS ▶

It is most important to distinguish Ehlers-Danlos syndrome from a condition known as *marfanoid hypermobility syndrome*. This entity will manifest the same hyperextensibility of joints, and individuals are able to accomplish contortions across all joints as seen in Ehlers-Danlos syndrome, but they lack the thin, hyperstretchable skin. Joint hypermobility without skin changes is also seen in *Marfan syndrome* and *osteogenesis imperfecta,* but these can be distinguished from Ehlers-Danlos syndrome by their other components.

HISTOPATHOLOGY ▶

In general, skin biopsies show no significant change. The raisin-like lesions that occur at the site of hematomas are fibrous masses with numerous capillaries and sometimes foreign-body giant cells. Subcutaneous nodules show partially necrotic fat tissue with dystrophic calcification surrounded by dense collagen.

In keeping with a generalized collagen defect, dentinal abnormalites occur. Vascular inclusions, numerous denticles, and irregular tubules are found, predominantly in the root. In addition, irregularities of the dentinoenamel and cementodentinal junctions as well as hypoplastic enamel have been described.

TREATMENT ▶

Ehlers-Danlos patients are not good surgical candidates because of bleeding tendencies, secondary infections, delayed wound healing, and dehiscences secondary to poor collagen formation and, therefore, minimal tensile strength. Generally, these patients are evaluated to assess the degree of their disease and observed. In particular, those with the ecchymotic form and severe forms are considered to be at risk for large vessel rupture and subcutaneous or gastrointestinal hemorrhages. Elective surgeries are avoided, and required interventions are limited in extent. They are also approached with preparations to support hemostasis and transfusions if necessary. Wounds are closed with long-term resorbable or nonresorbable sutures.

PROGNOSIS ▶

Patients with mild forms of the syndrome live full life spans. The ecchymotic form and the severe forms have variable life expectancies related to the severity of disease expression. Cardiovascular and gastrointestinal bleeding is the most significant complication and tends to occur in the late teens and early adult years.

Marfan Syndrome

CLINICAL PRESENTATION AND PATHOGENESIS ▶

Marfan syndrome is an autosomal-dominant trait. About 85% of cases result from transferred inheritance and 15% from new mutations in the sperm or oocyte prior to fertilization. The clinical features result from a basic defect in chromosome 15, which codes for a protein responsible for collagen's strength. Therefore, defective collagen that is more soluble and more elastic is formed and is incorporated into every organ that contains collagen, producing the widespread multiorgan manifestations of Marfan syndrome.

Individuals take on a distinctive "marfanoid" appearance characterized by a tall, slender build, long arms and legs, large hands, long fingers (called *arachnodactyly* because the fingers resemble the legs of a spider), and loose joints (Figs 4-43a and 4-43b). There is a disproportionate skeletal growth; the lower body segment (pubis to feet) is more elongated than the upper body segment (pubis to vertex of skull). It is speculated that Abraham Lincoln may have had Marfan syndrome.

The oral and maxillofacial area manifests the long face characteristics with a tendency toward prognathism. The palate is said to be highly arched and the arch form tapered. Malocclusion is an anticipated concern, and the teeth are often elongated.

The eyes will often be noted to have blue sclerae due to the defective collagen within the sclera revealing the choroidal plexus and retinal pigments (see Fig 4-43a). The suspensory ligaments of the lens

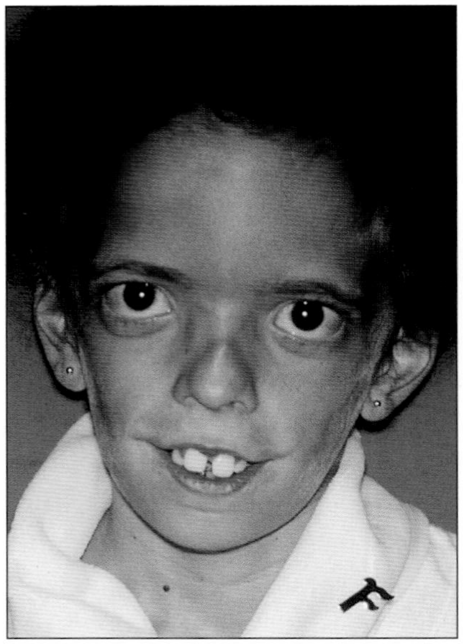

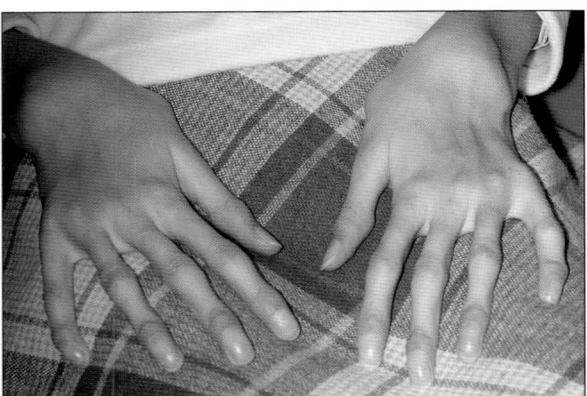

Fig 4-43a Prominent blue sclerae, exorbitism, hypertelorism, dolicephaly, and a "long face" are characteristic features of Marfan syndrome.

Fig 4-43b Arachnodactyly (spider-like fingers) is part of the disproportional skeletal growth in Marfan syndrome. Note also the increased length of the metacarpals.

break easily, resulting in the common finding of ectopic lenses (70% of cases) and lenses that are usually dislocated superiorly within the globe. Most patients are myopic, and detached retinas are common if individuals are physically active.

The skin will be stretchable in many individuals. Joints will also be hyperextensible and often lead to dislocations. Pectus excavatum is commonly seen.

The effects of defective collagen strength on the cardiovascular system pose the greatest risk and are the most common cause of sudden death in these individuals, occurring most commonly in their late teen years and early adulthood. All patients with Marfan syndrome have some degree of cardiovascular compromise. Mitral valve prolapse occurs in 80% of individuals. Some have mitral regurgitation due to severely "floppy" valves. Dilatation of the ascending aorta often creates aortic regurgitation and prevents complete filling of the coronary vessels, which in turn produces angina and ischemic electrocardiogram (ECG) changes as well as the potential for heart failure. Excessive aneurysmal dilatation may occur and, with rupture, lead to sudden death. The remaining cardiovascular system is also affected. Chordae tendinae are often incompetent, and renal artery changes lead to a high incidence of hypertension, which places the aortic dilatation at greater risk of an electrical malfunction of the heart or a catastrophic aneurysmal rupture.

Marfan syndrome occurs in about 2 per 100,000 births with an equal sex distribution. Because some of this syndrome is associated with sperm- and egg-related mutations, it is seen more commonly in children of older parents. Therefore, testing for chromosome 15 defects in older prospective parents can be of great value, as is prenatal testing of the fetus.

DIFFERENTIAL DIAGNOSIS ▶ The so-called marfanoid look is a feature of several syndromes and conditions. Some of the more apparent are *homocystinuria, multiple endocrine neoplasia syndrome type III,* and *Klinefelter syndrome.* Each can be distinguished from Marfan syndrome by the specific components seen in Marfan syndrome patients.

The blue sclerae and ectopic lens components are also common to *osteogenesis imperfecta* and *Ehlers-Danlos syndrome* and are part of homocystinuria findings. Each also can be separated from Marfan syndrome by its other components.

The diagnosis of Marfan syndrome is made from clinical findings. Urine hydroxyproline levels are elevated but are not usually needed to make a diagnosis. However, complete cardiovascular and ophthalmologic tests are required to assess the degree of involvement in each system and to predict risk.

Correction of these patients' associated malocclusions and prognathism is usually deferred because of the increased risks posed by their cardiovascular compromise and the greater priority of correcting correctable cardiovascular or ophthalmologic defects. If surgical procedures are performed for any reason, the American Heart Association's subacute bacterial endocarditis (SBE) prophylaxis regimen I is required (see Chapter 2, page 88, Table 2-2).

Today, alloplastic aortic valvular replacement and aortic arch replacements have greatly reduced the possibility of sudden death and are indicated wherever feasible. In patients not undergoing surgery, reduction of aortic vascular pressure with beta-blockers is indicated. (Note: Surgery subsequent to valvular–aortic arch replacement requires the AHA's SBE prophylaxis regimen II; see Chapter 2, page 88, Table 2-2).

Despite improvements in the correction of the cardiovascular defects, the prognosis remains poor. All vessels, including the great vessels of the heart and the heart itself, suffer from the same defect, which causes progressive and relentless dysfunction over time.

Mandibulofacial Dysostosis (Treacher Collins Syndrome)

Mandibulofacial dysostosis (MFD), also termed *Treacher Collins syndrome* after the individual who described its important components in 1900, is a distinct syndrome of known autosomal-dominant inheritance. Surviving individuals with MFD have a distinctive facial appearance (Fig 4-44a). It is characterized as "bird-like" or "fish-like" because of the convexity of the midface and underdevelopment of the mandible. The lower eyelid characteristically droops in the outer third, creating a downward sloping lateral canthus. The cheek prominences are flattened as a result of hypoplasia of the zygomas, and the pinnas of the ears are deformed. About 25% of affected individuals also have a tongue-shaped projection of hair over their zygoma as if it were an anteriorly positioned side burn.

The mandible is hypoplastic and creates an anteroposterior deficiency with an anterior open bite. The mandibular plane angle is very obtuse with prominent antegonial notching. The ramus and condyle are present but hypoplastic in all aspects. The maxilla is also hypoplastic but may show a posterior vertical maxillary excess, widely spaced teeth, and a highly arched palatal vault. The occlusion is usually a "scissors bite" type of malocclusion with rotated and lingually tipped teeth (Fig 4-44b).

Vision is normal, but the coloboma of the outer one third of the lower eyelid gives rise to a prominent "antimongoloid" slant, which is the prime recognition feature of this syndrome in 75% of individuals (see Fig 4-44a). In those with this feature, eyelashes medial to the coloboma are absent.

Hearing is abnormal. Conductive hearing loss is found to some degree in nearly all cases. This is most often due to sclerosis of the middle ear ossicles with fusion preventing transmission of vibratory energy. In some cases, one or more of the middle ossicles is absent or the oval window is absent. The external ear is deformed in about 80% of cases. The pinna may be hypoplastic, incomplete, crumpled, or displaced. The external ear canal is completely absent in about 30% of cases. In others, ear tags and skin pits occur in the cheek along the ala-tragal line (Fig 4-44c).

This syndrome does not seem to be directly associated with mental deficiencies, but learning disabilities exist and cognitive functions are secondarily impaired related to the hearing loss.

An associated cleft palate component is present in 30% of patients, and 15% have a lateral facial cleft created by elongation of one or both commissures. As part of the hypoplasia, the maxillary sinuses and the mastoid sinus usually are not pneumatized.

Mandibulofacial dysostosis is said to occur in half of cases as an autosomal-dominant trait and in the other half as a spontaneous mutation. This may be somewhat overstated because seemingly noninher-

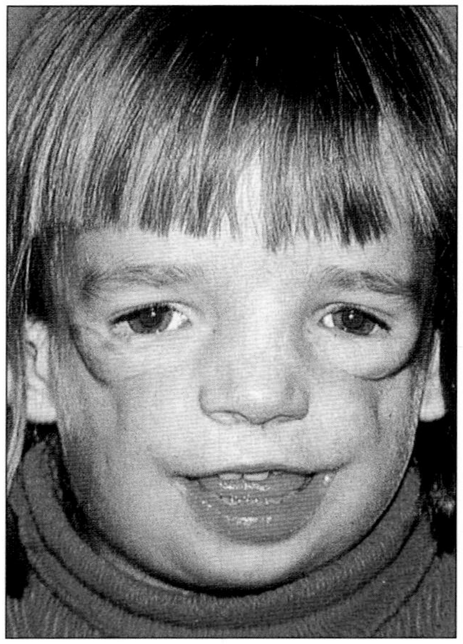

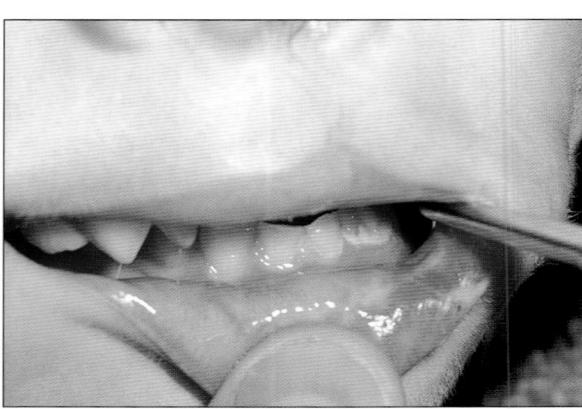

Fig 4-44a Distinctive "bird-like" facial appearance of mandibulofacial dysostosis (Treacher Collins syndrome).

Fig 4-44b Scissors-bite occlusion with lingually rotated teeth is common in mandibulofacial dysostosis (Treacher Collins syndrome).

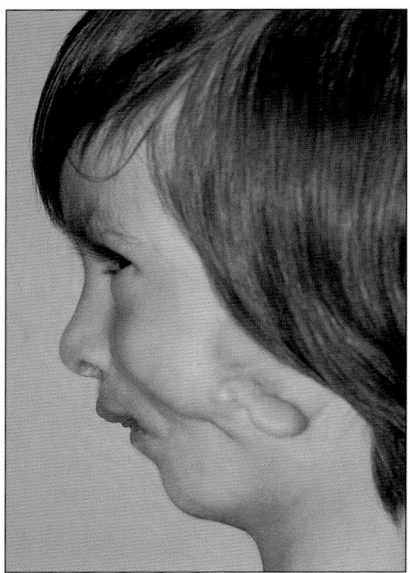

Fig 4-44c Syndromes such as Treacher Collins, Goldenhar, and hemifacial microsomia will often include malformed or absent external ears (pinnas).

ited cases may emerge from an existing inheritance that has a minimal or subclinical phenotypic expression. It is well-known that succeeding generations phenotypically express the defect as a more severe deformity. Today, rough statistics indicate that MFD occurs in 1 to 10 cases per 10,000 births, but this may be understated because the genetic defect is also associated with a high incidence of postnatal death (in addition to miscarriages and stillbirths).

The clinical disease is thought to be related to the absence or abnormality of the anterior portion of the fetal stapedial artery, which supplies the middle ear, maxilla, and the mandibular components of the first branchial arch; hence the location of the facial defects. Because the posterior branch of the stapedial artery is normal, the skull, scalp, and the area posterior to the ear are normal.

DIFFERENTIAL DIAGNOSIS ▶

Fully expressed MFD is distinctive. However, like most inherited deformities, a wide range of phenotypic expressions may be seen. Some cases will show only minimal signs and will, therefore, be difficult to recognize or seem to represent other syndromes. Other "mandibulofacial dysostoses" that cannot be easily classified, such as those described by François and Haustrate and by Peters and Hovels, among others, may represent only a minor variation of the same genetic defect.

One separate entity correctly belonging on a differential list with MFD of the Treacher Collins type is called *acrofacial dysostosis* as described by Nager and de Reynier. This syndrome is an autosomal-recessive trait that also manifests a "bird-like" facies due to mandibular hypoplasia, lower eyelid colobomas with a downward slope, and atresia of the external ear canal if lower eyelid colobomas are not present. This syndrome can be separated from MFD of the Treacher Collins type because of its additional components of hypoplastic or absent thumbs. There may also be fusion of the radius to the ulna or absence of either of these bones or of a metacarpal.

DIAGNOSTIC WORK-UP ▶

Mandibulofacial dysostosis of the Treacher Collins type is a diagnosis of clinical recognition. However, reconstructive surgical planning requires cephalometric tracings and CT scans in most cases. A complete audiologic examination is required.

TREATMENT ▶

The first priority in reconstructive surgery should be middle ear reconstruction to restore as much conductive hearing as possible. Hearing aids may also be required.

Orbital reconstruction and the zygoma deficiency are often approached with cranial bone grafts. Zygomatic osteotomies and Le Fort II–type osteotomies are other approaches that have been used to correct the midface and zygomatic maxillary complex. The lower eyelid can be improved with a cross eyelid flap and a lateral canthus repositioning.

The mandibular and maxillary hypoplasia usually requires extensive presurgical orthodontic arch coordination followed by a Le Fort I osteotomy and mandibular ramus osteotomies. Each case is different, but the general goal of orthognathic surgery is to impact and widen the posterior maxilla and autorotate and advance the mandible.

PROGNOSIS ▶

Reconstructive surgery can greatly improve the self-esteem and quality of life for these individuals. However, multiple staged surgeries followed by revisions are the rule, and the involvement of multiple specialists is required.

Hemifacial Microsomia–Oculoauriculovertebral Dysplasia (Goldenhar Syndrome Spectrum)

CLINICAL PRESENTATION AND PATHOGENESIS ▶

The term *hemifacial microsomia,* familiar to most oral and maxillofacial specialists, refers to varying degrees of hypoplasia or agenesis of mandibular condyle and ramus; hypoplasia of the temporal fossa, zygoma, and maxilla; lateral facial cleft; microtia (absence or remnants of ear structures); and variable ocular-dermoid hamartomas. An extended subset of findings occurs in some, representing a variant of hemifacial microsomia. This condition has been referred to as *oculoauriculovertebral dysplasia* or *Goldenhar syndrome.* In Goldenhar syndrome, findings also include vertebral abnormalities such as fusion of the atlas (C-1) to the occipital bone, hemicervical vertebrae, and cervical fusions. In addition, about 50% also have some type of cardiac abnormality.

There appears to be a 3:2 male-female predilection, and a reported 62% of cases are right sided. The specific facial malformations may include agenesis of the muscles of mastication and the parotid on the involved side. The hypoplastic to agenic temporal fossa-condyle-ramus complex results in deviation of the occlusion and symphysis to the affected side (Fig 4-45a). The maxilla, zygoma, and temporal bones are also hypoplastic. The maxillary dentition is often supraerupted on the unaffected side because of absence of occlusal contact and undererupted on the affected side because of both hypoplasia and an encroachment on the interarch space by the collapsed mandible (Fig 4-45b). About 10% of individuals also have a complete cleft lip and/or palate. The facial cleft is usually a mild extension of the ipsilateral commissure (Fig 4-46).

The ear malformations are similar to those seen in mandibulofacial dysostosis and are associated with conductive hearing loss extending to deafness in 50% of individuals. The hearing loss or deafness is due to absent or malformed middle ear ossicles. The pinna is involved in 100% of cases and will range from complete agenesis to residual ear-skin tags that are usually anterior to their anticipated location, some as far anterior as the midcheek or commissure (see Fig 4-44c).

The ocular dermoids, which are extraocular, are mostly in the lower outer quadrant of the orbit and create a soft tissue enlargement in the area (see Fig 4-46). A type of dermoid with some fat tissue within it (lipodermoid) has a propensity for the upper outer quadrant. Of those individuals with ocular dermoids, 60% have bilateral involvement. The 40% with unilateral involvement have the dermoid on the ipsilateral side of the facial malformations. Rare cases of microphthalmia or even anophthalmia have been reported. When either of these two findings is present, mental retardation occurs.

The vertebral anomalies occur in about 50% of cases. The common abnormality is fusion of the atlas to the occipital bone. Other vertebral abnormalities are hemivertebrae, fused vertebrae, supernumerary vertebrae, and spina bifida. While the cervical vertebrae are most affected, other vertebrae are also at risk.

About 50% of patients have an associated heart abnormality. The types are many, ranging from septal defects to tetrology of Fallot or any of its individual components.

The pathogenesis of hemifacial microsomia is unclear. Some evidence suggests a genetic factor, and the great variability of components suggests more than one factor and perhaps spontaneous mutations.

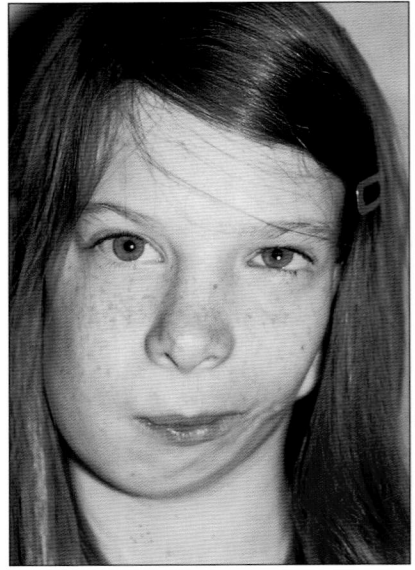

Fig 4-45a Mandibular and maxillary hypoplasia on the affected side with rotation of the mandible to the affected side is common in hemifacial microsomia.

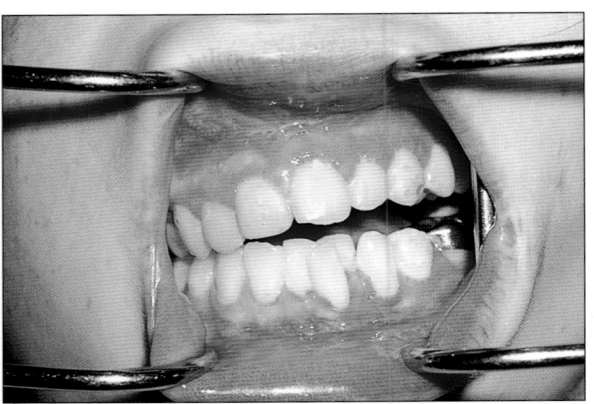

Fig 4-45b An open-bite deformity on the affected side is typical in hemifacial microsomia due to supraeruption of the teeth on the unaffected side and absent or delayed eruption on the affected side.

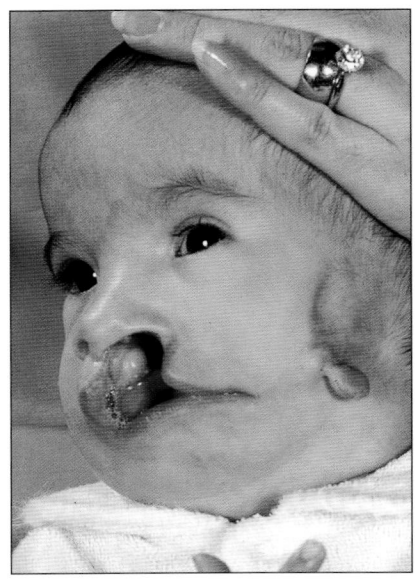

Fig 4-46 A unilateral facial cleft, complete cleft lip and palate, and ocular dermoids are often components of hemifacial microsomia.

Poswillo showed similar components in an animal model when he created hematomas related to the branchial arches in utero. It is, therefore, believed that this syndrome spectrum has several etiologies.

Extreme variability in severity and components is characteristic of this syndrome. Some patients may have only a single minor anomaly, such as a dysplastic ear or a hypoplastic ramus-condyle complex incidentally noticed on a panoramic radiograph (a forme fruste). Others may have an extensive array of anomalies consistent with what has been called *Goldenhar syndrome*, including heart defects and other internal organ defects.

DIFFERENTIAL DIAGNOSIS ▶

Hemifacial microsomia may appear similar to *mandibulofacial dysostosis* (Treacher Collins syndrome) except that hemifacial microsomia is unilateral, not bilateral, and mandibulofacial dysostosis frequently has characteristic bilateral downward displacements of the lateral one third of the lower eyelid (eyelid colobomas). Ear tags or misshapen ears may occur in the *Pierre Robin anomaly*, but the mandible in that anomaly is bilaterally symmetric, although very micrognathic. Extraocular dermoids are found in *frontonasal dysplasia,* but this malformation does not manifest ear tags or the hemifacial hypoplastic appearance of hemifacial microsomia. Teenaged and adult individuals with hemifacial microsomia may bear a resemblance to those with *hemifacial atrophy* (Romberg syndrome), but hemifacial atrophy occurs during the teen years in individuals who have to that point developed normally.

DIAGNOSTIC WORK-UP ▶

The diagnosis of this syndrome is one of clinical recognition. However, facial bone radiographs, CT scans, MRI scans, and echocardiography are often requested to assess for unnoticed components and/or to plan corrective surgeries.

TREATMENT ▶

Oral and maxillofacial surgery treatment focuses on correcting the components of the syndrome to improve the individual's function, development, and appearance. Children with agenesis of the condyle are often treated with a leveling osteotomy of the mandible combined with an autogenous costochondral graft at an early age (usually 18 months to 6 years). The maxillary occlusal cant is managed by serial splints, which guide eruption of the teeth to gain a level occlusion. The osteotomy should position the mandible in the midline and the costochondral graft should be placed with additional cancellous bone to fully reconstruct the ramus (Figs 4-47a and 4-47b). A costochondral graft will usually maintain a growth pattern on pace with the unaffected side until puberty. During that time, a rib will grow independently

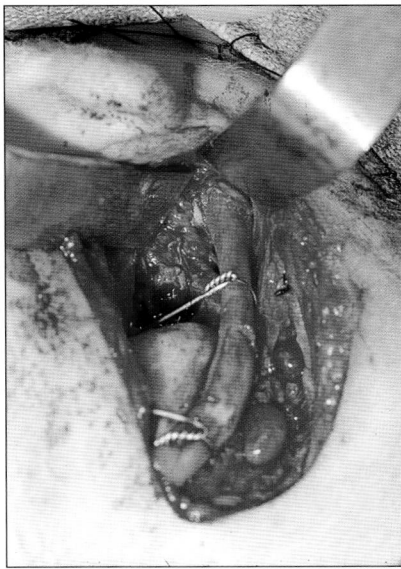 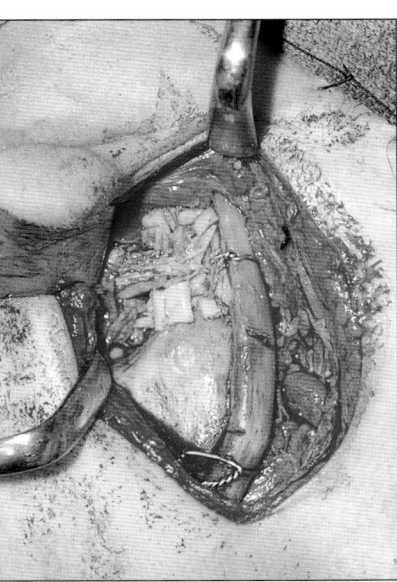

Fig 4-47a The costochondral rib graft is placed in the temporal fossa to reconstruct the articulation of the mandible on the affected side. Note that the costochondral rib graft alone does not fully reconstruct the ramus.

Fig 4-47b In children, a second rib graft can be harvested, particulated, and added to the costochondral graft to fully reconstruct the ramus.

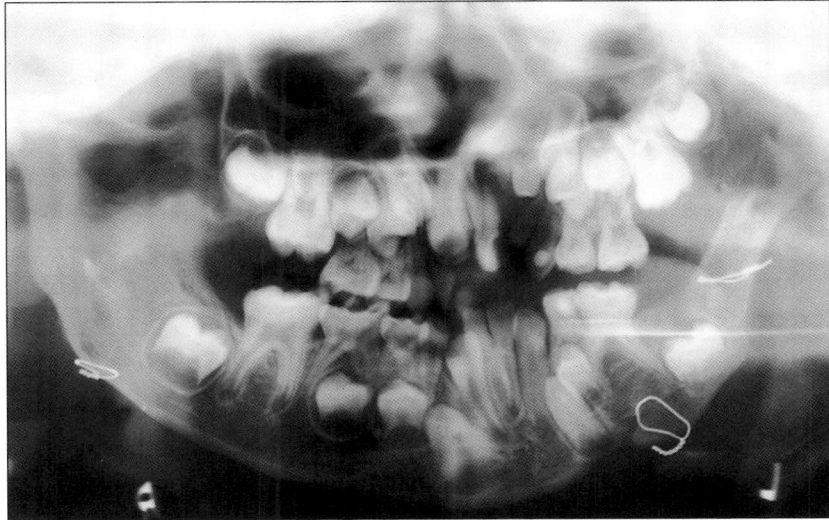 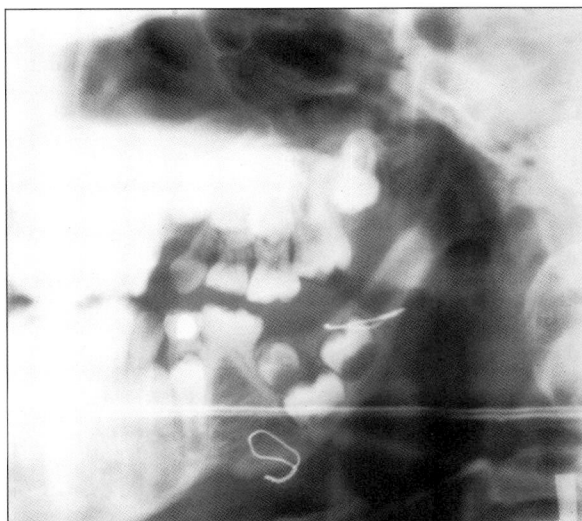

Fig 4-48a A costochondral rib graft will grow independent of the soft tissue matrix but proportional to chest growth. The rib graft originally placed at age 5 is seen here at age 10, having lengthened and maintained the symmetry of the mandible.

Fig 4-48b At age 13, after a somatic growth spurt brought on by puberty, the costochondral rib graft is shown to have lengthened to a point of overgrowth.

of these patients' deficient functional matrix by an endochondral growth plate mechanism at the cartilage-bone interface. Because rib growth roughly parallels mandibular growth during the prepubertal years, the mandible grows symmetrically. At puberty, about 60% of patients will begin to show an overgrowth consistent with the greater rib growth (chest development) related to puberty. The patient may then develop a lateral prognathism toward the opposite side and a flattened appearance on the affected side (Figs 4-48a and 4-48b). In such cases, the growth center must be removed in a condylectomy-like procedure and secondary osteotomies and bone grafts accomplished (Figs 4-48c to 4-48f).

In individuals who have only a hypoplastic ramus and condyle, the deformity is less severe. Before the eruption of permanent teeth, most can be treated with leveling ramus osteotomies of the mandible and serial maxillary splints. After eruption of the permanent teeth, most are treated by the same type of

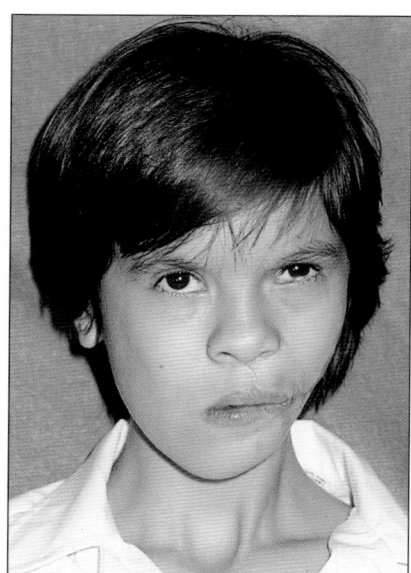

Fig 4-48c Overgrowth of a costochondral rib graft will displace the midline of the chin to the opposite side and flatten the contours of the affected side.

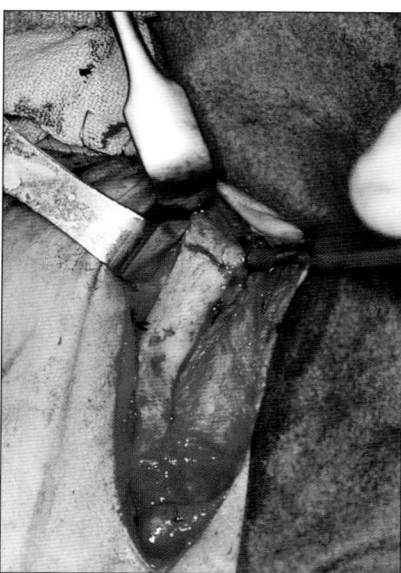

Fig 4-48d Upon exploration, a costochondral rib graft that has experienced overgrowth will resemble a natural rib with a hypertrophied costochondral junction. Here the excessive length of the costochondral graft is evident.

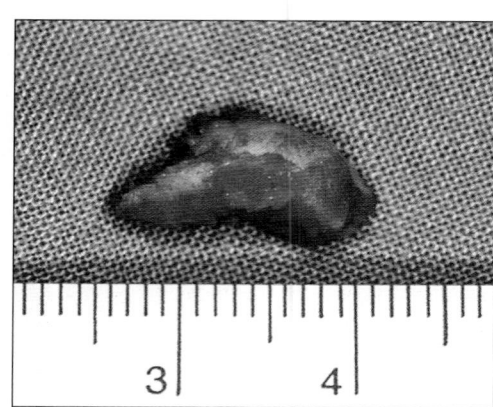

Fig 4-48e The costochondral junction of a costochondral rib graft that experienced overgrowth shows significant vertical and horizontal enlargement.

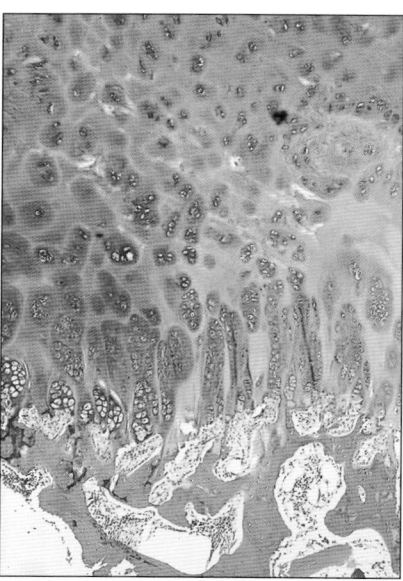

Fig 4-48f Histology from the costochondral junction of a costochondral rib graft that experienced overgrowth will show classic endochondral ossification similar to that of an epiphyseal growth plate.

osteotomies in the mandible and coordinated with a leveling Le Fort I osteotomy of the maxilla. Many also require a sliding osteotomy of the symphysis region to gain a midline chin point.

Because the ocular dermoids are extrabulbar, they may be excised or reduced via a lateral canthotomy approach. Patients with concomitant facial clefts or cleft lip and palate undergo surgery as is appropriate for each (lip and facial cleft at 2 to 3 months, cleft palate at 18 months to 2 years).

PROGNOSIS ▶

The components of the disease and their severity are established by the time of birth. Surgery can improve function and appearance and support better development, but it cannot achieve normalcy in any of these areas. Parents of children with hemifacial microsomia are best reminded of this and should know that initial corrective surgeries always require several additional surgeries and revisions.

Beckwith-Wiedemann Syndrome

CLINICAL PRESENTATION AND PATHOGENESIS ▶

Beckwith-Wiedemann syndrome is a syndrome of uncertain inheritance and multiple components, including prominent macroglossia and mandibular prognathism (Figs 4-49a, 4-49b, and 4-50). In addition, a nasal glabellar vascular malformation (which will diminish after the first year) and an omphalocele (abdominal cavity contents externalized through an umbilical defect) are usually present. In adults, the most prominent oral and maxillofacial features with which patients present will be macroglossia with prognathism together with a wide mandibular arch and an anterior open bite (due to the tongue size).

Additional components of the Beckwith-Wiedemann syndrome may include:

1. Neonatal hypoglycemia. Present in one third of cases, it is one of the most important and overlooked components of this syndrome. Unrecognized, it leads to mental deficiencies and mental retardation.
2. Ear lobe creases and pits. Seen best on the posterior aspect of the pinnas.

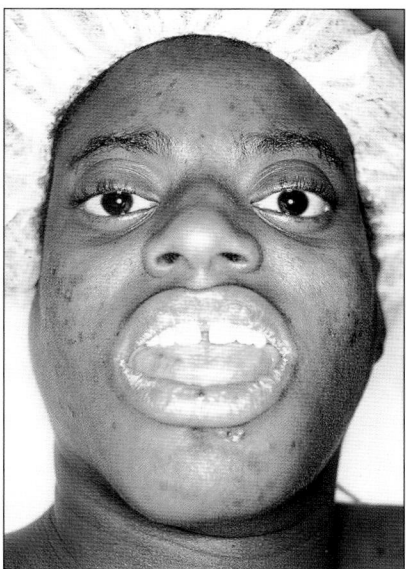

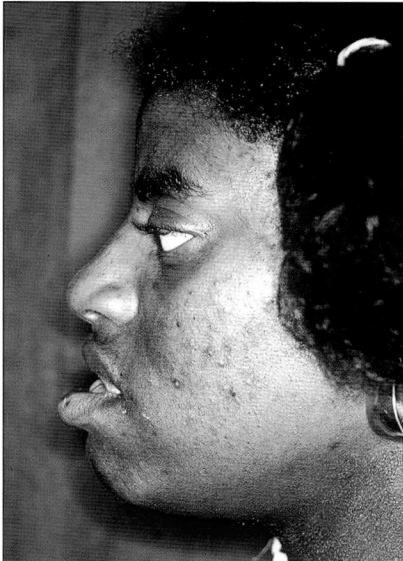

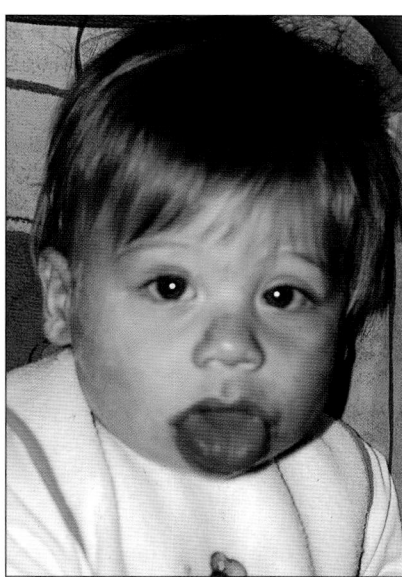

Fig 4-49a Prominent macroglossia produced lip incompetence and splaying of teeth due to Beckwith-Wiedemann syndrome. This patient underwent abdominal closure to correct an omphalocele as an infant.

Fig 4-49b Prognathism (mandibular anteroposterior excess) is a common component of Beckwith-Wiedemann syndrome.

Fig 4-50 The macroglossia in Beckwith-Wiedemann syndrome may develop in utero and is therefore seen in newborns and infants.

3. Cytomegaly of the adrenal cortex. Five percent of those affected later develop adrenal cortical carcinoma.
4. Renal medullary dysplasia. Five percent of those affected develop a Wilm tumor.
5. Skeletal enlargement (mild gigantism). Most patients will attain a height and weight above the 90th percentile.
6. Glandular hyperplasia. Hyperplasia of gonadal cells and of paraganglia, liver, thymus, and pancreas.
7. Diaphramatic elevations.
8. Visceral malrotations. Present in most cases with organ enlargement.

DIFFERENTIAL DIAGNOSIS ▶

The macroglossia, facial appearance, and slow mentation will initially be suggestive of *hypothyroidism, Hurler syndrome,* and *Sanfilippo syndrome,* the latter two being mucopolysaccharidosis I and III, respectively. To distinguish these from Beckwith-Wiedemann syndrome, one should seek signs of a repaired omphalocele or umbilic hernia, which would not be present in the other conditions.

DIAGNOSTIC WORK-UP ▶

The syndrome itself is diagnosed by its clinical components. However, a work-up that includes a serum glucose determination is important. In addition, serum cholesterol, triglycerides, and calcium have been noted as abnormal in many of these patients. These parameters as well as the response of insulin to glucose should be examined.

TREATMENT ▶

Most patients undergo abdominal repair of their omphalocele early in life. All hypoglycemic tendencies should be corrected. The macroglossia is difficult to manage. Glossoplasties are helpful, but the tendency of the tongue to re-enlarge continues after surgery. Corrective jaw surgery may also be indicated. In such cases, tongue size reduction before or during orthognathic surgery is often needed. Many cases will require two surgeries as the maxilla is often deficient in the anteroposterior direction.

Epidermolysis Bullosa

CLINICAL PRESENTATION AND PATHOGENESIS ▶

Epidermolysis bullosa is a set of hereditary diseases that result in defective components of collagen and other proteins of the basement membrane zone. There are several inheritance patterns and, therefore,

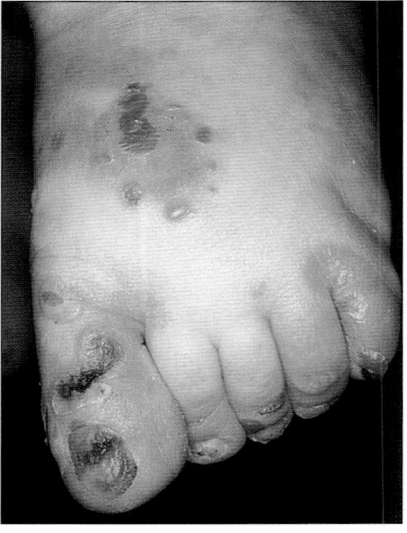

Fig 4-51 In infants, epidermolysis bullosa simplex oc- curs with small superficial bullae that heal without scar- ring. (Reprinted from Callen JP et al, *Color Atlas of Derma- tology*, with permission from WB Saunders and Co.)

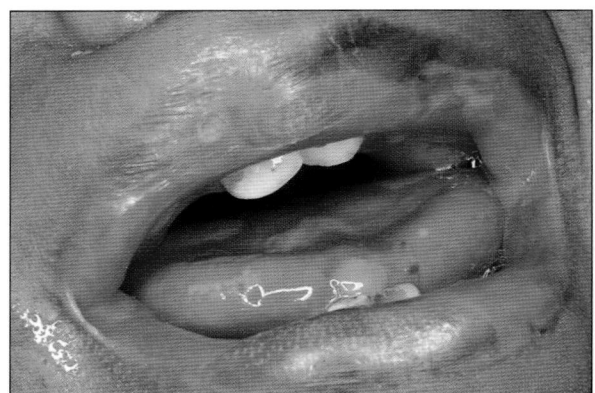

Fig 4-52 Epidermolysis bullosa simplex with muscular dystrophy frequently forms bullae of the oral mucosa. (Reprinted from Neville BW et al, *Color Atlas of Clinical Oral Pathology*, with permission from Lippincott Williams & Wilkins.)

several clinical presentations, but each will have the general manifestation of skin, oral, and sometimes other mucosal vesicles and bullae. The five recognized types are epidermolysis bullosa simplex, epider- molysis bullosa simplex with muscular dystrophy, epidermolysis bullosa atrophicans generalisata graves, epidermolysis bullosa dominant dystrophic/hypertrophic form, and scarring epidermolysis bullosa with dermolytic vesicles.

Epidermolysis Bullosa Simplex

Epidermolysis bullosa simplex clinically presents in neonates and infants. The nails, feet, hands, and neck develop vesicles and small bullae, presumably in response to friction. Oral vesicles are mild and small but do occur. The vesicles are located within the epithelium and, therefore, heal without scarring (Fig 4-51).

Epidermolysis Bullosa Simplex with Muscular Dystrophy

An autosomal-recessive disorder, epidermolysis bullosa simplex with muscular dystrophy appears at birth with multiple bullae and frequently includes oral mucosa. Extremities seem to develop more numerous bullae, which result in scarring and eventuate into muscular dystrophy with deformity (Fig 4-52). The mus- cular dystrophy may not be noted at birth but will be noted later with weakness and reduced strength.

Epidermolysis Bullosa Atrophicans Generalisata Graves

A severe clinical disease expression of autosomal-recessive inheritance, epidermolysis bullosa atrophi- cans generalisata graves develops in neonates within hours after birth and in infants. The nail beds are usually the first area of involvement; shedding of the nail is common. The remainder of the skin surface progressively develops bullae with the exception of the palms and soles. Many infants die within a few months. Survivors have nail distortion, growth retardation, anemia, scarring, and continued excoriated skin lesions. Oral lesions are found in almost all patients. Large, fragile vesicles and bullae are common, particularly on the posterior hard palate mucosa and soft palate. Teeth may be affected by enamel hypo-

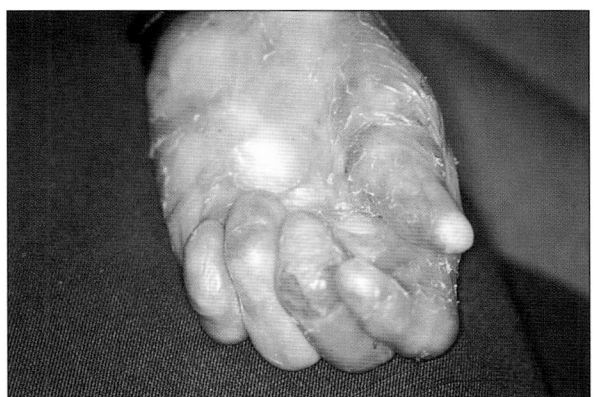

Fig 4-53 Epidermolysis bullosa dominant dystrophic/ hypertrophic form with dystrophic nails, prominent scarring and thick skin pads. (Reprinted from Laskaris G, *Color Atlas of Oral Diseases* 2nd ed, with permission from Thieme Medical Publishers.)

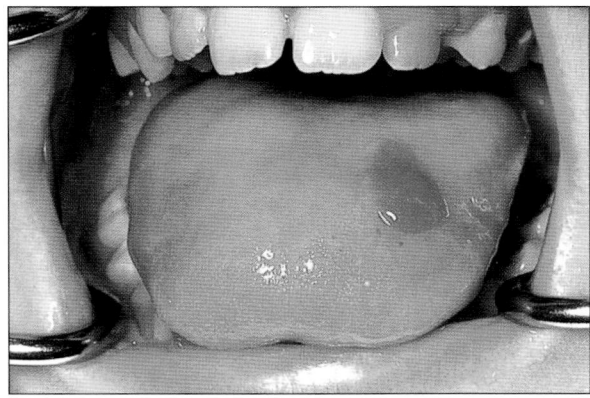

Fig 4-54 Vesicle on the tongue associated with skin bullae in scarring epidermolysis bullosa with dermolytic vesicles. (Reprinted from Strassburg M and Knolle G, *Diseases of the Oral Mucosa: A Color Atlas* 2nd ed, with permission from Quintessence Publishing Co.)

plasia and enamel pits, leading to caries. Perioral hemorrhagic and crusting lesions around the alar base and commissures are particularly noted to develop between 6 and 12 months of age.

Epidermolysis Bullosa Dominant Dystrophic/Hypertrophic Form

The dominant dystrophic/hypertrophic form of epidermolysis bullosa is a mild form of autosomal-dominant inheritance. It does not appear at birth, and only 20% of individuals develop manifestations before 1 year of age. Once vesicles or bullae begin to develop, they will gradually lessen with age. This type of epidermolysis bullosa is noted for scar formation. After bullae heal, they develop characteristically thick scars. Dystrophic nails also will develop. In addition, scarring of the skin at prominent areas of occurrence, such as the ankles, knees, hands, and elbows, will produce a thick skin pad in these locations (Fig 4-53). Teeth are not affected by this form of epidermolysis bullosa, but thick white mucosal pads and white mucosal-epithelial inclusion cysts may be seen on the tongue, buccal mucosa, and palatal mucosa.

Scarring Epidermolysis Bullosa with Dermolytic Vesicles

Scarring epidermolysis bullosa with dermolytic vesicles is autosomal recessive. It appears shortly after birth with skin bullae on the feet, fingers, buttocks, back, and occiput. Slight trauma or friction provokes bullae as it does in all forms of epidermolysis bullosa. This form seems to be somewhat more painful than most others and forms significant scarring, even keloid-like scars in some cases. This is thought to be caused by the deeper level of bullae formation, essentially on the dermal side of the basement membrane zone.

Oral vesicles (Fig 4-54) develop with the skin bullae and are just as prone to scar formation. Ankyloglossia or mucogingival scar bands in the vestibule may result. Commissures may develop scarring as well, causing a restriction of opening similar to that seen in scleroderma. Teeth will demonstrate pits and enamel hypoplasia, leading to caries.

DIFFERENTIAL DIAGNOSIS ▶

Epidermolysis bullosa is highly suggested by its familial inheritance, age of onset, and clinical picture. Only a few serious considerations on a differential diagnosis are warranted, including *bullous impetigo, dermatitis herpetiformis, pemphigus vulgaris,* and *erythema multiforme.* Any of these may form significant bullae and cause scar formation and may occur in infants and young children.

DIAGNOSTIC WORK-UP ▶

The diagnosis of epidermolysis bullosa is mostly by history and clinical presentation. However, a biopsy of a vesicle and adjacent normal tissue is needed to rule out specific autoimmune-based diseases such as pemphigus and to assess for the ultrastructural changes associated with some of the epidermolysis bullosa types. Therefore, the clinician should plan for a sufficient specimen size and prepare it for routine H&E sections, direct immunofluorescence, and electron microscopy.

HISTOPATHOLOGY ▶

The light microscopic findings of these diseases are nonspecific. They are all characterized by subepidermal bullae, which initially show little inflammation. Precise diagnosis requires electron microscopy and immunofluorescence mapping. From a histopathologic perspective, three types are recognized and will relate to certain clinical types:

Epidermal Type

Separation occurs through the basal cell layer. There is intracellular edema below the nuclei with subsequent vacuolation and disruption of the plasma membrane of the basal cell. This is seen in the simplex types.

Junctional Type

Separation occurs in the lamina lucida, secondary to decreased numbers of hemidesmosomes and abnormal hemidesmosomes due to poorly developed attachment plaques and subbasal dense plates. This is seen in lesional and nonlesional tissue. Affected teeth show abnormal enamel formation. The initial layer of enamel matrix is laminated, but the remainder is globular. The underlying problem is akin to that occuring in the skin, as vesicles form between the ameloblasts and the odontoblasts with the basement membrane remaining attached to the odontoblasts. It appears that ameloblasts develop normally or until the time of dentin formation when the cells form a little enamel matrix and then undergo squamous metaplasia. The dentin surface is irregular but not otherwise affected. This type is seen in epidermolysis bullosa atrophicans generalisata graves and the dominant dystrophic/hypertrophic types.

Dermal Type

Separation occurs deep to the lamina densa where the anchoring fibrils appear rudimentary and are decreased in number in both lesional and nonlesional tissue. In addition, fibroblasts form excessive amounts of collagenase, and a defect of a lamina densa protein has been noted. Milia that may form in oral mucosa are essentially epithelial cysts, derived from the epithelium that is detached during bulla formation. Dental findings are similar to those in the junctional form with enamel hypoplasia due to absence of the enamel's normal prismatic structure. Overproduction of poorly calcified cementum has also been described. This type is seen in the scarring types of epidermolysis bullosa.

Immunomapping

Immunomapping requires fresh, artificially induced blisters, such as suction blisters, as these are devoid of secondary changes. Cryostat sections of the tissue are then exposed to specific antisera against type IV collagen (found in the lamina densa and basal lamina), laminin (in the lower lamina lucida), and cutaneous pemphigoid antigen (BPAg) (in the upper lamina lucida). In the epidermal form, all antigens are at the base of the blister. In the junctional form, type IV collagen and laminin are on the floor, and BPAg is on the roof. In the dermal form, all of these antigens are on the roof.

TREATMENT ▶

Treatment is frustrating for the patient and clinician because at this time no treatment can alter the defective basement membrane zone proteins, which are produced by mutations in specific genes. Because these epidermolysis bullosa types are not autoimmune diseases, as is epidermolysis bullosa acquisita, systemic corticosteroids are not as effective. Systemic corticosteroid regimens such as regimen I, IIIA, and IIIB are used (see pages 205 to 206), but they only reduce secondary inflammation and scarring and do not alter the course of the disease. In addition, dapsone, 50 to 100 mg per day; retinoic acid-A, 30 to 60 mg per day; and beta carotene, 30 mg four times per day, may also have some beneficial results.

Ectodermal Dysplasia

CLINICAL PRESENTATION AND PATHOGENESIS ▶

Ectodermal dysplasia is a syndrome characterized by the clinical findings of hypodontia (missing and/or conical teeth), hypotrichosis (missing and/or sparse hair), and hypohidrosis (dry skin). It is primarily an inherited X-linked recessive trait associated with the repressed expression of a gene on the X chromosome in the positions from q13 to q21. Consequently, it is more common in men. Women often represent asymptomatic or only mildly affected carriers; however, some women have a fully expressed ectodermal dysplasia thought to be related to an autosomal recessive form indistinguishable from the more common X-linked form seen in men.

Essentially, the partial or complete loss of this gene function affects the number and complete development of ectodermal appendages, of which teeth, hair follicles, sweat glands, and sebaceous glands are the common targets. However, minor salivary glands, meibomian glands, and lacrimal glands may be affected as well.

The individual will be missing numerous teeth, especially the molar teeth, and may even be edentulous. The teeth that are present, most likely incisors and canines, will have conical crowns (Fig 4-55a) and roots and may also have shortened roots due to the effects of this gene loss on both the full development of the enamel organ and Hertwig root sheath. Because of these effects on the teeth, most individuals will have a reduced alveolar bone, a reduced vertical dimension, and consequently a pseudo-prognathism with an everted lower lip (Fig 4-55b). There may also be some xerostomia related to hypoplasia of minor salivary glands.

The facial appearance will be one of prognathism and prominent brow ridges (see Fig 4-55b). The eyebrows, facial hair, and scalp hair are usually thinned but may be absent in severe cases. The skin is soft, thin, and dry. There may be mild xerophthalmia if the lacrimal gland is hypoplastic, which will be worsened by the loss of meibomian glands. There is usually some corneal thinness as well.

The dryness of the skin and inability to sweat may produce fevers of unknown origin particularly in infants or children in whom the syndrome has not yet been diagnosed. Since both sweat and sebaceous glands are significantly reduced in about 65% of individuals, they will also develop eczema. The nails are usually normal.

DIFFERENTIAL DIAGNOSIS ▶

Ectodermal dysplasia is a distinctive clinical recognition diagnosis, particularly if all three components are present. However, it may be confused with other entities that resemble a single component of ectodermal dysplasia. *Isolated oligodontia* is the most apparent. The lip scarring of rhagades and the saddle nose deformity in *congenital syphilis* may resemble the facial picture of ectodermal dysplasia. Congenitally missing teeth are found in the rare *Witkop tooth-nail syndrome*, and conical teeth are found in *acrodental dysostosis. Trichodental syndrome*, an autosomal-dominant trait, produces congenitally missing teeth and fine, sparse hair and eyebrows, but no dry skin. This syndrome will resemble ectodermal dysplasia more closely than any other.

DIAGNOSTIC WORK-UP ▶

A panoramic radiograph is recommended to confirm the true absence rather than the lack of eruption of teeth and to assess their root shape and development. The remaining work-up consists only of a careful topographic examination. If the hypohidrosis is equivocal, it can be assessed by means of the starch-iodine test that is used on the face to detect sweating from aberrant reinnervation of sweat glands after surgery for Frey syndrome (see pages 28 to 30), using a 5-mg pilocarpine iontophoresis challenge.

HISTOPATHOLOGY ▶

Both hidrotic and anhidrotic types demonstrate hypoplasia of hair and sebaceous glands. Their numbers and size are reduced, and their maturation is affected. In the anhidrotic form, the eccrine glands are also affected. They may be completely absent or present in a few areas in a hypoplastic form.

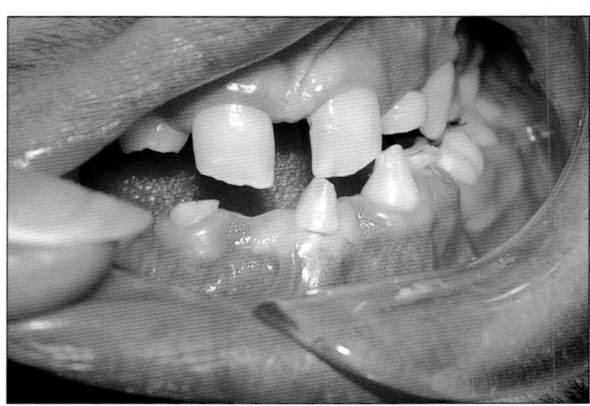

Fig 4-55a Some missing teeth, conical crowns, tapered and shortened roots, and excessive spacing between teeth are common oral manifestations of ectodermal dysplasia.

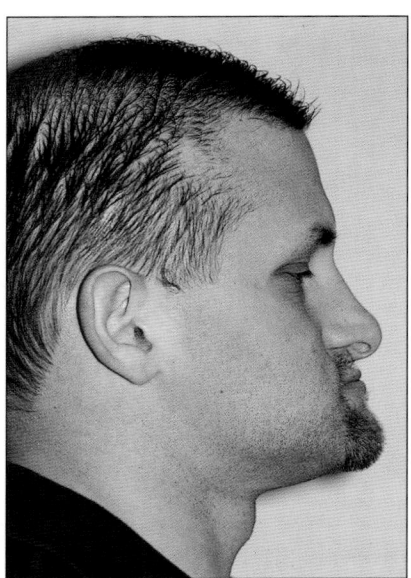

Fig 4-55b This individual's mandibular prognathism, thinned hair, and dry skin are typical of ectodermal dysplasia.

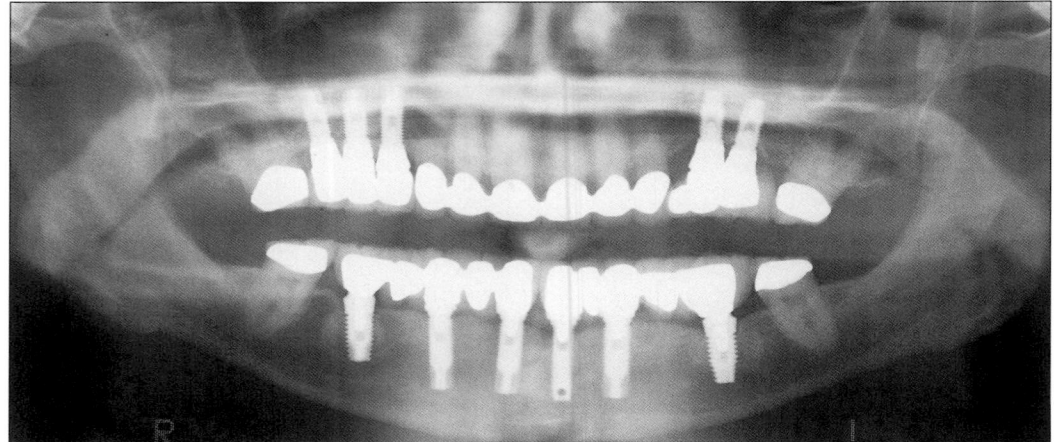

Fig 4-56 Since the bone is normal in individuals with ectodermal dysplasia, developmentally missing teeth or hypoplastic teeth lost because of incomplete root formation can be replaced with dental implant–supported restorations.

TREATMENT AND PROGNOSIS ▶

Salivary glands may be hypoplastic, and minor salivary glands may even be absent, resulting in xerostomia. Hypoplasia of nasal and pharyngeal mucous glands can cause rhinitis and pharyngitis.

Because of its genetic basis, there is no treatment to alter the course of ectodermal dysplasia. Symptom-related treatments that may be used include pilocarpine, 5 mg by mouth twice or three times a day, to improve xerostomia, xerophthalmia, and the ability to sweat in the facial skin area but not in other areas. This improved sweating ability from pilocarpine will be limited to the facial skin area because only the sweat glands located in the facial skin are innervated by sympathetic nerves, which have cholinergic receptors rather than the usual adrenergic receptors. The missing teeth may be replaced with overdentures or removable partial dentures if the conical teeth can be crowned to improve retention. Since the bone is normal, dental implants are an ideal dental replacement concept in individuals with ectodermal dysplasia (Fig 4-56).

Hyperplasias, Hamartomas, and Neoplasms: Their Biology and Its Impact on Treatment Decisions

CHAPTER 5

▶ *"The difficulty lies not in new ideas, but in escaping old ones."*
—John Keynes

The majority of the diseases found in a textbook of oral and maxillofacial pathology involve some type of cellular proliferation. Tissue masses are often generically referred to as tumors without distinguishing their specific pathology and their anticipated behavior or natural course. Therefore, simple growths such as the traumatic fibroma or pyogenic granuloma (pregnancy tumor) are considered as much of a "tumor" as an ossifying fibroma or a pleomorphic adenoma. Similarly, what are merely distorted attempts at tooth formation, such as odontomas and ameloblastic fibro-odontomas, have been elevated to "tumor" status on a par with the true odontogenic neoplasms represented by the ameloblastoma and the odontogenic myxoma. This chapter defines and separates the various broad categories of cellular proliferation according to their biologic behavior and describes the treatments necessary to resolve them. The separation of hyperplasias, hamartomas, choristomas, teratomas, benign neoplasms, and malignant neoplasms from each other is integral to the succeeding chapters, where specific surgical margins, contiguous tissue excisions, and adjunctive therapies are chosen based on an understanding of the dynamics of each disease category.

Hyperplasias

Hyperplasias may produce tissue masses referred to as tumors; however, they represent a limited cellular proliferation. Like hamartomas, they cease growth at some point and, unlike true neoplasms, they lack the capacity for autonomous growth. However, they may resemble neoplasms clinically and histologically by virtue of their increased cellularity, as demonstrated by the peripheral giant cell proliferation (Fig 5-1) and the common intraoral fibroma (Fig 5-2). The evolution of these lesions is usually initiated and controlled by an identifiable stimulus; however, the process stops when the stimulus is removed.

Hamartomas

Hamartomas represent a dysmorphic proliferation of tissue that is native to the area and does not have the capacity for continuous growth but merely parallels that of the host. The distinction between a hamartoma and a benign neoplasm is often arbitrary; in fact, most benign tumors of infancy and childhood are actually developmental hamartomas. Hemangiomas (Fig 5-3) and pigmented nevi are often cited as examples of hamartomas, as are odontomas, ameloblastic fibro-odontomas (Fig 5-4), and squamous odontogenic tumors. The salient features of hamartomas are that they cease growing at some point in their course and they do not infiltrate into surrounding tissues. Therefore, in bone they may be treated for cure by enucleation procedures and in soft tissue by local pericapsular excisions.

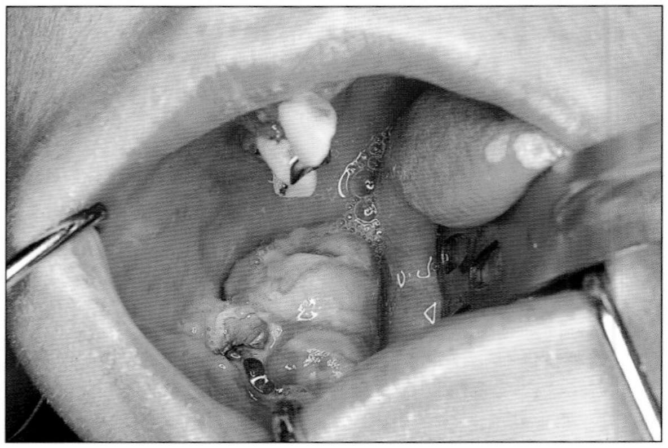

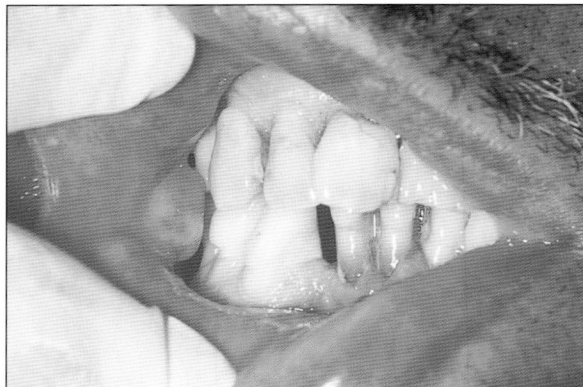

Fig 5-1 A peripheral giant cell proliferation represents a hyperplasia provoked by inflammation.

Fig 5-2 Although usually regarded as a neoplasia, the common intraoral fibroma more likely represents a hyperplasia initially provoked by a cheek-biting injury or a hamartoma of mucosal fibroblasts.

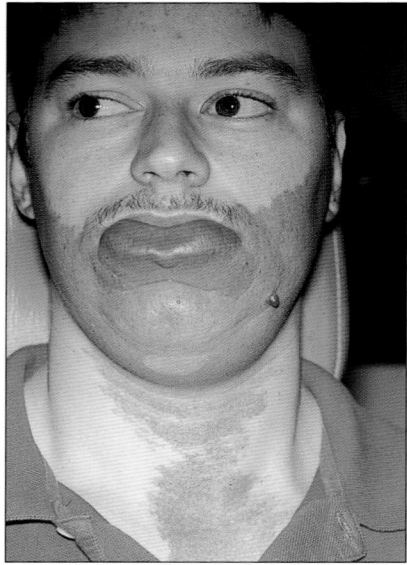

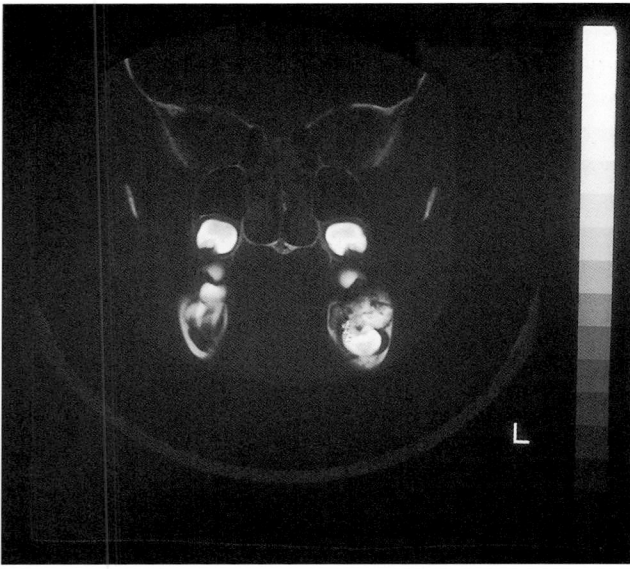

Fig 5-3 Although they may become large and cover a broad area, hemangiomas represent malformed blood vessels with limited growth potential.

Fig 5-4 This ameloblastic fibro-odontoma is little more than a disorganized attempt at tooth formation and thus represents a hamartoma rather than a true neoplasm.

Choristomas

Choristomas are similar to hamartomas except that they are dysmorphic proliferations of tissue that are not native to the site. Three examples are the rare heterotopic gastrointestinal cyst, which may be found in the tongue or floor of the mouth of infants and contains gastrointestinal glandular structures; the rare finding of bone or cartilage in the tongue (Fig 5-5); and the occasional development of thyroid tissue in the posterior tongue (Fig 5-6). The more commonly seen ectopic sebaceous glands known as Fordyce granules (Fig 5-7) and salivary gland tissue within lymph nodes may also be considered choristomas. Each has a limited proliferation.

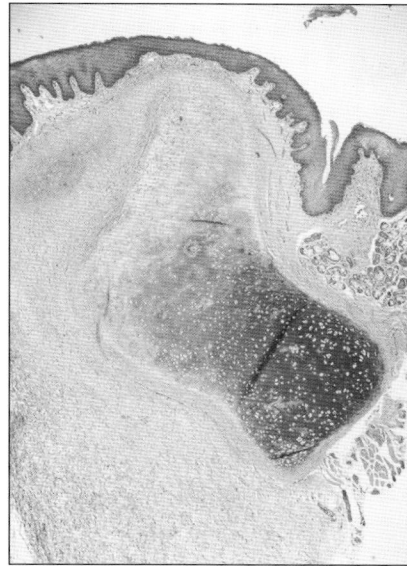

Fig 5-5 A well-defined mass of cartilage within the tongue representing a choristoma.

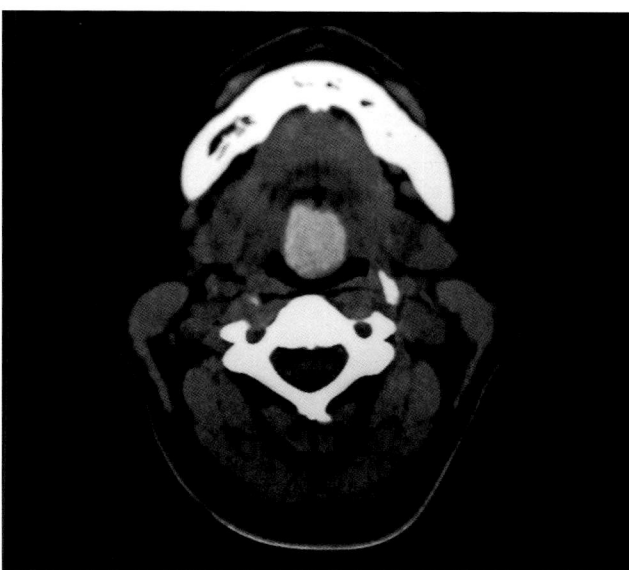

Fig 5-6 Formation of the thyroid gland in the tongue rather than in the neck is an example of a choristoma.

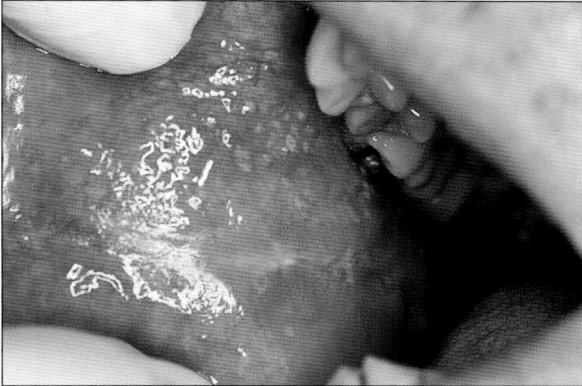

Fig 5-7 Ectopic sebaceous glands in the oral mucosa (Fordyce granules) are perhaps the most common example of choristomas.

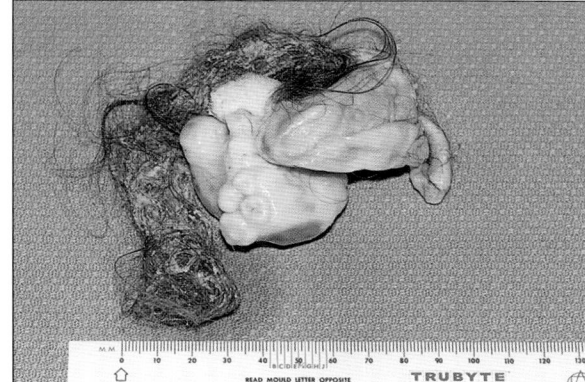

Fig 5-8 A teratoma such as this is a specific type of benign neoplasm that has structures from all three germ layers and a continuous growth potential.

Teratomas

Teratomas, which are often thought of as hamartomas or choristomas, are actually true neoplasms with the capacity for continual growth. They are neoplasias that arise from multiple germ layers and thus produce tissues that are foreign to the part in which they develop. They are distinct from other neoplasias that may also show tissue diversity, such as pleomorphic adenomas of salivary glands, which are derived from native tissue. The majority of teratomas occur within the ovary, where they are usually benign, or in the testes, where they are predominantly malignant. Teratomas also are seen in the neck, the jaws, and the floor of the mouth on rare occasions. One tumor of particular interest is the benign cystic teratoma of the ovary. Because of its origin from three germ layers, it will form various components of skin (including hair and sebaceous glands), teeth, and bone (Fig 5-8). The degree of differentiation and normal arrangement can be quite remarkable including bone with erupted teeth and even a fibrous periodontal ligament.

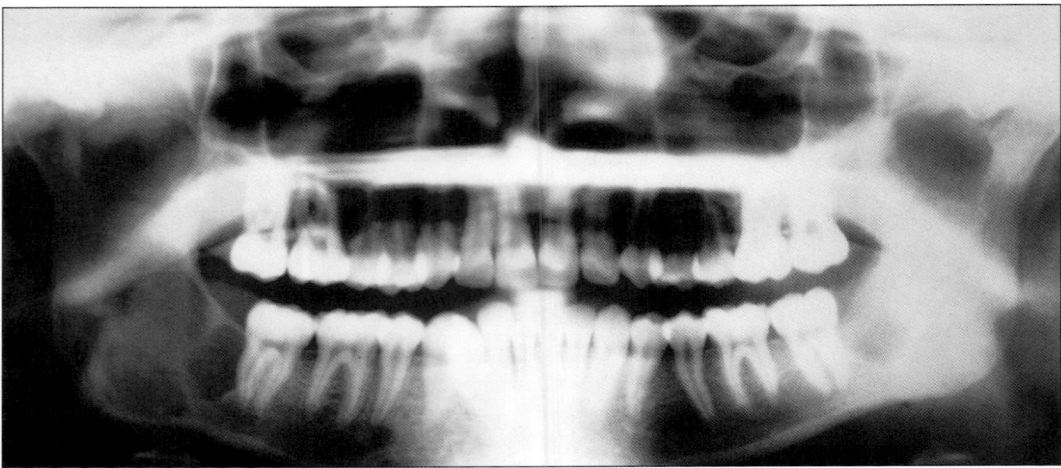

Fig 5-9 The ameloblastoma is typical of a true benign neoplasm by virtue of its continuous slow growth and its inability to metastasize.

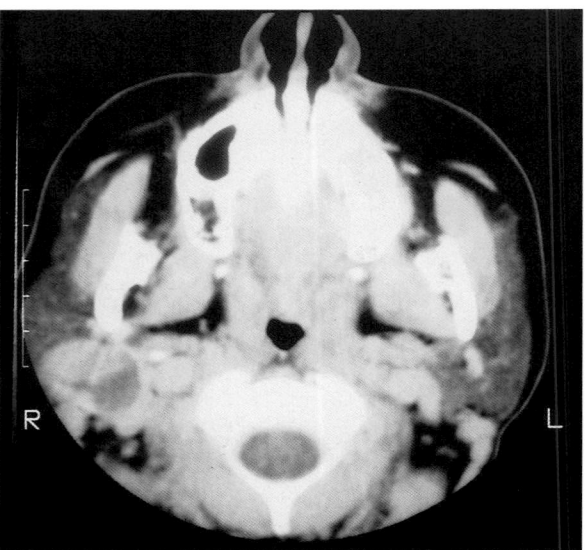

Fig 5-10 The pleomorphic adenoma, another example of a true benign neoplasm, will show slow but continuous growth and no metastatic ability. Note: A pleomorphic adenoma can transform into a malignancy, in which case it is termed a *carcinoma ex pleomorphic adenoma* and then has the ability to metastasize.

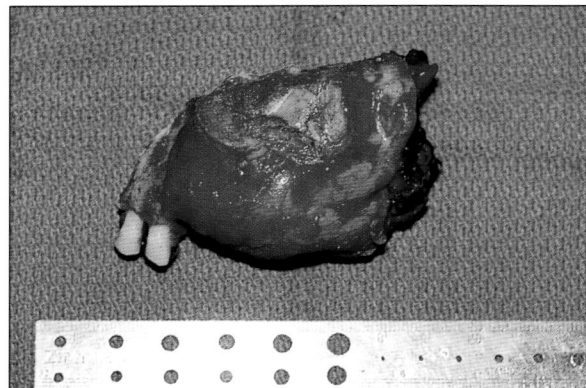

Fig 5-11 The ossifying fibroma is an example of a true benign neoplasm of bone.

Benign Neoplasms

Benign neoplasms also are dysmorphic proliferations of tissues, but they have the capacity for continuous autonomous growth. These neoplasms will continue to proliferate, albeit slowly in most cases, unless completely removed. Benign neoplasms are the result of genetic alterations that confer the property of continual autonomous growth, often including local tissue infiltration, but do not elaborate the enzymes and growth factors necessary for metastasis. Therefore, they require an en-bloc excision with tumor-free margins for cure.

The ameloblastoma of the jaws (Fig 5-9), the pleomorphic adenoma of salivary glands (Fig 5-10), and the ossifying fibroma of bone (Fig 5-11) are all examples of true benign neoplasms. These and other true neo-

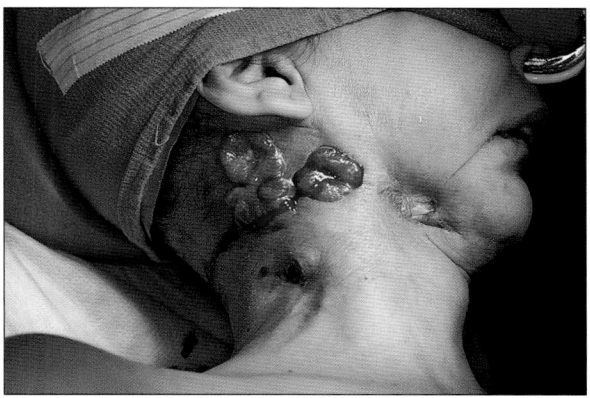

Fig 5-12 Squamous cell carcinoma is a good example of a malignant neoplasm owing to its continual infiltrative growth and its ability to metastasize to lymph nodes and distant organs.

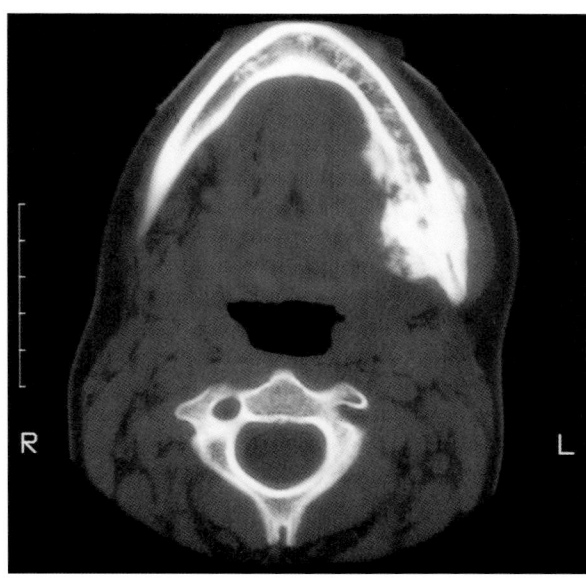

Fig 5-13 The osteosarcoma is the prototypical mesenchymal malignancy by virtue of its continuous infiltrative growth and ability to metastasize via the bloodstream.

plasms described elsewhere in this book are best characterized as continual proliferations with slow but unlimited growth potential. Hyperplasias are best characterized as limited cellular proliferations related to a stimulus that may have already disappeared or can be removed. Hamartomas are limited proliferations of tissue with no known stimulus and no truly invasive properties.

Malignant Neoplasms

Malignant neoplasms are dysmorphic proliferations of tissues that also have the capacity for continuous autonomous growth. However, they further elaborate the enzymes and growth factors necessary for metastasis and have a much higher spontaneous mutation rate so that they always have the potential to increase their growth rate, infiltrate native tissues faster than before, or metastasize after having shown no previous metastatic capability. Therefore, timely and complete removal is the first step in their treatment. Malignancies frequently require wide excisions with frozen section control of the margins and may often also require incontinuity excisions of adjacent anatomy and the known pathways of their spread (eg, the lymphadenectomy neck dissections associated with oral squamous cell carcinomas and the proximal neurovascular bundle excisions associated with adenoid cystic carcinoma). In addition, their propensity for regional and distant metastasis often necessitates adjunctive radiotherapy or chemotherapy.

Oral squamous cell carcinomas (Fig 5-12) and osteosarcomas of the jaws (Fig 5-13) both represent malignant neoplasms with the common features of continuous autonomous growth, metastatic potential, and mutagenicity to even more aggressive behavior.

Benign Epithelial Tumors of Mucosa and Skin

CHAPTER 6

▶ "I dressed the wound and God healed him."
—Ambrose Pare

This chapter discusses benign epithelial tumors of mucosa and skin. In this context the term *tumor* is used in the generic sense of an increase in cellular mass. The so-called tumors of this chapter primarily represent hamartomas, along with some hyperplasias and true neoplasms. The reader is referred to the definitions and elaboration of these forms presented in the preceding chapter.

Squamous Papilloma

CLINICAL PRESENTATION AND PATHOGENESIS ▶

Squamous papillomas are common lesions of the oral mucosa with a predilection for the mucosa of the hard and soft palate, including the uvula and the vermilion of the lips (Fig 6-1). It is an innocuous lesion that is neither transmissible nor threatening. As an oral lesion, it raises concern because of its clinical appearance, which may mimic exophytic carcinomas; verrucous carcinomas; or condyloma acuminatum, a viral disease that is transmissable.

The squamous papilloma is also noteworthy for its uncertain pathogenesis. Many oral and maxillofacial specialists accept its pathogenesis as being from the human papillomavirus (HPV). This is based on its similar appearance to cutaneous warts and the identification of HPV subtypes 2, 6, 11, and 57 in some oral squamous papillomas. However, despite extensive research, a definitive cause-and-effect relationship has not been established. If a DNA virus such as HPV were the stimulus, one would expect a direct contact transmission such as that seen with condyloma acuminatum and herpes. The squamous papilloma also shows no histopathologic signs of viral infections, such as internuclear inclusion bodies and vacuolated nuclei. Furthermore, HPV is not identified in most squamous papillomas. However, HPV types 1, 2, 4, 6, 7, 11, 13, 16, 18, 30, 32, 40, and 57 have been identified in other lesions containing oral squamous cells, suggesting that HPV may be merely an incidental finding unrelated to the development of a squamous papilloma. This is further suggested by the failure of tests to show HPV DNA in the squamous cells or basal cells of squamous papillomas.

Regardless of its pathogenesis, the squamous papilloma will usually present in one of the four sites of predilection, although it may occur on any oral mucosal surface. Usually appearing as asymptomatic single lesions without induration (clusters and multiple lesions occasionally develop), they generally have a sessile base but may sometimes have a stalk (Fig 6-2).

DIFFERENTIAL DIAGNOSIS ▶

Single squamous papillomas may resemble *verrucous carcinomas* or even *exophytic squamous cell carcinomas* if they have a sessile base. Certainly the finding of induration or ulceration would lead the clinician to suspect these two concerning lesions more strongly than a squamous papilloma. In addition, clustered or multiple squamous papillomas would suggest *focal epithelial hyperplasia (Heck disease)*. In addition, a *verruciform xanthoma* will clinically resemble squamous papilloma, but it is mostly seen on the gingiva or the edentulous alveolar ridge.

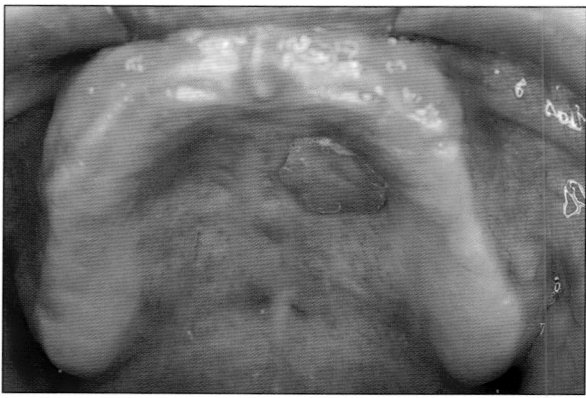

Fig 6-1 Oral squamous papilloma on the mucosa of the palate, a common location. This one has a broad sessile base.

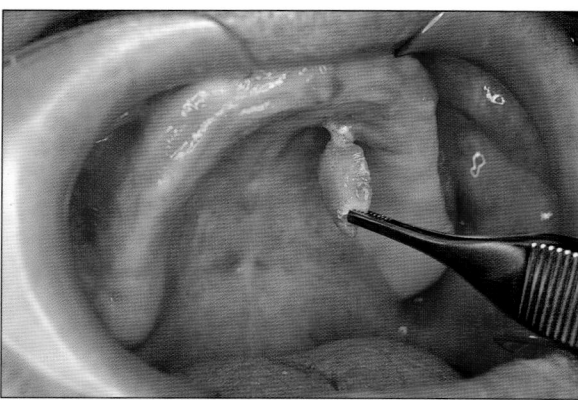

Fig 6-2 Oral squamous papilloma of the palate, this one with a stalk.

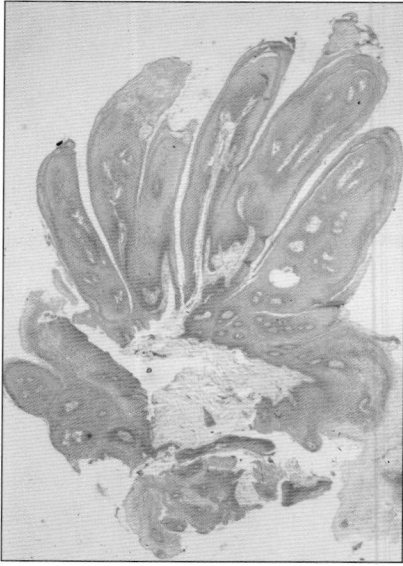
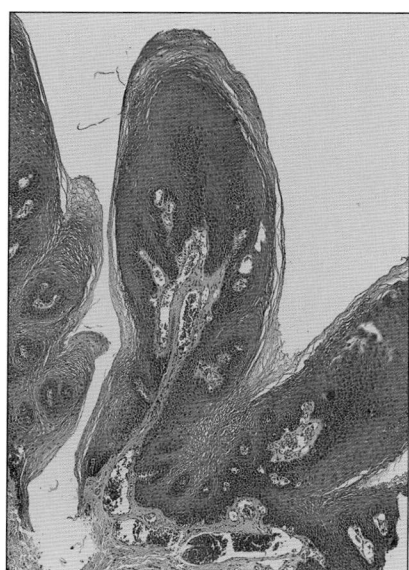

Figs 6-3 and 6-4 A squamous papilloma with finger-like projections. The fibrovascular cores are covered by stratified squamous epithelium.

HISTOPATHOLOGY ▶

The papilloma is a benign proliferation of squamous epithelium. With the epithelium's dependence for nutrition on the underlying fibrovascular tissue, the most efficient growth pattern is one of exophytic papillary projections, each with a fibrovascular core. The epithelium may show orthokeratosis, parakeratosis, and/or acanthosis. Mitoses may be numerous but are usually confined to the basal area. The prickle cells may have a clear glycogen-filled cytoplasm, particularly in lesions of the soft palate. Koilocytic cells (epithelial cells with pyknotic nuclei surrounded by a clear halo), which are often associated with viral disease, also may be present, but they can also be found in nonvirally infected oral mucosa. Their presence is not sufficient to confirm a viral etiology for any particular papilloma. The lamina propria frequently contains a chronic inflammatory infiltrate (Figs 6-3 and 6-4).

TREATMENT ▶

Because of the varied lesions on the differential diagnosis, most of which have a more concerning prognosis than that of the squamous papilloma, all lesions resembling a squamous papilloma are recommended for excision at the base (1-mm margin) to the depth of the submucosa. This excision should be curative. Recurrence or new lesions should raise suspicions of a possible retransmission of a condyloma acuminatum or of carcinoma.

Sinonasal Papillomas

CLINICAL PRESENTATION AND PATHOGENESIS ▶

Sinonasal papillomas are benign tumors that are found in three histologic types: the squamous papilloma, the inverted papilloma, and the cylindrical cell papilloma. Of these three types, the inverted papilloma has a 15% incidence of becoming a squamous cell carcinoma, while the cylindrical cell papilloma will histologically resemble an adenocarcinoma. Therefore, the histopathologic type of all sinonasal papillomas is of clinical significance and requires strict review. The clinician should also take care to note the location of any nasal papilloma because those on the septum are virtually always the innocuous benign squamous papilloma type, whereas those located on the lateral nasal mucosa (the medial wall of the maxillary sinus) are more likely to be of the inverted papilloma type, particularly if they are unilateral and present with epistaxis.

Most sinonasal papillomas are asymptomatic and found on routine examination. Others may be accompanied by a complaint of stuffiness or epistaxis. The benign squamous papilloma is usually translucent and may have a stalk; the cylindrical cell papilloma and the inverted papilloma have a broad base and are usually fixed.

DIFFERENTIAL DIAGNOSIS ▶

Sinonasal papillomas are somewhat distinct. However, a *nasal squamous cell carcinoma de novo* or a *squamous cell carcinoma developing in an inverted papilloma* are two important differential diagnoses. An *adenocarcinoma* may resemble a cylindrical cell papilloma clinically and histopathologically. In addition, a nasal *pyogenic granuloma* and a *juvenile angiofibroma* may produce a bleeding mass that will mimic the presentation of an inverted papilloma.

DIAGNOSTIC WORK-UP ▶

Septal papillomas may be locally excised without any specific work-up. Those that present on the posterior lateral nasal wall in a size greater than 1.5 cm or with epistaxis are best further reviewed by a computed tomography (CT) scan because of the potential for the inverted papilloma to recur if not excised with clear margins and its frequent presentation with sinus extension and bony destruction.

HISTOPATHOLOGY ▶

Squamous papillomas are exophytic lesions that present with the typical architecture of a papilloma, with fibrovascular cores supporting proliferating epidermoid cells. Mucous microcysts may occur.

Inverted papillomas grow endophytically with proliferating surface epithelium inverting into an underlying myxoid stroma, which may contain inflammatory cells (Fig 6-5). The epithelial cells are uniform and rarely produce keratin. Vacuolation, because of the presence of glycogen, is common, and occasional mitoses may be seen. Mucous cells with microcyst formation are not unusual. The surface of the papilloma can be lined by respiratory epithelium.

The growth pattern of cylindrical cell papillomas is the same as the inverted papilloma, with endophytic growth into a myxoid stroma. The proliferating cell, however, is more suggestive of respiratory epithelium with a pseudostratified arrangement of columnar cells and an eosinophilic granular cytoplasm. The surface may be ciliated and intraepithelial microcysts may occur (Figs 6-6a and 6-6b).

The sinonasal papillomas often show lateral spread of epidermal cells along the respiratory mucosa, indicating the need for wider excision to prevent recurrence. Because of their inverted pattern, there is sometimes difficulty in separating inverted papillomas from squamous cell carcinomas and cylindrical cell papillomas from adenocarcinomas. Inverted papillomas with numerous squamous cells and prominent keratin formation should be viewed with suspicion. Cylindrical cell papillomas consist of uniform, benign-appearing cells.

TREATMENT AND PROGNOSIS ▶

The routine benign squamous papilloma and the cylindrical cell papilloma are cured with a local excision. However, because it is reported to recur in 27% to 73% of cases treated by local excision, the inverted papilloma is usually treated with a medical maxillectomy via a lateral rhinotomy approach. Similar to a Weber-Ferguson approach without the infraorbital extension, this access will permit a wide excision using 1.0- to 1.5-cm margins, which should be supplemented with frozen sections. Alternatively, the midface degloving approach may be used with a transfixion incision to superiorly reflect the upper lip and nose. Some well-trained sinus endoscopic surgeons have removed inverted nasal papillomas with the

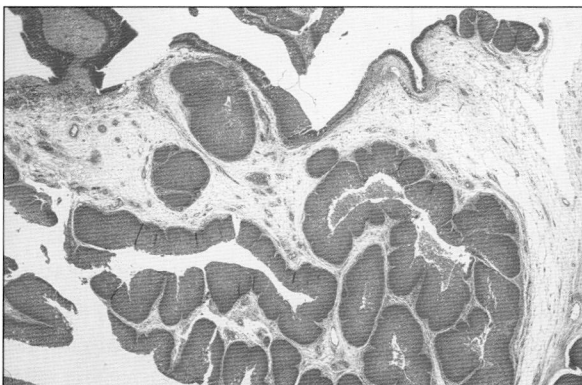

Fig 6-5 Inverted papilloma showing the downward growth of the acanthotic epithelium into a myxoid stroma.

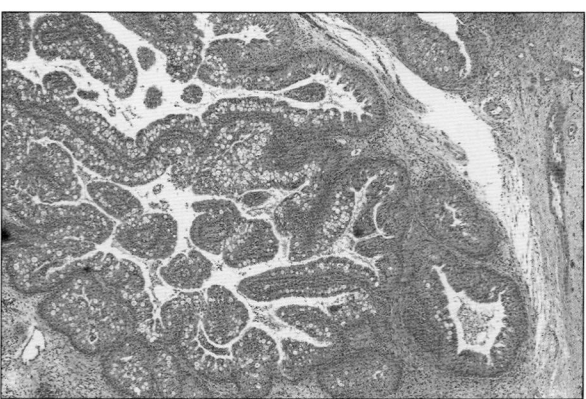

Fig 6-6a Cylindrical cell papilloma, which also shows endophytic growth.

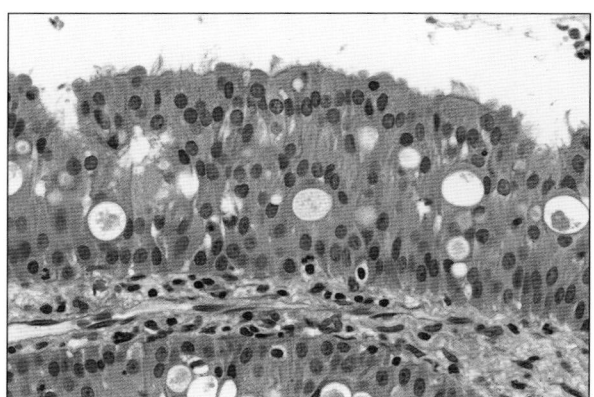

Fig 6-6b Cylindrical cell papilloma lined by a pseudo-stratified columnar epithelium. Cilia are present and microcysts can be seen.

endoscope. However, an insufficient number of controlled studies is available to fully recommend this approach without raising a greater concern for recurrence.

Verruciform Xanthoma

CLINICAL PRESENTATION AND PATHOGENESIS ▶

The verruciform xanthoma is a specific but rare lesion most commonly found on the attached gingiva (Fig 6-7), edentulous alveolar ridge, and sometimes the palate. Individuals are usually older than 45 years, and there is no sex or race predilection. The lesions are generally asymptomatic and will range in size from 2 mm to 2 cm. Their most common appearance is that of a slightly raised pebbly surface with a slightly pale or red color (Fig 6-8). However, variations of this presentation include a white surface, a depression rather than an elevation, and even ulceration.

The pathogenesis of the verruciform xanthoma is uncertain. One theory suggests that it is a focal proliferation of Langerhans cells, and it is supported by the immunohistochemical identification of Langerhans cells as part of these lesions. Another theory suggests that it is a local accumulation of lipid that subsequently becomes ingested by macrophages, which in turn secrete epithelial growth factors (EGFs) to stimulate a limited epithelial hyperplasia. The lack of an association with systemic hyperlipidemia states and the positive identification of Langerhans cells clearly favor the first theory over the second.

DIFFERENTIAL DIAGNOSIS ▶

Verruciform xanthoma is not usually the first consideration on the differential diagnosis. The more common *squamous papilloma* and the more concerning *exophytic squamous cell carcinoma* or *verrucous carcinoma* are more serious considerations. If the lesion is larger or more than one is present, consideration of either *condyloma acuminatum* or *focal epithelial hyperplasia* is appropriate.

HISTOPATHOLOGY ▶

This lesion has a very distinctive histology. It presents a verrucous surface covered by parakeratin, which extends into the epithelium in thick seams. The epithelium also exhibits acanthosis with equal elongation and extension of the rete ridges into the connective tissue (Figs 6-9a and 6-9b). Within the connective tissue papillae, numerous foamy cells are seen, which almost invariably are contained only within the papillae and rarely extend below the level of the rete ridges (Fig 6-9c). These xanthoma-type cells are macrophages that contain lipid and periodic acid–Schiff (PAS)–positive, diastase-resistant granules. There is evidence to suggest that the source of this material may be necrotic epithelial cells.

TREATMENT ▶

Local excision at the base of the lesion (1-mm margin) to the depth of the submucosa or to the supraperiosteal plane over bone is curative. There is no association with systemic lipid alterations, arteriosclerosis, or cardiovascular disease, and therefore blood studies related to this diagnosis are not required. Recurrence should be looked upon as suspicious for other diseases such as carcinoma or for a re-infection of condyloma acuminatum.

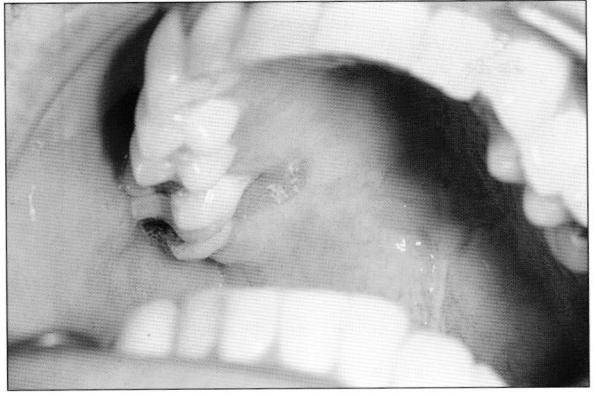

Fig 6-7 Verruciform xanthomas are most often seen on the gingiva. This one on the palatal gingiva has a characteristic pebbly surface and pale color.

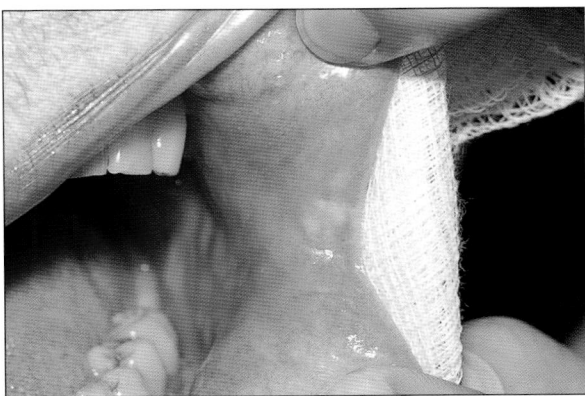

Fig 6-8 Verruciform xanthomas can also occur on the lips or buccal mucosa. This one also bears the characteristic features of a pebbly surface and pale color.

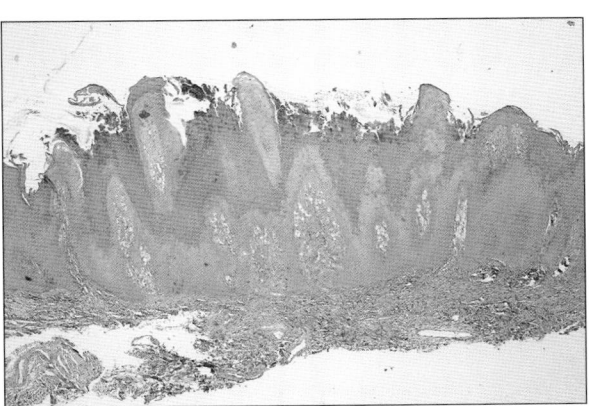

Fig 6-9a The verruciform xanthoma has a distinctive low-power appearance. The surface is verruciform. The rete ridges are elongated and of equal length, and there is a distinctive hyperparakeratosis.

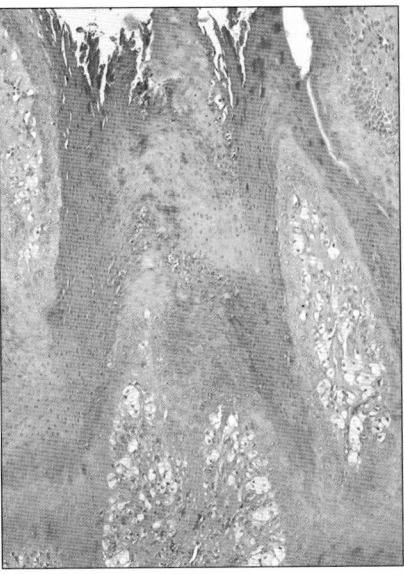

Fig 6-9b Higher-power view of Fig 6-9a showing the parakeratin seams and vacuolated cells representing foamy histiocytes in the connective tissue papillae.

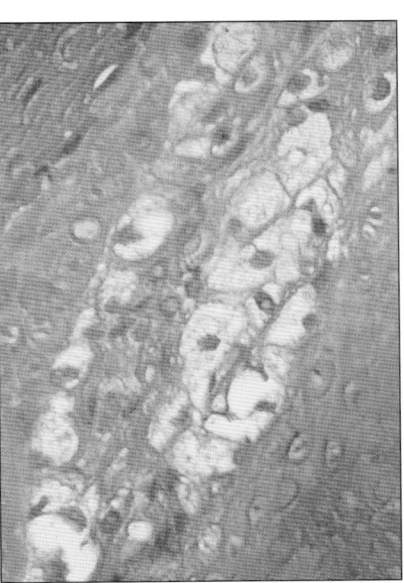

Fig 6-9c The same case as Figs 6-9a and 6-9b showing the foamy histiocytes within the papillae.

Seborrheic Keratosis

CLINICAL PRESENTATION AND PATHOGENESIS ►

Seborrheic keratosis is a benign proliferation of keratinocytes. Although the pathologist will refer to them as "basaloid cells" in the microscopic description, these are actually small keratinocytes with less cytoplasm and a darker-than-normal nucleus. They have several different clinical presentations and usually appear on the trunk and facial areas of individuals older than 40 years.

The most common clinical presentation is that of a solid, warty appearing, brown-black pigmented lesion with distinct borders raised above the skin surface. Most will be 1 to 3 cm, although some can be much larger. Those that develop on the cheek and other facial areas tend to be flatter and less pigmented, making them more difficult to distinguish from premalignant actinic keratosis, pigmented basal cell carcinoma, and early melanomas (Fig 6-10).

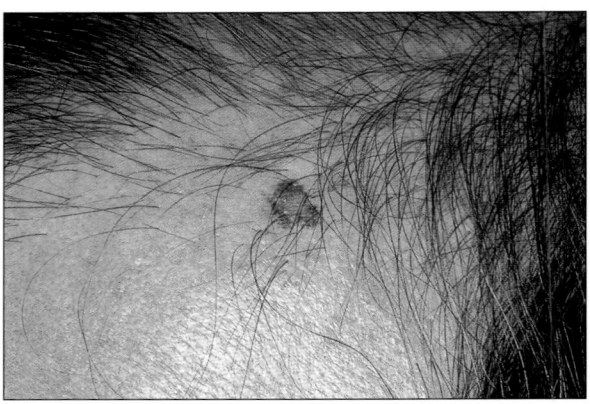

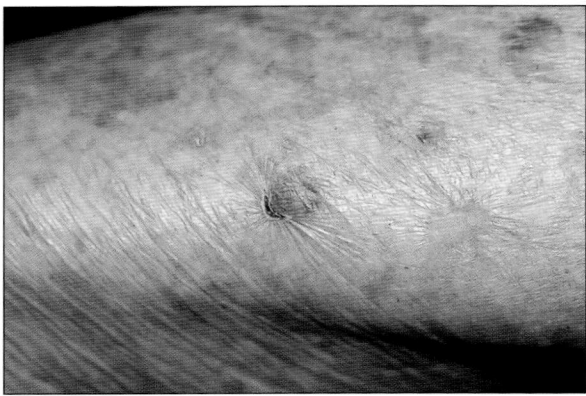

Fig 6-10 Seborrheic keratosis on the hairline of the scalp. Slightly raised and pigmented, it will mimic premalignant actinic keratosis and even melanoma.

Fig 6-11 This typical seborrheic keratosis is surrounded by a thin inflammatory area, which has given rise to the term *irritated seborrheic keratosis*.

Seborrheic keratoses may become irritated and develop an inflammatory base. Clinically, these seem to be more set into the skin and have thin, red, inflammatory rings around their circumference; they are often referred to specifically as *irritated seborrheic keratoses* (Fig 6-11). Nevertheless, the flat seborrheic keratosis of the face, the more common acanthotic type, and the irritated seborrheic keratosis are all variations of the same pathology, which seems to represent an age-related hamartomatous proliferation of altered keratinocytes.

DIAGNOSTIC WORK-UP ▶ No specific work-up or study is required other than a topographic search for other skin lesions. However, an association of the rapid appearance of multiple seborrheic keratoses with gastrointestinal malignancies has been noted. This association has been referred to as the *sign of Leser-Trélat* and may represent a coincidental occurrence of two pathologies known to occur at the same age, or a mutual proliferation derived from the emergence of a common oncogene or growth factor, or the loss of a common cell cycle regulator. Regardless, the prudent clinician should further assess the medical history for signs of such malignancies and consult a gastroenterologist or accomplish upper and lower gastrointestinal-contrast series.

DIFFERENTIAL DIAGNOSIS ▶ The flatter seborrheic keratosis, more common to the face and more likely to be observed by the oral and maxillofacial specialist, will be similar in appearance to premalignant *actinic keratosis*, the *lentigo-maligna–lentigo maligna melanoma–superficial spreading melanoma* series, and *skin squamous cell carcinomas* and *basal cell carcinomas*. In particular, the irritated seborrheic keratosis will bear a closer resemblance to both skin squamous cell and basal cell carcinoma as well as a *nodular melanoma*. The most distinguishing features of seborrheic keratosis that the clinician can use in the differential assessment are its abrupt delineation from normal adjacent skin, its general raised surface, and its frequent display of bumpy surface irregularities and pock marks, which are the result of pseudocyst formations in the epidermis.

HISTOPATHOLOGY ▶ Commensurate with its clinical appearance, seborrheic keratosis is an exophytic epithelial growth that is usually hyperkeratotic, acanthotic, and papillary (Fig 6-12). The base of the lesion is typically at the same level as the normal epithelium because the acanthosis occurs as an upward proliferation (Fig 6-13). Both squamous and basaloid cells comprise the tumor. The histologic appearance is quite variable, and several subtypes have been identified and may coexist.

The most common is the acanthotic type, which consists of basaloid cells (Fig 6-14) arranged in a broad network with intervening islands of connective tissue. Keratotic invaginations (pseudohorn cysts) as well as intraepithelial keratin cysts (true horn cysts) are present (Figs 6-12 and 6-15). There is increased melanin, usually confined to the deepest epithelial layers. An inflammatory component, which may have a lichenoid pattern, is often present.

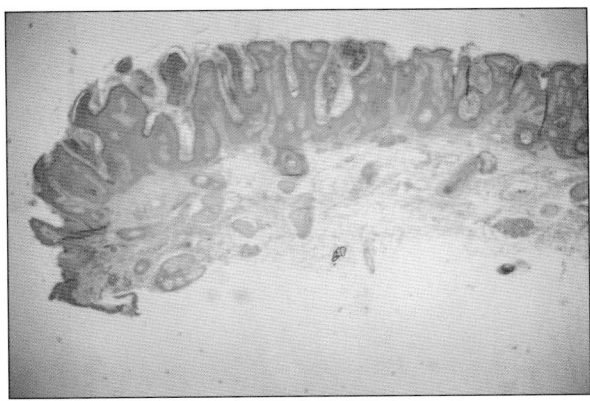

Fig 6-12 Seborrheic keratosis showing the exophytic, papillary proliferation. Horn cysts and pseudohorn cysts are present.

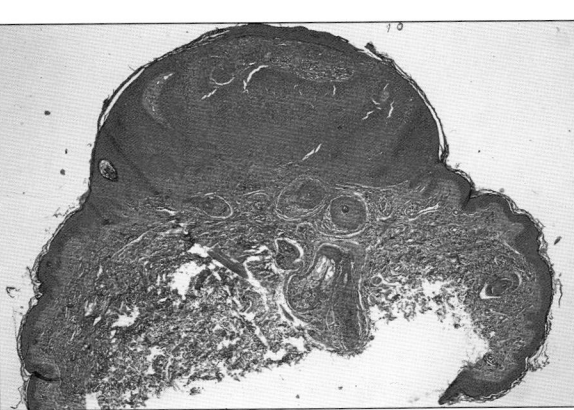

Fig 6-13 The exophytic growth of seborrheic keratosis gives it a "stuck-on" appearance clinically.

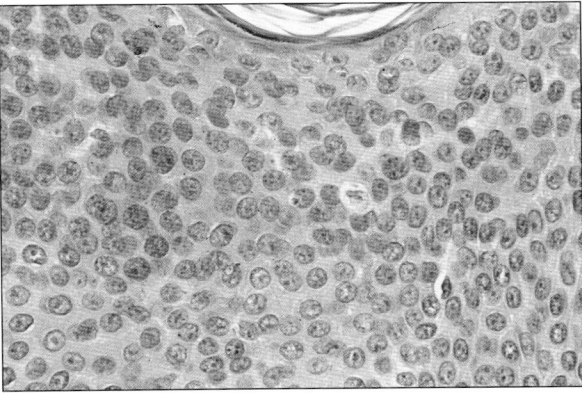

Fig 6-14 Basaloid cells comprise this seborrheic keratosis. The cells are very regular.

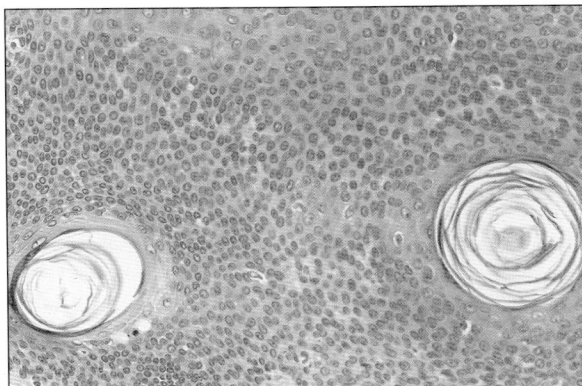

Fig 6-15 Horn cysts within seborrheic keratosis.

The adenoid or reticulated type consists of basaloid cells extending downward from the epidermis in a network of thin cords and strands. Intraepithelial keratin cysts are formed and there is usually marked pigmentation. The intervening stroma is highly eosinophilic and collagenous.

The irritated type is composed predominantly of squamous cells. Flattened eosinophilic squamous cells form "eddies" or whorls within the epithelium. They are numerous and small in size. There may be some downward proliferation of the lesion. Inflammation is mild to absent.

The hyperkeratotic or digitated type shows prominent hyperkeratosis with a verrucous surface in which the keratin covers spire-like projections. It is composed essentially of squamous cells.

There is also a cloning or nesting form in which nests of cells may resemble basal cell carcinoma.

TREATMENT ▶

Since seborrheic keratosis is not premalignant and only rarely is associated with symptoms, most can be left untreated. However, symptomatic lesions and those that are difficult to recognize or separate from premalignant and malignant skin diseases may be excised completely. Alternatively, an incisional biopsy may be accomplished to confirm the diagnosis, followed by destruction with laser, cryotherapy, or coagulation diathermy. It is not advisable to use any of these destructive techniques for a lesion for which the diagnosis is uncertain or in doubt because of the risk of recurrent disease.

Table 6-1 Classification of exocrine glands by mechanism and example

Type	Mechanism of secretion	Example
Merocrine	Secreting cell remains intact.	Salivary glands
		Pancreas
		Eccrine sweat glands
Apocrine	A portion of the secreting cell is pinched off and discharged but the base remains intact.	Apocrine glands in skin
		Mammary glands
Holocrine	Cell dies and is discharged with secretion.	Sebaceous glands

Skin Appendage Tumors

Although more than 25 different types of skin appendage tumors have been identified, their incidence is small. Because of the predilection of many of these tumors for the head and neck area, the increased awareness of skin conditions, and the greater number of facial skin surgeries being performed today, the oral and maxillofacial specialist has been increasingly involved in their diagnosis and treatment.

In general, skin appendage tumors have no distinguishing clinical features. Most present as a slow-growing subcutaneous nodule, which is diagnosed by histopathology once it has been removed. Like the vast majority of all skin appendage tumors, the tumors described in this chapter are benign. The less common, malignant tumors are discussed in Chapter 7.

Skin appendage tumors are divided into four categories based on their particular characteristics or their suspected histogenesis: eccrine sweat gland tumors, apocrine gland tumors, sebaceous gland tumors, and hair follicle tumors. Only those with a marked predilection for the head and neck regions are discussed in this chapter.

The Skin Appendages

To understand skin appendage tumors, it is helpful to review the structures that comprise skin appendages: sweat glands, apocrine glands, sebaceous glands, and the hair follicle complex. Their normal microscopic appearance, their location on the face and within the dermis, and their normal activity will explain much of the observed pathologies that arise from these structures (Fig 6-16).

Other than the hair follicle itself, skin appendages comprise three types of glands: eccrine sweat glands, apocrine oil-secreting glands, and sebaceous glands. Each gland has a different mechanism for secreting its product (Table 6-1).

1. Eccrine Sweat Glands

Location: Found everywhere on the skin except in areas where there are no skin appendages, such as the vermilion of the lip and the nail beds.

Type: Tubular (merocrine)

Structure: The basal coil consists of secretory and ductal portions. The secretory portion consists of clear cells that contain glycogen and dark cells that contain mucopolysaccharides. They secrete aqueous material with glycogen and sialomucin, respectively. The secretion is propelled through the duct by the contraction of myoepithelial cells. The intradermal duct is lined with a double layer of basophilic cuboidal cells and a luminal eosinophilic cuticle. The intraepidermal component (also called the *acrosyringium* because the cells are derived from dermal duct cells) has a single luminal layer and two to

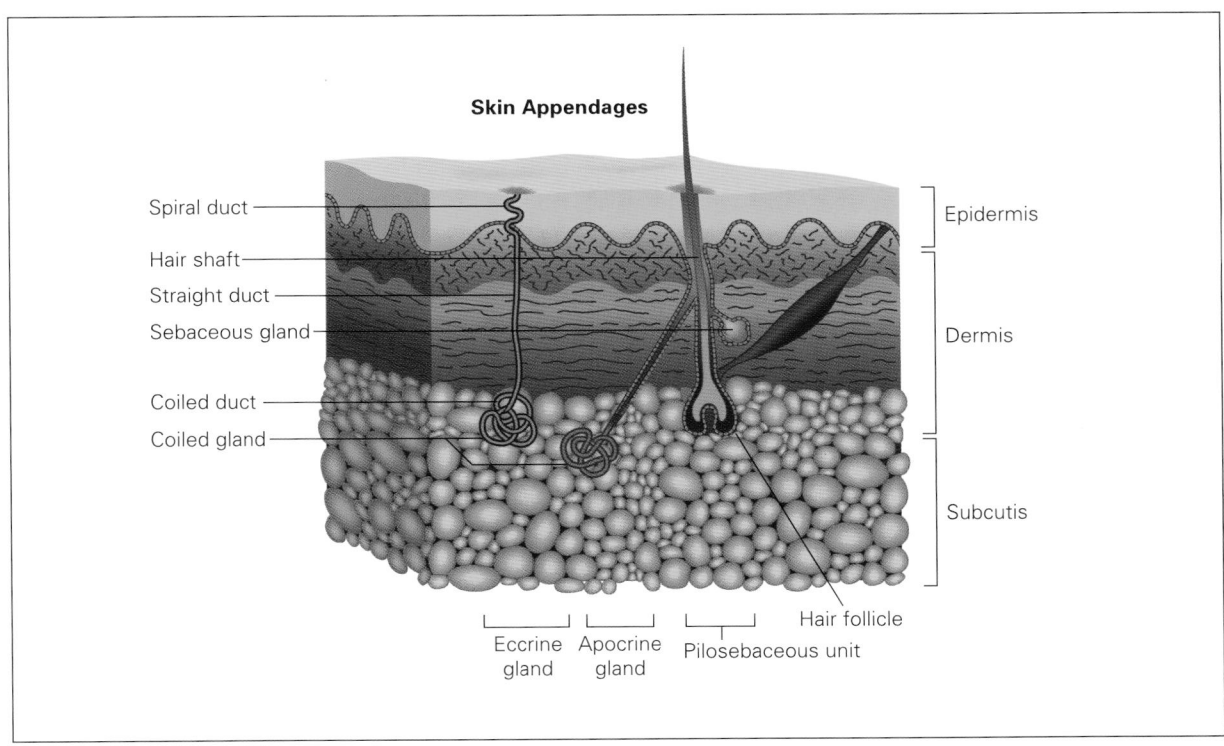

Skin Appendages

Spiral duct

Hair shaft

Straight duct

Sebaceous gland

Coiled duct

Coiled gland

Epidermis

Dermis

Subcutis

Hair follicle

Eccrine gland   Apocrine gland   Pilosebaceous unit

Fig 6-16 Cross section of human skin denoting the location of adnexal structures: hair follicles; sebaceous glands; and sweat glands and their ducts.

three layers of outer cells. Initially there is a luminal eosinophilic cuticle. The ductal cells undergo keratinization as they progress upward and the cuticle is lost.

2. Apocrine Glands

Location: Apocrine glands are limited in their distribution. In the head and neck area they are found in the external ear canal (ceruminous glands) and may also be present on the face and scalp.

Type: Tubular (apocrine)

Structure: These glands, like the pilosebaceous units, originate from the primary epithelial germ. Consequently, the glands will often empty into the pilosebaceous follicle above the level of the sebaceous duct. Occasionally, however, they may open directly on the skin surface.

The basal coil is entirely secretory with a single layer of secretory cells containing large granules and myoepithelial cells. The product is a sialomucin. The lumen of the secretory portion is approximately 10 times the size of the lumen of the eccrine glands.

3. Sebaceous Glands

Location: These are found throughout the skin with the exception of the palms and soles. They are associated with hair, with the notable exception of the so-called Fordyce granules, which are found in the vermilion of the lip as well as in the labial and buccal mucosa.

Type: Lobular (holocrine)

Structure: The gland is composed of lobules that lead to an excretory duct lined by stratified squamous epithelium. The lobules consist mainly of rounded cells with vacuolated cytoplasm that contains lipid. There may be degeneration of some of these cells, giving them a ghost-like appearance. The periphery of the lobules are composed of cuboidal cells that do not contain lipid.

4. Hair Follicles

These structures are much more complex than the glandular elements. The hair follicle has three basic zones: a lower portion that extends to the insertion of the arrector pili muscle, the isthmus that extends to the entrance of the sebaceous duct, and the infundibulum, which extends to the surface. The lower portion consists of the stem and the bulb. The bulb is composed of the dermal hair papilla, the hair matrix, the hair (composed of a medulla, cortex, and peripheral cuticle), an inner root sheath (composed of an inner root cuticle, Huxley layer, and Henle layer), and an outer root sheath. The histologic appearance of the hair follicle is variable because of changes associated with the hair cycle.

Hair Follicle Tumors

Trichofolliculoma

CLINICAL PRESENTATION AND PATHOGENESIS ▶

The trichofolliculoma is a hamartomatous process representing an aborted and disrupted attempt at hair follicle formation. This tumor is analogous to the odontoma or ameloblastic fibro-odontoma of the jaws, which represents an aborted and disrupted attempt at tooth formation. The trichofolliculoma arises from the midshaft area of the hair follicle and seems to mark a disturbance between the normal epidermal and dermal cell components of the hair follicle cycle (Fig 6-17).

Clinically, trichofolliculomas are usually irregular papules ranging from 1 to 4 cm that may have tufts of white hair emerging from their surface (Fig 6-18). Larger ones have a surface that is dome shaped with a reddened base and yellow surface crusting. Smaller ones have a normal surface color, a regular shape, and a central pore with a white or gray hair emerging from it.

DIFFERENTIAL DIAGNOSIS ▶

Depending on their size and shape, trichofolliculomas may resemble most of the common sun damage–related tumors: *keratoacanthoma*, *basal cell carcinoma*, and *skin squamous cell carcinoma*. Those with a reddened base and yellow crusting may mimic skin infections, particularly *folliculitis* and *infected sebaceous cysts*.

HISTOPATHOLOGY ▶

The architecture is of major significance and shows a dilated follicular structure with secondary follicles developing from it. The degree of differentiation of the secondary follicles is variable. There is a well-organized fibrous stroma (Fig 6-19).

TREATMENT AND PROGNOSIS ▶

Trichofolliculomas are treated with a local excision with 2-mm margins and should include the subcutaneous layer deep to the tumor. Such an excision should be curative without recurrence. Recurrences should raise suspicion of an unrecognized malignancy.

Trichoepithelioma

CLINICAL PRESENTATION AND PATHOGENESIS ▶

The trichoepithelioma is another hamartomatous proliferation of cells from the hair follicle. It seems to arise from cells deeper than the trichofolliculoma in the hair follicle apparatus (see Fig 6-17).

Clinically, trichoepitheliomas are firm subcutaneous nodules with a normal skin appearance. They may occur at any age but have a higher incidence in children and young adults. They occur most frequently on the forehead, nasolabial folds, upper lip, and nose (Fig 6-20). The overlying skin may be distended by the mass and shiny because of distension and convexity. Most are smaller than 2 cm (although larger ones

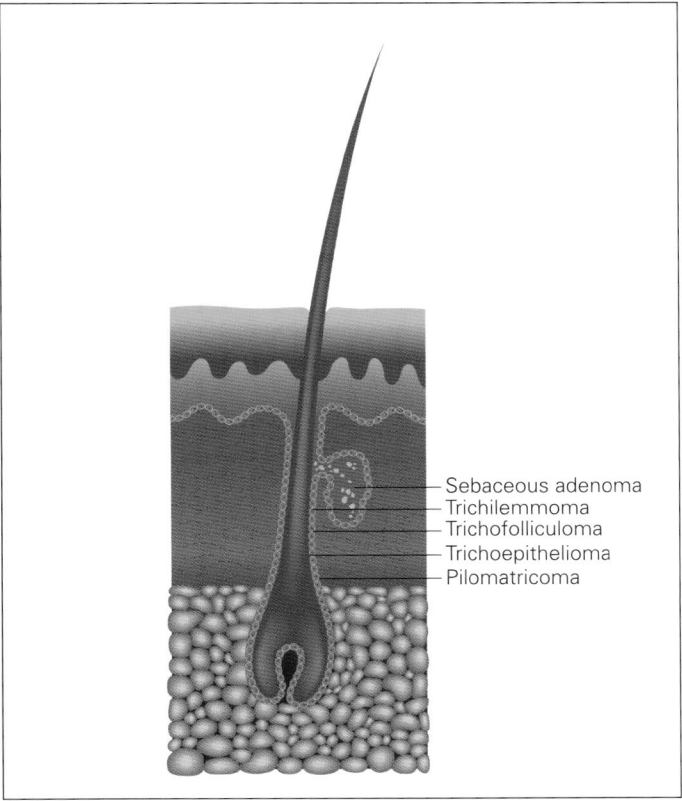

Fig 6-17 Anatomy of the hair follicle and its associated structures. Note the area of histogenesis of each tumor, which will correlate somewhat to its location in the skin and clinical presentation.

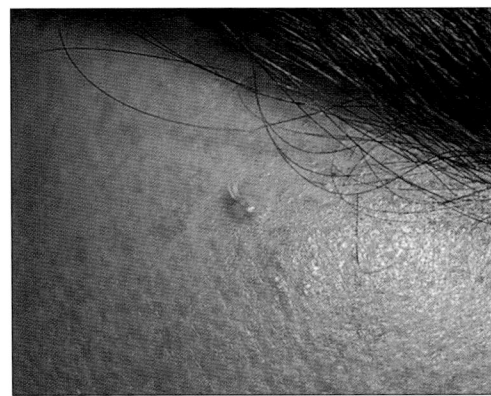

Fig 6-18 A trichofolliculoma will have an irregular surface that may also have a central pore and one or two white hairs emerging from it. (Reprinted from Callen JP, *Color Atlas of Dermatology*, with permission from WB Saunders Co.)

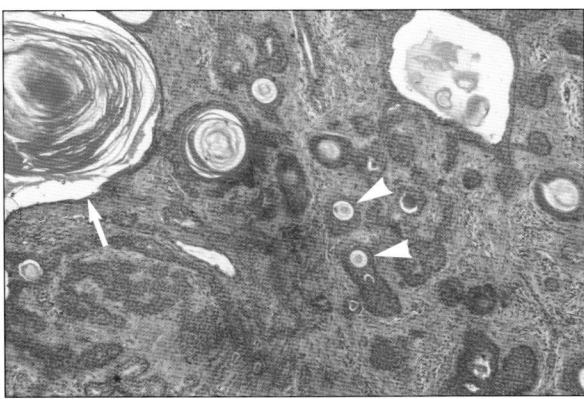

Fig 6-19 Trichofolliculoma showing a keratin-filled cyst lined by stratified squamous epithelium (the "primary" hair follicle [*arrow*] with adjacent "secondary" hair follicles [*arrowheads*]).

do occur) and appear as individual asymptomatic masses, but multiple nodules are known to occur from an autosomal-dominant inheritance. These are referred to as *epithelioma adenoides cysticum*, or *Brooke tumors*, by dermatopathologists. Multiple trichoepitheliomas occur as part of Cowden syndrome, in which multiple hamartomas (trichoepitheliomas and other skin appendage hamartomas, particularly the trichilemmoma) develop in the skin, the breast, the thyroid, and the gastrointestinal tract.

The desmoplastic trichoepithelioma is a clinical and histopathologic variant that often occurs on the face and is much more common in women. Because it is indurated, it strongly mimics a basal cell carcinoma or a skin squamous cell carcinoma.

DIFFERENTIAL DIAGNOSIS ▶

Although trichoepitheliomas are usually not ulcerated, the lesions they most resemble are *basal cell carcinoma*, *skin squamous cell carcinoma*, and *keratoacanthoma*. Multiple trichoepitheliomas, either of the Brooke type or as part of Cowden syndrome, may suggest the *basal cell nevus syndrome*, in which case the other specific components of each syndrome would need to be investigated. Early cases of the skin poxvirus infection *molluscum contagiosum* before the surface ulceration also may resemble multiple trichoepitheliomas.

HISTOPATHOLOGY ▶

These are circumscribed tumors whose predominant pattern is one of keratin cysts surrounded by basaloid cells (Fig 6-21). In addition, islands of basaloid cells with peripheral palisading may be present. The proliferation may be solid, reticular, or adenoid. The stroma is fibrovascular and can invaginate into the islands of basaloid cells to resemble a hair papilla. Sometimes, however, separation from basal cell carcinoma may be difficult.

271

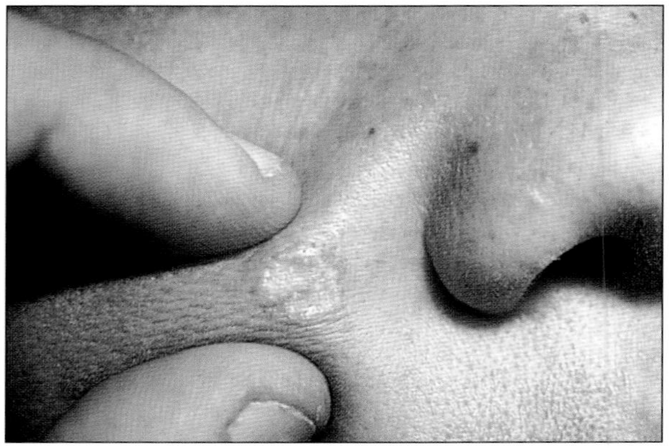

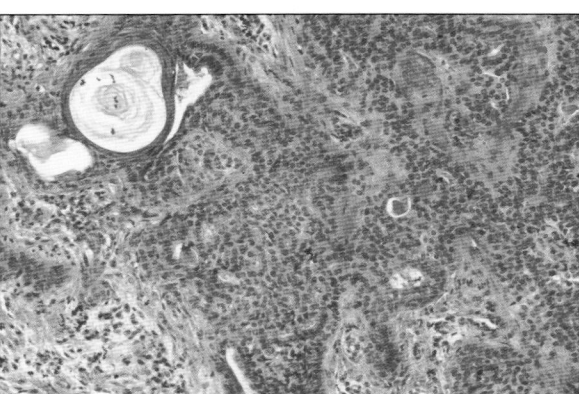

Fig 6-20 Clusters of subcutaneous nodules representing trichoepitheliomas are most often seen around the nasolabial folds in teenagers and young adults. (Reprinted from Callen JP, *Color Atlas of Dermatology*, with permission from WB Saunders Co.)

Fig 6-21 A trichoepithelioma showing keratin cysts surrounded by basaloid cells and areas resembling basal cell carcinoma.

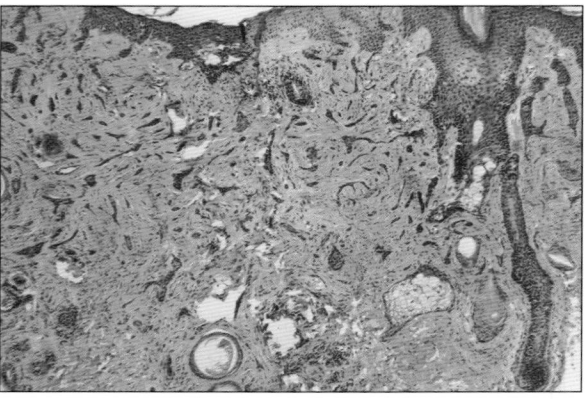

Fig 6-22a A desmoplastic trichoepithelioma with keratin cysts and strands of epithelial cells.

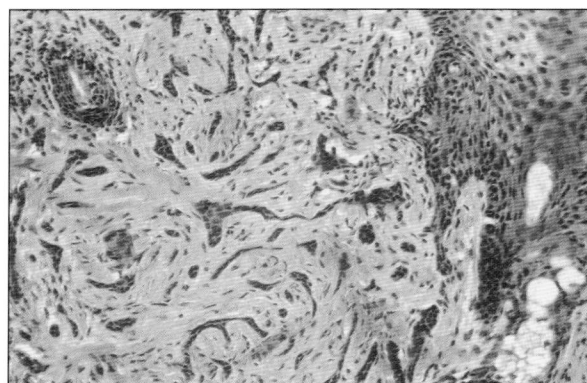

Fig 6-22b Higher-power view of Fig 6-22a showing the strands of epithelium in a well-collagenized stroma.

The desmoplastic trichoepithelioma consists of narrow strands of epithelial cells; a densely collagenized, hypocellular stroma; and keratin cysts (Figs 6-22a and 6-22b).

TREATMENT AND PROGNOSIS ▶

Solitary trichoepitheliomas are cured by local excision using 2-mm peripheral margins and excising the lesion deep to its subcutaneous extension. Multiple lesions may be left untreated with follow-up, recognizing their limited growth potential as hamartomas. However, it is best to remove all lesions if it is at all practical to do so. This may be accomplished by multiple local excisions, Mohs micrographic surgery (see Chapter 7), or a field excision requiring local flaps or skin grafting.

Trichilemmoma

CLINICAL PRESENTATION AND PATHOGENESIS ▶

The trichilemmoma is yet another hamartomatous proliferation arising from cells of the hair follicle. In this tumor, the cell of origin seems to be located in the superficial level of the hair follicle just below the basement membrane at the sebaceous gland level (see Fig 6-17).

Trichilemmomas may occur as solitary, independent tumors, but multiple lesions occur as the dominant feature of Cowden syndrome. In fact, multiple trichilemmomas are the most concise marker for the diagnosis of Cowden syndrome, which is an autosomal-dominant trait for multiple hamartomas (99%) as

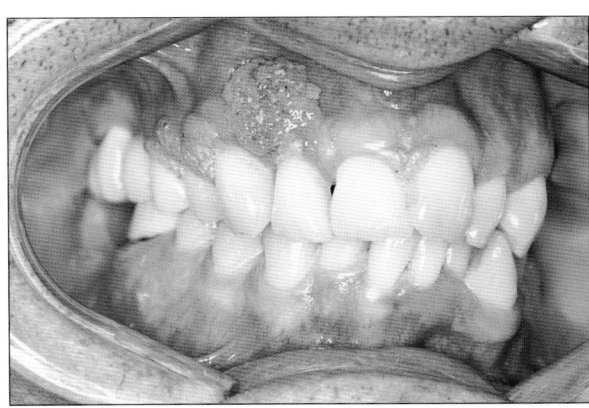

Fig 6-23 Cluster of oral papillomas in a patient with Cowden syndrome.

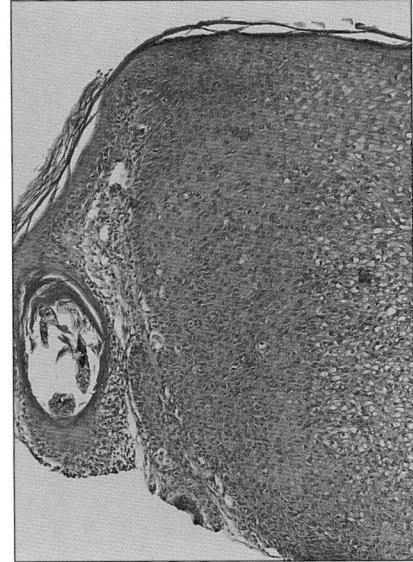

Fig 6-24 This trichilemmoma from the eyelid shows a lobular proliferation into the dermis with peripheral palisaded columnar cells. Clear, glycogen-containing cells also are present.

compared to breast tumors (75%), thyroid tumors (88%), and gastrointestinal tumors (70%). Pertinent to the oral and maxillofacial specialist, papillary lesions of the lips, gingiva, alveolar ridge, and tongue are seen in almost all patients with Cowden syndrome (Fig 6-23). These lesions produce a cobblestone appearance to the affected mucosa, which, when biopsied, will show multiple fibromas with epithelial hyperplasia. Larger numbers of trichilemmomas in Cowden syndrome correlate with the development of internal malignancies.

DIFFERENTIAL DIAGNOSIS

The eruption of multiple skin lesions in a teenager or young adult may raise suspicions for *basal cell nevus syndrome* as well as *Cowden syndrome*. As isolated lesions they will also resemble small *basal cell carcinomas*, *skin squamous cell carcinomas*, and *keratoacanthomas*. They may also resemble the early stages of an outbreak of *molluscum contagiosum* and, if only one or a few lesions are present, the common wart *verruca vulgaris*.

HISTOPATHOLOGY

There is a lobular proliferation of uniform small cells into the dermis from the epidermis. Glycogen-containing clear cells may be conspicuous. The peripheral cells are columnar and palisading. Keratinization occurs on the surface of the epidermis (Fig 6-24) and may be sufficient to form a cutaneous horn.

TREATMENT AND PROGNOSIS

Solitary trichilemmomas may be excised for cure using 2-mm peripheral margins and excision deep to the deepest extent of the tumor. Multiple lesions as part of Cowden syndrome are usually impractical to excise, and new ones frequently emerge after excision. Therefore, they are usually left untreated unless ulcerations or symptoms occur.

Pilomatricoma

CLINICAL PRESENTATION AND PATHOGENESIS

The pilomatricoma (previously termed the *calcifying epithelioma of Malherbe*) is the fourth and most common hair follicle–originating hamartoma pertinent to the oral and maxillofacial specialist. It arises from the deepest layer of the hair follicle shaft and hair follicle bud (see Fig 6-17). Therefore, the tumor will clinically present as a deep-seated subcutaneous mass (Fig 6-25) with a normal-textured and normal-colored or slightly yellow overlying skin (Fig 6-26). The pilomatricoma is most commonly seen in children

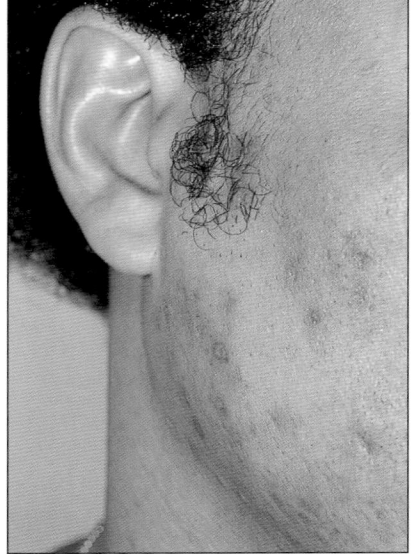

Fig 6-25 This pilomatricoma presents as a round, deep-seated, and freely movable mass that, in this location, may be confused with a parotid tumor. Pilomatricomas often are more deeply located in the skin.

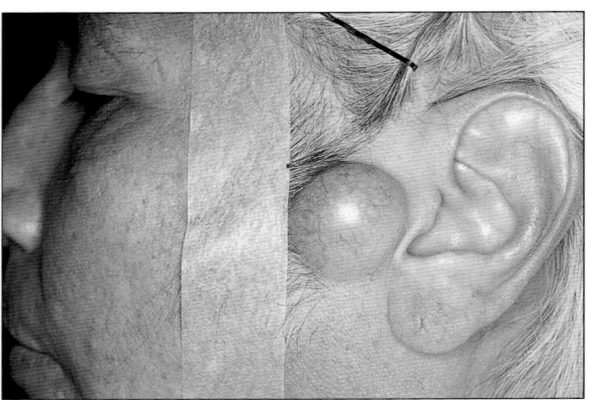

Fig 6-26 This more superficial pilomatricoma arose as a well-defined mass in the preauricular skin. Here the firm and uniformly hard consistency is more apparent, and it is therefore less likely to be confused with a parotid tumor. (Courtesy of Dr Drore Eisen.)

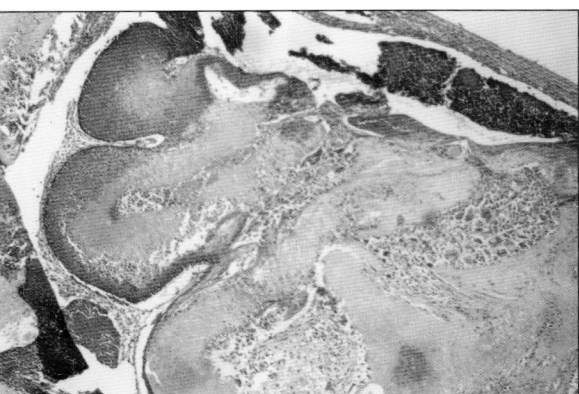

Fig 6-27a A pilomatricoma showing islands of basophilic cells and shadow cells. Some calcifications may be seen within the shadow cells.

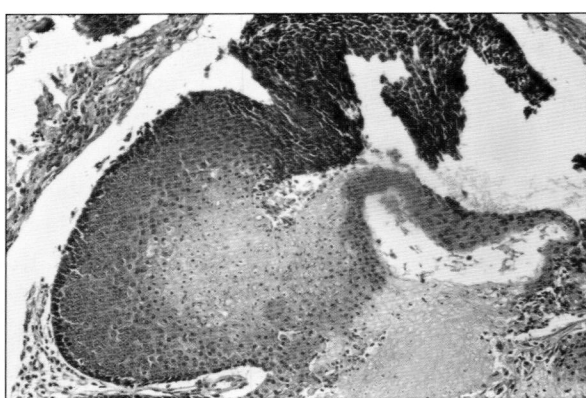

Fig 6-27b Higher-power view of Fig 6-27a showing the closely packed nuclei of the basophilic cells and the transition to shadow cells.

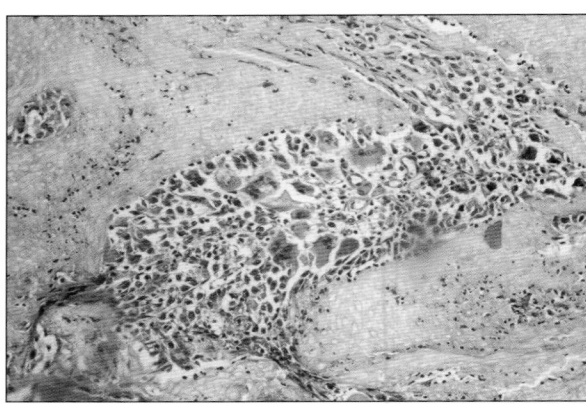

Fig 6-27c The same case as Figs 6-27a and 6-27b. The stroma contains numerous multinucleated giant cells.

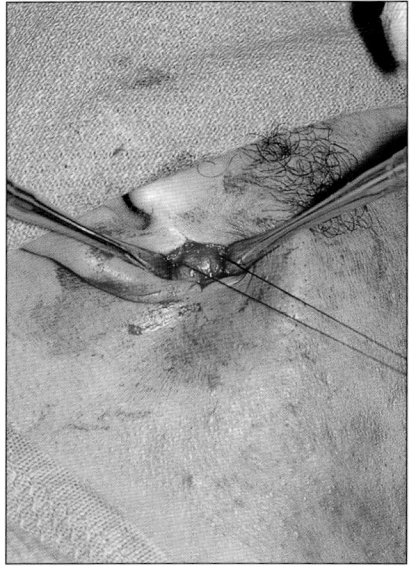

Fig 6-28 Because of its thin or absent capsule, a pilomatricoma is excised with 2-mm margins. The deep margin is usually the muscle fascia deep to this subcutaneous-level tumor.

and teenagers (60% to 80%). Most are solitary lesions, but rare multiple lesions do occur, some of which have demonstrated a familial inheritance. Most range in size from 0.5 to 4.0 cm, but very large pilomatricomas in excess of 10 cm also are possible. The mass will be very firm, presumably because of its internal calcification, and only slightly mobile as a result of its location deep in the dermis.

DIFFERENTIAL DIAGNOSIS ▶

The deep location of the pilomatricoma will be suggestive of cysts or other tumors arising from this level. Therefore, *dermoid cysts, sebaceous cysts,* and *nasolabial cysts* (for those that occur in nasolabial areas) are considerations. In addition, *fibromas, schwannomas,* and *granular cell tumors of the skin* present at the same level with an intact skin surface.

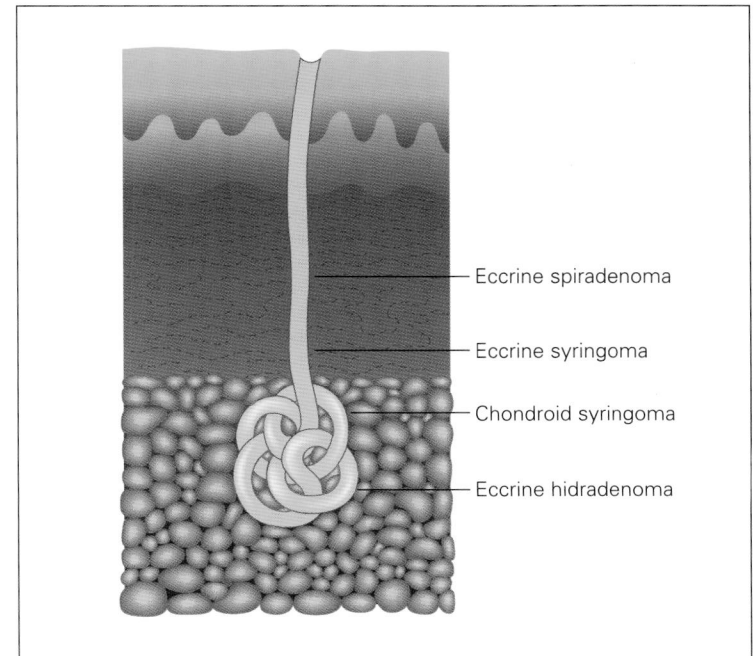

Fig 6-29 The anatomy of the sweat gland apparatus will explain much of the clinical presentations and locations of eccrine tumors as a function of the level of their histogenesis.

HISTOPATHOLOGY ▶ The pilomatricoma is a well-demarcated tumor consisting of epithelial islands with peripheral basaloid cells, which change into shadow cells (ghost cells) centrally (Figs 6-27a and 6-27b). The shadow cells may calcify. Small areas of keratinization may be seen within the islands. Multinucleated giant cells can be found in the stroma adjacent to the shadow cells (Fig 6-27c).

TREATMENT AND PROGNOSIS ▶ The pilomatricoma is excised for cure using 2-mm peripheral margins and a tumor-free deep margin. Because of its location in the deep layer of the dermis (reticular dermis) and its expansion into the subcutaneous layer, the deep margin of the excision is most often the underlying muscle fascia (Fig 6-28). Such locally excised tumors do not recur. Should a recurrence develop, concern for the rare malignant pilomatricoma is warranted and should prompt review of the original histopathology and a re-excision with at least 1-cm margins and frozen section guidance.

Eccrine Tumors

Eccrine Syringoma

CLINICAL PRESENTATION AND PATHOGENESIS ▶ The eccrine syringoma is believed to arise from the epithelium in the lower portion of the sweat duct or from the sweat gland itself (Fig 6-29). The most common clinical presentation is that of multiple small papules (1 to 3 mm) below the eyes in an adolescent or teenage girl (Fig 6-30). Less commonly, the eyelids, forehead, and neck may also be sites of multiple lesions. The lesions are mostly of normal skin color, although some may be yellowish or slightly brown. These lesions represent hamartomatous proliferations with limited growth potential.

DIFFERENTIAL DIAGNOSIS ▶ Multiple lesions of this kind are usually interpreted as *acne vulgaris*. The early stages of *molluscum contagiosum* and some other skin appendage tumors known to occur in the superficial skin in children and teenagers, such as *trichoepithelioma of the Brooke type* and *trichilemmoma* (alone or as part of *Cowden syndrome*), also bear some consideration. In addition, the multiple skin papillomas may suggest the small *basal cell carcinomas of the basal cell nevus syndrome*.

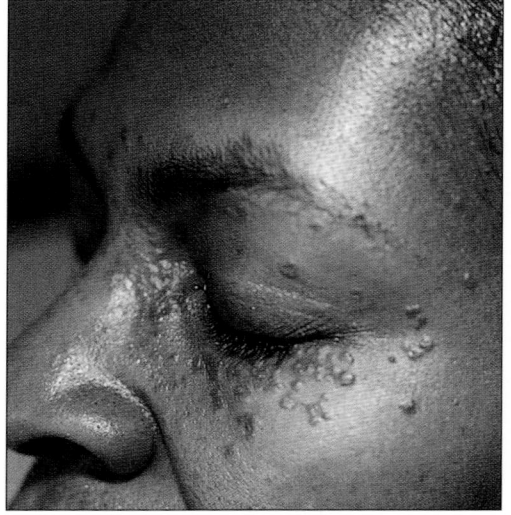

Fig 6-30 Eccrine syringoma typically appears as multiple small, flesh-colored, smooth papules around the eyes. (Reprinted from Callen JP, *Color Atlas of Dermatology*, with permission from WB Saunders Co.)

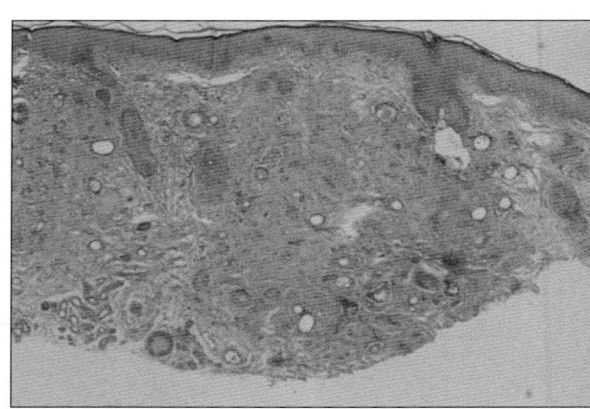

Fig 6-31a An eccrine syringoma showing ductal structures in a fibrous stroma.

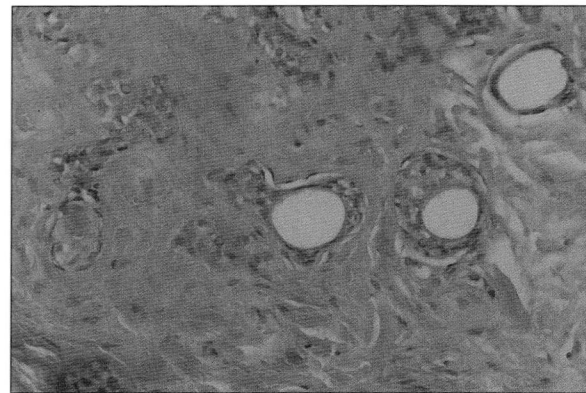

Fig 6-31b Higher-power view of Fig 6-31a showing solid and ductal structures, some of which have tadpole-like tails. Some cells have a clear cytoplasm.

HISTOPATHOLOGY ▶

The eccrine syringoma is a well-demarcated tumor in the superficial dermis. It consists of nests of polygonal cells in solid arrangement or with a central lumen, resembling ducts (Fig 6-31a) that may contain eosinophilic material. There is often a cord of tumor cells extending from the cell nest or the duct, giving it a tadpole- or comma-like appearance (Fig 6-31b). In some tumors, the cells have a clear cytoplasm.

TREATMENT AND PROGNOSIS ▶

Most eccrine syringomas are left untreated and accepted as a cosmetic imperfection. Since they are hamartomas, they are not likely to increase greatly in size. Cosmetic surgery procedures such as laser ablation and dermabrasion offer mild to moderate improvements. A dense coalescence of multiple lesions may require full excision and local flaps or skin grafting.

Chondroid Syringoma

CLINICAL PRESENTATION AND PATHOGENESIS ▶

The chondroid syringoma is another hamartomatous proliferation, this one originating from the base of the sweat gland (see Fig 6-29). It differs from the eccrine syringoma by its deeper location and its more solitary presentation as a single subcutaneous nodule. Like the eccrine syringoma, it has a predilection for the face, neck, and scalp, but unlike the eccrine syringoma it affects individuals of all ages. It presents as small, subcutaneous nodules between 0.5 and 3.0 cm in size (Fig 6-32). However, some can exceed 6 cm in size.

Although the chondroid syringoma does not contain true cartilage, it has been called the *mixed tumor of skin* with analogies drawn to the pleomorphic adenoma of salivary glands, which also is often called a mixed tumor. Neither mixed tumor designation is accurate with regard to true cartilage formation. The chondroid tissue is a reactive or inductive effect of what is essentially an epithelial tumor on the stroma, giving a chondroid appearance. The term *chondroid syringoma* should be used to describe this tumor of skin and the term *pleomorphic adenoma* should be used to describe the salivary gland tumor.

DIFFERENTIAL DIAGNOSIS ▶

The subcutaneous single nodular quality of the chondroid syringoma will liken it to a *sebaceous cyst* or a *dermoid cyst*. The *pilomatricoma*, described earlier in this chapter, presents in a similar fashion and location. In addition, some benign mesenchymal tumors such as a *schwannoma*, *fibroma*, and *granular cell tumor* will also present as subcutaneous nodules.

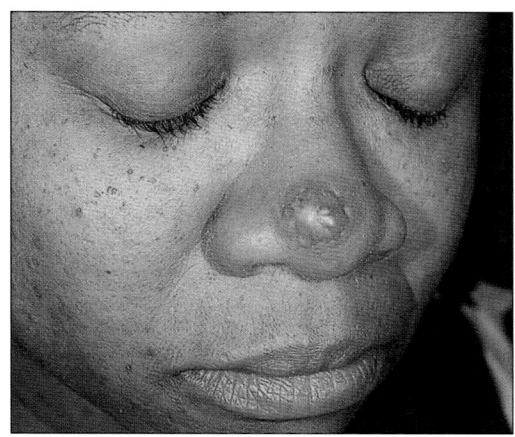

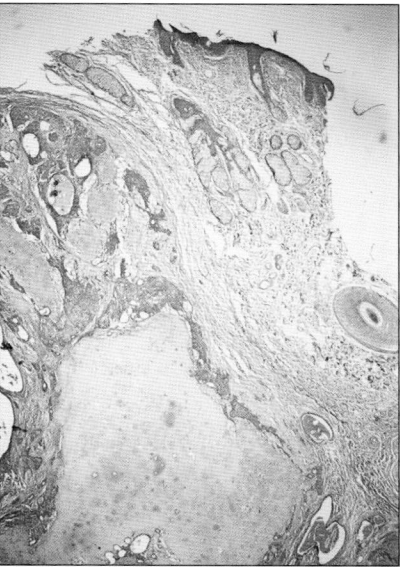

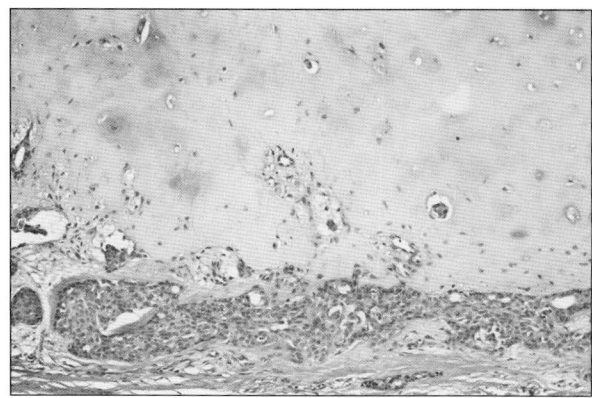

Fig 6-32 A chondroid syringoma will present as a small subcutaneous nodule that will distend the overlying skin. It has a predilection for the face and scalp. (Reprinted from Callen JP, *Color Atlas of Dermatology*, with permission from WB Saunders Co.)

Fig 6-33a A chondroid syringoma showing a well-demarcated tumor consisting of cellular islands and ductal structures as well as abundant basophilic, mucoid tissue.

Fig 6-33b Higher-power view of Fig 6-33a showing the epithelial islands and the myxochondroid tissue. These tumors bear a strong resemblance to the pleomorphic adenoma of salivary glands.

HISTOPATHOLOGY ▶

This cutaneous tumor is analogous to the pleomorphic adenoma of salivary glands. It is well demarcated and consists of epithelial cells arranged in nests, cords, and tubules together with a fibromyxochondroid stroma (Figs 6-33a and 6-33b).

TREATMENT AND PROGNOSIS ▶

As a solitary, firm, subcutaneous nodule, the chondroid syringoma is diagnosed after a local excision. Complete excisions should be curative. Such lesions should be excised with a pericapsular excision or an excision with about a 2-mm peripheral margin to the level of the underlying muscle fascia or to a level in the subcutaneous tissue below the extent of the tumor.

Eccrine Spiradenoma

CLINICAL PRESENTATION AND PATHOGENESIS ▶

The eccrine spiradenoma is a unique hamartomatous proliferation of sweat duct epithelium from the mid-duct level (see Fig 6-29), which, unlike most other skin appendage tumors, is painful both in the resting state as well as in response to palpation. It occurs at any body site and most frequently affects young adults. It usually presents as a single nodule within the dermis and will have an intact skin surface of normal color or a thinned and distended ashen surface with a reddened color (Fig 6-34).

DIFFERENTIAL DIAGNOSIS ▶

The painful nodular quality will be suggestive of a *sebaceous cyst*, a *secondarily infected dermal cyst*, or an *acne vulgaris* lesion. Painful nodules are also suggestive of a *glomus tumor*, although these occur in deeper locations. In addition, eccrine spiradenoma is clinically indistinguishable from its pain-associated sister eccrine tumor, the *eccrine hidradenoma*.

HISTOPATHOLOGY ▶

The tumor is composed of well-demarcated lobules within the dermis (Fig 6-35a). The lobules consist of two types of cells: a peripheral small dark cell and a more centralized larger, pale cell. These are often arranged as tubular structures that may be surrounded by hyalinized eosinophilic material. Tumor nests may similarly be surrounded by hyalinized material (Figs 6-35b and 6-35c). The adjacent stroma usually contains numerous dilated blood vessels and lymphatics.

TREATMENT AND PROGNOSIS ▶

Eccrine spiradenomas are usually excised for cure and for pain relief with a local excision using 2-mm peripheral margins and extending within the subcutaneous tissue to the depth of the tumor. Complete excision affords complete pain resolution and prevents recurrence.

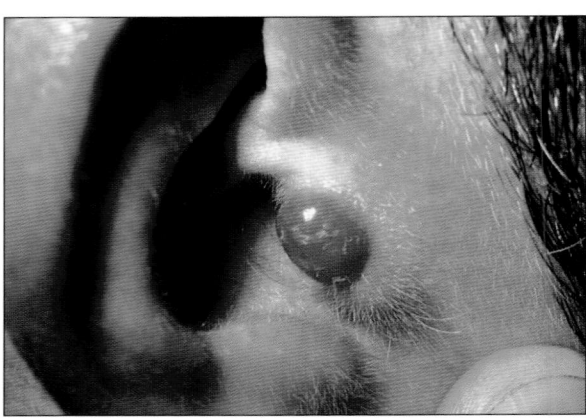

Fig 6-34 The eccrine spiradenoma originates within the dermis at the mid-duct level and will therefore have an intact skin surface of normal color. However, it is characteristically painful. (Reprinted from Mackie RM, *Skin Cancer* 2nd ed, with permission from WB Saunders Co.)

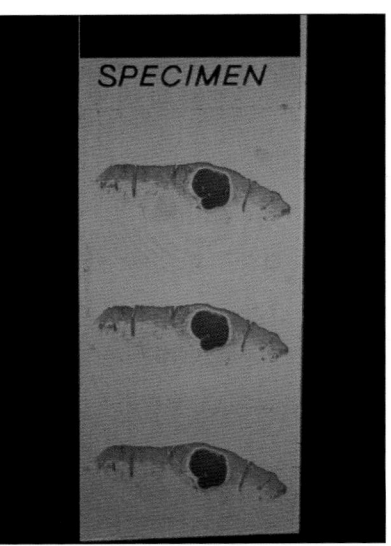

Fig 6-35a An eccrine spiradenoma consisting of a large, well-demarcated lobule within the dermis.

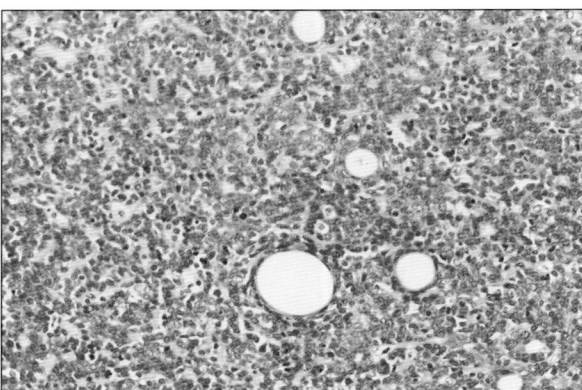

Fig 6-35b The eccrine spiradenoma is composed of intertwined cords of cells consisting of two types: some small dark-staining cells and larger cells with pale nuclei. Cytoplasm is scant. Some small cystic spaces are present.

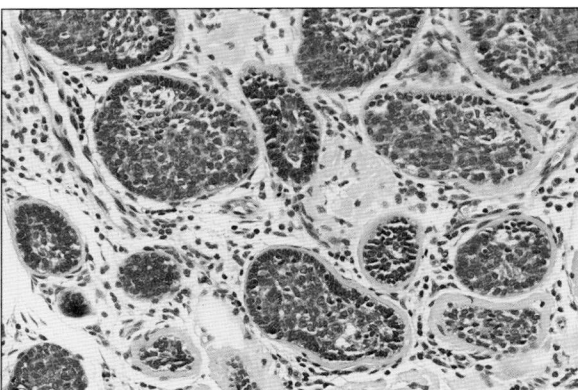

Fig 6-35c In this field, the eccrine spiradenoma shows discrete islands surrounded by hyaline material.

Eccrine Hidradenoma

CLINICAL PRESENTATION AND PATHOGENESIS ▶

The eccrine hidradenoma, like the eccrine spiradenoma, is associated with a painful presentation and represents a nodule in the dermis. Its histogenesis has been the subject of much debate because of the presence of two cell types histopathologically, one of which is a clear cell. However, staining for eccrine-associated enzymes clearly indicates that this tumor arises from ductal and/or sweat gland cells toward the base of the sweat gland–duct complex (see Fig 6-29).

Clinically, an eccrine hidradenoma can occur at any site in the young through older adult. It will usually appear as a single red or bluish nodule with spontaneous pain that increases in response to palpation (Fig 6-36). The overlying skin is usually thinned and distended.

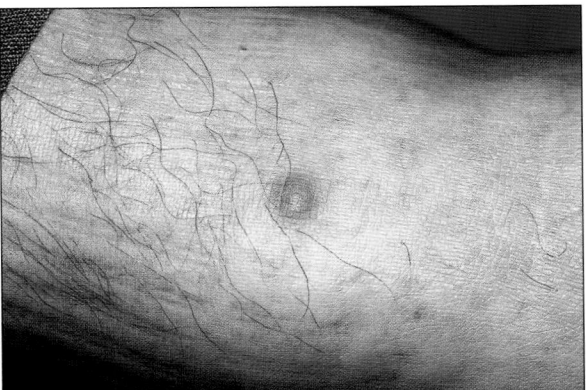

Fig 6-36 The eccrine hidradenoma is usually a red or blue nodule with a thin overlying skin. It is usually painful to palpation.

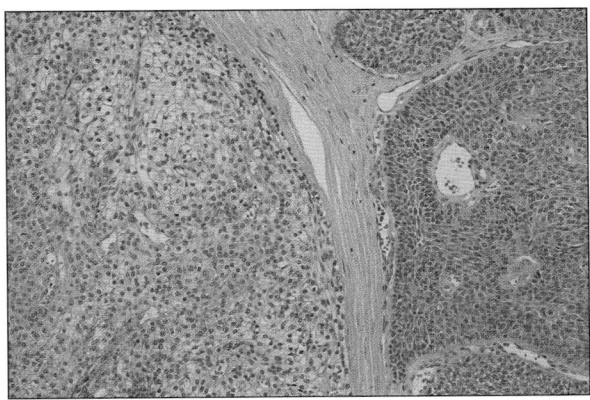

Fig 6-37 A clear-cell hidradenoma showing rounded clear cells on one side and more densely packed polygonal and spindled cells on the other.

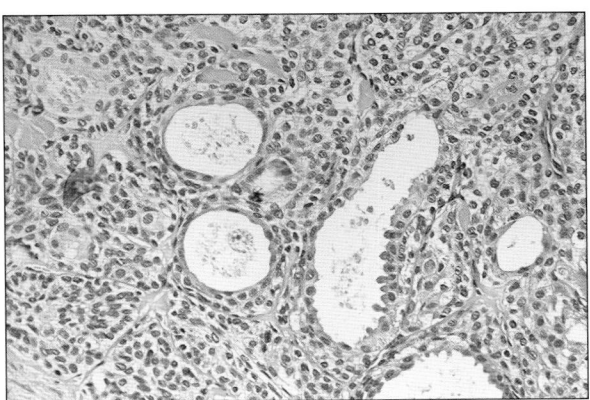

Fig 6-38 Lumina within a clear-cell hidradenoma.

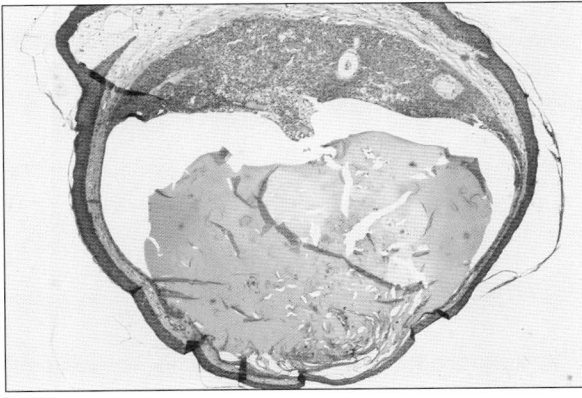

Fig 6-39 A large cystic space filled with eosinophilic material in an eccrine hidradenoma.

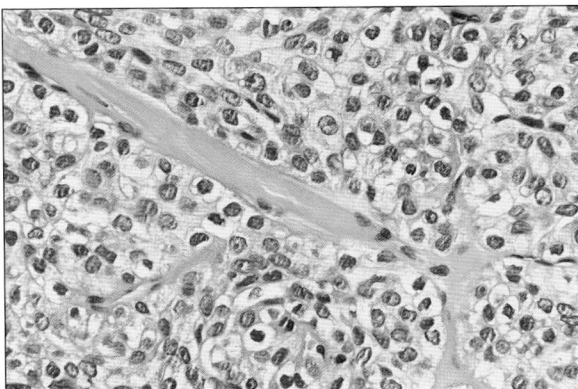

Fig 6-40 An eccrine hidradenoma showing an area of clear cells and a hyalinized septum.

DIFFERENTIAL DIAGNOSIS ▶

The differential diagnosis for eccrine hidradenoma is identical to that for and includes the *eccrine spiradenoma*. Thus, *infected acne lesions*, *sebaceous cysts*, and *dermoid cysts* are primary considerations, while a *glomus tumor* is a secondary consideration.

HISTOPATHOLOGY ▶

These are circumscribed, multilobulated dermal masses that may extend into subcutaneous fat. Occasionally there is attachment to the epidermis. The solid portions of the tumor consist of polygonal to fusiform cells and rounded cells with clear cytoplasm (Fig 6-37). Tubular lumina show varying degrees of prominence and are lined by cuboidal (ductal) or columnar (secretory) cells (Fig 6-38). There may be cystic spaces, some of which may be quite large. The lumen contains eosinophilic material (Fig 6-39) and is lined by tumor cells. Hyalinized collagen can form a pseudocapsule and extend into the tumor mass, forming septae (Fig 6-40).

TREATMENT AND PROGNOSIS ▶

Eccrine hidradenomas are locally excised to relieve pain and to obtain a diagnosis. They are completely excised using 2-mm margins and a depth of excision in the subcutaneous tissue beneath the extent of the tumor. Complete excisions will provide a cure without recurrence.

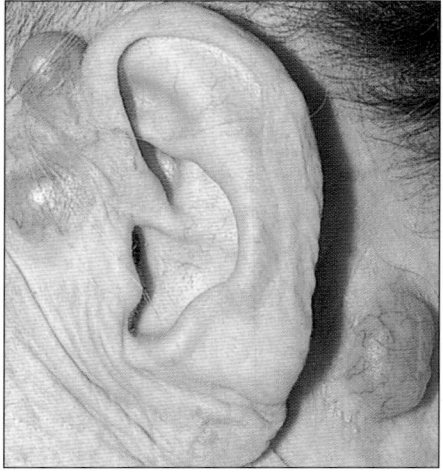

Fig 6-41 Single cylindromas are usually large protruding masses that may arise from the ear as well as from the scalp. (Reprinted from Cox NH and Lawrence CM, *Diagnostic Problems in Dermatology*, with permission from WB Saunders Co.)

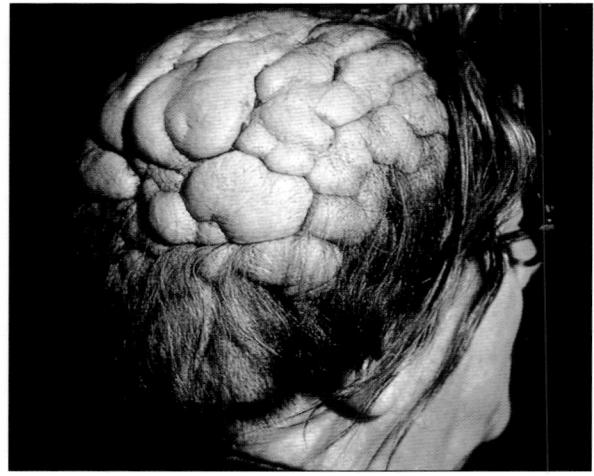

Fig 6-42 Multiple cylindromas of the scalp may coalesce to form a grid-like appearance of protruding square- or rectangular-shaped masses, often referred to as a *turban tumor*. (Reprinted from Mackie RM, *Skin Cancer* 2nd ed, with permission from WB Saunders Co.)

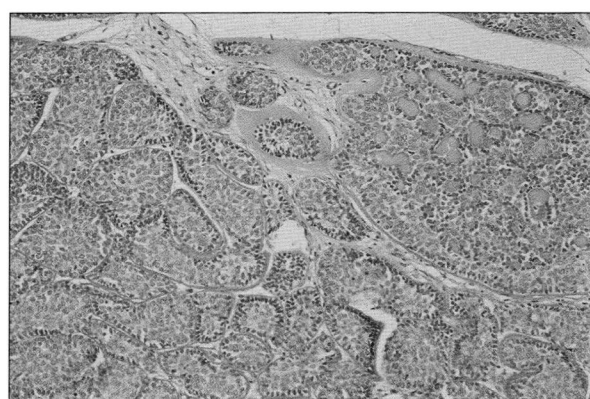

Fig 6-43 A cylindroma showing interlocking tumor islands, which are surrounded by hyaline material. Hyaline also is seen within the islands.

Apocrine Tumors

Cylindroma

CLINICAL PRESENTATION AND PATHOGENESIS ▶

The cylindroma of the skin and scalp has long suffered from a debatable histogenesis and confusion with the adenoid cystic carcinoma of salivary glands, known in the past also as cylindroma. For now, the enzyme reactions and the histopathologic identification of a decapitation secretion process, typical of apocrine cells, suggest that it is of apocrine origin. Regardless, this cylindroma is unrelated to any of the salivary gland tumors, least of all the malignant adenoid cystic carcinoma. Rather, it is a benign skin appendage tumor arising from apocrine glands. Most have no known inheritance pattern, although in some there will be a history of autosomal-dominant inheritance.

Clinically, the lesions may be single or multiple. New lesions will continue to grow and develop and may even coalesce. Lesions usually begin in the scalp or in the facial and neck tissues around the scalp and present as painless nodules in young adults. Single lesions may grow to large sizes (Fig 6-41), while multiple lesions may coalesce to cover a large area. When this occurs on the scalp, it is referred to as a *turban tumor* (Fig 6-42). Single as well as multiple lesions are nodular and will be pinker than normal skin. If they occur as a large scalp lesion they will produce a large area of alopecia and will have a cobblestone appearance that resembles the convolutions of the brain. In fact, these tumors may look like an exposed brain at first glance. In the fissures between coalesced scalp lesions, strands of hair may emerge.

DIFFERENTIAL DIAGNOSIS ▶

Single lesions will resemble several other *skin appendage tumors*. Since they occur around the scalp, *sebaceous cysts* and *dermoid cysts* are also considerations, as are some of the benign mesenchymal tumors such as the *schwannomas*, *granular cell tumors*, and *fibromas*.

The large multiple lesions of the scalp are usually clinically distinctive. However, multiple neurofibromas of *hereditary neurofibromatosis,* multiple lipomas of the rare *encephalocraniocutaneous lipomatosis syndrome,* and the numerous fibrous hamartomas of the rare *Proteus syndrome* may produce a similar appearance.

HISTOPATHOLOGY ▶

This tumor consists of irregularly shaped islands that fit together like a jigsaw puzzle. The islands are separated only by a hyaline sheath of variable thickness and a narrow band of collagen. A hyaline sheath

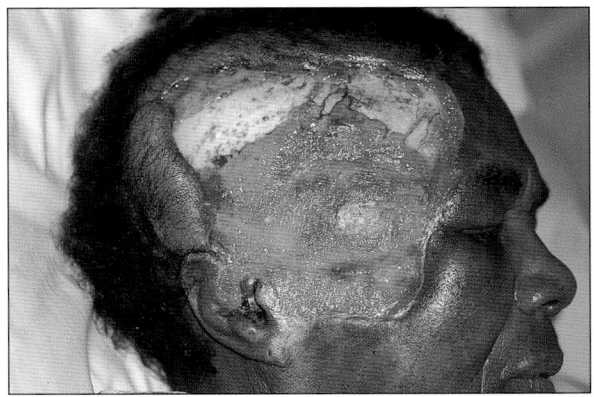

Fig 6-44a Excision of a cylindroma often results in a large scalp defect requiring a soft tissue flap reconstruction.

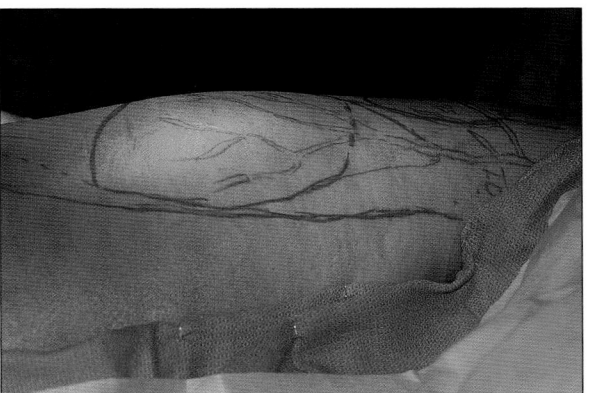

Fig 6-44b A free-vascular latissimus dorsi flap was required to reconstruct the large surface area of this defect.

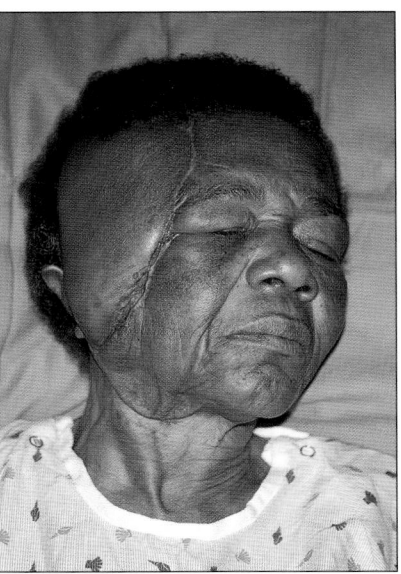

Fig 6-44c The healed flap successfully covered this large defect. A latissimus dorsi flap is one of the few flaps sufficiently large to cover a cylindroma turban tumor defect.

surrounds the islands, and hyaline droplets may be seen within the islands (Fig 6-43), and this component may be so prominent as to replace most of the epithelial cells.

The islands consist of smaller peripheral basalar cells and larger paler cells more centrally. Formation of lumina within the island may occur. There is a strong histologic resemblance to the eccrine spiradenoma, a tumor that sometimes occurs in combination with the cylindroma. These are dermal tumors that may extend into the subcutis.

TREATMENT AND PROGNOSIS ▶

Single lesions are locally excised, which establishes the diagnosis. Complete excision with 2- to 5-mm peripheral margins and to a depth in the subcutaneous tissue beneath the tumor extent should resolve the lesion. However, new primary lesions may develop later.

When large areas of the scalp are involved in the turban tumor appearance, the excision and reconstruction can be challenging, lengthy, and risky. Excising large areas of the scalp to the level of the subcutaneous tissues or more realistically the galea will incur significant potential blood loss. The surgeon should be prepared with Raney clips, electrocautery, topical hemostatic agents, and typed and cross-matched blood for potential transfusions. The excision need only incorporate 5-mm margins. However, because of its size, the tumor will leave a large surface area in need of cover (Fig 6-44a). Split-thickness skin grafting is a straightforward and practical method for reconstructing these defects. Other choices are the wide variety of fasciocutaneous or myocutaneous free vascular flaps (eg, the circumflex scapular flap, upper arm flap, and radial forearm flap) or the latissimus dorsi flap for the largest defects (Figs 6-44b and 6-44c).

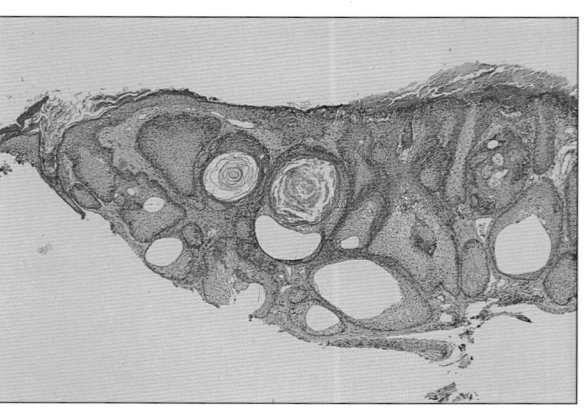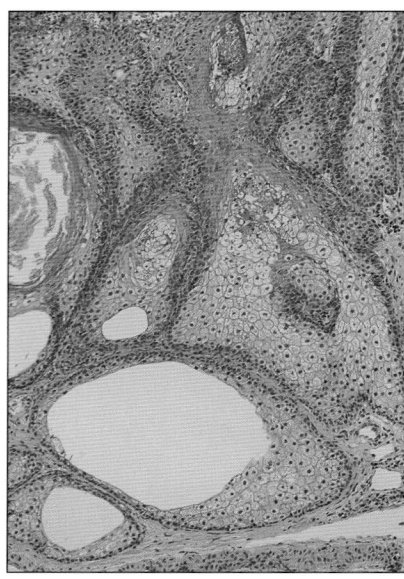

Figs 6-45a and 6-45b (*left*) Low-power view of a sebaceous adenoma. This demarcated lesion consists of islands of mature sebaceous cells with undifferentiated cells at the periphery, which are more visible at the higher power (*right*).

Sebaceous Tumors

Sebaceous Adenoma

CLINICAL PRESENTATION AND PATHOGENESIS ▶

Sebaceous adenomas are very rare, and when they are diagnosed Torre syndrome should be considered. In Torre syndrome, the sebaceous cell adenomas exhibit their usual hamartomatous or mere hyperplastic type of behavior, but they represent a marker for the syndrome noted to have a high preponderance of mainly colon carcinomas or other visceral or urogenital malignancies.

The sebaceous adenoma seems to arise within the sebaceous glands themselves but includes two undifferentiated cell lines along with mature sebaceous cells (see Fig 6-17).

Clinically, the lesions are solitary or are in groups of two or three clusters. They are slow-growing, pale yellow, raised nodules. Some may be slightly tender; most are 0.5 to 2.0 cm in size. They mostly occur on the face or neck in middle-aged and elderly individuals. The surface may be thinned and will occasionally crust or appear lobulated. A single sebaceous adenoma may be a marker for Torre syndrome, while multiple lesions increase the likelihood of this syndrome.

DIFFERENTIAL DIAGNOSIS ▶

The slightly elevated nature and their size suggest a *basal carcinoma*, a small skin *squamous cell carcinoma*, or a small *keratoacanthoma*. They may also appear as an *acne lesion* or a small *sebaceous cyst*.

HISTOPATHOLOGY ▶

These are well-demarcated lesions with a multilobular pattern. The tumor comprises two types of cells: undifferentiated germinal cells as seen at the periphery of normal sebaceous glands, and mature sebaceous cells (Figs 6-45a and 6-45b).

TREATMENT AND PROGNOSIS ▶

Like many of the other skin appendage tumors, sebaceous adenomas are excised because of their differential diagnosis potentials and are diagnosed from the excisional biopsy. Complete excision using 2-mm peripheral margins and a depth or excision in the subcutaneous tissue deep to the lesion's extent should be curative without recurrence. Recurrences should be looked upon as suspicious for sebaceous carcinoma.

When a diagnosis of a sebaceous adenoma is made, investigation for colonic or other visceral genito-urinary malignancies should be performed. Their association is too consistent to ignore. A lower gastrointestinal tract barium dye series and/or an abdominal-pelvic CT scan or MRI scan is recommended.

Premalignant and Malignant Epithelial Tumors of Mucosa and Skin

> "Always examine the chief complaint last; you will be surprised at what else you will find."
>
> —Joseph P. Welbourne

The Biology of Cancer

What Is Cancer?

Cancer is the end product of an unregulated proliferation of cells resulting from the accumulation of sequential genetic alterations (mutations) in a precursor cell. The resultant "cancer" is a population of cells that continue to mutate and that secrete self-perpetuating growth factors and angiogenic factors. Contrary to popular belief, cancer cells do not de-differentiate. Most tissues of the human body undergo a process of cellular renewal in which the loss of mature cells is followed by the proliferation of less mature precursor cells. The daughter cells of these precursor cells go on to differentiate into mature native tissues and are themselves incapable of cancer transformation. (This is evidenced by the observation that cancers do not arise from mature nerve, brain, or muscle tissue.) However, these remaining undifferentiated precursor cells in each tissue composite are vulnerable to a host of carcinogenic injuries to genes and are the source of most cancers. Malignant and even benign neural tumors such as astrocytomas, glioblastomas, schwannomas, and neurofibromas all originate from non-neural supporting tissues. Similarly, muscle tissue, which reduces its precursor cell population over time, forms rhabdomyosarcomas with the highest incidence in children and young adults. Oral squamous cell carcinoma is something of a misnomer since the cancer-generating cells are actually those within the basal cell layer of the mucosa. We call them squamous cell carcinomas only because the malignant squamous cell precursors (basal cells) undergo a partial squamous differentiation, making them look like squamous cells under the light microscope.

Evidence shows that cancers arise from the transformation of a single precursor cell into a clone consisting of many daughter cells with an accumulation of altered genes called "oncogenes." However, this does not mean that all cells within a cancer are alike. In fact, because each individual cell modifies its behavior and properties (mutates) with each cell division, cancer cells, even those within an early cancer, are a very heterogeneous population. The clinical impact is that over time, spontaneously, and as a response to treatment attempts, cancers can become resistant cell populations. The most resistant and fastest proliferating cell will become the dominant cell type of the tumor. This is observed in many cancers that initially grow slowly or do not metastasize and then transform into rapidly growing, invasive, and even metastasizing tumors (Fig 7-1). In particular, persistent tumors and tumors refractory to treatment are often seen to be histologically more anaplastic and clinically more aggressive.

What distinguishes a malignant tumor from a benign tumor is generally agreed to be the potential of a malignant tumor to metastasize. It is important to realize that the potential to metastasize is a property specific to each tumor related to the location and degree of its genetic alterations; it is independent

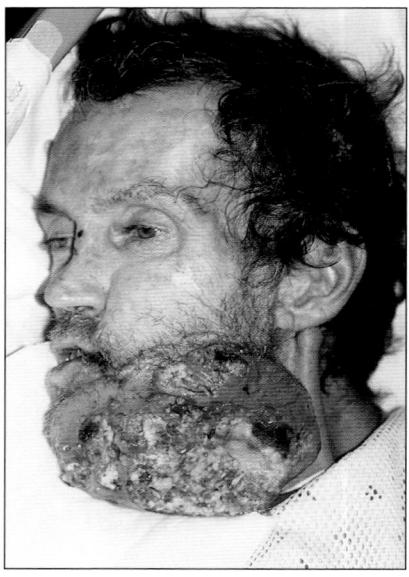

Fig 7-1 A large, fungating squamous cell carcinoma that underwent rapid proliferation after initial slow growth. Although it did not metastasize, it killed this individual by "tumor load."

of the histologic grade or the mitotic (growth) rate of the tumor. This explains the observation well recognized in oral squamous cell carcinoma that one moderately well-differentiated squamous cell carcinoma may metastasize early or widely from a relatively small (T_1 or T_2) lesion, yet another moderately well-differentiated or even a poorly differentiated squamous cell carcinoma may fungate and erode but not metastasize until very late. This principle is also well illustrated by the adenoid cystic carcinoma of salivary gland origin, which has a very slow growth rate of the primary tumor and a histology that contains only a few mitotic figures, but it expresses the property of perineural spread and bloodborne metastasis. It is a reminder that cancers are more than collections of cells with uncontrolled cell divisions. They also secrete enzymes, angiogenic factors, invasion factors, growth factors, and many other factors that confer on them the properties recognized as independent cell division, invasive growth, and often metastasis. Because their lethality is related to the elaboration of their growth factors more than to their state of differentiation, neither the light microscope nor the electron microscope nor even flow cytometry can accurately predict cancer behavior.

The Causes of Cancer

Epidemiologic studies have established associations between a number of environmental factors and the incidence of cancer. Some of these associations are so strong as to represent cause and effect roles. Some of the recognized causes of oral squamous cell carcinoma are tobacco-related products (particularly cigarettes), alcohol, several viruses (particularly human papillomaviruses 16, 18, and 32), irradiation, ultraviolet light, naturally occurring genetic defects such as are found in some syndromes, and random spontaneous genetic mutations. Cancer etiology is very complex and is related to the type of carcinogen, its dose, its frequency, and its application. It is also related to the synergistic or additive actions of two or more carcinogens, the susceptibility of the host, and most importantly, the length of time a carcinogen has interacted with host tissues.

To use oral squamous cell carcinoma as a model, the normal precursor cells in the basal layer are often exposed to the carcinogen of cigarette smoking and perhaps alcohol at an early age (too often at the age of 15 years or younger). The carcinogens benzopyrene and benzanthracene within cigarettes and either the alcohol itself or the nitrosamines found in many alcohol products damage the DNA of these cells by forming electrophilic intermediates. Like the intermediates formed by ionizing irradiation, these

Smoking and Carcinogenesis

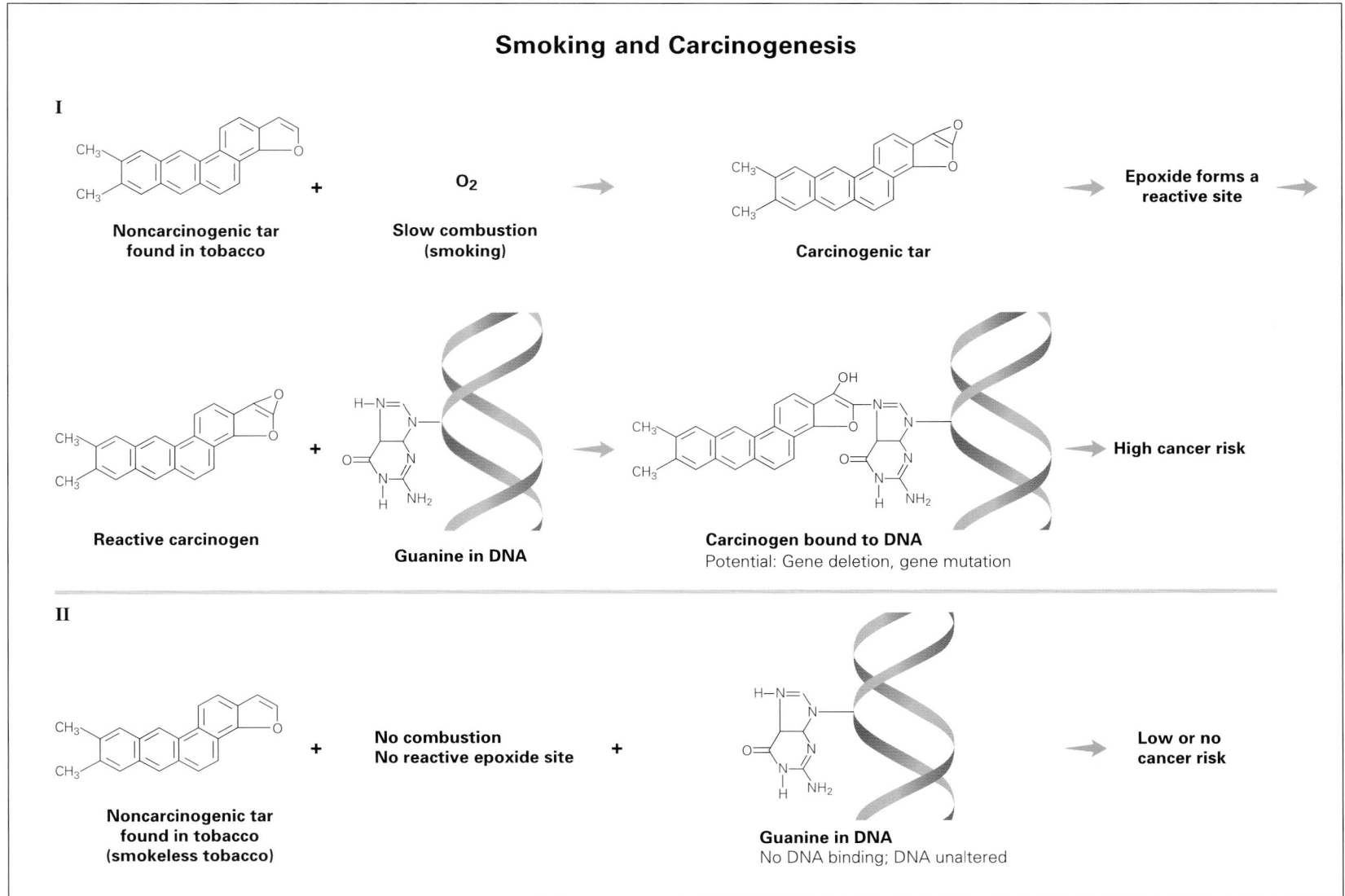

Fig 7-2 The carcinogens in tobacco are not actually carcinogenic until they are partially oxidized to an epoxide by the smoking process. Conversion of tobacco tars into their epoxide forms by the combustion of smoking allows them to bind to DNA.

electrophilic intermediates either pull electrons off the nucleotides within DNA, thereby damaging base pairs and base sequences, or become bound to DNA (Fig 7-2).

Cancers are not formed by a one-time exposure or by several exposures over a short period because the DNA is repaired by specific DNA polymerase enzymes. However, over time and with the synergistic or additive damage of several carcinogens, the sequential DNA damage exceeds the cells' DNA repair capability, leading to a permanently altered gene (mutation). Even then, the damaged basal cell is not necessarily destined to form a cancer. The DNA damage is usually severe enough so that the cell dies and, therefore, cannot pass on its cancer genetics. If the DNA-damaged cell does not die, it is often sterile and therefore cannot pass on its altered genes either. Even if the DNA damage is of the right type to confer viable unregulated growth, it may be lost in the normal slough of mucosal cells and never actually clone into a cancer.

For a cancer to become "initiated," a cell must accumulate at least six of these genetic mutations. Each mutation must be passed along to a daughter cell at the basement membrane, which retains this mutation and passes it on to its own daughter cells, which, if further bombarded by carcinogens, pick up another nonlethal, non–reproduction inhibiting, transferable mutation. Therefore, cancers are actually difficult to initiate and usually take years of repetitive carcinogen exposures before they develop. Because DNA turnover is greater during the growing years (0 to 20 years), DNA is more vulnerable to carcinogens in this time period. Once a cancer does develop, it represents a cell population with an unstable genome, which undergoes further self-initiated mutations, making it more aggressive, invasive, and increasingly more likely to metastasize.

Tobacco and Alcohol Combined

Clinicians have long recognized a strong association between oral squamous cell carcinoma and the combined use of cigarettes and alcohol, particularly so-called hard liquor such as whiskey. This combination may represent two associated lifestyle habits of which only cigarette smoking represents the true cancer-causing agent. Alternatively, this combination may represent an example of cocarcinogens working additively or synergistically to initiate a cancer sooner. Indeed, human papillomaviruses 16, 18, and 32 may play a similar cocarcinogenic role in some cases.

Cigarette Smoking and Cancer

Cigarette smoking is the primary risk factor for the development of oral cancer in the Western hemisphere. In order for electrophilic intermediates that damage DNA or become bound to DNA to be generated from tobacco products, the tobacco must be combusted (smoked). This burning of tobacco forms a partial oxidation (epoxide) in the benzopyrene and benzanthracene tars in tobacco, which in themselves are not carcinogenic, and transforms them into carcinogens. Thus, these epoxides of tobacco tars, not nicotine, are the actual DNA-damaging agents (ie, carcinogens) (see Fig 7-2). Nicotine is the addictive agent and is not by itself carcinogenic. Therefore, because these epoxides are not formed in "smokeless" tobacco, such tobacco products are not significantly carcinogenic and, despite the claims of several organizations, do not produce a higher incidence of oral squamous cell carcinoma than that which spontaneously occurs in the nonsmoking, nonusers of smokeless tobacco population. Certainly some individuals who have used "smokeless tobacco" have developed oral squamous cell carcinomas and have died from the disease. However, 9% of all squamous cell carcinomas in our major cancer center occurred in individuals with no direct tobacco history, indicating that "smokeless tobacco" history is coincidental rather than causative.

Exhaustive epidemiologic studies in the Division of Oral and Maxillofacial Surgery at the University of Miami School of Medicine have identified some specific associations between tobacco use, particularly cigarette smoking, and oral squamous cell carcinoma.

The first finding is the lack of association with smokeless tobacco. Snuff dipping and tobacco chewing create an inflammatory process and a clinical leukoplakia of hyperkeratosis (Figs 7-3a and 7-3b). However, long-term follow-up of these patches fails to show a significant number, if any, transforming into cancer. A few well-publicized cases of smokeless tobacco patients developing oral squamous cell carcinoma may be explained by concomitant cigarette smoking and non–tobacco-related squamous cell carcinomas, which account for about 9% of all oral squamous cell carcinomas, as noted above. Additionally, reviews of oral pathology files in regions of high smokeless tobacco use (eg, Texas, Colorado, North Carolina) do not reveal higher rates of either verrucous or invasive squamous cell carcinoma related to smokeless tobacco.

The second finding is based on a review of 2,632 oral squamous cell carcinomas, of which 236 (8.9%) were determined not to be associated with any tobacco products or with an obvious second-hand smoking history. This group represents those cancers that were initiated by spontaneous mutations from random errors during cell division, possibly other unrecognized carcinogens, and/or an inherited vulnera-

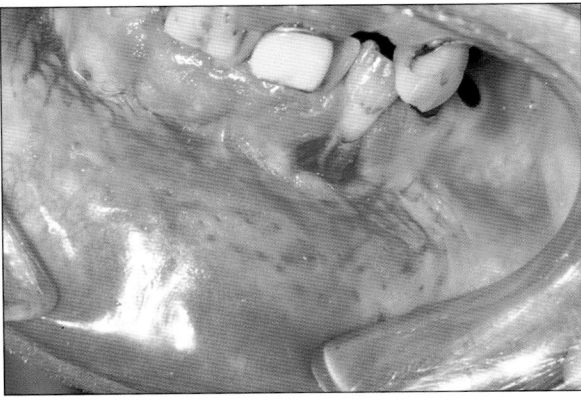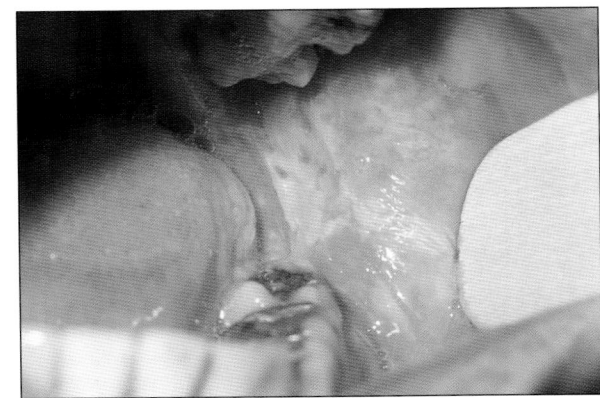

Figs 7-3a and 7-3b Smokeless tobacco will produce mucosal inflammation and hyperkeratosis but not dysplasia or carcinoma. The pinpoint red areas are inflamed minor salivary glands, not erythroplakia.

bility or predisposition to cancer development, which is found in breast cancer, pancreatic cancers, and others.

The third finding is an association with the frequency of smoking, the concentration of the tobacco-related tars, and the time of exposure from smoking habits to the development of oral squamous cell carcinoma. Animal studies using the standard topical carcinogen 9-12 dimethylbenzanthracine (DMBA) combined with human clinical studies have identified the following relationships: The probability of developing oral squamous cell carcinoma is proportional to the frequency of carcinogen exposure (packs per day) to the first power; the probability of developing an oral squamous cell carcinoma is proportional to the concentration of the carcinogen (amount of tars in the cigarettes) to the second power; and the probability of developing an oral squamous cell carcinoma is proportional to the time of exposure to the carcinogen (years of smoking) to the fourth power. Therefore, the time of exposure is the overwhelming controlling influence. In the oral squamous cell carcinomas related to cigarette smoking, it is more important to know the length of time the patient has been smoking than the number of packs per day. The traditional pack-year history becomes less predictive of risk than the knowledge of the age at which the individual first began smoking and the number of years of smoking. For instance, these findings indicate that the person who smoked two packs per day from ages 25 to 50 years (a pack-year history of 50 years) is at less risk than someone who smoked one pack per day from ages 15 to 50 years (a pack-year history of only 35 years). This is borne out by the histories of most squamous cell carcinoma patients who developed early-life cancers—that is, development in patients under age 50. In this group one finds lower cigarette consumption but earlier start dates, often at ages 12 to 15 years.

These data have yielded a useful probability equation for the development of oral squamous cell carcinomas:

$$P = K\,[f] \times [C]^2 \times [t]^{4.0}$$

where *K* is a constant greater than one and relates an individual's inherited susceptibility, *[f]* is the frequency of smoking in packs per day, *[C]* is the concentration of tars in the tobacco, and *[t]* is the time since beginning a regular smoking course (Figs 7-4a to 7-4c). This equation explains many clinical observations and is also somewhat predictive. Those who smoke more frequently generally develop more oral cancers (the [f] factor). Those who use unfiltered or less-filtered cigarettes and who smoke them to the butt seem to develop more oral cancers (the [C] factor). In fact, the [C] factor is also evidenced in those Central Americans who reverse smoke (ie, place the lit end of the cigarette into the mouth). These individuals regularly develop squamous cell carcinomas on the mucosa of the hard palate, which is a rare site for this cancer (Fig 7-5a). This reflects the close approximation of the smoke to the palatal mucosa

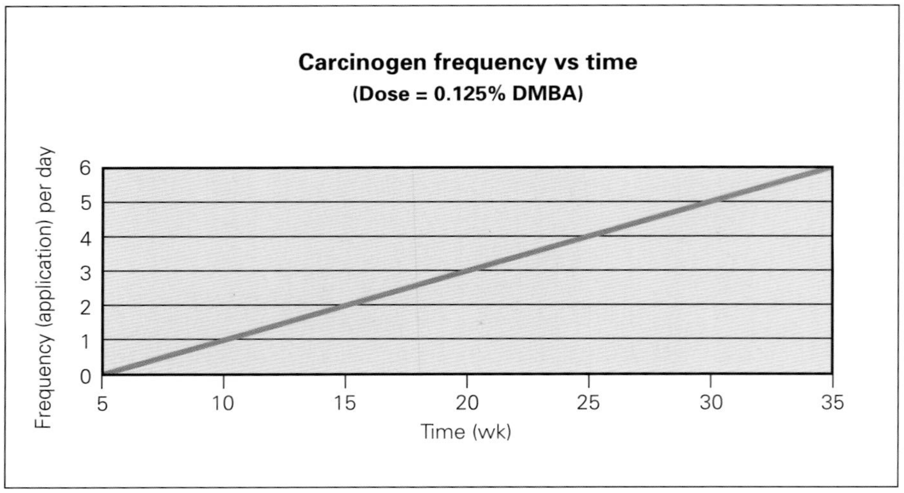

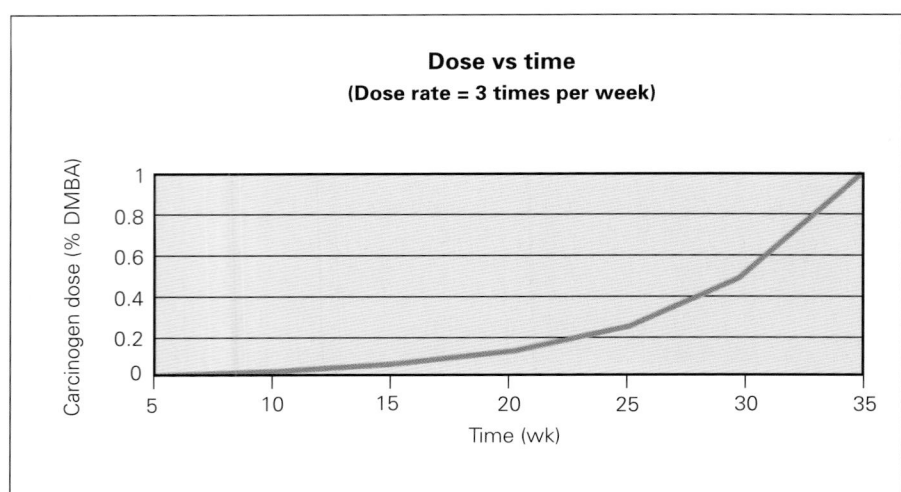

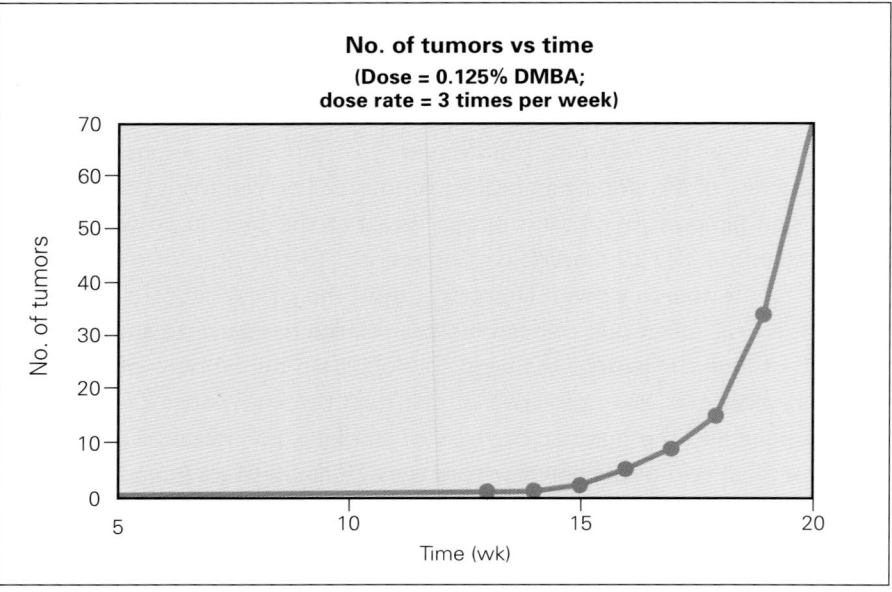

Fig 7-4a Laboratory oral cancer induction studies indicate that the rate of cancer formation has a linear relationship to the frequency of the carcinogen contact on a tissue surface.

Fig 7-4b Laboratory oral cancer induction studies indicate that the rate of cancer formation is related to the dose of the carcinogen by a squared function.

Fig 7-4c Laboratory oral cancer induction studies indicate that the rate of cancer formation is related to time by a t^4 function.

undiluted by the air space of the oral cavity; hence a higher concentration of carcinogens directly reaches the palatal mucosa. This [C] factor influence is further supported by the classic findings of Peto and Doll related to smoking and lung cancer. They essentially found that inhalers developed fewer lung cancers than noninhalers, the reverse of what one might expect. This was apparently due to the dilution of the heated smoke into the many air spaces within the lungs of inhalers. The noninhalers actually partially inhaled, introducing more concentrated smoke into the trachea and bronchi. The lung cancer that commonly developed in the noninhalers was bronchogenic squamous cell carcinoma due to a higher concentration of undiluted carcinogens in the bronchi.

The [t] factor explains the many patients who develop oral squamous cell carcinoma even after not smoking for more than 10 years (27%) and those who smoked for just 10 to 20 years and quit 30 years previously. These findings suggest that most of the cancer-causing cellular mutations occurred in their earlier years. This fact is supported by our data, which show that the mean induction time from first cigarette to oral cancer is 45 years for someone who begins smoking at age 20, but is only 41 years for

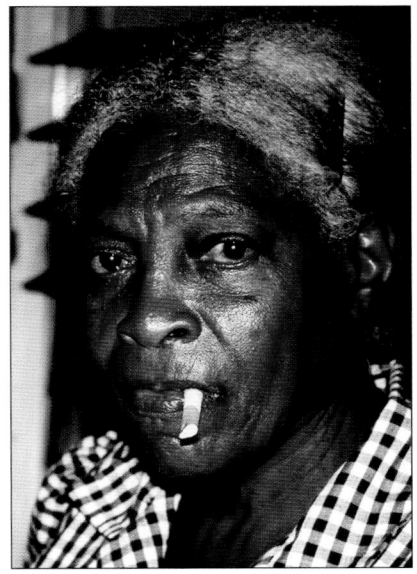

Fig 7-5a Reverse smoking, as has been observed in some cultures, results in a high incidence of palatal carcinoma due to a high concentration of the carcinogen striking the palatal surface in a focal area. (Courtesy of Dr Eustorgio Lopez.)

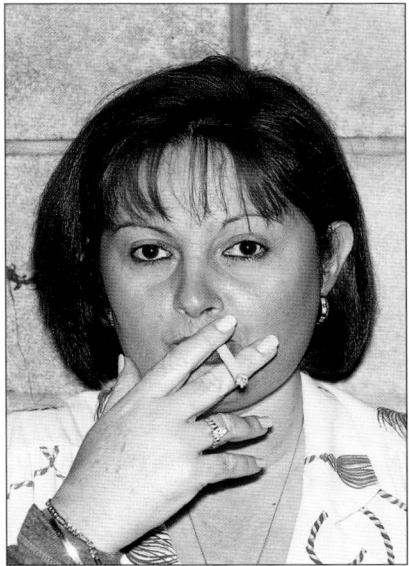

Fig 7-5b An individual's pattern of smoking is strongly correlated to the location of the oral cancer. Cigarette placement such as this would direct the smoke stream to the right tonsillar fossa/retromolar trigone area.

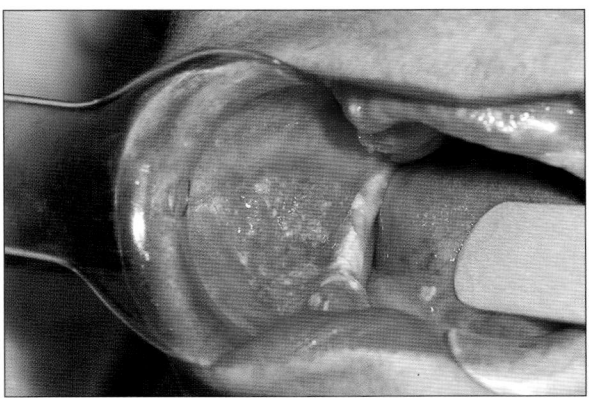

Fig 7-5c A buccal mucosa/retromolar trigone carcinoma that formed in the direct path of the smoke stream of the cigarette.

someone who begins smoking at age 18, 38 years at age 16, and 35 years at age 14. Therefore, the age at which the patient began smoking is the most significant risk factor because of the influence of time to the fourth power and the higher DNA turnover rate in youth.

The fourth finding is an association between the pattern of smoking in relation to the location of the cancer. Several patterns of smoking behavior have been identified related to how an individual holds a cigarette on the lips and in what direction the smoke stream is aimed. There is an 89% correlation between cancer location and the primary direction of the smoke stream (Figs 7-5b and 7-5c). The usual right-handed individual will place the cigarette on the right side of the lips and direct the smoke stream to the left side. These individuals tend to develop carcinomas on the left anterior tonsillar pillar, left retromolar trigone, left lateral border of the tongue, or left buccal mucosa. Other right-handed individuals will smoke in a crossover pattern, placing the cigarette on the left side of the lips and directing the stream to the same corresponding areas on the right side. These individuals develop right-sided cancers. Left-handed individuals will present an identical set of mirror-image patterns. Because more individuals are right handed than left handed, the overall occurrence of squamous cell carcinoma on the left side of the oral midline exceeds that on the right side (61% to 39%). It is also observed that floor-of-mouth carcinomas are seen in those individuals who manipulate the cigarette with their lips to direct the smoke stream downward into the floor of the mouth.

These patterns are consistent with the palatal occurrence of cancers in reverse smokers and the high incidence of bronchogenic carcinomas in noninhalers. The mucosa in the direct path of the smoke stream receives a higher concentration of carcinogens than any other site as well as a greater frequency over a longer time. Therefore, the pattern of smoking can be predictive of cancer location and provides some of the strongest evidence that cigarettes indeed cause oral cancer.

Cancer Progression

The single cancer-initiated cell will eventually develop into a clinical cancer. This process, often referred to as the *angiogenic mutation*, will occur when the last mutation confers invasive properties and the ability to recruit blood vessels to itself to sustain its expanded growth. Millions or even billions of cells will exist within the cancer, but not all of them will have the same properties. (This is also partially suggested in their histopathology: A so-called moderately well-differentiated lesion will have some very pleomorphic-looking cells and even some with bizarre mitotic figures, yet other areas in the same specimen slide will show keratin production and intercellular bridges indicative of a greater differentiation.) Therefore, to some extent the growth rate will be related to the fastest-growing cell, its radioresistance and/or chemoresistance, and the ability of one or a few cells to enter lymphatics or blood vessels and disperse to clone in another area (metastasis).

Metastatic potential is believed to be limited to a small percentage of the cells in a cancer. These cells must be able to adhere to vessel walls, invade through the walls, exist intravascularly, evade the immune system, transport viably to a distant organ, and clone in the new environment of that organ. Metastasis is a significant property since it may lead to death of the individual.

Oncogenes

Today it is believed that the multistep expression of cancer is carried through transformed genes (altered sequence of nucleotides in DNA) called *oncogenes*. Oncogenes may be conceptualized as "good genes gone bad." It has been shown that some tumor viruses contain genes that have a base sequence similar to that of normal mammalian cells but contain specific mutations that cause the expression of cancer in these cells; these are oncogenes. In addition, even rare genetic accidents such as chromosomal breakage, translocations, and gene deletions may occur in a statistical likelihood during cell replication unrelated to any carcinogen. Similarly, the DNA-damaging effects of chemical carcinogens (such as tobacco and alcohol) and energy-transfer carcinogens (such as ultraviolet light or irradiation) may confer a mutation and transform a normal gene into an oncogene. Further evidence of oncogenes as the biochemical center point of cancer development comes from syndromes such as multiple endocrine neoplasia syndrome, familial retinoblastomas, and even basal cell nevus syndrome, in which inherited DNA alterations or failure to repair DNA damage lead to oncogene expression of malignancy. Alternatively, carcinogens may delete or inactivate tumor-suppressor genes and thus allow expression of otherwise suppressed oncogenes.

Tumor-Suppressor Genes

Tumor-suppressor genes are the body's primary cancer surveillance system. These genes produce proteins, such as the well-known p53 and telomerase, that may repair damaged DNA or initiate a self-destruct sequence in a cell with abnormal DNA, causing cell death (apoptosis), as in p53. They may also repress or restrict the proliferation of cells such as telomerase. The loss of telomerase leaves telomeres on the ends of chromosomes. Telomeres signal cell replication. Their retention will confer the property of continued cell proliferation. In contrast to oncogenes, which essentially accumulate to produce a cancer, tumor suppressor genes produce or promote a cancer by their genetic loss or inactivation.

Biology of Metastasis

Although clinicians have traditionally accepted the concept that cancers metastasize through lymphatics and sarcomas through blood vessels, we now realize that both types of malignancy can metastasize by either means. Indeed, while squamous cell carcinoma of the oral cavity will most commonly metastasize to regional lymph nodes, it can and does sometimes metastasize through bloodborne routes to the lungs, brain, or bone.

Cancer's ability to metastasize is a complex biologic event requiring each of the following five steps:

1. Invasion through the basement membrane and between the endothelial cells of lymphatics or blood vessels. This of course requires enzymes such as collagenase, heparanase, and stromelysin, all of which degrade physiologic barriers.
2. Entrance into lymphatics or blood vessels to form a tumor embolus.
3. Survival of cancer cells within the lymphatics or blood vessels, where there are numerous immune surveillance cells and natural killer cells.
4. Escape from the circulation into a new tissue. This requires the elaboration of the same or similar enzymes as was required to enter the circulation.
5. Implantation in a new tissue area with establishment of a self-sustaining colony of cells (cloning). This requires angiogenic factors and numerous other growth factors to recruit blood supply, stimulate self-replication, down regulate some host cells, and activate other host cells (eg, osteoclasts to resorb bone).

One can see that metastasis requires one or a small number of cancer cells armed with diverse biochemical abilities beyond mere cell replication, and thus the odds are stacked against a successful metastasis. In fact, it is estimated that only 1% of a cancer's metastatic attempts are successful. This is why only cancers that inherently possess these advanced weapons (eg, adenoid cystic carcinoma of salivary gland origin, nasopharyngeal/base of tongue carcinoma, small cell carcinomas of the lung, etc) can metastasize early. Most cancers metastasize later or only after attaining a certain size and a more vast arsenal of metastatic weapons, and some never metastasize at all. Later metastasis is explained by the mutagenicity of the cancer. The longer the cancer goes untreated, the more likely one or more of the cancer cells will accumulate the additional genetic mutations (oncogenes) necessary to become a metastasis-capable cell. This understanding underscores the value of early diagnosis and prompt therapy.

Metastasis of oral squamous cell carcinomas is mostly to the regional lymph nodes of the neck (Fig 7-6). Cancers that have metastasized from the anterior floor of the mouth, anterior alveolar ridge between the mental foramen, and lower lip will first appear in the submental triangle lymph nodes along one of the anterior digastric muscles (level I, green). Cancers located more posterior in the floor of the mouth, in the oral tongue, the buccal mucosa, or the alveolar ridge between the mental foramen and the retromolar trigone will usually first appear in the submandibular triangle (level II, yellow). The submandibular triangle lymph node, which is located on the surface of the submandibular gland and just deep to the marginal mandibular branch of the facial nerve, is often called the *node of Stahr* after the German anatomist Hermann Stahr, who in 1909 noted that cancer of the tongue would settle in this node. Cancers that appear in the retromolar trigone, tonsillar fossa, and pharyngeal tongue will often first appear in the jugulodigastric lymph node located where the posterior digastric crosses the internal jugular vein (level III, orange). Squamous cell carcinomas arising from the nasopharynx area metastasize to the posterior digastric lymph nodes around the spinal accessory nerve (level V, pink). Each of these nodes is referred to as the *sentinel node* for its respective tumor location.

When a squamous cell carcinoma does metastasize via bloodborne routes, it will most often go to the lungs. When a single carcinomatous mass appears in the lung, it is unclear whether it represents a metastasis from the oral site or a second primary carcinoma in the lungs. The histopathology may be in-

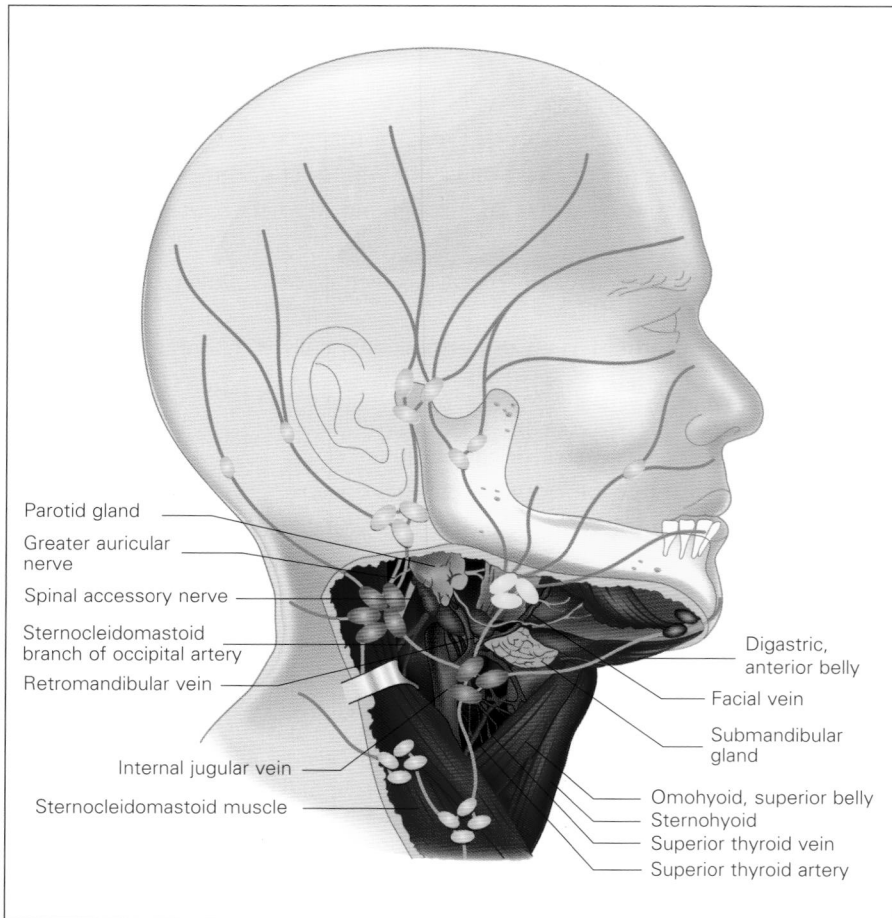

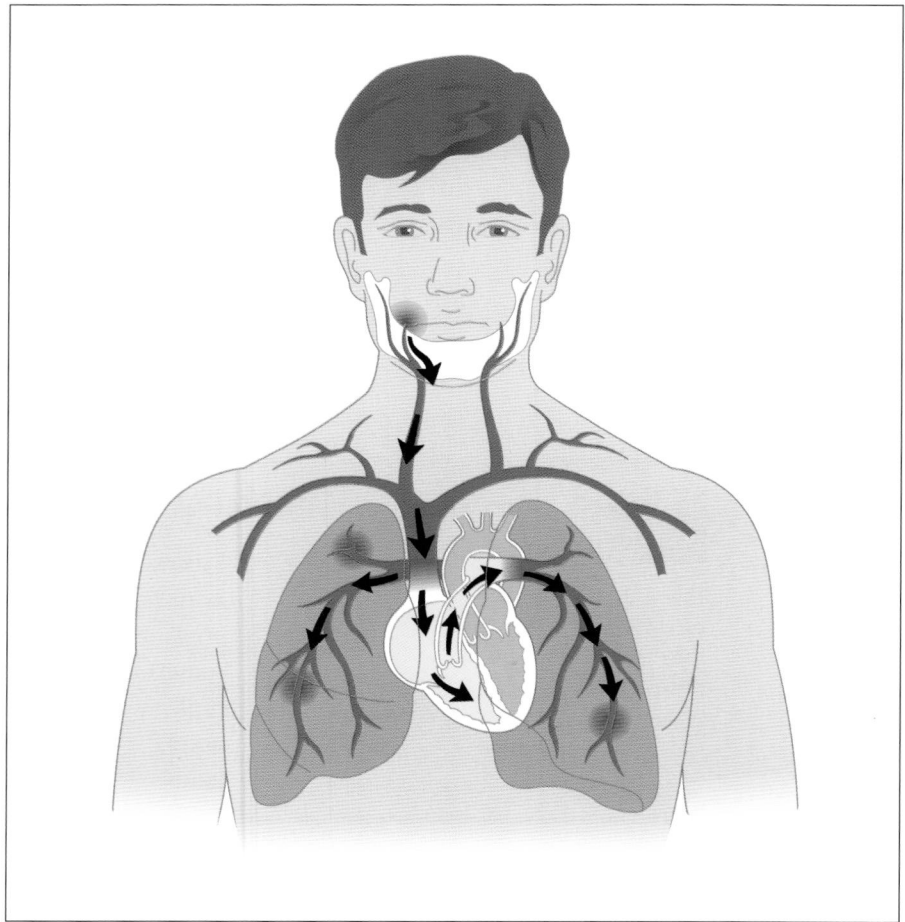

Fig 7-6 The lymphatic pathways in the neck explain much of the associations between the location of the oral primary carcinoma and lymph node metastasis. That is, tongue and lateral floor-of-mouth carcinomas usually metastasize to the submandibular nodes (node of Stahr, yellow); the anterior floor-of-mouth and midline areas metastasize to the nodes around the anterior digastric (green); tonsillar fossa and retromolar areas metastasize to the jugulodigastric nodes (orange). Base-of-tongue and nasopharynx carcinomas metastasize to the posterior digastric nodes around the spinal accessory nerve (pink).

Fig 7-7 Bloodborne metastasis to the lungs occurs via tumor emboli (often 25 to 100 µm in diameter) eroding into small veins that may drain into the pterygoid plexus, inferior alveolar vein, or facial vein, which in turn drains into the internal jugular or external jugular vein. The tumor emboli then flow downcurrent into the innominate (brachiocephalic) veins to the superior vena cava and right atrium. With each systole, the tumor emboli are pumped through the tricuspid valve into the right ventricle and then into the pulmonary artery system. As the tumor emboli are pumped further into the pulmonary vascular system, they wedge in small vessels to clone into metastatic deposits.

distinguishable. If numerous lung foci are found, then metastasis from the oral primary site is more likely. In fact, lung metastasis from an oral site is often multifocal.

The mechanism of oral cavity primary site metastasis to the lungs is via the venous system. The route begins with the intravasation of cancer cells into a small vein. This cancer embolus may then drain into the pterygoid plexus or another local vein. It then drains into the larger veins, such as the facial vein or retromandibular vein, and on into the internal jugular vein. It then flows through the brachiocephalic vein, which forms at the junction of each internal jugular vein and the respective subclavian vein. The cancer embolus next passes through the superior vena cava into the right atrium of the heart. As the heart contracts, the cancer embolus is pumped past the tricuspid valve into the right ventrical. From there, further cardiac contractions pump it through the pulmonary valve into the pulmonary artery. The cancer embolus then passes further into the branches of the pulmonary artery system, which progressively narrows, until it physically wedges into a small arteriole or capillary (Fig 7-7). Many cancer emboli contain less than 100 cells. One or several of these cells then lyse the arteriole wall to extravasate into the lung and replicate into a metastatic focus. The lung remains the most common organ for distant metastasis

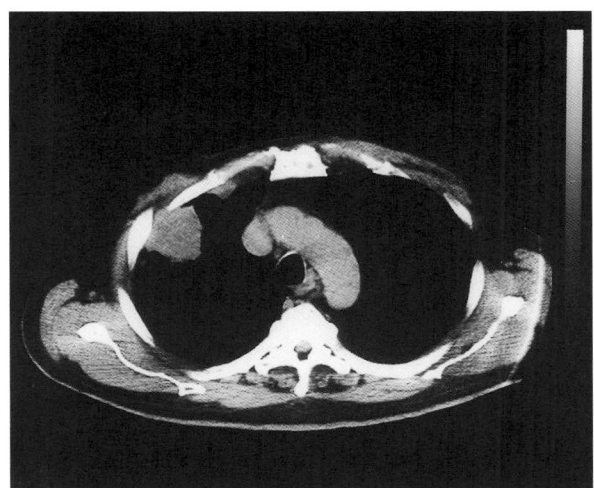

Fig 7-8 Metastatic deposits in the outer lung may not be distinguishable from primary lung cancers. However, they are generally seen in the lung parenchyma, whereas primary lung cancers are mostly bronchogenic or peribronchial and are therefore associated with the tracheobronchial tree.

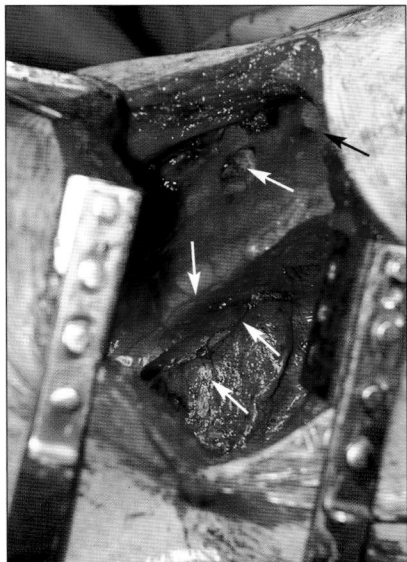

Fig 7-9 When a single metastatic deposit is identified through radiographic studies, numerous other microscopic deposits are usually present. Here a lung surgery shows numerous small deposits on the pleura and within the lung (*arrows*) that were not identified on the chest radiograph.

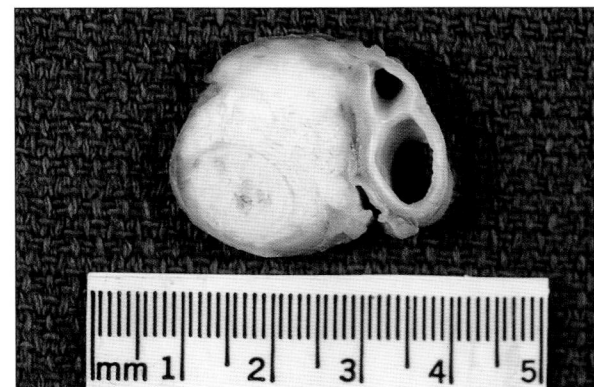

Fig 7-10 This large squamous cell carcinoma mass lies on the carotid arteries but shows no signs of erosion. Today "carotid blow-out" complications are very rare.

as a result of this mechanism, where the lung's pulmonary artery system serves as an effective filter (Fig 7-8). Therefore, metastatic foci will range from a single focus to multiple foci in a portion of one lung or disseminated throughout both lungs (Fig 7-9). In a similar fashion, the liver is the primary vascular filter of the abdomen via the portal vein, explaining why most abdominal cancers (ie, pancreas, colon, large bowel) metastasize to the liver.

How Cancer Kills

All cancers, including oral cancers, are life threatening. Oral squamous cell carcinoma in particular is recognized to have a 50% 5-year death rate. The death rate decreases when the cancer is diagnosed at an early stage and treated promptly, but it is still 50% for all cases. The American Cancer Society estimates the prevalence of oral cancer as 60,000 new cases each year. Accepting a death rate of 50% indicates that 30,000 US individuals succumb to oral cancer each year despite our best efforts to treat them.

Many clinicians mistakenly believe that the mechanism of death from oral cancer is a dramatic event such as an exsanguination from a "carotid blow-out" (Fig 7-10), an asphyxiation from a tumor mass obstructing the airway, a "stroke" from a large tumor mass in the brain, or occlusion of one of the internal carotid arteries. Today such events are very rare. Instead, the following are the mechanisms of death in order of their frequency.

Tumor Load

Tumor load is the most common, the slowest, and the gentlest pathway to death from oral cancers. Most patients lose weight, become weak, lapse into a coma, and die from a cardiorespiratory arrest. The weight

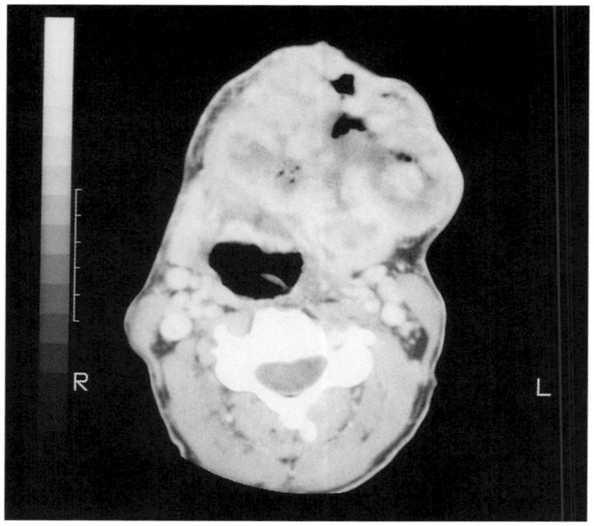

Fig 7-11 This extensive squamous cell carcinoma led to the patient's death from "tumor load." That is, despite gastrostomy tube feedings providing 5,000 calories per day and balanced nutrition, the cancer's systemic secretion of blocking factors prevented each cell's utilization of nutrients, causing the patient to lose weight. On autopsy, no metastasis was found.

loss and anemia of chronic disease develops despite gastric feeding tubes, iron and vitamin supplements, and even metabolic steroids. It has been observed that individuals will lose weight despite the intake of over 5,000 calories per day and otherwise normal bowel absorption (Fig 7-11). How is this possible? The very diabolic nature of cancer is not its replication rate, but the enzymes and growth factors it secretes. As the tumor load increases, the tumor secretes a greater amount of blocking factors and several vascular down-regulating enzymes, known as *anti-angiogenic factors*, which prevent normal cells from utilizing nutrients and metabolizing efficiently. These anti-angiogenic factors, which were first discovered in cancer cells, prevent normal tissues from recruiting new capillaries and instead promote the formation of new capillaries into the cancer.

It is important to note that this "tumor load" effect often is thought of as a failing immune system. Such a concept is incorrect. The white blood cell and immunoglobulin counts are usually normal and in proper function. Even when individuals progress to pneumonia, it is not caused by a tumor-related depression in their immune cells, but rather a loss of their protective reflexes and their physical barriers to infection or from medication-induced immune dysfunction.

Infection (Pneumonia)

As the tumor load increases and causes systemic weakness, infections, specifically pneumonia, become more likely. Individuals are often anemic, hypoproteinemic, and possibly malnourished by the secretory products of the tumor load (discussed above) and/or by the tumor-related dysfunction of the oral cavity and the effort required to eat or to be fed by someone else. This weakness and subsequent sedentary existence promotes atelectasis, which progresses to pneumonia. Many individuals are also prone to pneumonias via aspiration related either to the tumor itself, to surgery, or to radiotherapy. In addition, narcotic analgesics required for pain control both reduce the cough reflex and depress respiration, thus enhancing the likelihood for a pneumonia.

Complications of Treatment

A smaller percentage of patients die from direct complications of treatment or from side effects of therapy. Chemotherapy occasionally produces a severe marrow suppression, reducing white blood cell counts to less than $500/mm^3$ and resulting in a fatal systemic infection. Surgery has produced events such as the "carotid blow-out" or internal jugular vein exsanguination. It also poses the threat of upper airway obstruction, where patients die after the attachments of the tongue are removed or bulky flaps are placed in the airway. Even when tracheotomies are accomplished, obstruction can occur from dried secretions in the tracheotomy cannula or from displacement of the tracheotomy as a result of patient movement. More rarely, exsanguinations result from the tracheotomy cannula eroding through the trachea and then through the brachiocephalic vein. This is usually associated with long-term tracheotomies requiring ventilator support. Radiotherapy rarely produces life-threatening complications during its treatment. However, the delayed effects of radiotherapy can be a significant factor in the patient's death. Progressive later dysphagia from fibrosis in the pharyngeal musculature reduces nutritional intake and promotes aspiration. Osteoradionecrosis, limited jaw opening, xerostomia, caries, and secondary candidiasis commonly affect anyone who has had therapeutic radiotherapy over 6,000 cGy.

Progression of Comorbidities

The oral squamous cell carcinoma individual is often older and has a significant alcohol and smoking history. Many who present with an oral cancer also have hypertension, chronic bronchitis, emphysema, peripheral vascular disease, and ischemic cardiovascular disease. The physiologic impact of surgeries, chemotherapy, and radiotherapy often exacerbate these diseases, making them more difficult to control and increasing their rate of progression. It is not uncommon to have gained some control or even a potential cure of the oral cancer at 3 years only to have the patient die of a myocardial infarction or a cerebral vascular accident.

Paraneoplastic Syndromes

As discussed in the tumor load section above, cancers secrete a wide variety of enzymes, growth factors, and blocking factors. When a tumor secretes a growth factor or a hormone with a single physiologic response, it is often termed a *paraneoplastic syndrome*. One example of this is commonly seen arising from small cell (oat cell) lung carcinomas, but can also be seen rarely arising from some oral cancers. This is the tumor secretion of a parathyroid hormone–related peptide (PTHrp). This PTHrp is sufficiently close in its amino acid sequence and its active site conformation to native PTH that it has an identical effect. Such patients become significantly hypercalcemic, often with accompanying overt symptoms of confusion, constipation, and bone pain. Untreated, this leads to death. Similarly, some oral cancers will trigger a syndrome of inappropriate antidiuretic hormone (SIADH) by secretion of a small peptide chain nearly identical to ADH. These patients will have an independent cancer-related increase in ADH above the regulated native ADH levels, causing them to retain free water, develop hyponatremia, and undergo a characteristic decreased serum osmolality (less than 280 mOsm/kg) and an increased urine osmolality (greater than 150 mOsm/kg). Another example that may be seen in advanced cancers is a paraneoplastic pemphigus, in which the cancer secretes desmoplakin to which the immune system develops antibodies. These antibodies attack the intercellular bridge area, as often occurs in autoimmune pemphigus vulgaris, because of the similarity of the desmosomal antigen in pemphigus (desmoglein) to the cancer-related antigen desmoplakin. The result is the development of progressive, painful vesiculobullous lesions.

Principles of Cancer Treatment

The absence of any specific identifiable difference between a malignant cell and a normal cell remains the major barrier limiting the development of specific anticancer treatment. Today, surgery, radiotherapy, and chemotherapy are still the mainstays of cancer therapy. While immunotherapy, gene therapy, and antiangiogenic therapy hold hope for the future, as of this writing these therapies have not been firmly established and are not routinely used.

Each of the many malignancies occurring in the head and neck region may be managed by any one or by a combination of modalities. The protocol of therapy for each tumor depends on a multitude of factors, such as size, anatomic location, presence of metastasis, histologic grading, and general health of the patient. Unlike the use of antibiotics for infectious diseases, in which the treatment itself is rarely damaging to normal tissues, all existing types of cancer treatment cause significant damage to normal tissue. The general principles and limitations of each modality are described below.

Surgical Principles

Surgery remains the most successful therapeutic modality for oral squamous cell cancer. The surgical guidelines indicated for each malignancy are based on knowledge of the tumor's size, extent, anatomic location, history, and histologic appearance. For instance, it is an accepted principle that squamous cell carcinomas have a biologic behavior that is progressively more aggressive the more posterior the location in the foregut. A squamous cell carcinoma of the lower lip tends to be more exophytic, slow growing, and very late to metastasize. Squamous cell carcinomas of the tonsillar fossa tend to be less differentiated, exhibit early infiltrative spread, and are associated with early clinical or occult metastasis. The surgical approach to each is, therefore, quite different.

There are a number of accepted general principles of head and neck cancer surgery.

- Excision of the tumor must include excision of some normal tissue the amount of which depends on the characteristic invasion pattern of the particular tumor (eg, nerve resections and nerve canal resections may need to be part of the treatment for adenoid cystic carcinoma of minor salivary gland origin, and prophylactic neck dissection may be required in a tonsillar squamous cell carcinoma). En-bloc excision refers to removal of a tumor encased within a periphery of normal tissue. That periphery should appear normal clinically and on microscopic examination with frozen sections. In oral squamous cell carcinoma, the en-bloc principle often translates into removing the primary lesion with its draining lymphatics and lymph node chains contained within the fascial envelopes of the neck.
- The first approach to a tumor is associated with the best chance for cure. For instance, the recurrence rate for a facial basal cell carcinoma not previously treated is 3%. The recurrence rate of the same lesion if it has already recurred once is 18%. An old but true adage is "the first chance is the best chance, and it may be the only chance." Once a cancer has escaped therapeutic measures, the selection of resistant cells, the resultant injured hypoxic scar tissue, and the anatomic distortions make all forms of salvage treatment less successful.
- Combination therapy with chemotherapy and/or irradiation can improve results for most tumors. The use of combined therapy is a benefit-versus–side effect decision unique to each case.
- Host resistance should be improved as much as possible before and after surgery. Nutritional needs should be anticipated during the immediate and late postoperative course.
- Psychologic support of the patient should also be considered. Family members, friends, clergy, and members of the treatment team can help patients cope with the diagnosis, treatment, and their fears.
- Reconstruction and rehabilitation should be included as part of the overall treatment. Today's reconstructive approaches, which are predictable and have reduced morbidities, will improve most patients' functional and psychologic well-being.

The specific treatment approaches related to oral squamous cell carcinoma generally accepted for each lesion location follow each site discussion; however, some of the specifics of standard cancer approaches must be understood first.

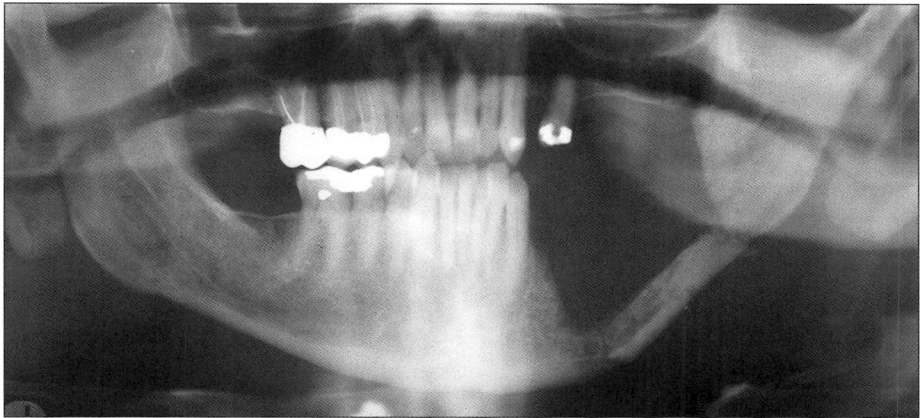

Fig 7-12a Peripheral resections of the mandible should avoid right angles and retain at least 1 cm of the inferior border. Otherwise a postoperative fracture, like the one seen here, may result.

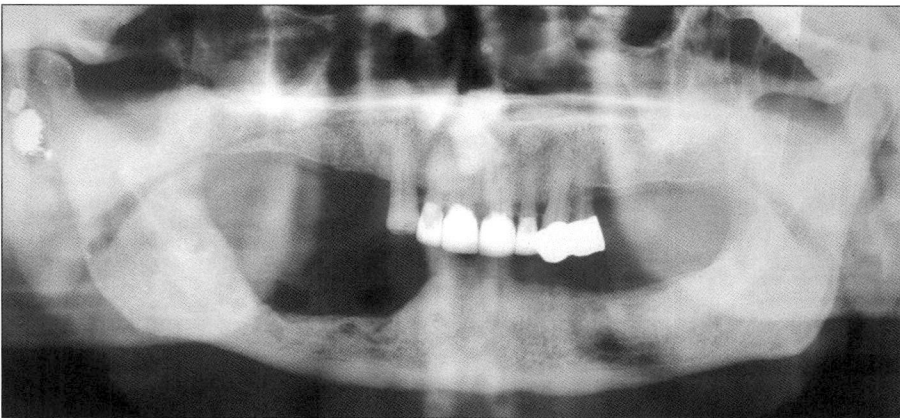

Fig 7-12b Peripheral resections that are rounded and retain more than 1 cm of the inferior border will not fracture.

Resections of the Mandible

When and how to resect the mandible is always controversial. When carcinomas show radiographic or scan evidence of bony invasion, the lesion becomes a T_4 lesion and a continuity resection is required. When the lesion is clinically adherent to periosteum, it is assumed to extend into the mandible through its many small foramina, and a continuity resection is again required. There is little indication for cortical plate removal without continuity resection because most believe that if the cancer truly extends to the cortex, it has microscopically infiltrated past the cortex into the medullary space. One possible exception is a tumor that approaches the cortex but is clinically separated from it. The removal of the cortex as an anatomic barrier is valid in this context.

Peripheral resections of the mandible are indicated in gingival carcinomas and less commonly in localized alveolar ridge carcinomas. Such peripheral resections have been the source of pathologic fractures if the inferior border is thinned too much. This is due to reflection of the vascular periosteum from the inferior border, which devitalizes osteocytes. As the inferior border is revascularized, resorption of mineral matrix precedes new bone apposition; therefore, the bone becomes maximally weakened at 3 weeks, the time when most fractures occur (Fig 7-12a). Most pathologic fractures in these situations occur at the junction of a resection's rectangular form, where a vertical wall meets a horizontal wall to which loading forces are directed. Therefore, when a peripheral resection is considered, at least 10 mm of inferior border should remain; if not, it is best to accomplish a continuity resection. The resection should not reflect soft tissue from the inferior border intended to be retained, and the design of the resection should create sloping walls rather than 90-degree right angles (Fig 7-12b).

When a portion of the mandible is resected with a continuity resection, the bony edges should be rounded and some form of stabilization provided to prevent displacement. Today, internal titanium stabilization plates serve this purpose well and have mostly replaced external skeletal pins of the Joe Hall Morris type (Fig 7-13).

Resections of the mandible in the area of the ramus include condylar extirpation more frequently than is truly required by the cancer invasion. Vertical subcondylar ostectomies of the ramus, which preserve the condyle and the posterior border of the ramus, are greatly preferred (Fig 7-14). Horizontal ostectomies, which also preserve the condyle but leave the coronoid process and temporal muscle pull to displace the proximal segment, are largely unnecessary and certainly require rigid internal fixation plates to prevent proximal segment displacement. Extirpations or ostectomies that leave less than 1 cm of the condylar neck result in too small a condyle to be useful. In such cases, a condylar extirpation is unavoidable (Fig 7-15).

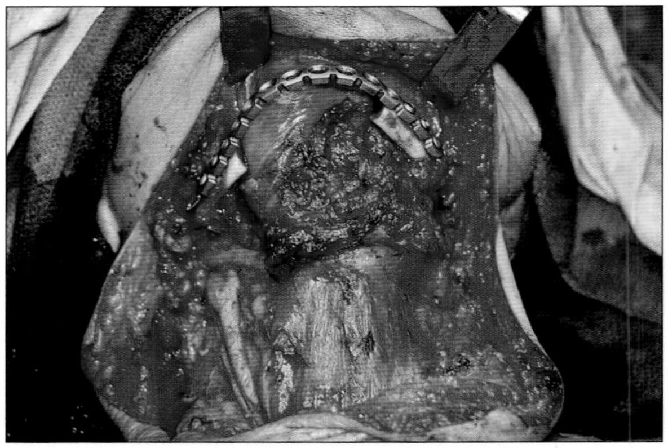

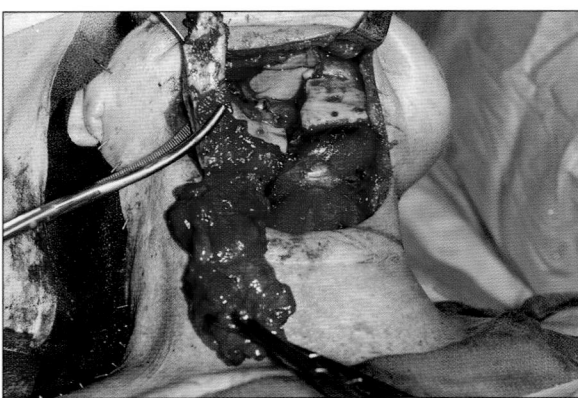

Fig 7-13 A rigid reconstruction plate stabilizes the proximal segments and restores continuity after a jaw–floor of mouth–bilateral neck resection, often referred to as a *commando procedure*.

Fig 7-14 Hemimandibular resections should include the coronoid process via a vertical subcondylar ostectomy to prevent displacement of the proximal segment and loosening of the plate screws on the proximal segment.

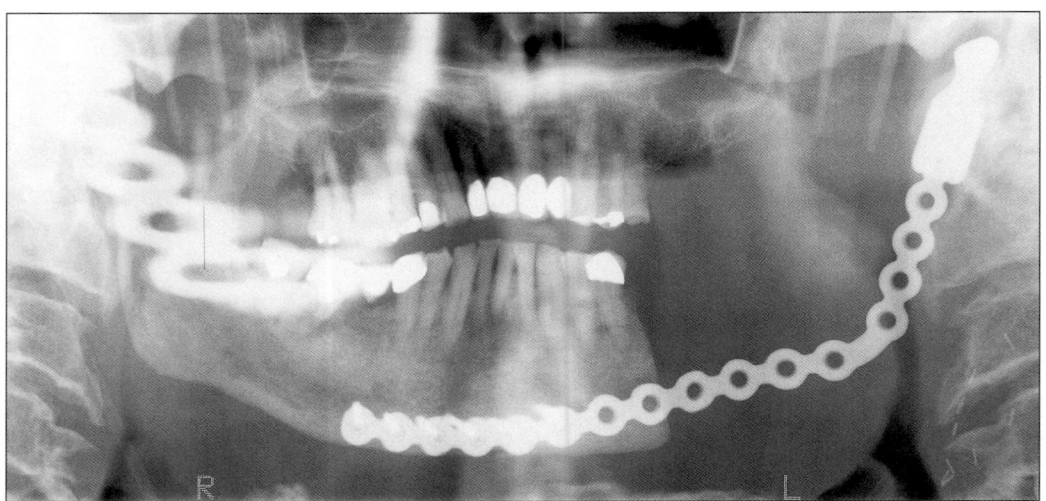

Fig 7-15 A rigid reconstruction plate bridges a hemimandibular defect and includes a condylar replacement. This patient can function without a bone graft for as long as the plate remains stable. Long-term follow-up indicates stability and absence of complications with this type of condylar replacement.

Neck Dissections

The biologic principle of an incontinuity neck dissection is that the lymphatics and lymph node chains in the neck are contained in the cervical fascia and in the fatty contents around the cervical fascia of the neck. The intent of any "modified" neck dissection is to remove this tissue composite of fascia. Today, two basic neck dissections of the many that exist represent the ends of a spectrum of approaches from most to least extirpative. Of these two neck dissections, the traditional full radical neck dissection is the most extirpative and the functional neck dissection of Bocca and Pignataro (often called the *Bocca neck*) the least extirpative.

Full Radical Neck Dissection

The full radical neck dissection includes the extirpation of the sternocleidomastoid muscle, the internal jugular vein, and the spinal accessory nerve in composite with the lymphatics contained in the cervi-

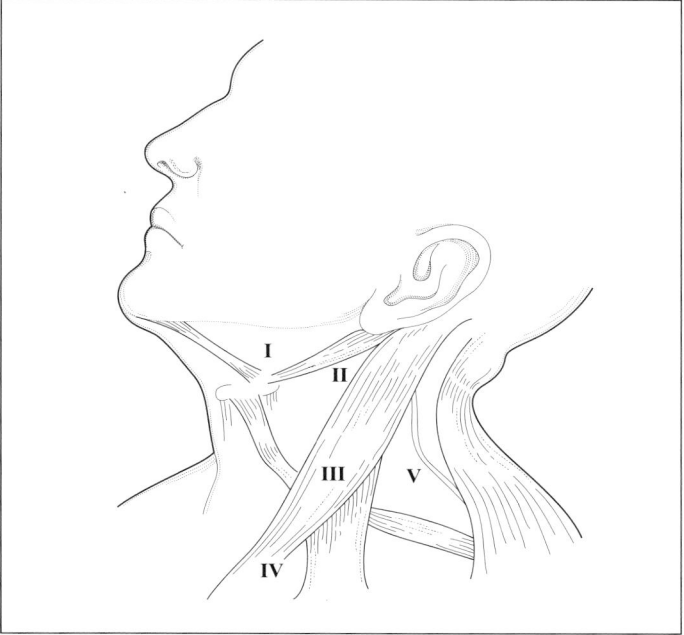

Fig 7-16 The five levels of the neck. The various cancer neck dissections can be described according to the removal of the contents in each level.

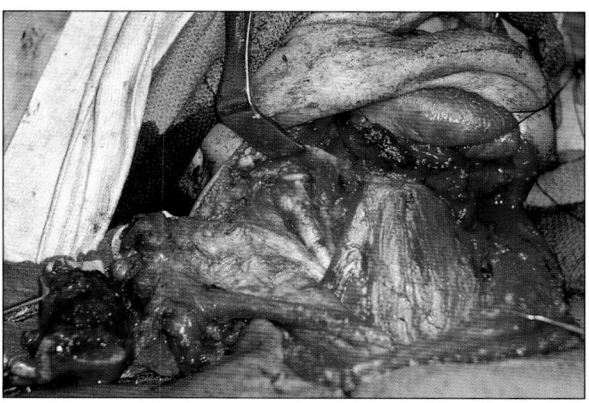

Fig 7-17 Modified neck dissection to remove the lymphatics at levels I through V, as well as the sternocleidomastoid muscle and the internal jugular vein. The spinal accessory nerve was preserved.

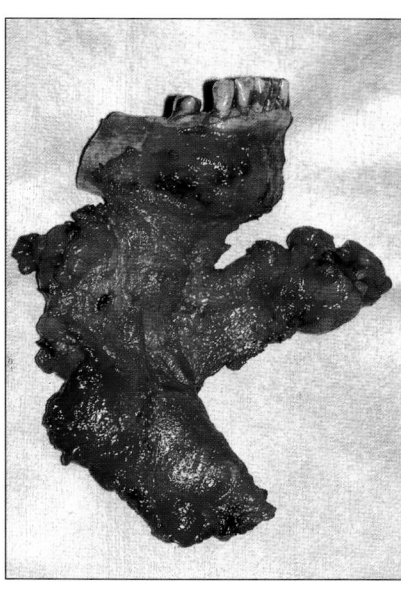

Fig 7-18 A so-called incontinuity dissection includes the primary tumor along with the neck contents as a single unit.

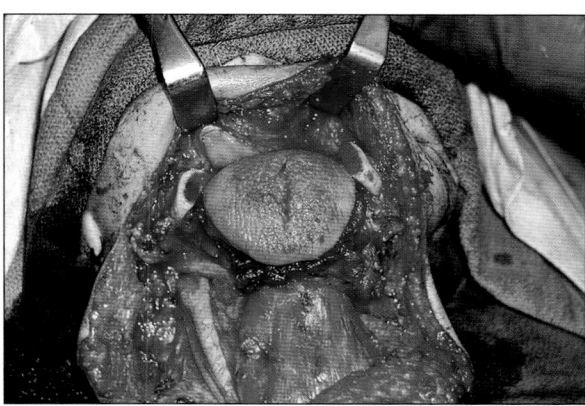

Fig 7-19 The defect resulting from a jaw and neck resection is significant. Here a midline defect of the mandible may compromise the airway via tongue displacement. A rigid reconstruction plate, as shown in Fig 7-15, will allow for tongue positioning to maintain the airway space. A pectoralis major myocutaneous flap is needed to reconstruct the soft tissue defect.

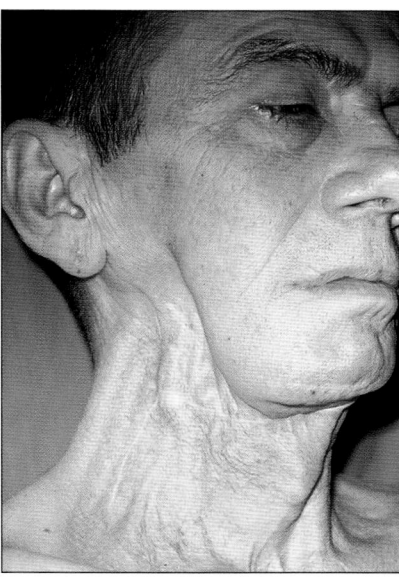

Fig 7-20 An unreconstructed jaw-neck resection will result in a functional compromise and visual deformity. Here the skin is fibrosed and adherent to the carotid artery.

cal fascia and fatty contents. This surgery extirpates the fascia from all five levels in the neck (Fig 7-16). It traditionally has also included extirpation of the tail of the parotid gland and the marginal mandibular branch of the facial nerve (Figs 7-17 to 7-20).

Functional Neck Dissection

In 1967, Bocca and Pignataro introduced the functional neck dissection with the correct assertion that the lymphatics of the neck do not enter the sternocleidomastoid muscle, the carotid sheath, or the epineurium of the spinal accessory nerve. This surgery literally peels the cervical fascia, carotid sheath, and fatty contents from these structures and preserves them. The functional neck dissection has since gained a firm place in cancer surgery (Figs 7-21a to 7-21e). It includes extirpation of the fascia in all five levels of the neck but preserves the important structures (functional contents) in each level. The supra-omohyoid neck dissection is a slight modification of the classic Bocca functional neck dissection that leaves the contents of the omohyoid triangle, also called level IV, and may or may not remove a portion of the fascia in level V. Level IV is anatomically bordered by the inferior belly of the omohyoid, the anterior border of the sternocleidomastoid, and the clavicle.

Modified Radical Neck Dissections

Since the introduction of the functional neck dissection, several neck dissections preserving some but not all of the three main structures preserved in the functional neck dissection have been developed; these are called *modified radical neck dissections*. The one most commonly in use today extirpates most of the same structures as the full radical neck dissection but preserves the spinal accessory nerve. Carcinomas that arise in the true oral cavity (the anterior tonsillar pillars to the lips) are associated with lymphatic spread into the posterior triangle of the neck only 0.9% of the time. Therefore, extensive dissection around or extirpation of the spinal accessory nerve as it courses through the posterior triangle of the neck usually is unwarranted.

Choice of neck surgeries is the surgeon's prerogative based on his or her experience and understanding of the literature. In general, the functional neck dissection is employed for prophylactic neck dissections—that is, treatment of the N_0 neck, indicating no regional lymph node metastasis—and for treatment of the N_1 neck, indicating limited regional lymph node metastasis. As the neck staging increases to N_2 or N_3, a modified radical or full radical neck dissection becomes preferred. This is due to the concern that N_2 and N_3 necks have sufficient escape of cancer cells beyond the capsule of the lymph nodes and that cancer cells will adhere to other structures in the neck, thereby reducing the effectiveness of the functional neck dissection.

Indications for Postsurgical Radiotherapy

Postsurgical radiotherapy is a better employment of radiotherapy than presurgical radiotherapy. With presurgical radiotherapy the tumor may have decreased macroscopically but not microscopically. Therefore, if the surgeon excises using the new radiation-shrunken clinical margin, there is a risk of leaving islands of cancer cells beyond the surgical margins. If the surgeon uses the pre-radiation clinical cancer margin, it will be gone, and an approximation as to where it was originally located will be required, making the excision less precise. In addition, extensive extirpative cancer surgery in previously radiated tissue inherits a high incidence of soft tissue dehiscence, wound infections, and osteoradionecrosis.

Postsurgical radiotherapy is designed to serve as "mop-up" radiotherapy, sterilizing a smaller population of cancer cells than would be required if used as a stand-alone therapy or as a presurgical therapy. Certainly radiotherapy is more effective if the cancer cell population is small and scattered across the treatment field rather than in a single large mass. Therefore, postsurgical radiotherapy is often used when resection margins are close or positive, when there is evidence of cancer cell spread outside of lymph nodes, or when the size of a tumor is sufficiently large as to raise suspicion of cancer cell escape beyond the margins of even the best surgery.

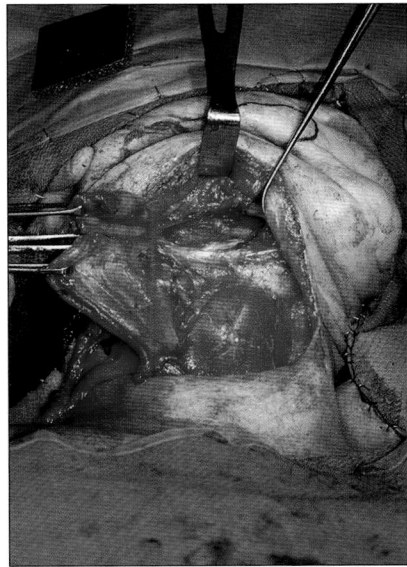

Fig 7-21a This functional neck dissection removed the fascial envelope in the anterior triangle of the neck. The carotid sheath is about to be opened so that it can be removed with the dissection, its contents can be preserved, and a continuation of the dissection around the sternocleidomastoid muscle and entry into the posterior triangle can be achieved.

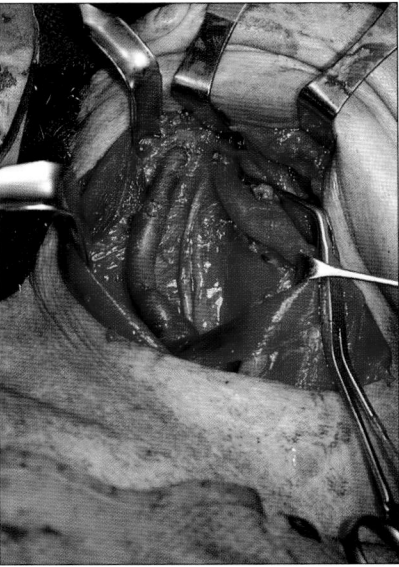

Fig 7-21b A functional neck dissection removes the neck lymphatics and the carotid sheath while preserving its contents, along with the sternocleidomastoid muscle and the spinal accessory nerve.

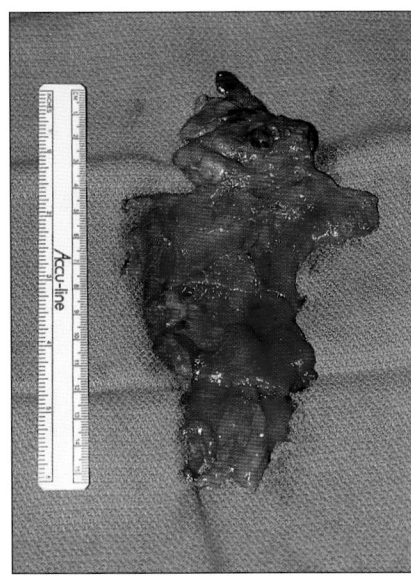

Fig 7-21c The specimen from a functional neck dissection lacks identifiable anatomic components. Sutures placed to orient the specimen will be an aid to the pathologist.

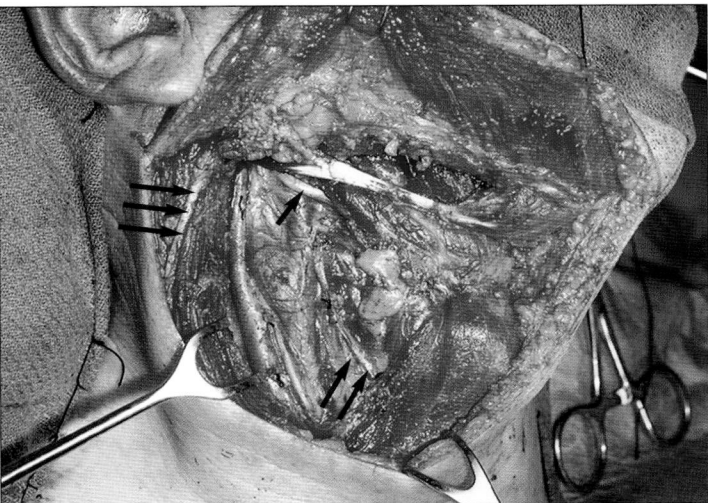

Fig 7-21d Anatomy of the neck after a functional neck dissection. Here, the carotid arteries, internal jugular vein, vagus nerve, hypoglossal nerve (*arrow*), superior laryngeal nerve (*double arrows*), and greater auricular nerve (*triple arrows*) can be easily seen.

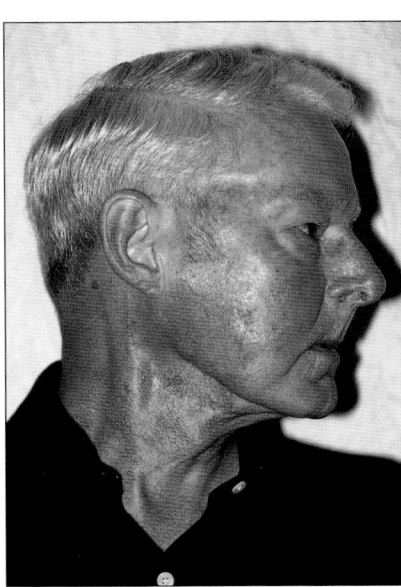

Fig 7-21e A functional neck dissection will thin the neck appearance but will prevent any significant concave deformity.

The indications and rationales for considering postsurgical radiotherapy are as follows:

- T_3 or T_4 lesions. There is a strong likelihood that even comprehensive and precise surgery cannot remove all cancer cells, either because of the large surface area of the tumor or because it has invaded anatomic barriers.
- Positive margins on the final pathology. Positive or even close margins as seen on a review of the final pathology indicate that at least some cancer cells have remained in the tissues.
- Extracapsular invasion. If the final pathology shows one or more than one lymph node positive for cancer, and the cancer cells are extending into or beyond the lymph node capsule, a high probability exists that cancer cells have escaped the fascial sheet and are now adherent to other neck structures.
- Four or more lymph nodes positive for cancer. This is evidence that the primary site has a strong propensity for regional metastasis. Because even thorough or full radical neck dissection usually leaves some small lymph nodes, these nodes may harbor residual cancer cells.

The use of postsurgical radiotherapy has its limitations. Radiotherapy cannot begin immediately after surgery because of the necessity for patient recovery and tissue healing. Therefore, it is best to begin postsurgical radiotherapy about 6 to 8 weeks following surgery, when the healing process is in an intermediate phase. Mature healing past 8 weeks is associated with an accumulation of scar tissue with less and less water. Since radiotherapy depends on ionizing the abundant water molecules in tissue into active free radicals, which in turn affects the DNA of cancer cells, a reduced tissue water content reduces the effectiveness of radiotherapy. Beyond 8 weeks, the value of postsurgical radiotherapy is diminished and is exceeded by its side effects.

Radiotherapy Principles

Radiotherapy involves a trade-off between normal tissue injury and effective tumor control. If radiotherapeutic doses sufficient to reduce cancer cell recovery were tolerated by the normal tissue and organ systems, all malignancies could be eradicated. The fact that the selective effects of radiotherapy are currently so narrow points to its limitations.

The radiosensitivities of tumors and various tissues involve the same trade-off of tumor injury versus normal tissue injury. The classic definition of a radiosensitive tumor is a tumor that is eradicated by irradiation in doses well tolerated by surrounding normal structures. Again, radiosensitivity is merely a ratio of tumor control to normal tissue injury (Table 7-1).

The tissue injury caused by irradiation is judged in levels. Cellular DNA is the main target. The energy transferred by direct linear energy transfer (LET) and secondary particle energy transfer produces activated electrophilic radicals such as •OH, H•, H••, •O+e− from the radiation beam striking the more numerous water (H_2O) molecules in the tissue. These, in turn, react with molecules of mainly DNA but also RNA and certain enzyme systems to induce sequence and structural changes (Fig 7-22). Damaged molecules like DNA may not replicate or may misreplicate with lethal cellular codes. Sometimes this can be observed microscopically as crosslinking, aborted mitosis, or chromosome breakage. If a sufficient number of target molecules are hit, cellular repair to functional or dysfunctional but survival status may result. The combination of these possibilities causes a certain percentage of cell deaths. Because the sensitivity of cancer cells to radiation is somewhat greater than that of normal cells, there is the possibility of sterilizing the entire cancer cell population while leaving the native tissue population reduced in cellular numbers and with injured cells, but recoverable to a viable state. The native tissue injury is manifested as hypocellularity and hypovascularity (fibrosis) (Fig 7-23). The tissue recovery is permanently altered by the reduction in replacement precursor cells and the reduced vascularity, limiting the building blocks of repair and the body's ability to use them. The organ involved undergoes clinical atrophy, fibrosis, and an ineffective healing response to injury.

Table 7-1 Relative tumor and tissue sensitivities

Tumor	Relative radiosensitivity	Normal tissues
Lymphoma	Very high	Lymphatics
Leukemias	Very high	Marrow
Seminomas	Very high	Ovarian follicle, spermatogenic tissue, intestinal mucosa
Oral squamous cell carcinoma	High	Oral mucosa
Skin squamous cell carcinoma	High	Skin
Esophageal carcinoma	High	Esophageal mucosa
Skin appendage carcinomas	High	Hair follicles
Transitional cell carcinomas	High	Bladder, ureters
Connective tissue elements within all tumors	Medium	Connective tissue fibroblasts
Astrocytomas	Medium	Glial cells
Adenocarcinomas of breast	Medium	Breast ductal cells
Salivary gland tumors	Low	Salivary ducts
Adenocarcinomas of kidney, pancreas, and colon	Low	Kidneys, pancreas, colon
Chondrosarcoma, osteosarcoma	Low	Bone, cartilage
Rhabdomyosarcoma	Very low	Striated muscle
Leiomyosarcoma	Very low	Smooth muscle

Radiotherapists describe a normal tissue minimum tolerance dose, which they define as the dose to which a given population of patients is exposed under a standard set of treatment conditions and that results in no greater than a 5% severe complication rate within 5 years (abbreviated TD 5/5). In addition, a maximum tolerance dose, TD 50/5, is defined as the dose to which a given population of patients is exposed under a standard set of treatment conditions and that results in a 50% severe complication rate within 5 years. Interestingly, oral mucosa TD 5/5 is judged to be 6,000 cGy in a 50 cm^2 area, while TD 50/5 is 7,500 cGy in a 50 cm^2 area. In a 10 cm^2 area, the TD 50/5 is 10,000 cGy. The presence of teeth and of dental and periodontal disease, combined with the necessity of jaw surgeries such as biopsies and tooth removals, appreciably reduce the practical TD 5/5 and TD 50/5, making the jaws (particularly the mandible) more likely to develop osteoradionecrosis than any other bone radiated to the same dose.

Recent efforts to increase the therapeutic ratio (ie, tumor lethal dose/normal tissue tolerance) have centered on modifying the radiotherapeutic type and dose schedules. Some of the more recent attempts are described.

Supervoltage Irradiation

Supervoltage irradiation is irradiation of 1 to 10 MEV (million electron volts). The rationale for supervoltage irradiation is that faster particles cause greater radiation injury to deep tissue tumors and less injury to skin. It was hoped that reduced scatter would allow greater focus of the irradiation path on the target tumor. It was also hoped that the increased particle penetration in dense tissue such as bone and teeth, combined with a reduction in secondary particles, would spare unnecessary damage in bone. However, this has not been found to be true in relation to osteoradionecrosis of the mandible.

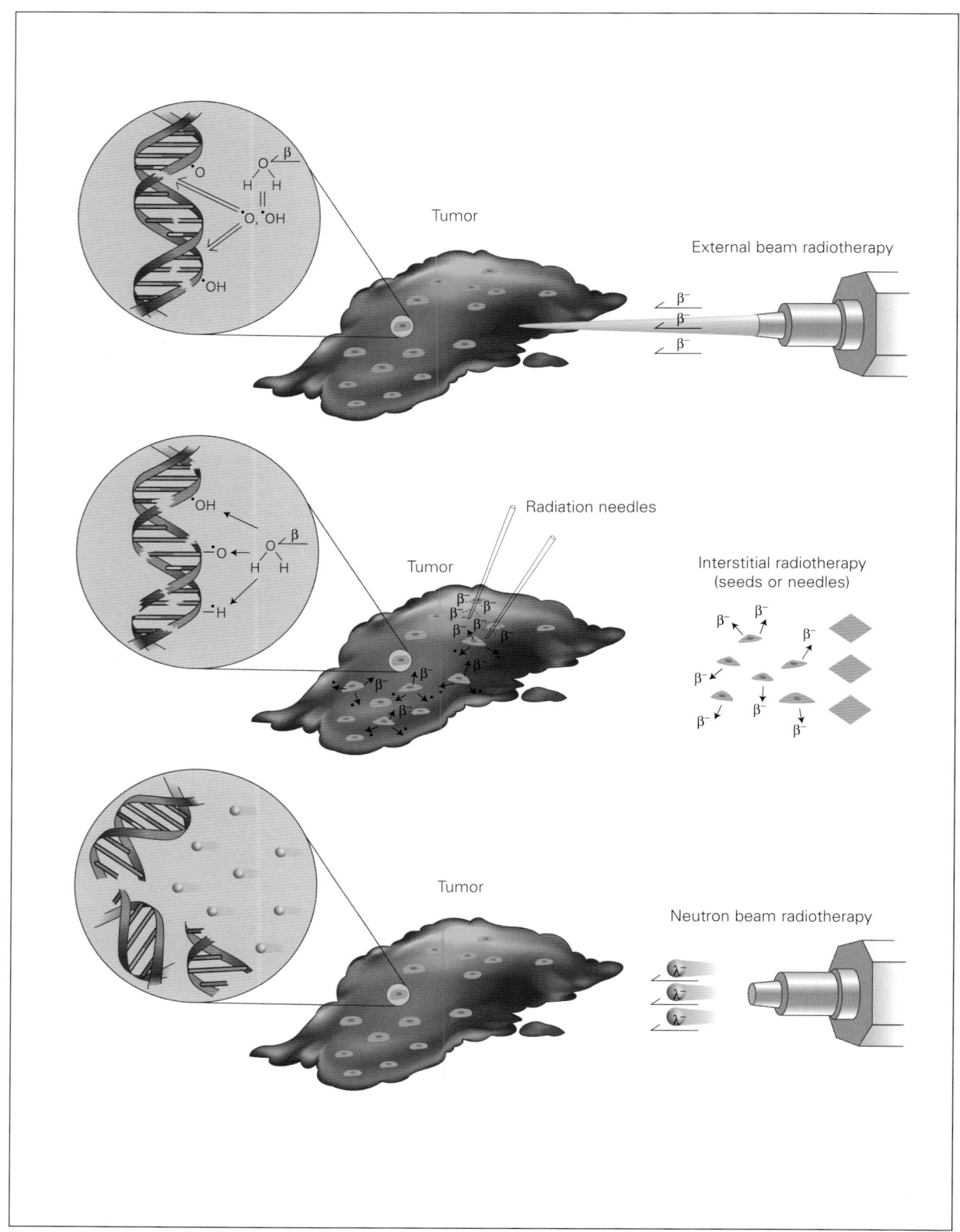

Fig 7-22 External beam and interstitial radiotherapy indirectly affect DNA by generating free radicals through the splitting of water molecules. Neutron beam radiotherapy directly affects DNA by virtue of its larger mass. Interstitial radiotherapy has a greater normal tissue injury effect than external beam radiotherapy, and neutron beam radiotherapy has a greater normal tissue injury effect than either of these.

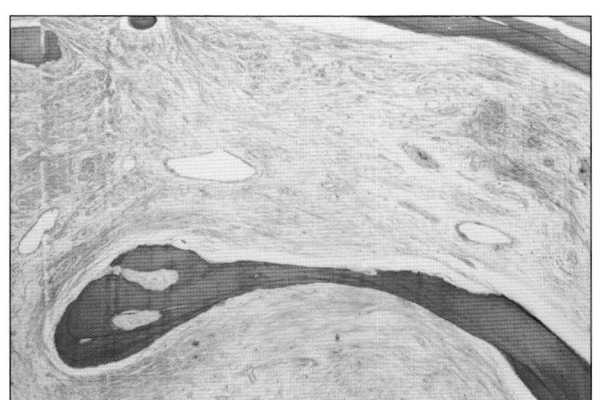

Fig 7-23 Radiotherapy diminishes cellular renewal. The radiated tissue becomes hypocellular-hypovascular-hypoxic (the 3-H tissue), as seen here.

Interstitial Radiotherapy (Brachytherapy)

Implanted radiation seeds or needles such as ^{226}Ra (radium) or ^{192}Ir (iridium) may be used in large, bulky tumors. They deliver a higher tumor kill per dose because their delivery is constant rather than intermittent or "fractionated," as is external beam radiotherapy. The tumor cells are therefore continually bombarded for the length of time the seeds are in place or over their decay time. Tumor cells cannot recover or repopulate, but neither can normal cells. Therefore, there is a higher incidence of radiation fibrosis and osteoradionecrosis with interstitial radiation (see Fig 7-22). This is particularly seen when interstitial radiation is used in the tongue or floor of the mouth, which results in severe damage to the lingual blood supply to the mandible and lingual cortex, creating a particularly widespread osteoradionecrosis along the curvature of the lingual cortex.

Neutron Beam Irradiation

Because high-speed neutrons are denser than the small particles of other radiation sources (electrons, B particles, etc), they transfer damaging energy to tissues more directly. They directly ionize DNA, RNA, and enzymes rather than ionizing water into •OH, H•, H••, and •O+e– radicals, which, in turn, must react with DNA, RNA, etc. Secondarily, fast neutrons are more effective in hypoxic tumors. Therefore, the use of neutron beam irradiation has been used in larger tumors and large neck metastases with large central hypoxic cores. However, neutron beam therapy is being abandoned because of a lack of increased tumor control and significant damage to normal tissue, particularly deep tissue fibrosis and osteoradionecrosis (see Fig 7-22).

Hyperfractionated Radiation

Hyperfractionated radiotherapy is a planned twice-per-day schedule of a somewhat lower dose per fraction. Rather than the usual 200 cGy per day, 5 days per week, the dosage may be modified to 150 cGy twice per day, 3 to 4 days per week. Schedules such as this one are designed to increase the tumor response rate and decrease the radiation necrosis rate. However, hyperfractionated radiation nonetheless results in many cases of osteoradionecrosis of the jaws.

Oxygen Enhancement

One of the known differences between neoplastic cells and normal cells is the ability of neoplastic cells to survive and proliferate in hypoxic environments. When exposed to the same amount of radiation, well-oxygenated cells will be two or three times more radiosensitive than hypoxic cells. Efforts to enhance the oxygenation of tumor cells have so far not produced an increased tumor response or patient cure. Although the theory is sound, the technical difficulty of enhancing the tumor oxygen tensions during irradiation is great. H_2O_2 tumor perfusion, hyperbaric oxygen therapy, and hyperbaric breathing with 5% $FICO_2$ have been studied, without conclusive results.

Drug Enhancement

Certain drugs, known as *radiosensitizers*, have the capacity to enhance the formation of free radicals in tissues being irradiated, which may enhance the tumor damage effect of radiation. Some known radiosensitizer drugs are methotrexate, 5-fluorouracil, actinomycin-D, and metronidazole. In addition, combining radiotherapy simultaneously with chemotherapy, immunotherapy, or hyperthermia has sometimes been used, but with no documented benefits.

In clinically practical terms, the two most important factors concerning radiation tissue damage to normal tissue as well as tumor tissue are total dosage and the distribution of dosage over time. This may be examined both at the cellular level and at the clinical level.

All human cells undergo a continual "cell cycle" that can be divided into four phases (Fig 7-24). After a mitosis, a new G_0 or resting phase begins. During late G_0 phase, enzymes necessary for DNA synthesis are themselves synthesized. During the S phase, actual DNA synthesis and replication of DNA occurs. During G_1, the mitotic apparatus is synthesized together with quantities of RNA. The M phase is the actual physical mitosis of cells with its own phases of prophase, metaphase, anaphase, and telophase. The other phase of mitosis sometimes described is called *interphase* and encompasses the G_1, S, and G_2 phases.

Cellular death has been shown to depend on the position of the cell in its replication cycle. The thickness of the shaded area in Fig 7-24 is proportional to the radiosensitivity of each phase. Known facts concerning cell radiosensitivities are:

1. Cells are most sensitive during mitosis. (Therefore, germinal cells and cancers with numerous mitotic figures are more radiosensitive.)
2. The G_0 phase is radioresistant; the longer the G_0 phase, the greater the radiation resistance. (Therefore, nerve cells, brain cells, and muscle cells are somewhat radiosensitive.)
3. The G_0-S phase border is as sensitive as the mitosis phase.
4. The S phase is generally resistant, though to a greater degree during the latter than during the earlier part.
5. In most cell lines, G_1 is sensitive. In a few lines, the resistance noted during the S phase extends into the G_1 phase.

At the clinical level, it is noted that less tissue damage occurs with the same total radiation dose if the interval between radiation exposures is lengthened; the reason for this is cellular recovery and attempts at normal cellular repair. Fortunately, normal cells recover more rapidly than cancer cells, and therein lies the advantage of fractionating the total dosage to widen the difference between cancer cell and normal cell damage. Therein also lies the contrast between external beam and implant radiation. Interstitial radiation even at a lower dosage will cause a much greater degree of cellular damage due to a constant radiation effect extending over their time in place or activity and the closeness of the radiation source to the target tissue. The constant radiation exposure of interstitial radiotherapy affects cells more often at their sensitive portions of the cycle. With fractionated external beam irradiation (usually 200 cGy per day, 5 days per week), the probability of catching the faster-proliferating tumor cells in sensitive portions of their cycles increases with the numbers of fractions. The separation of tumor kill versus normal tissue kill increases with the numbers of fractions (eg, 6,000 cGy at 200 cGy per day for 6

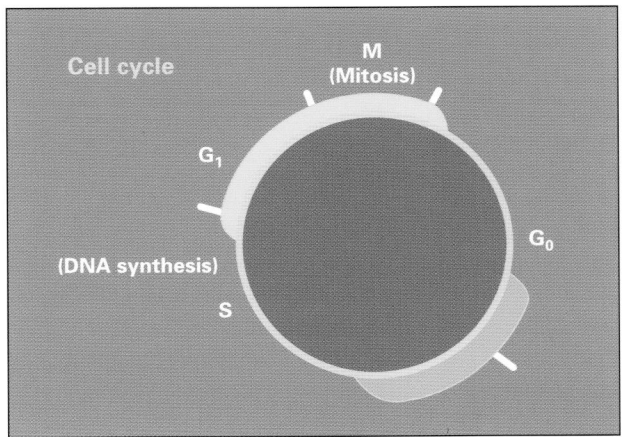

Fig 7-24 Because cells are vulnerable to radiation only during specific phases of their cell cycle, an increased radiation sensitivity is found in cell populations with higher turnover rates (mitotic indices) because of the cell's increased probability of being in a vulnerable phase of its cycle during the radiation exposure.

weeks causes more normal cellular damage than 7,200 cGy at 180 cGy per day for 8 weeks; the 7,200-cGy course over an extended time, although a greater total dose, would be slightly less damaging to normal tissues).

Chemotherapy Principles

The main problem faced in chemotherapy is similar to the one faced in radiotherapy, that is, the effective control of a tumor without inducing intolerable and even fatal toxicity. The limitation of chemotherapy is almost one of sheer numbers. A $T_2N_0M_0$ oral squamous cell carcinoma contains approximately 10^9 cells at diagnosis. Even a 99% effective cellular kill induced by chemotherapy leaves a residual 1% $\times$ 10^9 cells, or 10^7 cells. Even though this may shrink the tumor or even render it clinically unapparent, redevelopment of clinical disease is inevitable.

In bacterial infections, it is customary for antibiotics to achieve a kill of about the same magnitude, leaving as many residual microorganisms. In patients who are immunocompetent, the residual microorganisms are eliminated by a combination of several immune mechanisms. In cancer, no such immunocompetence exists, despite identification of certain antitumor immunoglobulins. In leukemias and lymphomas, cancer cell populations approach 10^{12} so that even 99.99% cell kills leave a residual tumor population of a billion (10^9) or more. For this reason, chemotherapy protocols require combination drug therapy to achieve maximum cellular kill and closely spaced induction doses, each of which may gain a 10^2 reduction in cancer cell populations, called a "log [logarithmic] kill." Treatment, whatever the drug combination, is therefore intensive and frequent in the attempt to achieve tumor cell kill at a greater rate than tumor cell repopulation. A major limitation to the success of drug treatment is the presence of drug-resistant cells that cause clinical tumor recurrence after an initial response.

Figure 7-25 illustrates the principle of log kill for chemotherapeutic agents. The solid-line chemotherapy log kill predicts a theoretic cure by closely spaced, intensive therapy. The downward slopes indicate a reduction in tumor cells; the upward slopes indicate a repopulation of tumor cells. The dashed lines illustrate the degree of further therapy required and the number of tumor cells that must be killed to achieve a cure. Therefore, one can see the theoretic advantage of treating smaller-sized tumors that begin with fewer tumor cells.

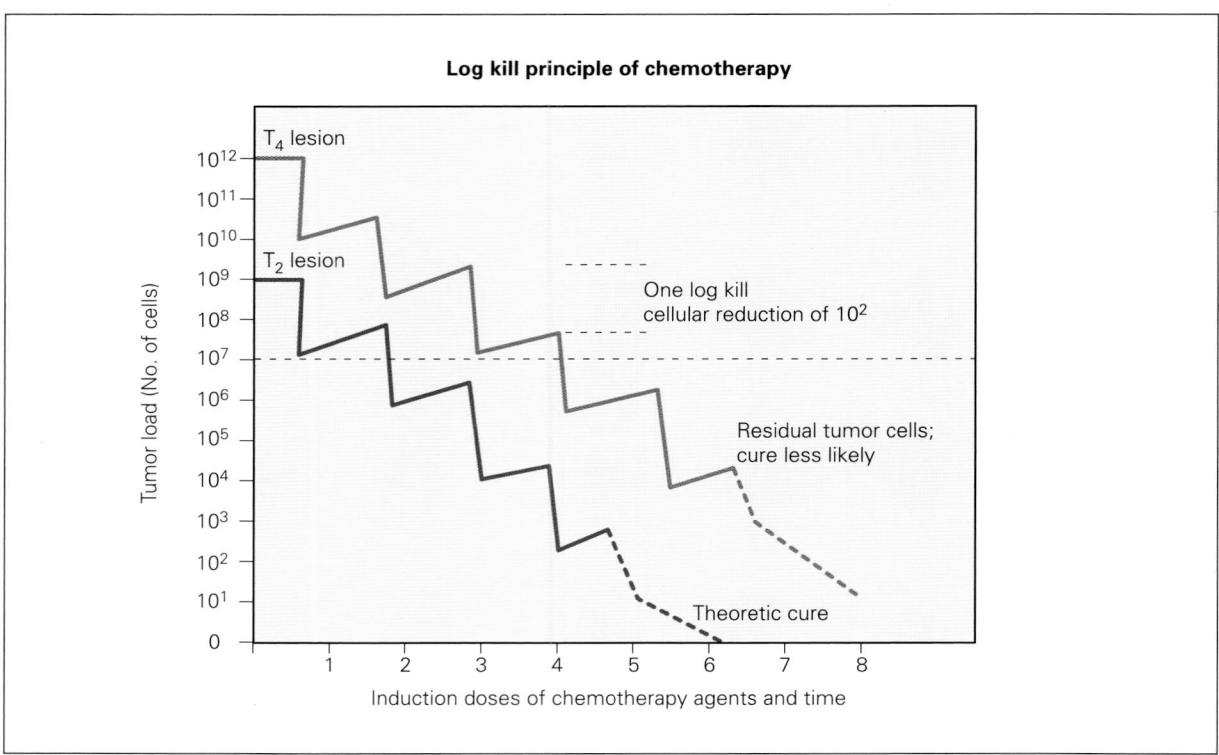

Fig 7-25 Chemotherapy reduces tumor cell populations by 10^2 (a log of 2) per induction cycle. Between cycles, the tumor cells attempt to repopulate. Therefore, serial induction cycles and combination drugs are used. The tumor becomes clinically undetectable at a size of about 10^7 cells.

Management of the Terminal Cancer Patient

Individuals in whom a cure is impossible can be maintained for extended periods with the goals of comfort, pain control, and preserved dignity. Some methods the oral and maxillofacial surgeon can use to attain these goals are outlined below.

Surgery

Selected patients may benefit from debulking surgeries to decrease tumor load, relieve pain, expand the airway, improve speech, etc. Some patients will require tracheotomies to prevent upper airway obstruction. Some will require removal of painful teeth, necrotic bone, or exposed plates or closure of fistulas, etc. Many patients will require placement of gastric feeding tubes (Fig 7-26).

Consultations

Palliative radiotherapy or chemotherapy should be considered to extend life and reduce pain. The side effects of these treatments must be weighed against the projected benefits for the individual. Consultations with internists or other medical specialists should be sought to control comorbid diseases, such as hypertension, pulmonary disease, and cardiovascular disease, and to manage anemias of chronic disease.

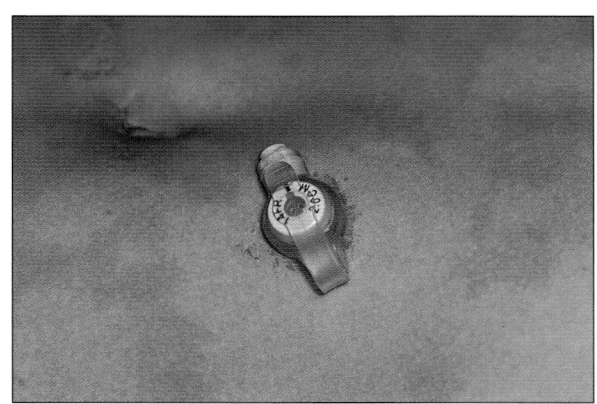

Fig 7-26 Gastrostomy feeding tubes or percutaneous esophageal gastrostomy (PEG) tubes are a valuable palliative measure because they are straightforward and well tolerated. The nutritional support and avenue for medications they provide extend life and permit an increased level of activity.

Pain Control

Addiction to narcotics should not be a barrier to adequate pain control. Indeed, most individuals with terminal cancer have developed a tachyphylaxis to narcotic-based analgesics and will therefore require high doses. It is often worthwhile to place an in-dwelling catheter for home health care–provided "patient-controlled analgesia" (PCA). Otherwise, relatively high and frequent doses of time-released morphine oral preparation or the more common oxycodone and hydrocodone compounds may be used.

Nutritional Support

Consultation with a dietician or bariatric surgeon may be required to overcome obstacles to food intake and to formulate the balance and consistency of food substances.

Home Health Care Support

Most individuals prefer the familiar surroundings of their own home. Nutritional support, analgesics, and other medications can be provided in the home. When possible, this is the preferred site of noninvasive health care.

Hospice Care

At times, the complexities of home health care and daily biologic functions will exceed the capabilities of family members and visiting nurses. Hospice care is an organized and complete service that may be provided in the home or in a special hospice facility by trained personnel who are able to manage an individual's complex needs. Nonetheless, whether using home hospice care services or a hospice facility, the orders related to pain control, medications, dressings, return visits, etc, should be clear and should include a contact number where the referring clinician can be reached.

Premalignant and Nonpremalignant Conditions

Erythroplakia-Leukoplakia

CLINICAL PRESENTATION AND PATHOGENESIS ▶

The lesions of erythroplakia-leukoplakia (Fig 7-27) often present a clinical dilemma. Their import is that any single lesion may represent one or the whole spectrum of diagnoses from benign hyperkeratosis to

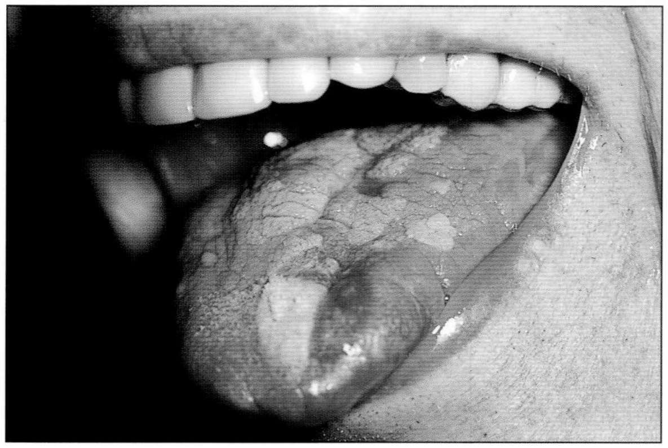

Fig 7-27 Erythroplakia-leukoplakia of the tongue that represented benign hyperkeratosis, various dysplasias, and carcinoma in situ.

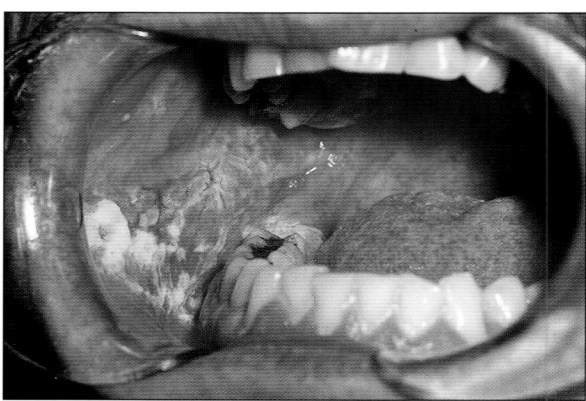

Fig 7-28 When examined closely most leukoplakias are revealed to be a mixture of leukoplakia and erythroplakia, termed *erythroleukoplakia*.

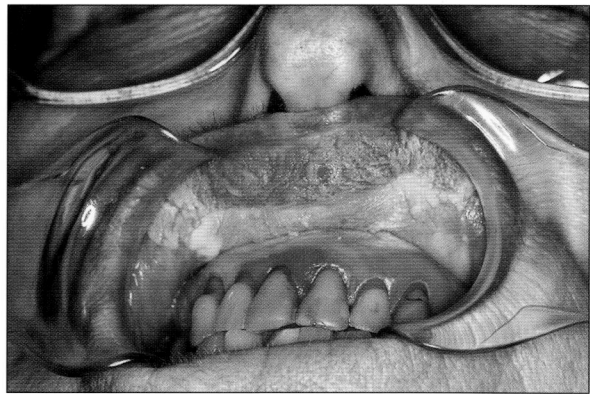

Fig 7-29 Proliferative verrucous leukoplakia is a premalignant condition that should be distinguished from other leukoplakia. Proliferative verrucous leukoplakia is clinically widespread and verrucous. Its reddened areas are friable and may demonstrate a surface slough when rubbed (Nikolsky sign).

invasive squamous cell carcinoma. They also clinically present in a diffuse pattern covering a wide surface area, making the choice of biopsy location difficult. The clinician is frequently concerned about the biopsy missing the most diagnostic area or about not being able to excise the entire lesion.

Lesions may appear solely as a white patch (leukoplakia) or as a white patch with red dots of thin mucosa within it (stippled leukoplakia) or as a mixed red-white patch (erythroleukoplakia) (Fig 7-28). They are almost always asymptomatic and do not rub off. However, the clinician is cautioned not to give too much significance to this overused observation. Many other white lesions, such as lichen planus, white sponge nevus, invasive carcinoma, and even the hypertrophic form of candidiasis, will not rub off.

Lesions can occur anywhere on the oral mucosa, but, in order of frequency, are seen most often on the buccal mucosa, mandibular buccal vestibule, maxillary and mandibular gingiva, tongue, and floor of the mouth. They can be associated with smokeless tobacco, cigarette smoking, other combustible smoking products, chronic frictional trauma, and alcohol and nutritional factors as suggested by the Plummer-Vinson syndrome. Many leukoplakias develop unassociated with any known stimulus, and these are the most risky of all; they have the highest incidence of being malignant at the time of biopsy and of evolving into a malignancy later. What was once primarily a male-associated entity now has an equal sex distribution presumably due to the increased numbers of women who smoke.

DIFFERENTIAL DIAGNOSIS ▶

White patches and red-white patches suggest the classic differential diagnostic spectrum ranging from *benign hyperkeratosis* to *dysplastic mucosa* to *carcinoma in situ, verrucous carcinoma,* and *invasive squamous cell carcinoma.* A clinical rule that is helpful to remember is that white oral lesions are white because of keratin, *Candida* infection, or fibrin. Lesions that are white or red-white are so because they produce varying amounts of keratin and have several areas of thinned mucosa with inflammation. Other oral keratotic lesions that may appear like a leukoplakia are *white sponge nevus, lichen planus,* and *chronic trauma–related hyperkeratosis.* Some *Candida* infections can be ruled out clinically by the rub-off test, but *hypertrophic candidiasis* cannot, and it is well to remember that *Candida* itself can cause a hyperkeratosis and, therefore, leukoplakia. It is also important to remember that *proliferative verrucous leukoplakia* (PVL) will present as a clinical leukoplakia initially and may continue to develop clinical leukoplakia in another area while the initial area transforms through the progressive phases toward invasive squamous cell carcinoma (Fig 7-29).

DIAGNOSTIC WORK-UP ▶

Approximately 5% of leukoplakias are found to be carcinomas at the time of first examination and another 5% will evolve into carcinomas. About 25% of erythroplakias are either dysplasia or invasive car-

Table 7-2 Ranking of leukoplakia probability related to occurrence and probability of leukoplakia representing dysplasia, by location*

Occurrence	Probability of dysplasia
1. Buccal mucosa	1. Floor of mouth
2. Mandibular vestibule	2. Tongue
3. Maxillary gingiva	3. Lower lip
4. Mandibular gingiva	4. Mandibular gingiva
5. Tongue	5. Buccal mucosa
6. Floor of mouth	6. Mandibular vestibule
7. Lower lip	7. Maxillary gingiva

*The areas most likely to develop leukoplakia are not necessarily the areas where the leukoplakia is most likely to represent a dysplastic lesion.

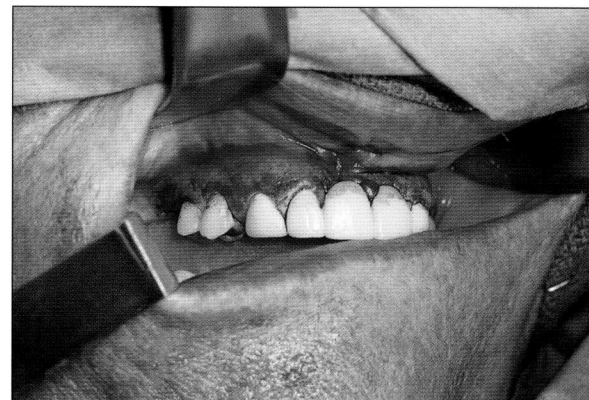

Fig 7-30 Increased staining of the gingiva around the central incisor with 1% toluidine blue directed the biopsy, which diagnosed a gingival carcinoma.

cinoma at the time of first examination and another 30% will become carcinomas. Therefore, stippled leukoplakia and erythroleukoplakia are believed to have a greater malignant potential.

The location of the leukoplakia/erythroplakia relates to its probability of representing a dysplasia or carcinoma. Table 7-2 indicates oral sites related to frequency of dysplasia or malignancy. Leukoplakia of the floor of the mouth, lateral border of the tongue, and lower lip have the highest association with dysplasia and development into malignancies.

Regardless of statistics, leukoplakia and erythroleukoplakia may be regarded as premalignant lesions in any location. Nearly all require a biopsy. Confusion and debate have emerged concerning the use of 1% toluidine blue, a vital in situ dye that is taken up to a greater extent by cells with higher turnover rates. The issue concerning toluidine blue has falsely focused on its use to help the clinician decide whether or not to biopsy the lesion. Nearly all lesions require biopsy; the purpose of toluidine blue is to direct the biopsy to the most likely area of dysplasia or carcinoma (Fig 7-30). To this end, toluidine blue can assist the biopsy in some cases. The computer-assisted oral brush biopsy (CDX) may allow a quick and convenient means of accomplishing a screening biopsy of multiple sites in a large surface lesion. This technique, while a much more accurate screening tool than exfoliative cytology, should not replace an incisional biopsy (see Chapter 1).

For the most part, areas that can be totally excised should be approached as an excisional biopsy. Otherwise, incisional biopsy of the erythroplakic areas, stippled areas, or areas of clinical atrophy are the most yielding. Multiple biopsies are frequently necessary.

The diagnostic work-up also should include mirror or fiberoptic examination of the laryngopharynx. Leukoplakia and erythroplakia are not limited to the oral mucosa. The pharynx and laryngeal mucosa also have a certain incidence of such lesions.

HISTOPATHOLOGY ▶ Lesions demonstrate a spectrum of histologic change within stratified squamous epithelium, ranging from simple hyperkeratosis to hyperparakeratosis and/or acanthosis to defective maturation. The latter changes may be minimal (mild epithelial dysplasia), moderate, or extensive (severe epithelial dysplasia or carcinoma in situ). Because there are no clearly defined histologic criteria to distinguish these groups, there may be considerable variation in diagnosis. The histologic changes may be appreciated from two perspectives—the overall architecture perceived at low magnification and the cytologic features viewed at higher magnification. It is critical that the lesion be properly assessed at low power, because isolated "atypical" cells may often be seen at high power that may have no pathologic significance in an architecturally normal epithelium.

Normal stratified squamous epithelium shows a smooth progression from cuboidal or columnar basal cells through polygonal prickle cells, which flatten as they approach the surface. Thus cells at any given level resemble their neighbors, and the epithelium tends to have a horizontal orientation (Fig 7-31a). A dysplastic epithelium, however, will often lose this stratification or polarity as the cells become elongated and appear to stream in a more vertical configuration (Figs 7-31b and 7-31c). A dysplastic epithelium will also lose its harmonious, orderly stratification, a feature that can be appreciated at low magnification (Fig 7-31d). The overall appearance may indicate hyperplasia and/or atrophy, but in either case there is often the formation of drop-shaped rete ridges (Fig 7-31e). Other distortions of the normal contour of the rete ridges may also occur.

Against this background, cytologic features may be put into context. Possible findings include basal cell replication; increase in nuclear-cytoplasmic ratio; cellular pleomorphism; hyperchromatism; increased number of mitoses; atypical mitoses; individual cell keratinization; prominent nucleoli; and lack of cellular adhesion (see Fig 7-47b).

The diagnosis is ultimately based on the assessment of these microscopic features together with clinical information and the pathologist's experience. The clinical situation has considerable influence on the diagnosis. Carcinomas of the floor of the mouth are frequently associated with epithelial dysplasia, whereas at other sites, such as the buccal mucosa, this relationship is not observed. Consequently, dysplasia of the floor of the mouth is likely to be looked on with greater suspicion than is dysplasia occurring elsewhere.

The clinical significance of the different categories of dysplasia is also debatable. The usual implication is that mild dysplasias are most likely reversible. However, when there is change from moderate to severe dysplasia, progression to carcinoma is increasingly likely. It has been shown, however, that carcinoma is not the inevitable outcome of a severe dysplasia, nor is there any assurance that a mild epithelial dysplasia will not advance to carcinoma.

The term *carcinoma in situ* has usually been reserved for lesions in which the epithelial changes occur throughout their entire thickness, but without violation of the basement membrane. There does not seem to be any reason, however, to distinguish carcinoma in situ from severe epithelial dysplasia (Fig 7-31f).

Some leukoplakias develop a papillary surface and may show broad rete ridges. These have been called *verrucous leukoplakias* and may be difficult to distinguish from verrucous carcinoma.

TREATMENT ▶ Erythroleukoplakias representing benign hyperkeratosis require only continued follow-up and an effort to eliminate any possible causative agents. Cases that show only mild dysplasia are believed to be reversible. These, along with the benign hyperkeratosis form, may be treated with isotretinoin (Accutane, Roche), 20 mg three times daily, or beta-carotene, 30 mg three times daily, which has shown improvement in some lesions and is now sometimes used as a chemoprevention agent in patients who have been treated for an oral carcinoma. The beta-carotene form is more tolerable for patients than tretinoin because of the latter's high incidence of causing mucositis, mood changes, and elevation of liver enzymes.

Erythroleukoplakias, which are graded as moderate dysplasia to carcinoma in situ, require excision of the entire lesion with a 1-cm margin regardless of size (Figs 7-32a and 7-32b). The excisional depth should extend into the submucosa, maximizing the possibility of removing a lesion before invasion occurs. This improves the eventual prognosis and could obviate the need for much more disfiguring and complex surgery or radiotherapy later. If at all possible, the resultant wound should be closed primarily by reasonable advancement of tissues. If it cannot be closed, a split-thickness skin graft for cover may be needed, or the wound may need to be allowed to granulate and then covered by secondary epithelialization.

The excised specimen should undergo multiple histologic sections to assess for areas of invasive malignancy. If a focal area of malignancy is discovered, the deep margin should be closely examined and the lesion staged to the full size of the original clinical lesion. If the tumor extends to the margin or what is deemed close to the margin, a re-excision, not observation, is recommended. If invasive malignancy is found to a depth greater than 3 mm, the N_0 neck may be considered for a functional neck dissection or radiotherapy of 5,000 cGy to 6,500 cGy. Because leukoplakias and erythroplakias often harbor areas of invasive carcinoma, laser ablation is discouraged and should be used with caution. The absence of a spec-

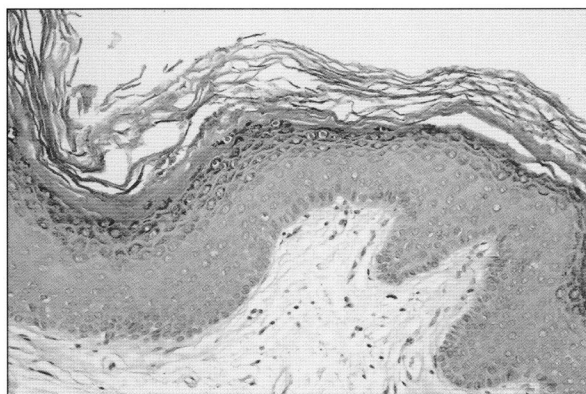

Fig 7-31a Benign hyperkeratosis showing a gradual progression from columnar basal cells through polygonal prickle cells with a flattening of these cells as they approach the surface. A striking granular cell layer that contains keratohyaline granules is characteristically seen in conjunction with the orthokeratinized surface.

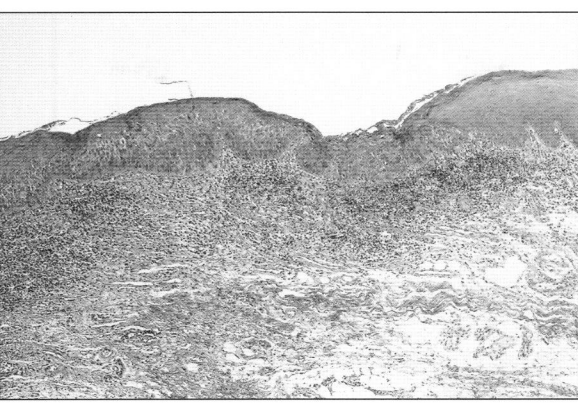

Fig 7-31b A specimen from the floor of the mouth shows a small portion of normal epithelium at one margin. The remainder of the epithelium is dysplastic. The dysplastic change is accompanied by an underlying chronic inflammatory infiltrate. Even at this power, a change in the normal arrangement of cells can be appreciated.

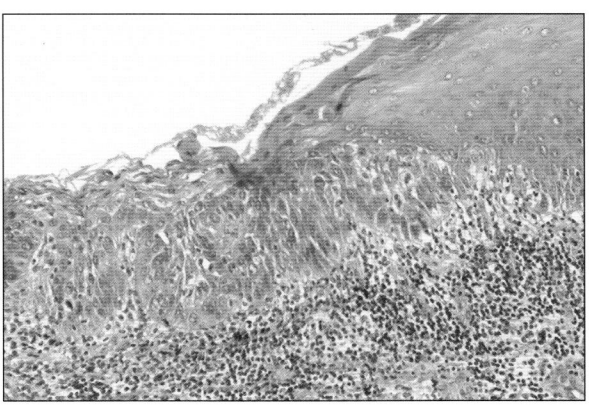

Fig 7-31c A higher-power view of Fig 7-31b shows the interface of the normal and dysplastic epithelium. The dysplastic component shows a vertical streaming of cells and loss of cellular adherence. This is also a lack of maturation, although some flattening of the cells can be seen near the surface.

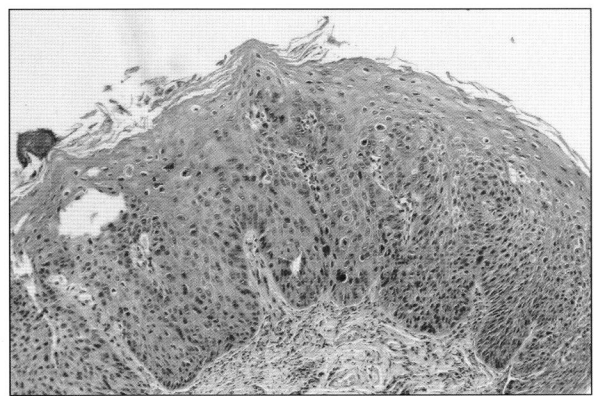

Fig 7-31d In this dysplastic epithelium, the harmonious arrangement of a benign stratified squamous epithelium seen in Fig 7-31a is not present. There are scattered atypical and hyperchromatic cells.

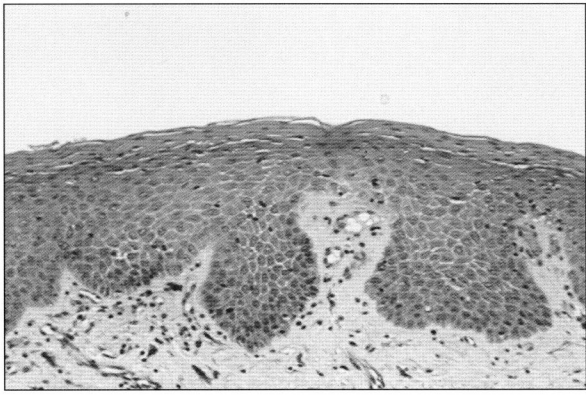

Fig 7-31e Formation of drop-shaped rete ridges in dysplastic epithelium is a precursor for imminent invasive carcinoma.

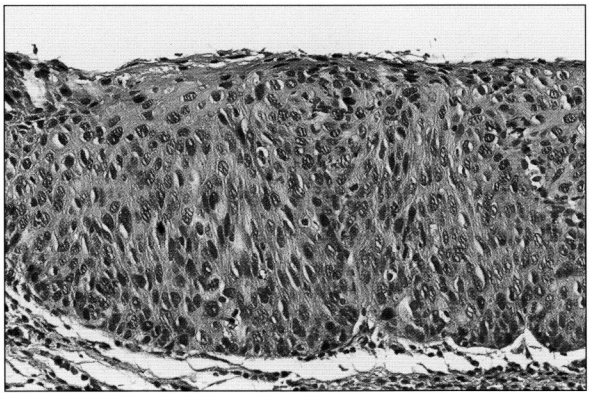

Fig 7-31f The term *carcinoma in situ* is typically used for cases in which there is no differentiation and little difference between the deepest and the most superficial cells, as is the case here.

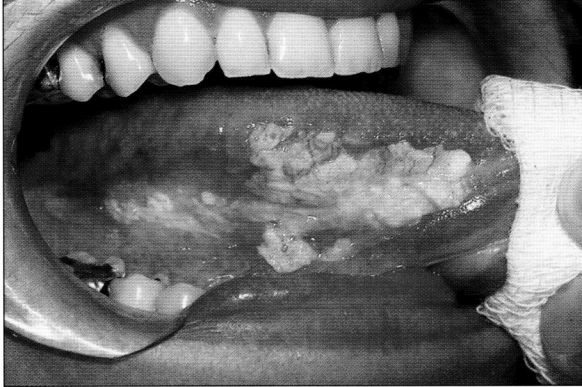

Fig 7-32a This leukoplakia of the tongue should undergo a scalpel excision rather than either several incisional biopsy samplings, which can miss the most diagnostic areas, or excision with a laser, which does not provide a microscopic assessment of the adequacy of the margins.

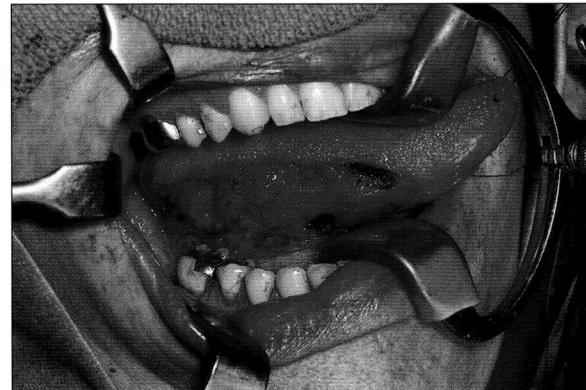

Fig 7-32b Excision of a large leukoplakia with 1-cm margins revealed dysplasia and carcinoma in situ. A wound defect of this size can still be closed primarily.

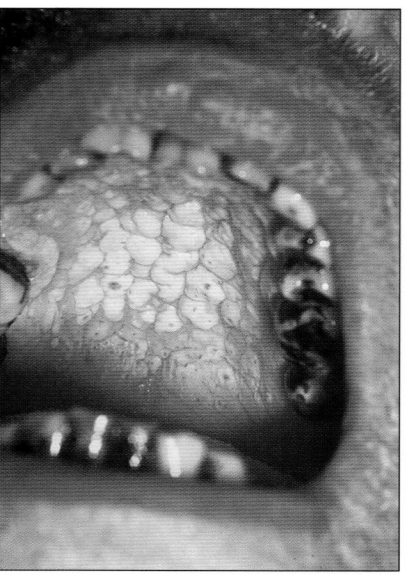

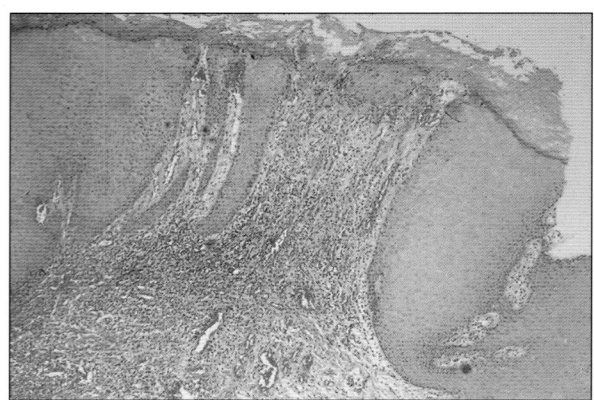

Fig 7-33a Nicotinic stomatitis appears as a leukoplakia with focal inflammatory points, which are inflamed minor salivary gland openings. This is not a premalignant condition.

Fig 7-33b Nicotinic stomatitis showing the marked epithelial hyperplasia that corresponds to the clinically white areas and the central area of chronic inflammation that corresponds to the red areas.

imen to examine deep margins or peripheral margins runs the risk of allowing recurrences that often extend deep within the tissues and may produce regional neck metastasis.

PROGNOSIS AND FOLLOW-UP ▶

Close follow-up is required. Frequent biopsies and laryngopharyngeal mirror or fiberoptic examinations are included together with the oral examination. During the first 2 years, examination every 4 months is advisable. If the area of the lesion is stable, follow-up may be extended to every 6 months.

Nicotinic Stomatitis

CLINICAL PRESENTATION AND PATHOGENESIS ▶

The typical nicotinic stomatitis patient is an adult man who is a frequent pipe smoker or, less commonly, a cigar smoker. The condition itself and the degree of its clinical appearance is directly proportional to the frequency of either of the two smoking habits. It is not seen in those who smoke only cigarettes. The condition is localized to the hard palate mucosa, although a small portion may extend onto the soft palate mucosa. The mucosa will appear white and thickened because of acanthosis and hyperkeratosis. There will be thin red lines of normal mucosa separating and circumscribing the hyperkeratotic areas. In the middle of the white hyperkeratotic areas, one or more small red dots, which correspond to inflammation around the openings of minor salivary gland ducts, will be noticeable (Fig 7-33a).

The cause of this tissue reaction is suspected to be tobacco insult to the palate. However, repeated exposures of the palate to hot liquids will cause a similar appearance. The combination of the heat and the specific tobacco products related to pipe and cigar tobacco probably incite this unique tissue reaction.

DIFFERENTIAL DIAGNOSIS ▶

Nicotinic stomatitis is clinically diagnostic. Few lesions or conditions resemble its presentation.

DIAGNOSTIC WORK-UP ▶

No work-up is required. The diagnosis remains a history-related clinical diagnosis.

HISTOPATHOLOGY ▶

Corresponding to the clinically white areas is hyperplasia of the epithelium characterized by hyperkeratosis and acanthosis. Corresponding to the centrally located area of erythema is a chronic inflammatory infiltrate, typically associated with a ductal orifice (Fig 7-33b). The ducts themselves may show hyperplasia and squamous metaplasia, but dysplasia is not a feature of this condition.

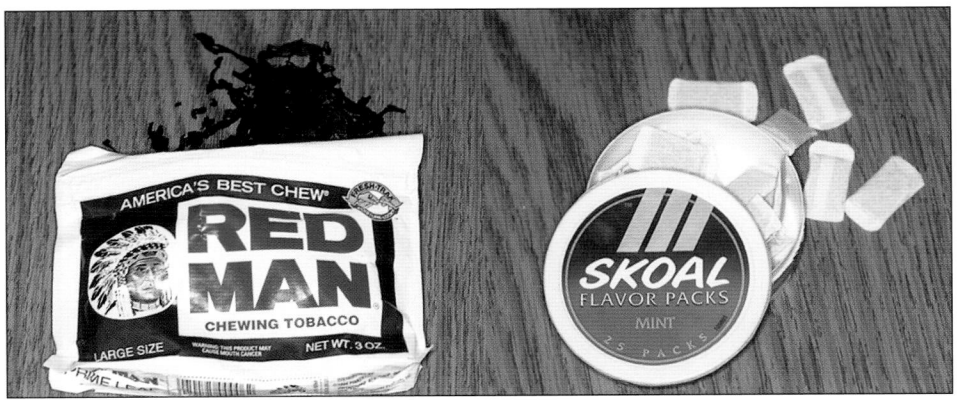

Fig 7-34 The common smokeless tobacco products in the United States are weak carcinogens at their worst. They produce an inflammatory patch with hyperkeratosis, termed a *snuff-dipper's patch*, wherever they are placed, but they rarely produce an invasive carcinoma.

TREATMENT ▶

No specific treatment is required. Cessation of smoking will cause the clinical appearance to improve over several months. Only infrequent cases will completely recover a normal appearance.

PROGNOSIS ▶

Nicotinic stomatitis of the palate is not a premalignant disease. In most cases, however, the individual has a significant tobacco insult to the other tissues of the oral cavity, which are more prone to respond with a malignancy. Therefore, the significance of nicotinic stomatitis is mostly as a marker for a smoking history and relates a need to thoroughly examine all other areas of the oral cavity.

Smokeless Tobacco Keratosis

CLINICAL PRESENTATION AND PATHOGENESIS ▶

Smokeless tobacco in the form of chewing tobacco (leaf tobacco) and dips and snuff (ground tobacco) are popular forms of tobacco use. These are only potential carcinogens because of their low propensity for spontaneously oxidizing to an epoxide form (Fig 7-34; see also Fig 7-2). Because of their use in a noncombustion fashion, benzopyridine epoxides do not form and therefore their incidence of invasive cancer induction and even verrucous carcinoma is no higher than that of a control population. Nonetheless, they do produce a clinically identifiable keratosis that appears as a white patch with an irregular, sometimes leathery surface often called a *snuff-dipper's pouch*. The lesion will outline the size and location of the tobacco product. It is asymptomatic and is slowly reversible if the smokeless tobacco is discontinued (see Figs 7-3a and 7-3b).

Another form of smokeless tobacco, a much more potent carcinogen associated with a high incidence of oral squamous cell carcinoma, is used in parts of China, India, Sri Lanka, and some other Asian countries. Betel nuts with slake lime or other related tobacco products are used as a form of oral gratification from an early age. Slake lime and spice combinations mixed with tobacco, in a form called a "quid" or a "pan," are placed in the buccal vestibule for long periods. Slake lime, a turpentine-like compound, not the betel nut, is the actual carcinogen. With the use of this form of smokeless tobacco, the buccal mucosa reacts with chronic inflammation and resultant submucosal fibrosis. Carcinoma occurs at a higher incidence and with a shorter induction time than with cigarette smoking. In India and Sri Lanka, oral carcinomas account for 50% of all malignancies due to these carcinogens; in the United States, oral carcinomas account for only 2% of all malignancies and are mostly due to the carcinogens in cigarettes. Induction times range from 15 to 30 years as opposed to 25 to 50 years for cigarette-related carcinogens. In addition, the submucosal fibrosis frequently leads to limited mouth opening from scar contracture of the oral mucosa and buccinator muscles.

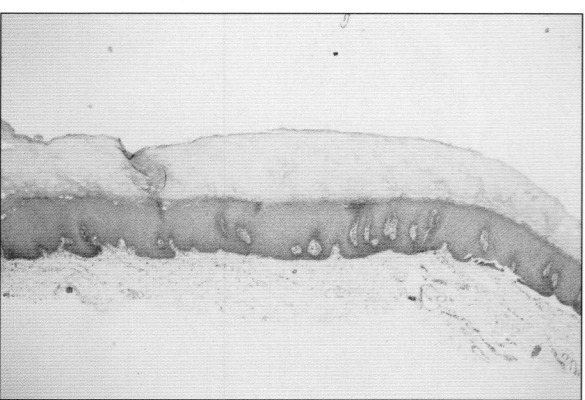

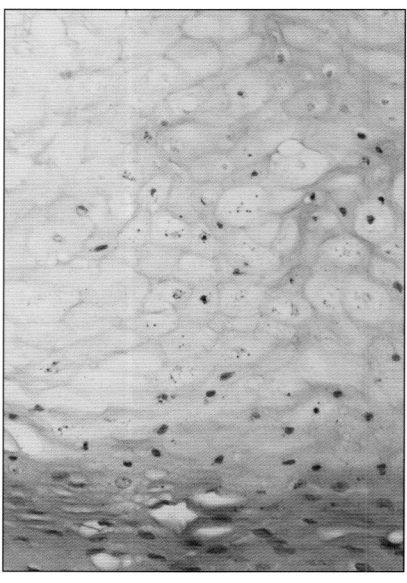

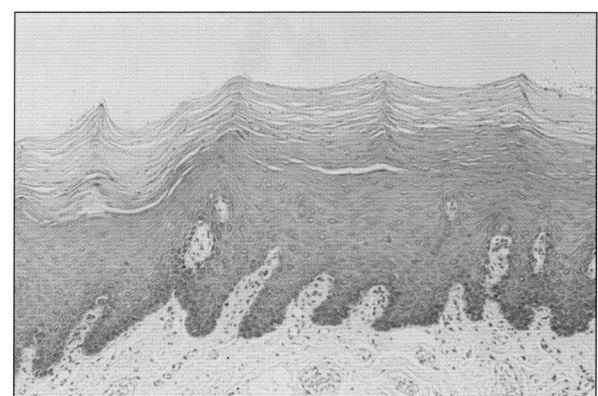

Fig 7-35a A lesion associated with the use of smokeless tobacco. A thick, pale surface layer can be seen, but there is no dysplasia.

Fig 7-35b Higher-power view of Fig 7-35a shows the change in the superficial cells. Pale and hypertrophic, they appear to be a reactive change to the presence of tobacco.

Fig 7-35c The spire-like pattern within the keratinized layer is often associated with the use of tobacco products.

Smokeless tobacco of any type is alkaline (pH 8.0 to 9.4) and may contain spices and flavorings that evoke inflammation. The epithelial response to persistent inflammation is hyperkeratosis (causing a white appearance); the local salivary glands respond with periductal hyperemia (the pinpoint red dots within the white areas); and the submucosa responds with the end product of inflammation, which is repair via collagen deposition known as *scar*. Therefore, depending on the specific form of smokeless tobacco used and the duration of exposure, there will be a variable amount of scar clinically identified as a thickened and inelastic mucosa.

Extreme scar accumulation, termed *submucous fibrosis*, is associated with the use of betel nut–slake lime preparations. This entity may be severe and produce a significant limitation of jaw opening. It is thought to be due to the *Areca catecha* component in the betel nut, which is known specifically to stimulate collagen synthesis.

DIFFERENTIAL DIAGNOSIS ►

Because smokeless tobacco keratosis resembles a premalignant lesion, it must be distinguished histologically from *dysplastic mucosa, verrucous carcinoma*, and *invasive carcinoma*.

DIAGNOSTIC WORK-UP ►

All lesions require biopsy to assess for histologic dysplastic changes and to rule out carcinoma.

HISTOPATHOLOGY ►

A variety of histologic changes may be encountered, with snuff producing a greater change than chewing tobacco. In general, epithelial hyperplasia is seen with varying degrees of hyperparakeratosis and hyperorthokeratosis, the thickness correlating with the amount of tobacco used. Hyperplasia of basal cells may be found. A superficial zone of pale, washed-out cells is one of the most consistent findings (Figs 7-35a and 7-35b). Epithelial dysplasia may be seen but is uncommon and is usually noted in the presence of an inflammatory reaction. A chevron or spire-like pattern of keratin formation may be seen (Fig 7-35c) but appears to be more strongly associated with smoking of tobacco.

TREATMENT ►

Smokeless tobacco keratosis requires only discontinuation of the product. Excision is not recommended unless the histopathologic characteristics are unclear or unless the patient has discontinued the use of smokeless tobacco without a resulting clinical change. If the patient identifies a lesion to be the result of a betel nut–slake lime preparation used in the noted Indo-Asian cultures, the lesion should be regarded as truly premalignant or as an invasive carcinoma and must be biopsied. If an invasive carcinoma is identified in association with betel nut–slake lime use, a wide local excision (2-cm margins) without a prophylactic neck dissection is required. Carcinomas arising from betel nut–slake lime use seem to lack the ability to undergo lymphatic spread until very late in their course.

PROGNOSIS AND FOLLOW-UP ▶

If the smokeless tobacco is discontinued, the prognosis is excellent. Reversion of the affected mucosa to clinical and histologic normalcy is the rule. If the habit continues, the leathery patch will persist and thicken. If the amount used is high, the frequency is high, and its use continued over a long period of time, a carcinoma induction at some future time is remotely possible. Therefore, long-term follow-up and patient education are required.

Submucous Fibrosis

CLINICAL PRESENTATION AND PATHOGENESIS ▶

Submucous fibrosis will usually present as a limited jaw opening (trismus) (Fig 7-36a). Early or less severe forms may have a near normal opening but will present with a thickened inelastic buccal mucosa that will have a thin white surface. It is mostly seen in the East Indian, Sri-Lankan, South Asian, and Southeast Asian cultures because of their use of betel nut with slake lime for oral gratification and recreation. The *Areca catecha* component in betel nut is thought to be the main pathogenesis via its stimulatory effects on collagen synthesis (up to 170%), but the chronic inflammatory reaction provoked by the alkalinity and spice components adds to the accumulation of scar tissue (collagen). Patients with a limited jaw opening experience a higher incidence of caries and periodontitis due to restriction of access for oral hygiene and dental care. Indeed, access for routine dental care in such patients is severely limited and sometimes impossible.

DIFFERENTIAL DIAGNOSIS ▶

The presentation of a restricted jaw opening is suggestive of *radiation fibrosis* if there is a history of radiotherapy of over 5,000 cGy. Previous surgeries or injuries in the masseter, buccopharyngeal raphe, and anterior tonsillar fossa may develop a *vertical scar band* that will also be tight and inelastic. Chronic infections, particularly *actinomycosis*, are well-known to induce a fibrosis and may also present with a limited jaw opening with a firm and inelastic quality. In addition, *temporomandibular joint bony ankylosis* and *fibrous ankylosis* from injuries or foreign bodies, *juvenile rheumatoid arthritis*, and both *traumatic and progressive myositis ossificans* can produce a limited jaw opening. However, in each the oral mucosa will be supple and of normal color and texture.

DIAGNOSTIC WORK-UP ▶

No specific test will confirm a suspected diagnosis of submucous fibrosis. The diagnosis is made from a history of repetitive exposures to betel nut or a similar substance, the clinical appearance, and the texture of the tissue. An incisional biopsy will reveal a thinned epithelial surface and the excessive deposition of otherwise normal collagen in the submucosa. Indeed, a biopsy of the most severe area or of an area of ulcerations is recommended to rule out squamous cell carcinoma because the slake lime in the betel nut–slake lime preparation is a known carcinogen, and submucous fibrosis is considered to be a premalignant sign.

HISTOPATHOLOGY ▶

In submucous fibrosis, the characteristic change is within the connective tissue, where very dense avascular collagenous tissue is deposited (Fig 7-36b). Adjacent skeletal muscle may atrophy. Some chronic inflammatory cells may be present. There are also epithelial changes ranging from atrophy with hyperkeratosis to dysplasia to squamous cell carcinoma.

TREATMENT ▶

The only two effective approaches to submucous fibrosis are (1) no treatment with follow-up and discontinuation of the betel nut–slake lime habit (behavior modification), and (2) total excision with soft tissue myocutaneous or free microvascular flaps transposing viable elastic skin. Approaches using injections of steroids, chymotrypsin, hyaluronidase or alcohol, and surgeries using mucosal or nonvascularized split-thickness skin grafts have not only been ineffective but have often worsened the condition with added scar tissue.

Mild cases or cases with limited jaw opening that still permit reasonable eating abilities and access for oral hygiene and dental care may be treated without intervention but with a focus on quitting the betel

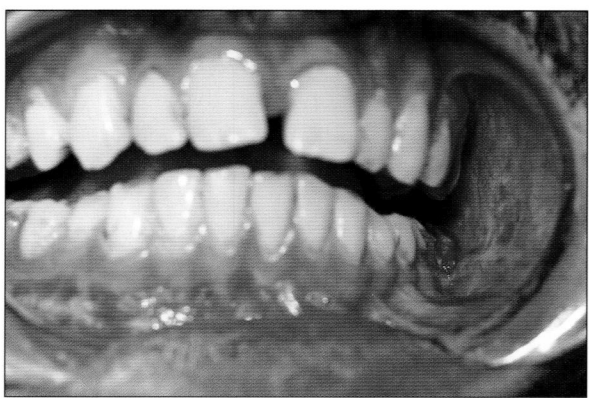

Fig 7-36a This maximum jaw opening of only 3 mm of interincisal distance is the result of submucous fibrosis of the buccal mucosa caused by betel nut–slake lime use.

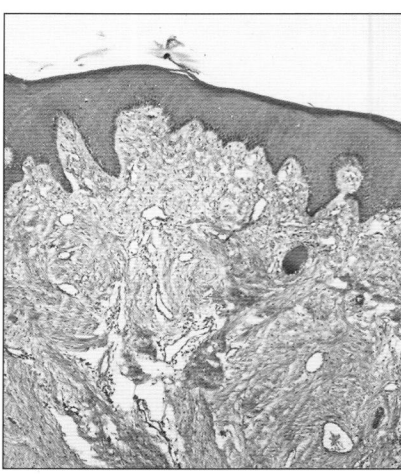

Fig 7-36b Submucous fibrosis is a loss of elastic fibers and fibroblasts, which are replaced by extracellular collagen.

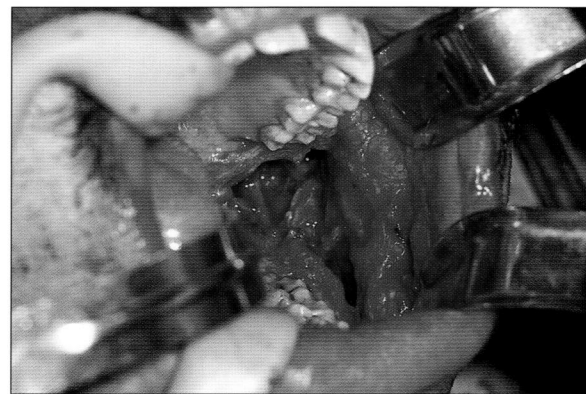

Fig 7-36c The submucous fibrosis must be completely excised to regain a full opening. This will result in a large defect requiring a sufficiently large skin paddle from either a myocutaneous or a free microvascular flap.

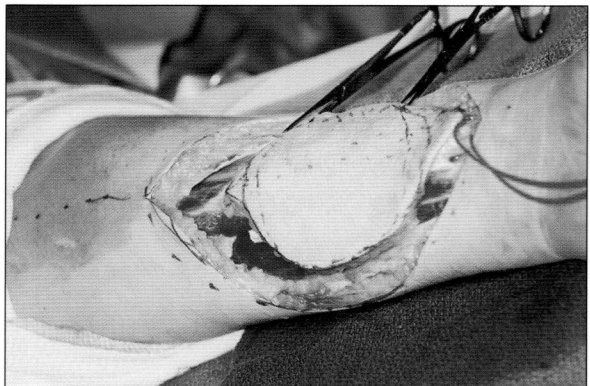

Fig 7-36d Harvesting of a radial forearm free vascular fascio-cutaneous flap to replace the unresilient submucous fibrosis with viable stretchable skin.

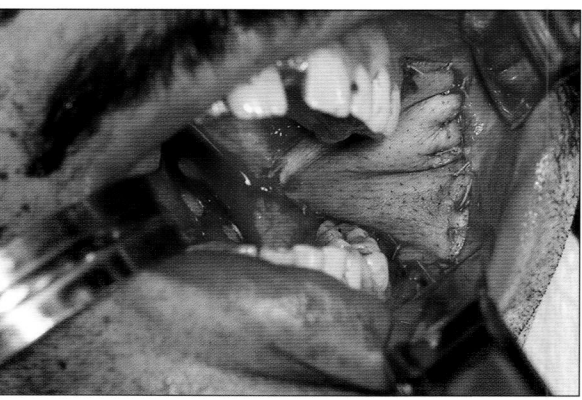

Fig 7-36e The viable skin paddle from the flap is sutured into the buccal mucosa while the mouth is in an open position.

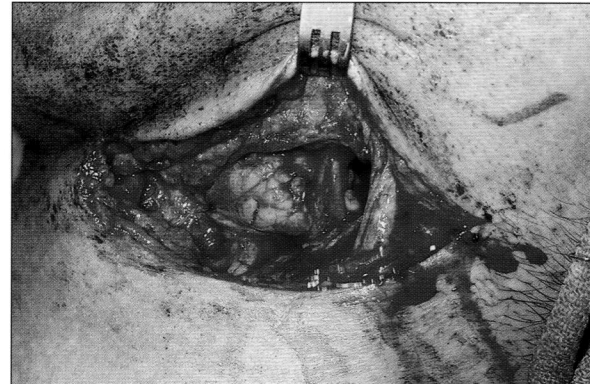

Fig 7-36f The vessels of the free vascular flap can be anastamosed to the facial artery and vein, respectively.

nut–slake lime habit. Severe cases can be successfully treated to a permanent near-normal jaw opening with complete excision and replacement surgery of the affected areas. Some cases will be unilateral, but most are bilateral and therefore require two flaps.

Because the submucous fibrosis is due to the absorption of the fibrosis-producing agents through the surface epithelium, the most severely involved levels are in the lamina propria and upper submucosa. These are excised with a wide field excision in the area of clinical involvement until the soft tissue release is sufficient to gain an opening in excess of 35 mm between erupted incisors (Fig 7-36c). In longstanding cases some muscle fibrosis is also present, requiring excision of at least a portion of the involved muscle. This usually requires excision of the buccinator, but in the most severe cases the medial pterygoid muscle and the anterior border of the masseter muscle may require release.

Once the submucous fibrosis is excised, a viable, size-matched skin paddle, which will retain its elastic fibers, must be placed into the defect. In such defects, free microvascular flaps consisting of skin and subcutaneous tissue layers are the best choice because of their size and thickness match. Here the radial forearm microvascular flap (Figs 7-36d and 7-36e) or the circumflex scapular flap are the flaps of choice and can be directly anastamosed to the facial artery and vein (Fig 7-36f). A pectoralis major or a

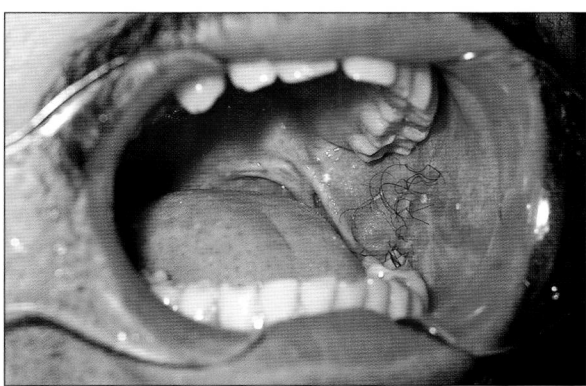

Fig 7-36g Replacement of each fibrosed buccal mucosa with a viable and stretchable skin paddle results in a permanent increase in jaw opening.

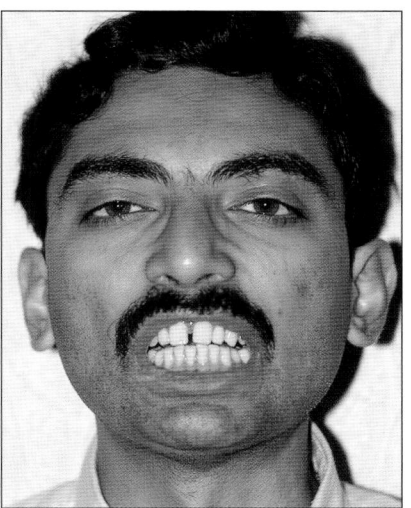

Fig 7-36h This individual with bilateral submucous fibrosis had a maximum jaw opening of 3 mm.

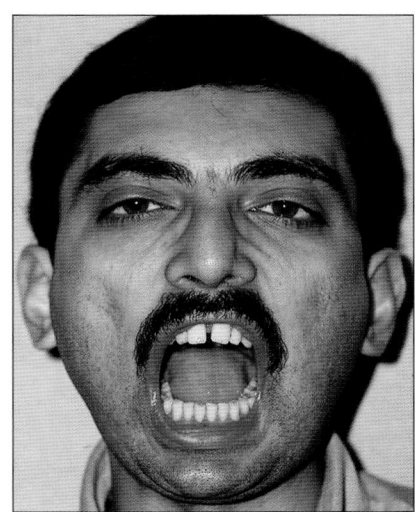

Fig 7-36i After grafting of bilateral free vascular flaps from the radial forearms, an unrestricted opening is achieved.

trapezius pedicled myocutaneous flap can also serve the same purpose; however, these flaps are less ideal because of the added bulk of the muscle pedicle and the thicker subcutaneous layers in the chest and back as compared to the radial forearm. A superior-based platysma flap with a supraclavicular skin paddle is a less common myocutaneous flap but one that may be used in this situation.

PROGNOSIS ▶

When an individual continues the betel nut–slake lime habit, the prognosis of an untreated submucous fibrosis is one of progressive fibrosis to a complete trismus and a high risk for squamous cell carcinoma development. In individuals who go untreated but quit the habit, the fibrosis may be arrested, or it will progress only slightly and confer a reduced risk for carcinoma development. In those cases that are treated with aggressive excision and flap reconstruction, the increased opening is maintained long term (Figs 7-36g to 7-36i). However, if the exposure to betel nut or similar agents is resumed, the skin paddle itself and/or surrounding tissue will become fibrosed and a limited jaw opening will recur.

Verrucous Carcinoma

CLINICAL PRESENTATION AND PATHOGENESIS ▶

Verrucous carcinoma is a separate and distinct form of oral carcinoma. It suggests a superficially spreading but nonmetastasizing, noninvasive type of papillary and exophytic cancer, but this is true only of a true verrucous carcinoma. Like many cancers, it evolves from premalignant forms and may further evolve into more invasive forms. The premalignant form of verrucous carcinoma seems to be the recently described entity verrucous hyperplasia. As verrucous carcinomas evolve, a certain percentage will become invasive squamous cell carcinomas.

The true verrucous carcinoma will present as a rough-textured, exophytic, white-to-red papillary lesion. It is most often found on the buccal mucosa (60% of cases) and the gingiva (30% of cases), of which the maxillary gingiva is more frequently involved than the mandibular gingiva (Fig 7-37). There is a slight male predilection, and those affected are usually older than 50 years. The lesions are slow growing and will be reported to be asymptomatic. The surrounding tissue may show satellite lesions, particularly posterior to the primary lesion, but is otherwise normal and is not indurated (Fig 7-38).

DIFFERENTIAL DIAGNOSIS ▶

Verrucous carcinoma can be reliably distinguished from *invasive squamous cell carcinoma* only histopathologically. Some invasive squamous cell carcinomas are clinically papillary and quite exophytic, thus

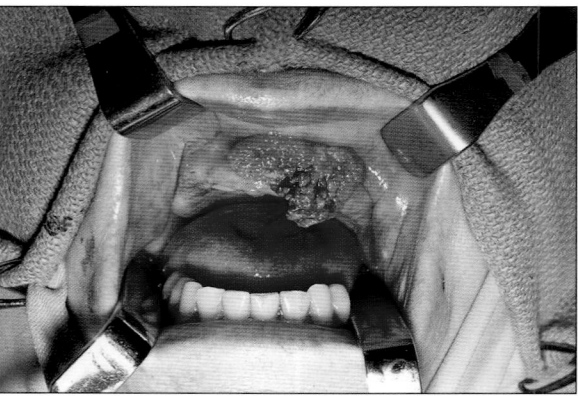

Fig 7-37 Verrucous carcinoma involving the maxillary gingiva and labial vestibule. This patient smoked cigarettes but did not use smokeless tobacco.

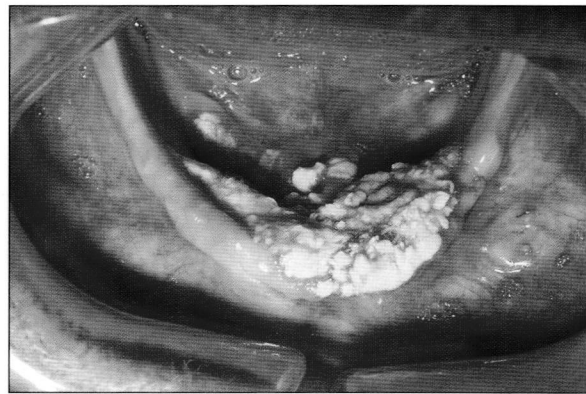

Fig 7-38 Verrucous carcinoma of the alveolar ridge–floor of the mouth. Note the satellite lesions in the posterior floor of the mouth on each side. This patient also smoked cigarettes but did not use smokeless tobacco.

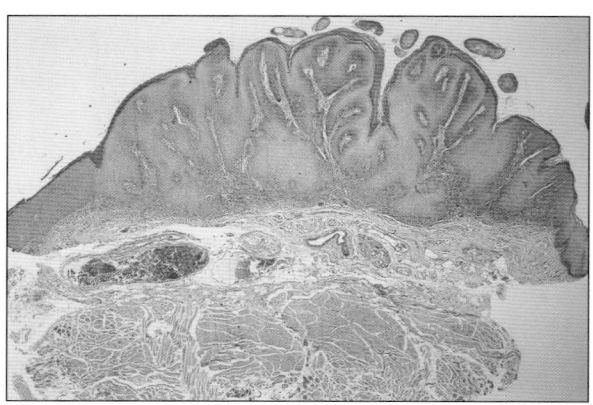

Fig 7-39a A low-power view of a verrucous carcinoma shows the exo-endophytic growth pattern with the verrucous surface, and the "pushing" tumor margin with a subjacent inflammatory infiltrate. The tumor is well demarcated, and the tumor mass is seen to push below the level of the adjacent normal epithelium.

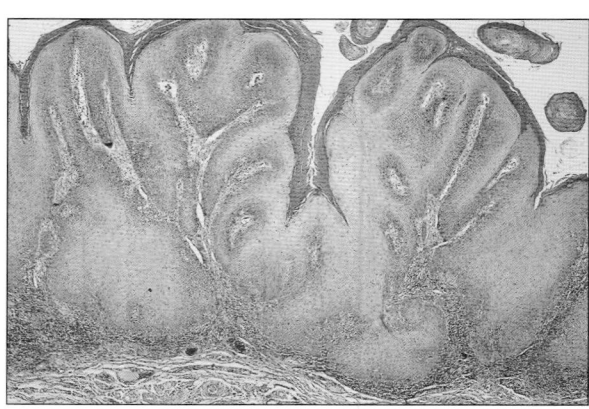

Fig 7-39b A higher-power view of Fig 7-39a shows the parakeratinized clefts and the broad rete ridges.

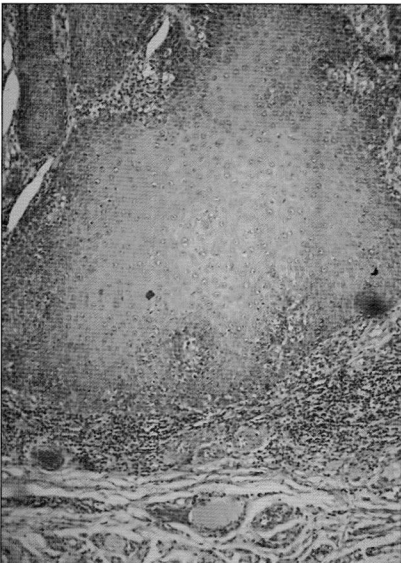

Fig 7-39c The same verrucous carcinoma as shown in Figs 7-39a and 7-39b lacks cellular atypia. Note the absence of infiltration.

closely resembling a verrucous carcinoma. *Clinical leukoplakia (benign hyperkeratosis)*, which is not dysplastic, or an oral *verrucous hyperplasia* lesion are common. Cases of abundant hyperkeratosis will have a texture similar to that of verrucous carcinoma. Verrucous hyperplasia is both clinically and histologically verrucous. It is a consideration on the differential diagnosis and may need to be treated in the same fashion as verrucous carcinoma. Small lesions may also be confused with *squamous papillomas*, and multiple small satellite lesions may resemble *focal epithelial hyperplasia (Heck disease)*.

DIAGNOSTIC WORK-UP ▶

The presence of additional lesions or the extension of the suspicious lesion into the pharynx is a concern with verrucous carcinoma. It is, therefore, important to consider a mirror or fiberoptic examination of the nasopharynx and laryngopharynx. In addition, a panoramic radiograph and even periapical radiographs in those areas where the lesion approaches bone are recommended to assess for invasive squamous cell carcinoma. Although a TNM staging is not pertinent to verrucous carcinoma, it is recommended at the time of biopsy in case histopathologic studies identify a squamous cell carcinoma. An incisional biopsy of the lesion will rule out the other entities on the differential list and establish the diagnosis.

An adequate biopsy specimen is necessary for accurate diagnosis, since it is primarily the architecture of this tumor that is diagnostic. An adequate specimen is one that includes at least one normal margin to a depth within the submucosa.

Low-power views show a lesion that demonstrates an exo-endophytic growth pattern. The surface is papillary with a thick, parakeratinized covering that extends into the deep, cleft-like interpapillary spaces. The rete ridges are broad and bulbous and exhibit a "pushing" border, which extends deep to the level of the adjacent normal epithelium. A subepithelial chronic inflammatory infiltrate is present (Figs 7-39a and 7-39b). At high power, the acanthotic epithelium shows little atypia (Fig 7-39c). The hyperplasia may cause some cellular crowding, but pleomorphism and mitoses are rare or absent. There is no infiltration of the connective tissue by the epithelium. The verrucous carcinoma thus has deceptively benign histologic features; inadequate biopsies that fail to allow for an appreciation of the overall architecture may lead to the erroneous diagnosis of a benign epithelial hyperplasia. It should also be understood, however, that verrucous carcinoma may harbor foci of invasive squamous cell carcinoma.

The histologic features of verrucous carcinoma include:

• Exo-endophytic growth pattern
• Verrucous surface with parakeratinized clefts
• Bulbous rete ridges
• Pushing border with no infiltration
• Subepithelial inflammatory infiltrate
• Cytologically benign characteristics

TREATMENT ▶

True verrucous carcinoma is noninvasive. Therefore, bony resection and neck dissections are not among the treatment considerations. However, verrucous carcinomas are very serious cancers because of their peripheral spread. Excision to a depth of the full thickness of mucosa is appropriate. In the buccal mucosa, the excisional depth would be to the buccinator fascia. In the gingival area, excision should be to the supraperiosteal plane. The peripheral margins are most important since recurrences arise mostly from this area or from new clinical lesions emerging from clinically and histologically normal-appearing but genetically altered mucosa. One-centimeter margins are the rule, but 2-cm margins are needed for the posterior and floor-of-the-mouth margins because many verrucous carcinomas have been known to spread in this direction and will follow the salivary flow channels.

PROGNOSIS AND FOLLOW-UP ▶

The prognosis for verrucous carcinoma of the oral cavity is excellent because lesions are identified early and the access for excision is straightforward. Verrucous carcinoma of the nasopharynx and the supraglottic larynx are much more difficult to treat because of access limitations and size, which is generally large at the time of diagnosis. Oral cavity verrucous carcinoma has about an 80% cure rate. Of the remaining 20%, a large number represent verrucous carcinoma that either is too extensive to resect or is indicative of a "field cancer" phenomenon in which normal-appearing mucosa progressively develops verrucous hyperplasia–verrucous carcinomas over a wide area. Management of such cases often requires radiotherapy either as a sole modality (6,000 cGy to 7,200 cGy) or combined with surgery. The concern about verrucous carcinoma transformation into invasive and anaplastic malignancies has been overstated. Large series indicate that the incidence of invasive carcinoma after radiotherapy for a verrucous carcinoma is less than 6%. Even these cases may represent spontaneous malignant transformation or misdiagnosis. Therefore, there is no absolute contraindication to radiotherapy for these lesions in select cases of extensive disease.

Follow-up should include a mirror or fiberoptic examination of the nasopharynx and laryngopharynx in addition to a clinical examination. Recommended follow-up intervals are every 4 months for the first 2 years followed by every 6 months thereafter.

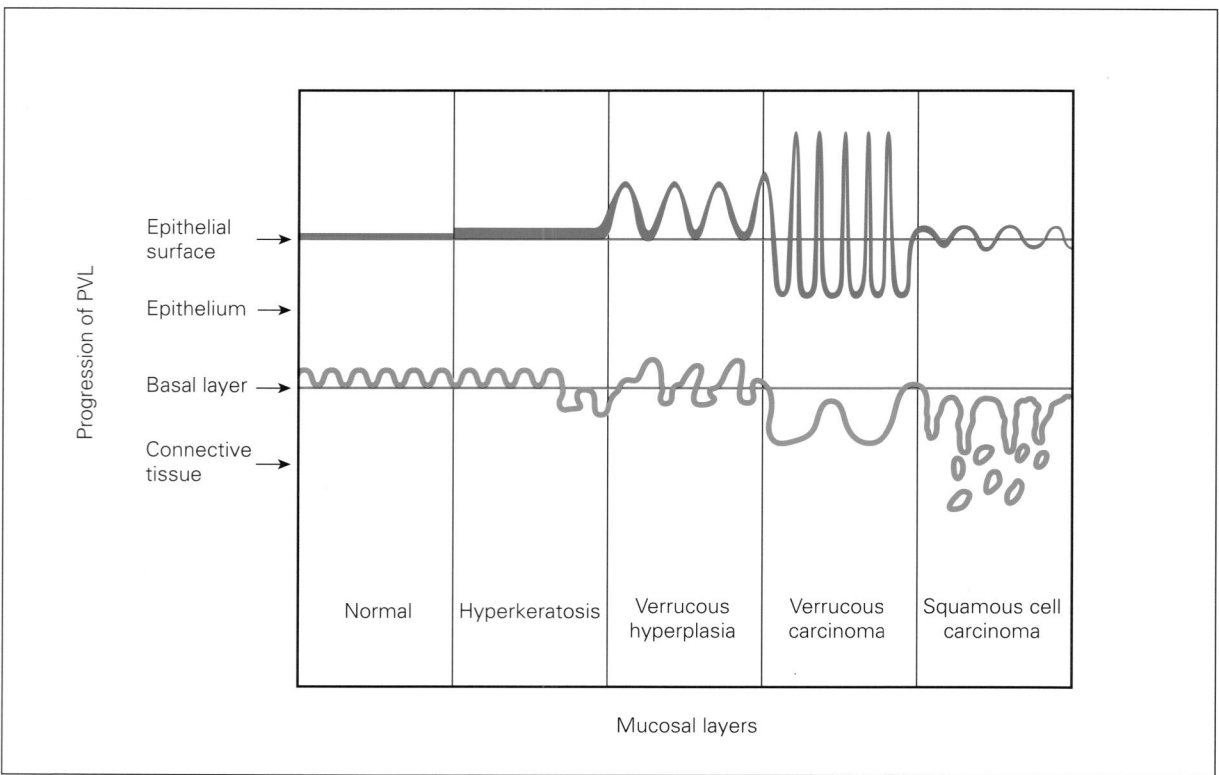

Fig 7-40 Progression of PVL through advancing stages. Note the surface changes and those at the basement membrane level over time.

Proliferative Verrucous Leukoplakia

CLINICAL PRESENTATION AND PATHOGENESIS ►

Proliferative verrucous leukoplakia (PVL) is a field cancer development phenomenon where clinically normal-appearing oral mucosa slowly transforms through advancing stages of clinical leukoplakia, verrucous hyperplasia, and verrucous carcinoma, and then into invasive squamous cell carcinoma. Histopathologically normal mucosa is observed to undergo a cellular transformation through various forms of dysplasia into verrucous hyperplasia, then into verrucous carcinoma, and finally into various differentiated patterns of invasive squamous cell carcinoma (Fig 7-40).

Proliferative verrucous leukoplakia is more common in women (4:1) and with advancing age. It is rare before the age of 45 years and has a peak incidence around 65 years. Most patients (78%) are nonsmokers. Initial lesions appear as relatively innocuous asymptomatic clinical leukoplakia of the attached gingiva, buccal mucosa, labial mucosa of the lips, or tongue. The lesions will strongly mimic benign hyperkeratosis, lichen planus, or hypertrophic candidiasis. Indeed, there is a strong association with *Candida* organisms. In these authors' experience, various *Candida* species were identified in 92% of cases. The relationship may be incidental where the verrucoid surface texture traps *Candida* organisms as a colonization phenomenon only; or, on the other hand, it may be causative, where products of chronic *Candida* colonization or *Candida* infections act as topical carcinogens, which produce the observed transformations into dysplasia and malignancy. *Candida* may also represent an unrelated component of an age- or genetic-related loss of telomeres or other such tumor-suppressor proteins, which would dysregulate oral epithelium toward dysplasia and at the same time reduce the normal tissue's resistance to *Candida* (Figs 7-41a to 7-41c). Some evidence of telomerase alterations has been found, and about 40% of individuals with PVL also have skin fungal lesions or vaginal candidiasis, findings that support this concept.

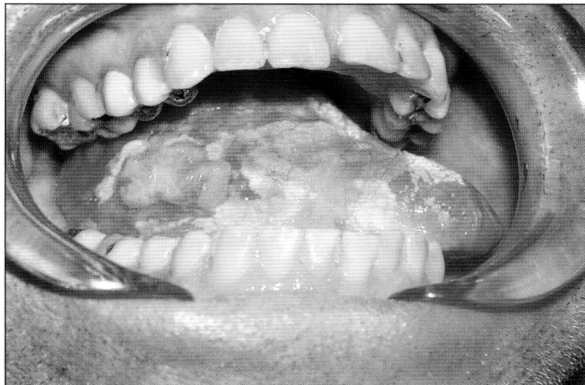

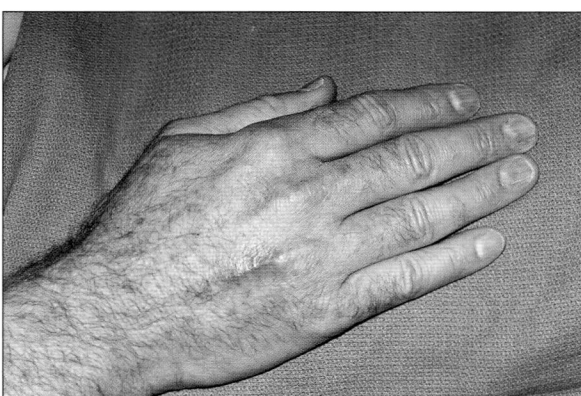 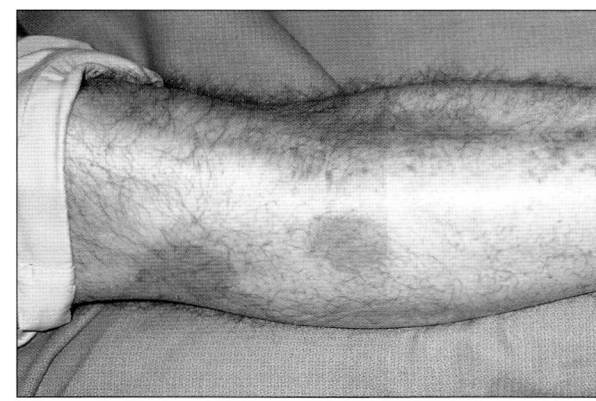

Fig 7-41a Proliferative verrucous leukoplakia of the tongue with a focal area of microinvasive squamous cell carcinoma on the right lateral border. This patient had chronic oral candidiasis for several years prior to the finding of PVL.

Figs 7-41b and 7-41c Concomitant fungal lesions on the skin of the hand, the arm, and other locations support the suspicion of some genetic alteration that increases the risk for both epithelial proliferation/dysplasia and superficial fungal infections.

Early lesions will be white, irregular, asymptomatic surface lesions, appearing either singly or in small clusters (Figs 7-42a and 7-42b). As they continue over several months, adjacent surfaces develop identical lesions while the original lesion is observed to enlarge in a creeping surface phenomenon. The base may become reddened, and pain may develop over time. When left untreated, large surface areas become involved and the older lesions develop a more verrucous appearance. These advances occur over several years and may come to involve nearly the entire oral mucosa and may even extend into the pharynx. The lip vermilion also becomes involved, often with brownish-black exophytic lesions that will encroach onto the skin edge of the vermilion (Fig 7-42c). Some of the verrucous lesions will develop 3- to 5-cm-long strands, creating a grotesque appearance (Fig 7-42d). Eventually, untreated cases will develop induration and/or ulceration indicative of the final transformation into invasive carcinoma. The invasiveness and rate of tissue destruction also increases with time and will progress into an anaplastic and clinically fungating tumor, which will often cause death by debilitation and tumor load (Fig 7-42e).

DIFFERENTIAL DIAGNOSIS ▶

The earlier stages of PVL will appear as *benign hyperkeratosis, lichen planus,* or *hypertrophic candidiasis.* Indeed, biopsies of these early lesions are often misdiagnosed as one of these. Therefore, the clinician should be alert to the possibility of PVL should the lesions "spread out" or fail to respond to treatment regimens aimed at either lichen planus or candidiasis.

Other considerations may include *dysplasia* or *verrucous carcinoma* unrelated to PVL or perhaps related to smoking habits. *Hereditary benign intraepithelial dyskeratosis* (HBID) or coalesced lesions of *condyloma acuminatum* will also appear as multiple or coalesced areas of clinical leukoplakia.

DIAGNOSTIC WORK-UP ▶

White oral lesions in general are strong considerations for a biopsy, and the potential for PVL is one of the reasons for this. Biopsies should be excisional if the lesion is small. Incisional biopsies in larger lesions should be placed within the confines of the clinical lesions. The biopsy should be to a depth into the submucosa or to the supraperiosteal plane over bone.

Since candidiasis is part of the differential diagnosis and may be seen along with PVL, a periodic acid–Schiff (PAS) stain may be requested. In addition, since a PVL-related squamous cell carcinoma or one that is unrelated to PVL may be diagnosed, a complete head and neck examination and a TNM classification are recommended.

HISTOPATHOLOGY ▶

The diagnosis of PVL is not an isolated histologic diagnosis; rather, it is a sequence of combined clinical and histologic events. In the early part of the disease, the histologic picture is consistent with a simple benign hyperkeratosis, but over time the picture changes, often evolving through verrucous hyperplasia to verrucous carcinoma and ultimately to infiltrating squamous cell carcinoma. Verrucous hyperplasia histologically is broad-based and shows the exophytic projections covered by hyperparakeratotic stratified

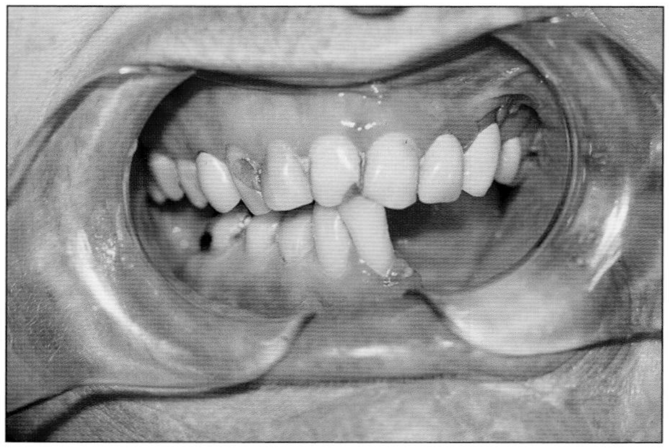

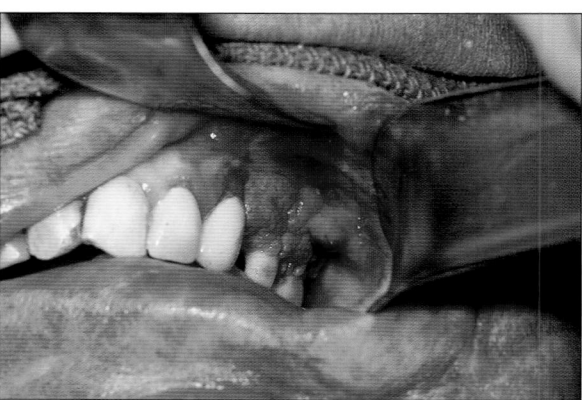

Fig 7-42a Small area of clinical leukoplakia in a non-smoker representing verrucous hyperplasia as part of PVL. Note the normal lip and gingival areas at this time.

Fig 7-42b Initial PVL lesions were excised, but no chemoprevention protocol was followed. Margins of the excised specimen were clinically and histologically normal.

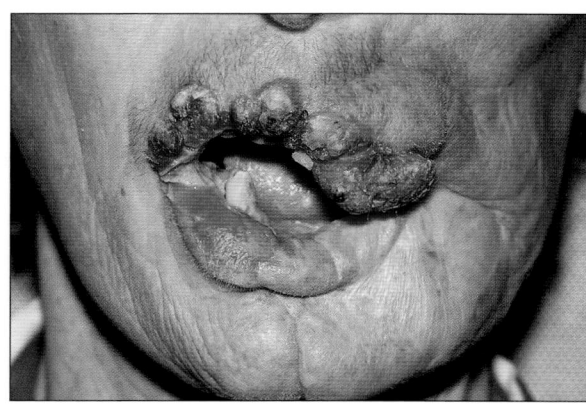

Fig 7-42c Development of extensive verrucous carcinomas and invasive carcinomas 1 year later.

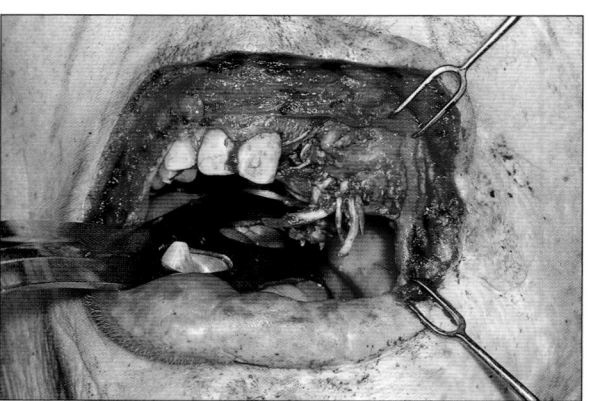

Fig 7-42d Extensive excision of the upper lip lesions was required. Note the elongated strands of verrucous carcinoma and the involvement of the gingiva, which also was normal 1 year earlier.

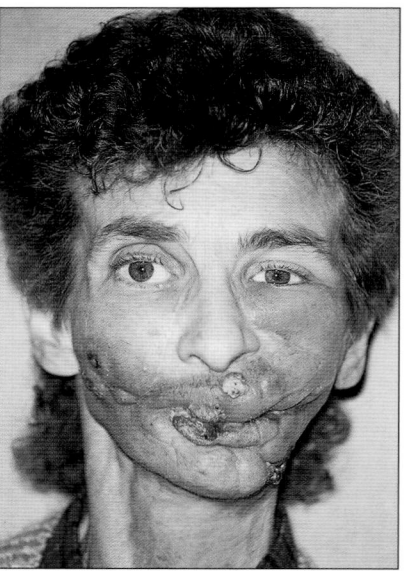

Fig 7-42e The final phase of PVL is a transformation into an aggressive and erosive type of squamous cell carcinoma that results in an excessive tumor load leading to death. Metastasis rarely occurs even in the presence of extensive local disease.

squamous epithelium with deep intervening clefts as is seen in verrucous carcinoma. It is often difficult to make a clear distinction between verrucous hyperplasia and verrucous carcinoma. The major difference is that verrucous hyperplasia does not exhibit the "pushing border" of verrucous carcinoma. It is essentially an exophytic lesion as opposed to an exo-endophytic lesion. An inflammatory infiltrate is variably present, and cellular atypia is sometimes noted (see Fig 7-40).

TREATMENT ▶

The goal of PVL treatment is to slow down or prevent the relentless transformation to more advanced premalignant conditions and, eventually, invasive carcinoma. It is advisable to inform the patient from the outset that the cause of PVL is unknown and therefore is not related to any previous oral procedures, medications, diet, or habits, and that it is incurable but can be treated to slow its progression and transformation. In doing so, PVL is usually compatible with longevity but several surgeries and ongoing medications are likely to be necessary.

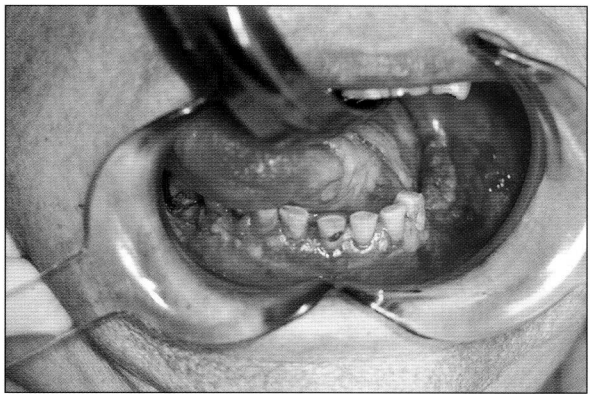 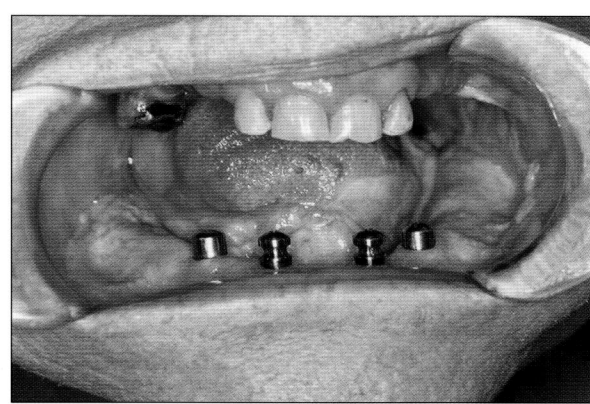

Fig 7-43a This PVL presented with numerous widespread erythroleukoplakias. The excised lesions evidenced all degrees of dysplasia, including carcinoma in situ, verrucous hyperplasia, and verrucous carcinoma.

Fig 7-43b The PVL lesions of Fig 7-43a were excised and skin grafted. Use of the chemoprevention protocol prevented the progression and extension of the few remaining lesions for 9 years, when the patient died of unrelated causes.

Excision is recommended for all lesions that are either symptomatic or suspicious for verrucous or invasive carcinoma, and/or where size and location make excision practical without creating undue morbidity or deformity. The principles of PVL excisions will differ somewhat from those of other leukoplakias. First, clear peripheral margins, either grossly or microscopically, are not necessary because of its diffuse nature and the fact that even microscopically clear and normal margins may be genetically altered or biochemically already on their way to dysplasia. Second, the areas of excision often cover a very large surface. It is common to graft these areas with split-thickness skin grafts of 0.015 to 0.020 inches in thickness and to bolster or splint them to the wound base so as to obtain the best adaptation. The excisional depth is relatively superficial unless invasive carcinoma is diagnosed. The usual PVL represents a spectrum of dysplasia, verrucous hyperplasia, and verrucous carcinoma, all of which are noninvasive beyond the basement membrane. Therefore, excisions to the level just into the submucosa or to the periosteum over bone are adequate (Figs 7-43a and 7-43b).

The second stage of treatment is medical and is often described as chemoprevention. The following regimen of medications has proven effective in slowing PVL progression or arresting it in a particular phase: betacarotene, 30 mg (50,000 IU) four times daily (ongoing); fluconazole (Diflucan, Pfizer), 100 mg every day for 2 months; nystatin (Mycostatin, Westwood), oral suspension 100,000 U/mL, one tsp (5 mL) four times daily swish and spit (ongoing); and selenium, 100 mcg every day (ongoing).

The betacarotene in this regimen is thought to enhance the maturation of epithelial cells and to down regulate their response to epidermal growth factors. Some practitioners will substitute retinoids such as isotretinoin (13-*cis*-retinoic acid) (Accutane, Roche) at 60 to 80 mg every day, but most adults find the skin and mucosal drying and chapping effect too great to tolerate long term. The fluconazole and nystatin are of course to treat candidiasis. Fluconazole's initial course of 2 months is designed to be coupled with nystatin to cover all species of *Candida* and to gain an initial complete suppression, after which nystatin alone can be used ongoing without fear of the complications and side effects that may result from long-term fluconazole therapy. The fluconazole can be reintroduced as needed later. Selenium is an antioxidant, which is thought to suppress the formation of free radicals that alter cells.

At times, griseofulvin ultramicrosized (Fulvicin P/G, Grispeg-Schering), 125 mg three times daily, may be used instead of fluconazole or nystatin. Griseofulvin is a drug that is both antifungal (used mostly for skin fungal infections) and enhances maturation of epithelial cells.

Laser ablation is not recommended for excision of PVL. Its use has been associated with rapid redevelopment, perhaps because of its lack of precise depth control, which leaves altered basal cells at the

PROGNOSIS ▶

depth of the wound to repopulate the area. In addition, radiotherapy has minimal effect on PVL and should be reserved for cases that have progressed into invasive carcinoma and then mostly after an ablative cancer surgery.

The natural course of PVL is a slow but relentless progression from clinical leukoplakia to extensive invasive carcinoma over 5 to 15 years. Selective surgeries, the chemoprevention protocol described, and close follow-up every 2 months will prevent most cases from transforming into an uncontrolled carcinoma and will improve the individual's function and quality of life in the process. Nevertheless, some individuals will indeed progress to uncontrolled disfiguring cancers, which will be refractory to most treatments and lead to death (see Fig 7-42e). However, regional lymph node metastasis is very rare and distant metastasis is almost never seen even in advanced cases or on autopsy. This underscores the differences between cancers that evolve from PVL and those that arise from smoking-related carcinogens. Although they both are squamous cell carcinomas, they have somewhat different genetic mutations and therefore somewhat different biologic potentials.

The natural course of PVL is an ever-increasing rate of progression toward dysplasia and into cytologically anaplastic cancers. If radiotherapy were employed during the verrucous hyperplasia or verrucous carcinoma stage of PVL, it would be blamed for this transformation. Yet untreated PVL-related verrucous lesions progress to anaplastic cancers without radiation exposures. It is likely that in the past many "anaplastic transformations" were correlated to the radiotherapy where radiotherapy was only coincidental to the natural course of this disease. Therefore, radiotherapy is no longer contraindicated in the treatment of verrucous carcinomas, nor is it contraindicated in the treatment of PVL. However, it should be reserved only for chemoprevention—refractory cases and those in which size or location make them unresectable.

Mucosal Squamous Cell Carcinomas

Diagnostic Considerations

For all lesions suggestive of mucosal squamous cell carcinoma, there is a recommended work-up designed to stage the present disease, search for synchronous lesions (other separate and simultaneously occurring cancers) or associated pathologies, and establish the diagnosis without compromising future treatment.

Examination

The oral cavity, neck, and pharynx should be thoroughly examined. This should include thorough palpation for neck and oral masses and a visual examination of all oral tissues after all removable appliances have been removed, since these can obscure difficult-to-visualize areas such as the lateral floor of the mouth, pterygoid notch, posterior tongue, and tonsillar fossa. A panoramic radiograph should be taken and the dentition examined. The examination should also include a visual inspection of the pharynx and air passages to the level of the vocal cords. This may be accomplished by a mirror exam (indirect laryngoscopy) or a fiberoptic exam (nasopharyngoscopy) (Fig 7-44). Both of these procedures are easier with the use of topical anesthesia.

Staging

Suspicious lesions must be clinically staged prior to biopsy (Table 7-3). The biopsy itself and potential wound scarring or infection may distort the lesions and confuse later staging. A biopsy may also induce

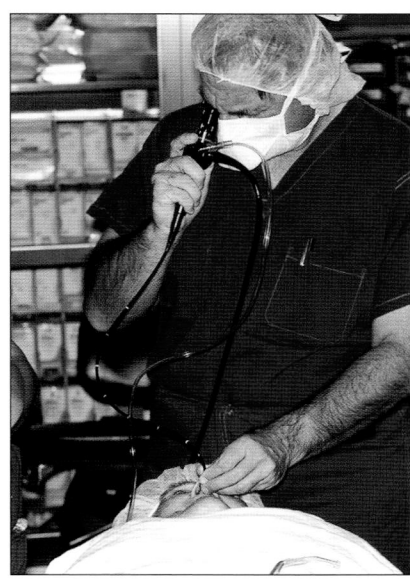

Fig 7-44 A fiberoptic nasopharyngoscopy under topical anesthesia is an excellent technique to examine for second primary carcinomas or recurrent carcinomas.

inflammation within regional lymph nodes, which would be included in the staging and thus falsely stage the neck.

To note the size (T), the visible lesion is crudely measured in centimeters with a ruler. The greatest dimension of the lesion is recorded, and only clearly visible boundaries are used.

The appreciation of palpable nodes (N) is by clinical feel and a rough ruler estimation of size. All palpable nodes must be included. The classification is strictly clinical. No allowance is made for the subjective bias for anticipating the node to be of an inflammatory nature. Computed tomographic (CT) or magnetic resonance imaging (MRI) scans, which may identify normal but nonpalpable nodes, are not currently used to clinically stage these lesions.

The scientific basis for advancing the N staging to N_2 when a node exceeds 3 cm is the understanding that clinically palpable nodes that are greater than 3 cm are usually two or more nodes fused by tumor growing out of the capsule of each node. The advance to N_3 when the clinical node exceeds 6 cm is based on the understanding that such large masses represent extranodal cancer masses and thus cancer cells out of the fascial envelope of the neck.

The metastatic work-up (M) usually includes a general physical examination and a chest radiograph since squamous cell carcinoma is more likely to spread to the lung via hematogenous routes than to any other distant organ. This portion of the staging is performed after the biopsy results confirm the diagnosis. Some practitioners also use a skull CT scan and/or a technetium-99 methylene diophosphate (^{99}TcMDP) scan to assess for brain metastasis or bone metastasis, but this is not part of the required testing for staging. These additional studies, although reasonable, are not sufficiently yielding other than in advanced or recurrent tumors. More important is a continued search in the aerodigestive tract for a metachronous primary tumor. Prior to definitive management of a confirmed oral squamous cell carcinoma, either a triple endoscopy, a barium swallow, or a CT scan including the neck and esophagus is highly recommended.

Once the TNM staging is accomplished and the biopsy confirms the diagnosis of squamous cell carcinoma, a stage grouping is recommended for reporting results and for prognostication (Table 7-4).

Biopsy

After staging is biopsy. It is recommended that a biopsy be performed at the initial visit before any work-up other than examination, staging, and in-office radiographs. Patients with squamous cell carcinoma are

Table 7-3 TNM classification for oral squamous cell carcinoma according to the American Joint Commission on Cancer Staging

T	Primary tumor size
T_S	Carcinoma in situ
T_1	Tumor size 0 to 2 cm
T_2	Tumor size 2 to 4 cm
T_3	Tumor size > 4 cm
T_4	"Massive" tumors or tumor invading bone or intrinsic muscles of the tongue, floor of the mouth, suprahyoids, or muscles of mastication

N	Regional lymph node
N_0	No clinically palpable nodes
N_1	Clinically palpable ipsilateral node < 3 cm
N_{2A}	Clinically palpable ipsilateral node 3 to 6 cm
N_{2B}	Two or more clinically palpable ipsilateral nodes 3 to 6 cm
N_3	Bilateral or contralateral palpable node OR any clinically palpable node > 6 cm

M	Distant metastasis
M_X	Metastasis not assessed
M_0	Metastasis assessed: none found
M_1	Metastasis present

Table 7-4 Oral squamous cell carcinoma staging

Stage	Primary tumor size	Regional lymph node	Distant metastasis
0	T_S		
I	T_1	N_0	M_0
II	T_2	N_0	M_0
III	T_3	N_0	M_0
	T_1	N_1	M_0
	T_2	N_1	M_0
	T_3	N_1	M_0
IV	T_4	N_0	M_0
	T_4	N_1	M_0
	Any T	N_2	M_0
	Any T	N_3	M_0
	Any T	Any N	M_1

often not the most compliant patients. They have a fear of what their diagnosis may be. Delaying biopsy often results in denial of their disease until it becomes painful or fungating and less curable.

Incisional biopsies for lesions suspicious for squamous cell carcinoma should be biopsied within the clinical confines of the lesion. Although some authors have suggested the inclusion of the lesion's edge and a margin of normal-appearing tissue in the biopsy specimen, as is valid for mucocutaneous and vesiculobullous disease, this practice in oral squamous cell carcinoma adds little to the diagnosis and extends the surgical tumor margins into planes and areas that may compromise treatment and prognosis. It is more important to take a sufficiently deep biopsy to include underlying muscle. Knowledge of the depth of invasion is pertinent to treatment planning and to prognosis.

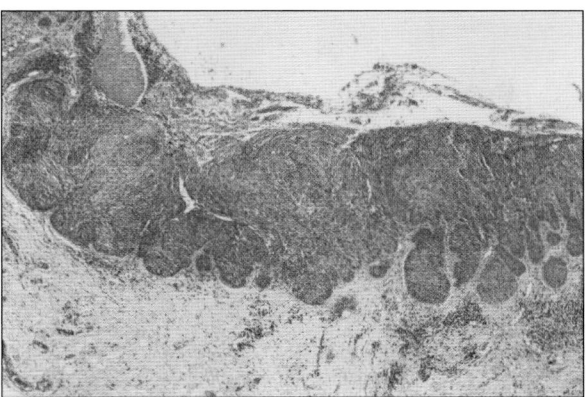

Fig 7-45a Squamous cell carcinoma showing superficial infiltration into the connective tissue.

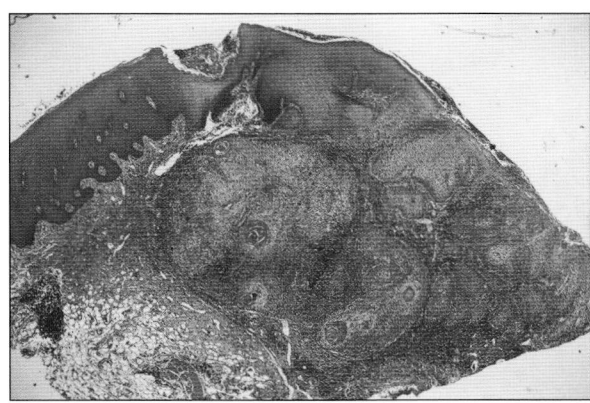

Fig 7-45b Squamous cell carcinoma showing extensive invasion into the underlying tissue. Note the inflammatory response.

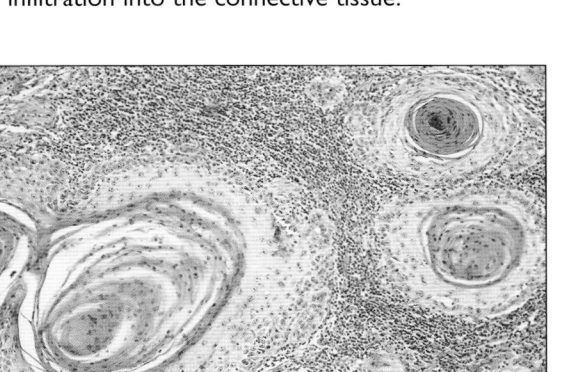

Fig 7-46a A well-differentiated squamous cell carcinoma with prominent keratin formation. The tumor islands show differentiation from the periphery to the center.

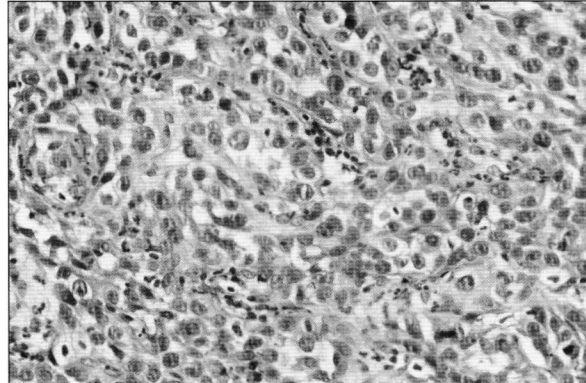

Fig 7-46b A poorly differentiated squamous cell carcinoma lacking any obvious keratin formation or organization.

Histopathology

There may be considerable range in the histologic appearance of oral squamous cell carcinoma. The commonality is that the basement membrane of the surface epithelium has been violated and that the neoplastic epithelium infiltrates the connective tissue. The extent of the infiltration may range from a few small islands to strands, broad sheets, and large islands that may obliterate the supporting tissue (Figs 7-45a and 7-45b). The appearance of the invading epithelium is variable. In some lesions, the islands may show an almost normal maturation process from the basal cells at the periphery to the keratin mass in the center. These are well-differentiated tumors, and cellular atypism and mitotic activity may be minimal (Fig 7-46a). At the other end of the spectrum are the poorly differentiated lesions in which keratin formation is not seen and maturation of tumor cells cannot be appreciated (Fig 7-46b). In these instances, mitoses are usually more prevalent and cellular atypism is more marked. In the poorly differentiated carcinomas, it may be necessary to use immunohistochemistry to identify cytokeratins for accurate diagnosis. Pleomorphism, prominent nucleoli, reversal of nuclear/cytoplasmic ratio, individual cell keratinization, and both normal and abnormal mitoses are features noted in varying combinations in different tumors (Figs 7-47a and 7-47b).

The stroma typically contains an inflammatory infiltrate of lymphocytes, plasma cells, and macrophages. Particularly when there is infiltration of skeletal muscle, large numbers of eosinophils may be

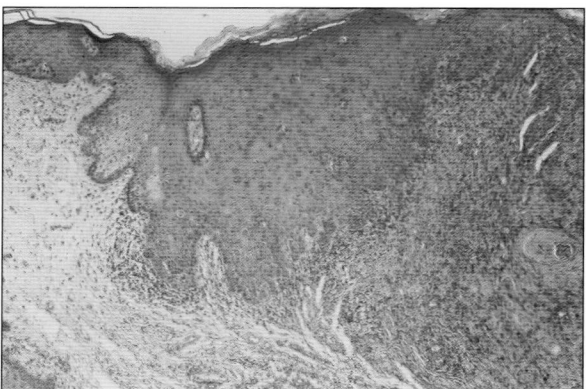

Fig 7-47a In this section from the tongue, a progression of change can be appreciated. On the left side, the epithelium appears normal. In the middle section, the epithelium is dysplastic with individually keratinized cells and bud-like extensions at the base. Accompanying this is underlying chronic inflammation, which is absent in the area of normal epithelium. Finally, on the right side, an infiltrating squamous cell carcinoma is present.

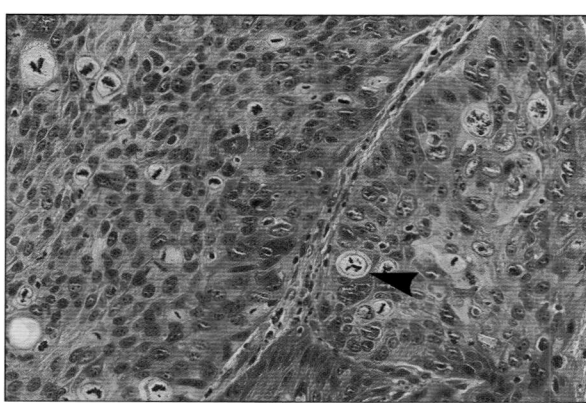

Fig 7-47b Squamous cell carcinoma in which there are numerous mitoses, many of which are atypical. A tripolar mitosis (*arrowhead*) can be seen. In addition, pleomorphism, hyperchromatism, and prominent nucleoli are present.

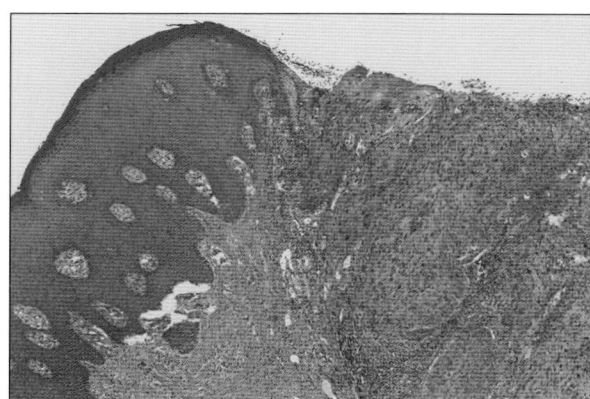

Fig 7-48 In this squamous cell carcinoma, there is no apparent progression from a dysplastic epithelium. The epithelium adjacent to the tumor is normal in appearance.

seen. Neutrophils will often aggregate within keratin pearls, and sometimes liberation of keratin will induce a giant cell response. The stromal inflammation appears to be a host response to the tumor, and infiltrating islands will often be surrounded by inflammatory cells. While many carcinomas have dysplastic epithelium at their margins, a considerable number show a normal adjacent epithelium (Fig 7-48).

Squamous Cell Carcinoma of the Lips

CLINICAL PRESENTATION AND PATHOGENESIS ▶

Squamous cell carcinoma occurs much more frequently on the lower lip than on the upper lip. Together, they account for 25% to 30% of oral squamous cell carcinomas. It has often been noted that upper lip carcinomas behave more aggressively than lower lip carcinomas, and that lower lip carcinomas have two general presentations, the most common being an exophytic, slow-growing mass and the less common an eroding and destructively invasive ulceration. This appears to be related to the two different carcinogenic mechanisms. The slow-growing, exophytic mass is generally related to sun exposure and occurs on the paramidline lip pout of the lower lip (Fig 7-49). It behaves like cutaneous squamous cell carcinoma by its slow growth and minimal metastatic potential because the oncogene stimulation of ultraviolet light usually does not confer the enzymatic properties necessary for regional metastasis. The specific carcinogenic portion of ultraviolet light is thought to be UVB light. UVB light at 290 to 320 nm is a more complete carcinogen than UVA light that is 320 to 340 nm. The erosive and infiltrating carcinomas, including those of the upper lip, seem to be related more to pipe and cigarette smoking. In these, the oncogene expression is more like traditional mucosal squamous cell carcinoma, with its greater invasive potential and propensity for lymph node metastasis (Fig 7-50).

DIFFERENTIAL DIAGNOSIS ▶

The more common exophytic lower lip cancer will look similar to a *keratoacanthoma*, which is also associated with sun exposure. The clinical history of a squamous cell carcinoma, however, will be longer (often 6 months to 1 year) than that of the keratoacanthoma (6 weeks to 2 months). Exophytic masses on the lower lip may also represent salivary gland tumors, particularly *mucoepidermoid carcinoma*. Inflammatory conditions such as an infected trauma site, which is a *pyogenic granuloma*, and another more unusual entity that is seen after trauma and has a noted occurrence in the lip, a *traumatic eosinophilic granuloma*, will appear similar to a squamous cell carcinoma of the lip. Rarely, an identical-looking mass

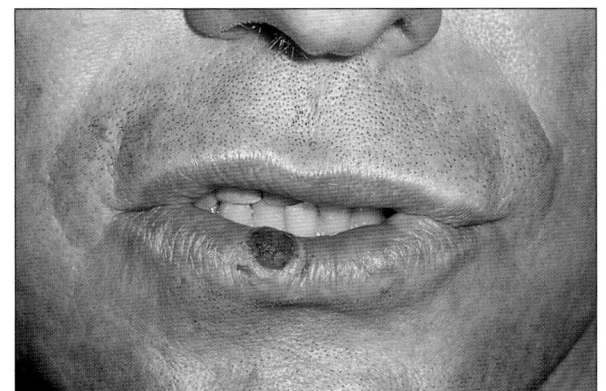

Fig 7-49 Most squamous cell carcinomas of the lower lip are caused by the ultraviolet spectrum in sunlight. They are usually localized and exophytic masses.

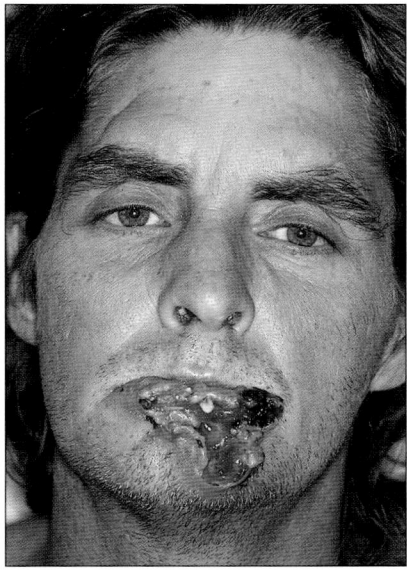

Fig 7-50 Lower lip squamous cell carcinomas will present less commonly as large ulcerative lesions with extensive local destruction.

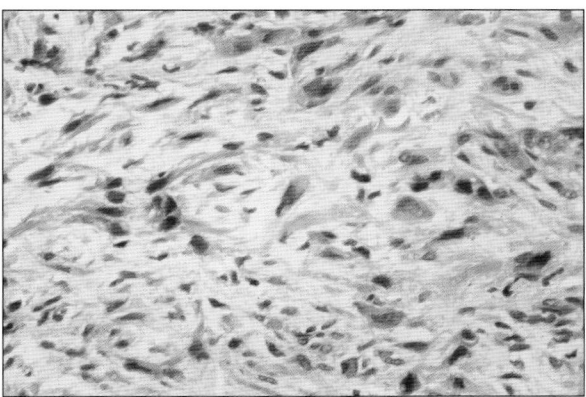

Fig 7-51a A spindle cell carcinoma showing spindle cells with atypical hyperchromatic nuclei.

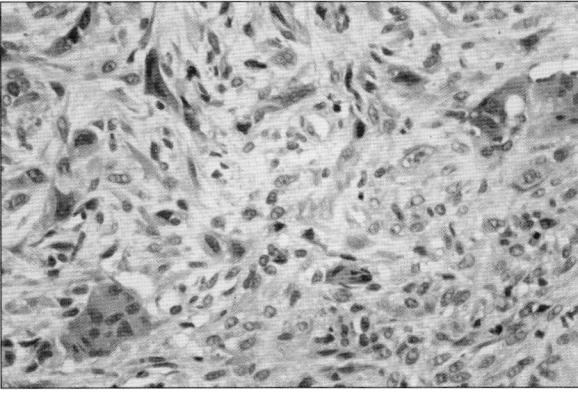

Fig 7-51b Another field from the tumor shown in Fig 7-51a in which multinucleated giant cells are present.

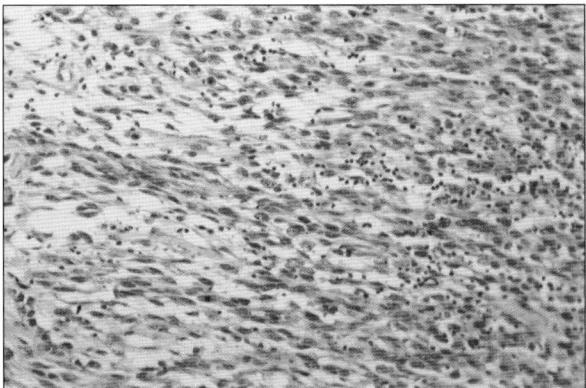

Fig 7-51c A spindle cell carcinoma in which there is little atypia.

called a *Merkel cell tumor* may emerge from the skin portion of the lower lip. This tumor arises from neuroendocrine cells located in skin epithelium. This is particularly a consideration in patients older than 60 years.

The differential diagnosis for the erosive and destructive type would include all of the above with the exception of the keratoacanthoma.

DIAGNOSTIC WORK-UP ▶ Complete examination and staging are required. The exophytic, slow-growing carcinoma of the lower lip may be excised as the diagnostic biopsy and the treatment. If an incisional biopsy is accomplished, it should be performed vertically within the lesion to avoid extending it laterally toward the uninvolved lip. Erosive lesions should undergo incisional biopsy.

HISTOPATHOLOGY ▶ Carcinomas of the lip are usually well differentiated. One less common variant that has a predilection for the lip is spindle cell carcinoma, which has a sarcomatous appearance. Although in some cases intercellular bridges, early keratinization, or evolution from surface epithelium may be observed, these clues are most often absent. The spindle cells may be anaplastic and intermingled with collagen (Fig 7-51a). Neoplastic giant cells may be seen (Fig 7-51b). Other tumors show little cellular atypia (Fig 7-51c).

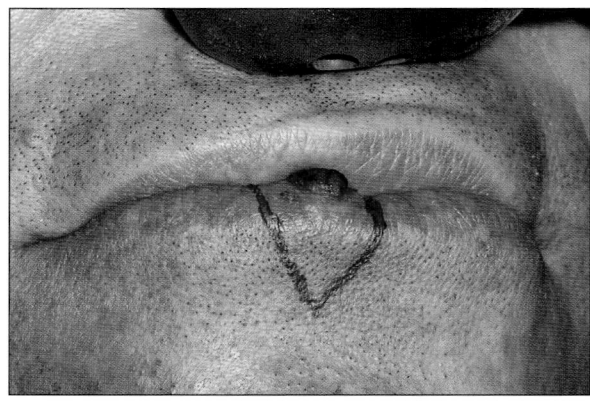

Fig 7-52a Exophytic localized lower lip carcinomas are excised with 0.5-cm margins in either a V-shaped or shield-shaped excision that ends short of the mentolabial crease.

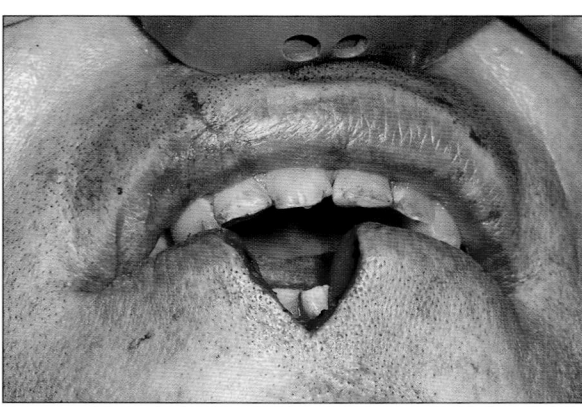

Fig 7-52b The through-and-through excision defect of the lower lip can be primarily closed if it represents less than 40% of the lip length.

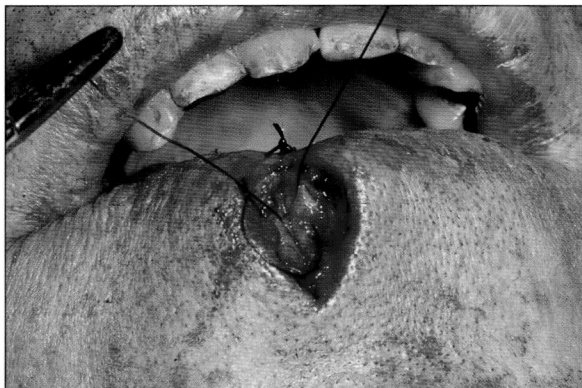

Fig 7-52c The lip defect closure should precisely align each anatomic layer and be closed from the oral mucosa outward to the skin.

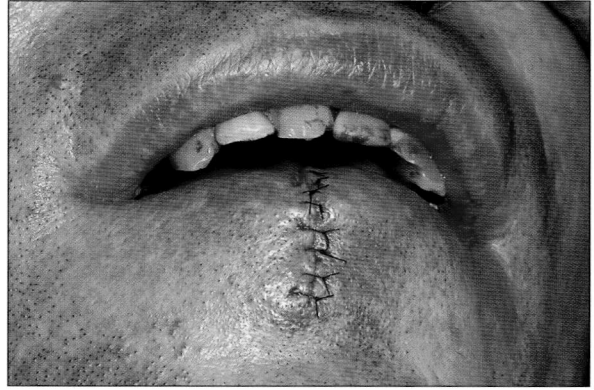

Fig 7-52d The completed lip closure should have precisely aligned the vermilion-cutaneous junction and have everted the lip surface to prevent notching from vertical scar contraction.

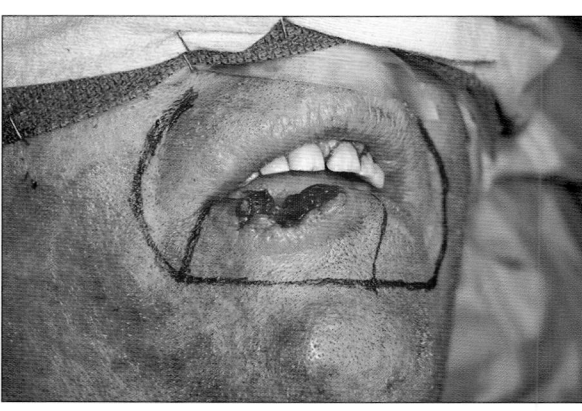

Fig 7-53a Lower lip carcinomas involving more than 40% of the lip cannot be adequately closed primarily. Here a Karapandzic flap is outlined to close the defect from this planned excision.

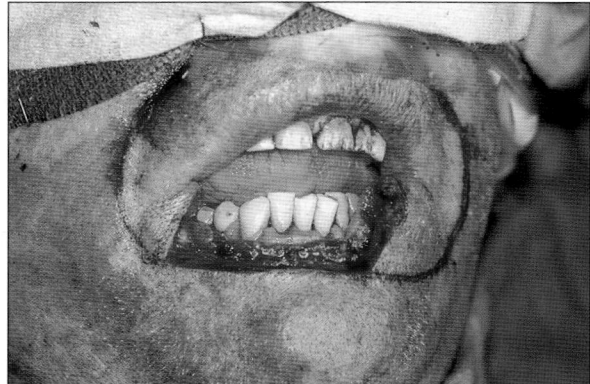

Fig 7-53b To accommodate the Karapandzic flap, the tumor excision is rectangular in shape.

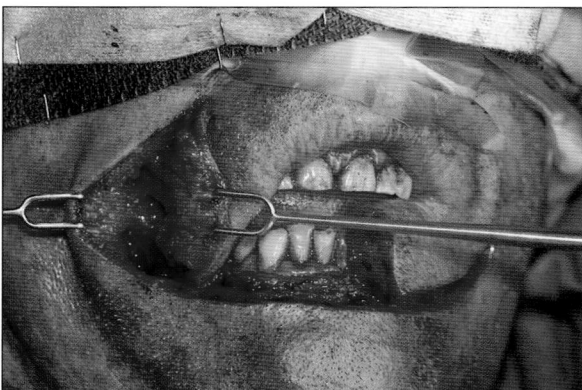

Fig 7-53c The Karapandzic flap extends through the full-thickness excision base toward the commissure, where the incision is then made only through skin so as to preserve the function of the commissure.

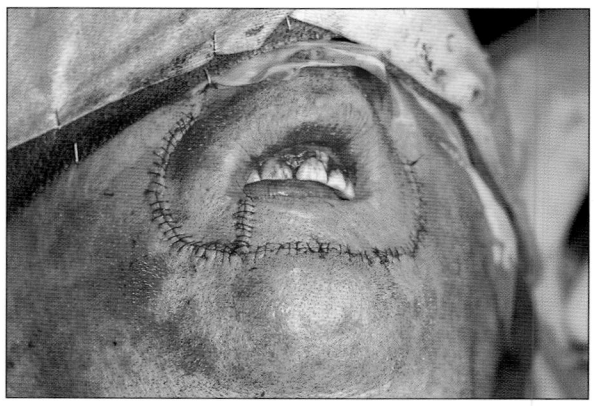

Fig 7-53d The lateral edges of the Karapandzic flap are rotated to align the vermilion and closed, thereby rounding the commissures and decreasing the oral stoma diameter while maintaining its elasticity and function.

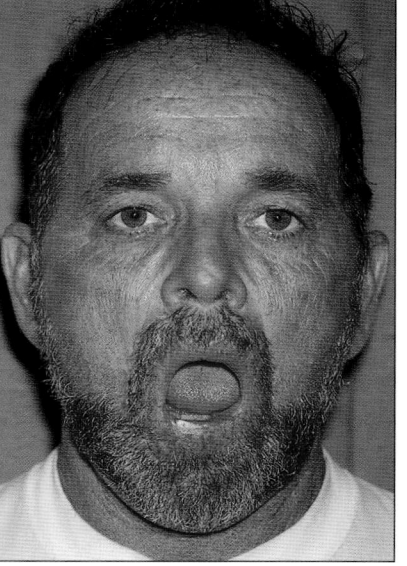

Fig 7-53e The result of a Karapandzic flap is a somewhat reduced opening that can still be stretched open and even accommodate the insertion of dental appliances without secondary procedures.

Ultrastructural identification of desmosomes and tonofilaments is certainly helpful, but on a more practical level the identification of cytokeratins by immunohistochemistry is the most useful modality for diagnosis.

TREATMENT ▶

The exophytic, slow-growing carcinoma that occupies 40% or less of the lower lip area is managed by a V- or shield-shaped excision through the full thickness of the lip. Five-millimeter margins are appropriate but should be assessed with frozen sections (Fig 7-52a). The length of the excision is usually short of the mentolabial crease. Lip closure is very important for function and appearance. The lip is closed from the mucosal surface outward in five layers: the oral mucosa, the fascia of the orbicularis oris on the lingual side, the fascia of the orbicularis oris on the labial side, the dermis, and the skin surface (Figs 7-52b and 7-52c). The surgeon is cautioned to minimize sutures within the orbicularis oris muscle itself because tight sutures will lead to necrosis of small segments of muscle, and this will lead to scarring. The surgeon should also align the vermilion-skin junction precisely to prevent a noticeable step defect of this line (Fig 7-52d).

A prophylactic neck dissection is not indicated. However, if palpable nodes exist, bilateral functional neck or supraomohyoid neck dissections are indicated (see the section on functional neck dissection on page 300). Because these types of lip carcinomas are related to sun damage, many patients have concomitant actinic keratosis of the lower lip vermilion. If the vermilion appears to be atrophic, shows crusting in areas, and has a history of ulcers, consideration of a simultaneous vermilionectomy is reasonable (see the section on actinic keratosis surgery on page 355.)

The erosive and infiltrative lesions often occupy more than 40% of the lip. In such cases, the excision is accomplished in a rectangular shape with 1-cm margins and frozen section control (Fig 7-53a). Lip rotation flaps, particularly the Karapandzic flap or the modified Estlander-type flaps, are excellent (Figs 7-53b to 7-53e). In some cases, distant pedicled flaps such as the radial forearm free vascular flap or the pectoralis major pedicled flap are needed because of near total lip and chin involvement. Such rare large lesions are also possible indications for bilateral functional neck dissections or supraomohyoid dissections.

PROGNOSIS AND FOLLOW-UP ▶

Squamous cell carcinoma of the lower lip has a 92% 5-year survival rate with local excision without neck surgery. Follow-up should consist of an oral and head and neck examination every 4 months for 2 years, and thereafter every 6 months.

Squamous Cell Carcinoma of the Oral Tongue

CLINICAL PRESENTATION ▶

Carcinoma of the oral tongue—that is, that portion of the tongue anterior to the circumvallate papillae—is distinguished from carcinoma of the base of the tongue (pharyngeal tongue) by their differing behaviors, treatments, and prognoses. Carcinoma of the oral tongue encompasses 75% of all tongue cancers and is the most common intraoral malignancy (excluding the lip, which is generally not considered to be intraoral and in which the carcinogen is different). Oral tongue carcinomas account for 20% to 30% of all intraoral cancers.

The most common location is the lateral border in the area of the lingual tonsils. The left side is more common than the right (61% to 39%), ostensibly because the greater number of right-handed smokers aim the smoke stream toward the left side. The lesions will be red-white in color but may appear only as clinical leukoplakia (all white), be exophytic (Fig 7-54), or be ulcerated (Figs 7-55a and 7-55b). Some lesions will be indurated (firm to palpation), which is indicative of tumor cells infiltrating between the muscle fibers of the tongue. About 60% are painless, as cancer by itself is indeed painless. However, 40% present with pain due to the advanced stage of the disease. Painful cancers are painful not because they invade nerves per se, but because they invade and expose areas of high nerve-end density, such as periosteum, or become secondarily infected.

DIFFERENTIAL DIAGNOSIS ▶

An ulcerated lesion on the tongue is a classic differential diagnosis. Certainly squamous cell carcinoma is the primary consideration, but other diseases can also be represented by a tongue ulcer. In particular,

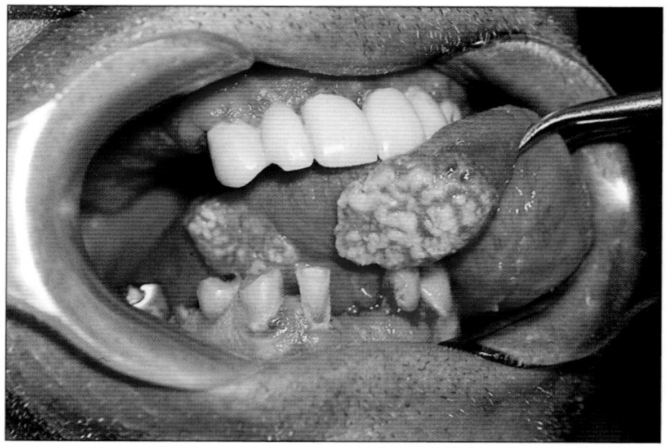

Fig 7-54 Two synchronous primary carcinomas on the lateral border of the tongue.

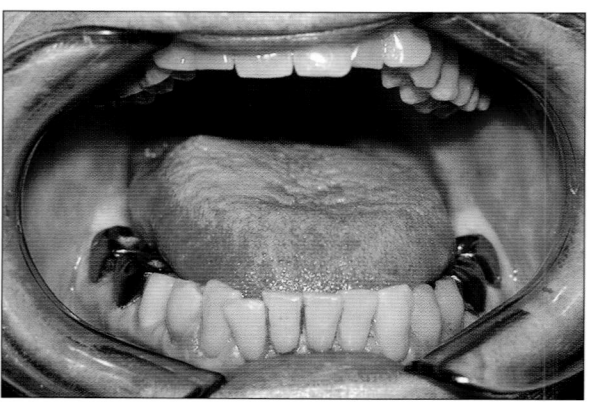

Fig 7-55a Initial view of the oral cavity during a routine dental examination.

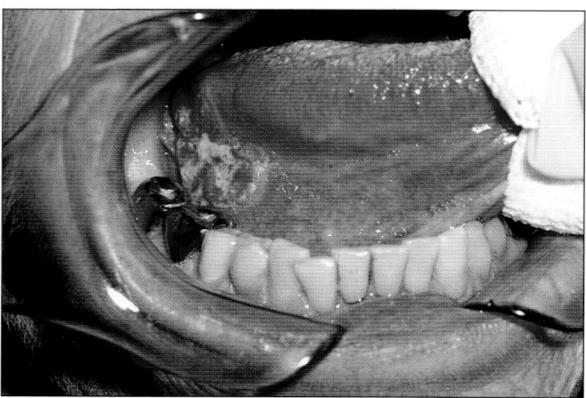

Fig 7-55b A thorough oral examination should include visualization of the posterior tongue via tongue retraction and protrusion. During such an examination of the area shown in Fig 7-55a, a significant unsuspected carcinoma was discovered.

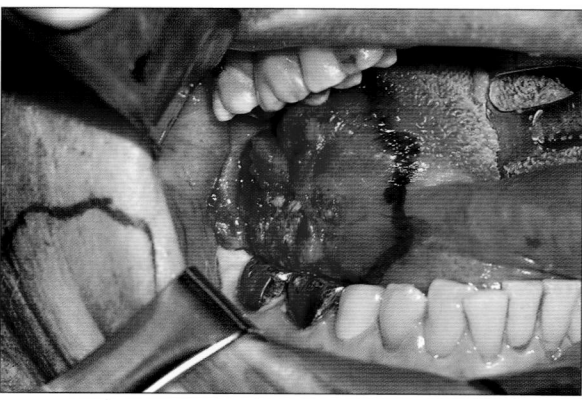

Fig 7-55c Carcinoma of the tongue requires excision with 1.5- to 2.0-cm margins and assessment with frozen sections.

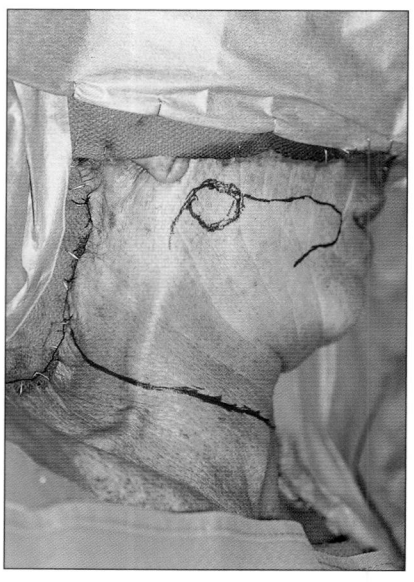

Fig 7-55d Lateral border of tongue carcinoma planned for excision with an incontinuity functional neck dissection via a visor incision/apron flap approach.

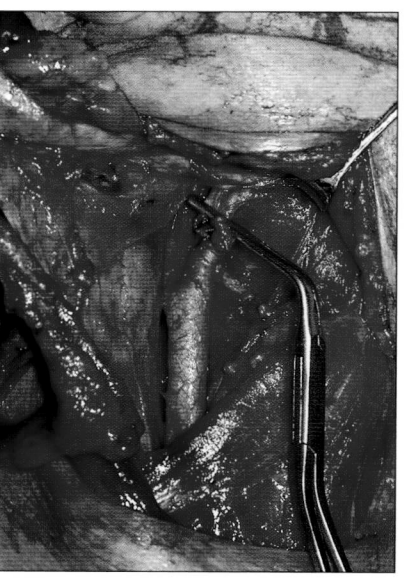

Fig 7-55e Here partial completion of the functional neck dissection permits a temporary clamping of the external carotid artery, which will reduce the bleeding when the tumor is excised from the tongue.

oral tuberculosis (TB)–associated ulcers related to pulmonary TB, and systemic fungal diseases such as *histoplasmosis* and *coccidioidomycosis* originating from a lung focus may produce a tongue ulcer as well. *Trauma* remains a common cause of tongue ulcers. The rare *traumatic eosinophilic granuloma* occurs most often on the tongue and will also present with induration. Some cases of *primary syphilis (chancre)* may also mimic a red-white patch or ulcer suggestive of carcinoma.

DIAGNOSTIC WORK-UP ▶ A clinical oral and head and neck examination should be followed by a mirror or fiberoptic examination of the laryngopharynx and then a TNM staging and incisional biopsy.

TREATMENT ▶ Debate exists about the best primary mode of therapy—surgery or radiation. Either one, when handled correctly, is as effective as the other for tumor control. The debate more or less involves side ef-

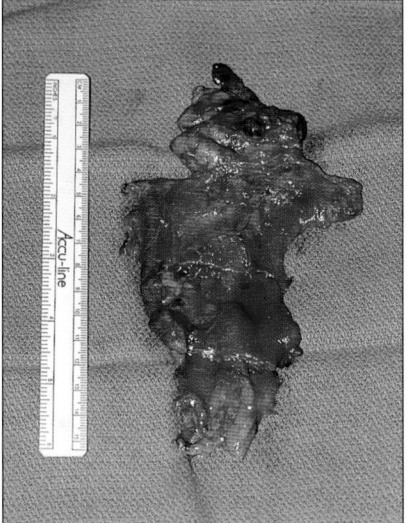

Fig 7-55f Incontinuity resection of tongue carcinoma and neck lymphatics via a functional neck dissection.

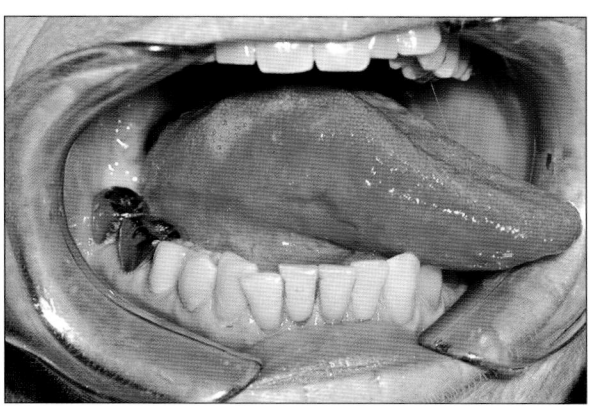

Fig 7-55g A 5-year postoperative view of the tongue shows a minimal defect and normal function.

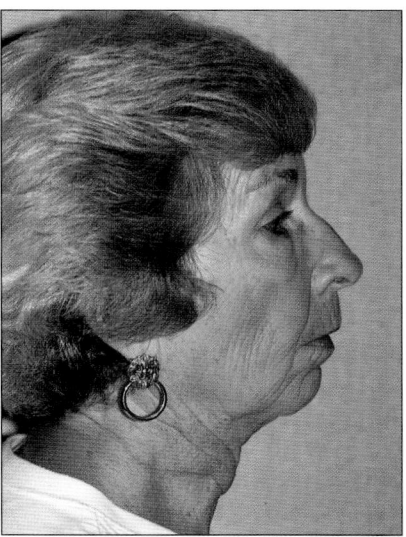

Fig 7-55h A 5-year postoperative profile shows absence of deformity after curative cancer surgery.

fects and morbidity. It is our opinion that surgery is the preferred modality and that postoperative radiotherapy is a distinct consideration in many cases. The type of surgery performed, the decision to use radiotherapy postoperatively or even preoperatively, and whether or how to treat the neck depend on many factors such as the clinical staging, the patient's ASA risk, the thickness of the tumor, the histologic grade, and histologic features related to perineural or perivascular spread, among others. Generally, the primary tumor is excised with 1.5-cm margins for $T_1N_0M_0$ lesions. For $T_2N_0M_0$ and more advanced stages, treating the neck prophylactically with either an incontinuity functional neck dissection or radiotherapy in a dose of 5,000 cGy to 6,500 cGy is recommended if the incisional biopsy shows greater than 3-mm depth of invasion. For nodal disease of N_1, a functional neck dissection is recommended. For nodal disease of N_2 or N_3, most believe that a modified radical neck dissection is preferred, followed by postoperative radiotherapy from 5,000 cGy to 6,500 cGy (Figs 7-55c to 7-55h).

PROGNOSIS AND FOLLOW-UP ▶

The prognosis for oral tongue squamous cell carcinoma varies according to many factors, particularly the TNM staging, the thickness of the primary tumor, evidence of perineural spread, lymph node capsular invasion, and intralymphatic emboli. In all, adjusted 5-year survival rates are between 40% and 60%.

Patient follow-up, which is critical, varies among practitioners. For the most part, re-examination occurs every 4 months for the first 2 years followed by every 6 months thereafter. Follow-up should include a chest radiograph once a year and a mirror oropharyngeal examination.

Squamous Cell Carcinoma of the Pharyngeal Tongue

CLINICAL PRESENTATION ▶

The portion of the tongue posterior to the circumvallate papillae is referred to as the pharyngeal tongue. Carcinomas that develop in this location, which have a propensity for early regional lymph node metastasis, are the main cause of the "unknown primary" phenomenon. In these situations, the patient will present with a unilateral or sometimes bilateral neck mass. Unfortunately, much of the time the mass is an N_3 presentation and is fixed. In these situations, the primary tumor is asymptomatic (Figs 7-56 and 7-57). Alternatively, patients with base-of-the-tongue carcinomas will present with pain, dysphagia, or mouth-/throat-bleeding histories.

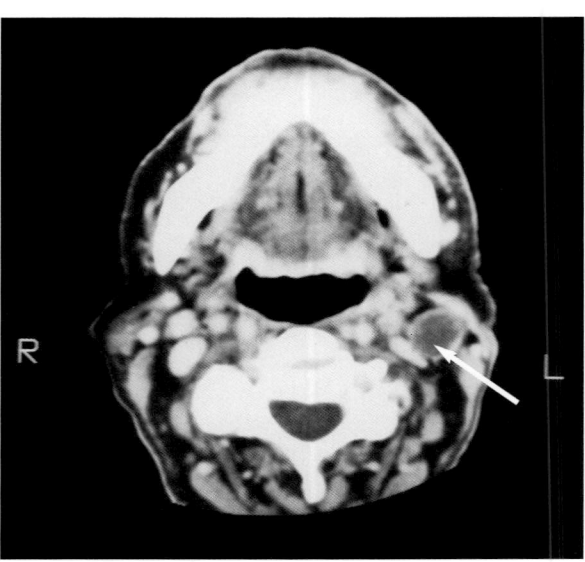

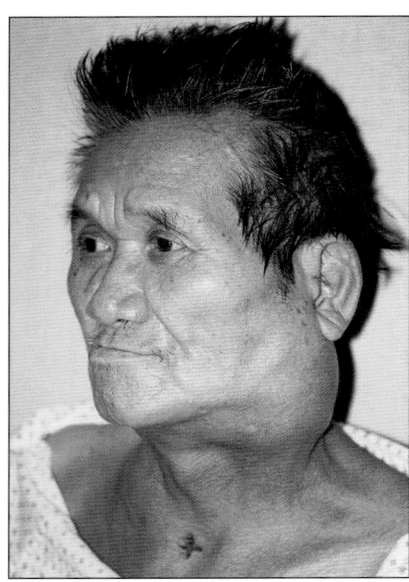

Fig 7-56 Clinically subtle squamous cell carcinoma metastasis to a jugulodigastric lymph node from a base-of-the-tongue primary carcinoma is more easily detected by a CT scan. The hypodense center with a hyperdense ring at the periphery is typical of metastatic cancer in a lymph node (*arrow*).

Fig 7-57 This large, clinically apparent metastasis arose from an unknown primary carcinoma probably somewhere in the pharynx or base of the tongue.

DIFFERENTIAL DIAGNOSIS ▶

The neck mass presentation from an unknown primary tumor can be confusing because the primary tumor may be so small as not to be visible by laryngoscopic examination, and biopsies may not confirm the diagnosis. Large, firm neck mass presentations are seen in *cervical TB adenitis* (scrofula), *cat-scratch disease, branchial cysts, non-Hodgkin lymphoma* (usually in those older than 40 years), and *Hodgkin lymphoma* (usually in those younger than 40 years).

DIAGNOSTIC WORK-UP ▶

Direct laryngoscopy with random biopsies of the pharynx and base of the tongue is often required. In addition, a fine needle aspiration (FNA) of the mass often facilitates diagnosis. Failing to establish a diagnosis by these means may make it necessary to perform an open lymph node biopsy. Although open cervical lymph node biopsies are required to diagnose lymphomas and many infectious diseases, they are used only as a last resort in situations where the index of suspicion for squamous cell carcinoma is high. The issue of an open neck biopsy affecting prognosis is unresolved. Because these patients have a poor prognosis in any event, an open biopsy is acceptable if the diagnosis cannot be attained by any other means; if carcinoma is identified, the neck is treated with a cancer neck dissection, usually followed by radiotherapy.

If cancer is confirmed, a triple endoscopy and/or a barium swallow and CT scan of the esophagus are recommended.

HISTOPATHOLOGY ▶

Squamous cell carcinomas in this area are usually more poorly differentiated. One particular variant that occurs in this location, as well as in the hypopharynx and larynx, is the basaloid squamous cell carcinoma. This is a poorly differentiated, highly aggressive tumor. It is biphasic. The squamous component may be a carcinoma in situ or an invasive lesion, while the connecting basaloid portion proliferates as invasive lobules, nests, or cords with pseudoglandular spaces. There is comedo necrosis and considerable mitotic activity (Figs 7-58a and 7-58b). The basaloid cells are often surrounded by basal lamina–like material. The stroma may be myxoid, and perineural invasion occurs. This tumor must be distinguished from the solid type of adenoid cystic carcinoma. Muscle-specific actin can be helpful here, as it is negative in the basaloid squamous cell carcinoma.

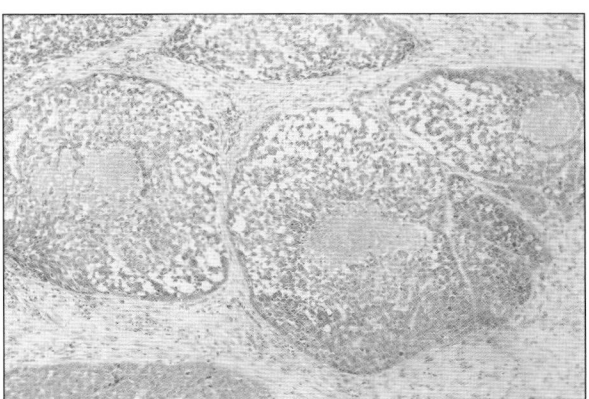 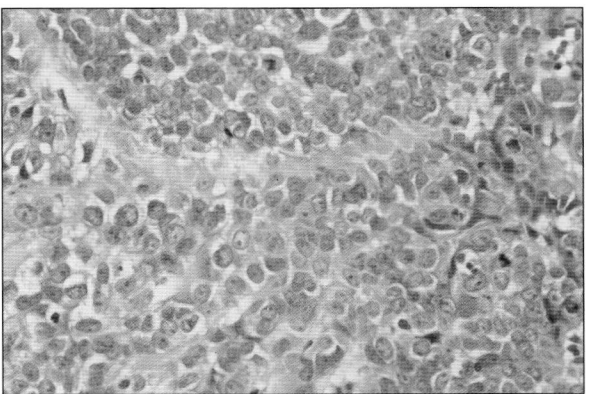

Fig 7-58a A basaloid squamous cell carcinoma in which the islands show prominent comedo necrosis.

Fig 7-58b The cells of the basaloid squamous carcinoma are relatively bland but have a high mitotic rate.

TREATMENT ▶ Cases in which the primary tumor is unassociated with regional lymph node metastasis are treated mostly with bilateral high-dose radiotherapy of the primary tumor and the neck in the range of 6,400 cGy to 7,200 cGy. If the neck mass is large, surgery in the form of a full radical neck dissection or a modified radical neck dissection (see pages 298 to 300) is often combined with postoperative radiotherapy in the same dose range.

PROGNOSIS AND FOLLOW-UP ▶ The general prognosis for carcinomas in this location is poor. Considering all TNM classes, the overall adjusted 5-year survival rate is about 15% to 25%. Follow-up consisting of nasopharyngoscopy or indirect laryngoscopy in addition to clinical examinations is carried out every 4 months for the first 2 years and every 6 months thereafter. An annual chest radiograph is recommended.

Squamous Cell Carcinoma of the Floor of the Mouth

CLINICAL PRESENTATION ▶ Carcinomas of the floor of the mouth (Fig 7-59) follow tongue cancer as the most common intraoral location for squamous cell carcinoma, accounting for 15% to 20% of cases, and more in African Americans. Most cases present as a red-white patch or ulcer. Induration is present if the lesion has infiltrated into underlying tissue. Many present with palpable regional neck metastasis, which is often bilateral because of the thinness of the floor-of-the-mouth tissues and the abundant crossover lymphatics in this region.

DIFFERENTIAL DIAGNOSIS ▶ A floor-of-the-mouth ulcer in an adult has a narrower differential diagnosis than a similar ulcer on the lips or tongue. The floor of the mouth is not an anticipated site for a keratoacanthoma, as is the lip, nor is it an anticipated site for a TB ulcer, as is the tongue. In addition, the rare but cancer-mimicking lesion of a traumatic eosinophilic granuloma, which occurs on tongue or lips, does not seem to occur in the floor of the mouth. Instead, *traumatic ulcers* and *syphilis chancres* are realistic entities, as are *premalignant dysplasias* and *verrucous carcinomas* in the nonulcerated lesions.

DIAGNOSTIC WORK-UP ▶ Work-up requires clinical oral and head and neck examinations, including a mirror or fiberoptic examination of the laryngopharynx followed by a TNM staging and an incisional biopsy.

HISTOPATHOLOGY ▶ Carcinomas of the floor of the mouth frequently evolve from a dysplastic epithelium. Because many cases develop around the orifice of Wharton duct, it should be recognized that the dysplastic process will often extend into the ductal epithelium (Fig 7-60).

TREATMENT ▶ Surgery and radiotherapy claim equivalent results in treatment of floor-of-the-mouth lesions. Surgery is our preference because of the high incidence of severe osteoradionecrosis when radiation to the floor

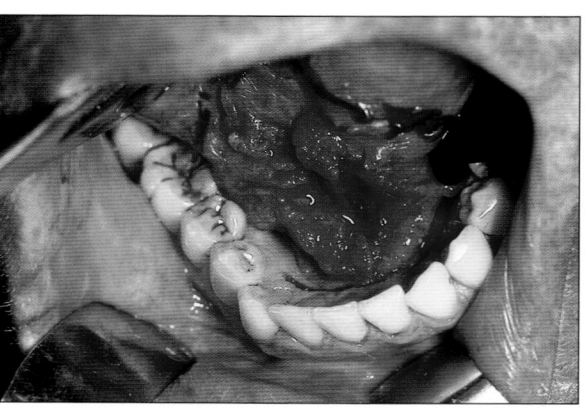

Fig 7-59 Carcinoma in the midline of the floor of the mouth. Note the central ulceration, the rolled and indurated margins, and the satellite lesion opposite the first molar. Because of crossover lymphatics, both sides of the neck require treatment.

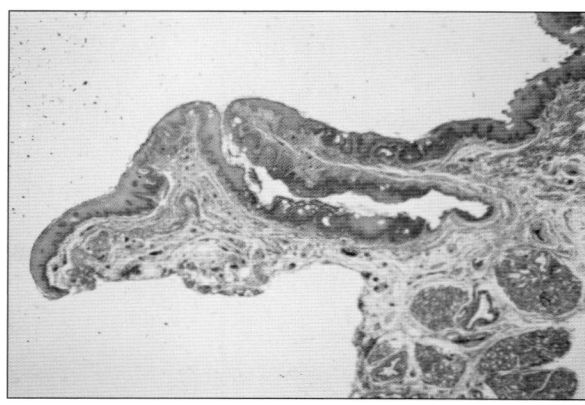

Fig 7-60 This lesion in the floor of the mouth was dysplastic and had areas of carcinoma. Note that the adjacent Wharton duct also shows dysplastic changes.

of the mouth exceeds 6,800 cGy. Because the adult mandible becomes more perfused with age from the lingual periosteal vascular plexus than from the inferior alveolar system, radiotherapy to the floor of the mouth affects this critical blood supply, creating some of the most refractory cases of mandibular osteoradionecrosis.

Microinvasive $T_1N_0M_0$ lesions less than 3 mm in thickness may be excised with frozen section–controlled margins of at least 1.5 cm. Although some surgeons and oncologists disagree, $T_1N_0M_0$ lesions greater than 3 mm in thickness, $T_2N_0M_0$ lesions, and $T_3N_0M_0$ lesions require prophylactic neck treatment. This may take the form of bilateral functional neck dissections or radiotherapy in the range of 5,000 cGy to 6,500 cGy. Bilateral neck therapy is an especially strong consideration in floor-of-the-mouth lesions because crossover lymphatics cause a high incidence of contralateral spread.

Those with N_2 or N_3 neck presentations are candidates for combined surgery-radiotherapy treatment, in particular surgery followed by radiotherapy within 6 to 8 weeks.

PROGNOSIS AND FOLLOW-UP ▶

Survival statistics for floor-of-the-mouth carcinomas are similar to those for the oral tongue and will vary according to the same factors. Overall adjusted 5-year survival ranges between 40% and 60%.

Follow-up consisting of examination, including a mirror or fiberoptic examination of the laryngopharynx, is indicated every 4 months during the first 2 years and every 6 months thereafter. A chest radiograph is indicated annually.

Squamous Cell Carcinoma of the Buccal Mucosa

CLINICAL PRESENTATION ▶

Carcinoma of the buccal mucosa accounts for 10% of all intraoral cancers. It presents as a red-white patch and sometimes as an exophytic mass (Fig 7-61). The lesions often are part of a diffuse area of clinical leukoplakia-erythroplakia and may extend onto the anterior tonsillar pillar or the retromolar trigone. They are usually asymptomatic but will produce an induration of the cheek or a limited jaw opening if infiltration into the masseter or temporalis occurs (Fig 7-62).

DIFFERENTIAL DIAGNOSIS ▶

The main differentials for carcinomas of the buccal mucosa are a *verrucous carcinoma* and *erosive lichen planus*. The buccal mucosa is a common site for each of these entities. Verrucous carcinoma should not be truly ulcerated but may appear similar to an exophytic but invasive squamous cell carcinoma. Erosive lichen planus should be more painful and show bilateral lesions, but it can mimic dysplasia and carcinoma clinically. Other considerations are a *syphilis chancre, candidiasis,* and a *cheek-biting traumatic ulcer,* particularly one that is secondarily infected.

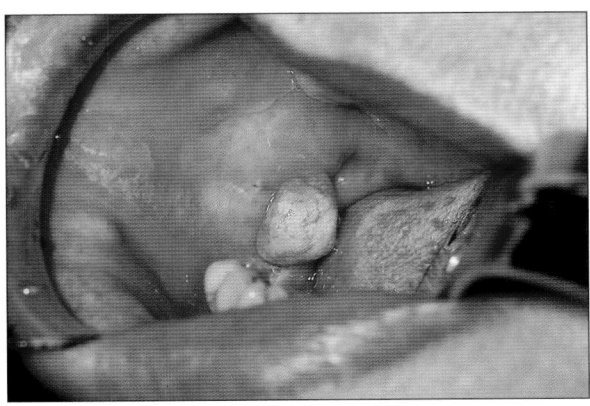

Fig 7-61 Exophytic localized squamous cell carcinoma on the buccal mucosa.

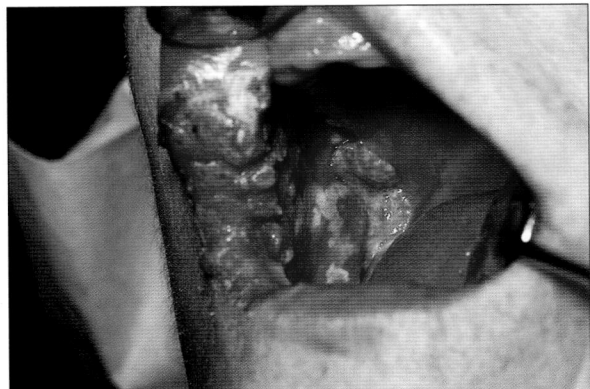

Fig 7-62 This squamous cell carcinoma involved the entire buccal mucosa and extended from the vermilion and commissure area to the retromolar trigone.

DIAGNOSTIC WORK-UP ▶ An oral and head and neck examination is required, including a mirror or fiberoptic examination of the laryngopharynx followed by a TNM staging and an incisional biopsy.

TREATMENT ▶ Because of the location of carcinomas in the buccal mucosa, a true incontinuity resection together with the fascia in the neck is impossible. Such resections can also create a through-and-through cheek defect. These factors, combined with the often more diffuse surface area involved in buccal mucosa lesions, favor radiotherapy as the primary mode of therapy. Most are treated with a general field radiation of 5,000 cGy to the primary tumor and to the ipsilateral neck. The primary tumor then often receives a "boost" of between 1,000 cGy and 2,200 cGy, resulting in a primary tumor dose totalling between 6,000 cGy and 7,200 cGy.

PROGNOSIS AND FOLLOW-UP ▶ Invasive carcinoma of the buccal mucosa does not have meaningful statistics associated with it as does carcinoma of the tongue and floor of the mouth. Many other entities such as verrucous carcinoma and carcinoma in situ have been included with buccal mucosa carcinoma data, skewing the statistics. In general, the overall 5-year adjusted survival ranges between 40% and 60%.

Follow-up consists of an oral and head and neck examination, including mirror or fiberoptic examination of the laryngopharynx, every 4 months for the first 2 years and every 6 months thereafter. An annual chest radiograph is advised.

Squamous Cell Carcinoma of the Retromolar Trigone/ Tonsillar Pillar

Carcinoma of the retromolar trigone area, including the buccopharyngeal raphe and anterior tonsillar pillars, accounts for about 15% of intraoral cancers. It will present as a red-white patch or sometimes as an exophytic mass. The lesions may also be part of a diffuse leukoplakia-erythroplakia (Fig 7-63). Most are asymptomatic, but many will present with a limited jaw opening due to infiltration into the pterygoid, masseter, or temporalis muscles.

DIFFERENTIAL DIAGNOSIS ▶ If pain and swelling are present, a *tonsillitis* or a *peri-tonsillar abscess* may be considered. However, both of these considerations usually occur in younger individuals and have more significant pain and dysphagia. *Verrucous carcinoma* may look like the exophytic type of invasive carcinomas. *Lichen planus* can involve these areas as well but should be mostly bilateral and show more of a presentation on the buccal mucosa. Other inflammatory diseases such as *Candidiasis,* a *chancre of syphilis*, a *TB ulcer*, or one of the two more prevalent systemic fungal diseases, *histoplasmosis* or *coccidioidomycosis,* are also considerations.

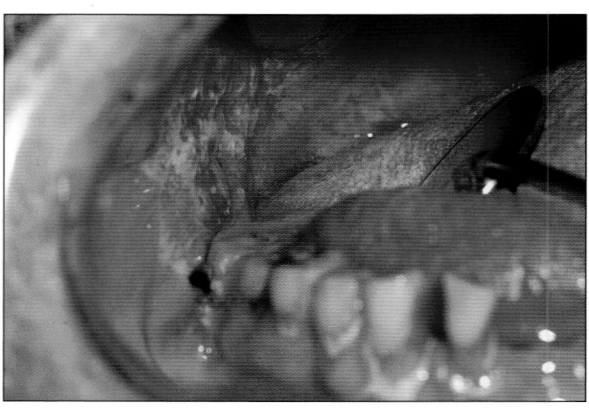

Fig 7-63 Squamous cell carcinoma of the retromolar trigone frequently extends onto the buccopharyngeal raphe and the anterior tonsillar pillar.

DIAGNOSTIC WORK-UP ▶ An oral and head and neck examination is required, including a mirror or fiberoptic examination of the laryngopharynx followed by a TNM staging and an incisional biopsy.

TREATMENT ▶ In contrast to carcinomas primary to the buccal mucosa, retromolar-trigone/tonsillar pillar primary carcinomas can be treated with excision and incontinuity neck dissections. The resection margins are 1.5 to 2.0 cm in soft tissue. Because the mandible and/or the internal pterygoid muscle are often invaded, a composite resection of the tumor along with the posterior mandible is frequently required. Because of the posterior location of these cancers, the depth of invasion and/or the presence of palpable nodes usually require some type of neck dissection. The resultant mucosal defect is best reconstructed with a myocutaneous flap. A pectoralis major flap or a trapezius flap with a skin paddle is most often used. The continuity defect is bridged and stabilized with a titanium reconstruction plate using three or four bicortical screws on each native bone segment.

This approach is the most predictable and has the lowest risk for wound-healing delays or complications. Once again, the posterior location of this tumor and the frequent invasion into the mandible or pterygoid spaces often require postoperative radiotherapy of 5,000 cGy to 6,500 cGy.

PROGNOSIS AND FOLLOW-UP ▶ Survival statistics for retromolar trigone/tonsillar pillar carcinomas vary with size and local lymph node metastasis. Five-year survival for all patients ranges from 40% to 60%.

Follow-up, consisting of an examination of the oral cavity and neck as well as a mirror or fiberoptic examination of the laryngopharynx, is indicated every 4 months during the first 2 years and every 6 months thereafter. An annual chest radiograph is also indicated.

Squamous Cell Carcinoma of the Gingiva

CLINICAL PRESENTATION ▶ Gingival carcinoma (Fig 7-64) is an indolent, slow-growing carcinoma that has a low propensity to metastasize. Accounting for a little less than 10% of all intraoral carcinomas, it will present as a red-white thickening of the marginal and interdental gingiva. It will often have a history of several years and is frequently confused with various periodontal conditions. This carcinoma may not be very infiltrative, but its surface spread may be extensive. Frequently, the entire gingiva on each side of the midline is involved, but it includes only the attached gingiva.

DIFFERENTIAL DIAGNOSIS ▶ The most common condition from which to differentiate gingival carcinoma is chronic persistent *periodontitis*. In addition, *lichen planus* of the attached gingiva and the *pemphigoid* forms that involve the attached gingiva may each mimic gingival carcinoma by their red-white appearance and scar formation. Because gingival carcinoma is usually not ulcerated but appears as a thickened red-white gingiva, *verrucous carcinoma* and the benign hyperkeratosis form of clinical *leukoplakia* are also distinct considerations.

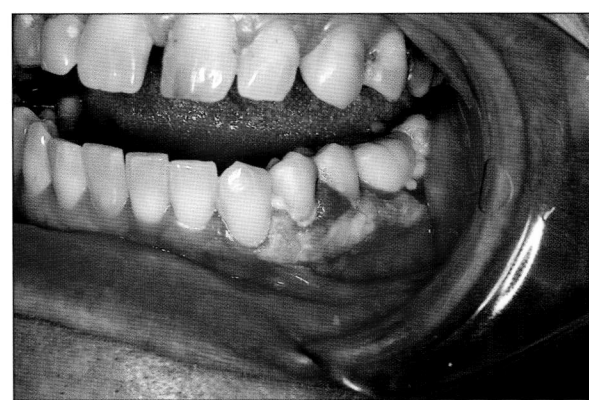

Fig 7-64 Gingival carcinoma is slow growing and limited to the attached gingiva. It is nevertheless a treacherous carcinoma because of its diffuse extension along the attached gingiva, its inclusion of both the buccal and lingual gingiva, and its potential to invade the crestal bone through the abundant local lymphatic and blood vessels.

DIAGNOSTIC WORK-UP ▶

An oral and head and neck examination is required, including a mirror or fiberoptic examination of the laryngopharynx followed by a TNM staging and an incisional biopsy. It is important to biopsy such lesions to include the periosteum. Because of the thick epithelium and the thinness of the connective tissue in this area, biopsies that do not include the periosteum will be difficult to assess for the presence and depth of invasive carcinoma. Periapical radiographs and a panoramic radiograph are also required to assess areas of possible bony invasion.

HISTOPATHOLOGY ▶

Carcinomas of the gingiva are typically well differentiated; however, distinguishing a hyperplastic response from a carcinoma may be particularly difficult at this site unless a sufficiently deep biopsy is taken. This is primarily due to the lack of marked cellular atypia and the thinness of the tissue, which makes evidence of infiltration difficult to appreciate.

TREATMENT ▶

Gingival carcinoma is treated with a specific type of surgical excision. The surgeon must resist the temptation to perform only a soft tissue gingivectomy. While the carcinoma rarely extends beyond the attached gingiva, the abundant lymphatics and vasculature of the alveolar bone–gingival complex necessitate an excision of soft tissue including the alveolar bone (Fig 7-65a). The excision must include both buccal and lingual gingiva. The bone is resected to the level of the root apices superior to the mandibular canal in the posterior mandible and short of the sinus floor or nasal floor in the maxilla. Frozen sections are extremely important because of the diffuse spread along the marginal gingiva. In fact, even if clear margins are established, biopsy of the gingiva posterior to the clear margins is recommended because of satellite lesions and "skip" areas of uninvolved gingiva with this cancer. Because of the low propensity of gingival carcinoma to undergo local lymph node metastasis, a prophylactic neck dissection is not recommended.

The excision of bone and soft tissues will obliterate the vestibule for future prosthetic use (Fig 7-65b). Most patients require a secondary vestibuloplasty for prosthetic rehabilitation. The remaining bone is also sufficient in health and height for osseointegrated implants, which can be placed at the time of resection (Figs 7-65c and 7-65d).

PROGNOSIS AND FOLLOW-UP ▶

The prognosis associated with gingival carcinoma is excellent compared to other areas where intraoral carcinoma may occur. Adjusted 5-year survival rates are between 85% and 90%.

Follow-up is the same as that for the other locations of intraoral carcinoma because its purpose is to detect not only recurrence from disease re-emergence, but new primary tumors.

Squamous Cell Carcinoma of the Alveolar Ridge

CLINICAL PRESENTATION ▶

Carcinoma of the alveolar ridge may be confused with gingival carcinoma because their anatomic location is similar (Fig 7-66). The major difference is that alveolar ridge carcinoma is not limited to the attached gingiva. It will enter into either the buccal or lingual vestibule (Fig 7-67), the floor of the mouth

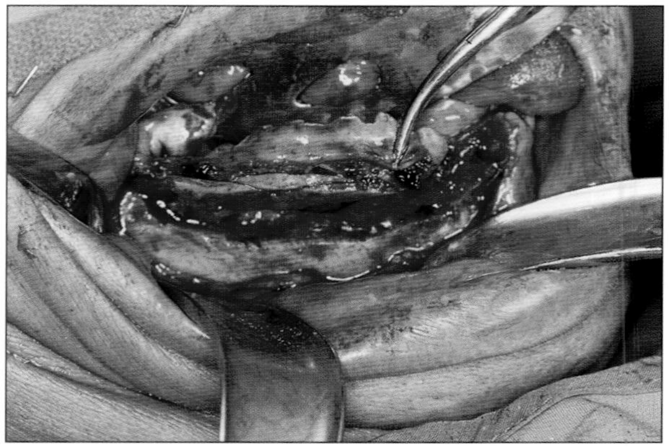

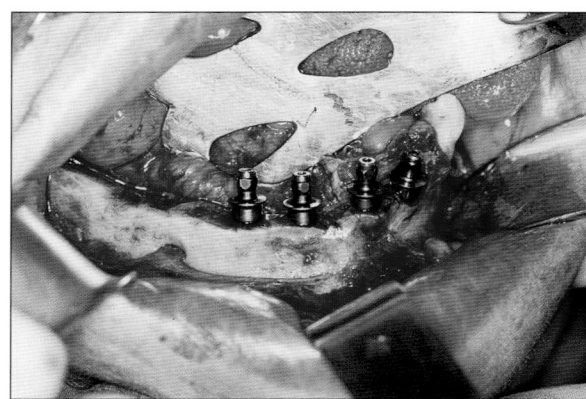

Fig 7-65a Excisions of gingival carcinoma must include the attached gingiva and alveolar bone to at least the mid-root level.

Fig 7-65b Since excision of gingival carcinoma includes teeth and some alveolar bone, immediate placement of dental implants is a feasible option that results in early dental rehabilitation. Dental implants may be placed whether or not postoperative radiotherapy is planned provided its onset is at least 6 weeks after surgery.

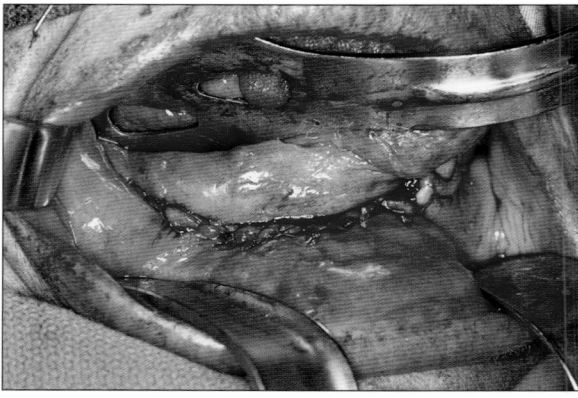

Fig 7-65c Excision of the attached gingiva will cause an obliteration of the buccal and lingual vestibules upon closure. A vestibuloplasty 3 to 4 months later is usually required.

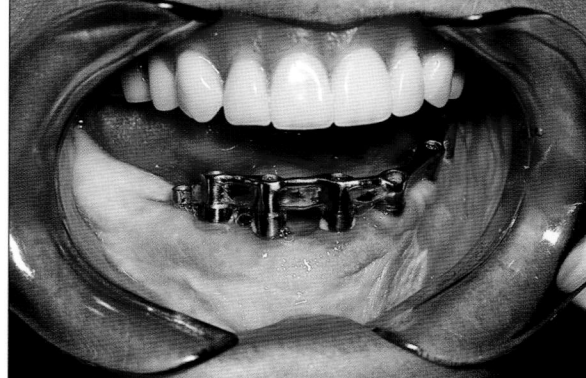

Fig 7-65d Fully osseointegrated dental implants and a healed split-thickness skin graft create an ideal situation for a functional and retentive prosthesis.

(Fig 7-68) if the tumor is on the mandibular alveolar ridge, or the palate if the tumor is on the maxillary alveolar ridge. This distinction is important because alveolar ridge carcinoma is more infiltrative and faster spreading than gingival carcinoma. It also has a greater propensity for bony invasion and regional lymph node spread.

The lesions will appear as red-white patches with ulceration. As in other intraoral locations, the lesion is usually painless unless it becomes secondarily infected or infiltrates a significant area of periosteum. Alveolar ridge carcinoma accounts for a little less than 10% of all intraoral carcinomas and includes those that are often termed *retromolar pad carcinomas*.

DIFFERENTIAL DIAGNOSIS ▶ When systemic fungal disease occurs in the oral cavity, it is usually found on the gingiva-vestibule area and is a friable red granulation tissue or an ulcer. The presentation of systemic fungal disease is very similar to that of alveolar ridge carcinoma. Therefore, *histoplasmosis* and *coccidioidomycosis* oral lesions from lung foci are serious considerations. A *traumatic ulcer* from occlusion or a dental appliance and a *chancre of primary syphilis* are also considerations. In the retromolar area, the presence of a partially impacted third molar may give rise to a *pericoronitis* or *scarring from a postpericoronitis* episode, which may resemble a carcinoma.

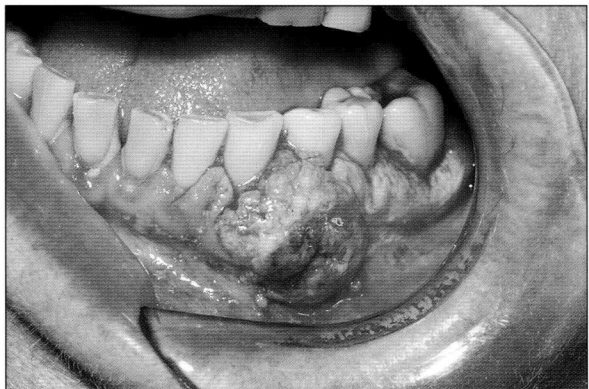

Fig 7-66 Alveolar ridge carcinoma is similar to gingival carcinoma but can be distinguished by its extension beyond the attached gingiva. This is an important distinction because of its greater aggressiveness and propensity to metastasize to regional lymph nodes.

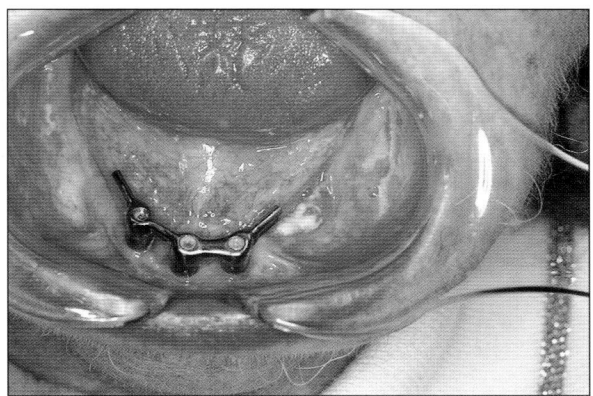

Fig 7-67 Dentures can hide alveolar ridge carcinomas; therefore, appliances should be removed before the start of an examination. In cases such as this, the suggestion is often raised of denture irritation provoking the development of carcinoma. However, there is no evidence to support this, and it thus remains a coincidental occurence.

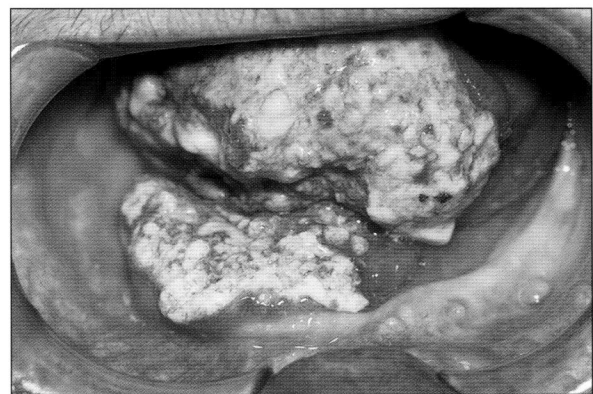

Fig 7-68 Alveolar ridge carcinoma extending into the floor of the mouth and onto the tongue.

DIAGNOSTIC WORK-UP ▶

An oral and head and neck examination is required, including a mirror or fiberoptic examination of the laryngopharynx followed by a TNM staging and an incisional biopsy. A panoramic radiograph and a CT scan to assess for the presence and degree of bony invasion are recommended.

TREATMENT ▶

The proximity of alveolar ridge carcinoma to bone and its propensity to invade bone often require that the excision include bony resection. Because radiotherapy does not greatly affect tumor cells within bone, surgery is the principle treatment modality. In mandibular alveolar ridge carcinoma of $T_2N_0M_0$ or more advanced stages, a mandibular resection with 2-cm bony margins is included as part of the soft tissue excision with 1.5- to 2.0-cm soft tissue margins. A prophylactic functional neck dissection is performed in most cases. Treatment of N_1 necks is also usually accomplished with a functional neck dissection, and N_2 and N_3 necks by a modified or full radical neck dissection. Postoperative radiotherapy is a consideration in more advanced cases. Treatment of alveolar ridge carcinoma of the maxilla is similar to that for palatal carcinoma.

The resultant bony defect and soft tissue defect require stabilization and reconstruction. Two general approaches are common today. One approach is to reconstruct immediately with a composite bone–soft tissue free vascular transfer from either the fibula or the ilium; the other is to stabilize the mandible with a titanium reconstruction plate and reconstruct the soft tissue with a myocutaneous pedicled flap from the pectoralis major or trapezius and accomplish definitive bony reconstruction secondarily after further radiotherapy and/or chemotherapy and a tumor-free interval. We prefer the latter approach because of the added morbidity and the inadequate bone contours and volume associated with a free vascular transfer. In addition, free vascular transfers often delay postoperative radiotherapy because of a prolonged hospital course or complications.

PROGNOSIS AND FOLLOW-UP ▶

The prognosis varies greatly depending on the tumor's size, location, and infiltration into bone or adjoining tissue spaces. Overall adjusted 5-year survival rates range between 40% and 60%, the same as for oral tongue and floor-of-the-mouth carcinoma but in distinct contrast to gingival carcinoma.

Follow-up is the same as for tongue and floor-of-the-mouth carcinoma, which is an oral and head and neck examination including a mirror or fiberoptic examination of the laryngopharynx every 4 months for the first 2 years, then every 6 months thereafter. An annual chest radiograph is recommended.

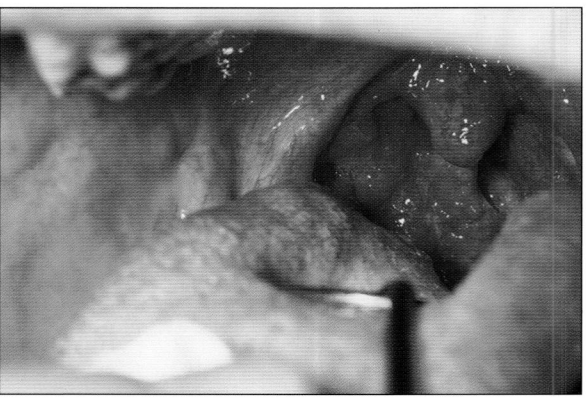 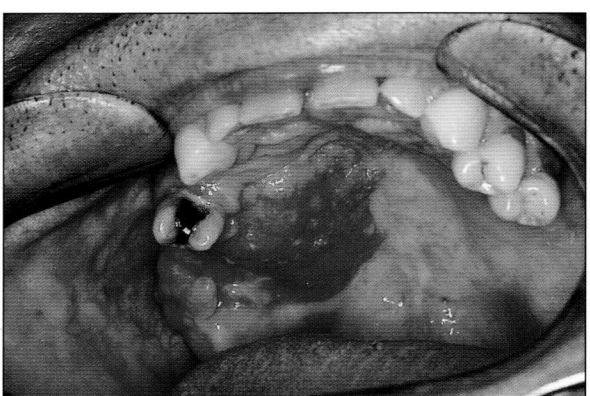

Fig 7-69 Squamous cell carcinoma of the soft palate is more common than that of the hard palate. It too is a dangerous location because of crossover lymphatics and a diagnosis that is often delayed by confusion with a "sore throat."

Fig 7-70 Squamous cell carcinoma of the hard palate in a patient who practiced reverse smoking. This type of tumor is uncommon. It frequently extends onto the alveolar ridge and will infiltrate alveolar bone sooner than the bony palate.

Squamous Cell Carcinoma of the Palate

CLINICAL PRESENTATION ▶ Squamous cell carcinoma of the soft palate (Fig 7-69) is more common than that of the mucosa over the hard palate. Carcinoma of the soft palate accounts for 10% to 15% of intraoral carcinomas. Carcinoma of the hard palate accounts for less than 5%, but many alveolar ridge carcinomas extend onto the mucosa of the hard palate. Carcinoma of the hard palate is a common finding in those who practice reverse smoking (because of the close proximity of the carcinogen in high concentrations). Reverse smoking is common in Panama and some other Central American countries, all of which see a higher incidence of palatal carcinoma (Fig 7-70).

Soft palate lesions are rarely ulcerated. Most appear as red-white patches, sometimes with induration reducing the mobility of the soft palate musculature. On the hard palate, the lesions are more often ulcerated as part of a red-white patch.

DIFFERENTIAL DIAGNOSIS ▶ Carcinoma of the palate includes three unique differential diagnostic considerations not found in other locations. In particular, *extranodal non-Hodgkin lymphoma* has a predilection for the palate and for patients 50 years or older. It will present as a reddish soft tissue enlargement that is soft and boggy rather than indurated but that may still resemble carcinoma. If the lesion is ulcerated and the duration is unknown, *necrotizing sialometaplasia* becomes a serious consideration. The third unique consideration is that of a *primary carcinoma arising in the maxillary sinus* and eroding onto the palate. In addition, minor salivary gland malignancies, particularly *mucoepidermoid carcinoma* and *adenoid cystic carcinoma*, must be considered. As in other locations, systemic fungal diseases, particularly *histoplasmosis* and *coccidioidomycosis*, as well as a *chancre from primary syphilis,* can mimic a carcinoma in this location.

DIAGNOSTIC WORK-UP ▶ An oral and head and neck examination, including a mirror or fiberoptic examination of the laryngopharynx, is required, followed by a TNM classification and an incisional biopsy. If carcinoma is confirmed by the biopsy, a chest radiograph is required, as is a CT scan or MRI scan. Scans are of great value for carcinomas in this location. Spread into the sinuses, orbit, or nasal cavity, as well as the presence or degree of invasion into the maxilla, must be assessed (Figs 7-71a and 7-71b).

TREATMENT ▶ Squamous cell carcinoma of the soft palate is best treated by radiotherapy. The primary tumor and bilateral neck fields are usually treated with a field dose of 5,000 cGy followed by a boost to the primary tumor of another 1,000 cGy to 2,200 cGy to bring the total primary dose to a range between 6,000 cGy and 7,200 cGy. Surgery for soft palate cancers is not generally indicated because of the lack of

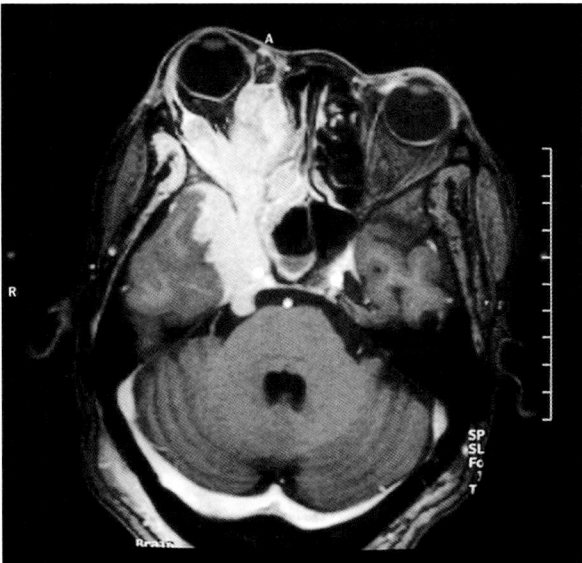

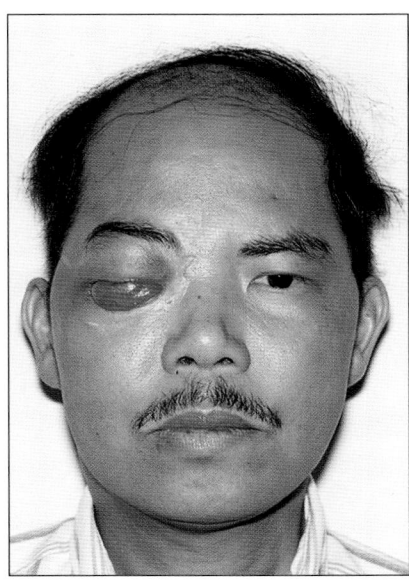

Fig 7-71a Squamous cell carcinoma in the retro-orbital space, the posterior ethmoids, and the middle cranial fossa. This tumor extension advanced from a soft palate carcinoma and is now unresectable and terminal.

Fig 7-71b Clinical photograph of patient whose CT scan is shown in Fig 7-71a. Note the periorbital edema and cheek swelling due to carcinoma blockage of lymphatics. The right eye was blinded because of carcinoma invasion into the optic nerve.

anatomic compartmentalization, the inability to perform a resection in continuity with the necks, and the functional deformity of unreconstructable soft palate loss.

Squamous cell carcinoma of the hard palate mucosa is best treated by surgery because of the potential and actual invasion onto bone or sinuses. The most common surgery is a type of hemimaxillectomy, since hemimaxillectomies differ somewhat among surgeons. The principles include 2-cm soft tissue and bony margins controlled with frozen sections. Most hemimaxillectomies are best accomplished with a transoral approach (Fig 7-72a). The lip split of a Weber-Ferguson type of approach will provide improved access if the tumor has extended into the orbit, ethmoids, or posterior to the posterior sinus wall and into the pterygomaxillary space. Otherwise, this approach offers no significant advantage over a transoral approach. If the scans identify orbital extension or if orbital extension is apparent clinically, an orbital exenteration must be included.

In hemimaxillectomy surgery, some prosthetic considerations must be incorporated into the surgery. One is the anterior resection margin. Many surgeons adhere to the term *hemimaxillectomy* precisely and resect through the midpalatal suture and the maxillary midline between the incisors. It is better to resect through the thin portion of either the ipsilateral or contralateral nasal floor as a barrier against tumor extension to the opposite side. It is also best to avoid a resection between the maxillary incisors. A maxillary prosthesis will fit and look better if the resection is accomplished through the lateral incisor tooth socket and 5 mm (one-half socket width) is left as a ledge onto which an appliance can be attached. In addition, an obturator prosthesis should be placed immediately to reduce nasal air escape, hypernasal speech, and nasal regurgitation (Figs 7-72b to 7-72e). The prosthesis should seal the oral cavity from the sinus and nasal cavities during eating and swallowing. A premade appliance is modified with the addition of a soft tissue conditioner and fixed to the maxilla with wires or screws. In the past some hemimaxillectomy defects had a split-thickness skin graft placed on the lateral side in order to produce an intentional scar band. Such scar bands created undercuts to assist in the retention of a prosthesis. However, this is rarely used today because of improvements in materials that can take advantage of the natural undercuts of the defect. Such split-thickness skin grafts were dry and flaked keratin into the mouth, an an-

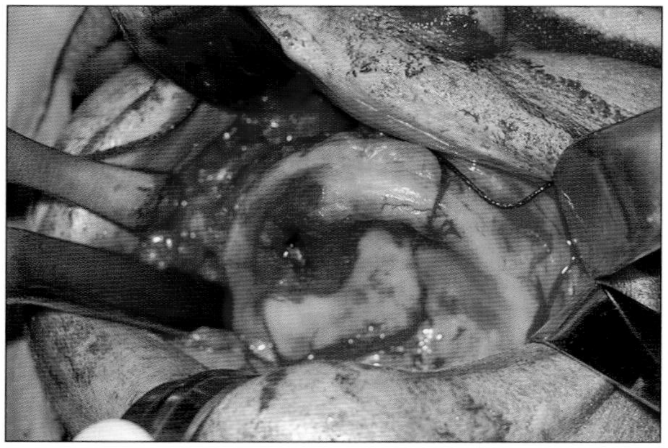

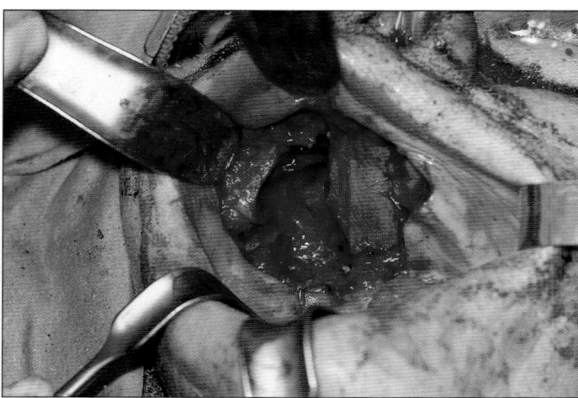

Fig 7-72a Hemimaxillectomy with 2-cm soft tissue and bony margins is recommended for a maxillary carcinoma. Most can be accomplished via a transoral approach.

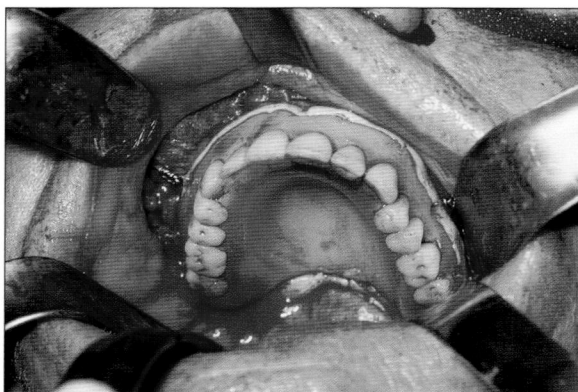

Fig 7-72b The defect resulting from a maxillary cancer resection will include a large oro-antral and oronasal communication.

Fig 7-72c Maxillary defects are initially managed with a soft tissue reline of the patient's denture or a premade splint. The denture-obturator splint will require fixation with zygomatic buttress, circumzygomatic wires, or a palatal screw.

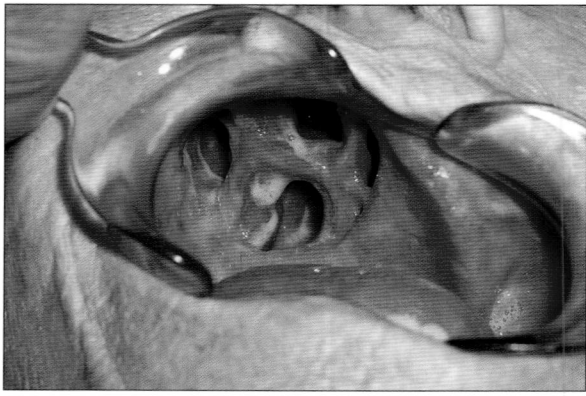

Fig 7-72d After 6 months, the surgical defect has become dimensionally stable and is ready for a permanent obturator prosthesis. A mucosalized surface, as seen here, is better than a skin-grafted surface, which has the disadvantages of dryness and the slough of keratin.

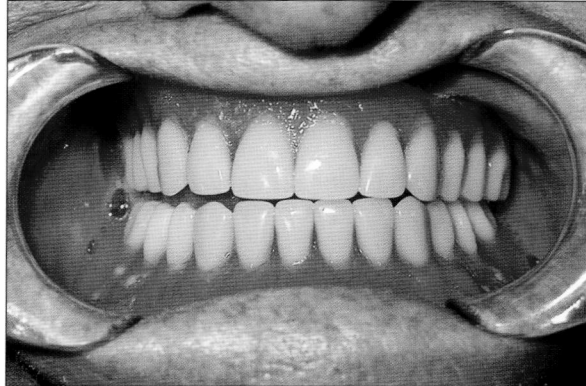

Fig 7-72e A permanent obturator prosthesis can be retained by undercuts in the surgical defect, as was accomplished here. However, retention via implants placed into the remaining bone is preferred because it will permit a more balanced occlusion and better stability.

noyance to patients. A moist, natural mucosal surface in the defect is preferred. The surgeon should consult a maxillofacial prosthodontist before surgery to coordinate this planning.

Hemimaxillectomy for carcinoma does not permit incontinuity neck surgery. Because of the propensity for maxillary cancers to undergo regional lymph node spread, N_0 necks are best treated with either surgery or radiation. Often, the postsurgical wound bed, lymphatic drainage fields, and the neck are irradiated as a single comprehensive plan.

Prognosis and Follow-Up ►

The prognosis of maxillary cancers in general is poorer than those of the mandible, tongue, and floor-of-the-mouth areas. Adjusted 5-year survival statistics generally show a 25% to 40% survival rate. For this reason, prosthetic management of the maxillary defect should be continued for a minimum of 2 years, and longer if the patient has regained sufficient function with the prosthesis. Surgical closure of the large oral-antral-nasal communication is possible and predictable with a temporalis flap or a radial forearm free vascular transfer, but its closure will obscure examination and visualization of recurrent disease. After 2 years, 90% of recurrences will have become evident. At that time, a surgical closure may be considered if the obturator prosthesis is inadequate (see Figs 7-72d and 7-72e).

Follow-up is the same as for tongue and floor-of-the-mouth carcinoma with the addition of a CT or MRI scan annually for the first 2 years to assess for recurrence within the orbit or pterygomaxillary space.

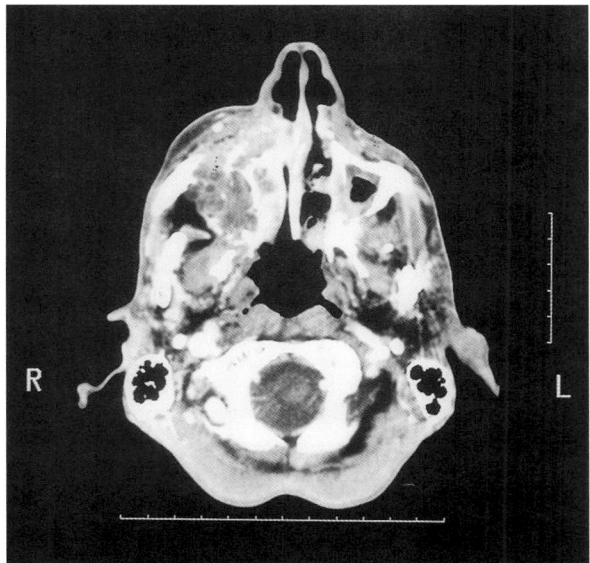 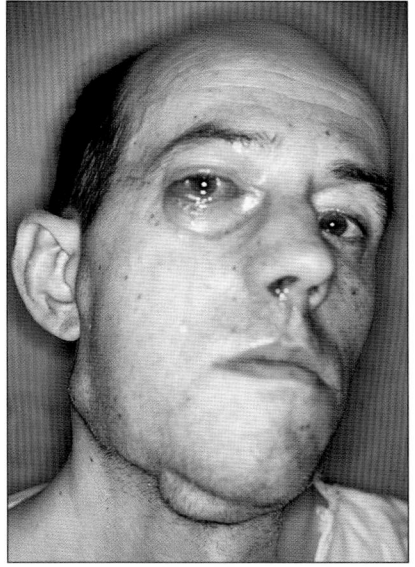 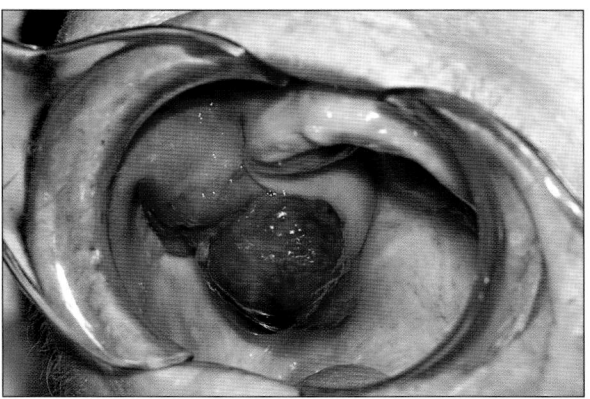

Fig 7-73a A squamous carcinoma arising in the maxillary sinus may reach a significant size before it produces sufficient signs and symptoms for the individual to seek care.

Fig 7-73b Extensive spread from a maxillary sinus carcinoma producing signs and symptoms of epistaxis, diplopia, epiphora, and evident neck metastases.

Fig 7-73c Maxillary sinus squamous cell carcinoma protruding into the oral cavity.

Squamous Cell Carcinoma of the Maxillary Sinus

CLINICAL PRESENTATION ▶ Squamous cell carcinoma arising in the maxillary sinus (Fig 7-73a) usually goes unnoticed until its erosion or size produces symptoms (Fig 7-73b). Therefore, it may present with any one of many signs and symptoms. In order of frequency, these include nasal stuffiness, swelling over the cheek, pain in the area, chronic sinusitis, epistaxis, and ocular symptoms (usually epiphora and diplopia). Many such cancers will present with a mass bulging into the oral cavity or into the nasal cavity (Fig 7-73c). Because they erode the sinus floor, early mobility of the maxillary teeth may be a presenting sign. Many patients have undergone removal of maxillary teeth for what was believed to be periodontal disease only to manifest a bulging mass through the socket wounds over the next few weeks. In about 5% to 10% of cases, paresthesia or anesthesia of some branch of the maxillary division of the trigeminal nerve is found.

A panoramic radiograph or facial bone series will show a soft tissue mass in the sinus and usually bony erosion of one or more walls of the sinus.

DIFFERENTIAL DIAGNOSIS ▶ The usual presentation of nasal stuffiness and a mass-related enlargement of the maxilla suggests other malignancies that may arise in the maxillary sinus. The most common of these is an *adenoid cystic carcinoma* of salivary gland origin. Others include *mucoepidermoid carcinoma* and a *lymphoepithelioma*, which is itself a variant of squamous cell carcinoma. Inflammatory sinus disease such as *chronic sinusitis* with granulation tissue accumulation or *osteomyelitis of the maxilla* may also produce the same signs and symptoms. Specific sinus diseases such as *mucormycosis*, if the patient is an insulin-dependent diabetic or is otherwise immunocompromised, and *sarcoidosis* are rare, but remain considerations. In addition, sarcomas of bone such as *fibrosarcoma* and *malignant fibrous histiocytoma* are realistic though uncommon. In younger patients, *rhabdomyosarcoma* may also be considered.

DIAGNOSTIC WORK-UP ▶ Maxillary sinus carcinomas require a CT or MRI scan as part of their work-up in addition to the routine oral and head and neck examination with a mirror or fiberoptic examination of the laryngopharynx. Incisional biopsy can be performed through a Caldwell-Luc approach to the antrum. It is important to

Table 7-5 Specific TNM clinical classification for maxillary sinus carcinoma

T–Primary tumor of maxillary sinus

T_X	Primary tumor cannot be assessed
T_S	Carcinoma in situ
T_1	Tumor limited to the antral mucosa with no erosion or destruction of bone
T_2	Tumor causing bone erosion or destruction, except for the posterior antral wall, including extension into hard palate and/or middle nasal meatus
T_3	Tumor invades any of the following: bone of posterior wall of maxillary sinus, subcutaneous tissues, skin of cheek, floor or medial wall of orbit, infratemporal fossa, pterygoid plates, ethmoid sinuses
T_4	Tumor invades orbital contents beyond the floor or medial wall including apex and/or any of the following: cribriform plate, base of skull, nasopharynx, sphenoid sinus, frontal sinus

N–Regional lymph nodes

N_0	No clinically palpable nodes
N_1	Clinically palpable ipsilateral node < 3 cm
N_{2A}	Clinically palpable ipsilateral node 3 to 6 cm
N_{2B}	Two or more clinically palpable ipsilateral nodes 3 to 6 cm
N_3	Bilateral or contralateral palpable node OR any clinically palpable node > 6 cm

M–Distant metastasis

M_X	Metastasis not assessed
M_0	Metastasis assessed; none found
M_1	Metastasis present

note that the TNM classification for sinus tumors differs from the classification for the oral cavity. In this TNM classification, scans are required to assess disease extent and contribute to the staging. The pertinent TNM classification for carcinoma of the maxillary sinus is presented in Table 7-5.

TREATMENT ▶ Carcinoma of the maxillary sinus is a serious disease because of its generally late diagnosis, its usually aggressive behavior, and the surrounding anatomy where perforation through the thin walls of the sinus allows it to enter other important anatomic compartments. Treatment almost always requires aggressive hemimaxillectomy or maxillectomy surgery through a Weber-Ferguson type of incision. At times it may also require a lower lip–split incision and a midline mandibulotomy to retract the mandible laterally to gain access to the pterygomaxillary and infratemporal spaces. Lesions that encroach on the orbit require an orbital exenteration, and those that invade the ethmoid sinuses require an extension of the Weber-Ferguson incision around the medial canthus. The neck should be treated concomitantly either by surgery or radiation. Usually a functional neck dissection for N_0 or N_1 necks and a full radical neck dissection for N_2 or N_3 necks is required as well. Combination surgery and radiotherapy improve tumor control and prognosis.

The resultant defect is treated initially and in the long-term using an obturator prosthesis in a fashion similar to that described for carcinoma of the palate.

PROGNOSIS AND FOLLOW-UP ▶ The prognosis for maxillary sinus cancer remains poor despite new and aggressive surgical and radiation approaches. The overall adjusted 5-year survival rates are between 15% and 25%.

Follow-up requires direct examination and a mirror or fiberoptic examination of the laryngopharynx every 4 months for 2 years, and then every 6 months thereafter. A CT or MRI scan is also valuable at yearly intervals over the first 2 years.

Undifferentiated Nasopharyngeal Carcinoma (Lymphoepithelioma)

CLINICAL PRESENTATION AND PATHOGENESIS ▶

Undifferentiated nonkeratinizing squamous cell carcinomas account for 75% of malignancies in the nasopharynx. One common and peculiar histologic type has been termed *lymphoepithelioma* because of the intimate association of cancer cells with T lymphocytes in a syncytial pattern. Nevertheless, this cancer and the others in this group represent a rapidly proliferating and metastasizing type of cancer of squamous cell origin. Many of these patients will be 10 to 20 years younger than the average oral carcinoma patient. Individuals in their 30s, 40s, and early 50s are at the highest risk.

Essentially a rare tumor, it has a greatly increased incidence in southern China and Taiwan, and an intermediate incidence in those who emigrate to the US. There is a male predilection. A strong association with Epstein-Barr virus has been noted, although no clear cause and effect has been established.

Most patients will present with symptoms or signs of a tumor mass. Nasal obstruction, epistaxis, dysphagia, and the "feeling of something in the throat" are common findings. Unilateral or bilateral cervical lymphadenopathy is not uncommon at the time of presentation. The majority of tumors arise from the lateral nasopharyngeal wall (fossa of Rosenmüller) (Fig 7-74).

DIFFERENTIAL DIAGNOSIS ▶

The suspicion of malignancy of some type is very high with the usual presentation of this carcinoma. Therefore, the differential diagnosis encompasses a small subset of other aggressive malignancies found in this area, in particular, *non-Hodgkin large cell lymphoma* and aggressive salivary gland malignancies such as *adenoid cystic carcinoma, high-grade mucoepidermoid carcinoma,* and *malignant pleomorphic adenoma.* Because of the generally younger age range associated with this type of squamous cell carcinoma, *rhabdomyosarcoma,* which has a predilection for the facial area, is also a consideration.

DIAGNOSTIC WORK-UP ▶

In addition to a complete oral, nasal, and head and neck examination, these patients require a fiberoptic or mirror examination of the nasal vault and laryngopharynx. A CT or MRI scan is also needed, as direct visualization of these tumors is often difficult. Because biopsy access is often difficult, general anesthesia may be required. Depending on the location of the tumor mass, a biopsy specimen may be obtained via a transnasal, transantral, or transoral approach.

HISTOPATHOLOGY ▶

Most nasopharyngeal carcinomas are squamous cell carcinomas that arise from respiratory mucosa and manifest a spectrum of differentiation levels. There are two major categories. The first is the keratinizing tumors, which demonstrate intercellular bridging and/or keratin production and may range from well to poorly differentiated lesions. Most are poorly differentiated. The second group comprises the far more numerous nonkeratinizing tumors in which evidence of squamous differentiation cannot be appreciated by light microscopy. Some consist of large polyhedral cells with defined cell margins in a plexiform pattern. A pavementing pattern may be seen. Others are undifferentiated; the cells have round to oval nuclei, prominent nucleoli, and undefined cell margins, so that there is often a syncytial arrangement. Mitoses may be abundant (Figs 7-75a and 7-75b). The cells can also be spindle shaped. Squamous differentiation can be appreciated only ultrastructurally by the presence of desmosomes and tonofilaments. Immunohistochemistry will reveal the presence of cytokeratins. The connective tissue stroma is scant in these tumors. Some nasopharyngeal carcinomas, which have been called *lymphoepitheliomas,* are infiltrated by large numbers of lymphocytes (see Fig 7-75a). These lymphocytes are not neoplastic, however, and appear to be reactive in nature.

TREATMENT ▶

The location and usual anatomic size of these lesions preclude surgery. Almost all lesions of this type are treated with radiotherapy alone or combined with a chemotherapy protocol. The response to radiotherapy in the dose range of 6,000 cGy to 7,200 cGy is one of tumor shrinkage to a clinically undetectable status and improvement in the signs and symptoms produced by the tumor. However, this response is representative of tumor cell population kinetics and selection of resistant cells. Such tumors may weigh up to 10 g and contain about 10^{10} cells. The radiotherapy imparts a 99% tumor cell kill, rendering the tumor undetectable visually or by radiographic means. The residual 1% of tumor cells, which

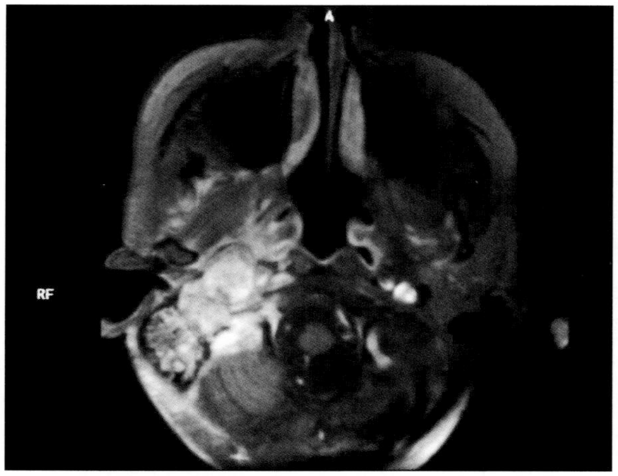

Fig 7-74 This nasopharyngeal carcinoma presented with only a complaint of a "funny feeling" in the throat, yet was diffusely invasive around the base of the skull. Note the relatively small bulge into the nasopharynx that produced the patient's symptom.

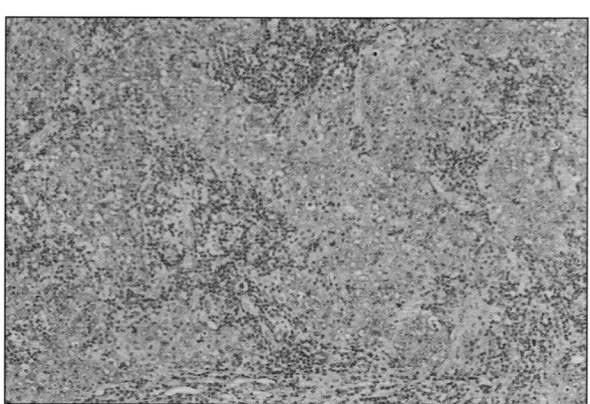

Fig 7-75a A nonkeratinizing squamous cell carcinoma of the nasopharynx in which the tumor cells form broad, pale sheets and in which foci of lymphocytes can be seen.

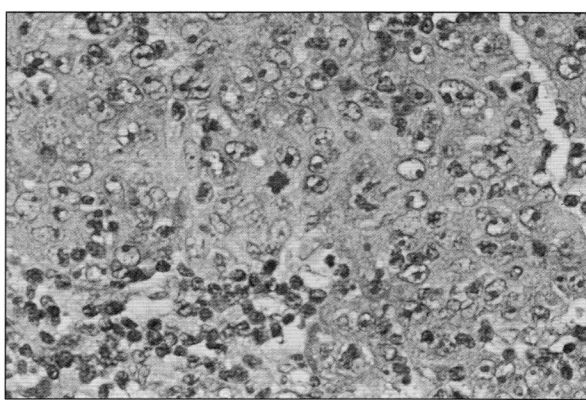

Fig 7-75b A higher-power view of Fig 7-75a. The tumor cells have a syncytial arrangement, and numerous mitoses are present.

represents a population of 10^8 (a tumor becomes visible at about 10^8 cells), is composed of radioresistant or at least radiotolerant cells. Therefore, the remission is not permanent in these cancers; recurrences usually occur and progress to a fatal outcome.

In other tumors and in smaller tumors, the reduction in viable cell numbers may be more complete and translate into a complete cure. The problem in particular with these cancers is that the maximum tolerated dose causes remission, not cure. Curative doses for this tumor are usually beyond normal tissue tolerance.

PROGNOSIS AND FOLLOW-UP ▶

The prognosis is very poor. Adjusted 5-year survival rates are 10% to 15%. Recurrences representing re-emergence of the original tumor often occur within 6 months to 1 year. Therefore, follow-up must be very close; it is usually every 2 to 3 months over the first 2 years and then every 6 months thereafter. Follow-up consists of direct examination and mirror or fiberoptic examination of the area. In addition, CT or MRI scans are required at periodic intervals.

Premalignant Conditions and Malignancies of Skin

Actinic Keratosis

CLINICAL PRESENTATION AND PATHOGENESIS ▶

Actinic keratosis is a common sun-induced premalignant lesion found on the more sun-exposed surfaces of the skin and the lower lip (it is not found on the upper lip). The correlation of light complexion and a reduced ability to tan is characteristic of individuals with blonde or red hair and blue or green eyes who thus compose the major population who develop the spectrum of sun-damage–related pathologies. Actinic keratosis is histologically dysplastic and is premalignant. It is the skin corollary to dysplastic erythroleukoplakia of the oral mucosa.

Early lesions will present as atrophic, indurated red plaques, sometimes with surface crusting (Fig 7-76). More mature lesions will appear yellow and scaly (Fig 7-77). Occasionally, keratin accumulation will occur, producing a yellow-green build-up called a *cutaneous horn* (Figs 7-78a and 7-78b). Most importantly, lesions will be set against a background of atrophic skin with areas of hypo- and hyperpigmentation. The most common sun-exposed regions are the top of the pinna, the forehead, the infraorbital skin, the dor-

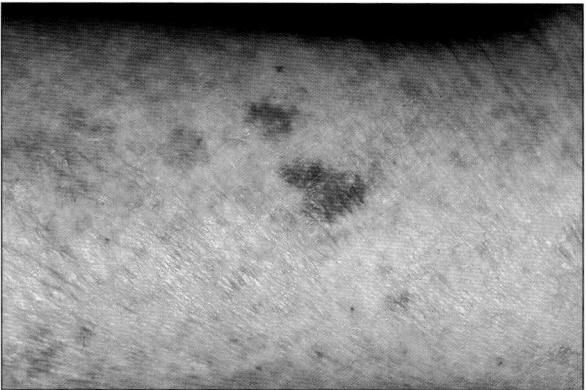

Fig 7-76 Actinic keratosis of the forearm, manifested here as a thickened pigmented plaque, is a premalignant condition.

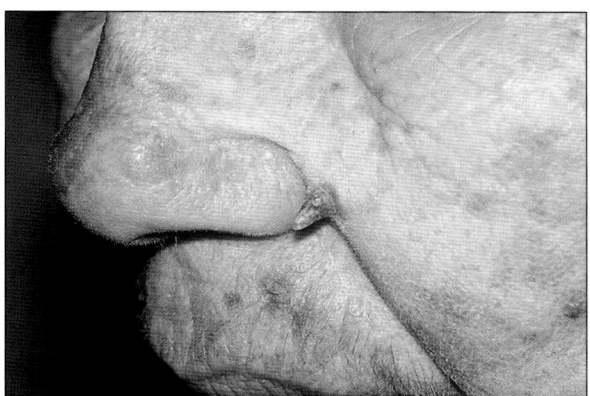

Fig 7-77 Multiple actinic keratoses on severely sun-damaged facial skin including a cutaneous horn, which is frequently associated with actinic keratosis.

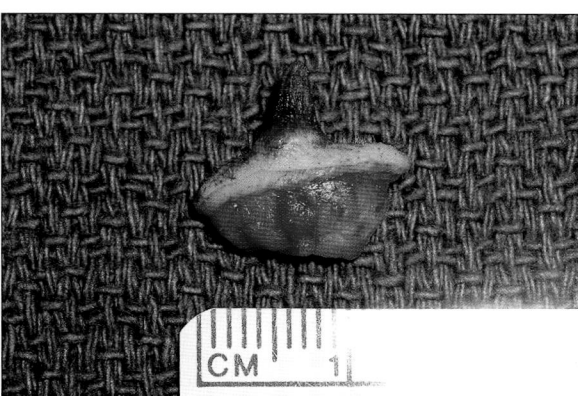

Fig 7-78a A cutaneous horn should be excised with a superficial excision. Like the horn of an animal, which it resembles, the cutaneous horn is a product of compacted keratin.

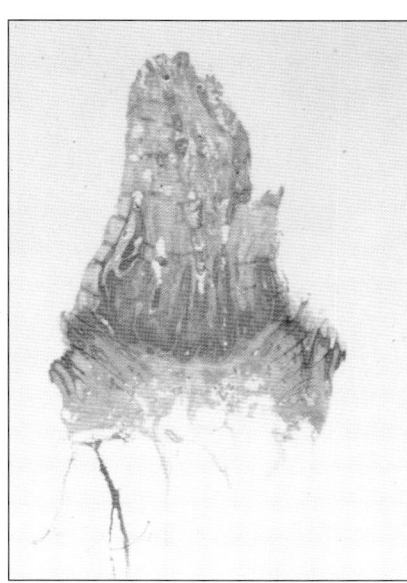

Fig 7-78b The excised cutaneous horn represents a layer of dysplastic epithelium on which compacted keratin forms a horn-like projection.

sum of the nose, the dorsum of the hands, the shoulders, and the vermilion of the lower lip. Lower lip actinic keratosis occurs along the entire vermilion but is usually more severe in the lower lip pout, which is the most everted portion of the lower lip (see Fig 7-88).

DIFFERENTIAL DIAGNOSIS ▶

Actinic keratosis of skin, a premalignant form of skin squamous cell carcinoma, will appear like an early *basal cell carcinoma*. There is always the possibility that any one of many actinic keratoses may progress to a malignancy. While it is not a premalignant form of melanoma, because of the skin texture and pigmentation changes it causes, actinic keratosis resembles the spectrum of *various nevi, lentigo maligna melanoma,* and *melanoma.*

Actinic keratosis on the vermilion of the lower lip may also be termed *actinic cheilitis* and has a more focused differential, mainly *squamous cell carcinoma* and *habitual lip-biting or lip-wetting*.

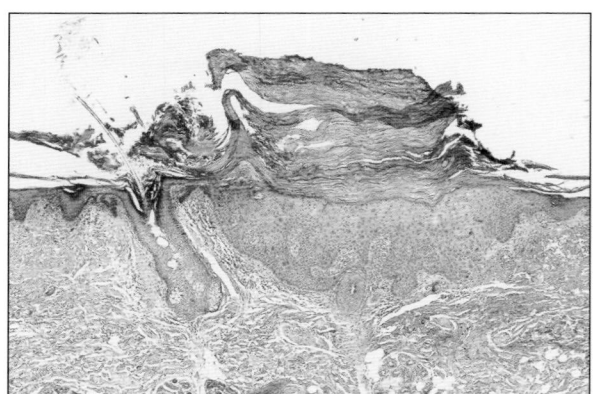

Fig 7-79a Actinic keratosis with a thickened parakeratinized scale.

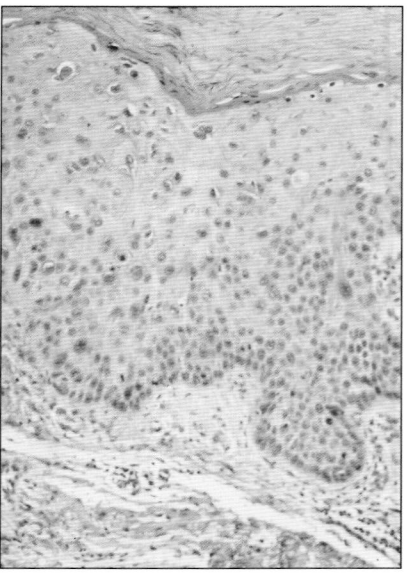

Fig 7-79b A higher-power view of Fig 7-79a shows epithelial dysplasia.

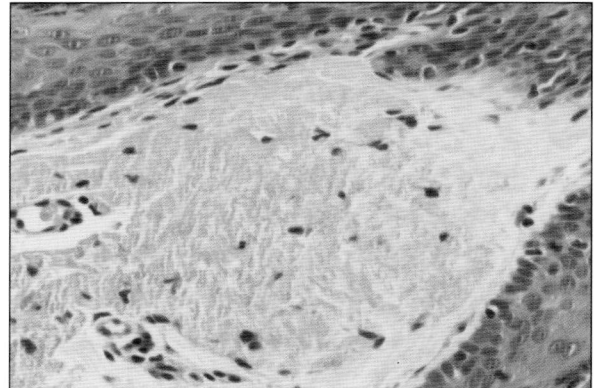

Fig 7-80 Solar elastosis showing replacement of normal fibrous tissue by amorphous basophilic material. Sun-damaged skin will typically show such changes.

DIAGNOSTIC WORK-UP ▶ Excisional biopsy should be performed. If there are multiple lesions, excision of the most clinically advanced or ulcerated lesions is preferable.

HISTOPATHOLOGY ▶ Actinic keratosis is characterized by epithelial dysplasia that may affect the basal cells only or may progressively involve the prickle cell layers. The changes include increased cell size with hyperchromatic nuclei, pleomorphism, and atypical mitoses. A parakeratinized scale will typically form on the surface, and it may contain neutrophils. In more extreme cases, a cutaneous horn may form. This is defined as a keratotic mass in which the height is at least half of its greatest diameter. Although most are usually seen in conjunction with actinic keratosis, this reactive lesion may also overlie seborrheic keratosis or squamous cell carcinoma (Figs 7-79a and 7-79b).

Some histologic variants are observed. In conjunction with the parakeratinized surface, the lesion may show atrophy; hyperplasia with a basaloid proliferation of bud-like cords into the dermis (proliferative actinic keratosis); or dermal lymphocytic infiltrate (lichenoid actinic keratosis). Melanin pigmentation may occur with melanocytes within the dysplastic epithelium and melanophages in the dermis. Focal areas of acantholysis can develop.

The superficial dermis will show solar elastosis manifested by the presence of blue-gray material with hematoxylin & eosin (H&E) stain (Fig 7-80). This is due to altered elastic fiber synthesis by sun-damaged fibroblasts. The material is positive for elastin.

Actinic cheilitis shows epithelial atrophy and flattening of the epithelial–connective tissue interface. Early lesions may lack cellular atypia. The connective tissue contains a banded inflammatory infiltrate with many plasma cells, and blood vessels are widely dilated.

TREATMENT ▶ Actinic keratosis is considered a reversible lesion. The goal in treatment of a field of what seems to be actinic keratosis is to resolve or control as many as possible nonsurgically and to selectively excise the unresponsive lesions (which, by their unresponsiveness, may indicate that they have progressed to an early squamous cell or basal cell carcinoma).

Treatment may take any one of the following forms.

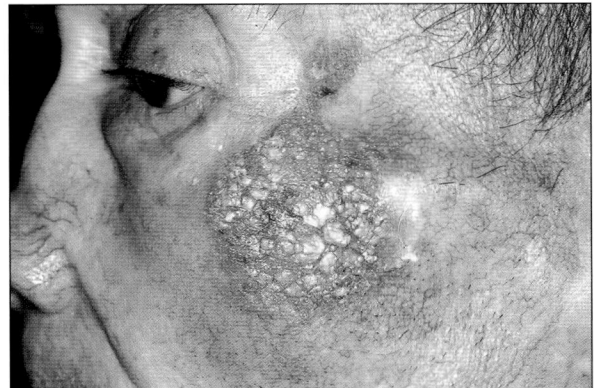

Fig 7-81 Overuse of topical 5-FU, use of 5% 5-FU creams instead of 2% 5-FU creams, or use without a topical steroid cream may result in either a painful inflammation or an actual chemical burn.

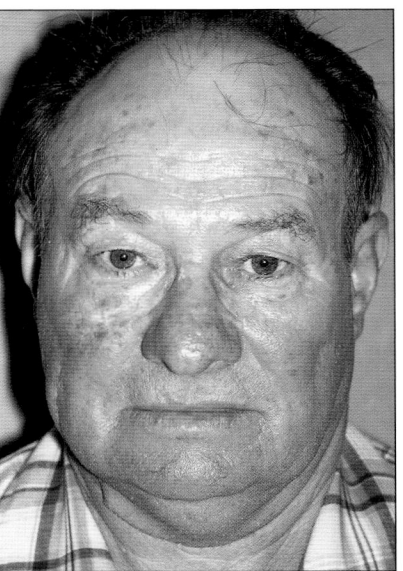

Fig 7-82a Numerous actinic keratoses on severely sun-damaged facial skin treated with intermittent courses of 2% topical 5-FU and 0.05% fluocinonide cream (Lidex, Medicis).

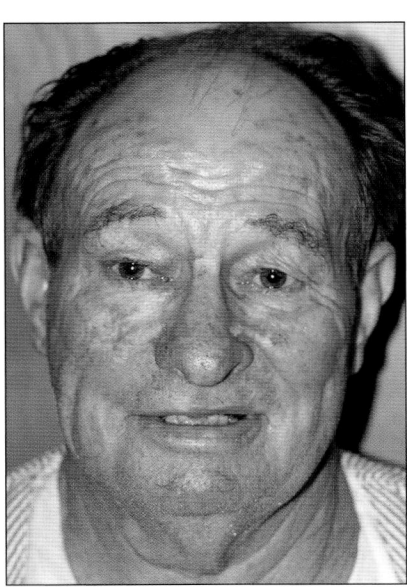

Fig 7-82b Twelve years later, areas of actinic keratosis either have resolved or have not progressed. However, a new basal cell carcinoma has formed at the right medial canthus where these topical agents were not applied.

Sun Screens

Spontaneous remissions are possible if sunlight exposure is severely curtailed. Use of sun screen with a sun protection factor (SPF) of 15 or higher combined with protective clothing is a valid treatment approach.

Tretinoin

Tretinoin topical cream 0.05% (Retin-A, Ortho Biotech), used alone in mild and early cases, has shown resolution. It is applied once daily or at most twice daily over 2 to 4 months. Unresponsive lesions are considered for topical 5-fluorouracil treatment or surgery.

Topical 5-Fluorouracil

5-Fluorouracil (5-FU) is an effective topical chemotherapeutic drug for actinic keratosis that may help identify lesions that have evolved into skin squamous cell carcinoma or actually represent basal cell carcinomas. 5-FU is used on facial skin and on the lip vermilion as a 2% topical cream twice daily for a period of 3 weeks. It will cause an uncomfortable skin or lip inflammation, which begins within 3 to 5 days and persists throughout treatment (Fig 7-81). It may be intense enough to cause a superficial slough or a set of crusty ulcerations, particularly on the lower lip vermilion. Because of the discomfort and appearance, some patients will curtail the 3-week course, drastically reducing therapeutic efficacy. An excellent recommendation is to combine the topical 5-FU with a topical corticosteroid cream such as 0.05% fluocinonide (Lidex cream, Medicis Dermatologics) or 1% hydrocortisone (Topicort cream, Aventis) (Figs 7-82a and 7-82b). Two-percent topical 5-FU (Efudex, ICN) may also be combined with tretinoin for enhanced effect of each agent.

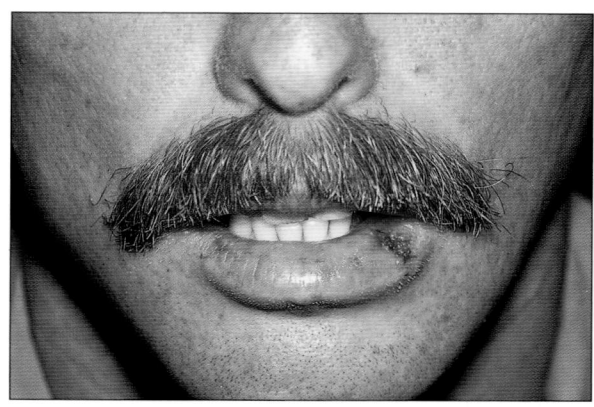

Fig 7-83a Small lower lip squamous cell carcinoma. The lip vermilion also has extensive sun damage consistent with actinic keratosis.

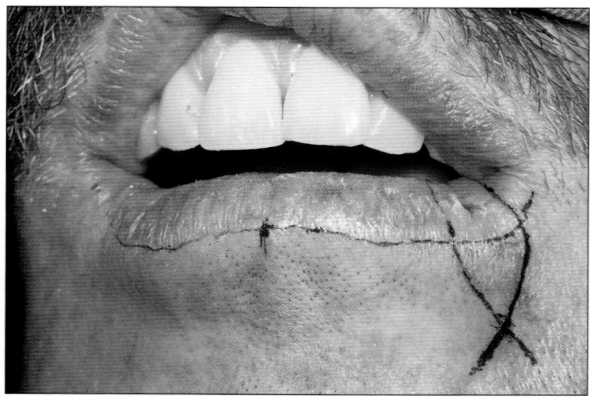

Fig 7-83b Outline of a combined excision of the lip carcinoma and a vermilionectomy. The vermilionectomy outline follows the gentle curve of the vermilion cutaneous line and includes 1 to 2 mm of skin.

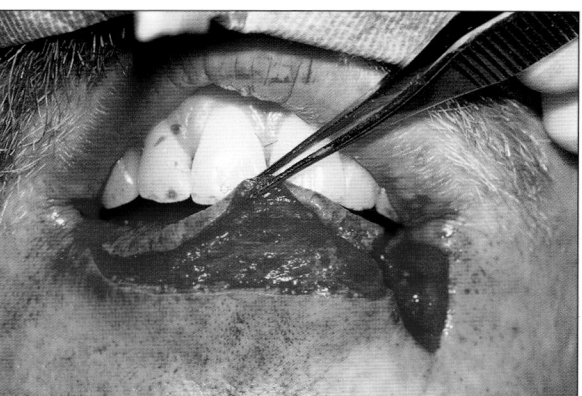

Fig 7-83c The vermilionectomy excises the vermilion at the level of the orbicularis oris fascia after the V-shaped excision of the carcinoma is accomplished and tumor-free margins are documented.

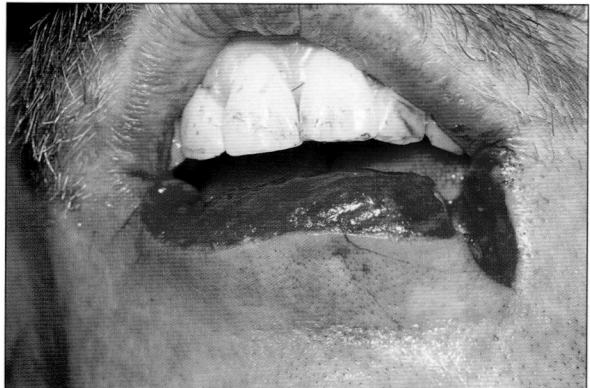

Fig 7-83d Absolute hemostasis is required before the mucosa can be advanced. The skin margin should be well defined and symmetrical.

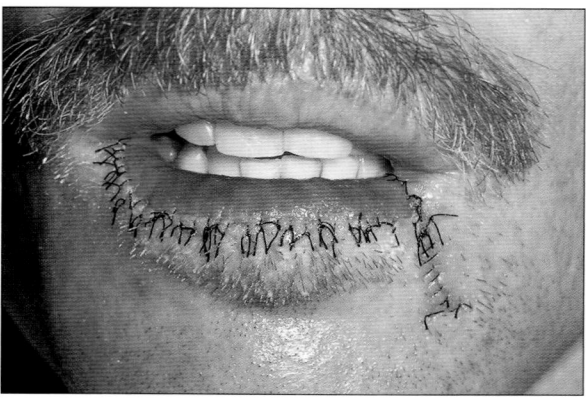

Fig 7-83e After all the minor salivary glands have been removed from the labial mucosal, it should be evenly advanced to the skin edge. Ideally, the vermilionectomy and advancement flap should include the entire length of the vermilion or a slight color mismatch will result, as shown here.

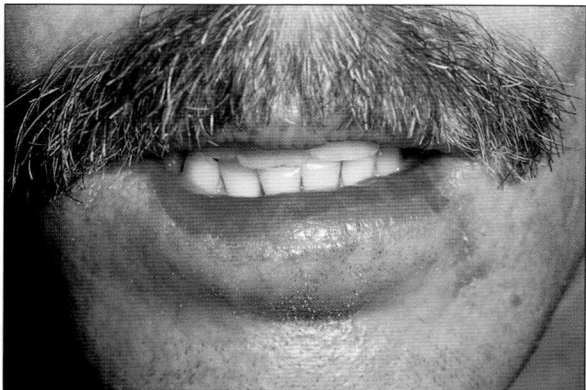

Fig 7-83f The initial results of a vermilionectomy reconstructed with a mucosal advancement flap will be resolution of the actinic damage but a reddened lip that must be protected from sun exposure for 6 months. Note the color mismatch at the left commissure due to the natural vermilion left in that area.

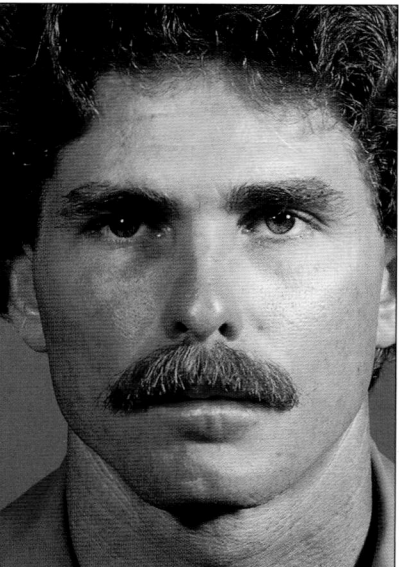

Fig 7-83g After 6 months to 1 year, the vermilion color and shape normalize.

Surgery

Facial lesions unresponsive to topical 5-FU are candidates for local excision. Electrodessication or cryosurgical removal by those experienced in such techniques is also effective.

For persistent lower lip actinic keratosis, a vermilionectomy (often referred to as a "lip shave," a term that should be discarded) with a mucosal advancement flap for lip reconstruction is required (Fig 7-83a). The vermilionectomy should excise the vermilion thickness up to but not including the fascia overlying the orbicularis oris fibers (Figs 7-83b and 7-83c). The vermilionectomy should also include the vermilion from commissure to commissure since partial vermilionectomies usually result in an irregular lip shape with poorly matched color. Excision of 1 to 2 mm of skin margin is advised to compensate for the healing contraction, which tends to invert the lip. The oral mucosal resection edge should be just into clinically uninvolved tissue. The specimen of lip vermilion should be oriented with sutures relating right-left and skin-oral side for frozen section assessment to rule out areas of invasive squamous cell carcinoma. If identification of an area of focal carcinoma is made, a small V-shaped excision should be accomplished.

The mucosal advancement flap is developed by a full-thickness undermining of the labial mucosa. The labial mucosal flap is then advanced and precisely sutured to the skin edge. For this flap, there are five critical elements that must be considered for an ideal result. First, the flap must be able to be advanced without stretching, or the lip will become inverted. Second, minor salivary glands adherent to the flap must be removed, or a lumpy lip will result. Third, absolute hemostasis must be achieved, or a subflap hematoma will cause loss of the flap and a scarred, contracted lip (Fig 7-83d). Fourth, the excision of the vermilion must duplicate the curvilinear contour of the lower lip vermilion–skin junction, particularly the paramidline lip pout. If it does not, a straight unesthetic lip contour will result (Fig 7-83e). Fifth, the patient must absolutely refrain from exposing the lip to any sun for 6 months. It is especially critical during the first 3 months, as the labial mucosa has no natural protection from sun damage and may burn excessively and completely necrose, resulting in a so-called fish-mouth deformity.

It is also important to inform the patient that the reconstructed lip will look reddened and lipstick-coated initially and to some extent for about 1 year (Fig 7-83f). After 1 year, the color more closely matches a normal vermilion and the edema resolves to eliminate the "full lip" look (Fig 7-83g). Paresthesia of the lower lip is common but is usually tolerable and affects the reconstructed vermilion only at its surface.

PROGNOSIS AND FOLLOW-UP ▶ Actinic keratosis requires a constant vigilance for the appearance of new lesions and the evolution of skin cancers. Repeated treatments are often necessary, and patients must take precautions to control their sun exposure. Follow-up examinations are recommended every 6 months.

Keratoacanthoma

CLINICAL PRESENTATION AND PATHOGENESIS ▶ Keratoacanthomas are tumorous skin lesions that bear a close relationship to well-differentiated squamous cell carcinomas of skin. They are most often related to sun exposure and are most commonly found on the heavily sun-exposed surfaces of the face, shoulders, and dorsum of the hands. Isolated keratoacanthomas may emerge after a penetrating trauma even in sites not exposed to sun. True oral cavity keratoacanthomas may not exist at all or, at the very most, are extremely rare. However, lower lip keratoacanthomas emerging in the paramidline lip pout are well-known (Fig 7-84a).

The keratoacanthoma is classically described to emerge from a normal surface over 6 weeks, undergo a 6-week period of dormancy, and then undergo extrusion of its central keratin plug and involute into a dimpled scar over another 6 weeks; unfortunately, only 40% of cases conveniently follow this sequence. The remaining 60% either involute only partially, remain the same size, or increase in size after a period of quiescence. A fully developed keratoacanthoma will be an elevated mass with a central crater of brown or black keratin. The edge will be elevated and rolled in a sharp border with adjacent skin. The adjacent skin will often show a 1- to 2-mm band of erythema (Fig 7-84b).

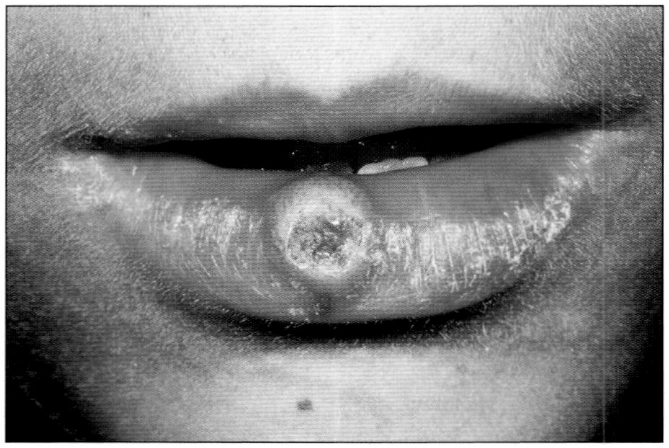

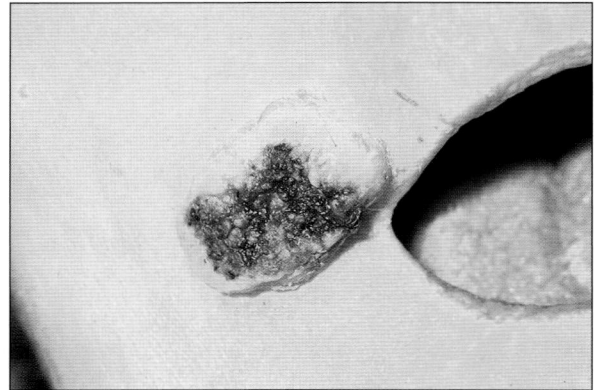

Fig 7-84a Keratoacanthomas of the lower lip will occur in the same paramidline area as lip carcinomas. Like keratoacanthomas on skin, those on the lip will usually have a central keratin plug and distinct rolled, elevated margins.

Fig 7-84b Keratoacanthomas of the facial skin will often have a blackened central keratin plug and distinct rolled and elevated margins.

A keratoacanthoma can arise at any age, but adults with a history of sun exposure are the most common group affected. Most keratoacanthomas will be isolated lesions, but there are two syndrome-like complexes in which the lesions can be multiple. One, called the *Ferguson-Smith type*, is found in children, often in numbers ranging from 5 to 20; in this group, the lesions almost always involute completely. The other, called the *Grybowski type*, is found in adults; in this group, the lesions are small and may number well over 100. They are also found as a component in Torre syndrome, which also consists of low-grade visceral carcinomas and sebaceous neoplasms.

The variability in clinical course between different keratoacanthomas is probably related to the cell line from which they arise. The hair follicle epithelium (also referred to as the pilosebaceous unit) normally undergoes cycles of proliferation and resting phases. Sun damage to its DNA structure stimulating a neoplastic growth may very well be expected to result in the same types of phasic growth and even extrusion of a central keratin plug (analogous to shedding of the hair shaft). Like well-differentiated skin squamous carcinomas that produce some of their usual product, keratin, and do not metastasize, a keratoacanthoma also is a well-differentiated type of skin squamous cell carcinoma that produces some keratin in the form of hair protein and also does not metastasize.

DIFFERENTIAL DIAGNOSIS ▶ A mature keratoacanthoma may so closely resemble a *skin squamous cell carcinoma* clinically and histopathologically that the conditions may be indistinguishable. In fact, keratoacanthomas may represent a squamous cell carcinoma arising from hair follicle epithelium. Other sun-damage–related lesions that may clinically resemble a keratoacanthoma include *basal cell carcinoma* and *melanoma*, both of which may themselves generate a dark-brown to black crateriform center. Some skin squamous cell carcinomas and basal cell carcinomas produce a central brown-black core due to keratin production. The *pigmented type of basal cell carcinoma* in particular produces a brown-black color due to melanin dispersal and uptake by macrophages, which are termed melanophages. The melanoma appears brown-black because it produces melanin from melanocytes. In addition, the virus-related skin lesions of *molluscum contagiosum* may also produce one or more small skin nodules that express a central plug. However, this plug is whitish, and the lesions are neither elevated nor have rolled edges as is characteristic of a keratoacanthoma.

DIAGNOSTIC WORK-UP ▶ Suspected keratoacanthoma lesions should be excised. Incisional biopsies may suffice but are of limited value because they do not provide a sufficient amount of tissue or the best orientation for an unequivocal diagnosis.

HISTOPATHOLOGY ▶ As with verrucous carcinoma, the diagnosis of keratoacanthoma relies strongly on the architecture of the lesion, so an appropriate biopsy specimen is necessary. An excisional biopsy is preferred, but a

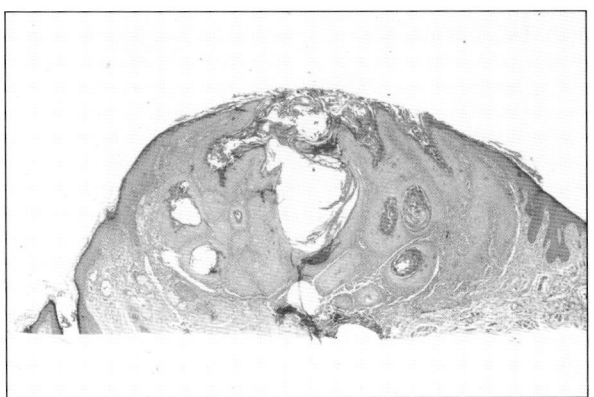

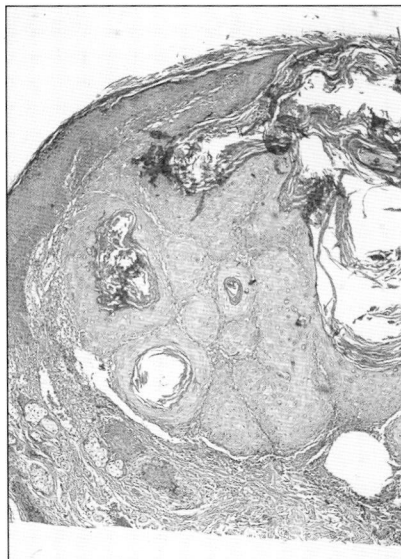

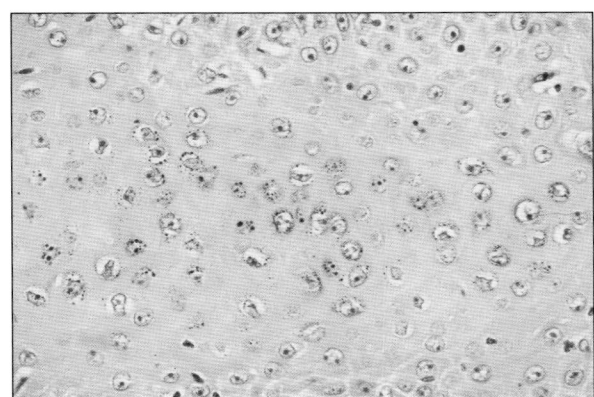

Fig 7-85a A keratoacanthoma showing a well-demarcated, keratin-filled, crater-like lesion. There is an exo-endophytic growth pattern and an inflammatory infiltrate at the base.

Fig 7-85b A higher-power view of Fig 7-85a shows the buttress or lip at the tumor margin formed by the normal adjacent epithelium.

Fig 7-85c A high-power view of cells within a keratoacanthoma shows the keratinization that occurs and the resultant glassy appearance.

fusiform incisional biopsy through the center of the lesion, incorporating one and preferably both margins, can suffice. The most diagnostic phase of the solitary keratoacanthoma is its fully developed stage. Under low-power magnification, the lesion appears as a cup-shaped, keratin-filled crater around which the normal adjacent epithelium abruptly changes into a proliferative acanthotic epithelium showing pseudoepitheliomatous hyperplasia (Fig 7-85a). This epithelium exhibits an exo-endophytic growth pattern. At the periphery, the normal epithelium is lifted upward and forms a lip or "buttress" over the crater (Fig 7-85b). At the base, a dense inflammatory infiltrate rich in lymphocytes is present. Examination at higher power indicates that the epithelial cells undergo keratinization, a process that may extend through all layers. The cytoplasm is eosinophilic and glassy in appearance (Fig 7-85c). Occasional mitoses and atypical cells may be visible but are not prominent.

The early stages of keratoacanthoma are more proliferative. Strands of epithelium may extend into the connective tissue, and there may be more atypia. Perineural invasion has been observed, but this does not indicate metastatic potential or a change in biologic behavior.

Later stages of keratoacanthoma, when involution is occurring, no longer show proliferation. Most epithelial cells have undergone keratinization, and shrunken, necrotic cells may be seen. The latter process, known as *apoptosis*, appears to contribute to the involution. As healing occurs, the crater flattens. The base undergoes fibrosis, which is ultimately responsible for scarring, and the keratin plug is extruded.

The marked similarity of these lesions to well-differentiated squamous cell carcinoma is obvious. In a reclassification study by Kern and McCray, it was found that in only 81% of cases of keratoacanthoma could squamous cell carcinoma be ruled out, and in only 86% of cases of squamous cell carcinoma could keratoacanthoma be ruled out. Although many studies have been undertaken, as yet no absolute criteria distinguish the two entities.

Both solitary mucosal keratoacanthoma and lesions of multiple keratoacanthomas show the same histologic features as lesions of the skin. In the eruptive form, however, the lesions are much less crateriform.

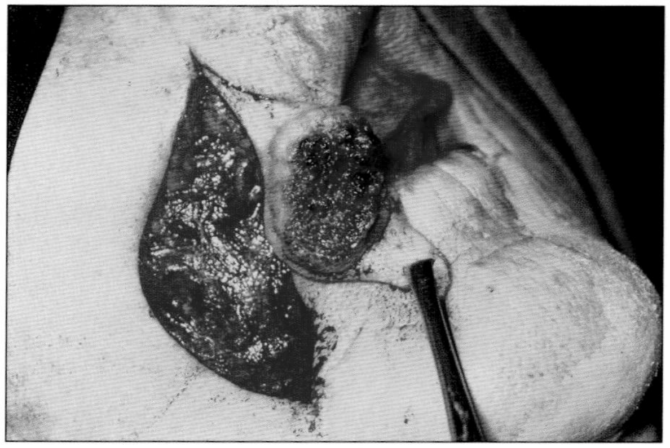

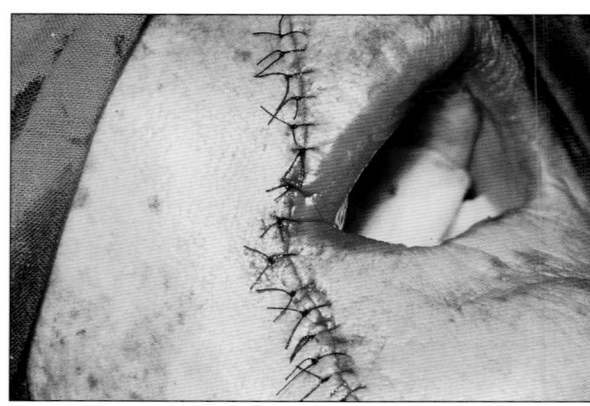

Fig 7-86a Excision of a keratoacanthoma on the facial skin shown in Fig 7-84b requires only 2- to 3-mm peripheral margins and a depth into the upper subcutaneous layer.

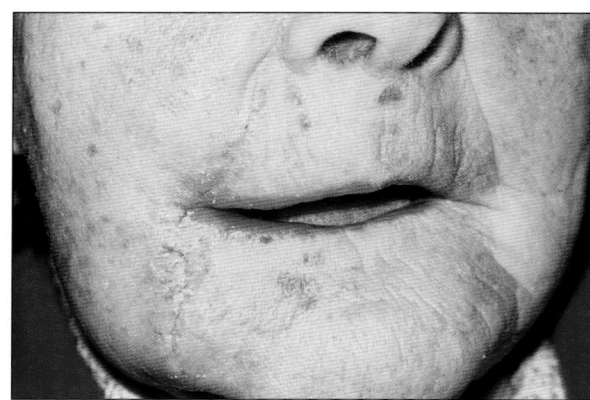

Fig 7-86b Most keratoacanthomas of skin can be closed primarily. Since keratoacanthomas are localized masses, the incision design can be made with consideration for natural skin folds (here the nasolabial crease) and for functional anatomic units (here the commissure).

Fig 7-86c The healed excisional area has blended into the nasolabial crease. The commissure remains undistorted.

TREATMENT ▶

Keratoacanthomas require excision because less than half involute on their own, and those that do result in a more obvious and depressed scar than those that are excised. Excision also provides the most reliable diagnosis and a cure for keratoacanthomas, as well as for the other serious considerations in the differential diagnosis.

The excision of a keratoacanthoma of skin requires only 2 to 3 mm of peripheral margins (Fig 7-86a) and a depth into the subcutaneous fat layers. Most excisional wounds can be closed primarily (Figs 7-86b and 7-86c). On the lower lip, lesions are excised with a V-shaped through-and-through excision with peripheral margins of 2 to 3 mm. The lip is closed in multiple layers from the mucosa outward to the skin, and special care should be taken to align the orbicularis oris muscle fibers with muscle fascia sutures (sutures through the muscle itself will cause necrosis of small portions of muscle) and to align the vermilion-cutaneous junctions from each side.

PROGNOSIS ▶

Excised keratoacanthomas rarely recur. New lesions may develop, however, in adjacent or other sun-exposed areas.

Basal Cell Carcinoma

CLINICAL PRESENTATION AND PATHOGENESIS ▶

Basal cell carcinoma (BCC) is the most common skin neoplasm. The ratio of basal cell carcinomas to squamous cell carcinomas of skin in sun-damaged skin is 5:1. Like squamous cell carcinoma of skin, BCC is found on the sun-exposed areas of the face, shoulders, and extremities. However, it is not seen on the lower lip, and it is less common on the forehead or pinna of the ear compared to squamous cell carcinoma of skin.

Correlation of BCC to ultraviolet light (particularly UVB 290 to 320 nm) as the primary carcinogen is related both to time and degree of exposure. Therefore, an increased incidence is found with advancing age, particularly after the age of 40 years. However, greater numbers of young people are developing BCC, ostensibly related to increased populations in the sunbelts (some have attributed the trend to depletion of the ozone layer, but this has not been proven).

Basal cell carcinoma is considered a malignant lesion by convention, yet it does not have metastatic potential. Nevertheless, it remains a dangerous lesion because of its subtle and relentless growth potential that may cause it to present as either a small scaly ulcer or as a large destructive lesion destroying

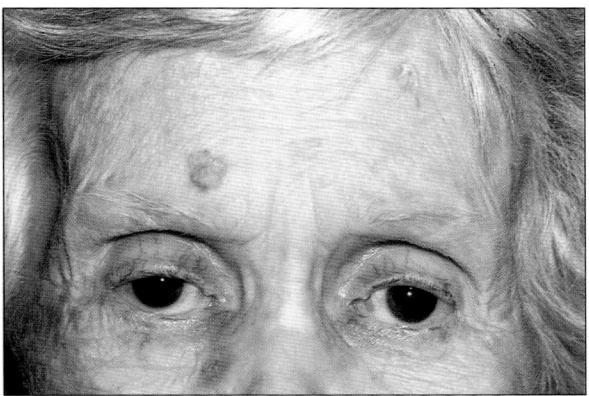

Fig 7-87 The nodular-ulcerative type of basal cell carcinoma is the most common. This one appears as a pearly dome-shaped mass.

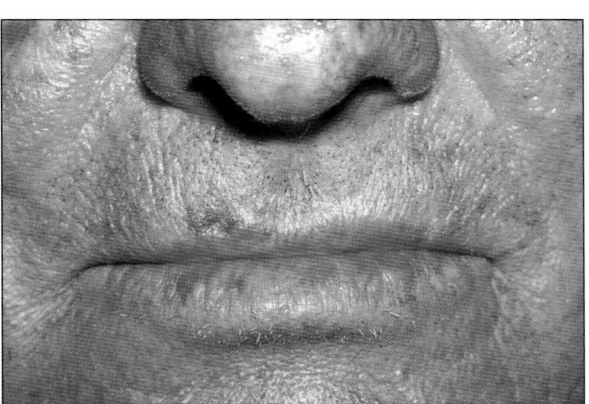

Fig 7-88 This nodular-ulcerative type of basal cell carcinoma on the upper lip produced an irregular ulcer with rolled edges (the so-called rodent ulcer). Note the areas of actinic keratosis on the lower lip.

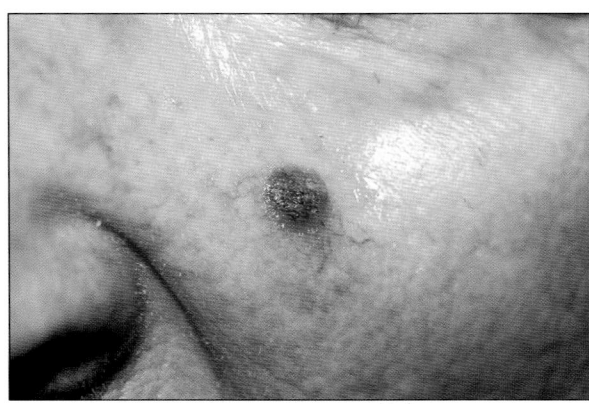

Fig 7-89 A pigmented basal cell carcinoma may be brown, black, or even blue. It may resemble a melanoma.

an entire side of the face. There are several histopathologic subtypes of basal cell carcinoma. However, the one that is most deeply infiltrative and destructive is the basosquamous cell subtype, which has features of both a basal cell carcinoma and a squamous cell carcinoma.

Today, there are five recognized clinical types of BCC, each with its own growth pattern and implications for treatment.

Nodular-Ulcerative Basal Cell Carcinoma

Nodular-ulcerative BCC is the most common type of BCC (Fig 7-87). It will appear as a pearly, dome-shaped papule. It may have small telangiectatic vessels within it, and it may ulcerate in the center. Usually irregular in shape, the ulceration has been termed the *rodent ulcer* because of its appearance of having been chewed by rodents (Fig 7-88). The growth pattern is irregular, and the lesion may form a multilobular mass. When ulcerations occur, the area often heals with some scarring, giving the false impression of a noncancerous condition. This cycle of ulceration, healing, growth, and re-ulceration has been known to create enormously destructive lesions.

Pigmented Basal Cell Carcinoma

Nodular BCC may also contain melanin from local melanocytes stimulated by the BCC and from dispersed melanin that is taken up by macrophages, which are then called melanophages. This imparts a black, brown, or blue color to the lesion depending on the depth of the melanin deposition (more superficial melanin appears black, deeper melanin transitions into brown and then blue) (Fig 7-89). Because this may make the lesion appear to be a melanoma, biopsy should be performed. However, close examination will show pigmented BCC retaining a pearly white, translucent surface and margin.

Cystic Basal Cell Carcinoma

Cystic BCC is merely a variant of the nodular-ulcerative type of BCC that has undergone subsurface cellular breakdown (Fig 7-90). Therefore, rather than creating an ulcer by surface necrosis, it creates a small cystic space through subsurface necrosis.

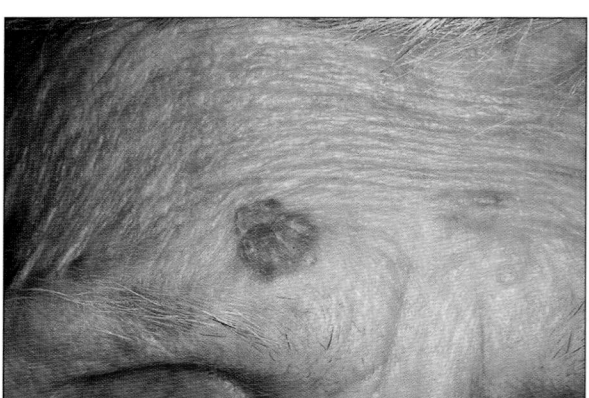

Fig 7-90 This histologically cystic basal cell carcinoma clinically appeared with an irregular elevated surface suggestive of vesicles.

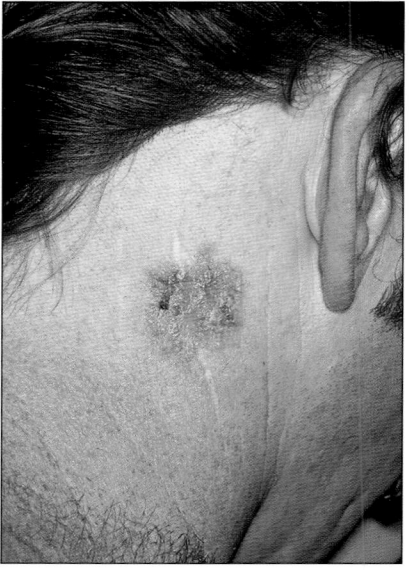

Fig 7-91 This large, flat, recurrent sclerosing basal cell carcinoma shows hypopigmentation, hyperpigmentation, and very irregular margins. Note the linear scar within its center resulting from a previous attempt to excise it.

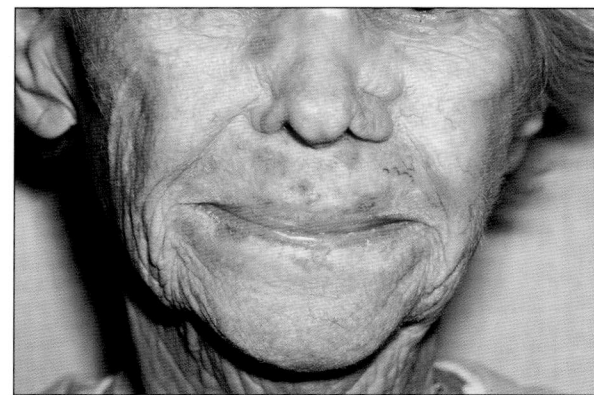

Fig 7-92 Superficial basal cell carcinomas will present as flat, red, scaly plaques.

Sclerosing or Morpheaform Basal Cell Carcinoma

Sclerosing or morpheaform BCC is a more serious form of BCC because its wide extension and deep invasion are masked by a nonulcerated, innocuous appearance (Fig 7-91). This lesion will appear as a pale white to yellowish flat scar or area of hypopigmentation. Its borders to normal skin are indistinct, showing gradual blending. The texture is firm, resembling scar tissue, and suggests the dermal extensions, which average 7.2 mm from the lesion's clinical border.

Superficial Basal Cell Carcinoma

Superficial BCC, the least aggressive form, is at the opposite end of the infiltrative growth spectrum from the sclerosing or morpheaform BCC (Fig 7-92). Superficial BCC spreads outward for several centimeters at a superficial level but does not show vertical invasive growth until very late. Therefore, it may cover a large surface area but is usually not indurated or ulcerated. Superficial BCCs usually manifest well-demarcated, red, scaly plaques that blanch under finger pressure like a hemangioma.

DIFFERENTIAL DIAGNOSIS ►

Basal cell carcinomas, in general, are one of a subset of skin lesions related to sun damage. The other lesions include *actinic keratosis, skin squamous cell carcinoma, keratoacanthoma*, and *melanoma*. The nodular-ulcerative type, in particular, will show the surface irregularity and ulcerations seen in actinic keratosis and skin squamous cell carcinoma. The pigmented BCC resembles a melanoma, but so does the cystic BCC, suggesting a nodular melanoma by its raised nodular quality. The sclerosing/morpheaform BCC may easily be confused with a *scar* or an area of *atrophic hypopigmented skin*. The superficial type may resemble a *vascular malformation* or *lymphangioma*.

HISTOPATHOLOGY ►

Basal cell carcinomas are usually well-demarcated lesions (Fig 7-93a), but some may be infiltrative, particularly the sclerosing type (see Fig 7-97). The nodular-ulcerative lesion, which is by far the most common form of BCC, usually consists of well-defined nests of basaloid cells within the dermis. Nests may

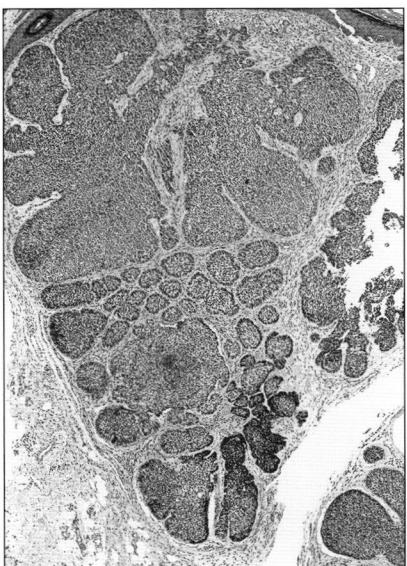

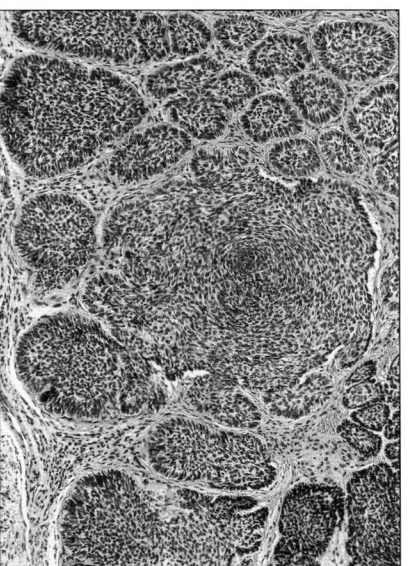

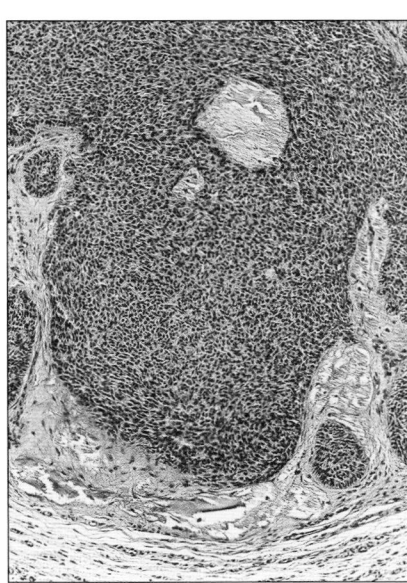

Fig 7-93a A basal cell carcinoma forming broad sheets and islands of uniform cells.

Fig 7-93b A higher-power view of Fig 7-93a. The smaller islands show peripheral palisading of cells. This is not apparent in all areas. Some squamous differentiation can be seen, and some artifactual separation of islands from the connective tissue is present.

Fig 7-94 This high-power view of a basal cell carcinoma shows the mucinous material adjacent to the tumor island.

originate from the basal cell layer of the overlying epidermis or from follicular epithelium. The cells have round to oval nuclei and scant cytoplasm. Intercellular bridges are typically absent. The cells at the periphery of the nest are often palisaded (Figs 7-93a and 7-93b). Degeneration secondary to ischemia may occur and give rise to cyst formation, which may be extensive. The resemblance to ameloblastoma may be striking, although the BCC may show individual cell necrosis and mitoses, which are not seen in the ameloblastoma.

The stroma of the BCC is an important component of the tumor. The area adjacent to the tumor islands is often mucinous (Fig 7-94), and retraction of the stroma from the islands is often seen (Fig 7-95a). It had been thought that this is a result of fixation artifact, but this does not seem to be the case. The absence of bullous pemphigoid antigen in these areas may be a factor. This phenomenon can be helpful diagnostically. Collagenases and proteases within the tumor are thought to contribute to the expansion of the lesion. Their absence in seborrheic keratosis is thought to be responsible for the exophytic growth of the basaloid cells in that lesion.

Many histologic variations may occur, some expressing differentiation to skin appendages. Clear cells, due to the presence of glycogen, recapitulate the outer root sheath of hair follicles. Squamoid changes and keratin cysts also are an expression of differentiation toward hair follicles and, when extensive, are called keratinizing BCCs. The adenoid BCC suggests a glandular pattern, and small cystic spaces surrounded by small basaloid cells are seen (Figs 7-95a and 7-95b). The pigmented BCC differs histologically only in the presence of numerous pigment-laden melanocytes and melanophages (Fig 7-96).

Of greater clinical significance are the superficial and sclerosing types of BCC, which are ill-defined, diffuse tumors and thus more subject to recurrence. The superficial type occurs predominantly on the trunk, but the sclerosing type has a predilection for the face. In the sclerosing tumor, there is a proliferation of cuboidal to fusiform basal cells as ill-defined cords within a cellular stroma (Fig 7-97). Consequently, identification of the tumor cells within the stroma is difficult, and to define the margin of the tumor it may be necessary to resort to immunohistochemistry for cytokeratin identification.

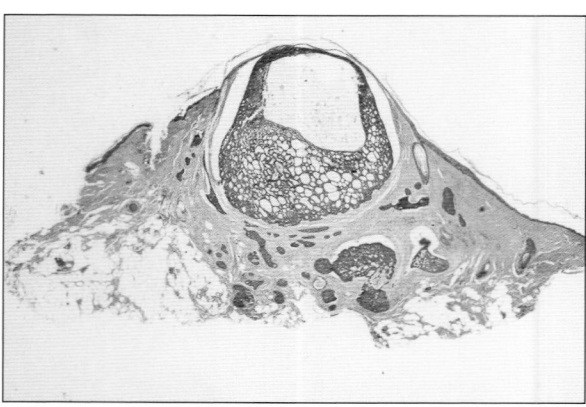

Fig 7-95a This basal cell carcinoma shows lack of encapsulation. There is cyst formation and an adenomatous arrangement of cells in addition to the more typical tumor islands. Retraction of stroma around some islands can be seen.

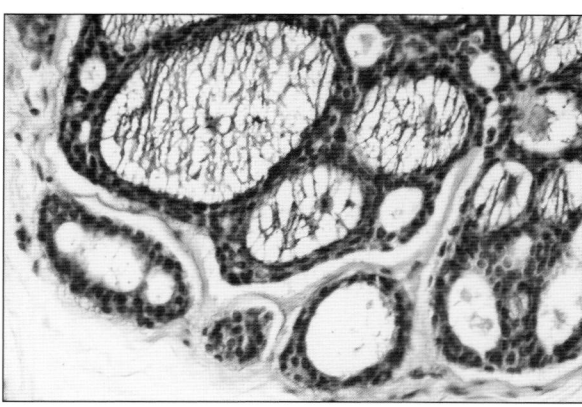

Fig 7-95b A higher-power view of Fig 7-95a showing glandular differentiation with a cribriform pattern.

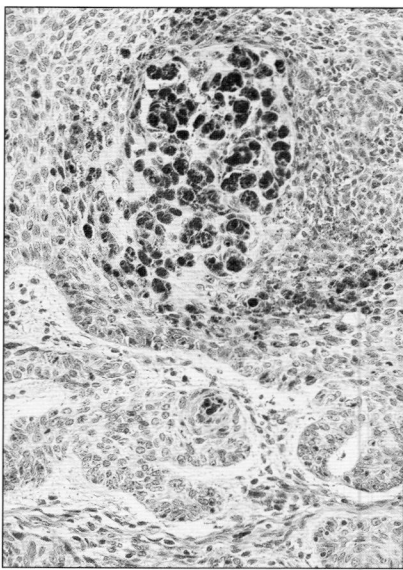

Fig 7-96 A pigmented basal cell carcinoma in which large numbers of melanophages are present. Melanocytes can usually be found intermingled with the tumor cells. They can be identified by means of a silver stain.

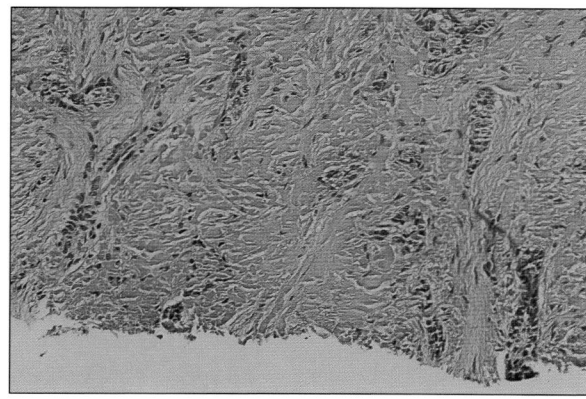

Fig 7-97 From the deep margin of a biopsy of a sclerosing basal cell carcinoma. There are infiltrating cords of cuboidal epithelial cells in a dense, abundant stroma.

The basosquamous cell carcinoma is essentially a basal cell carcinoma in which there is a significant squamous proliferation. Whether this represents a single entity is unclear. Some may represent a basal cell carcinoma with squamous metaplasia, while others may represent a collision tumor of a basal cell carcinoma and a squamous cell carcinoma.

The BCCs within the basal cell nevus syndrome are usually well-differentiated tumors. The base of the keratin pits in this syndrome demonstrates basaloid hyperplasia and sometimes even small basal cell carcinomas.

TREATMENT ▶ Most BCCs are clinically recognized and treated for cure at the first opportunity. If there is uncertainty about the diagnosis or type, an incisional biopsy from within the confines of the lesion is recommended.

The common nodular-ulcerative BCC that is less than 2 cm and not around the eyes or ears may be treated by electrodessication and curettage, excision, cryosurgery, or Mohs micrographic surgery with

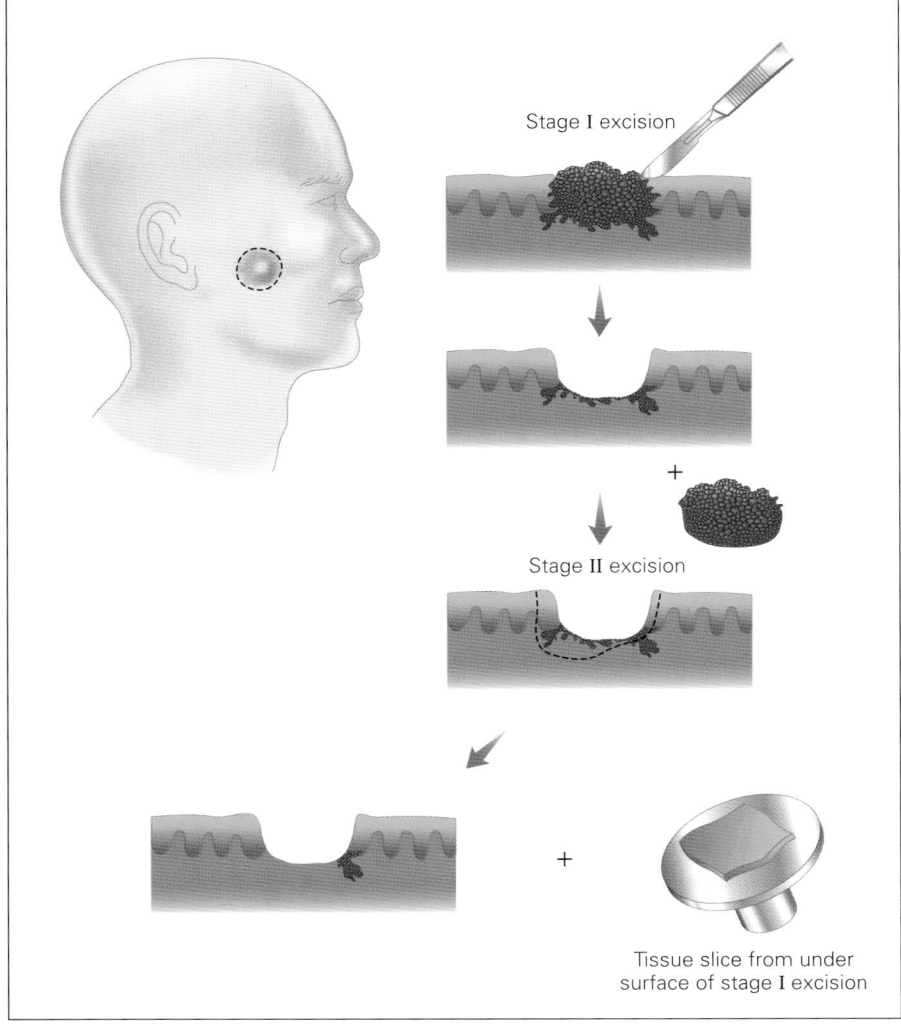

Fig 7-98a Mohs stage I excision excises the visible lesion to its anticipated depth of invasion. The specimen is mounted for frozen assessment. (Redrawn from Leffell DJ and Brown MD, *Manual of Skin Surgery*, with permission from John Wiley-Liss Publishers.)

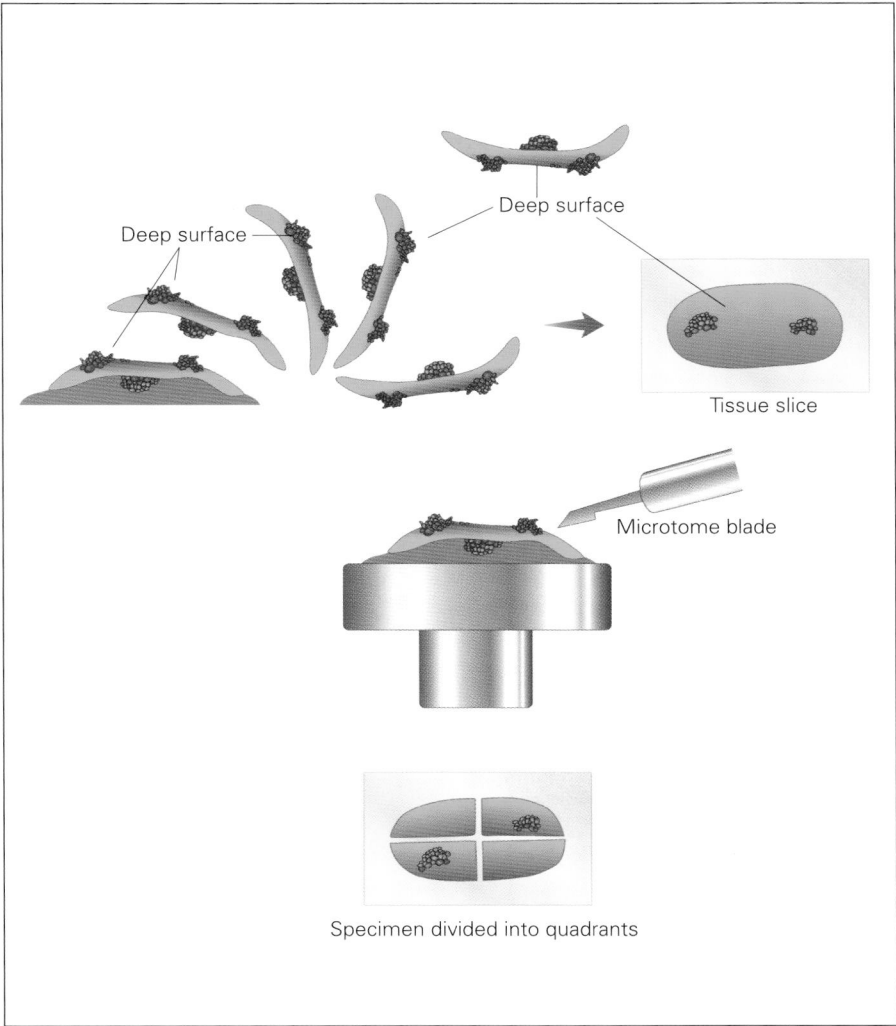

Fig 7-98b The first excised specimen is mounted on the microtome with a deep surface facing upward. In this diagram, the frozen section–processed slide identifies two areas of residual tumor. (Redrawn from Leffell DJ and Brown MD, *Manual of Skin Surgery*, with permission from John Wiley-Liss Publishers.)

equal outcomes. A 98% cure rate is recognized for surgery of lesions of this size if 4- to 5-mm margins are employed.

Selection of treatment modality is often related to the clinician's training and experience. Some of the principles that must be considered include the following.

Cryosurgery

Cryosurgery is limited by the depth of freezing achievable. Unless specialized thermocouples are used, it is limited to the superficial BCC with less than 3 mm of invasion.

Electrodessication and Cautery

Electrodessication and cautery are limited to the nodular-ulcerative type and the superficial type of BCC because of absolute need for margin assessment by frozen sections of the other types.

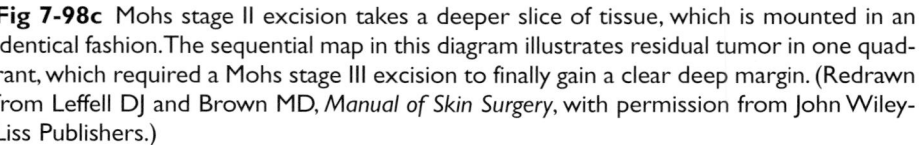

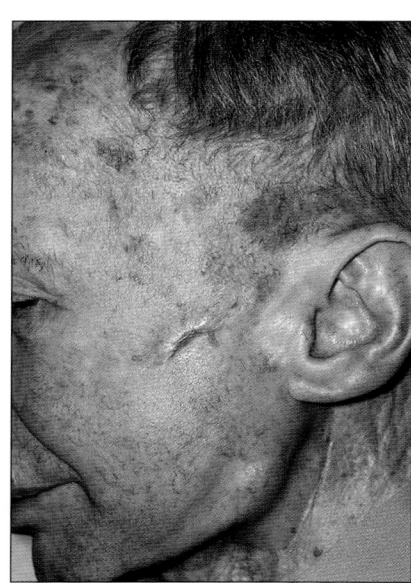

Fig 7-98c Mohs stage II excision takes a deeper slice of tissue, which is mounted in an identical fashion. The sequential map in this diagram illustrates residual tumor in one quadrant, which required a Mohs stage III excision to finally gain a clear deep margin. (Redrawn from Leffell DJ and Brown MD, *Manual of Skin Surgery*, with permission from John Wiley-Liss Publishers.)

Fig 7-98d Because the Mohs technique allows the area of excision to heal by secondary intention, it often leaves an unacceptable scar that requires revision.

Mohs Micrographic Surgery

Mohs micrographic surgery enables fine control of the margins of excised tissue, providing greater assurance of complete excision with minimal excision of normal tissue. Mohs micrographic technique is particularly advantageous in the sclerosing/morpheaform type and all types of BCC around the eyelids and canthal areas. It was first described in 1941 by Fredrick Mohs, who used zinc chloride ($ZnCl_2$) as an in situ tissue fixative. Mohs's concept involved mixing $ZnCl_2$, which was being used in dentistry of the era, to accomplish a chemical gingivectomy as a treatment for periodontal disease. It was placed in a vehicle paste (stibinite) and applied to skin lesions over 24 hours. Because of its dehydrating effects, the $ZnCl_2$ fixated the tissue to a depth of 2 to 3 mm. Mohs then excised the lesion in layers and examined each layer microscopically. Each visit excised the lesion to bleeding edges or to the patient's report of pain. He progressed with several such outpatient visits until he obtained tumor-free margins and a tumor-free base. The procedure has since been modified to a 1-day procedure using unfixed fresh tissue and

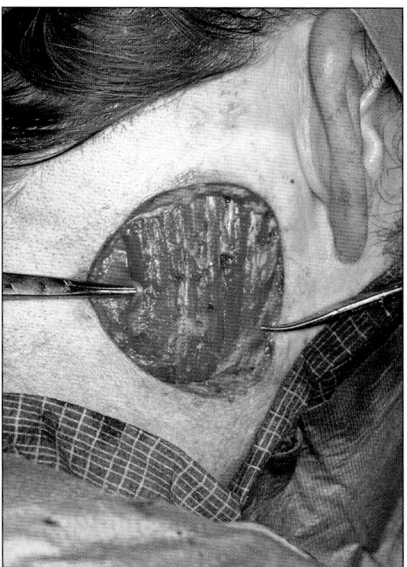

Fig 7-99a The sclerosing basal cell carcinoma shown in Fig 7-91 required a wide excision with 1.5-cm margins at a depth to the muscle fascia of the sternocleidomastoid muscle. Here the lesser occipital nerve and greater auricular nerve are pointed out.

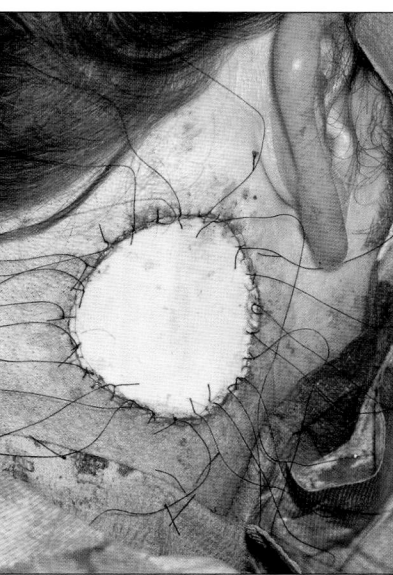

Fig 7-99b A split-thickness skin graft is a practical reconstruction that will not obscure a recurrence. Here the skin graft is sutured to the wound periphery.

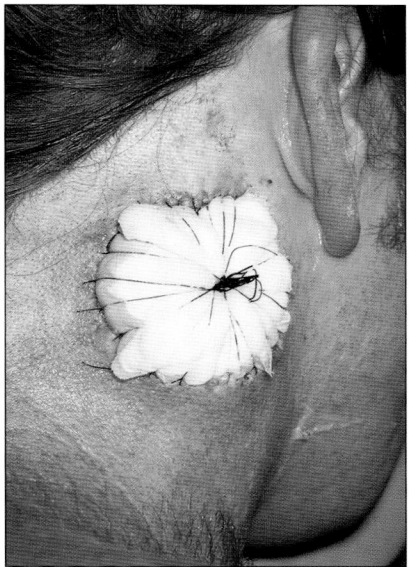

Fig 7-99c A bolster dressing will promote healing to this type of an irregular wound base. Here the initial layer is Vaseline gauze (Kendall Health Care) followed by sterile cotton and 3-0 silk tieover sutures, which apply downward pressure when tightened.

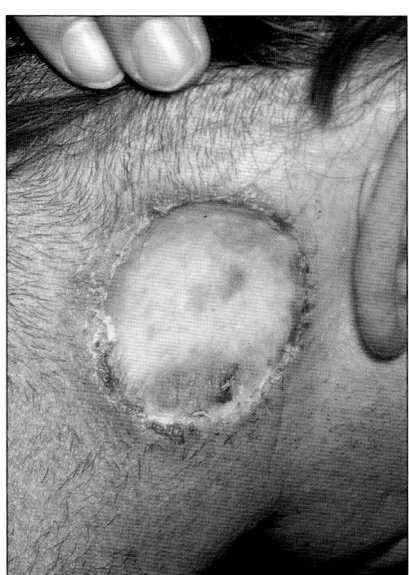

Fig 7-99d Bolster dressings achieve a nearly 100% take of the skin graft. A skin graft such as this will contract and become less noticeable over 1 or more years. If there is no recurrence, it can then be excised and a revision accomplished to improve the appearance.

cryostat-generated frozen sections. The lesion is accurately mapped by scalpel excision in thin layers, which are cut into quadrants before frozen section preparation (Fig 7-98a). Elimination of persistent tumor may be observed in any location by means of serial layers oriented to the same quadrants. Drawings may facilitate construction of a three-dimensional model indicating the excisional block and the tumor with all of its projections within it (Figs 7-98b and 7-98c).

The Mohs technique can be tissue sparing and, when strictly applied, is associated with a high cure rate. However, since the wound is left to heal by secondary intention, it often leaves an unacceptable scar (Fig 7-98d).

Local Excision

Surgical excision with frozen section assessment is not greatly different from Mohs micrographic surgery. Each is indicated primarily for larger tumors and for recurrent tumors, although they can be used to eradicate the other types as well.

Local excision has not been entirely replaced by Mohs micrographic surgery and remains a reliable and time-honored method for treating BCCs. Local excision with routine frozen section control may be more practical in recurrent BCC, in larger or deeper lesions, and in sclerosing/morpheaform types of lesions. Smaller lesions and those located in areas that can be readily closed should be closed primarily. Larger excisions can be practically managed with split-thickness skin grafts (Fig 7-99a). For best results, the skin graft should be adapted with an overlying pressure bolster (Figs 7-99b to 7-99d). Other large excisions may require local rhomboid or rotation flaps (see Figs 7-105a to 7-105g) or more rarely myocutaneous or free vascular flaps (Figs 7-100a to 7-100f).

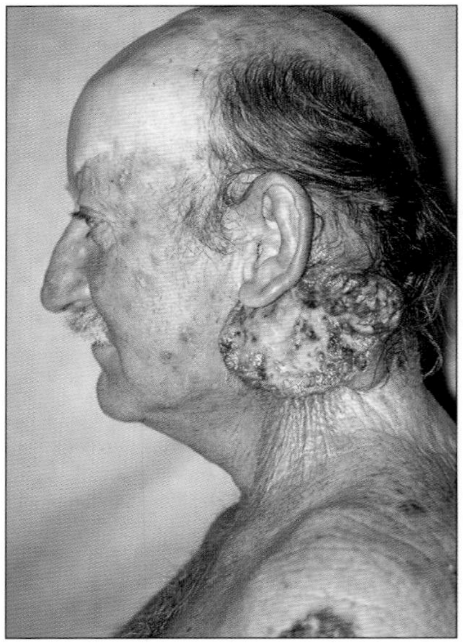

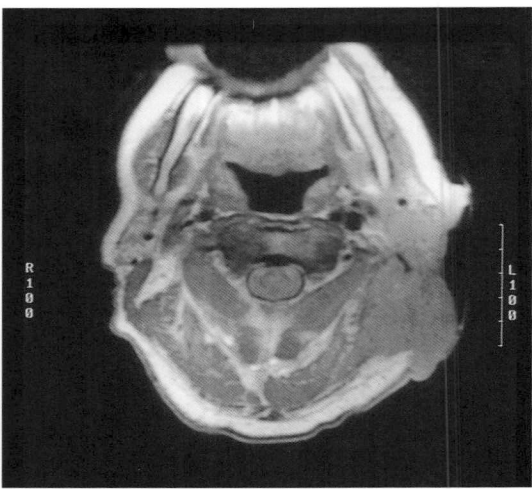

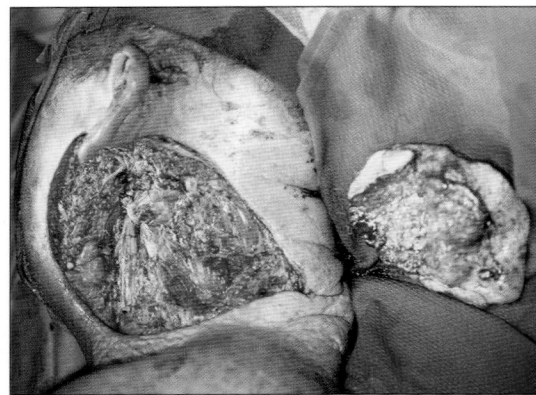

Fig 7-100a Some basal cell carcinomas are of the basosquamous type and will be deeply infiltrating, extensive, and very necrotic.

Fig 7-100b Infiltration of this basosquamous cell carcinoma extends into the splenious capitus muscle, the transverse process of the atlas (C-1), and the prevertebral fascia.

Fig 7-100c This basosquamous cell carcinoma required a wide excision using 2.5-cm margins and a direct neck dissection down to the prevertebral fascia.

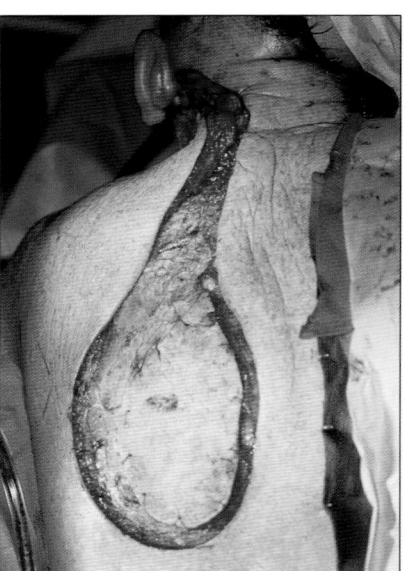

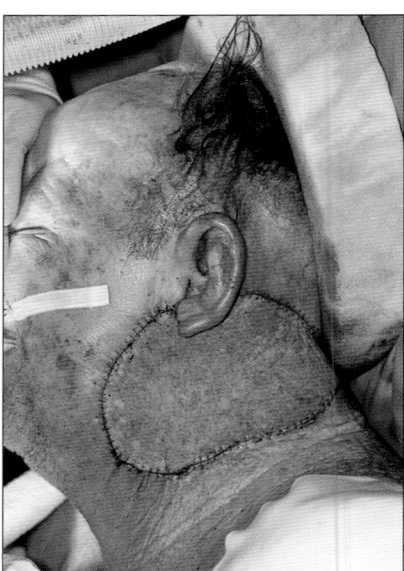

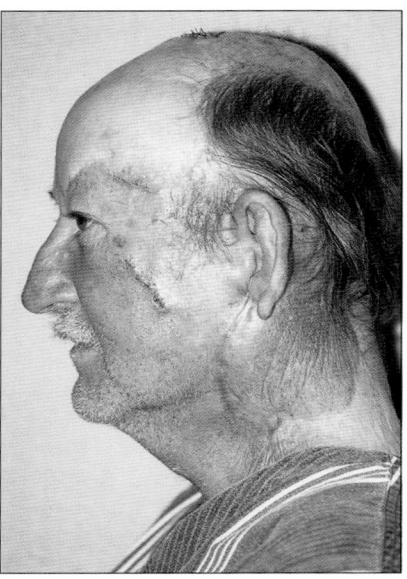

Fig 7-100d Some large defects of skin and underlying muscle created by the excision of skin cancers require myocutaneous or free vascular tissue flaps. Here a large skin paddle on a trapezius myocutaneous flap is being developed.

Fig 7-100e The trapezius myocutaneous flap is ideally suited to reconstruct defects in the posterior triangle and nape of neck areas.

Fig 7-100f The healed trapezius myocutaneous flap is an excellent color and thickness match. Excising this necrotic tumor protected the carotid artery from erosion and eliminated the significant odor and unsightly appearance of the tumor.

Radiotherapy

Radiotherapy is a necessary and useful treatment modality for elderly patients or for those who cannot tolerate the required surgery or anesthesia. It may also be a consideration in areas around the eyelids and canthus, where surgery of any type can cause dysfunction of eyelid closure or epiphora. Usually, BCCs treated by radiotherapy receive 5,000 cGy to 6,500 cGy of electron beam radiotherapy, which is preferred over the usual beta particle source for its reduced depth of penetration.

Generally, the prognosis for BCC is excellent. Recurrences are related to several factors: (*1*) Identification of tumor cells at the margins of an excision is strongly associated with recurrence. When tumor cells are found at an excision margin, the recurrence rate rises to 30% from the overall rate of 3%. Therefore, for all patients with questionable margins, techniques using frozen section margin assessment, as well as re-excision, are preferred over a "wait and see" approach. (*2*) Recurrent lesions develop after a second treatment 18% of the time, compared to 3% for a first treatment approach. Therefore, aggressive initial treatment is recommended. It is also noted that many of the disfiguring types of BCC started as small, recurrent lesions. (*3*) The sclerosing/morpheaform type has a high recurrence rate due to its diffuse lateral and deep infiltration. These lesions require more aggressive initial therapy and close follow-up. (*4*) Recurrences are related to depth of invasion and location. Basal cell carcinomas around the nose, eyes, and ears, where tumor cells readily migrate along the tarsal plate or perichondrium, are the most recurrent.

It must also be recognized that new primary BCCs will arise in sun-damaged skin. Sun exposure precautions, the use of sunscreens, and frequent examinations are part of overall management (see also the section on actinic keratosis treatment, pages 352 to 355).

Squamous Cell Carcinoma of Skin

The classic description and the most common form of squamous cell carcinoma of skin is a small ulcer or exophytic mass emerging from an area of actinic keratosis or sun-damaged skin. These carcinomas are like basal cell carcinomas in their appearance, their relationship to sun-damaged skin, and their causative carcinogen, ultraviolet light (UVB 290 to 320 nm, in particular). However, there are distinctions in distribution. Squamous cell carcinoma will occur in most areas of sun-damaged skin, including the scalp, top of the pinnas, dorsum of the hands, and lower lip vermilion, areas where basal cell carcinomas rarely develop.

Most squamous cell carcinomas of the skin behave much less aggressively than their counterparts on oral mucosa. Although they will sometimes ulcerate and proliferate into exophytic masses (Fig 7-101), they will usually not invade deeply until late and usually not metastasize to regional lymph nodes. They are usually less than 4 mm in thickness and are not invasive beyond the upper dermis. Their incidence of regional lymph node metastasis is about 1%. There are two important exceptions to this general biologic behavior. The first is a form often called the *basosquamous cell carcinoma*, which at the time of presentation usually has invaded through the dermis and is more than 6 mm in thickness. These tend to erode into underlying tissues including bone, have a greater recurrence potential, and will frequently metastasize to regional lymph nodes, increasing the overall regional lymph node metastasis incidence for all skin squamous cell carcinomas to 7% (Fig 7-102). The other exception is the rare skin squamous cell carcinoma that arises in areas of skin irradiation damage, burn injury, chronic ulcers, or from what has been called *Bowen disease of skin*, which is actually carcinoma in situ. The carcinogen causing these exceptions in squamous cell carcinoma of the skin is either different from ultraviolet light or synergistic with it to more severely damage DNA and create a more aggressive oncogene expression.

Squamous cell carcinoma of skin is a subset of sun-damage–related skin cancers and premalignancies that have an overlapping general clinical appearance. These include *actinic keratosis, basal cell carcinoma, lentigo maligna melanoma, melanoma,* and *keratoacanthoma.*

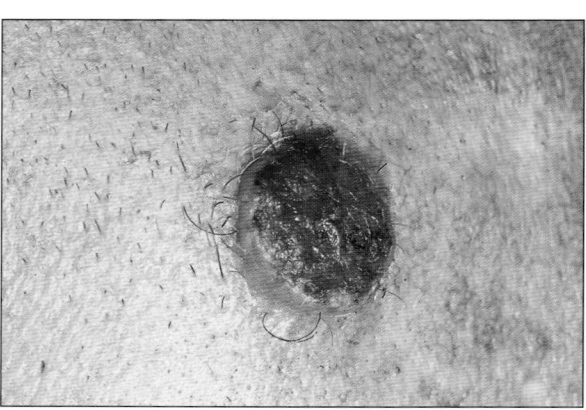

Fig 7-101 Although most squamous cell carcinomas of skin are exophytic and slow growing, because of neglect some may nevertheless become ulcerative, infiltrating, and very necrotic.

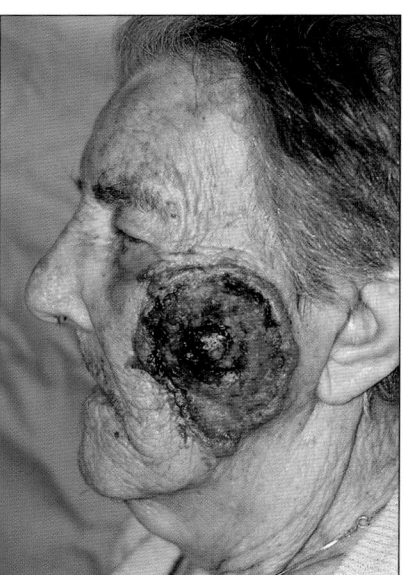

Fig 7-102 The basosquamous cell carcinoma is larger, grows faster, and infiltrates deeper structures.

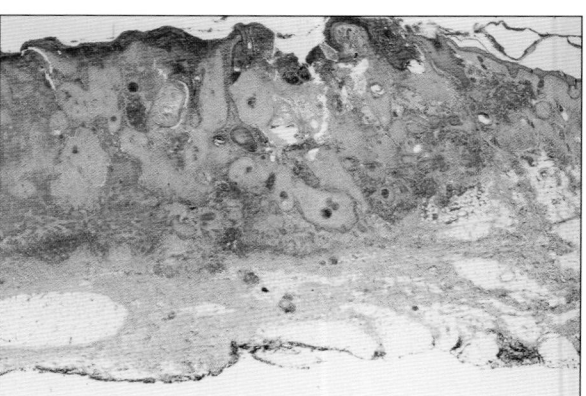

Fig 7-103 A squamous cell carcinoma of the skin that is typically well differentiated. Numerous keratin pearls can be seen.

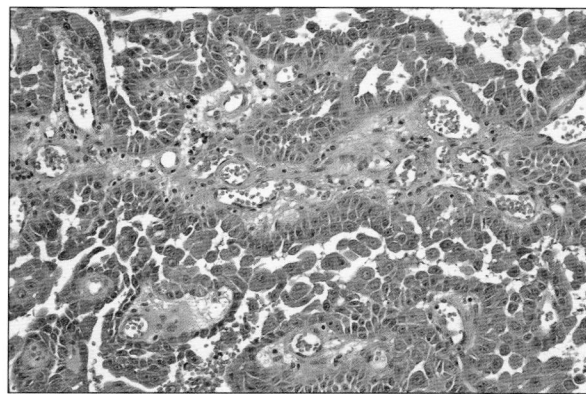

Fig 7-104 This adenoid squamous cell carcinoma shows prominent acantholysis, which results in a pseudoglandular appearance.

HISTOPATHOLOGY

Squamous cell carcinomas of the skin typically are well-differentiated, keratin-producing tumors (Fig 7-103) that are histologically identical to their oral mucosa counterparts.

There is a variant known as *adenoid* (or *acantholytic*) *squamous cell carcinoma* that also tends to occur in sun-damaged skin and sometimes the lower lip. This type is characterized by marked acantholysis, which creates a gland-like pattern (Fig 7-104).

TREATMENT

Lesions unresponsive to topical 2% 5-fluorouracil or clinically suggestive of squamous cell carcinoma of the skin should be excised with 5-mm margins and the margins assessed with frozen sections (Fig 7-105a). If the margins are free of tumor and the tumor thickness is less than 4 mm, no further excision is required (Figs 7-105b and 7-105c). In most cases, a primary closure can be accomplished. In the moderately sized excisions, local advancement flaps are recommended (Figs 7-105d to 7-105f). Local advancement flaps have the advantage of ideal color match and thickness match as compared to distant flaps (Fig 7-105g). Lesions that exhibit dermal invasion into the reticular dermis and are 4 to 8 mm in

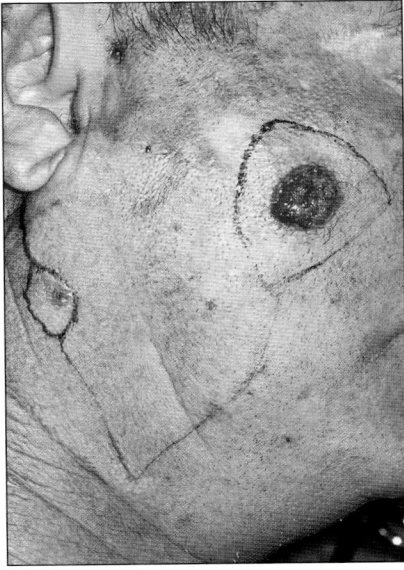

Fig 7-105a Localized skin squamous cell carcinomas are excised with 0.5 mm to 1.0-cm margins. Here the excision is outlined to include a local rotation flap to reconstruct the anticipated defect.

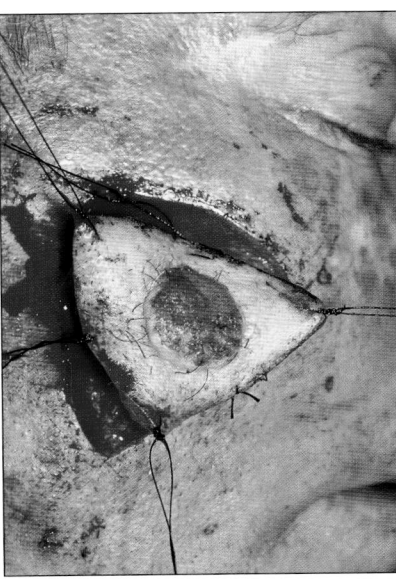

Fig 7-105b The excision includes the subcutaneous layer but is superficial to the muscles of facial expression and hence the facial nerve fibers, which enter the muscles on their deep surface.

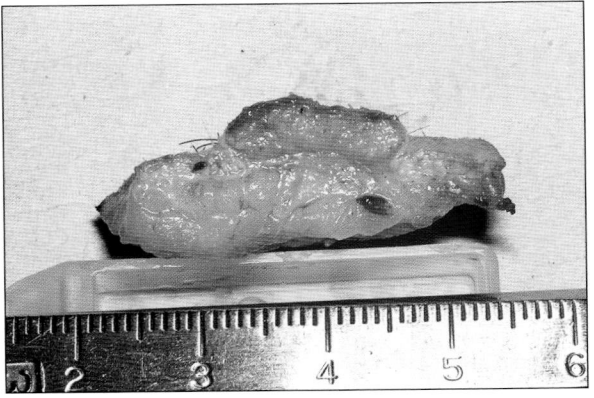

Fig 7-105c A bisection of this skin squamous cell carcinoma shows grossly uninvolved deep and peripheral margins. The depth of excision into the subcutaneous layer (about 1 cm) includes the papillary and reticular dermis.

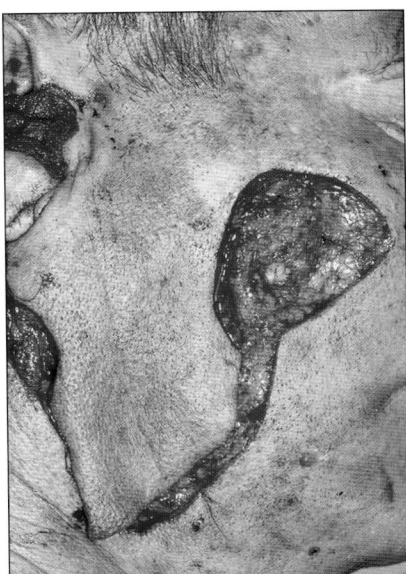

Fig 7-105d This local flap is partially a random-pattern skin-subcutaneous flap and is partially based on the transverse facial artery.

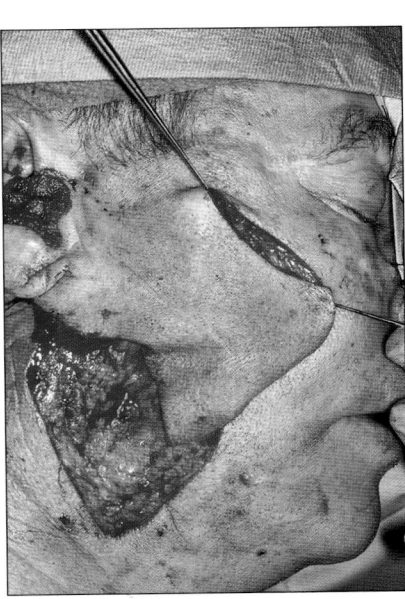

Fig 7-105e The skin flap must be sufficiently mobilized to rotate into the defect without tension.

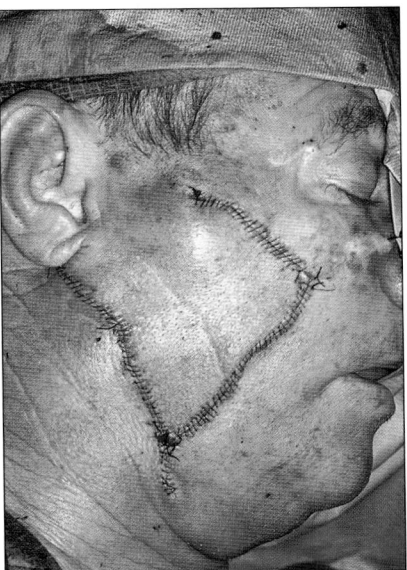

Fig 7-105f Local skin flaps take advantage of the redundancy of skin in this age group, which allows for undermining and a tension-free closure of the donor area.

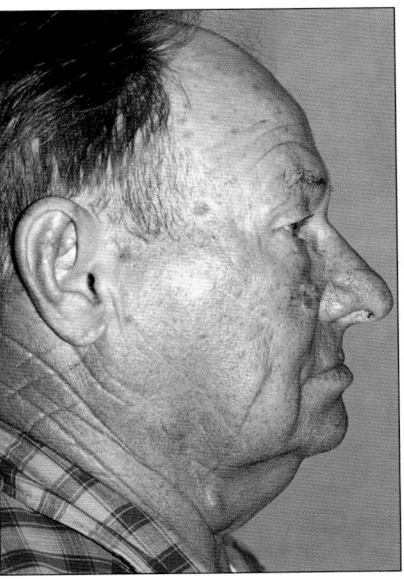

Fig 7-105g Local skin flaps are ideal because of their color and thickness match as well as the ability to design the flap in natural skin folds or resting skin tension lines.

thickness require excision with margins of 1.5 cm with frozen section assessment even if the original margins were tumor free. Tumors that penetrate through the dermis into the subcutaneous fat or exceed 8 mm should undergo a wide field excision with at least 2.5-cm margins and a prophylactic functional neck dissection if the neck is staged N_0. Clinical evidence of lymph node involvement requires either a functional neck dissection if the neck is staged N_1 or a type of radical neck dissection if the neck is staged N_2 or N_3. Large excisions such as these usually require myocutaneous or free vascular flaps as illustrated in Figs 7-100c to 7-100f.

The primary squamous cell carcinoma of skin may be treated with the technique of Mohs micrographic surgery (see pages 364 to 365) as an alternative to scalpel excision with frozen section control. This technique is considered when lesions occur around the eyes and for some larger tumors.

PROGNOSIS AND FOLLOW-UP ▶

Isolated skin squamous cell carcinomas from sun-damaged skin have a 95% cure rate. However, many occur in a field of sun-damaged skin, actinic keratosis, basal cell carcinomas, and other skin squamous cell carcinomas. Many affected individuals need ongoing follow-up, sunscreen use, sun exposure precautions, and periodic treatment courses of isotretinoin or topical 2% 5-fluorouracil.

The skin squamous cell carcinoma exceptions—those that are more erosive, infiltrating, and associated with a higher metastatic potential—have a reduced cure potential to about 60% and often involve multiple disfiguring recurrences until the tumor is unreachable and threatens brain or vital neck structures, eventuating in death.

Merkel Cell Tumor

CLINICAL PRESENTATION AND PATHOGENESIS ▶

Merkel cells are specialized neurotactile dermal cells in skin derived from neuroepithelium and known to contain abundant neurosecretory granules. Although rare, when these cells form tumors, the tumors may mimic aggressive skin basal cell carcinomas clinically (Fig 7-106). This skin cancer was first described by Toker in 1978 as a "trabecular carcinoma." Since the identification of numerous secretory granules in its cytoplasm, it has been recognized as a neuroendocrine cell carcinoma.

Clinically, the tumors represent aggressive skin cancers. They can occur at almost any age but have a distinct predilection for the elderly (60 to 100 years). They will present mostly as large, indurated mass lesions that may have small surface ulcerations. Early tumors will be acne-like or violaceous or purple nodules, but these will soon enlarge into the more commonly observed firm, indurated mass. The primary lesion has a predilection for the facial skin and the skin portion of the lips. Early lymph node metastasis is common (50% to 90% have lymph node spread at the time of diagnosis).

DIFFERENTIAL DIAGNOSIS ▶

It would be statistically unrealistic for a clinician to readily diagnose a Merkel cell tumor when faced with an indurated skin cancer. Most cases suggest the more common skin cancers: *squamous cell carcinoma of the skin, basal cell carcinoma, melanoma,* and, less likely because of its absence of peripheral extension, *keratoacanthoma*. More rarely, a *non-Hodgkin lymphoma* or a *metastasis to skin* from a distant site will create a similar appearance. If the lesion occurs on the lip, as some Merkel cell carcinomas do, an additional consideration would be a *traumatic eosinophilic granuloma*.

DIAGNOSTIC WORK-UP ▶

Work-up requires incisional biopsy within the confines of the lesion. There is also an elevation of serum neuron–specific enolase levels, which is not specific but suggestive of this tumor.

HISTOPATHOLOGY ▶

This is a monotonous, round cell tumor consisting of rather closely packed cells in sheets, clusters, or trabecular arrangement. The tumor is found in the dermis and infiltrates the subcutis with entrapment of fat cells and vascular invasion. A grenz zone separates the tumor from the epidermis (Fig 7-107a). The cells have round to oval nuclei with evenly distributed chromatin and inconspicuous nucleoli. There is a striking degree of mitotic activity (Fig 7-107b), and the cytoplasm is scanty and poorly defined. Although argyrophilic granules are present, their sparsity can make silver nitrate staining unreliable for identification. The stroma is very vascular, contributing to the often reddish color of these tumors clinically.

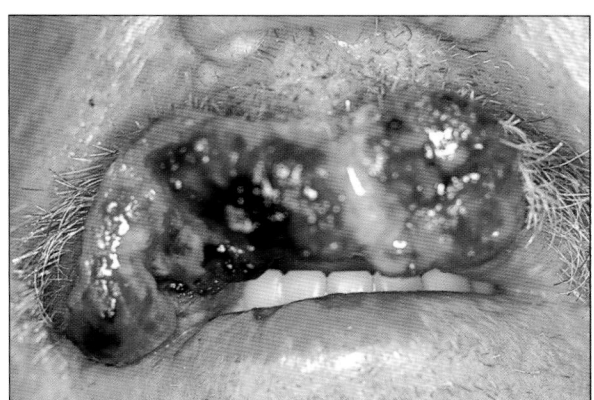

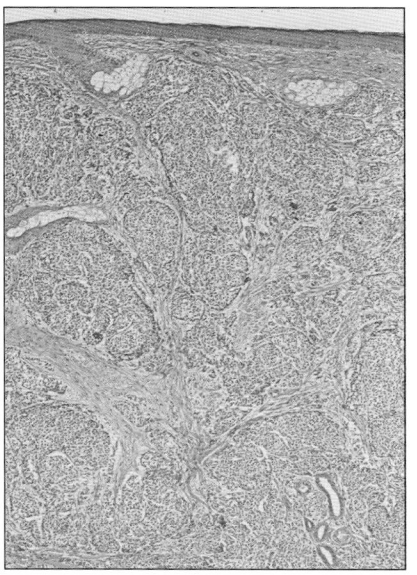

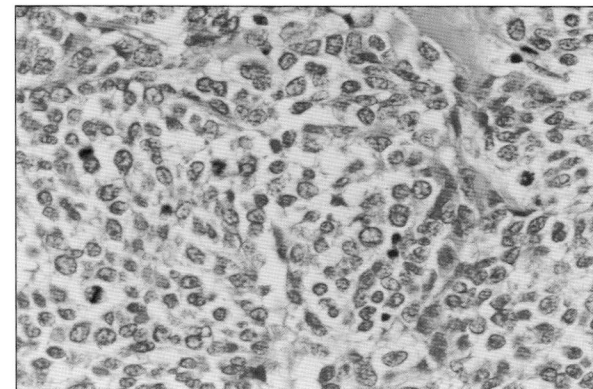

Fig 7-106 This extensive ulcerative Merkel cell tumor clinically resembles an erosive basosquamous cell or basal cell carcinoma.

Fig 7-107a A Merkel cell carcinoma showing a pattern of clusters of cells and a grenz zone (tumor-free zone) below the epithelium.

Fig 7-107b A higher-power view of Fig 7-107a shows a rather uniform population of cells and a high rate of mitotic activity.

Merkel cell carcinoma must be histopathologically distinguished from malignant lymphomas and metastatic carcinoma, particularly small cell carcinoma of the lung. The nuclei in malignant lymphoma are not usually as uniformly rounded as in Merkel cell carcinoma, and while lymphomas are positive for leukocyte-common antigen, this is lacking in Merkel cell tumors. Distinction from metastatic small cell carcinoma is more difficult. Both are cytokeratin positive with a paranuclear distribution, but small cell carcinomas are usually positive for carcino-embryonic antigen, while Merkel cell carcinoma is not. Ultrastructurally, Merkel cell carcinomas are characterized by the presence of cytoplasmic dense-core, neurosecretory, membrane-bound granules and perinuclear intermediate filaments arranged in whorls (fibrous bodies).

TREATMENT ▶

Too few cases of Merkel cell carcinoma have been reported to determine the most reliable treatment modalities. There is good evidence that wide local excision with 2-cm margins and, depending on the location, ipsilateral or bilateral neck dissections are preferred. It would also seem prudent to consider postoperative radiotherapy in the dose range of 6,000 cGy to 6,800 cGy in elderly patients who are not candidates for more aggressive surgery.

PROGNOSIS AND FOLLOW-UP ▶

Merkel cell tumors have a high recurrence rate (30% to 60%) by re-emergence of the original tumor, a metastasis incidence of 50% to 90%, and a death rate of 15% to 50%, all indicating a poor prognosis. Follow-up should be at 3-month intervals for the first 2 years and every 6 months thereafter.

Malignant Tumors of Adnexal Structures

Malignant skin appendage tumors are very rare and almost never anticipated. The oral and maxillofacial specialist may diagnose one when excising a small lesion presumed to be a cosmetic imperfection or a benign adnexal tumor or by accomplishing an incisional biopsy of a large, fungating, neglected lesion. In any of these situations, the five malignant adnexal tumors included here—microcystic adnexal carcinoma, ductal eccrine carcinomas, mucinous eccrine carcinoma, pilomatrix carcinoma, and sebaceous carcinoma—are true malignant counterparts of the benign skin adnexal tumors discussed in Chapter 6.

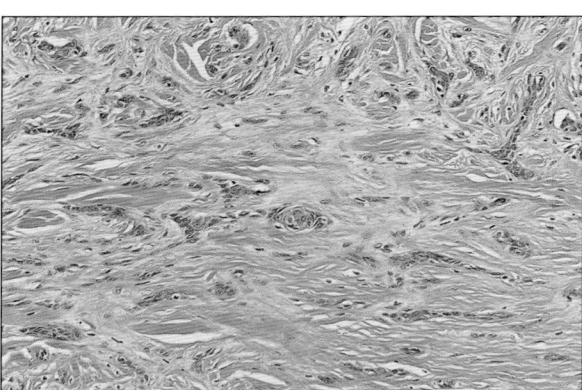

Fig 7-108 Microcystic adnexal carcinoma demonstrating extensive infiltration by the tumor islands in a dense, hyalinized stroma.

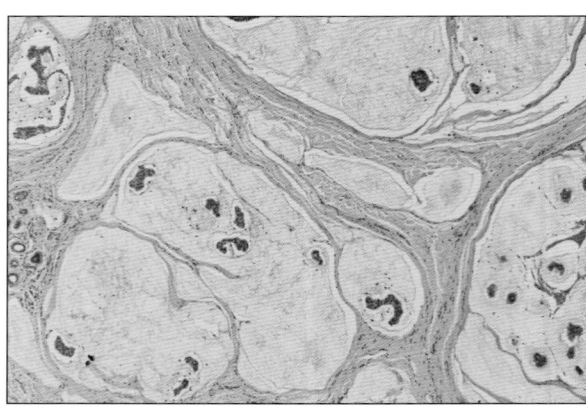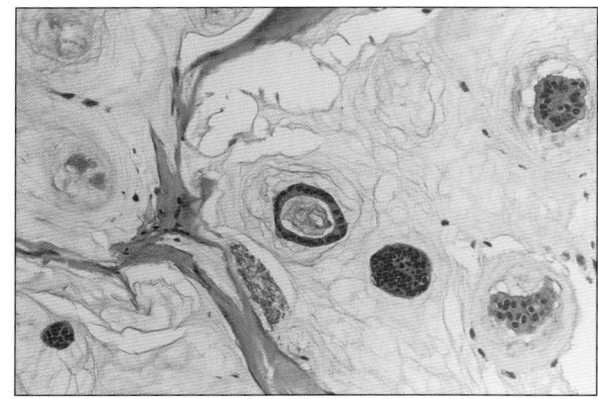

Figs 7-109a and 7-109b A mucinous eccrine carcinoma showing pools of mucin within which are found small islands of tumor cells.

Microcystic Adnexal Carcinoma (Malignant Syringoma)

CLINICAL PRESENTATION

Microcystic adnexal carcinoma has a marked predilection for the nasolabial fold and upper lip. It is usually slow growing and appears as a tan-to-pink, indurated plaque-like lesion or as a nodular or cystic lesion. Numbness of the lip has been associated with this tumor. These neoplasms occur over a wide age range. Some have developed in patients previously irradiated for acne.

HISTOPATHOLOGY

Cytologically bland and uniform cells form nests and cords that may be attached to each other, resulting in a branching appearance. Tail-like extensions, as seen in syringomas, may be present. Some tumors have ductal structures and some show keratinization. Infiltration of the subcutaneous tissue and perivascular invasion are common. The stroma is dense and hyalinized. Bland cytology with extensive infiltration are the characteristic features (Fig 7-108).

TREATMENT

Local excision with 1.5- to 2-cm tumor-free margins is indicated. Frozen section control is necessary because of the tumor's perivascular spread. Prophylactic neck dissection is not required.

Ductal Eccrine Carcinoma

CLINICAL PRESENTATION

Ductal eccrine carcinoma is a slow-growing but infiltrating tumor with a propensity to undergo lymph node metastasis. Tumors of ductal eccrine carcinoma appear as skin-colored or reddish nodules that slowly increase in size over several years. About half are ulcerated. Middle-aged and elderly individuals are most frequently affected.

HISTOPATHOLOGY

The tumor is infiltrative, and mitoses are present. The cells proliferate in anastomosing cords and nests. Tubular structures with a small lumen lined by one or two layers of cells may be seen. Although these lesions may mimic metastatic carcinoma, their slow growth argues against that diagnosis.

TREATMENT

Since this is an infiltrating tumor with a propensity to undergo lymph node metastasis, excision with 1.5-cm, tumor-free margins is indicated, and a lymph node neck dissection is recommended. Radiation is not effective. About 50% of cases metastasize to regional lymph nodes, although distant metastasis to lung, liver, and bone occur as well. Local recurrence occurs in 70% to 80% of cases.

Mucinous Eccrine Carcinoma

CLINICAL PRESENTATION

Mucinous eccrine carcinoma is similar in clinical appearance to ductal carcinoma but is less infiltrative and less likely to undergo lymph node metastasis. It has a marked predilection for facial skin.

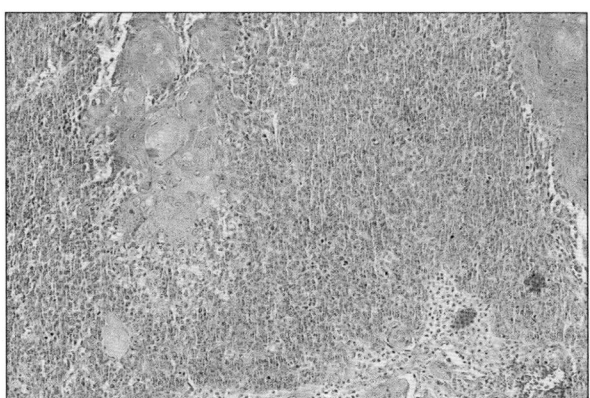

Fig 7-110 Pilomatrix carcinoma showing some shadow cells and the presence of frequent mitoses. This mitotic activity is a key factor in classifying this lesion as malignant.

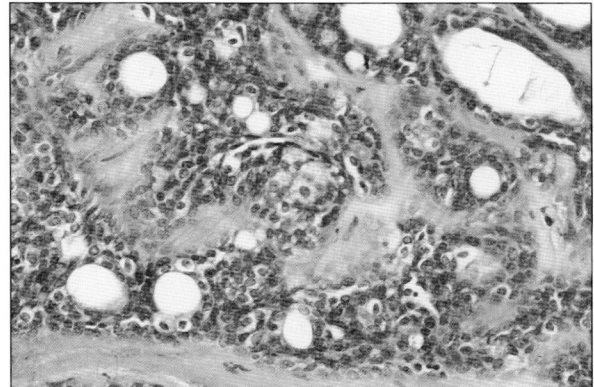

Fig 7-111 A sebaceous carcinoma in which a few mature sebaceous cells can be seen among the dark-staining tumor cells.

HISTOPATHOLOGY ►

This tumor is characterized by pools of mucinous material surrounding nests of polygonal cells (Figs 7-109a and 7-109b).

TREATMENT ►

Mucinous eccrine carcinoma is a low-grade tumor. It requires a complete local excision without a prophylactic neck dissection.

Pilomatrix Carcinoma

CLINICAL PRESENTATION ►

Pilomatrix carcinomas are nodular, sometimes exophytic lesions, pink in color and usually less than 3 cm in diameter. They are usually seen in adults and show a predilection for females.

HISTOPATHOLOGY ►

Clusters of large polygonal cells are seen in a dense collagenous stroma. The central areas contain shadow cells. There is cellular atypism and frequent mitoses. The tumor is infiltrative and invades blood vessels (Fig 7-110).

TREATMENT ►

This tumor is locally aggressive, and distant metastases have been reported as well. Wide surgical resection using 1.5- to 2.0-cm tumor-free margins is the usual treatment. A prophylactic neck dissection is not required.

Sebaceous Carcinoma

CLINICAL PRESENTATION ►

Sebaceous carcinoma has a predilection for the eyelid, but other areas of the face are also commonly affected. On the eyelids, the origin is mainly from the meibomian glands, and the carcinoma may mimic chronic blepharoconjunctivitis or a chalazion. Skin lesions occur as nodules, which grow rapidly and may ulcerate. Patients are usually elderly. Some cases have arisen as a component of Torre syndrome.

HISTOPATHOLOGY ►

The tumor consists of lobules of varied size that contain undifferentiated cells and sebaceous cells (Fig 7-111). Many cells are atypical and pleomorphic. The tumor margins are poorly defined. In lesions of the eyelid, the tumor cells may permeate the surface epithelium in pagetoid fashion.

TREATMENT ►

In both ocular and extraocular tumors, the behavior is aggressive. One third of these lesions recur or metastasize. Wide surgical excision that includes clinically involved lymph nodes is the treatment of choice. Although ocular lesions may undergo distant metastasis, skin lesions undergo regional spread. However, tumors that arise in Torre syndrome do not metastasize.

Management of Irradiated Patients and Osteoradionecrosis

> "The surgeon of today must enlist the forces of healing and repair, lest he be a surgeon of the last century who somehow stumbled into a modern operating room."
> —Walton Van Winkle and Thomas K. Hunt

Radiation Injury to Tissues

Radiation is high linear energy transferred to tissue with the intent to kill cancer cells. Normal cells are also damaged or killed, however. Because cancer cells replicate more frequently than normal cells, they are more likely to be irradiated at a vulnerable time in their cell cycle. However, many normal cells are also caught at vulnerable times in their cell cycle, thereby creating the well-known radiation-sensitivity spectrum (Fig 8-1). Germinal and lymphoreticular cells are the most sensitive, endothelial cells and fibroblasts are of intermediate sensitivity, and muscle and nerve have little sensitivity to radiation. It is the intermediate group of endothelial cells and fibroblasts that is important to the clinician because they are the primary cells involved with healing.

When radiation energy passes through normal tissue, it kills a small number of cells immediately. Most cells survive but incur internal damage to their DNA, RNA, enzyme systems, and cell membranes. These cells, mainly the vascular endothelial cells and healing-related fibroblasts, can be considered impaired. Although they live out their normal life spans or shortened life spans, these impaired cells often are not replaced by daughter cells when they die. Consequently, the tissue becomes less cellular, less vascular, and less oxygenated over time. The well-known "three-H tissue" (hypocellular, hypovascular, hypoxic) develops, which progresses and therefore worsens with time. This explains why irradiated tissue heals slowly or not at all (Fig 8-2).

Clinically, irradiated tissue develops an initial erythema and dermatitis as an acute response to the radiation damage. Caused by vascular hyperemia indicative of vascular damage and tissue inflammation (Fig 8-3a), these conditions will subside and the tissue will normalize clinically over the next 4 months. Subclinically, however, the damaged endothelium induces thrombosis, and fibroblasts die without being replaced by daughter cells, leaving behind extracellular collagen (three-H tissue). The tissue becomes fibrotic and inelastic, radiation hyper- and hypopigmentation of skin often develop, and radiation telangiectasias become apparent (Fig 8-3b). It is this type of tissue, involving skin, mucosa, and bone, that is at risk of nonhealing if wounded by an injury or from surgery. Such tissue is more likely to become an avascular, nonhealing wound such as osteoradionecrosis of bone or soft tissue radiation necrosis several years after radiation.

The Pattern of Radiation Injury

The pattern of radiation injury is important because it explains physiologically why irradiated tissue worsens over time without the normal healing seen with most other injuries. In addition to direct cellular and vascular damage, radiation creates a concentric pattern of radiation injury resembling a target.

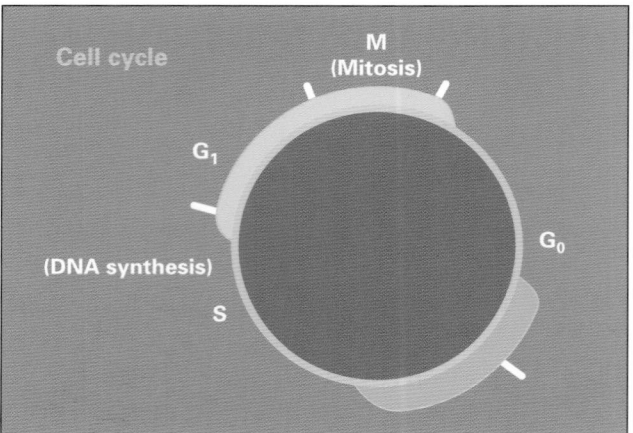

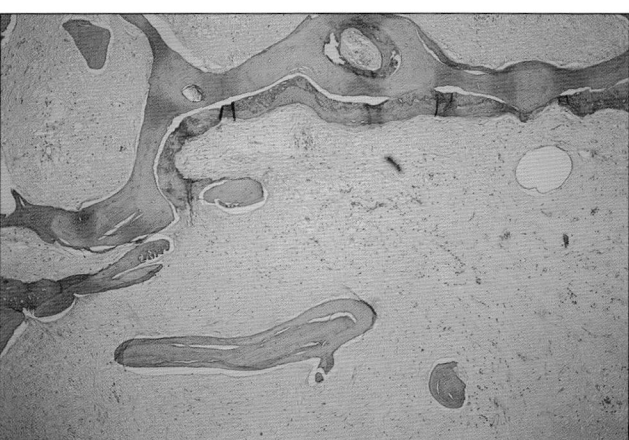

Fig 8-1 There are specific times in the cell cycle when a cell is vulnerable to radiation. Cells with high turnover rates will be within a vulnerable time in the cycle more frequently than cells with low turnover rates, and therefore will be more susceptible to radiation injury.

Fig 8-2 Radiation will induce a hypovascular, hypocellular, hypoxic tissue, which has a reduced capacity for healing.

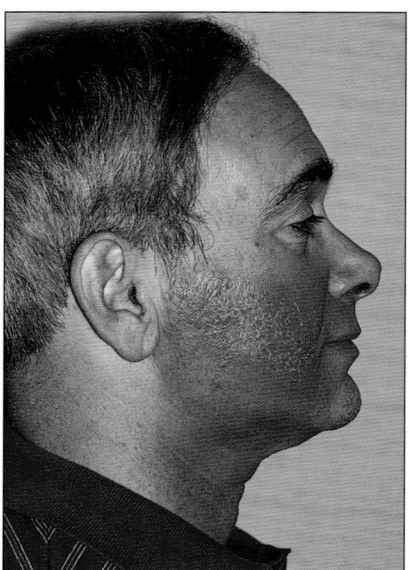

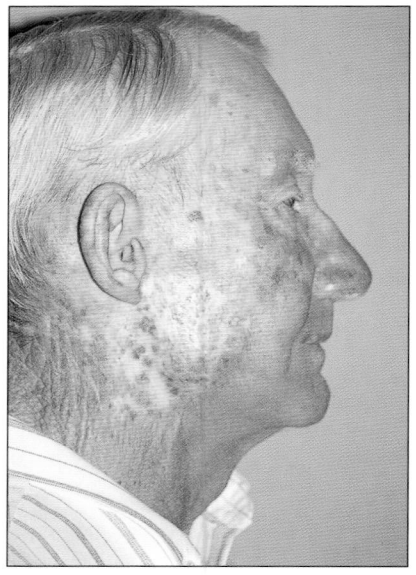

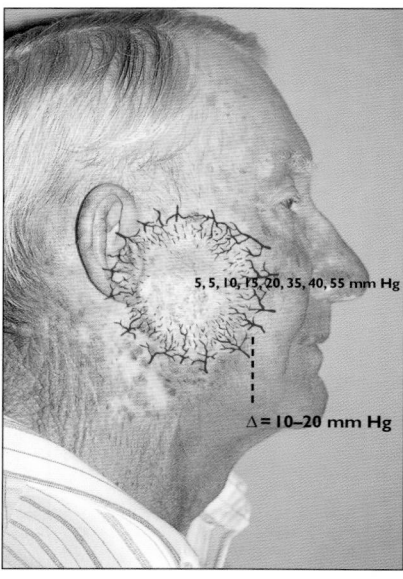

Fig 8-3a Three weeks after radiotherapy, hyperemia, acute inflammation, and skin exfoliations (the so-called sunburn effect) are seen in the form of a reddened area with white flakes.

Fig 8-3b Twelve years after radiotherapy in a field similar to that shown in Fig 8-3a, hypopigmentation, a tight inelastic skin quality, and atrophy are the clinical manifestations of "three-H" tissue. Note the transition zone at the edge of the irradiation field.

Fig 8-3c Oxygen tension measurements of the irradiated field will show a shallow oxygen gradient ranging from normal outside or at the edge of the irradiation field to the most hypoxic at the center of the field.

At the center of the irradiated field is the greatest damage. From this center the radiation damage slowly lessens until it becomes nonexistent outside of the irradiated field (Fig 8-3c). This pattern is established by the isodose lines of external beam radiotherapy, by which means the tumor's center, which has the greatest diameter, receives the greatest dose. Away from the tumor's center, the isodose lines plot a lesser radiation dose because of the tumor's smaller mass. This establishes an injury pattern in which the oxygen gradients from outside the irradiated field to inside the irradiated field as well as within the irradiated field toward its center are very gradual (see Fig 8-3c). These oxygen gradients are on the order of only 2 to 7 mm Hg. Because the wound-healing macrophage can respond only to oxygen gradients on the order of 20 mm Hg, irradiated tissue never benefits from macrophage-directed revascularization (angiogenesis) as do other tissues. This pattern of injury is similar to that seen in diabetic ulcers of the leg. Because of the microangiopathy associated with diabetes, a gradual or low oxygen gradient is established, resulting in failure of wound healing in this disease as well.

When interstitial radiation sources are used, the pattern of radiation injury remains the same, but it occurs through a different mechanism. With interstitial radiotherapy, the gradual damage and, therefore, the low oxygen gradient field is established by the distance from the radiation seeds or needles. Because radiation energy decreases with distance from the radiation source by a power of four, tissue that is farther away from the center receives less damage by a power of four. Therefore, a gradual tissue damage gradient is established.

Radiotherapy Protocols

Three basic types of radiotherapy protocols have been used over the past few decades. External beam radiotherapy is the most common, followed by interstitial or implant seed radiotherapy. Neutron beam radiotherapy is now rarely if ever used because of serious radiation fibrosis and radiation necrosis complications.

External Beam Radiotherapy

External beam radiotherapy is usually cobalt-60 radiation, which emits the electron encased within the element's central neutron called a *beta particle*. The beta particle is, therefore, small and negatively charged. Beta particles affect cells not by directly damaging DNA or RNA, but rather by killing or damaging cells from their collisions with the more abundant water molecules in them. The transferred energy splits water (HOH) into free radicals such as superoxide O and hydroxyl OH. These free radicals, with an exposed electron orbit, in turn react with DNA, RNA, enzyme systems, and cell membranes (Fig 8-4).

Standard electron beam therapy is administered at 200 centiGray (cGy) per day. (A centiGray is equivalent to the term it replaced, the rad.) Today, typical tumoricidal doses range from 6,000 cGy to 7,600 cGy and average around 7,000 cGy. A common protocol is to "field radiate" the neck and the tumor or surgical bed to 5,000 cGy and to provide an additional 2,000-cGy to 2,200-cGy "boost" at the primary site or surgical site.

A variation of this standard protocol is hyperfractionated radiotherapy. Each daily dose is referred to as a fraction. Instead of delivering a daily dose of 200 cGy for 5 days per week, various schedules have been developed to deliver 150 cGy or 180 cGy twice daily 3 or 4 days per week. Although this scheme was primarily used to reduce the incidence of osteoradionecrosis, its track record has shown that it has not. Nevertheless, external beam radiotherapy is less damaging to normal tissues than the other types of radiotherapy.

Interstitial Radiotherapy

Interstitial radiotherapy, often called *brachytherapy* in the head and neck region, involves the use of radioactive seeds or needles. The half-life of [226]radium is about 1,600 years. It also gives off high-energy gamma rays and radon gas. The high-energy gamma rays are very damaging to normal tissues, and its long half-life, together with its radon gas by-product, makes it difficult to store safely. Therefore, [192]iridium, which has a half-life of only 74 days and no gaseous by-product, is preferred. Interstitial radiotherapy, regardless of the isotope, is more damaging to normal as well as tumor cells because of its placement directly into the tissue and its continuous energy emissions. When interstitial radiotherapy is used, the time between fractions, enabling normal cells (and tumor cells as well) to recover, is not present. Therefore, interstitial

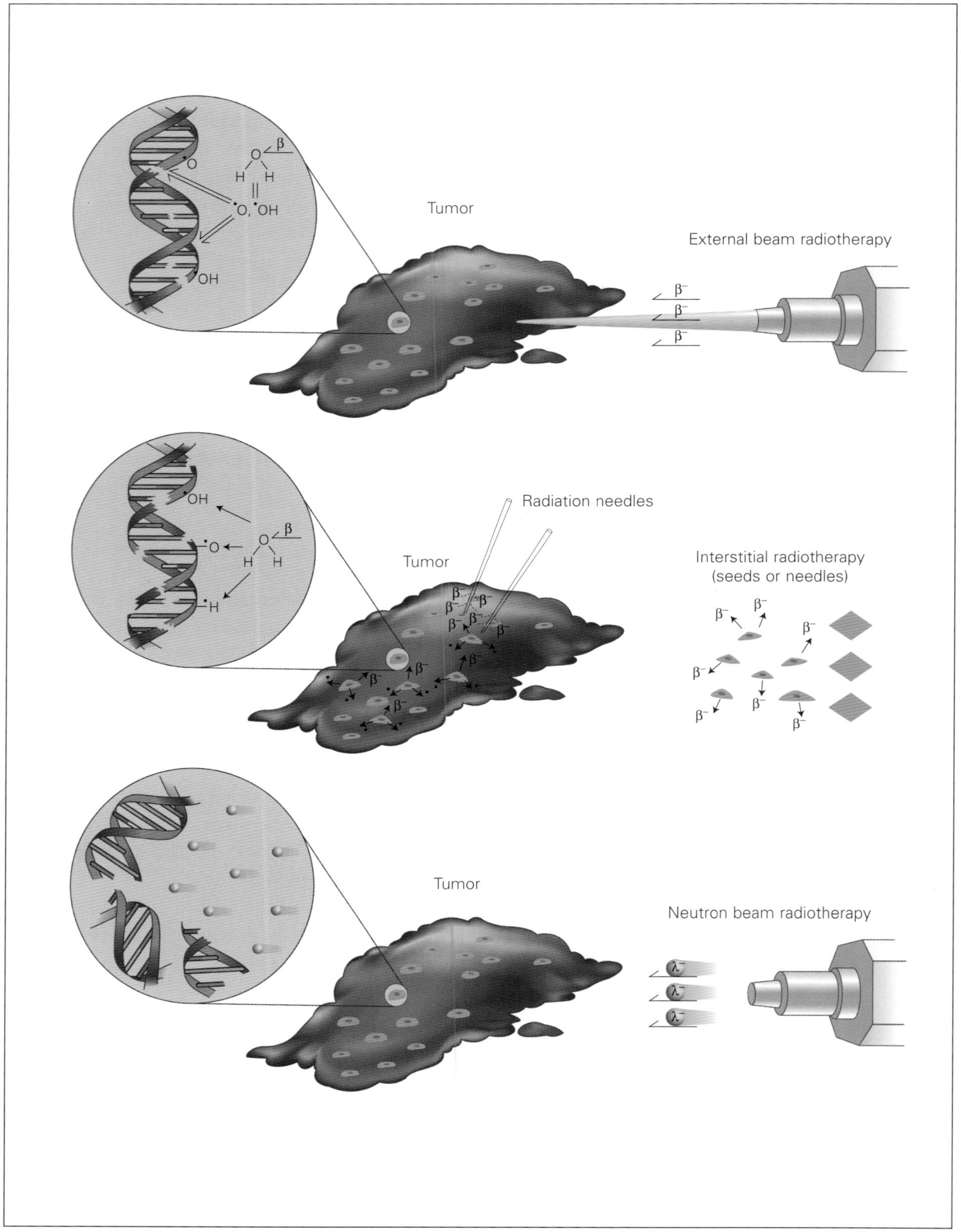

Fig 8-4 External beam radiotherapy causes DNA damage indirectly by generating free radicals from water molecules. Interstitial radiotherapy also generates free radicals from water molecules, but it is more damaging because it is within the tumor. Neutron beam radiotherapy causes the greatest DNA damage because of the neutron's greater mass (1,865 times that of a beta particle), which therefore directly damages DNA.

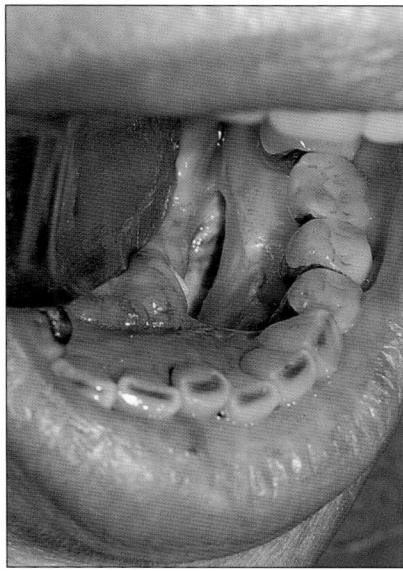 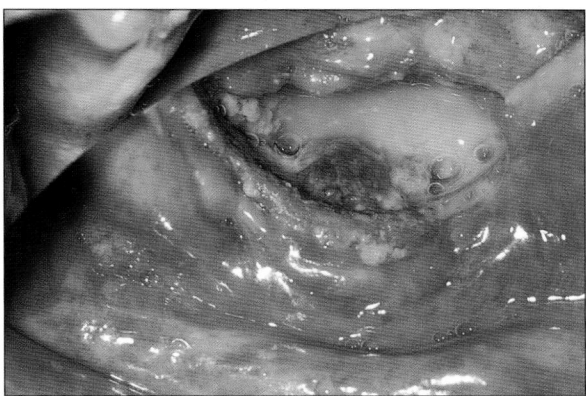

Fig 8-5 Exposed nonviable lingual cortex from the alveolar crest to the inferior border resulted from floor-of-the-mouth interstitial radiotherapy. This is an example of stage III osteoradionecrosis. Note the necrotic mylohyoid muscle and the absent periosteum.

Fig 8-6 An edentulous mandible manifests stage III osteoradionecrosis after floor-of-the-mouth interstitial radiotherapy similar to that shown in Fig 8-5, indicating that the radiation damage is independent of the presence of teeth.

radiotherapy is more damaging to normal tissues and poses a higher risk for the development of osteoradionecrosis. Another increased risk factor for osteoradionecrosis occurs when interstitial radiotherapy is used to treat floor-of-the-mouth or tongue carcinomas, where it is placed close to the lingual cortex of the mandible (Fig 8-5). Because the adult mandible receives a significant portion of its blood supply through the lingual periosteum, radiation to this area is most damaging and is associated with a higher incidence of osteoradionecrosis (Fig 8-6).

Neutron Beam Radiotherapy

Neutron beam radiotherapy, the radiation therapy most damaging to normal cells as well as tumor cells, is rarely used today because of its complications. A neutron is 1,865 times the mass of a beta particle and, therefore, penetrates deeper into tissues, directly damaging DNA, RNA, enzymes, and cell membranes (see Fig 8-4). Patients who receive this type of radiation present with significant muscle and deep tissue fibrosis and are at the highest risk for osteoradionecrosis.

Radiotherapy Complications and Their Management

Radiation Mucositis

Radiation mucositis is the oral mucosa's response to acute radiation injury. It will present as a diffuse erythema with pain or mucosal ulcerations and a fibrinous exudate. This condition, which is self-limiting, may develop in the last 3 weeks of radiotherapy and may extend for about 1 month after radiotherapy.

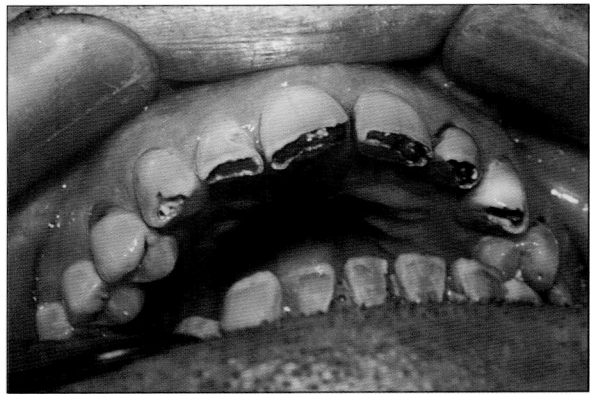

Fig 8-7 Incisal radiation caries on the maxillary teeth and lingual radiation caries on the mandibular teeth (but no pit and fissure caries in the posterior teeth) after floor-of-the-mouth radiotherapy, indicating that the cause is related more to radiation damage to the pulp than to xerostomia.

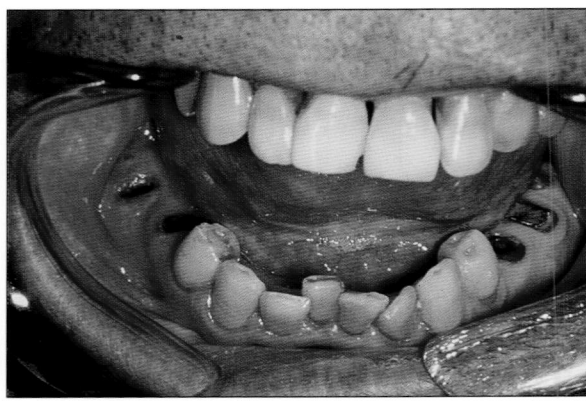

Fig 8-8 External beam radiation to the posterior mandible for treatment of a tonsillar carcinoma caused severe radiation caries in the posterior teeth but spared the anterior teeth, which were outside the radiation field.

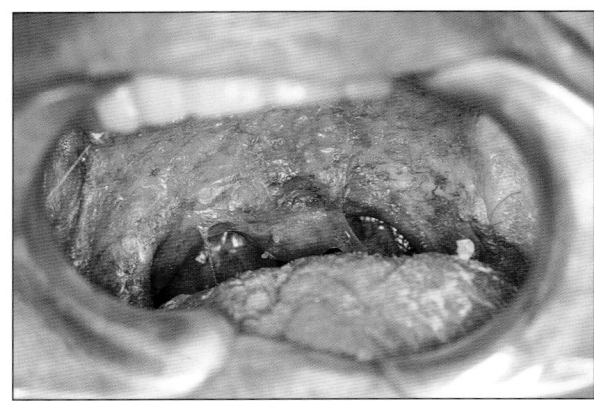

Fig 8-9 Severe mucositis and xerostomia after radiotherapy.

During this acute painful phase, topical viscous 2% xylocaine gel as well as systemic analgesics may be needed to control pain. Antibiotics are not required unless there is an associated lymphadenitis or systemic toxicity represented by fever, chills, or a skin erythema. Nevertheless, patients will benefit from chlorhexidine gluconate rinses, if tolerated, to reduce bacterial colonization of the ulcers. Nutritional support may be needed in some cases. In severe cases, it is reasonable to provide intravenous fluid therapy and nasogastric tube feeding for a short time. Reassurance that this condition and accompanying pain will subside is welcomed by patients.

Radiation Caries

The old dogma concerning radiation caries is that it results from xerostomia, which permits cariogenic bacteria to proliferate unopposed by the usual lysosomes and IgA immunoglobulins in saliva and causes the loss of the saliva's natural buffering capacity. Although this mechanism contributes to radiation caries, it is not its only or most significant cause. Caries in nonirradiated individuals occurs in pits, in fissures, and interproximally. It is also chalky and soft from dissolved tooth structure. Radiation caries, by contrast, is hard and black. It occurs at the gingival margin, cusp tips, and incisal surfaces (Fig 8-7). It would, therefore, be unrealistic to accept radiation caries as a mere extension of nonradiation caries from reduced salivary flow. Moreover, radiation caries is either present only in the irradiated field or is more severe in the irradiated field, while the entire mouth is affected by xerostomia (Figs 8-8 and 8-9).

Radiation caries is mainly due to pulpal necrosis and odontoblast death, which causes deterioration of both the dentin and the dentinoenamel junction. The enamel is subsequently lost from the dentin because of dentinal dehydration and dentinoenamel junction deterioration (similar to dentinogenesis imperfecta). The exposed dentin becomes black or brown and hard and deteriorates further. Pulp testing teeth with radiation caries may or may not produce a response. Yet when the pulp is examined, it is avascular and resembles the three-H tissue of radiation damage. The problem is that the dental profession deems a tooth "vital" if it responds to pulp testing, which reflects nerve enervation. However, vitality of any tissue is a matter not of nerve enervation but of blood supply and perfusion. Because nerves are the most radiation-resistant tissues and because pulpal nerve endings arise from cells in the gasserian ganglion, the tooth with radiation caries may have a responsive pulp but is actually nonvital due to avascular necrosis of the vascular pulpal tissues, including the odontoblasts.

It is now possible to predict which teeth are most at risk of developing radiation caries: those in the direct path of 6,000-cGy or greater radiation (see Fig 8-8). Even the best oral hygiene, dental care, and fluoride carriers will not prevent all radiation caries.

Once developed, radiation caries should be treated promptly using restorative techniques appropriate for the degree of lost and involved tooth substance.

Radiation-Induced Xerostomia

Radiation-induced xerostomia is caused by the direct damaging effects of radiation on both major and minor salivary gland structures located in the radiation path (see Fig 8-9). Glandular tissue in general is very sensitive to radiation. Following radiation therapy, the mouth becomes dry as a result of the loss of salivary gland acini. The skin becomes dry as well because of loss of sweat and sebaceous glands. A histopathologic study of irradiated glands will show the three-H tissue replacement of the acini but preservation of the ducts. Ductal epithelium is somewhat radiation resistant.

Because most radiation ports leave some areas of mucosa untouched, there is an opportunity to stimulate the remaining glands to overproduce. Although it improves mouth moisture in only about 70% of irradiated patients, pilocarpine (Salagen, MGI Pharma), 5 mg by mouth three times daily, often improves eating, speaking, and swallowing functions. However, it should be taken regularly to gain and maintain an improvement, and it must be given with caution to individuals with heart diseases associated with brachycardia, heart block, or other medications that may slow heart rate or conduction.

Additionally, sports water bottles are used by many individuals, and Evian atomized water spray has been found to be beneficial to many.

Radiation Dysphagia

One of the most troubling and least treatable later complications of radiotherapy is radiation dysphagia. Many patients will report difficulty swallowing (food "getting stuck" in the hypopharynx) and will aspirate on swallowing after radiotherapy. This condition is caused by radiation fibrosis within the pharyngeal constrictors, which makes these series of three muscle pairs stiff and unable to contract in the coordinated fashion that is necessary to propel food into the esophagus. There is, unfortunately, little that can be done directly to correct this. Occasionally, swallowing therapy helps. Improving mouth moisture and increasing the liquid content of the diet helps indirectly. Esophageal dilations do not improve this condition unless the esophagus itself was included in the radiation ports.

Radiation Effects on Jaw Growth and Developing Teeth

Radiation during the growth and development years will create a dose-related hypoplasia of the mandible as well as partial or complete agenesis of teeth within the portals of radiotherapy. These effects are primarily manifested as an anteroposterior deficiency of the mandible (retrognathia) (Fig 8-10a) and a general reduction in the size of the ramus and body of the mandible, creating a severe chin deficiency appearance. The teeth within the radiated bone will generally be smaller and will usually exhibit arrested root development (Fig 8-10b). Since the crowns will be affected to a lesser degree, many teeth will appear radiographically to have a normal crown size with no roots, mimicking an exfoliating primary tooth. Some teeth will fail to form altogether (agenesis) (see Fig 8-10b).

The teeth may be replaced with removable partial dentures or with implant-supported fixed dental appliances, provided that all remaining growth has been completed and the patient has undergone the

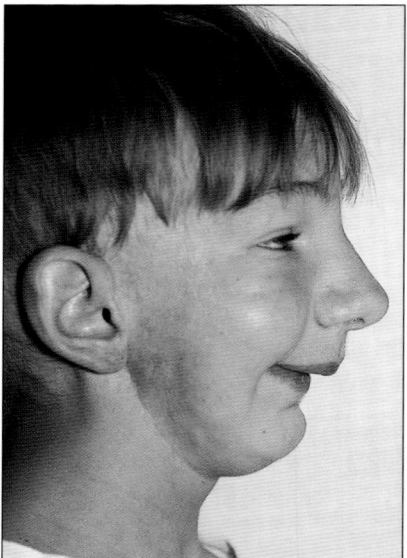

Fig 8-10a Radiotherapy at age 2 months affected the growth and development of the mandible in the ramus and body areas, which now at age 10 is manifested as a significant anteroposterior deficiency.

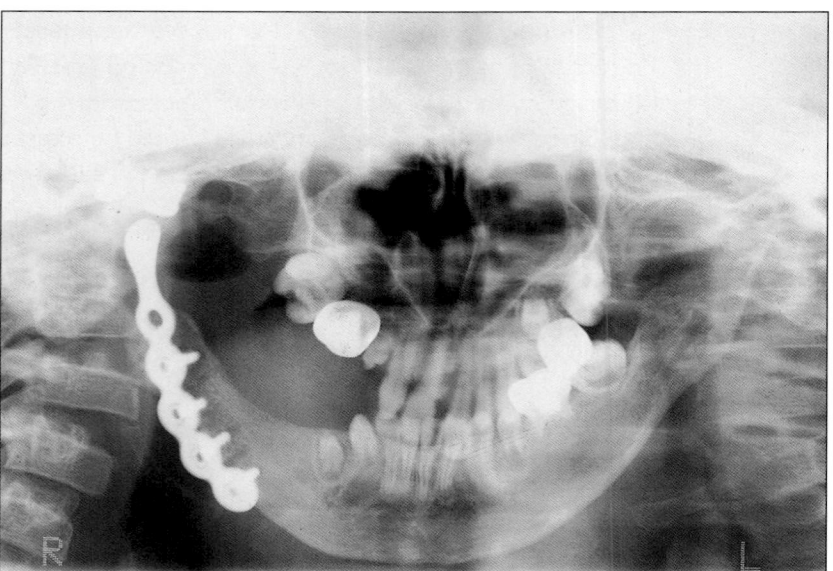

Fig 8-10b The radiation effects on the rami of the mandible are evidenced by an irregular morphology. Note the reconstruction of the joint; this was necessitated by the radiation fibrosis, which produced a limited jaw opening. Also note the absence of root formation and hypoplasia of the teeth, which becomes progressively less severe further from the radiotherapy ports (anteriorly).

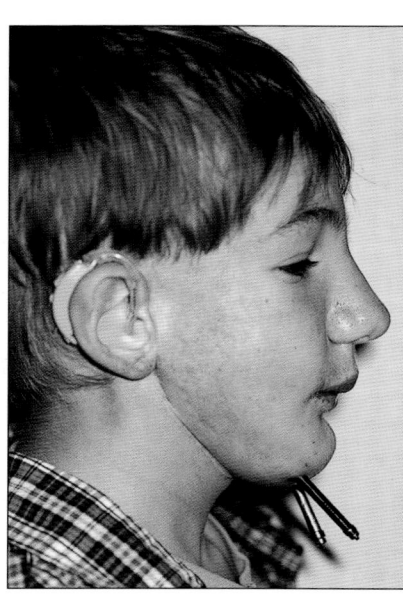

Fig 8-10c This boy's mandible was successfully lengthened using distraction osteogenesis and HBO therapy.

20/10 hyperbaric oxygen (HBO) protocol (20 sessions at 2.4 ATA for 90 minutes on 100% oxygen prior to surgery and 10 sessions after surgery). In cases of significant anteroposterior deficiency, osteotomies advancing the jaw using rigid fixation techniques and bone grafting can be accomplished, again provided that the patient has completed the 20/10 HBO protocol. As an alternative, distraction osteogenesis in what usually is a young patient can also be successful provided that an appropriate distraction device can be adapted to the hypodeveloped jaw and that the patient has undergone the 20/10 HBO protocol (Fig 8-10c).

Radiation-Induced Trismus

Radiation-induced trismus is a condition that frequently accompanies osteoradionecrosis in the posterior body and ramus region of the mandible and is usually improved with the successful treatment of the osteoradionecrosis. However, radiation-induced trismus without osteoradionecrosis is a unique and difficult problem. The trismus is not a consequence of the effects of radiation on the temporomandibular joint but instead is due either to radiation fibrosis within the masseter and medial pterygoid muscles or to restrictive fibrosis in the mucosa of the anterior tonsillar pillar and retromolar areas (Fig 8-11).

If the trismus is due to tight and unresilient mucosal restrictions in the tonsillar and/or retromolar areas, a significant increase in opening may be achieved by excising this tissue and replacing it with a viable skin paddle from either a myocutaneous or a free microvascular flap (Figs 8-12a to 8-12e). If the trismus is the result of radiation fibrosis in the pterygomasseteric sling, the prognosis is much worse. Such fibrosis cannot be effectively excised without risking the blood supply to the ramus and thus precipitating an osteoradionecrosis. The fibrosis also cannot easily be replaced by viable flap tissue, thus limiting the clinician's options. Modest gains can be achieved with bilateral coronoidectomies or partial excisions of the fibrosis in the masseter or medial pterygoid muscles. These also must be followed with intensive jaw-opening exercises using a device such as the Therabite (Therabite), by tongue blade exercises, or by the chewing of soft, sugarless gum.

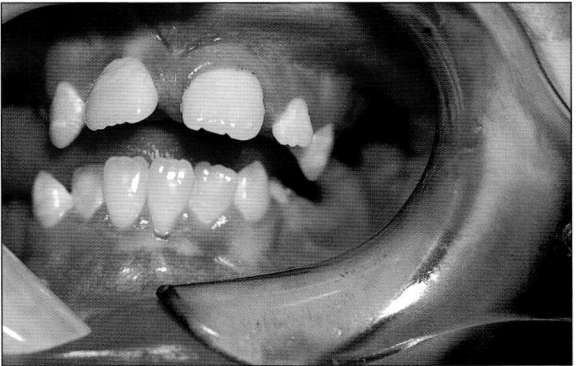

Fig 8-11 The limited jaw opening in this young patient was due to radiation fibrosis of the buccal mucosa and anterior tonsillar pillar areas.

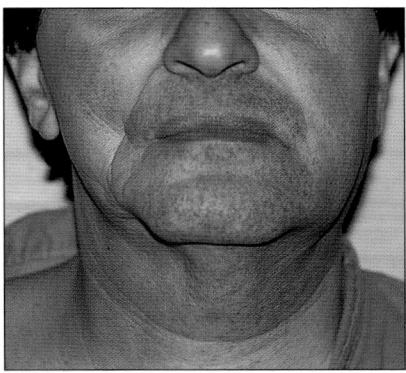

Fig 8-12a Significant radiation fibrosis of the soft tissues of the cheek and upper neck. A restricted opening of only 1 mm was primarily due to fibrosis of the buccal mucosa and buccopharyngeal raphe.

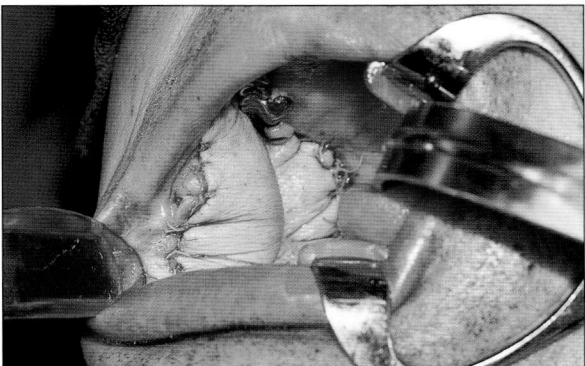

Fig 8-12b Excision of the radiation fibrosis in the buccal mucosa obtained an increased opening. This must be maintained by the placement of viable skin or mucosa that retains its elastic (stretchable) properties. Here a skin paddle from a radial forearm microvascular flap is sutured into place.

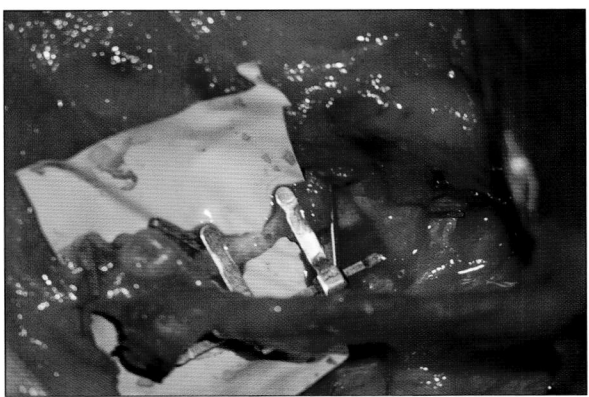

Fig 8-12c To retain the elastic quality of the skin paddle, a vascular re-anastomosis (shown here) must be accomplished or a flap that retains its pedicle (eg, a myocutaneous flap) must be used.

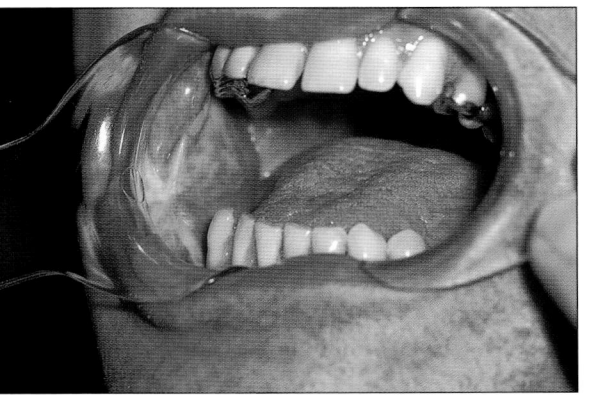

Fig 8-12d Healed skin paddle of the flap, which can accommodate an improved oral opening because of its ability to stretch.

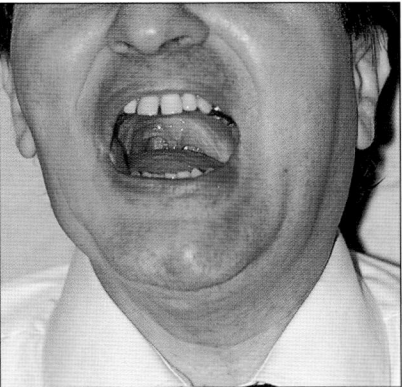

Fig 8-12e Postoperative opening of 33 mm was achieved and permanently maintained by the replacement of radiation fibrosis with viable elastic skin.

Managing the Irradiated Patient Before Radiotherapy

Patients should be seen by trained dental personnel before beginning radiotherapy. Because radiotherapy usually begins within 1 month of a cancer diagnosis, the dentist should evaluate the individual as soon as possible to accomplish caries control, prophylaxis, and impressions for fluoride carriers. Teeth with apical pathosis or advanced periodontal disease should be planned for removal, as should any clinically sound teeth in the mandible that will be in the direct path of radiation of 6,000 cGy or greater. Fluoride carriers and otherwise good dental care and hygiene will not prevent all radiation caries, and many

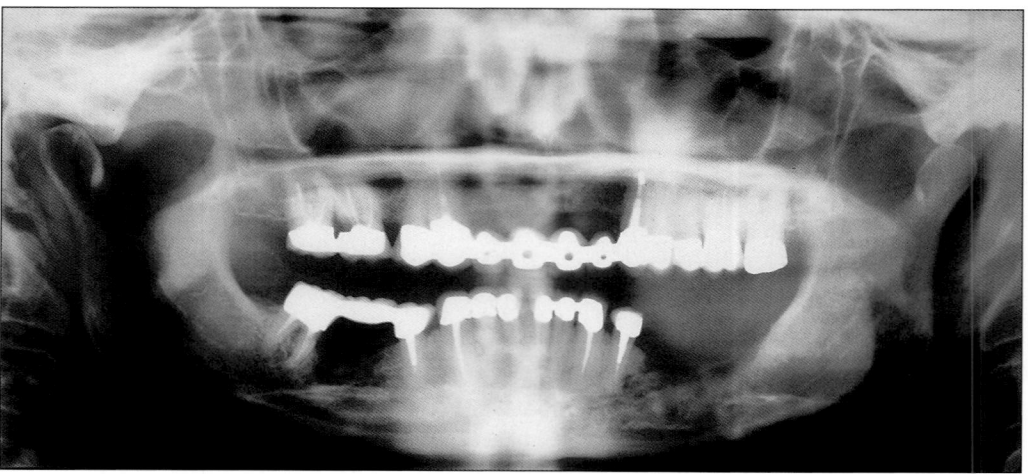

Fig 8-13a Bilateral osteoradionecrosis in extraction sites where the extractions were accomplished 3 years after radiotherapy and without the support of HBO. Note the slow development and progression of osteoradionecrosis, evidenced by the fixed prosthesis over the osteoradionecrotic area on the right side. Both of these areas of osteoradionecrosis could have been prevented by the preradiation removal of the mandibular molars.

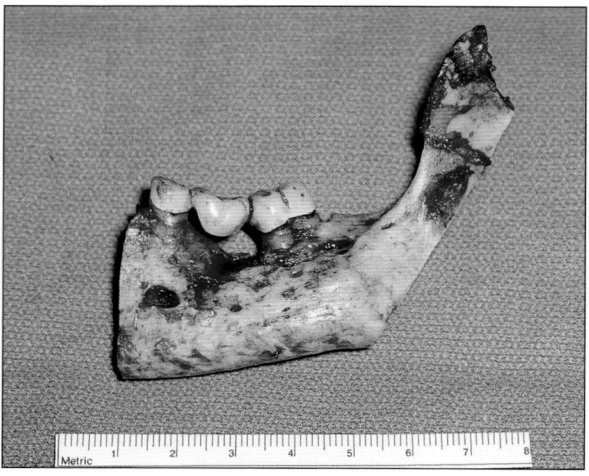

Fig 8-13b Resection specimen of osteoradionecrosis shows nonvital bone and bone loss at a nonhealed extraction site and around each abutment tooth.

postradiation extractions are performed for periodontal failure rather than for caries. Maxillary teeth do not require preradiation removal unless they are otherwise indicated for removal. This is because the greater blood supply and thinner bone in the maxilla makes osteoradionecrosis in this bone a rare event. If the dentist and patient elect to retain mandibular teeth in the direct path of radiation of 6,000 cGy or greater, informed consent should be obtained, outlining the increased risk of osteoradionecrosis (Figs 8-13a and 8-13b).

The timing of preradiation tooth extraction is important. Studies have shown that 21 days is the recommended time for bone revascularization and healing to take place before radiotherapy can begin without a significant risk for osteoradionecrosis. Certainly the risk decreases at 14 days. However, cases of osteoradionecrosis will best be prevented by allowing 21 days between tooth removal and onset of radiotherapy. If the radiotherapy must begin prior to 21 days, informed consent should be obtained from the patient to show that he or she accepts an increased risk for development of osteoradionecrosis.

Managing the Irradiated Patient During Radiotherapy

Although a good pre-radiotherapy dental evaluation and care should prevent the necessity of managing dental disease during radiation therapy, an occasional toothache or a dental abscess during the radiation course does occur. In such cases, the radiation therapist may volunteer to temporarily suspend the radiotherapy so that the clinician may treat the patient. However, this is usually contraindicated because if the radiation therapy is temporarily stopped, the cancer cells will repopulate, often with more radiation-resistant cells, which may in turn worsen the prognosis, necessitating an increased radiotherapy dose from what was originally planned. In addition, combining tooth extraction tissue injury with ongoing radiation injury invites osteoradionecrosis (Fig 8-14). Instead, the patient's pain should be controlled with noninvasive methods. Alternatives to tooth extraction in these cases include pulpotomies, pulpectomies, endodontic treatment, and analgesics. If a dental abscess has developed, a soft tissue incision and drainage in addition to endodontic therapy and antibiotics is recommended. No interruption in the radiation

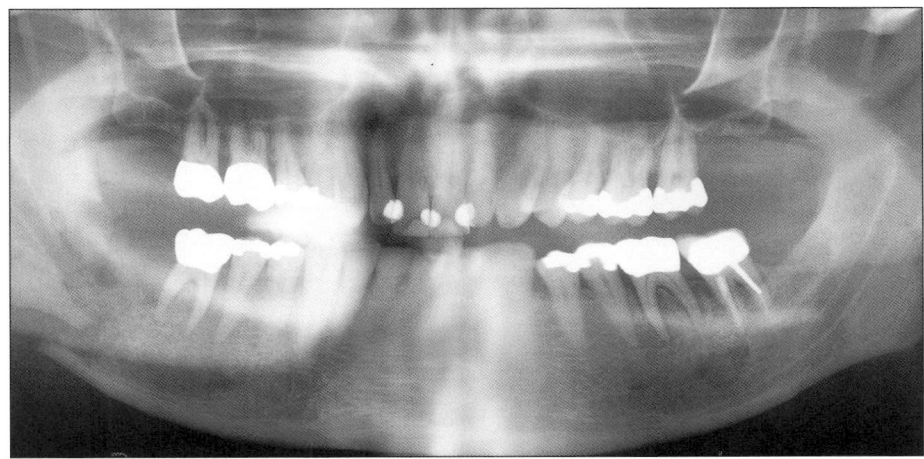

Fig 8-14 A second molar tooth was removed during radiotherapy, which rapidly led to a stage III osteoradionecrosis with a pathologic fracture.

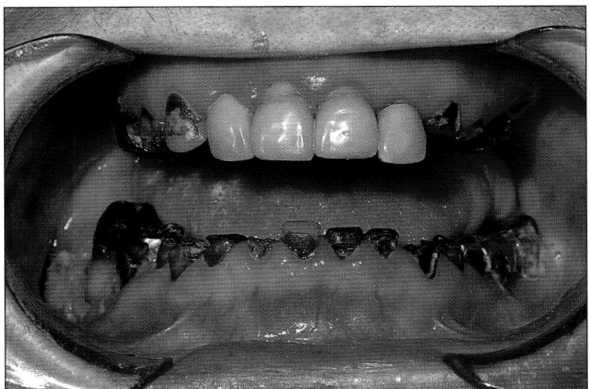

Fig 8-15a Numerous nonrestorable teeth with radiation caries, which were removed after using the 20/10 HBO protocol.

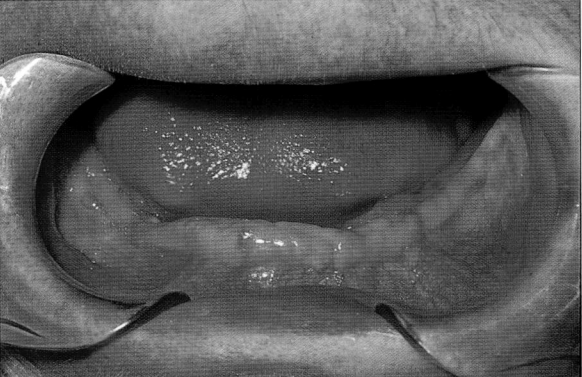

Fig 8-15b The patient shown in Fig 8-15a healed without developing osteoradionecrosis after receiving the 20/10 HBO protocol.

sequence should be necessary. Within the first 4 months after radiation, the so-called "golden window" will allow for definitive follow-up care, including tooth extraction without the need for HBO. During this time, the irradiated tissues will have recovered from the acute radiation hyperemia, and inflammation will not yet have developed the three-H tissue associated with nonhealing.

Managing the Irradiated Patient After Radiotherapy

The first 4 months after radiotherapy represent a time of tissue recovery without the accumulation of the three-H tissue effects. It offers a short but useful period in which to accomplish necessary oral surgery procedures without the need for HBO. After 4 months, development of the three-H tissue will begin to affect healing. After this time, the standard protocol of HBO is recommended for elective surgery in irradiated tissues. That protocol consists of 20 sessions at 2.4 atmospheres of absolute pressure (ATA) for 90 minutes on 100% oxygen prior to surgery and 10 sessions after surgery. Daily sessions are conducted 5 or 6 days per week. Specifically related to tooth extraction years after radiotherapy, this protocol has shown a dramatic reduction in the development of osteoradionecrosis (Figs 8-15a and 8-15b). This protocol is also indicated when any other surgery is performed on irradiated tis-

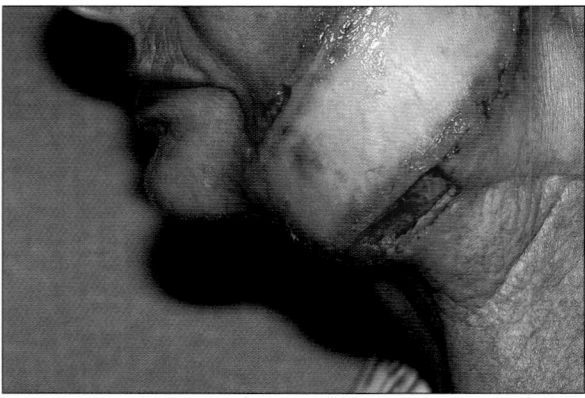

Fig 8-16a A viable vascularized flap (myocutaneous or free vascular transfer) with excellent blood supply of its own nonetheless fails to heal into irradiated tissue unsupported by preoperative HBO. Here dehiscence of the irradiated tissue from the flap is apparent.

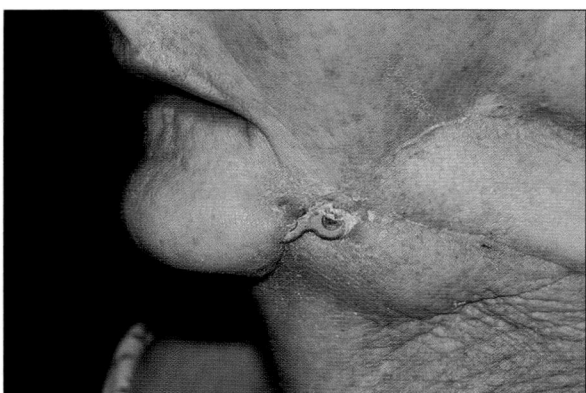

Fig 8-16b Plate exposures and fistulae at the edge of a vascularized flap are common if HBO is not used.

sue. Even vascularized or pedicled vascular flap surgery requires this protocol. Although the flap may be vascular, the tissue into which it is placed is not. Frequent dehiscences, tissue necrosis, and infections occur adjacent to vascularized flaps that have been placed into irradiated tissues unsupported by HBO (Figs 8-16a and 8-16b). Today, this protocol has also allowed the placement of osseointegrated dental implants in irradiated patients without a significant incidence of osteoradionecrosis.

Hyperbaric Oxygen Therapy

Hyperbaric oxygen is oxygen used as a pharmaceutical drug. The dosage and absorption is regulated by the pressure in the chamber and the established protocols of the Undersea and Hyperbaric Medicine Society. As with any drug, too small a dose will provide no therapeutic value and too high a dose will produce toxicity. The two protocols described in this text are scientifically and time proven to be effective and safe.

Hyperbaric oxygen is delivered in either a single person (monoplace) chamber or a multiperson (multiplace) chamber. Each type of chamber is capable of meeting the parameters of the radiation tissue elective surgery protocol and the osteoradionecrosis treatment protocol discussed later in this chapter. The 100% oxygen breathed at 2.4 ATA dissolves oxygen in physical solution in interstitial tissues and blood. This oxygenation of tissues outside the hemoglobin delivery system is able to generate enhanced oxygen gradients throughout the irradiated tissue and especially between the irradiated and nonirradiated tissue (Fig 8-17a). This permits wound-healing macrophages to migrate into the area and secrete several cytokines, including vascular endothelial growth factor (VEGF), that stimulate capillary angiogenesis and fibroplasia (Figs 8-17b and 8-17c). The result is that the three-H tissue that begins at about 30% of normal vascularity realizes an increase to about 75% of normal vascularity. The protocol of 20 HBO sessions prior to elective surgery in irradiated tissue followed by 10 sessions after surgery creates this angiogenesis, which is permanent. Therefore, repeated or follow-up surgeries in the irradiated area would not require repeated HBO protocols (Fig 8-17d).

Hyperbaric Oxygen and Cancer

The most common application of HBO therapy for oral and maxillofacial indications is in irradiated patients with a history of cancer, particularly squamous cell carcinoma. Some clinicians have been concerned about the potential of HBO to stimulate dormant cancer cells or accelerate growth of existing, unrecog-

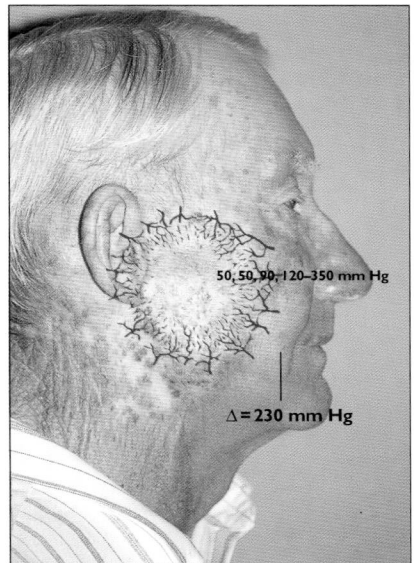

Fig 8-17a During HBO, the oxygen tensions in the irradiated and normal tissues, as shown in Fig 8-3c, are increased seven- to tenfold, thereby increasing the oxygen gradient and stimulating the macrophages to secrete angiogenic factors.

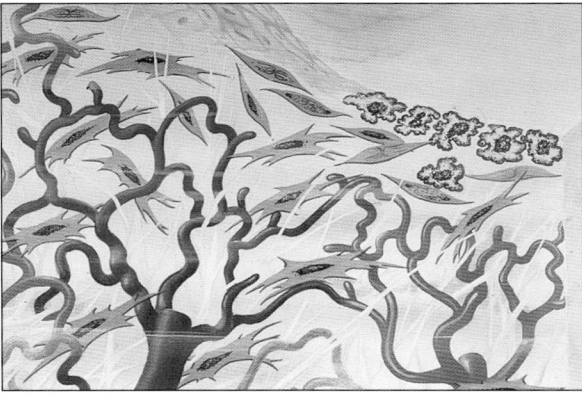

Fig 8-17b Macrophages are attracted to the irradiated tissue when oxygen gradients exceed 20 mm Hg. They then secrete angiogenic factors, which produce the observed neo-angiogenesis in irradiated tissues.

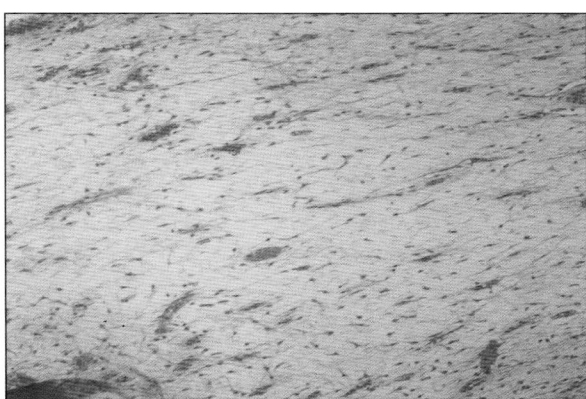

Fig 8-17c Irradiated tissue response to HBO is evidenced by capillary angiogenesis and increased cellularity.

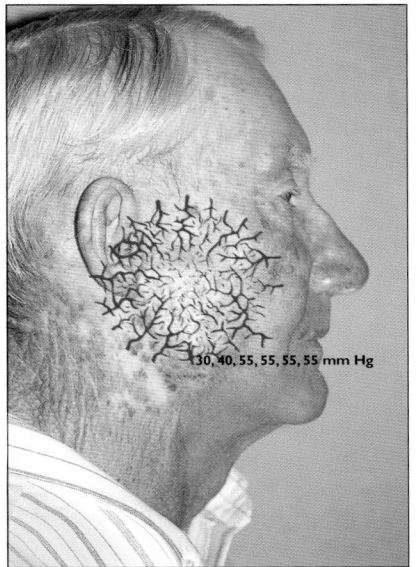

Fig 8-17d The HBO-induced angiogenesis in irradiated tissues is shut off at approximately 75% to 80% of normal tissue vascularity because of vessel ingrowth, reducing the oxygen gradient to less than 20 mm Hg during an HBO session.

Table 8-1 Recurrence of oral squamous cell carcinoma

Stage*	Without HBO	With HBO
I	7/35 (20%)	6/33 (18%)
II	12/48 (25%)	12/57 (21%)
III	22/66 (33%)	27/78 (35%)
IV	57/94 (61%)	53/89 (60%)

*Stage of TNM classification according to the American Joint Commission on Cancer Staging.

nized cancers. However, to date, several well-performed animal studies and one human trial have shown no promotion of cancer growth or emergence of new primary carcinomas in patients who have undergone HBO therapy. This is most likely because cancers are autonomous mutating cell populations expressing abnormal genes. They proliferate as facultative anaerobes by producing their own set of cytokines and growth factors independently of normal growth factors. Hyperbaric oxygen works through wound macrophages, not on epithelial cells, and causes these macrophages to express normal gene functions related to angiogenesis (VEGF) and collagen synthesis (bFGF). For the clinician and the patient, it is important to understand that HBO does not expose one to a higher risk of recurrent or new primary carcinomas (Table 8-1).

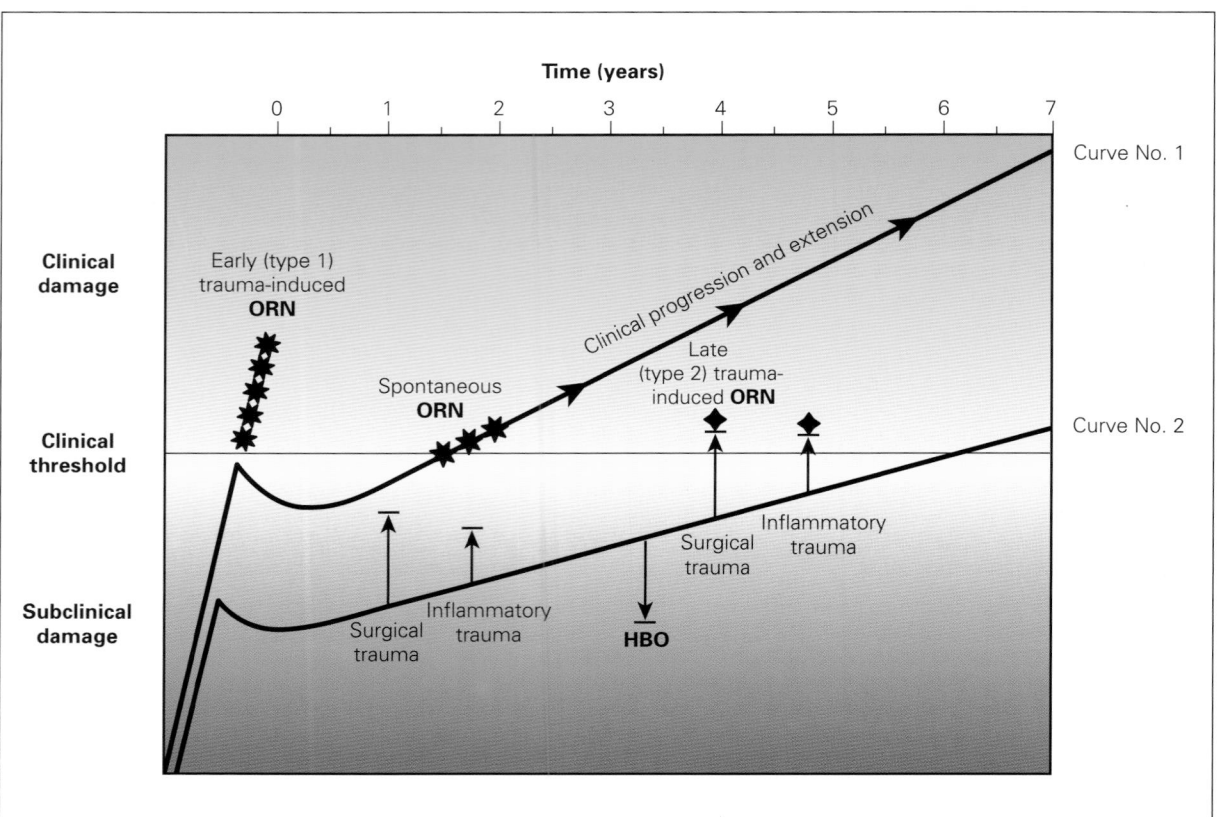

Fig 8-18 These curves plot damage resulting over time from two radiation doses: one extremely high (curve no. 1) and the other more moderate (curve no. 2). The clinical threshold is a line of subclinical radiation damage above which development of clinically exposed nonviable bone (osteoradionecrosis [ORN]) begins.

Osteoradionecrosis

Osteoradionecrosis is bone death caused by radiation injury. It is not an infection of compromised bone, as had previously been thought, but an avascular necrosis of bone caused by the three-H tissue effects of radiotherapy. Infections associated with osteoradionecrosis are secondary infections due to the exposure of bone and deep tissue planes.

There are three types of osteoradionecrosis (Fig 8-18): early trauma-induced osteoradionecrosis, spontaneous osteoradionecrosis (unassociated with any traumatic event), and late trauma-induced osteoradionecrosis. Figure 8-18 depicts the normal tissue injury curve over time. The radiation injury is intended to stay below a threshold. Below this threshold is subclinical injury recognized as three-H tissue. Above this threshold, soft tissue or bone death (osteoradionecrosis) or both occurs. High-dose radiotherapy (above 7,200 cGy) brings the injury vector closer to the clinical threshold than does a more moderate dose of radiotherapy (6,000 cGy to 6,400 cGy). If radiotherapy should continue indefinitely, osteoradionecrosis would occur acutely at about 10,000 cGy to 12,000 cGy. This has happened, though rarely, when radiotherapy miscalculations have been made or desperate clinical situations have necessitated such high doses.

Early Trauma-Induced Osteoradionecrosis

Early trauma-induced osteoradionecrosis results from combining radiation injury with surgical injury and thereby extending the injury vector above the clinical threshold. The clinical scenarios are when invasive dental procedures (eg, tooth removal) are performed during radiotherapy; when teeth are removed before radiotherapy but radiotherapy begins shortly thereafter; and when surgery involves sectioning the mandible to access a tumor (mandibulotomy), reflecting periosteum, or placing a wire or plate, and radiotherapy follows shortly thereafter. In these scenarios, osteoradionecrosis develops either during radiotherapy or in the first few months thereafter.

The normal tissue injury vector is deflected downward (recovery) during the first 4 months after radiotherapy for each dose. This "golden window" represents cellular survival and resolution of inflammation. However, each curve then depicts an upward deflection, which is due either to the normal life span or to a shortened life span of healing fibroblasts and vascular endothelial cells, ending in cellular death without cellular replacement. Essentially, this is the beginning of three-H tissue development. The slope of this upward deflection depends not only on the initial radiation dose and type of radiotherapy but on numerous other factors, such as concomitant chemotherapy or hyperthermy and a patient's associated diseases, age, nutrition, and smoking and alcohol habits. Therefore, the slope of this progressive tissue injury to normal tissue will always progress toward a more advanced state but at a different rate (indicated by the slope of the curve) for each individual.

Spontaneous Osteoradionecrosis

Spontaneous osteoradionecrosis develops when the dosage of radiotherapy is very high, bringing the injury vector close to the threshold. Then, after the 4-month recovery time, the vascular damage and stromal damage advance at a faster rate so that, between 6 months and 2 years, the injury vector crosses the threshold. The most common clinical scenario is one in which an individual receives 7,400 cGy or more; after 6 to 18 months, a bone exposure of the lingual cortex develops or what seems to be rapidly advancing periodontal bone loss occurs. Both represent nonvital bone due to the initial high radiotherapy dose.

Late Trauma-Induced Osteoradionecrosis

Moderate radiotherapy dosages produce tissue injury well below the clinical threshold. After the first 4 months of recovery, a more gradual upward slope of three-H tissue occurs, which maintains the tissue injury below the clinical threshold. Even continuing tissue injury from periodontal disease or a short-term injury from a tooth removal may not precipitate the development of osteoradionecrosis if it occurs within the first 2 years. However, because of the progression of the radiation-induced injury, the same injury at 3, 4, or 5 years will result in osteoradionecrosis (extend the injury vector over the threshold). The common clinical scenario of this pathophysiology is an individual who received radiotherapy 5 or 10 years previously. No complications from the radiotherapy developed except for some xerostomia and radiation caries. A tooth may have been removed 6 months after the radiotherapy without healing complications. However, now a tooth is removed without the support of HBO and the socket fails to heal. The bone continues to be exposed over several months as pain begins and an osteolytic process is seen on radiographs. This is late trauma-induced osteoradionecrosis (see Figs 8-13a and 8-13b).

Prevention of Osteoradionecrosis

Many cases of osteoradionecrosis can be prevented by the preradiation management recommendations discussed in the first portion of this chapter. Additional cases of osteoradionecrosis can be prevented by

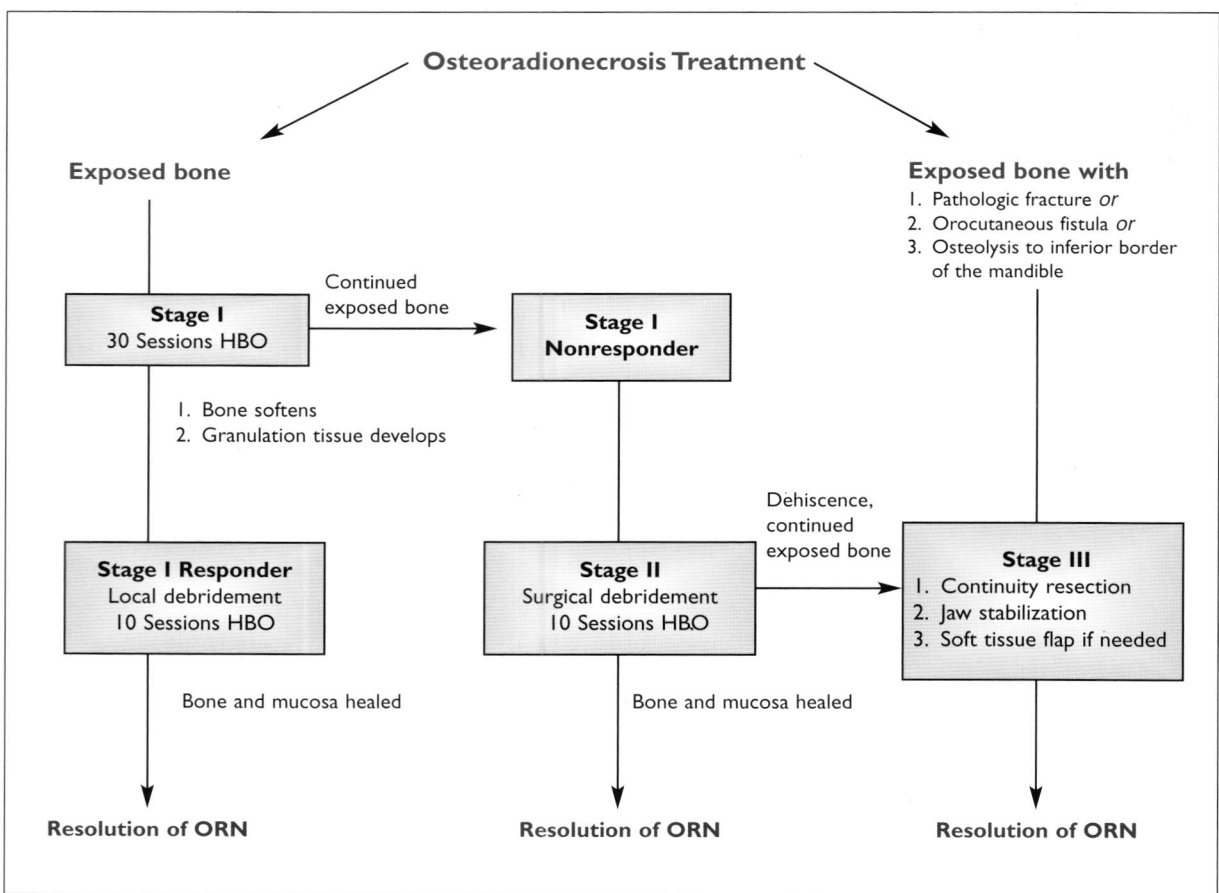

Fig 8-19 Osteoradionecrosis (ORN) of any type may be resolved with the staged protocol using hyperbaric oxygen and selected surgery.

using the 20/10 HBO protocol when any elective surgery, especially tooth extraction or dental implant placement, is performed on irradiated tissue.

However, it is important to remember that HBO increases the vascularity to only 75% of the vascularity of nonirradiated tissue, not 100%. Therefore, tooth removals should be accomplished with minimal reflection of the periosteum in order to maintain blood supply to the mandible. It is counterproductive to significantly reflect periosteum to gain a primary closure or to accomplish a "radical alveolectomy." Instead, minimal reflection of the buccal periosteum to remove only sharp, bony projections and maintenance of the lingual periosteum will best maintain bone vitality. A similar minimal soft tissue periosteal reflection approach should also be used when placing dental implants into HBO-improved irradiated mandibles.

Treatment of Osteoradionecrosis

Established osteoradionecrosis with exposed bone represents an advanced radiation tissue injury. A specific protocol using hyperbaric oxygen combined with selective surgeries when required has proven effective in resolving osteoradionecrosis (Fig 8-19). This protocol is recommended by the Undersea and Hyperbaric Medicine Society and endorsed by the National Cancer Institute through a consensus conference. It uses 30 sessions of hyperbaric oxygen at 2.4 ATA for 90 treatment minutes of 100% oxygen followed by 10 sessions after an assessment or surgery. This protocol not only uses hyperbaric oxygen to develop a capillary angiogenesis in the three-H tissue, but uses the individual's response to it as a

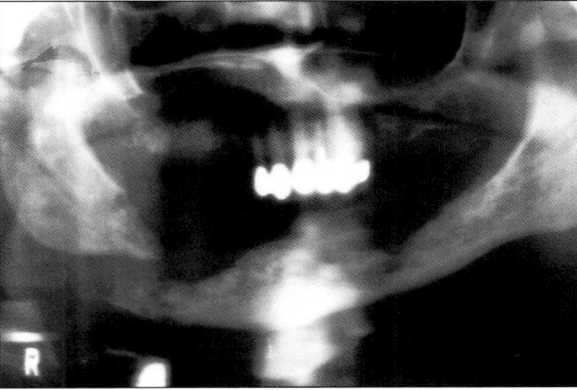

Fig 8-20 Stage III osteoradionecrosis due to a pathologic fracture. Note the bilateral osteolysis and an incipient fracture in the parasymphysis area on the opposite side from the obvious fracture.

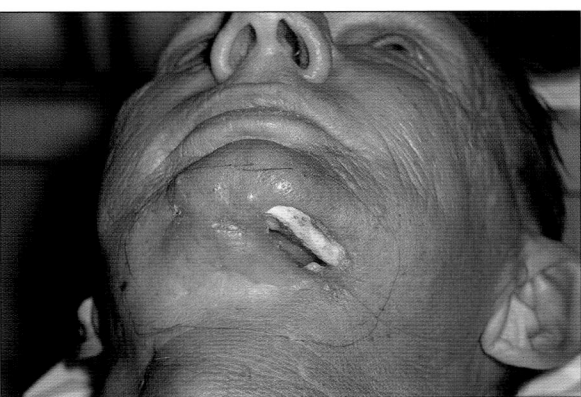

Fig 8-21 Stage III osteoradionecrosis due to an orocutaneous fistula. Note the loss of skin, platysma, and floor-of-the-mouth contents in addition to the obviously nonvital bone.

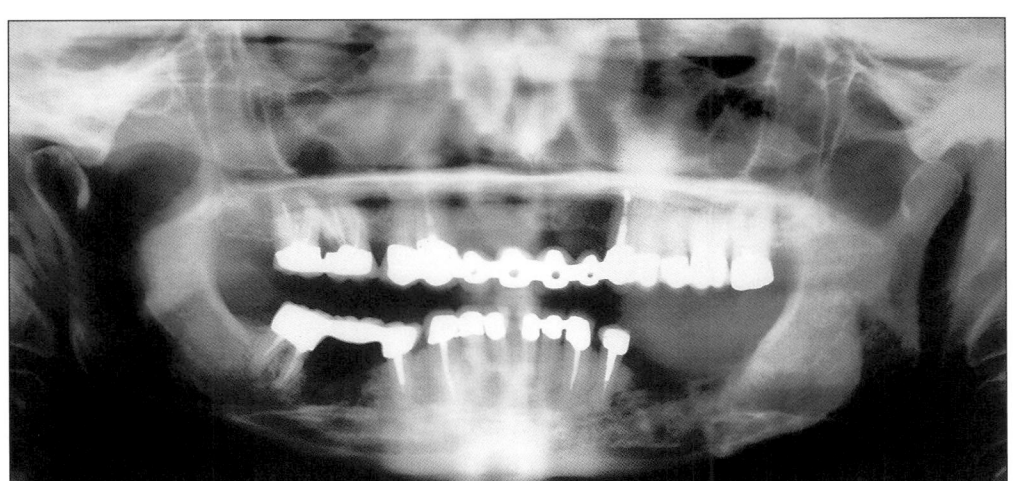

Fig 8-22 Bilateral osteoradionecrosis. There is osteolysis to the inferior border in the body of the mandible on each side. Each would represent a stage III osteoradionecrosis.

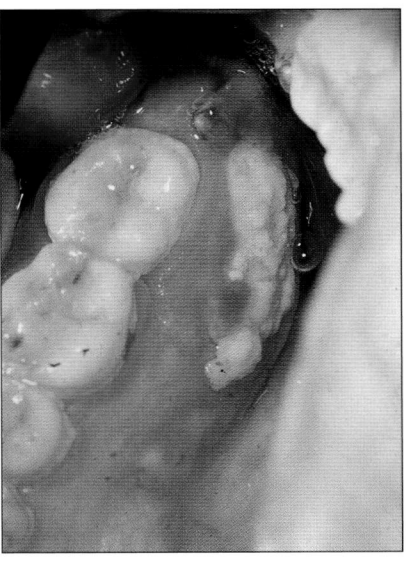

Fig 8-23a Osteoradionecrosis responding in stage I. The exposed bone has softened after 30 sessions of HBO and granulation tissue is undermining it.

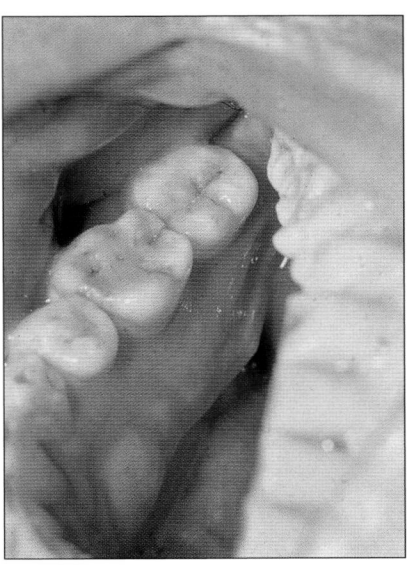

Fig 8-23b A response in stage I will heal with no further exposed bone once the original nonviable bone has sequestered or is removed.

guideline to select the correct degree of adjunctive surgery. The focus of hyperbaric oxygen in the treatment of osteoradionecrosis is not on the dead bone; it is on the radiation-injured tissue that is not yet dead. Only surgical removal can manage the dead bone.

Osteoradionecrosis that presents with a pathologic fracture (Fig 8-20), an orocutaneous fistula (Fig 8-21), or osteolysis to the inferior border of the mandible (Fig 8-22) represents an advanced stage (stage III). Other individuals with osteoradionecrosis are placed into stage I of the protocol. In stage I, individuals receive an initial 30 sessions of hyperbaric oxygen. After 30 sessions, the wound is assessed for a response. A stage I responder will evidence granulation tissue and a softening of the exposed bone. At this time, the soft exposed bone is debrided and the final 10 sessions of hyperbaric oxygen are completed. If successful, exposed bone will become covered with mucosa over the following 1 to 2 months (Figs 8-23a and 8-23b).

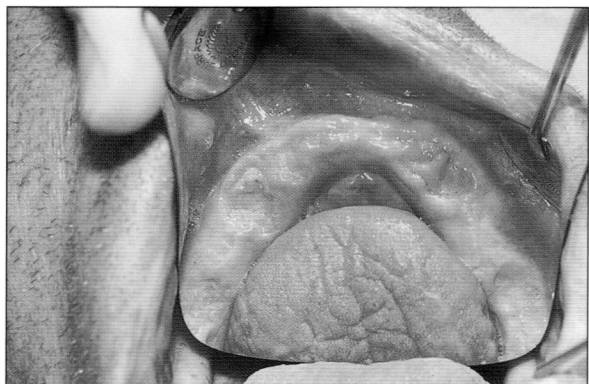

Fig 8-24a A stage I nonresponder is advanced to stage II. Exposed bone remains in the anterior tooth sockets after 30 sessions of HBO.

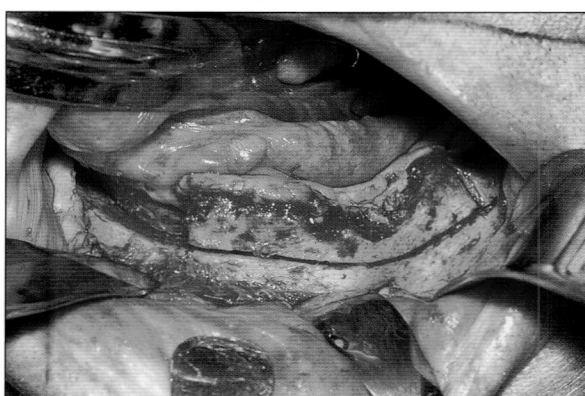

Fig 8-24b In stage II, the exposed nonviable bone is excised with saline-cooled saws and minimal reflection of the periosteum, which supplies the majority of the blood to the mandible.

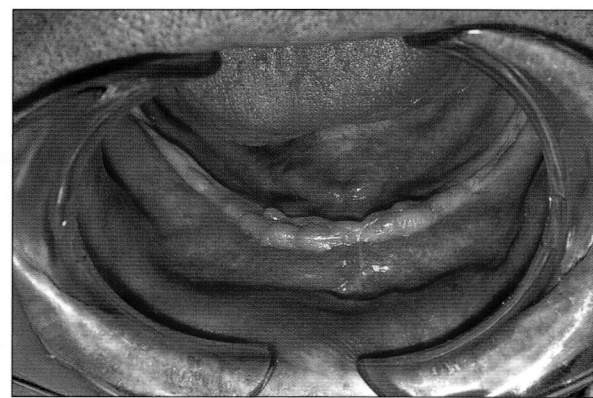

Fig 8-24c A stage II responder will heal and evidence a complete soft tissue cover without any dehiscence or further exposure of bone.

If the exposed bone is unchanged after 30 sessions of hyperbaric oxygen and no granulation tissue is present, the individual represents a stage I nonresponder and proceeds to stage II (Fig 8-24a).

In stage II, the exposed bone is surgically removed with minimal reflection of the vascular periosteum over vital bone. If the exposed bone is a tooth socket, the bony excision is an alveolectomy (Fig 8-24b). If the exposed bone is buccal or lingual cortex, the bony excision takes the form of a decortication. A primary closure over the remaining bleeding viable bone should be achieved. After this surgery, the individual goes on to complete the final 10 sessions of hyperbaric oxygen therapy.

Stage II responders will heal to resolution of their osteoradionecrosis without a dehiscence and without further exposed bone (Fig 8-24c). Stage II nonresponders will develop dehiscences and further exposed bone indicative of a greater amount of dead bone than was clinically or radiographically evident. Stage II nonresponders are advanced to stage III.

Because of nonresponse in stage II, individuals in stage III usually will have received their complete 40 sessions of hyperbaric oxygen. These individuals are then directly treated with stage III surgery. Individuals in stage III who present with a pathologic fracture, an orocutaneous fistula, or an osteolysis to the inferior border of the mandible undergo their first 30 sessions of hyperbaric oxygen prior to stage III surgery (Fig 8-25a).

Stage III surgery consists of a continuity resection back to bleeding bone margins (Fig 8-25b). The bony edges of the host bone should be rounded to prevent penetration through thin tissues, and there should be minimal reflection of the vascular periosteum on the remaining host bone. If a soft tissue defect is present, soft tissue flaps such as myocutaneous or free vascular flaps are accomplished at this time (Figs 8-25c and 8-25d). The defect is best stabilized with a rigid titanium reconstruction plate or with external pin fixation. If the individual has not received the full course of 40 hyperbaric oxygen sessions, the final 10 sessions are performed in the postoperative phase.

Once the tissues have healed and matured (about 3 to 4 months) (Figs 8-25e and 8-25f), bony reconstruction can be accomplished without the need for additional hyperbaric oxygen (Fig 8-25g). Such individuals can then undergo dental rehabilitation if required with split-thickness skin graft vestibuloplasties and/or dental implant placement.

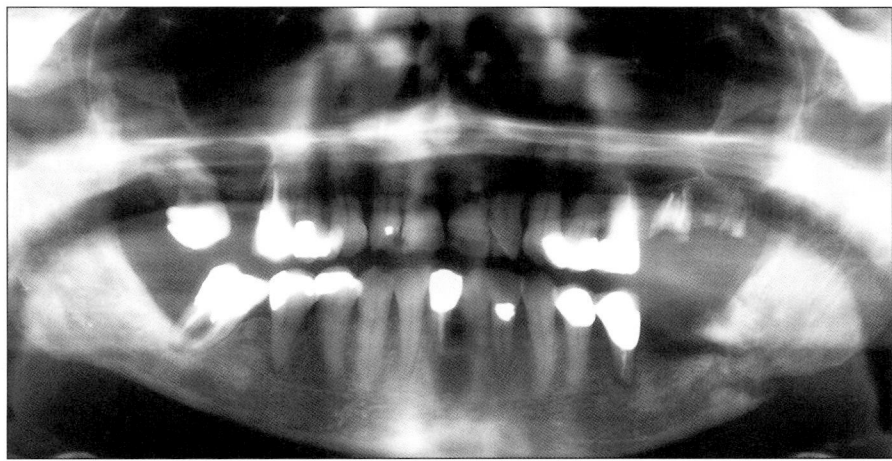

Fig 8-25a Pathologic fracture at the left angle of the mandible through a third molar root establishes this as stage III osteoradionecrosis.

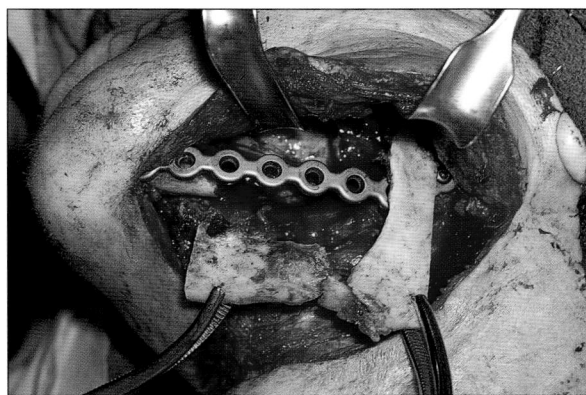

Fig 8-25b Stage III osteoradionecrosis requires a resection and usually a rigid plate reconstruction of the mandible. Here the resection included the pathologic fracture and the coronoid process. The resection margins are bleeding bone.

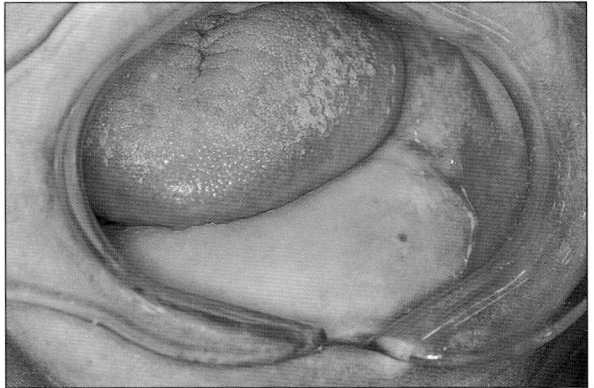

Fig 8-25c Healed skin paddle from a myocutaneous flap replaces the radiation-damaged soft tissue and provides a covering over a titanium reconstruction plate and the remaining native mandible.

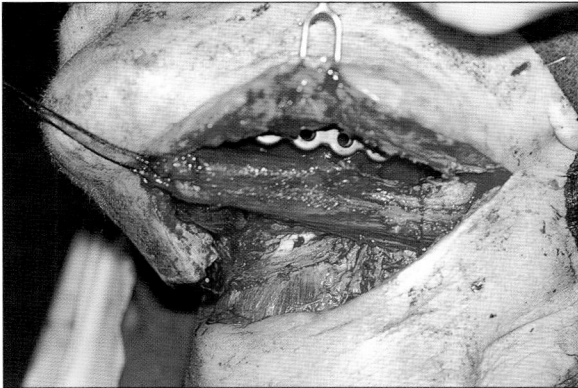

Fig 8-25d Many stage III osteoradionecrosis patients also have significant soft tissue loss, requiring some type of a myocutaneous flap. Here a sternocleidomastoid muscle flap is used to fill the wound dead space and add soft tissue.

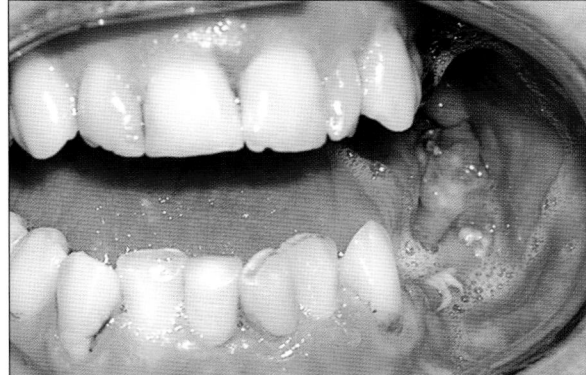

Fig 8-25e Osteoradionecrosis showing exposed nonvital bone prior to surgery and HBO.

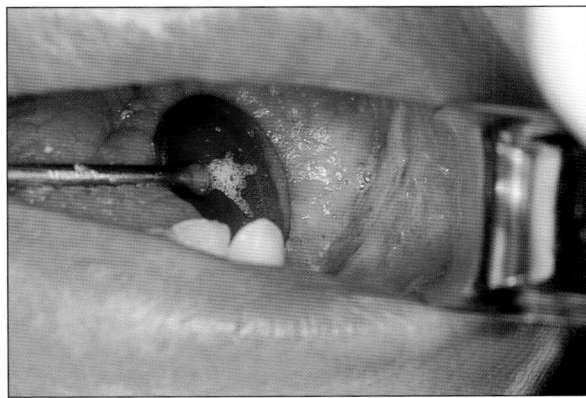

Fig 8-25f Osteoradionecrosis resolved as indicated by complete soft tissue healing without further exposed bone.

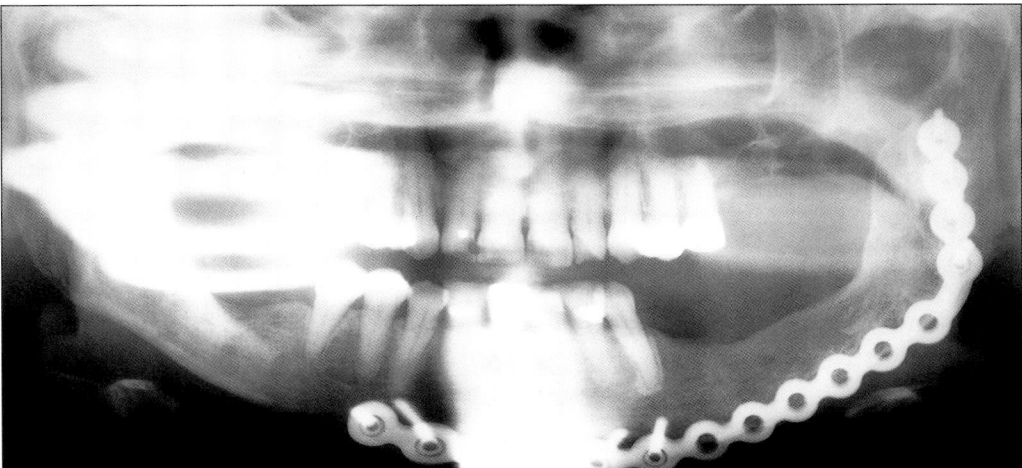

Fig 8-25g The osteoradionecrosis defect in Figs 8-25a to 8-25f can be reconstructed with excellent results using standard cancellous marrow grafts after 3 months of initial healing and without the need for further HBO.

Table 8-2 Cost analysis of osteoradionecrosis*

Treatment	No. of patients	Average 1-year cost	Average total cost	Resolution rate
No HBO	141	$47,000	$153,000	9%
HBO without surgery	92	$38,000	$91,000	18%
HBO protocol with surgery	536	$51,000	$51,000	98%

*January 1, 2001, US dollars.

Cost of Treating Osteoradionecrosis

Because it is a chronic disease, osteoradionecrosis can become extremely costly if unresolved (Table 8-2). Office visits, antibiotics, analgesics, minor surgeries, and hospitalizations for a 3-year course of unresolved osteoradionecrosis average more than $153,000. The protocol to resolve osteoradionecrosis recommended by the Undersea and Hyperbaric Medicine Society and discussed in this text is also expensive. Hyperbaric oxygen, osteoradionecrosis surgery, hospitalizations, reconstructive surgery, etc, are expensive as well. However, because this protocol resolves the osteoradionecrosis rather than allowing it to continue, its accumulated costs are only $51,000 including reconstructive surgery and dental rehabilitation. Aside from the obvious value of pain resolution, improved function, and improved appearance, disease resolution is far more cost-effective than the ongoing accumulated costs of chronic disease.

Benign Soft Tissue Tumors of Mesenchymal Origin

CHAPTER 9

▶ *"Small incision—big mistake."*
"See well what you do so you can do well what you see."
—*Stuart N. Kline*

Predominantly Fibrous Tumors

Fibroma

CLINICAL PRESENTATION AND PATHOGENESIS ▶

The fibroma is not a true neoplasm because its growth potential is limited. Since it ceases to grow once it reaches about 2 cm in diameter, it probably represents a reactive hyperplasia of fibroblasts or a hamartoma. It presents as a painless, firm mass that protrudes from the submucosa. The overlying mucosa is intact with mature epithelium unless some form of trauma has caused surface ulceration secondarily. It is generally rounded, does not blanch, and is not painful to palpation. Most are found on the buccal mucosa in the areas adjacent to the occlusal plane and are thus believed to be related to tooth abrasion, cheek biting, or sucking trauma (Fig 9-1a). In the past these have been referred to as traumatic fibromas or irritation fibromas; however, a traumatic stimulus is not always apparent. Other locations include the lateral border of the tongue and the labial mucosa.

DIFFERENTIAL DIAGNOSIS ▶

A mass with benign characteristics within the submucosa can be almost any benign tumor arising from native cells within the submucosa. Therefore, a *schwannoma*, *lipoma*, or benign minor salivary gland tumor such as a *pleomorphic adenoma*, *canalicular adenoma*, or *basal cell adenoma* is possible. A neurofibroma is not likely to clinically present as a fibroma because of its unencapsulated nature, which usually imparts an irregular and, if severe, a "bag-of-worms" consistency. On the other hand, a schwannoma is well encapsulated and will present as a submucosal bulging mass.

DIAGNOSTIC WORK-UP AND TREATMENT ▶

These lesions and most of the serious considerations on the differential list are diagnosed and treated by local excision. The mass with its overlying mucosa is excised with 1- to 2-mm margins to the depth of the underlying muscle fascia (Figs 9-1b and 9-1c). The resultant wound can be closed by undermining and advancing the edges. If the lesion is in the buccal mucosa close to the commissure, it is best to excise it with the long axis oriented anteroposteriorly. A vertical excision may scar in such a manner as to restrict the oral opening.

HISTOPATHOLOGY ▶

A fibroma usually appears as a well-defined mass of hypocellular collagenized tissue. Cellularity is variable, however, as is the degree of vascularity. If an inflammatory component is present, it is usually found adjacent to the overlying epithelium or perivascularly. The epithelium is often attenuated and may be hyperkeratinized (Fig 9-1d). Most of these lesions are reactive rather than neoplastic, and only their circumscription separates them diagnostically from fibrous hyperplasia.

PROGNOSIS ▶

Local excision is curative. If left untreated, fibromas will remain with little change. However, excision is recommended to rule out more serious neoplasms.

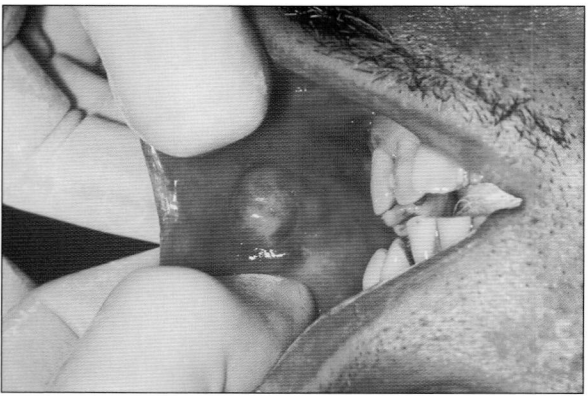

Fig 9-1a The buccal mucosa adjacent to the occlusal plane is a common location for a fibroma. Note the broad base and smooth surface.

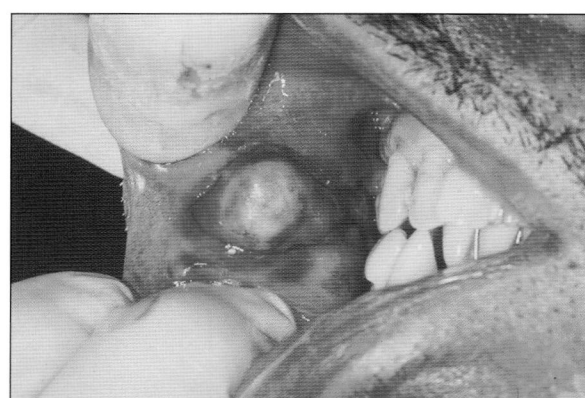

Fig 9-1b Oral fibromas are excised with 1- to 2-mm peripheral margins.

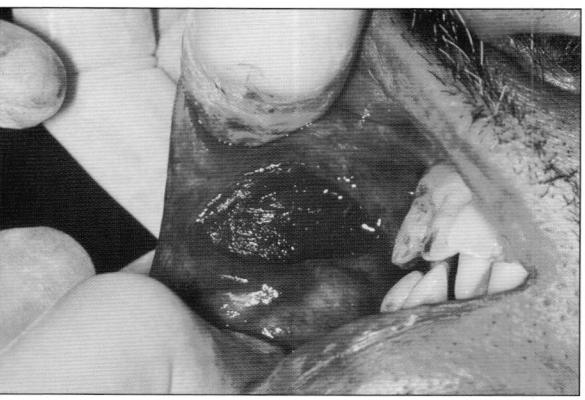

Fig 9-1c The depth of excision for a fibroma is to the level of the muscle fascia. At this level, the edges can be undermined for a primary closure.

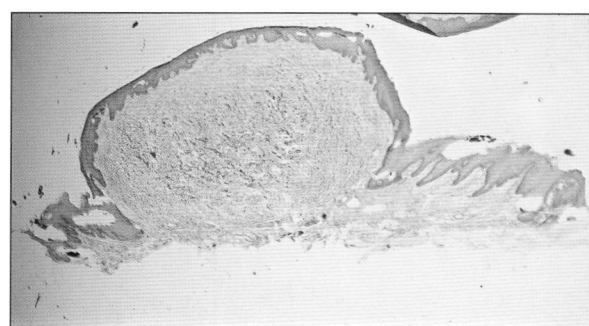

Fig 9-1d Fibroma showing a demarcated mass of dense collagen covered by an attenuated stratified squamous epithelium.

Giant Cell Fibroma

CLINICAL PRESENTATION AND PATHOGENESIS ►

Occasionally the clinician may be confused by a pathology report diagnosing a "giant cell fibroma" in what seemed to be a routine intraoral fibroma. Indeed, the two are nearly identical except for the histopathologic finding of multinucleated but stellate-shaped giant cells in the giant cell fibroma. Both the intraoral fibroma and the giant cell fibroma represent a focal fibrous hyperplasia that has limited growth potential and is usually static when first seen. Both are curable by local excision around their clinical periphery and into the submucosa.

This lesion should not be confused with the *giant cell fibroblastoma*, a term often used by general pathologists and dermatopathologists. This lesion, a true benign neoplasm, is a distinctive subcutaneous/dermal mass of 2 to 6 cm seen mostly in young boys. It is not related to the giant cell fibroma of the oral cavity.

HISTOPATHOLOGY ►

These fibromas may have smoothly rounded or verruciform surfaces (Figs 9-2a and 9-2b). Within a fibrous mass are large stellate and angulated cells, some of them multinucleated (Fig 9-2c). The stellate cells often have dendritic processes. Ultrastructurally, these cells appear to be atypical fibroblasts and may contain melanin.

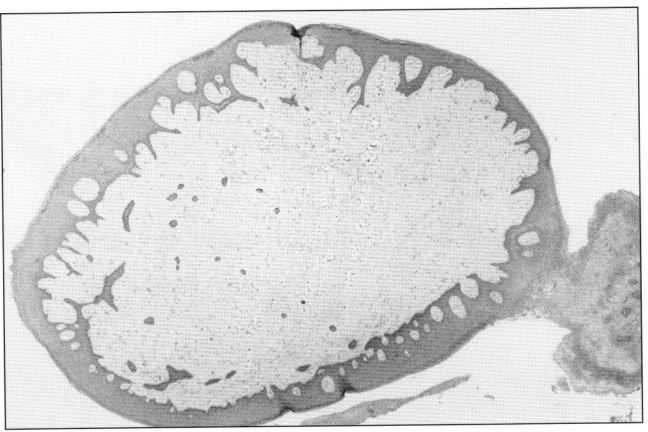 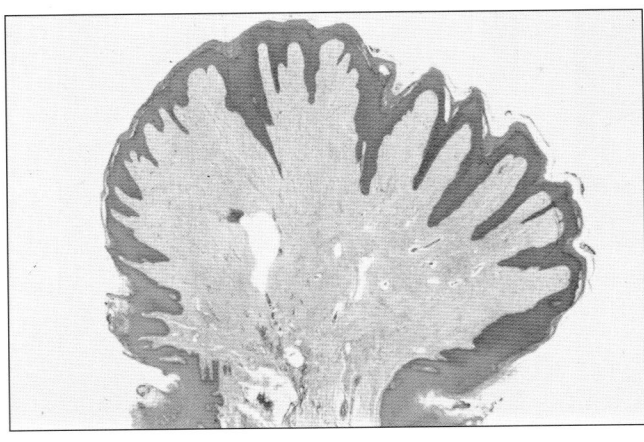 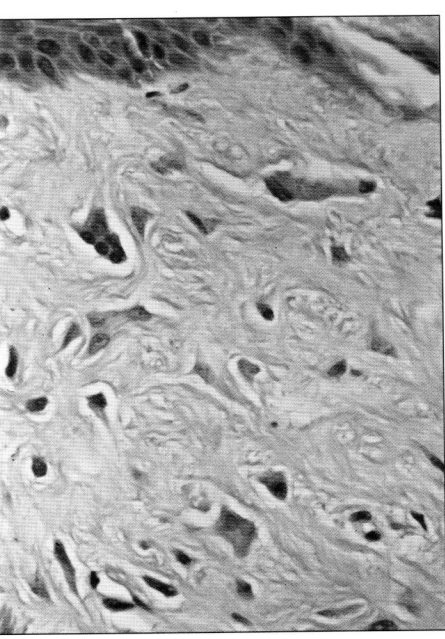

Figs 9-2a and 9-2b Low-power views of two giant cell fibromas, one having a smooth appearance (*left*) and the other a verruciform surface (*right*).

Fig 9-2c The angulated and multinucleated cells of the giant cell fibroma.

Nodular Fasciitis

CLINICAL PRESENTATION AND PATHOGENESIS ▶

Nodular fasciitis is an apparently benign reactive lesion that mimics fibrosarcoma so closely that about one half are mistakenly reported as a fibrosarcoma. The lesion emerges from the subcutaneous fascia or the submucosa and grows rapidly for about 2 weeks; it gives the impression of a rapidly infiltrating fibrous mass that is often suggestive of a malignancy. In about half of the cases dull pain is present. The mass will be firm and indurated, and in the head and neck area it will be located most commonly over the bony prominences of the angle of the mandible (Figs 9-3a and 9-3b), the symphysis, zygoma, or skull.

Although common in the upper extremities, nodular fasciitis in the maxillofacial area and oral cavity is rare. Those that develop in this area usually arise in children or adolescents; in the more common sites, the patient's age is 20 to 35 years. In about 15% of cases, a preceding incident of trauma to the area is documented. In the maxillofacial region, in particular, the mass will often be adherent to periosteum and may cause an erosion of the outer cortex (Fig 9-4). This phenomenon is even more commonly noted in what is termed *cranial fasciitis*, which is a nodular fasciitis that occurs during the first year of life and arises from the galea of the scalp. It will frequently erode the outer table of the skull and sometimes the inner table as well.

Despite its infrequent association with trauma, nodular fasciitis is thought to represent an overexuberant reaction to innocuous injury or inflammation. Therefore, even partial excision seems to deactivate the lesion, resulting in resolution. In some cases, spontaneous regression occurs, further suggesting the reactive nature of this lesion.

DIFFERENTIAL DIAGNOSIS ▶

The clinical presentation, rapid growth, infiltration, pain, and adherence to surrounding tissue of this lesion are strongly suggestive of a malignancy. Therefore, fibrous malignancies and fibromatoses (eg, *fibrosarcoma*, *malignant fibrous histiocytoma*, *aggressive fibromatosis*, and a *desmoid tumor*) make up the prime differential considerations. In children, this same rapid proliferation and firm mass adherent to periosteum can be created by some inflammatory diseases, particularly *Garré osteomyelitis with proliferative periostitis* and an *early cellulitis*.

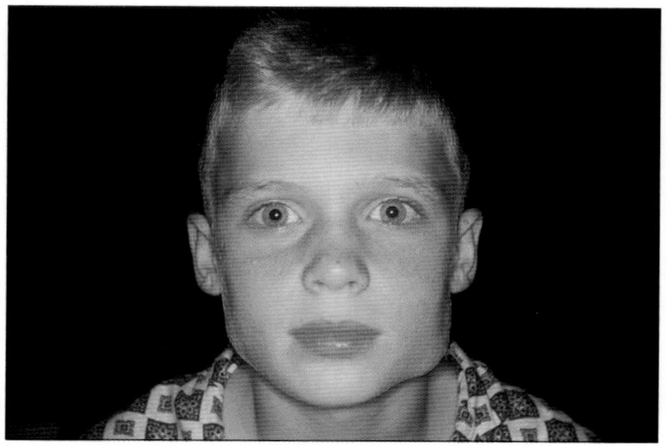

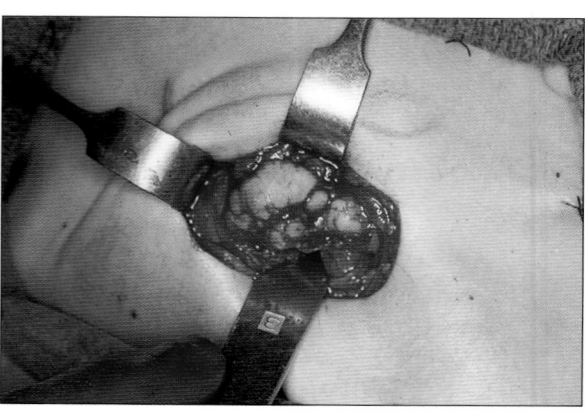

Fig 9-3a Nodular fasciitis in the head and neck area often occurs at the angle of the mandible as a firm fixed mass.

Fig 9-3b Nodular fasciitis in this area will arise from periosteum or from the parotid masseteric fascia and will infiltrate local muscles.

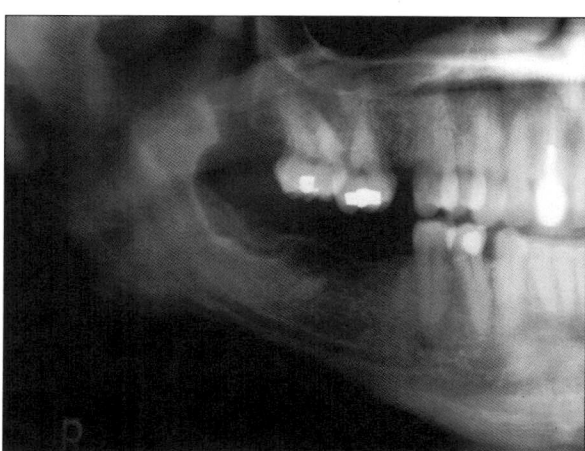

Fig 9-4 Since nodular fasciitis often arises from periosteum, it may cause a resorption of the cortex.

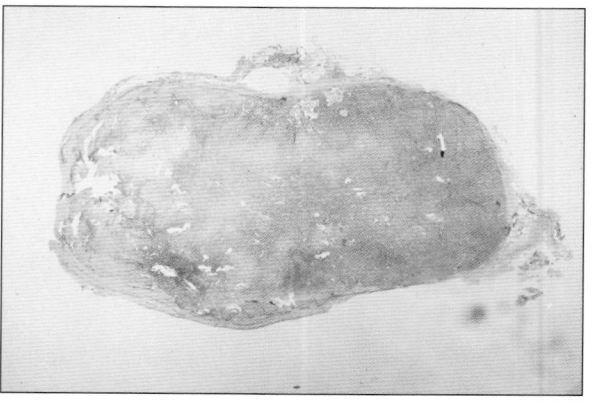

Fig 9-5a The well-defined nodular appearance of nodular fasciitis.

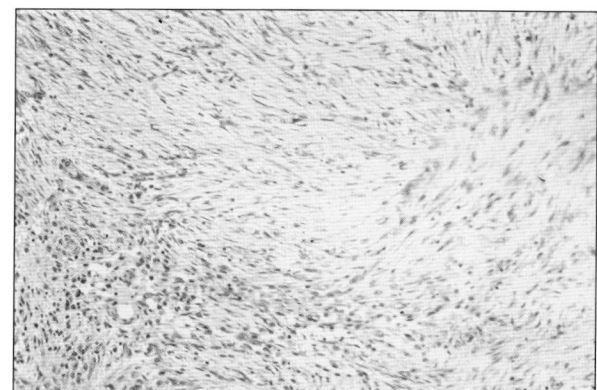

Fig 9-5b The typical feathered appearance seen in nodular fasciitis. Note also the inflammatory foci.

DIAGNOSTIC WORK-UP ▶

Because of the concern about and the need to rule out a malignancy, an incisional biopsy is recommended. It is important to note that the most diagnostic area of nodular fasciitis, and of all fibrous malignancies, is the deep tissue. A biopsy that is too superficial may lead to an incorrect diagnosis and treatment.

HISTOPATHOLOGY ▶

Fascial tumors are often infiltrative and diffuse; however, most intramuscular and subcutaneous tumors are well demarcated and circumscribed (Fig 9-5a). The tumors consist of plump, immature fibroblasts forming short bundles and fascicles. An abundant ground substance results in a feathered appearance, which is characteristic of this lesion (Fig 9-5b). Capillaries may be prominent and are concentrated at the periphery. Scattered inflammatory cells and erythrocytes are present.

TREATMENT ▶

The clinician is best advised to discuss a diagnosis of nodular fasciitis with the pathologist and to seek additional opinions if there is any uncertainty. On one hand, one would not want to treat a nodular fasciitis with the aggressive extirpative surgery required of a fibrosarcoma or a malignant fibrous histiocytoma. On the other hand, one would not want to seed tumor cells and delay extirpative surgery for fibrosarcoma or malignant fibrous histiocytoma misdiagnosed as nodular fasciitis.

If nodular fasciitis is confirmed, local excision to eradicate the bulk of the lesion without the need to gain tumor-free margins will result in resolution.

PROGNOSIS ▶

Recurrence occurs in only 1% to 2% of nodular fasciitis even with incomplete removal.

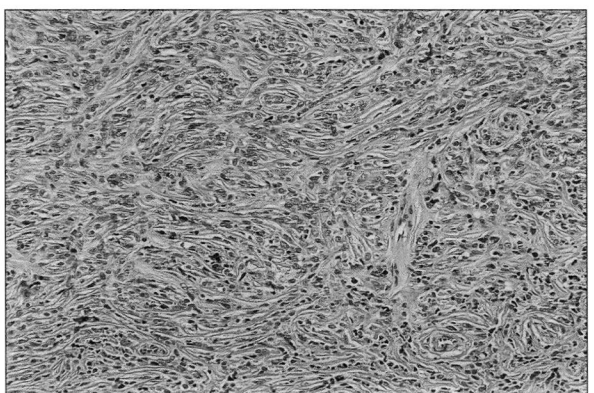

Fig 9-6 A fibrous histiocytoma with a storiform pattern.

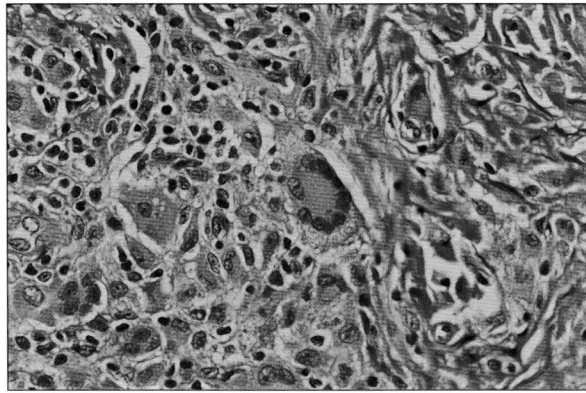

Fig 9-7 A Touton giant cell with a wreath-shaped arrangement of nuclei beyond which can be seen some pale cytoplasm containing lipid vacuoles in a fibrous histiocytoma.

Fibrous Histiocytoma

CLINICAL PRESENTATION AND PATHOGENESIS ▶

A benign fibrous histiocytoma is a common skin tumor but a very rare oral tumor. On skin, it occurs as a slow-growing, painless red nodule that is sometimes black because of hemosiderin accumulation. Tumors range in size from 2 mm to 2 cm and are most commonly found on the skin of the extremities in adults 20 to 40 years of age. Deeply situated fibrous histiocytomas are less common but grow to a larger size. Most reach a size ranging from 5 to 8 cm.

Too few oral lesions have been reported to determine preferred sites. Those that have been reported arose from the submucosa of the tongue, floor of the mouth, or buccal mucosa. Rarely, lesions have occurred centrally within the mandible. In such cases, they have produced a radiolucency with indistinct borders and only slight expansion.

The pathogenesis seems to be that of a true neoplasm with continued but slow growth and a limited capacity for invasion. The controversy as to its histogenesis (fibroblasts vs histiocytes) may be an academic point since the histiocytic-appearing cells as well as fibroblasts originate from the same precursor cell.

DIFFERENTIAL DIAGNOSIS ▶

In the past, cutaneous lesions often were called *dermatofibromas*. Their single unencapsulated nodularity is nonspecific and may suggest several benign skin tumors such as *neurofibroma*, *granular cell tumor*, *lipoma*, and *nodular fasciitis*. Those that appear black from hemosiderin accumulation may resemble a *nevus* or *melanoma*. Infrequently, a benign-appearing fibrous histiocytoma turns out to be a small or early *malignant fibrous histiocytoma*.

On oral soft tissue, the nodular red appearance and often ulcerated surface is more suggestive of a *pyogenic granuloma*, a *hemangioma*, or a *traumatic eosinophilic granuloma* than of a fibrous histiocytoma. Owing to its rarity, it is doubtful that fibrous histiocytoma would be on a differential list; it would more likely be a surprise finding.

DIAGNOSTIC WORK-UP AND TREATMENT ▶

Cutaneous and mucosal tumors are diagnosed and treated by local excision with 5-mm margins. Bony lesions may be resolved by a local resection using 5-mm margins.

HISTOPATHOLOGY ▶

Fibrous histiocytomas are unencapsulated masses consisting of fascicles of fibroblastic cells with some histiocytic cells. There is often a storiform pattern (Fig 9-6). Touton or foreign body giant cells may be present, and areas of hemorrhage are common (Fig 9-7). The overlying epithelium is often hyperplastic and may show pseudoepitheliomatous hyperplasia.

PROGNOSIS ▶

Local excision is expected to be curative. Recurrence rates are less than 5%.

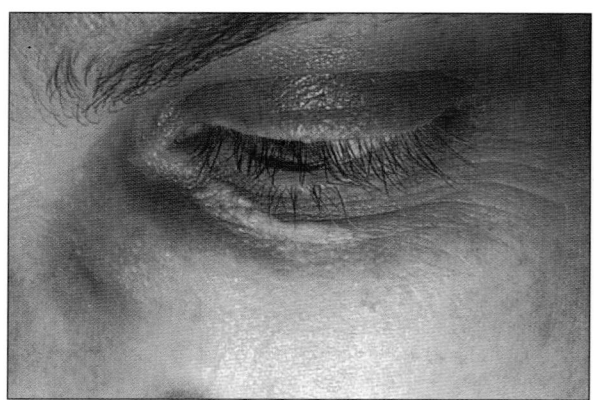

Fig 9-8 Multiple subcutaneous elevations representing xanthelasmas. (Reprinted from Callen JP, *Color Atlas of Dermatology*, with permission from WB Saunders Co.)

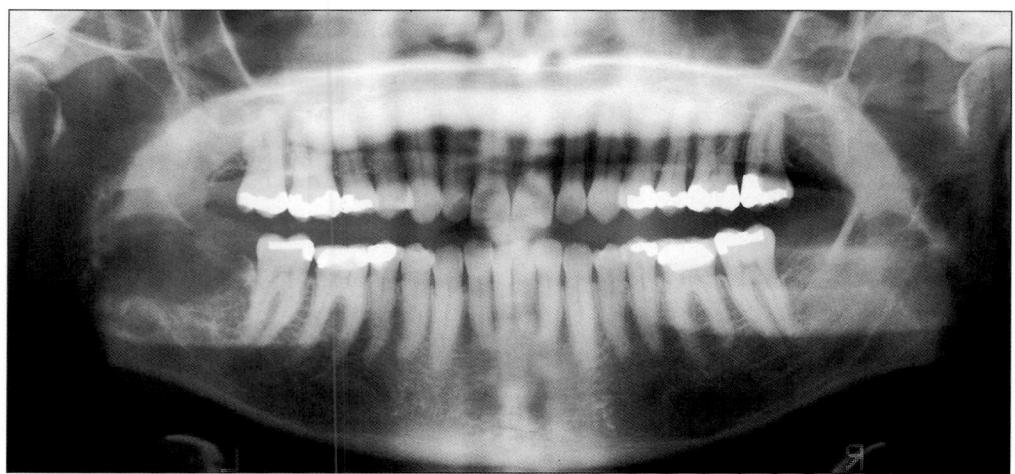

Fig 9-9 A central deep xanthoma in the mandible will appear as an irregular radiolucency with little or no expansion.

Xanthomas

CLINICAL PRESENTATION AND PATHOGENESIS ▶

Xanthomas are not true neoplasms but aggregates of lipid-containing histiocytes. Most xanthomas occur on skin surfaces and are related to any one or several of the five known subtypes of systemic hyperlipidemia (see the section on hyperlipidemia states and their relation to xanthomas on pages 401 to 402). The verruciform xanthoma of the oral mucosa has no known association with hyperlipidemic states.

Cutaneous Xanthomas

The cutaneous xanthomas are divided into four types.

Eruptive Xanthoma
These lesions are small yellow papules found mostly in the gluteal area. They are associated with hypertriglyceridemia and hyperlipidemia types I, III, IV, and V.

Tuberous Xanthoma
These large flat lesions occur subcutaneously on the buttocks, elbows, fingers, and knees. They are associated with hyperlipidemia types II and III.

Plane Xanthoma
These flat lesions occur in skin creases. They are seen in hyperlipidemia types II and III and may be associated with biliary cirrhosis. When they occur in normolipidemic individuals, there is often an associated malignancy.

Xanthelasma
These are the common subcutaneous elevations that occur on the eyelids of elderly normolipidemic individuals (Fig 9-8). They also occur early in hyperlipidemia types II and III.

Table 9-1 Fredrickson and Lees classification of the primary hyperlipidemias*

	Phenotype†					
	I	IIa	IIb	III	IV	V
Cholesterol		+	+	+		
Triglycerides	++		+	+	+	+
HDLs						
LDLs		+	+			
VLDLs			+	abn	+	+
Chylomicrons	+					+

*Plus sign denotes increased concentration; abn, abnormal; HDLs, high-density lipoproteins; LDLs, low-density lipoproteins; VLDLs, very-low-density lipoproteins.
†Types IIa and IIb carry a markedly increased risk, and types III and IV a moderately increased risk of coronary artery disease. Types IV and V are associated with an increased incidence of pancreatitis. Type I is rare.

Deep Xanthoma

The deep xanthoma, which usually occurs in tendons or synovium, may also occur in bone. In the mandible, the lesion produces a poorly demarcated radiolucency with irregular borders and minimal to no expansion of the cortices (Fig 9-9). The radiographic appearance resembles that of an idiopathic bone cavity but is somewhat less radiolucent. These xanthomas occur in normolipidemic individuals or may be associated with hyperlipidemia types II and III.

Hyperlipidemia States and Their Relation to Xanthomas

Because cutaneous or deep xanthomas often share a relationship with hyperlipidemic states, a brief review of hyperlipidemic forms and types is in order. The primary form of hyperlipidemia is genetic and is classified according to plasma triglyceride and cholesterol levels; these are the forms associated with some xanthomas. The secondary form of hyperlipidemia affects patients with various medical conditions, including diabetes, alcoholism, chronic renal failure, chronic liver failure, hypothyroidism, and estrogen therapy; these are not associated with xanthomas.

The primary or genetic form of hyperlipidemia is divided into five types based on Fredrickson and Lees classification (Table 9-1). Briefly, type I is characterized by hypertriglyceridemia and chylomicrons; type IIa, by hypercholesterolemia with increased low-density lipoproteins; type IIb, by both hypertriglyceridemia and hypercholesterolemia with increased low-density lipoproteins and very-low-density lipoproteins; type III, by both hypertriglyceridemia and hypercholesterolemia and by abnormal very-low-density lipoproteins; type IV, by hypertriglyceridemia and increased very-low-density lipoproteins; and type V, by hypertriglyceridemia, chylomicrons, and an increase in very-low-density lipoproteins.

Tuberous xanthomas, which form large plaque-like lesions on the buttocks, elbows, fingers, and knees, are associated with hyperlipidemia types II and III. Plane xanthomas, which occur in skin folds, are associated with hyperlipidemia types II and III. The xanthelasma, which affects the face and eyelids, may be seen in types II and III but is mostly seen in normolipidemic individuals. Deep xanthomas that may be seen in bone, including the mandible, are often associated with type II or type III and very rarely type IV (Table 9-2).

The collection of lipid-laden histiocytes, extracellular lipid, and fibrosis represents progressive stages of the pathologic process. The mechanism begins when excess lipoproteins leave the serum and traverse the vessel wall to be taken up by tissue macrophages. The macrophages break down the lipid protein in

Table 9-2 Xanthoma types, hyperlipidemic states, location, and histologic appearance

Type	Association with hyperlipidemia	Location	Histologic appearance
Eruptive xanthoma	Types I, III, IV, and V	Predilection for buttocks	Sheets of nonfoamy and foamy histiocytes
Tuberous xanthoma	Types II and III	Subcutis of elbow, buttocks, knees, and fingers	Sheets of xanthomatous histiocytes; large extracellular cholesterol deposits; significant fibrosis, modest inflammation
Plane xanthoma	Types II (primary biliary cirrhosis) and III, and normolipidemic persons	Skin creases, particularly of palms	Sheets of foamy histiocytes; little fibrosis and inflammation
Xanthelasma	Types II and III and normolipidemic persons	Eyelids	Sheets of foamy histiocytes; little fibrosis and inflammation
Deep xanthoma	Types II and III; rarely type IV; also associated with cerebrotendinous xanthomatosis	Tendons of hands and feet; achilles tendon; less commonly bone	Similar to that of tuberous xanthoma

their cytoplasm to lipid and component amino acids. Some of the lipid is released into the surrounding extracellular space, thereby creating the light microscopic picture of foamy histiocytes and extracellular lipid collections. The presence of extracellular lipid, especially cholesterol, induces inflammation followed by a fibroblastic reaction in the surrounding tissue and will thus result in fibrosis. Some such lesions have been called *fibroxanthomas*.

DIFFERENTIAL DIAGNOSIS ▶

The differential diagnosis of cutaneous xanthomas is a moot question because of their distinctive presentation. When a deep xanthoma occurs in the mandible, it may not be recognized as a xanthoma at first because of its rarity. The radiographic picture will mostly resemble that of an *idiopathic bone cavity* or a *chronic osteomyelitis*. Other radiolucent lesions that may have indistinct borders such as a *central hemangioma* or a *metastatic tumor focus* are also considerations.

DIAGNOSTIC WORK-UP AND TREATMENT ▶

Cutaneous xanthomas do not necessarily require surgical removal. Diagnosis of the correct hyperlipidemic state by a complete serum triglyceride and cholesterol profile is required. If control to a normolipidemic state or something close to it is achieved, many lesions will slowly regress over several years. If the lesion is surgically excised and the hyperlipidemic state controlled, recurrence is unlikely. If the lesion is excised and the hyperlipidemic state persists, the xanthoma will slowly recur.

A xanthoma of the mandible is discovered on exploration. The mandible will contain a yellow friable substance (loose histiocytes, cholesterol, and lipid deposits), which will be curettable. There may also be small amounts of fibrous connective tissue. A lateral decortication with a thorough curettage and preservation of the inferior alveolar nerve is recommended. The outcome of this treatment is usually bony regeneration unless there is persistent uncontrolled hyperlipidemia.

HISTOPATHOLOGY ▶

Xanthomas consist of collections of histiocytes that contain lipid (Fig 9-10). The different clinical types of xanthoma show differing histologic characteristics (see Table 9-2), but those affecting the head and neck area, particularly lesions affecting the eyelids, usually consist simply of foamy histiocytes with little inflammation or fibrosis.

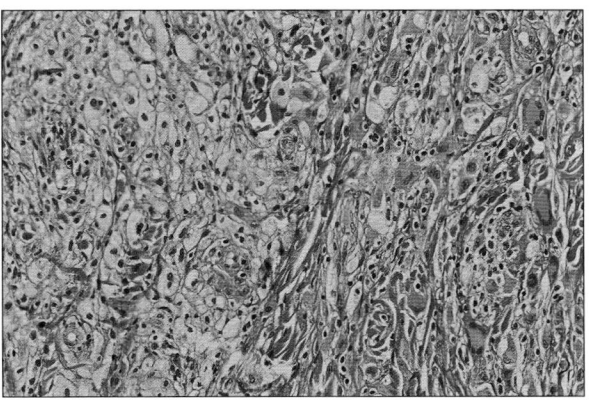

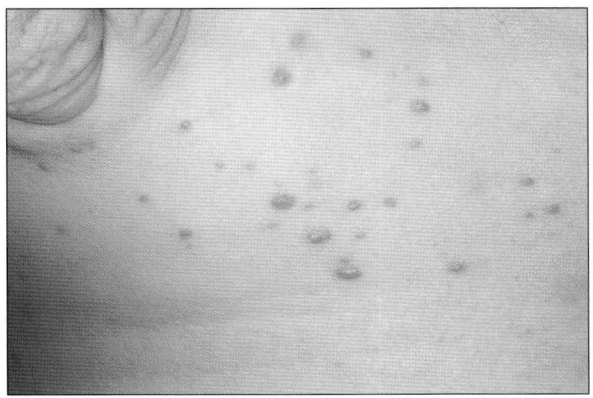

Fig 9-10 Xanthoma containing foamy histiocytes, some fibrous tissue, and Touton giant cells.

Fig 9-11 Juvenile xanthogranulomas appear as small orange to yellow nodules. Frequently multiple, they may also occur singly. (Courtesy of Dr Drore Eisen.)

Juvenile Xanthogranuloma

CLINICAL PRESENTATION AND PATHOGENESIS ▶

The juvenile xanthogranuloma is a cutaneous or, in rare cases, a deep soft tissue reactive lesion that gradually regresses. Small cutaneous papules usually develop shortly after birth; in 20% of cases, they are present at birth. Another 10% of cases first develop lesions in or after the teenage years.

The lesions are usually small (2 mm to 2 cm) red papules. Older lesions are white or yellow. The facial skin, head and neck, and extremities are the most common sites (Fig 9-11). Oral lesions are rare. Despite its name, there is no association with hyperlipidemia or lipid abnormalities. The lesions are asymptomatic but occur in groups of at least several scattered over a wide area at one time.

The natural course of this disease is one of spontaneous regression over several months. The regressed lesion will frequently leave a depressed, hyperpigmented scar. Therefore, some cases will show lesions during different stages of development and regression.

The pathogenesis of juvenile xanthogranuloma is uncertain. It seems to be a reactive set of lesions rather than multiple neoplasms or hamartomas. Because a similar set of virus-related tumors has been found in animals, a viral etiology is probable but unconfirmed.

DIFFERENTIAL DIAGNOSIS ▶

The child will present with a paradoxical picture of multiple skin lesions suggesting an infectious disease, but no other signs or symptoms of an infection. Therefore, one of the more important considerations is a cutaneous presentation of *Langerhans cell histiocytosis*. Other diseases that may show cutaneous nodules without signs of an infectious disease include *neurofibromatosis*, *Gardner syndrome (multiple sebaceous cysts)*, and even *basal cell nevus syndrome (basal cell carcinomas)*. However, in each of these entities, the age would be somewhat older than infancy and early childhood. The child would more likely be older than 8 years, an age at which 75% of juvenile xanthogranuloma cases would already have occurred. *Pediatric xanthomas* associated with hyperlipidemic states may also cause multiple skin lesions that are flat but may be slightly raised because of a collection of lipid-laden histiocytes.

One infectious disease worthy of including on a differential list is *molluscum contagiosum*, a viral disease known to produce 2- to 4-mm self-regressing skin lesions and few systemic toxic symptoms. However, as these mature lesions regress, they form a white waxy plug, which represents virally altered epithelial cells.

DIAGNOSTIC WORK-UP ▶

Excision of a representative lesion will confirm the diagnosis, although obvious clinical lesions can be diagnosed without biopsy.

HISTOPATHOLOGY ▶

The lesions are usually defined but unencapsulated masses composed of histiocytes with some scattered lymphocytes and eosinophils (Fig 9-12a). Over time, the histiocytes become foamy because of the presence of lipid, and Touton giant cells are seen. These are characterized by a peripheral wreath-like

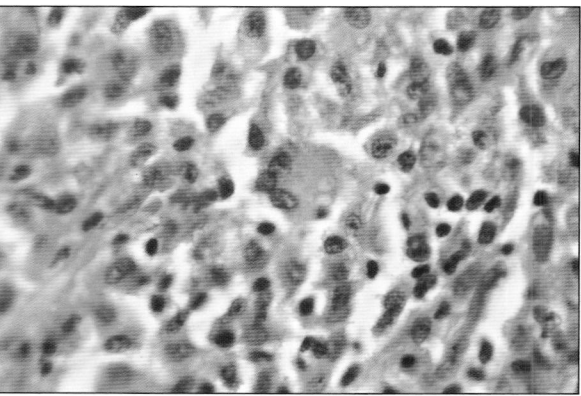

Fig 9-12a A juvenile xanthogranuloma with giant cells and inflammatory cells, including eosinophils.

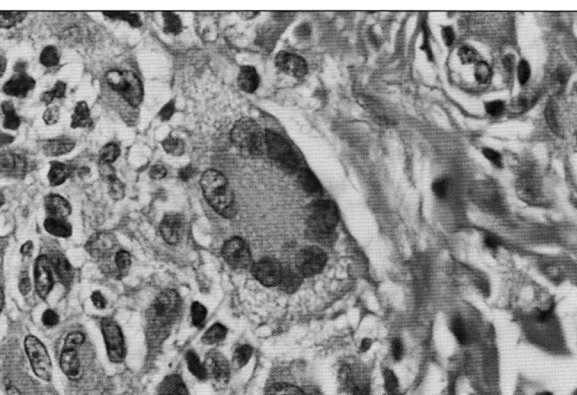

Fig 9-12b Touton giant cell with nuclei in a wreath-like arrangement, beyond which is a lipid-containing foamy cytoplasm.

arrangement of nuclei surrounded by a rim of foamy cytoplasm (Fig 9-12b). Subsequently, interstitial fibrosis takes place, such that the lesion may resemble a fibrous histiocytoma.

TREATMENT ▶

No specific treatment is required except parental reassurance of the anticipated regression of even the larger, deep-seated lesions. Information about residual scarring and some hyperpigmentation is advised. Follow-up facial skin resurfacing procedures may be necessary.

PROGNOSIS ▶

Once lesions regress, they do not recur. Regression occurs over several months to a year for each lesion.

Tumors Containing Fat

Lipoma and Lipoma Variants

CLINICAL PRESENTATION AND
PATHOGENESIS ▶

Lipomas are usually hamartomatous proliferations of mature fat cells. They are a common tumor of skin but less common in the oral cavity, accounting for only 2% to 4% of benign neoplasms. They occur most frequently in mature adults aged 40 to 60 years. In the head and neck region, they are noted to arise from the superficial subcutaneous layer or from the submucosa. Oral lesions are most commonly found in the buccal vestibule around the mental foramen, floor of the mouth, and tongue (Fig 9-13). A so-called deep-seated lipoma will arise deep to the platysma in the neck or within the fascial spaces around the jaws (Fig 9-14).

A lipoma will present as a soft, slow-growing, asymptomatic mass. When it is displaced, the overlying skin or mucosa can often be seen to dimple. Additionally, applying ice to the mass will cause a lipoma to harden. The overlying mucosa or skin is usually of normal color. The yellow color of a lipoma will not show through the overlying epithelium unless it has been greatly thinned. Lipomas may also occur within the parotid gland and will have a clinical presentation similar to that of a benign salivary gland neoplasm (Fig 9-15).

Traditionally, lipomas have been subdivided into several variants based primarily on histopathologic differences. However, there are some important clinical implications in most of these variants.

Solitary Lipoma

The solitary lipoma is the most common type in general and among those found in the oral mucosa and head and neck region.

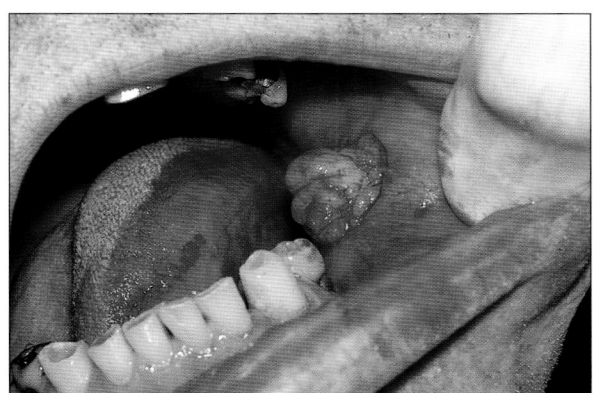

Fig 9-13 The buccal vestibule in the mental foramen region is a common location for oral lipomas.

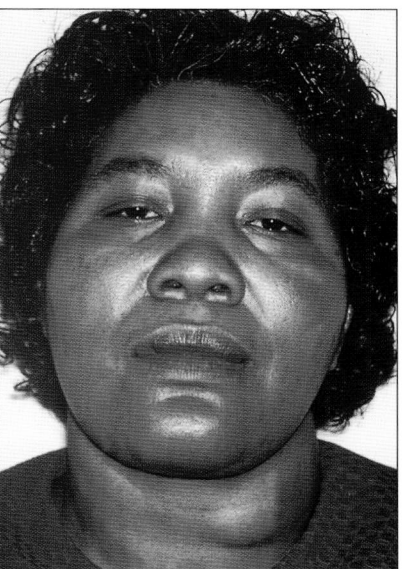

Fig 9-14 Lipomas are often located in the anterior neck deep to the platysma, where they will present as a soft, well-demarcated, movable mass.

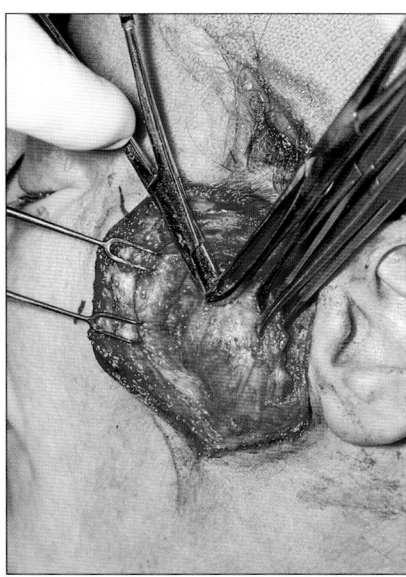

Fig 9-15 Lipomas may also occur within the parotid gland as a discrete encapsulated tumor mimicking a benign salivary gland neoplasm.

Multiple Lipomas

Approximately 5% of all patients with a lipoma have multiple solitary-type lipomas unrelated to a syndrome. Familial lipomatosis is a hereditary disease associated with multiple lipomas. A congenital syndrome of multiple lipomas with macrocephaly and hemangiomas is called *Bannayan-Zonana syndrome*.

Angiolipoma

This is the only lipoma that is symptomatic: It is characteristically painful and tender, particularly during its early growth phases.

Spindle Cell Lipoma

Histologically noted for its replacement of fat cells by spindle-shaped fibroblast-like cells, this lipoma is noted to occur mainly in the posterior triangle of the neck and shoulder area.

Pleomorphic Lipoma

Noted for its bizarre giant cells and hyperchromatic nuclei, pleomorphic lipomas, like spindle cell lipomas, have a predilection for the posterior triangle of the neck and shoulders.

Benign Lipoblastoma

Benign lipoblastoma occurs exclusively in infants and young children. Histologically, it closely resembles a myxoid liposarcoma, but it is a benign tumor.

Angiomyolipoma

Angiomyolipoma is a specific hamartomatous proliferation of perirenal fat.

Myelolipoma

Myelolipoma is a specific hamartomatous proliferation of mature fat and bone marrow cells found in the adrenal glands or pelvic soft tissues.

Intramuscular-Intermuscular Lipoma

This is a significant variant of lipomas because it is often large, deep-seated, and infiltrates into deep tissue, often muscle. Also called *infiltrating lipoma*, it frequently causes muscle soreness. It seems to represent a true neoplastic growth more than a hamartomatous proliferation.

Liposarcomas arise independently rather than from pre-existing benign lipomas. The spectrum from the hamartomatous proliferations of solitary lipomas to the pleomorphic and infiltrating lipoma to finally a liposarcoma indicates that these separate tumors are due to the serial and cumulative genetic damage required to manifest progressively less-controlled cellular proliferations. The solitary lipoma is not a threatening lesion, but it does represent a collection of altered cells. With normal weight gain, the size of a lipoma increases, but in even severe weight loss, the size stays the same. Lipoma cells are therefore autonomous to normal cellular regulations.

DIFFERENTIAL DIAGNOSIS ▶

Solitary lipomas of the upper neck or oral mucosa will overlap clinical presentations and pathogeneses with several benign lesions. In the oral mucosa, a *minor salivary gland tumor*, *schwannoma*, *neurofibroma*, *vascular malformation*, and *lymphangioma* are most likely. In the neck, these same considerations are valid with the exception of the minor salivary gland tumor, but would also include a *lymph node enlargement* from many possible diseases, *sebaceous cyst*, *dermoid cyst*, and either a *branchial cyst* or a *thyroglossal tract cyst* depending on location.

DIAGNOSTIC WORK-UP AND TREATMENT ▶

Solitary lipomas require an exploration and a local excision (Fig 9-16a). The fatty nature of the tumor is readily apparent as it will bulge out of the wound. There is usually a thin capsule around the lobulated tumor (Figs 9-16b and 9-16c). A pericapsular excision is adequate. When placing a lipoma specimen in formalin, the clinician will note that the specimen floats. Because fat is less dense than formalin (or water), it will float, confirming the fat content and suggesting the diagnosis of lipoma (Fig 9-16d).

HISTOPATHOLOGY ▶

The solitary lipoma consists of lobular, circumscribed masses of mature fat cells, which may have a thin capsule and contains delicate fibrovascular trabeculae (Figs 9-17 and 9-18). The lesions are well vascularized. In some instances the fibrous component is more apparent, so that they may be more appropriately called "fibrolipomas."

There are several variants of lipoma, the major significance of which is that they may resemble liposarcomas histologically. The angiolipoma consists of mature fat cells separated by numerous small blood vessels, which may contain thrombi. In some instances, the vascular component may almost completely dominate the tumor. The spindle cell lipoma consists of a combination of mature fat cells and uniform spindle cells. One may dominate the other. These are circumscribed or encapsulated tumors. The pleomorphic lipoma is a circumscribed tumor that consists of mature fat cells and pleomorphic and multinucleated giant cells, often with chronic inflammatory cells in a loose myxoid stroma (Fig 9-19a). The giant cells are characterized by marginally arranged, often overlapping nuclei, which resemble the petals of a flower, hence the term *floret giant cell*. The central cytoplasm is eosinophilic (Fig 9-19b). The relative quantities of giant cells and fat cells are highly variable. These tumors must be distinguished from liposarcomas.

PROGNOSIS ▶

Excision is expected to be curative; recurrence rates are less than 5%. Malignant transformation does not occur.

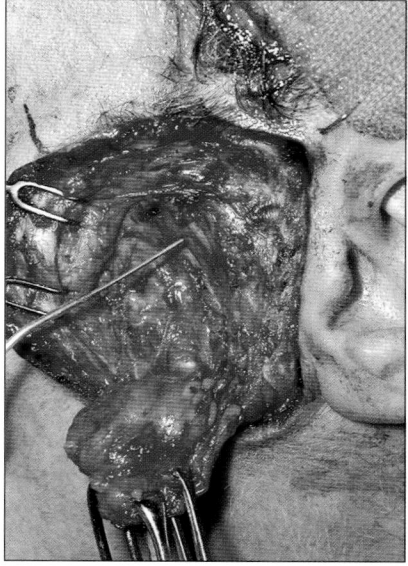

Fig 9-16a A parotid gland lipoma is excised with pericapsular dissection in the superficial lobe, preserving the branches of the facial nerve.

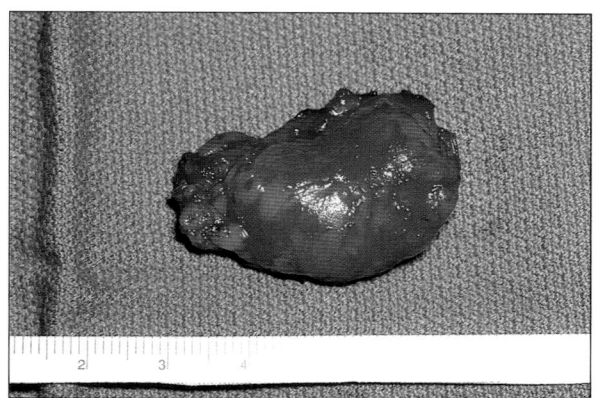

Fig 9-16b Lipomas are discrete tumors with a thin capsule.

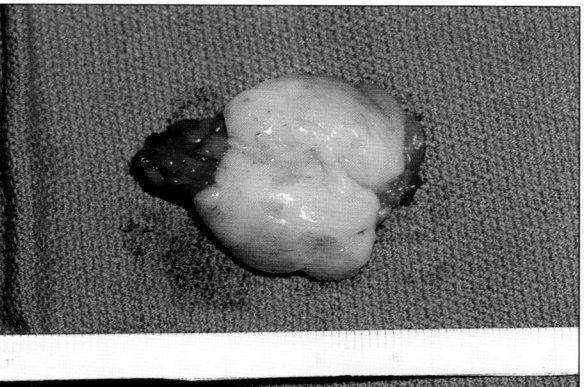

Fig 9-16c A bisected gross specimen reveals the thinness of the capsule and the solid yellow color of the tumor.

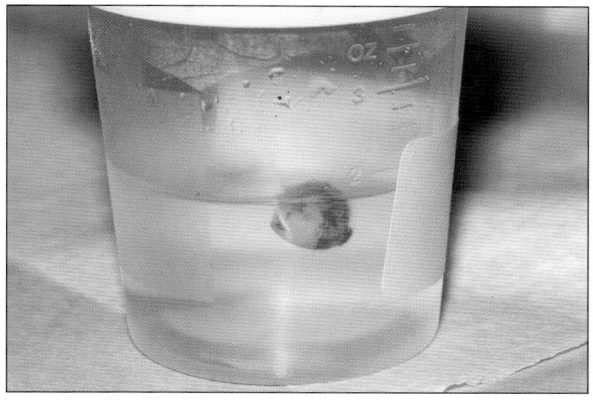

Fig 9-16d Because fat has less density than water or formalin, it will float in the specimen container.

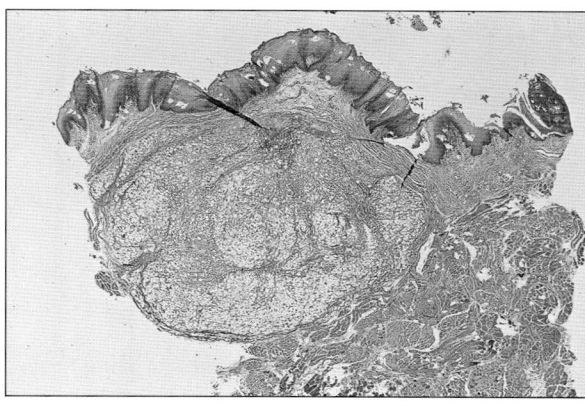

Fig 9-17 A lipoma of the tongue showing a well-demarcated mass of fat divided into lobules by fibrovascular trabeculae.

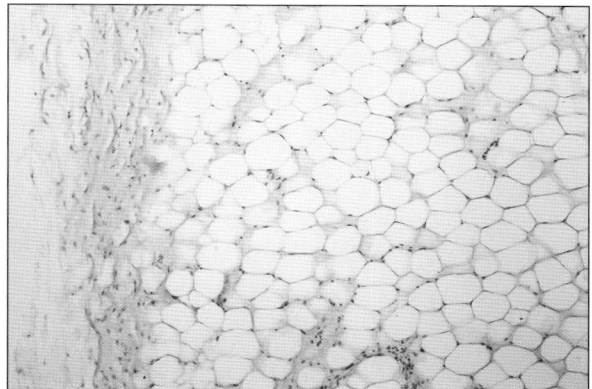

Fig 9-18 The normal-appearing mature cells of the typical lipoma. Note the thin fibrous capsule.

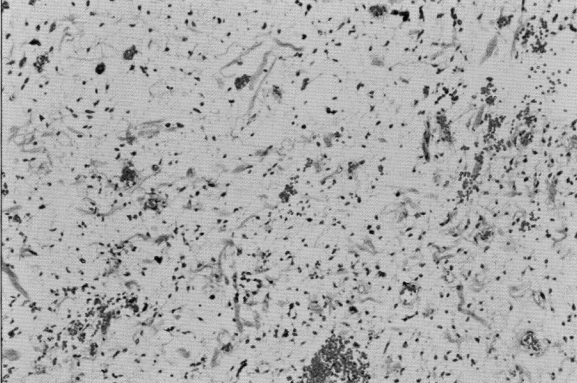

Fig 9-19a This pleomorphic lipoma presents a very different picture from the usual lipoma. Its myxoid appearance suggests the possibility of a malignant neoplasm.

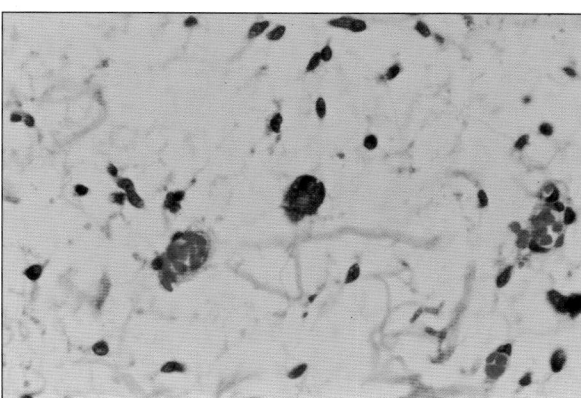

Fig 9-19b A high-power view of Fig 9-19a shows a floret giant cell with its overlapping, peripherally placed nuclei and central eosinophilia.

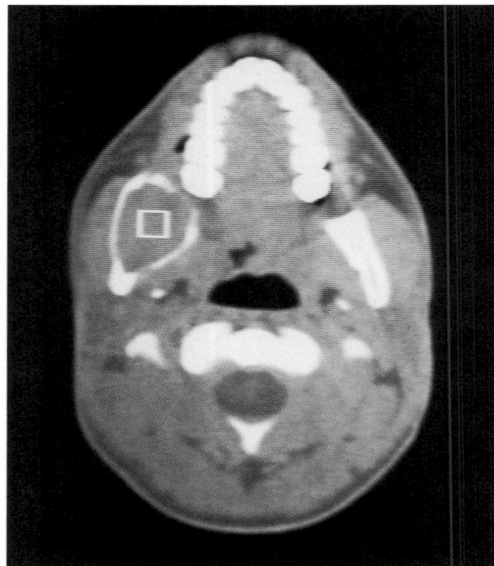

Fig 9-20 The rare schwannoma that occurs centrally within the jaws will present as an expansile unilocular radiolucency.

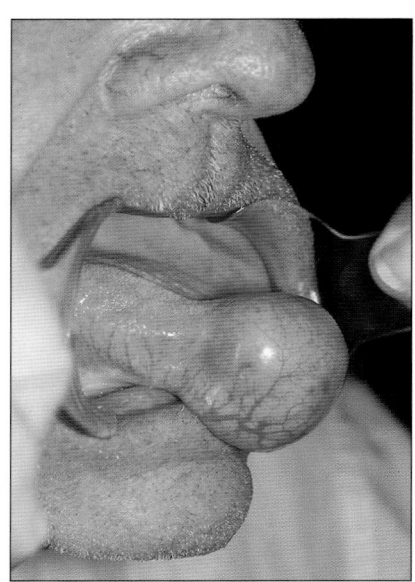

Fig 9-21 This schwannoma in the tongue is a freely movable, well-delineated mass that expanded and thinned the mucosa.

Neurogenic Tumors

Schwannoma

CLINICAL PRESENTATION AND PATHOGENESIS ▶ The schwannoma is a benign tumor arising from and consisting solely of Schwann cells. Comparisons between schwannomas and neurofibromas are frequent, but these tumors can be readily separated clinically and usually histologically. Unlike schwannomas, neurofibromas are a mixed-cell population that includes Schwann cells.

Schwannomas can occur at any age but are most common between 30 and 50 years. Neurofibromas have a predilection for the teen and 20-year groups. Schwannomas occur most commonly in the head and neck area and the flexor areas of the extremities. In the oral cavity, the tongue and floor of the mouth are the most common sites. They rarely will occur centrally within the mandible or maxilla and give rise to a unilocular expansile radiolucency (Fig 9-20). Soft tissue tumors will present as discrete, freely movable masses and seem to have a smooth surface (Fig 9-21). Neurofibromas, on the other hand, are integrated into the surrounding tissue and have a lobulated, irregular surface. Both tumors are usually painless and very seldom cause paresthesia or anesthesia. Schwannomas are usually single tumors; however, some are occasionally seen as multiple lesions as part of neurofibromatosis type I, which is almost always otherwise associated with neurofibromas alone.

DIFFERENTIAL DIAGNOSIS ▶ A schwannoma in the floor of the mouth or tongue has an intact overlying epithelium and, therefore, resembles several other benign lesions known to occur in this region, such as the *granular cell tumor*, *lipoma*, *salivary gland neoplasm*, and lymph node enlargements associated with a variety of diseases, among them *sarcoidosis* and *lymphoma*. A *neurofibroma* may be considered on the differential list, but its diffuse extension and lobulated surface usually distinguishes it from a schwannoma.

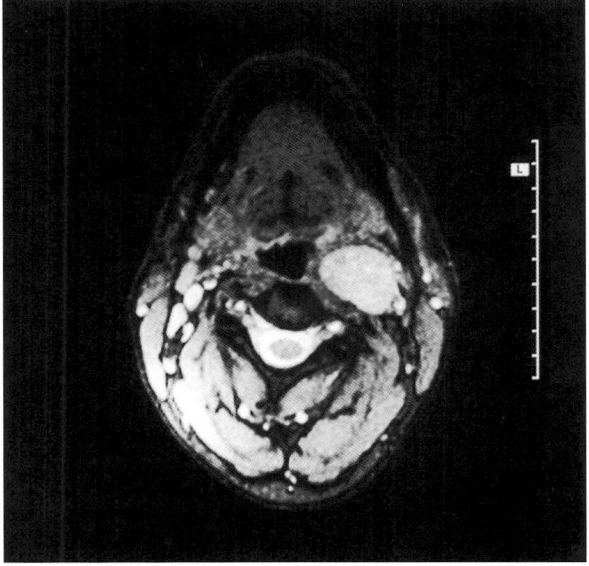

Fig 9-22a This schwannoma developed in the lateral pharyngeal space apparently from the glossopharyngeal nerve and presented as a bulge in the tonsillar fossa.

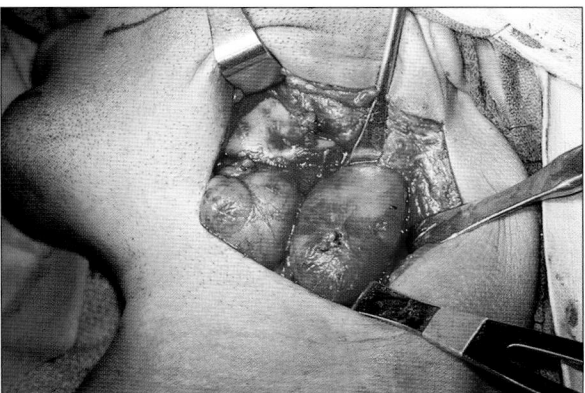

Fig 9-22b A schwannoma can be removed with a pericapsular dissection. This large schwannoma is removed from the lateral pharyngeal space by direct access.

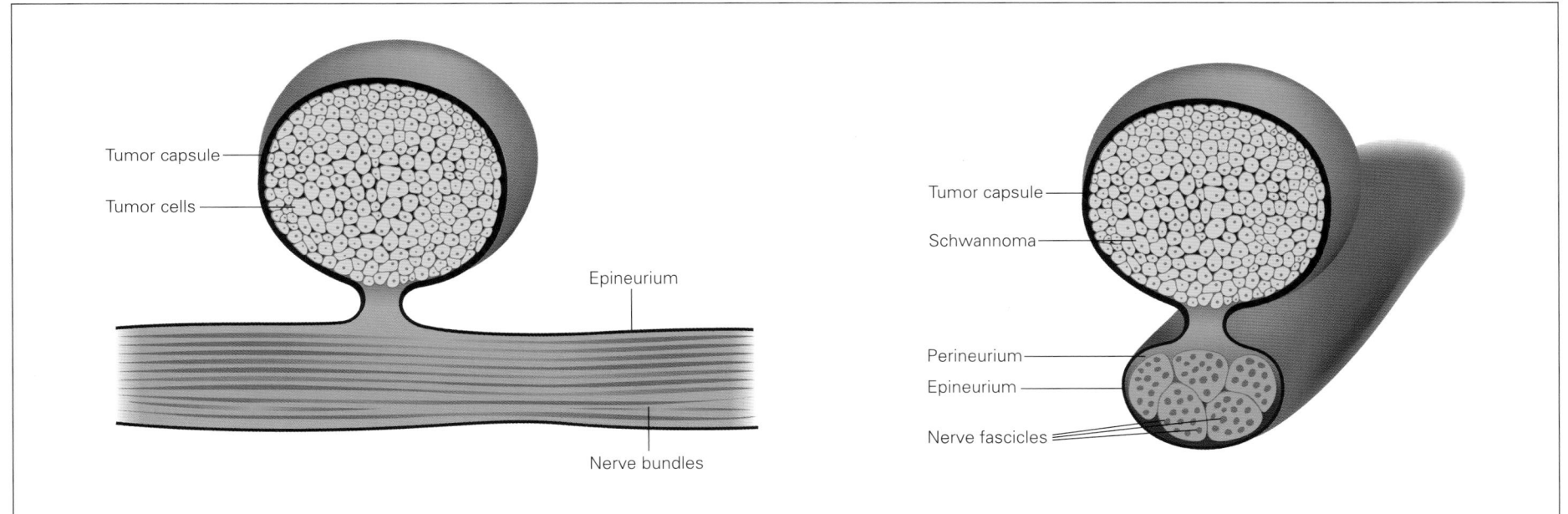

Fig 9-23 A schwannoma develops from epineurial Schwann cells and will therefore arise from a stalk connected to the parent nerve. Excision of the tumor at the stalk will allow for preservation of the parent nerve when the schwannoma develops from a nerve trunk rather than from a small branch.

DIAGNOSTIC WORK-UP AND TREATMENT ▶

Most tumors are approached with exploration and pericapsular excision (Fig 9-22a). At the time of exploration, a prominent smooth capsule is usually found (Fig 9-22b). The tumor seems to emanate from the nerve trunk surface (epineurium) if it arises from a medium-sized or large nerve. In such situations, the tumor can be excised from the nerve at its single thin stalk, thereby preserving the nerve. If the tumor arises from or close to nerve endings, no identifiable nerve will be found (Fig 9-23).

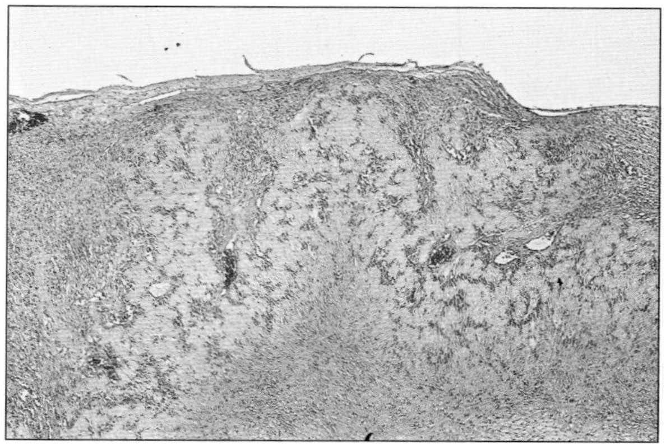

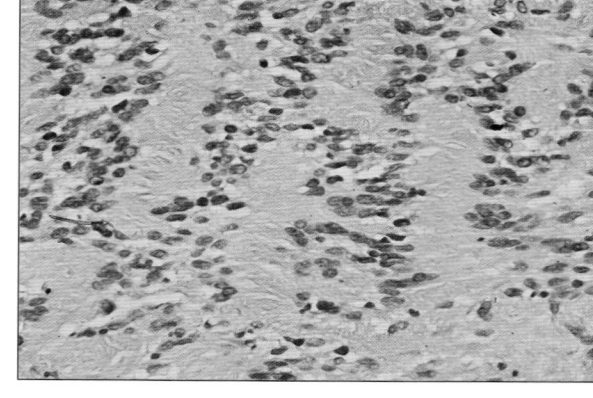

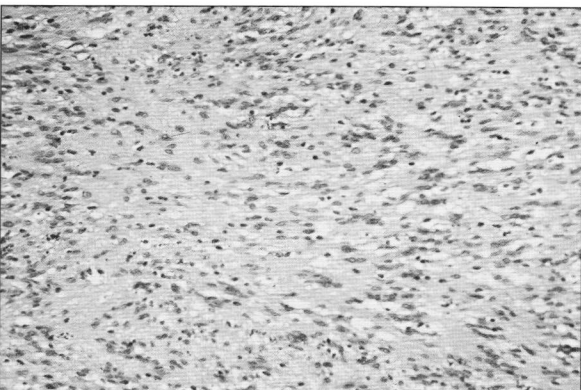

Fig 9-24a This schwannoma shows a well-demarcated neoplasm with a thin fibrous capsule. At this low-power view, the appearance of the Antoni A pattern can be appreciated. The adjacent pattern is Antoni B. The vascularity of these tumors can also be appreciated.

Fig 9-24b Verocay bodies with parallel stacks of Schwann cell nuclei and the centrally placed eosinophilic cytoplasm.

Fig 9-24c Antoni B pattern with a haphazard arrangement of Schwann cells and a vacuolated stroma.

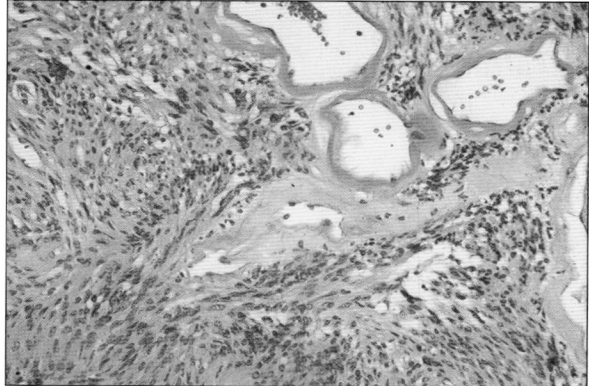

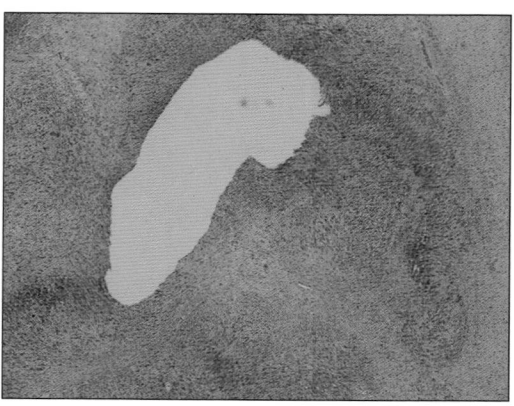

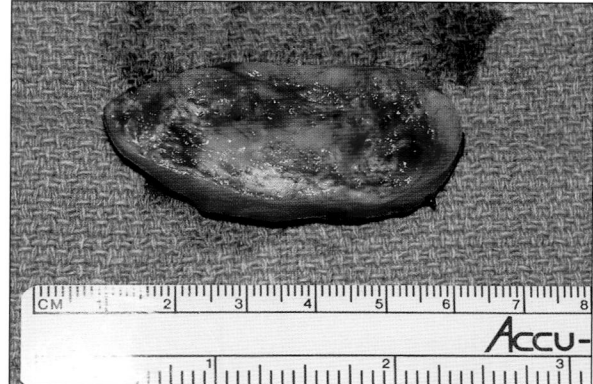

Fig 9-24d Vessels in schwannomas often have wide, irregular lumina; fibrotic walls; and adjacent hyalinization.

Fig 9-24e Cystic change in an intraoral schwannoma measuring 2 cm. The "cyst" is lined by Schwann cells and not by epithelium.

Fig 9-25 A bisected gross specimen of a schwannoma will show a thin capsule and a soft textured mass with some hemorrhagic foci.

If the tumor occurs centrally in bone, it is usually an unexpected finding. In the mandible, it can be excised from the inferior alveolar nerve and the nerve can be preserved. When it occurs within bone, the tumor mass itself is also well encapsulated, lending it to an enucleation and curettage procedure.

HISTOPATHOLOGY ▶

These are encapsulated tumors composed of spindle cells, which are Schwann cells. The capsule is epineurium (Fig 9-24a). The tumor cells are arranged in two patterns. In the Antoni A pattern, the more distinctive and better organized pattern, the nuclei lie in palisaded clusters. When two such clusters occur around an eosinophilic mass, the resultant structure is called a *Verocay body* (Fig 9-24b). The eosinophilic area consists of cytoplasmic material and replicated basal membrane. The spindle cells may also be arranged in bundles and interlacing fascicles. The Antoni B pattern shows a haphazard arrangement of Schwann cells in a loose stroma, which contains small vacuoles (Figs 9-24a and 9-24c). Schwannomas often have a prominent vascular component with dilated, irregular vessels and thick, fibrotic walls (Figs 9-24a and 9-24d).

These tumors may undergo degenerative changes, although this is not usual in the relatively small intraoral lesions. When the changes are pronounced, the tumors have been called *ancient schwannomas* and may show cyst formation, hyalinization, calcification, hemorrhage, and nuclear atypism (Fig 9-24e). These tumors are nonetheless benign. Neurites are not a component since schwannomas develop peripheral to the nerve.

PROGNOSIS ▶ Excision of schwannomas is associated with a nearly 100% cure rate. Although schwannomas and neurofibromas both arise ostensibly from Schwann cells, the tumors are very different in clinical presentation, histopathology, ultrastructural features, treatment approaches, and prognosis. The schwannoma is a benign outgrowth of Schwann cells that is straightforward to excise, does not recur, and does not undergo malignant transformation. In contrast, a neurofibroma is a mixed outgrowth of Schwann cells, neurites, and "epithelioid Schwann cells." It is unencapsulated with prominent integration into normal tissue; difficult to excise; recurs or at least persists from incomplete excision; and, in hereditary neurofibromatosis, can transform into a malignancy.

Schwannomas grow slowly, and many plateau in their growth, perhaps indicating that the tumor represents a hamartoma. As the tumor matures, it will become less cellular because of cellular degeneration. Stromal hyalinization, cyst-like formations (Fig 9-25), and calcifications may also occur within the tumor, particulary in large tumors of long duration. This has been termed an *ancient schwannoma* but is not associated with malignant transformation and has no real clinical or behavioral importance.

Solitary Neurofibroma

CLINICAL PRESENTATION AND PATHOGENESIS ▶ A solitary neurofibroma is a single neurofibroma that occurs in an individual who does not have hereditary neurofibromatosis. The condition may at first be difficult to identify because a single neurofibroma may be the first sign of neurofibromatosis, and the hereditary history of neurofibromatosis may be lacking because of the high incidence of new cases due to spontaneous mutations. Nevertheless, solitary neurofibromas account for 90% of cases of neurofibroma (the other 10% are associated with neurofibromatosis).

A neurofibroma will present as an asymptomatic mass within the subcutaneous or submucosal tissues. The mass will be diffuse. The edges will gradually blend into normal tissue without a clear distinction (Fig 9-26). Similarly, the mass will infiltrate into and incorporate normal tissues such as muscle, glands, and lymph nodes. Its palpable quality will be that of a lobulated surface, the so-called bag of worms feeling.

Occasionally, neurofibromas will develop centrally within the jaws (Fig 9-27) or within difficult-to-access spaces, such as the infratemporal space, the lateral pharyngeal space, or the pterygomandibular space (Fig 9-28).

DIFFERENTIAL DIAGNOSIS ▶ The diffuse, soft nature of the neurofibroma will give the same tactile impression as that of a *lipoma*, a *vascular malformation*, a *lymphangioma*, and a *rhabdomyoma*. Vascular malformations and lymphangiomas especially are seen more commonly in the same young age group as are neurofibromas.

DIAGNOSTIC WORK-UP AND TREATMENT ▶ A neurofibroma is usually diagnosed by incisional biopsy. Once a neurofibroma is confirmed, a computed tomography (CT) scan is recommended to assess its relationship to nearby anatomy. If the tumor is small and accessible, it should be excised with 1-cm margins and frozen section control of the margin. If the tumor is large, it may be unresectable or resectable but associated with a greatly increased morbidity. Such large tumors present a treatment dilemma, which is further compounded by the vascular nature of neurofibromas. This compromises visualization, which in turn compromises the surgery and also adds expectations of increased blood loss, which may require transfusions. Neurofibromas are unencapsulated tumors, making their complete removal more difficult (Fig 9-29), and since they bear a close histologic resemblance to normal connective tissue, frozen section assessments at the margins are not reliable. Radiotherapy is not an option because of the possibility of radiation sarcomas developing in future years. Therefore, some neurofibromas are not treated or are treated with intentionally incomplete removal in a debulking type of procedure. Other large tumors undergo radical excision, for which reconstructive surgery is required.

In contrast to the schwannoma, a neurofibroma arises from the internal portion of a nerve clinically. In most cases the parent nerve is not identifiable. In some cases the nerve can be seen to enter the

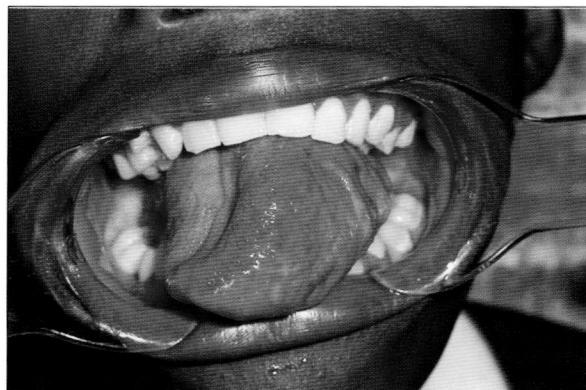

Fig 9-26 A neurofibroma is unencapsulated and diffuse within the tissue of origin. Note the large, dilated vein, indicating the typical vascular nature of neurofibromas.

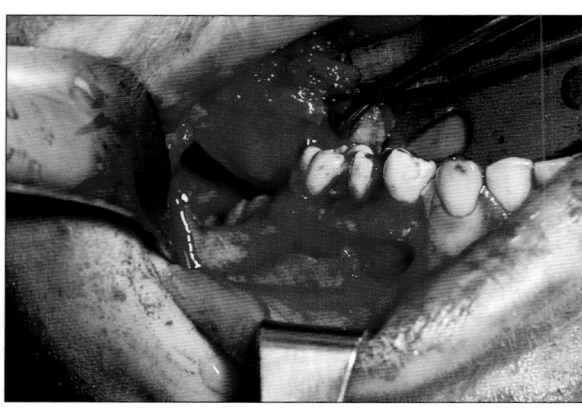

Fig 9-27 Removal of a central neurofibroma of the mandible. Intraosseous bone neurofibromas are more localized than those in soft tissue.

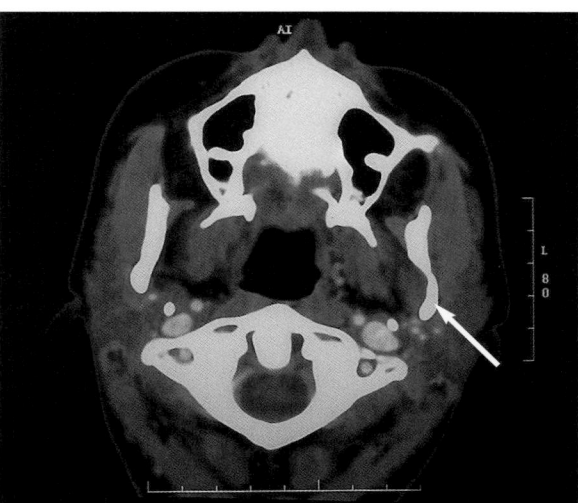

Fig 9-28 Deeply located neurofibroma in the pterygomandibular space inducing a resorption in the area of the lingula (*arrow*).

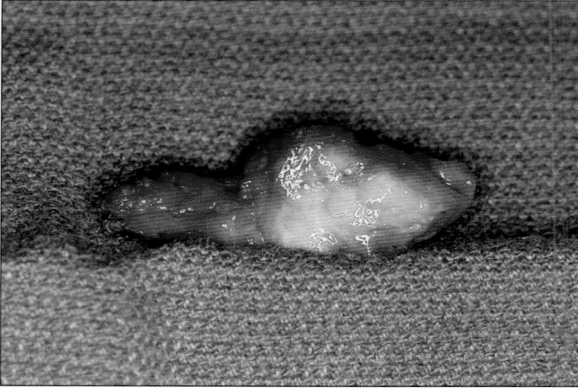

Fig 9-29 Excised neurofibroma with the parent inferior alveolar nerve. Note its unencapsulated nature. The tumor arises from the nerve so that no remaining parent nerve is identifiable.

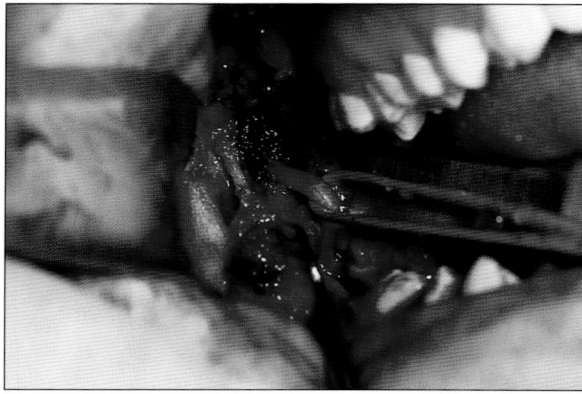

Fig 9-30 The inferior alveolar nerve can be seen entering the neurofibroma and becoming part of the tumor.

proximal end of the tumor (Fig 9-30). Because the nerve is incorporated into and is actually part of the neurofibroma, it cannot be preserved (Fig 9-31).

HISTOPATHOLOGY ▶

The lesions are unencapsulated, consisting of interlacing bundles of spindle cells that typically have wavy or "serpentine" nuclei (Figs 9-32a and 9-32b). The stroma is often fibrillar and eosinophilic but may have mucoid areas (Fig 9-32c). Mast cells and scattered lymphocytes are usually present, and neurites may be found within the tumor. The solitary neurofibroma and the usual neurofibroma of neurofibromatosis do not differ histologically. Cellular atypia may be seen in benign neurofibromas, but mitotic activity indicates malignant change. This phenomenon is more likely to be seen in neurofibromatosis.

Although Schwann cells appear to be a major component of neurofibromas, other cells, such as fibroblasts, are also present.

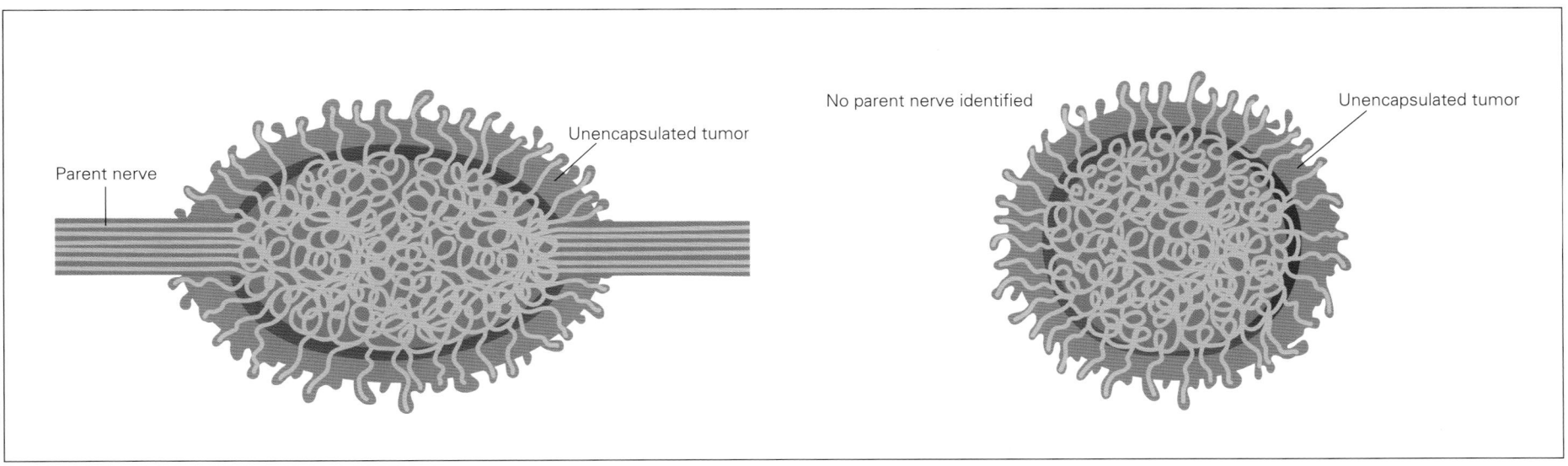

Fig 9-31 A neurofibroma is unencapsulated and infiltrates surrounding tissues. It arises from perineurial fibroblasts so that the parent nerve is caught up within and is part of the tumor.

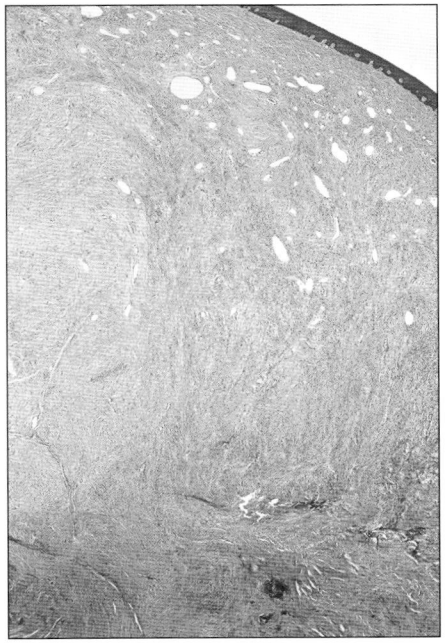

Fig 9-32a Low-power view of a neurofibroma. Note the lack of encapsulation, in contrast to a schwannoma, which is encapsulated.

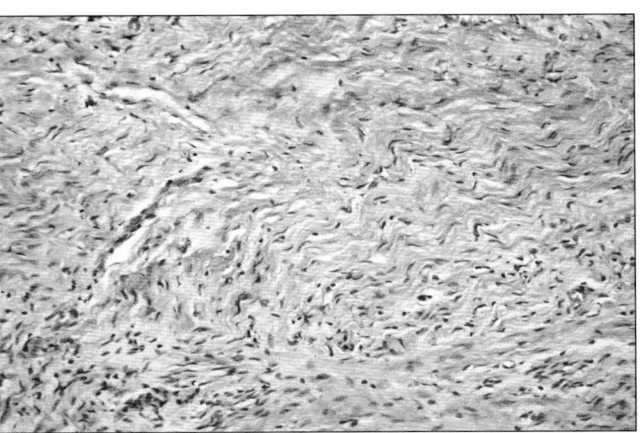

Fig 9-32b A neurofibroma showing the wavy pattern of the collagen fibers as well as the serpentine nuclei.

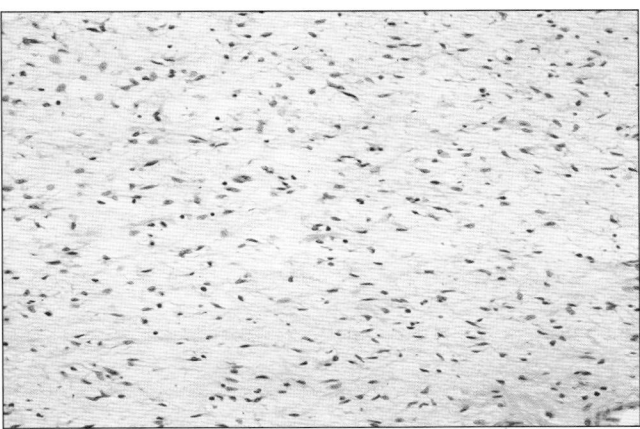

Fig 9-32c This portion of a neurofibroma shows myxoid areas.

PROGNOSIS ▶ For patients with small lesions excised with tumor-free margins, the prognosis is excellent. Even in tumors that are incompletely excised, the residual lesion grows back so slowly that a lasting gain is attained. Solitary neurofibromas do not exhibit a spontaneous transformation to malignancy. It seems only those that are irradiated or those that are part of hereditary neurofibromatosis have a known malignant potential.

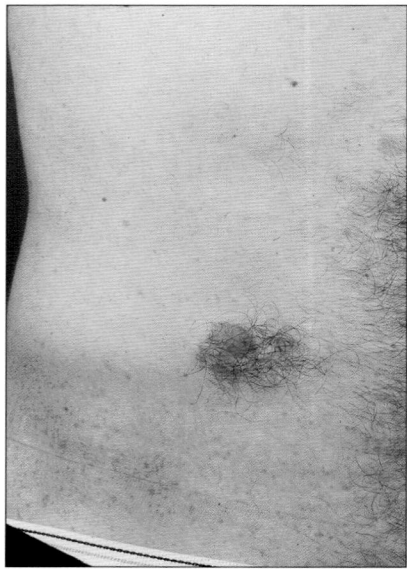

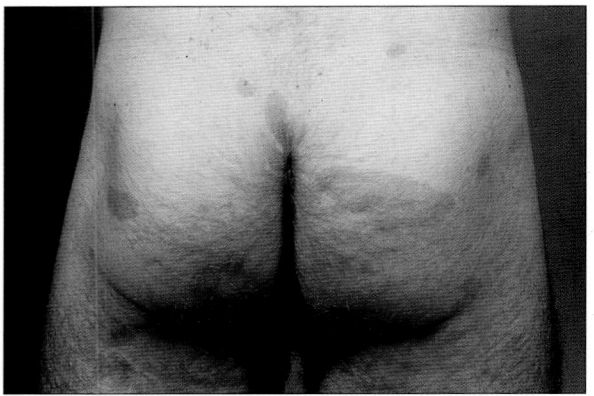

Fig 9-33 In neurofibromatosis type I, café-au-lait macules usually precede the development of neurofibromas. They will mostly occur in areas not exposed to the sun.

Fig 9-34 In neurofibromatosis type I, café-au-lait macules usually appear in multiple areas and have smooth, rounded edges likened to the map contour of the coast of California.

Neurofibromatosis

Neurofibromatosis is divided into two forms: a peripheral form (type I) and a central form (type II).

Neurofibromatosis Type I (Von Recklinghausen Neurofibromatosis)

CLINICAL PRESENTATION AND PATHOGENESIS ▶ Neurofibromatosis type I (NF-I) is an autosomal-dominant trait recently shown to be related to a mutation in the pericentromeric proximal gene locus on chromosome 17. About one half of all cases have a hereditary etiology; the other half represent new mutations. Neurofibromatosis has an incidence of 1 in every 5,000 live births.

This syndrome-like disease is associated with several varied findings, but multiple neurofibromas and so-called café-au-lait pigmented macules are its prime characteristics.

Although NF-I is related to a single genetic abnormality, the neurofibromas that form do not arise from a single cell line. Either the genetic defect affects several types of Schwann cells or a single abnormal cell line induces other cells to contribute to the neoplasm. However, when malignant transformation occurs, the malignancy is always from a single cell line (a monoclonal proliferation). Thus, NF-I has been conceptualized by some as a polyclonal hamartoma or as a hyperplastic proliferation of several Schwann cell types with malignant transformation representing a further mutational event in a single cell line leading to a monoclonal malignancy.

NF-I is the form most clinicians associate with neurofibromatosis. It begins in the first few years of life with the development of café-au-lait macules, which may go unnoticed or be dismissed as freckles. Café-au-lait macules almost always develop years before neurofibromas. They can be distinguished from a freckle (ephelis) by their larger size and their occurrence on areas not exposed to the sun (Figs 9-33 and 9-34). One of the most characteristic locations for an NF-1–related café-au-lait macule is the axilla, which is specifically examined in suspicious cases (called the "axillary freckle sign" or "Crowe sign"). NF-I can be diagnosed early in many cases from a biopsy of a café-au-lait macule. Such café-au-lait macules

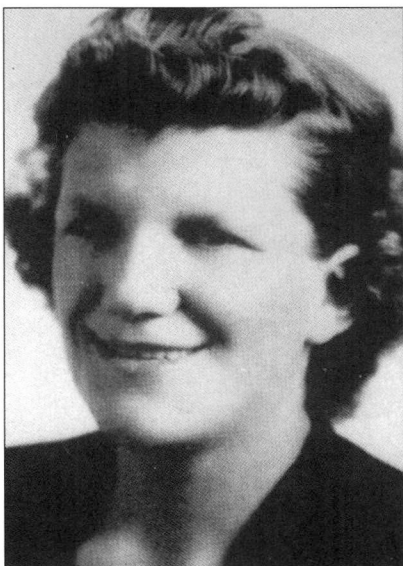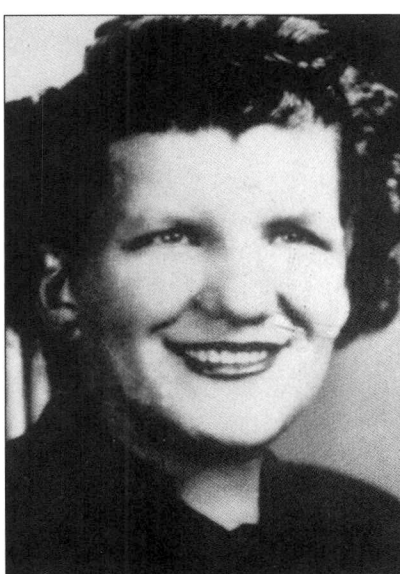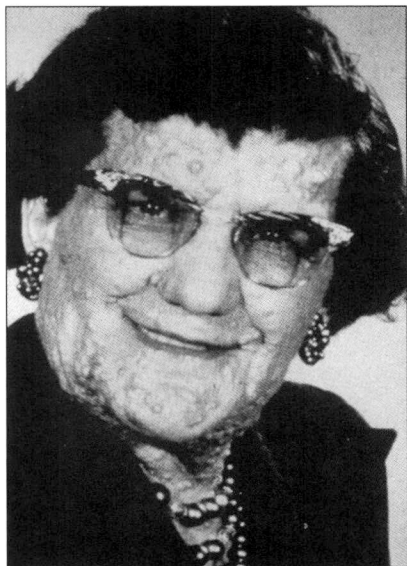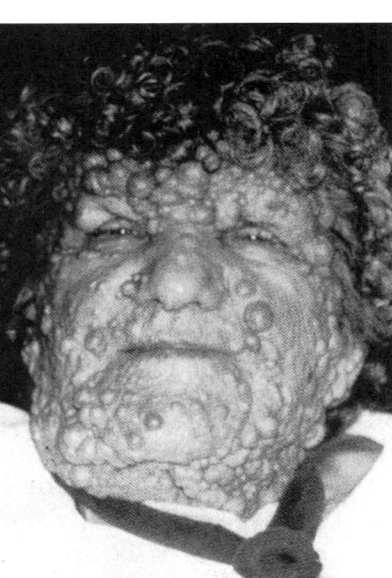

Figs 9-35a to 9-35d In these facial photographs, taken about 10 years apart, the gradually advancing progress and number of cutaneous neurofibromas can be seen. (Reprinted from Reynolds RL, Pineda CA. Neurofibromatosis: Review and report of a case. JADA 1988;117:735–737. Copyright 1988 American Dental Association. Reprinted by permission of ADA Publishing, a Division of ADA Business Enterprises, Inc.)

often accumulate pigment in giant melanosomes called *macromelanosomes* and are somewhat unique to NF-I. Clinically, café-au-lait macules must be 1.5 cm or larger in the adult and 0.5 cm or larger in children before they are considered diagnostic. By convention, the finding of six or more café-au-lait macules of 1.5 cm or larger in adults (12 years or older) establishes the diagnosis of NF-I even if no neurofibromas are yet present.

Neurofibromas, which are the hallmark of NF-I, usually become apparent during the preteen and teenage years after the appearance of café-au-lait macules. These neurofibromas are slow-growing lesions primarily of skin, but they are also sometimes found on oral, pharyngeal, or laryngeal mucosa. Tumors increase in number and size throughout the years (Figs 9-35a to 9-35d). Most tumors in the skin fail to exceed 4 to 5 cm, although adjacent tumors can coalesce. There is usually an acceleration of the tumor growth rate at puberty and during pregnancy.

Oral neurofibromas occur mostly on the tongue, floor of the mouth, buccal mucosa, and palate (see Fig 9-26). Gingival enlargement occurs in NF-I and is due to the development of neurofibromas in the gingiva (Fig 9-36).

NF-I is also associated with brown pigmented spots on the iris called *Lisch nodules* (90% of cases) and with skeletal abnormalities (40% of cases). The skeletal abnormalities are either external erosive defects changing the morphologic characteristics of the bone, or they are internal osteolytic defects. Some of the external cupped-out resorptive defects are due to neurofibroma impingement, while others are developmental defects unrelated to any direct neurofibroma effect (Fig 9-37). The internal resorptive defects are frequently seen in the zygoma, orbit, and ramus of the mandible. Some produce a noticeable enlargement of the mandibular canal and foramen (Fig 9-38). In most cases, the defects do not represent central neurofibromas; when explored, they reveal nonneural fibrous tissue or a fibrous cortical defect. Some contain vascular malformations, which produce a prominent bleeding episode. Skeletal abnormalities of the vertebrae and other bones are well-known in NF-I. These include vertebral resorption leading to angular scoliosis, shortening of long bones, and pseudoarthrosis (Table 9-3).

In adolescent boys, hyalinization of breast tissue produces a pseudogynecomastia. (True gynecomastia is an enlargement of native breast tissue rather than a thickening due to fibrous hyalinization.)

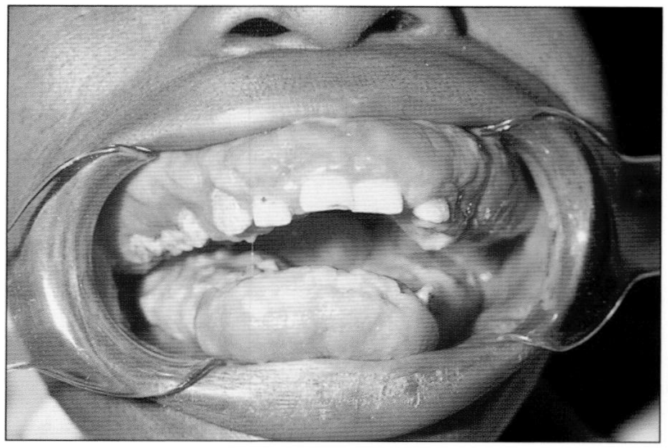

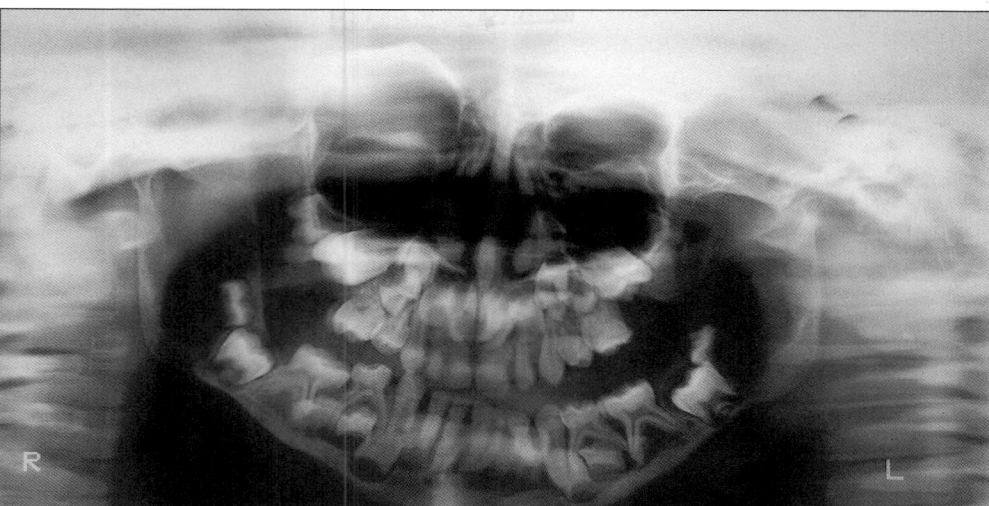

Fig 9-36 Neurofibromatosis type I is one of only a few conditions that produces gingival enlargement. In NF-I it is due to the development of neurofibromas in the gingiva.

Fig 9-37 Developmental defects in each ramus related to neurofibromatosis type I.

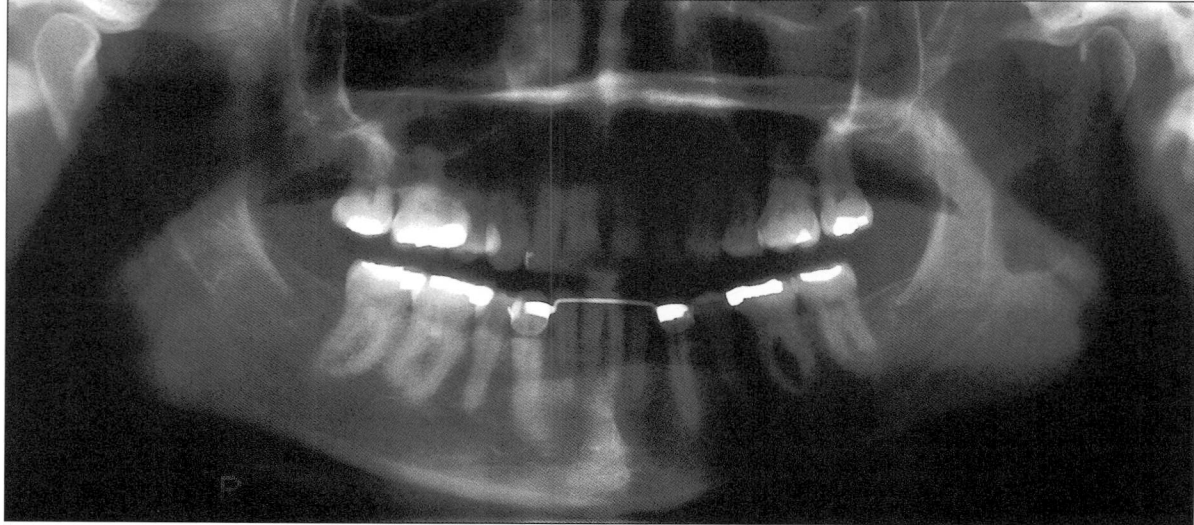

Fig 9-38 Enlargement of the mandibular canal at the lingula and a round radiolucency of the ramus produced by a neurofibroma.

Neurofibromatosis Type II

CLINICAL PRESENTATION AND PATHOGENESIS ▶

Neurofibromatosis type II (NF-II) is less common than NF-I (NF-II, 1:50,000; NF-I, 1:5,000) and may have no or few peripheral signs. Instead, these individuals develop intracranial and intraspinal neural tumors rather than neurofibromas. They form schwannomas, astrocytomas, meningiomas, and ependymomas. The most common tumor is the schwannoma, which most often occurs as an acoustic neuroma but can be associated with the intracranial portion of the trigeminal nerve. In fact, bilateral acoustic neuromas are considered sufficient evidence to establish the diagnosis of this form of neurofibromatosis (Table 9-4). The most common clinical presentation of NF-II is unilateral or bilateral hearing loss, which may be accompanied by some tinnitus or dizziness associated with vestibular dysfunction. The inheritance pattern of NF-II is also autosomal dominant but arises from a mutation on a distal gene locus in chromosone 22.

Table 9-3 Diagnostic criteria for neurofibromatosis type I

NF-I is present in an individual with at least two of the following:
Six or more café-au-lait macules greater than 5 mm in children and greater than 15 mm in teenagers and adults
At least two neurofibromas of any type or one plexiform neurofibroma
Freckling in axillary or inguinal regions
Optic nerve glioma
Two or more iris hamartomas (Lisch nodules)
A distinct osseous lesion, eg, sphenoid wing dysplasia, thinning of long bone cortex with or without pseudoarthrosis
A first-degree relative (parent, sibling, child) with NF-I according to above criteria

Table 9-4 Diagnostic criteria for neurofibromatosis type II

NF-II is present in an individual with:		
Bilateral VIII nerve tumors	*OR*	A first-degree relative with NF-II and *EITHER*
		A unilateral VIII nerve tumor *OR*
		Two of the following:
		Dermal or subcutaneous neurofibromas
		Plexiform neurofibroma
		Schwannoma
		Glioma
		Meningioma
		Juvenile posterior capsular lenticular opacity

DIFFERENTIAL DIAGNOSIS ▶

In the early childhood years before the onset of neurofibromas, NF-I may appear to be similar to the *Jaffe type of fibrous dysplasia* or to the fully expressed form with precocious puberty, *Albright syndrome.* However, even at this time, NF-I may be distinguished by the pattern of café-au-lait macules. Café-au-lait macules of NF-I have smooth edges (often likened to the coast of California) whereas café-au-lait macules of fibrous dysplasia syndromes are craggy and irregular (often likened to the coast of Maine).

As neurofibromas develop in the skin, NF-I may appear like *Gardner syndrome,* in which some patients develop multiple sebaceous cysts, or *Madelungs syndrome,* in which patients develop multiple subcutaneous lipomas. If the neurofibromas in NF-I are large and diffuse, they may also resemble the tissue enlargements seen in *Klippel-Trenaunay-Weber syndrome.*

Many individuals with NF-II will be asymptomatic; the diagnosis will be suspected only by the incidental finding of an intracranial mass on a CT or magnetic resonance imaging (MRI) scan. Others may be diagnosed by the gradual onset of unilateral or bilateral hearing loss. Occasionally sudden hearing loss may occur as well. The overall effect of other intracranial tumors, such as *meningiomas, epidermoid cysts,* or *vascular malformations,* will present a hearing loss suggestive of an acoustic neuroma and therefore NF-II. In addition, *cholesteatomas, mastoiditis,* and *Ménière disease* each may produce a hearing loss and/or a vestibular dysfunction suggestive of NF-II.

DIAGNOSTIC WORK-UP ▶

Diagnosis of NF-I is best confirmed by biopsy of a neurofibroma. Biopsy of a melanotic macule will contribute to or confirm the diagnosis if it shows macromelanosomes. Diagnosis of NF-II is best made with a CT or MRI scan, auditory testing, a search for subcutaneous nodules, and an ophthalmologic examination.

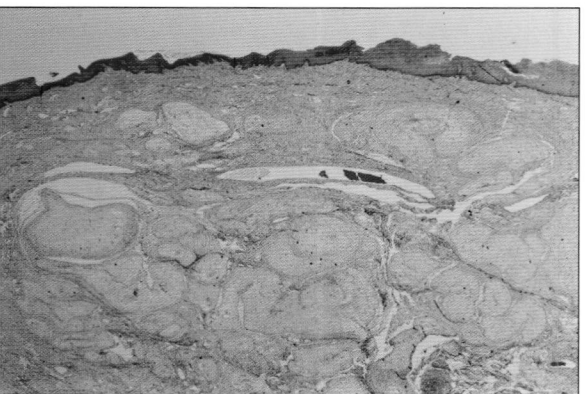

Fig 9-39a A plexiform neurofibroma appearing as numerous lobules.

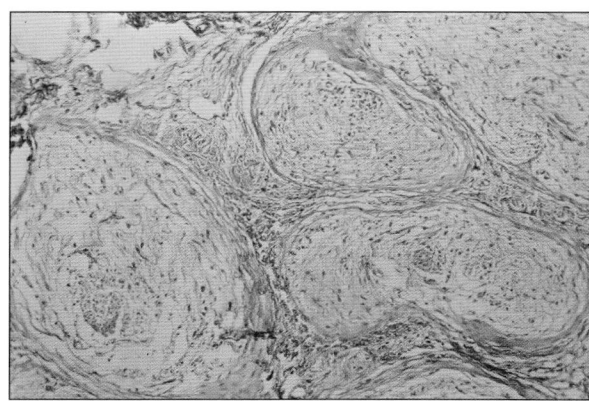

Fig 9-39b High-power view of a portion of a plexiform neurofibroma showing the distinct nerve bundles.

HISTOPATHOLOGY ▶

The usual neurofibroma of NF-I is identical to that seen in patients who do not have neurofibromatosis. The plexiform neurofibroma, however, is virtually pathognomonic of neurofibromatosis. It consists of a tortuous arrangement of hypertrophic nerve, which appears as lobules or discrete bundles within the connective tissue (Figs 9-39a and 9-39b). Over time, the nerve is replaced by Schwann cells and thick wavy collagen. It should be remembered that pleomorphism may be seen in neurofibromas, but mitoses signify malignant change.

The café-au-lait macules show an increase in melanin pigment in the basal cells of the skin. Typically, but not invariably, the melanin is in the form of giant melanosomes. Their presence may be related to the age of the lesion.

Bone lesions are often an erosive defect due to impingement by a tumor mass, but the cystic bone lesions show fibroblasts in short intersecting fascicles with occasional giant cells. This resembles the fibrous cortical defect.

In NF-II, the diagnostic lesions are bilateral vestibular schwannomas that have the usual appearance of a Schwannian proliferation as seen in other schwannomas. Other neural neoplasms affecting other central nerves may also be present. These include small schwannomas, neurofibromas, meningioma-like lesions of cranial nerves, and meninges of the temporal bone.

TREATMENT AND PROGNOSIS ▶

In NF-I, the large number of lesions makes complete surgical therapy nearly impossible. Therefore, surgery is reserved for large neurofibromas, symptomatic neurofibromas, and those located in areas where their presence compromises function. As with large solitary neurofibromas, large neurofibromas associated with NF-I are hamartomas and thus when incompletely removed may not grow back or will grow slowly. Incomplete removal, even if accomplished multiple times, is not believed to hasten a transformation to malignancy.

In NF-I, the spontaneous malignancy transformation rate is between 2% and 13%. Because such high incidences are reported by tertiary centers to which recurrent and complicated cases are referred, it is probably closer to 2% than 13%. The risk of spontaneous malignant transformation is related to the length of time the disease has been present. It is almost never seen within the first 5 years and only rarely before 10 years. The transformation to malignancy may be suspected when a lesion undergoes a rapid enlargement or becomes painful. Once a malignancy is noted, it should be removed with wide (3- to 5-cm) margins. Unfortunately, the malignancies that arise (neurosarcomas) are very aggressive ones. In such cases, the 5-year survival rate is less than 20%.

NF-II is usually treated by specifically trained otologic surgeons or neurosurgeons. Masses of the internal auditory canal and cerebellopontine angle are consistent with acoustic neuromas and actually represent the encapsulated slow-growing biology of a schwannoma. Therefore, some are left to follow-up if

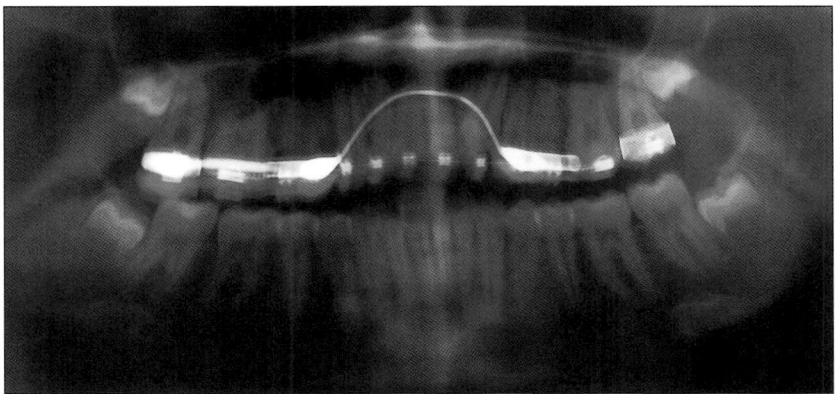

Fig 9-40 A nonexpansile, cyst-like radiolucency of the anterior mandible proved to be a C-fiber (traumatic) neuroma. There was a history of trauma followed by pain.

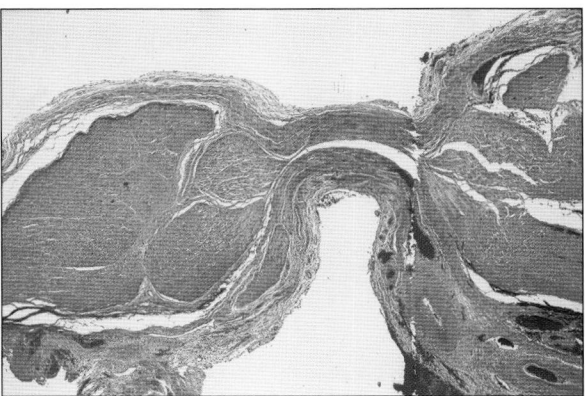

Fig 9-41 Selective regeneration of C fibers from a transsected inferior alveolar nerve, creating a C-fiber (traumatic) neuroma.

there are no or only mild symptoms. Most, however, are treated with microsurgical inner ear/cranial surgery. Rare cases, in which surgical morbidity is enhanced because of systemic disease or advanced age, may be treated by gamma knife radiosurgery or stereotactic radiotherapy.

The Elephant Man Mistake

A popular movie entitled *The Elephant Man* portrayed the story of a tragic individual with hideous facial and scalp tissue proliferations as arising from an extreme case of hereditary neurofibromatosis. The well-known individual was Joseph (John) Merrick, who reportedly died of an airway compromise related to the weight of these tissue proliferations. Yet, the study of archived tissue from this man showed not neurofibromas but rather hyalinized connective tissue more consistent with Proteus syndrome. Moreover, his preserved skull showed bony expansions with irregular ridges, a feature not seen in neurofibromatosis, and a plaster cast of his foot showed the pathognomonic "moccasin" appearance of Proteus syndrome. Indeed, Joseph Merrick did not actually have neurofibromatosis but Proteus syndrome, a much rarer hereditary syndrome of harmartomas causing overgrowth of numerous tissues. The importance of this distinction is that individuals with the more common neurofibromatosis have unnecessarily endured greater anxiety and a heavier psychologic burden since this Hollywood mistake.

Neuromas

C-Fiber Neuromas and Deafferentation Neuropathies

CLINICAL PRESENTATION AND PATHOGENESIS ►

The oral and maxillofacial specialist is often called upon to examine, advise, and treat patients with severe postsurgical or postinjury pain responses that linger well beyond the immediate postoperative period. Most of these individuals have a nerve injury that previously would have been diagnosed as a so-called traumatic neuroma. Upon exploration, however, most injury sites reveal not a neuroma formation but an epineurial injury and/or a partial nerve trunk separation with scar formation (Fig 9-40). In those that do reveal a nodule interpreted as a neuroma, the nodule consists almost exclusively of small, unmyelinated C fibers (Fig 9-41).

C-fiber neuromas and deafferentation neuropathies are the two most common responses to a nerve injury that causes long-term pain for the patient. They are often caused by overinstrumentation of root canal files, overdrilling during dental implant placements, or removal of an impacted tooth, or as a result

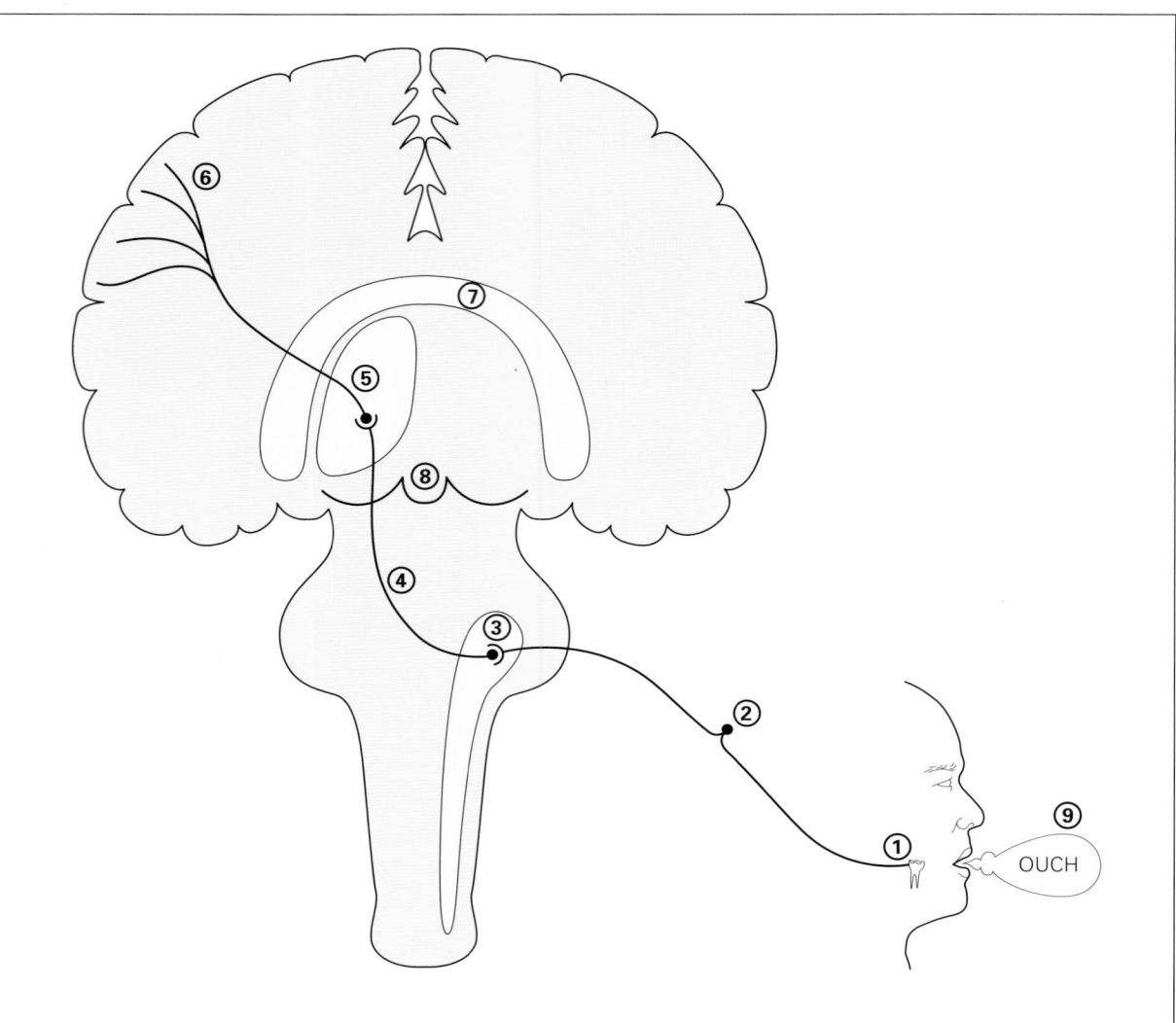

Fig 9-42a Neuroanatomy of the sensory portion of the trigeminal nerve: (1) pain perception; (2) Gasserian ganglion (neurons of the first order); (3) Nucleus caudalis (center of gate) (neurons of the second order); (4) Ventral central trigeminal tract (crossed); (5) ventral central posterior medial nucleus (VPM) of thalamus (neurons of the third order); (6) Cortex (pain evaluation) (cortical conscious modulation of gate); (7) Limbic lobes (emotional modulation of gate); (8) Midbrain periaqueductal gray matter (production + control of endorphins); (9) Pain reaction and affect.

of fractures, and they can occur during almost any surgery performed in close approximation to a sensory nerve. The patient will often complain that a partial numbness will accompany the pain, which will be burning in nature. The patient will further relate that the pain is always present at some level but fluctuates in intensity throughout the day and from one day to the next. The finding of a classic traumatic neuroma, that is, a nodule that is painful only when compressed, is rare and may even be a normal nerve impinged upon by an appliance. The actual pain responses of C-fiber neuromas and deafferentation neuropathies are much more constant, severe, and variable.

Neuroanatomy of the Trigeminal Nerve

To understand each entity, a review of the anatomy and physiology of the sensory portion of the trigeminal nerve is necessary (Fig 9-42a).

The sensory portion of the trigeminal nerve is a three-neuron system. The nerve endings that receive a painful stimulus are in the pulps of teeth, periosteum of the jaws, oral mucosa, temporomandibular joint (TMJ), facial skin, etc. Their cell bodies are located in the Gasserian ganglion in the middle cranial fossa. These are unipolar cells that receive the painful action potential from the periphery via their afferent arm and send the signal unchanged to the nucleus caudalis in the medulla, pons, and upper cervical segments of the spinal cord via their efferent arm. These neurons in the Gasserian ganglion are called *neurons of the first order*.

In the nucleus caudalis, neurons of the first order synapse with nerve cell bodies in this nucleus called *neurons of the second order*. However, many other nerve fibers from various subconscious and conscious levels of the brain also synapse with these neurons of the second order. The nucleus caudalis therefore serves as the "gate" for the trigeminal nerve and is analogous to the substantia gelatinosa in the spinal cord, where the synapses of somatic noncranial nerves take place.

In the nucleus caudalis, the signal is greatly modified by these subconscious and conscious levels of influence, which synapse in the nucleus. Some are said to be *inhibitory* (closing the gate), while others are *excitatory* (opening the gate). The final modified signal that leaves the nucleus caudalis dictates the intensity of the pain but not the cerebral cortex evaluation of the pain. This modified signal ascends in the ventral central trigeminal tract for about 2 to 4 cm before it crosses the midline to ascend further and synapse in the ventral central posterior medial nucleus (VPM) of the thalamus. Here the neuron of the second order synapses with a neuron of the third order. There are no other known influencing synapses on the neuron of the third order in the VPM, which seems to be primarily a relay station. This neuron of the third order leaves the VPM to project its fibers to the postcentral gyrus of the cerebral cortex. Here the signal is interpreted as pain, the intensity of which has been defined by the signal leaving the nucleus caudalis, but now the cerebral cortex evaluates the pain against the individual's expectations, past life experiences, and social values into a final pain reaction.

The Gating Mechanism of Pain

The gate control theory of pain, as first described by Melzack and Wall, while not perfect, does at least explain the clinical observation of painful responses in most injuries and diseases. It asserts that pain is transmitted by small (1- to 3-μm-diameter) unmyelinated fibers (C fibers) and that touch, temperature, and proprioception are transmitted by larger (20- to 25-μm-diameter) myelinated fibers (A fibers). These larger myelinated fibers act as a counterbalance to pain and are inhibitory to the gate, while the smaller unmyelinated C fibers, which are evolutionarily more primitive, are slower conducting and, because they lack myelination, more resistant to injury and more regenerative. The A fibers evolved more recently, are faster in conduction, and, because of the complex synthetic machinery necessary to synthesize myelin, less regenerative, and they actually die off as a result of injury.

These two "pre-gate" influences normally remain in balance, but they can be thrown into imbalance by certain conditions, which can influence the intensity of perceived pain in one direction or the other. The common practice of shaking the cheek during a local anesthetic injection, for example, excites the myelinated A fibers, which have an increased conduction velocity, causing inhibition of the gate. Since this inhibitory signal arrives before the painful stimulus of the needle injection transmitted by unmyelinated C fibers, the patient feels little or no pain. Transcutaneous nerve stimulation and acupuncture essentially rely upon the same principle to dampen pain signals.

This pre-gate function of the neurophysiologic system also explains the pain from a C-fiber neuroma, except that in this case, the nerve damage injures both C-fiber and A-fiber populations. However, the C fibers, with their greater capacity to regenerate, undergo proliferation, whereas the more fragile A fibers undergo atrophy. Consequently, the neuroma contains unmyelinated C fibers almost exclusively and is therefore painful. The pain of herpes zoster and its postherpetic neuralgia complication can be explained by a similar mechanism. In the case of herpes zoster, the DNA viruses selectively infect and destroy the

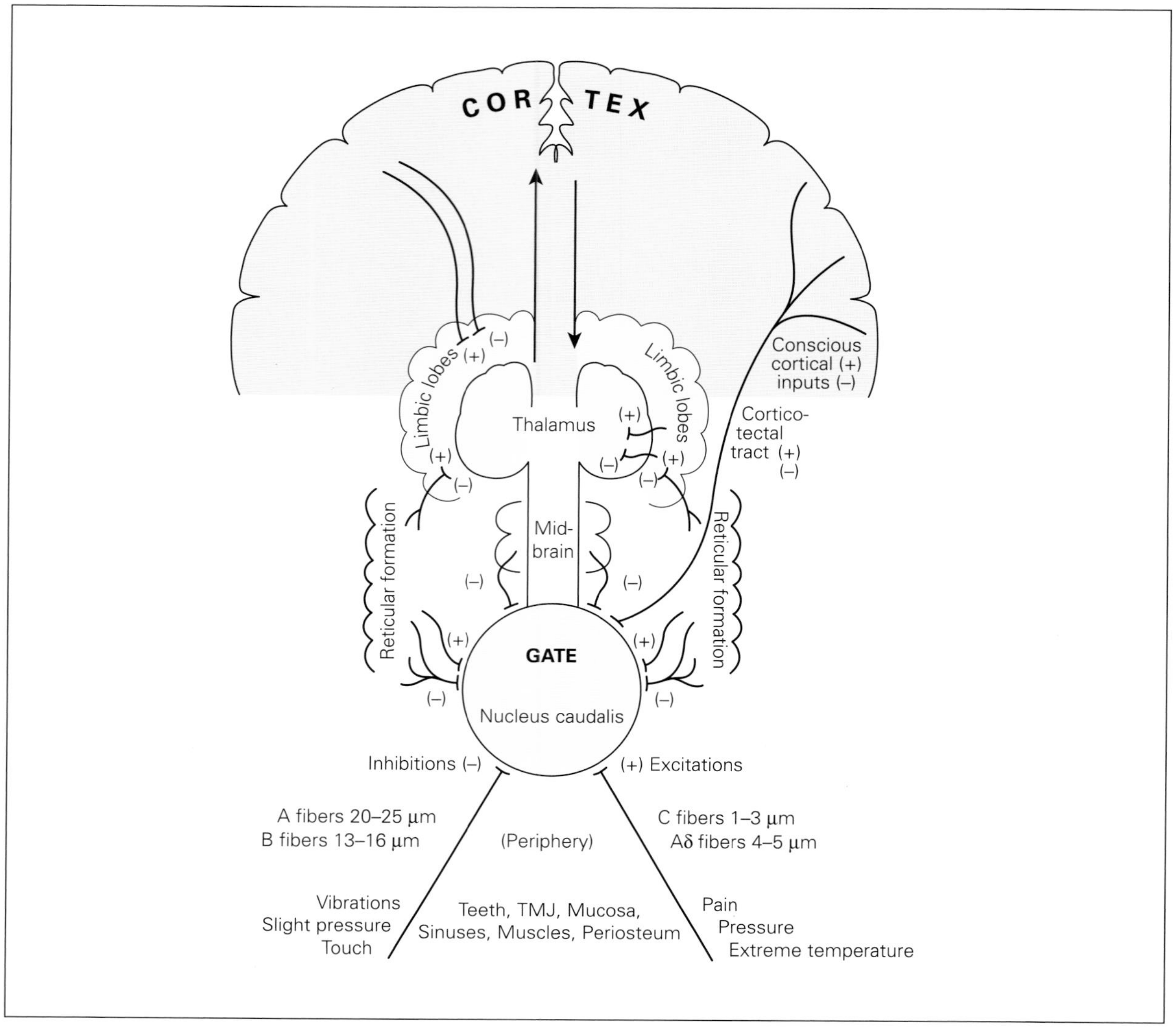

Fig 9-42b Gate control theory of pain modulation related to the trigeminal nerve.

larger A fiber–related cell bodies in the Gasserian ganglion, creating an imbalance between C fibers and A fibers. The pain related to both C-fiber neuromas and herpes zoster is due to a relative increase in the number of pain-transmitting C fibers and a relative decrease in the number of so-called anti-pain A fibers. The difference is that in the case of a C-fiber neuroma, pain is due to a selective regeneration of C fibers; in the case of herpes zoster, it is due to a selective destruction of A fibers.

Once the modified signal enters the nucleus caudalis, it synapses with the neuron of the second order, which also receives synapses that will modify the pain signal from other brain sectors (Fig 9-42b). One of these influencing areas is the reticular activating system, where sleep and rest, etc, will inhibit and close the gate while sleeplessness, fatigue, etc, will excite and open the gate. Another influencing area is the midbrain, where the endogenous endorphins usually send an inhibitory influence to the gate. However, if chronic illness, for example, has depleted the endorphin supply or if drug use has increased endorphin midbrain receptors, the midbrain inhibitory influence may be diminished, resulting in a more open gate. Similarly, narcotics will bind to the midbrain endorphin receptors to inhibit them, producing their well-known pain-relieving effects. Another area that projects fibers to the gate is the limbic lobes, from which emotions are said to arise and where tricyclic mood elevators such as amitriptyline (Elavil) and sedatives such as benzodiazepines (Valium and Versed) are said to act. Therefore, mood elevators and sedatives can reduce pain while emotional stress has been observed to exacerbate pain. In addition, the conscious cerebral cortex can project fibers to the gate, which helps to explain stoic individuals as well as the cultures in which acceptance of pain is valued and encouraged versus some social cultures in which a secondary gain and sympathy are received from pain.

C-Fiber Neuroma

TREATMENT AND PROGNOSIS ▶

The C-fiber neuroma is a recognized but rare entity that will produce focal pain in the area of injury, which may radiate to adjacent areas and be referred to other distributions of the trigeminal nerve. When the nerve is blocked with a local anesthetic proximal to the neuroma, nearly complete pain relief is achieved. In such cases, exploration of the injured site and excision of the C-fiber neuroma can be expected to produce pain relief. In such cases, the patient may opt to leave the parent nerve transsected in return for 100% anesthesia of that nerve distribution or to undergo a nerve-grafting procedure, which will achieve a maximum return of sensation of only 60% to 75% and will produce a 100% anesthesia in an area around the donor site.

Deafferentation Neuropathy

TREATMENT AND PROGNOSIS ▶

Most postnerve injury pain syndromes unfortunately represent a deafferentation neuropathy that is not usually amenable to surgery. A completely transsected nerve usually does not produce a deafferentation neuropathy but rather a painless anesthetic area. However, a partially transsected or an abraided nerve more readily results in a deafferentation neuropathy in which the patient relates intense pain and often a paresthesia as well.

When a nerve is injured without transsection, the more hardy C fibers recover and a greater number of the more fragile A fibers die off. As the area of nerve injury heals, avascular scar tissue is formed, which further favors the loss of A fibers since they require a greater amount of nutrients and oxygen to synthesize myelin, and eventually leads to the classic imbalance in the types of fibers ascending to the gate. This clinical pain syndrome is worsened by the centralization of the pain. In such cases the cell bodies in the Gasserian ganglion do not die off but remain as injured cells, producing pain mediators such as substance P, which enhances and perpetuates the pain. When the nerve is blocked with a local anesthetic proximal to the injury site, the patient will report little or no relief of pain. Therefore, surgery cannot be expected to gain pain relief. Instead, these individuals are best treated with central-acting systemic medications such as Tegretol, Trileptal, Neurontin, Depakote, Elavil, etc. These may also be supplemented with physical therapy, biofeedback, transcutaneous nerve stimulation, and other pain-management therapies commonly employed in pain clinics. Carbamazepine (Tegretol, Novartis) is the primary drug used in the medical management of pain. A starting dose of 200 mg every day is recommended; this can be increased by up to 200 mg every day as tolerated against side effects, to a maximum of 800 mg per day. The dosage of Tegretol must be regulated for best therapeutic effect, and a baseline complete blood count is recommended because of its dose-related effect of bone marrow suppression. To keep the Tegretol dose low and reduce side effects if they occur, gabapentin (Neurontin, Parke-Davis), 300 mg three times daily, or divalproex sodium (Depakote, Abbott), 50 mg every day, and/or amitriptyline (Elavil, AstraZeneca), 50 mg by mouth at bedtime, may be added to the Tegretol. In such cases, neurectomy, alcohol blocks, and even gamma knife radiosurgery to the Gasserian ganglion have not proven effective in reducing the pain and have even been known to worsen the pain.

HISTOPATHOLOGY ▶

Neuromas consist of densely collagenized fibrous tissue, representing scarification, intermingled with nerve fascicles (Fig 9-43).

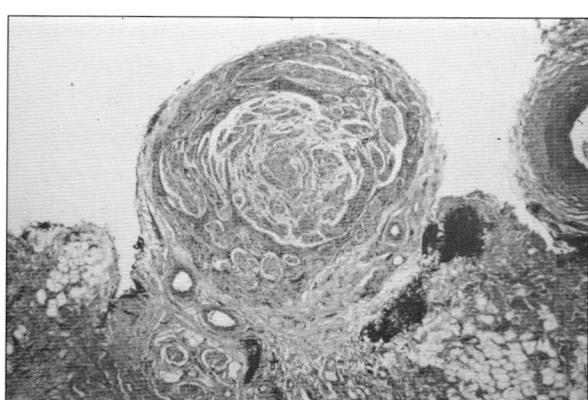

Fig 9-43 This C-fiber neuroma is characterized by a discrete nodule that is composed of nerve bundles surrounded by collagen.

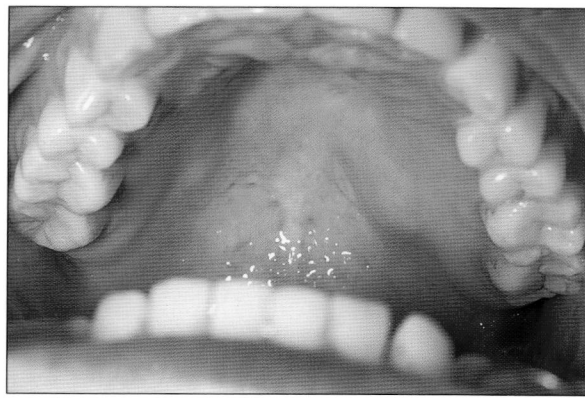

Fig 9-44 Nodule in palate that was diagnosed as a palisaded encapsulated neuroma.

Palisaded Encapsulated Neuroma

CLINICAL PRESENTATION AND PATHOGENESIS

The palisaded encapsulated neuroma may be more common than once thought owing to its frequent misidentification, usually as a schwannoma because of its palisading histopathologic appearance, and sometimes as a neurofibroma. Unlike a schwannoma, however, it lacks Verocay bodies.

The palisaded encapsulated neuroma is of importance to the oral and maxillofacial specialist because of its predilection for the perioral facial skin and for the palate (Fig 9-44). It will usually present as a non-painful submucosal or intradermal mass with an intact overlying surface epithelium. Most individuals are between 40 and 60 years of age.

The palisaded encapsulated neuroma has no association with neurofibromatosis or with any neuroendocrine syndrome. In fact, electron microscopic studies suggest this entity to be the result of reactive axonal regeneration attempts, and therefore it may represent a nonpainful, non–C fiber traumatic neuroma. Its small size (less than 1 cm) and limited growth are consistent with a disturbance in nerve regeneration and hence a hyperplasia rather than a neoplasm.

DIFFERENTIAL DIAGNOSIS

Because of its rarity, a palisaded encapsulated neuroma would not warrant inclusion on most differential lists. It will usually be a histopathologic finding. On the perioral facial skin, a round subcutaneous mass would suggest a *sebaceous/epidermal cyst* or one of the more deeply located skin appendage tumors such as a *pilomatricoma, eccrine syringoma, chondroid syringoma,* and especially the dermally located *eccrine spiradenoma.* If the nodule is within the area of the nasolabial crease, one might consider a *nasolabial cyst.*

On the palate, a submucosal nodule with an intact surface is most suggestive of a *minor salivary gland neoplasm.* Therefore, a *pleomorphic adenoma,* a *canalicular adenoma,* or even early malignancies such as *adenoid cystic carcinoma* or *mucoepidermoid carcinoma* may be considered. In addition, a true *schwannoma* or a *neurofibroma* may present in the palate in a similar fashion.

DIAGNOSTIC WORK-UP AND TREATMENT

Small nodules in either the skin or palate location are diagnosed and treated with a local excision including the surface epithelium. Margins at the lesion's periphery need be only 1 to 2 mm.

HISTOPATHOLOGY

These are well-circumscribed lesions with a complete or partial capsule. They consist of spindle cells arranged in fascicles, which show some nuclear palisading. They do not form Verocay bodies, however. The capsule may be continuous with the perineurium of a peripheral nerve. Immunohistochemistry suggests that the lesion consists of Schwann cells (S-100 protein positive) and axons (positive neurofilament staining) and that the capsule is most likely perineurium since it stains positive for epithelial membrane antigen.

PROGNOSIS

This has not been known to be a recurrent tumor; excision as described is expected to be curative.

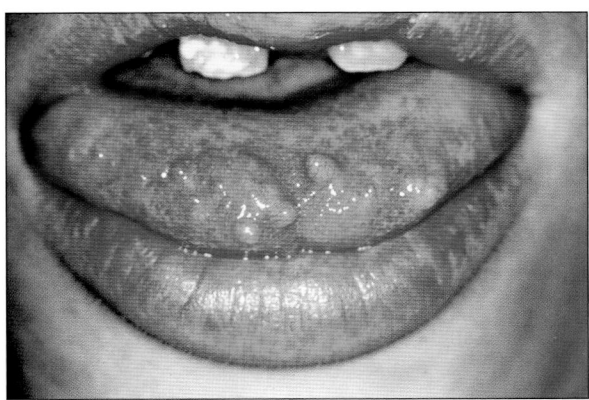

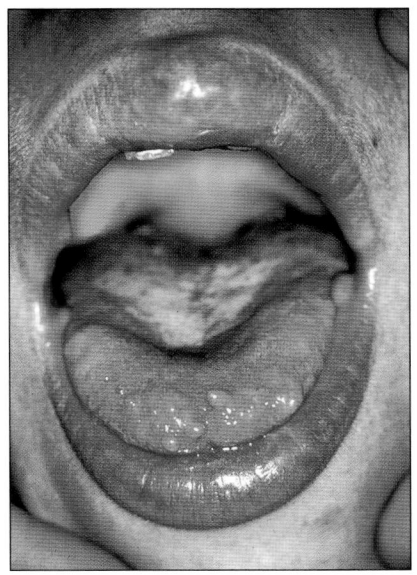

Fig 9-45a Multiple mucosal neuromas in the submucosa of the tongue is one component of multiple endocrine neoplasia syndrome III.

Fig 9-45b The oral neuromas in multiple endocrine neoplasia syndrome III are most commonly seen on the anterior tongue and lips.

Multiple Endocrine Neoplasia Syndrome III

CLINICAL PRESENTATION AND
PATHOGENESIS

Multiple endocrine neoplasia syndrome III is important to the oral and maxillofacial specialist because the first manifestation of this syndrome is multiple mucosal neuromas, which, if recognized, offer a potentially life-saving diagnosis.

Besides these painless multiple mucosal neuromas, the other components of this syndrome are medullary thyroid carcinoma, pheochromocytoma, and a long face or marfanoid facial appearance. All of these components arise from a deletion of a gene in neural crest primordia, which induces either hyperplasia or neoplasia in cells of neural crest derivation. The syndrome has autosomal-dominant inheritance, but about 50% of cases result from new mutations in utero.

The mucosal neuromas are nonpainful submucosal proliferations of both myelinated and unmyelinated fibers. They are usually small nodules of about 5 mm in diameter and occur on both oral and ocular mucosa. Intraorally, they are mostly found within the upper and lower lips and on the anterior dorsum of the tongue (Figs 9-45a and 9-45b). They may also be seen on the gingiva, palate, and buccal mucosa. Ocular neuromas, which are more common on the upper lid, will give it a characteristic thickening and eversion. Oral neuromas appear first; about 50% are noticed in the first year of life and the others before the age of 10 years. Occasionally, submucosal neuromas may also be found in the nasal, laryngeal, or bronchial mucosa.

Medullary carcinoma of the thyroid is the most life-threatening component of this syndrome, and more than 90% of individuals develop this aggressive metastasizing malignancy. Medullary thyroid carcinoma develops after the appearance of mucosal neuromas; most are diagnosed between the ages of 18 and 25 years and 95% have at least one metastatic deposit when diagnosed. Most metastases occur in regional lymph nodes of the neck or mediastinum. The term *medullary thyroid carcinoma* itself refers to a histogenesis from the parafollicular cells (C cells) that originate from the ultimobranchial body in the embryo. This body is a neural crest component, explaining the inclusion of medullary thyroid carcinoma in this neural crest–related syndrome.

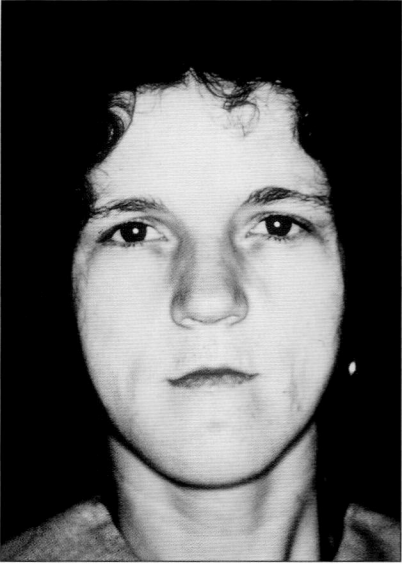

Fig 9-45c A vertical maxillary excess facial appearance, temporal muscle wasting, and thinness of the facial skin are characteristics of the multiple endocrine neoplasia syndrome III.

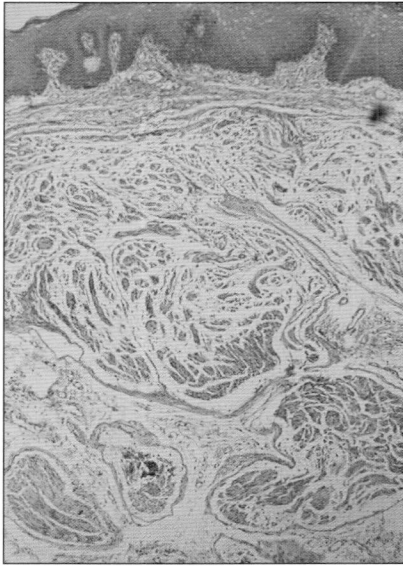

Fig 9-46 A neuroma of the tongue from a patient with multiple endocrine neoplasia syndrome III. Shown are nerve bundles with a prominent perineurium.

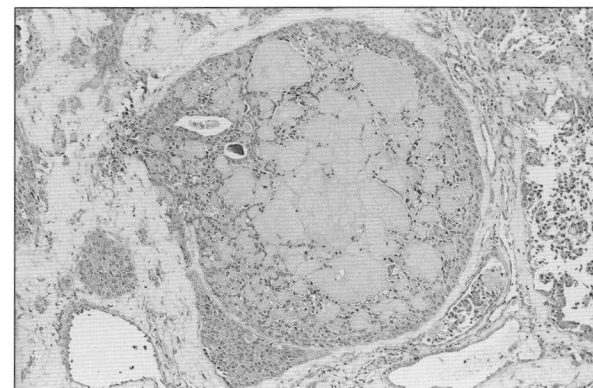

Fig 9-47 Medullary thyroid carcinoma showing epithelial cells with abundant amyloid and some calcification.

A pheochromocytoma occurs in about 50% of cases. Its incidence increases with age. Ninety percent of those that survive the medullary thyroid carcinoma (average age of death is 21 years) go on to develop a pheochromocytoma, sometimes as separate bilateral tumors over several years. Most are less than 4 cm in diameter; those greater than 4 cm are suspected to be malignant.

The long facial appearance that is familiar to oral and maxillofacial surgeons who treat individuals with vertical maxillary excess is found in an accentuated form in multiple endocrine neoplasia syndrome III. This includes temporal muscle wasting and a generalized thinness of the facial skin (Fig 9-45c). Sometimes the proximal extremity muscles have atrophied and exhibit weakness as well.

DIFFERENTIAL DIAGNOSIS ▶

It is hoped that the oral and maxillofacial specialist will observe and recognize the oral or ocular neuromas well in advance of development of the thyroid and adrenal tumors. Oral mucosal nodules in a child may merely represent *neuromas unrelated to any syndrome.* They may also appear similar to the mucosal thickenings in *focal epithelial hyperplasia* (HECK disease). Finally, they may appear like a *mucocele* or *mucus cyst in the lips* or as *swollen papillae from a nonspecific inflammation* in the tongue.

Ocular neuromas may appear as an *infected meibomian gland* (sty) or as an outcropping of *molluscum contagiosum.*

DIAGNOSTIC WORK-UP ▶

Whether single or multiple, submucosal nodules in individuals of any age should be excised for a histopathologic diagnosis. If a neuroma is diagnosed, a CT scan of the neck and abdomen should be undertaken to assess for the presence of thyroid or adrenal tumors. It may also be of value to test for serum calcitonin levels, which are usually elevated in medullary thyroid carcinomas, and for urinary vanillylmandelic acid, which is elevated when a pheochromocytoma is present. Ultrasound may also be useful for suspected tumors in cases in which the CT scan is equivocal or cannot be performed.

HISTOPATHOLOGY ▶

The neuromas of this syndrome consist of Schwann cells and axons surrounded by perineurium. The adjacent connective tissue is normal, lacking the fibrosis of the C-fiber neuroma. This lesion represents a hamartoma rather than a neoplasm (Fig 9-46).

Medullary thyroid carcinomas consist of clusters of epithelial cells with granular eosinophilic cytoplasm in a hyalinized, amyloid stroma. Calcifications, often resembling psammoma bodies, are frequently present (Fig 9-47).

TREATMENT AND PROGNOSIS ▶

The mucosal neuromas require no specific treatment unless excision would alleviate an encumbrance of lip or eyelid closure. Because of the nearly universal development of medullary thyroid carcinoma in these patients, a prophylactic thyroidectomy is almost always recommended. The pheochromocytomas are excised only when evidence of their development is found.

If the thyroid is removed before a medullary thyroid carcinoma develops, the long-term prognosis is good. If a thyroid carcinoma is present at the time of diagnosis, the prognosis is reduced to less than 50% survival due either to early infiltration into the neck or lymph node metastasis and extension into the mediastinum. Total thyroidectomy followed by radiotherapy of 5,000 cGy to 6,800 cGy is recommended. If the individual survives and later develops a pheochromocytoma, usually in the teenage years, an adrenal resection is required. However, there is a 10% death rate from a cardiovascular hypertensive crisis either just before or just after this surgery.

Congenital Granular Cell Tumor

CLINICAL PRESENTATION AND PATHOGENESIS ▶

The congenital granular cell tumor is a specific lesion representing a hamartomatous proliferation of granular cells rather than a true neoplasm. It is present at birth as a mass arising from the anterior maxillary or mandibular gingiva. It is more common in females than in males (9:1) and more common in the maxillary gingiva than in the mandibular gingiva (3:1). The lesions seem to be painless and will almost always arise from a narrow stalk (Fig 9-48). Even so, some can reach very large sizes (that of an adult's fist) and interfere with feeding (Fig 9-49a). Most will be 2 to 4 cm and brought to the clinician's attention by neonatal nursing personnel or the parents. Occasionally, two (or more) will appear in the same area or one may appear on each jaw.

Although the granular cells of this tumor are identical to those of the granular cell tumors of adults and those of some ameloblastomas under light microscopy, they seem to be of a different origin. The granular cells in this congenital tumor fail to show the suggestive neural elements ultrastructurally or the S-100 protein immunohistochemically as do adult granular cell tumors. Therefore, it is suspected that the congenital lesion arises from vascular pericytes or smooth muscle rather than Schwann cells as is believed to be the histogenesis of adult tumors.

DIFFERENTIAL DIAGNOSIS ▶

Several serious tumors can arise from the anterior jaws (particularly the maxilla) in neonates. However, the congenital granular cell tumor is a clinically recognizable tumor if the clinician identifies a stalk and an intact surface epithelium and confirms that the tumor was present at birth. The *melanotic neuroectodermal tumor of infancy (MNETI)* is the primary differential that can easily be eliminated if the parents or obstetrician can confirm the presence of the mass at birth. The MNETI is not a congenital lesion; it will arise between 2 and 11 months of age. The MNETI will also show clinically black to blue pigmentation and destruction of the anterior maxilla. Malignancies such as a *rhabdomyosarcoma* or a *neuroblastoma* are also serious considerations, but each will be destructive masses and will not have an associated stalk. Benign lesions common to newborns, such as *hemangiomas* and *lymphangiomas*, are also considerations, but these also will not emerge from a single stalk.

DIAGNOSTIC WORK-UP AND TREATMENT ▶

There are some anecdotal reports that these lesions will regress, but regression is not a constant finding. Small lesions can be excised in the neonatal period and closed with a simple suturing. Before the excision, it is well to educate the neonatal staff and reassure parents that the tumor is not a dangerous one and that the child should not be permanently affected in any way. It is also wise to inform the neonatal staff and parents that the baby will cry during the procedure because of fear, not because of pain, and that a small amount of local anesthesia will assure that.

Large lesions (greater than 4 cm) have a significant blood supply, all of which flows into the mass and out of the mass through its stalk (Fig 9-49b). Excision through the stalk may create a rapid blood loss in a neonate such that transfusion is required. Such blood loss can easily be prevented. Before the lesion is excised, the stalk should be stretched slightly and two hemostats placed on the stalk. The stalk should

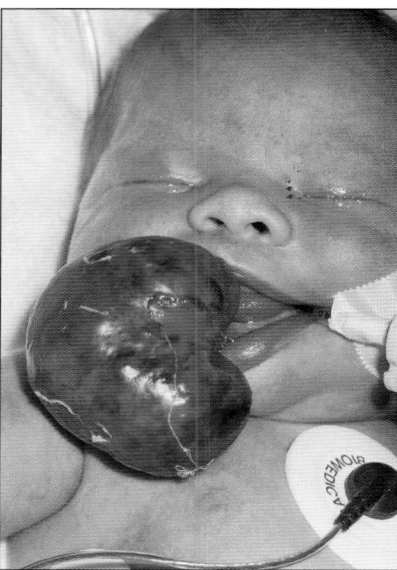

Fig 9-48 A congenital granular cell tumor is present at birth and will arise from a stalk connected to the gingiva.

Fig 9-49a Some congenital granular cell tumors will reach a very large size and may thus be thought to represent other conditions, particularly malignancies.

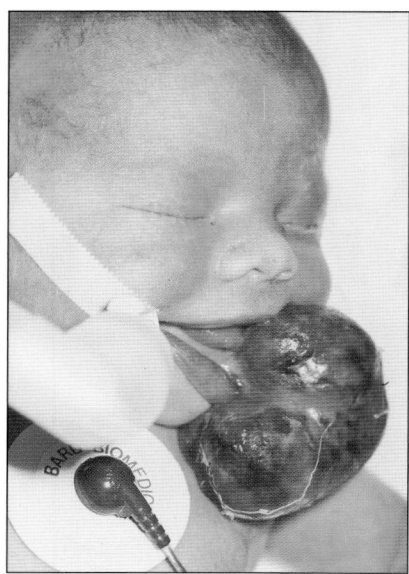

Fig 9-49b Despite its very large size, the congenital granular cell tumor always arises from a stalk. In large tumors, the stalk will contain blood vessels of significant size that may cause excessive bleeding if they are not clamped prior to excision.

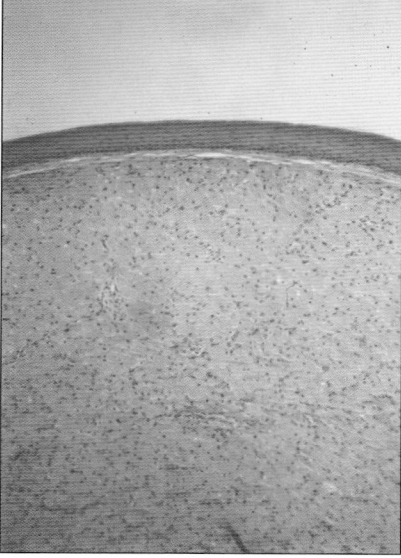

Fig 9-50a A congenital granular cell tumor is covered by a thin stratified squamous epithelium. Pseudoepitheliomatous hyperplasia is not seen in these lesions.

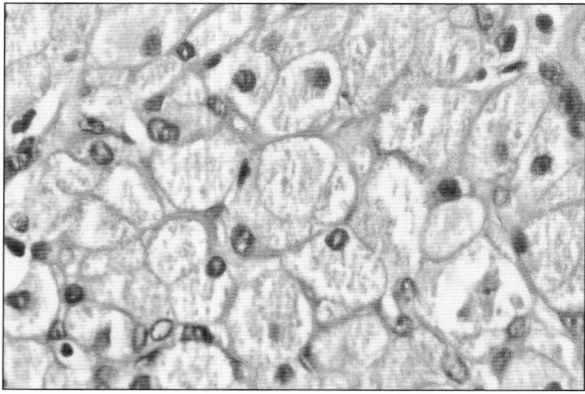

Fig 9-50b The granular cells of this congenital granular cell tumor are identical in appearance to the cells of the noncongenital granular cell tumor.

be cut between the hemostats, the tumor mass delivered on one hemostat and the other hemostat used to gain a tissue vascular tie. In this manner, the tumor can be removed with no blood loss.

 HISTOPATHOLOGY

The histologic appearance of the cells composing this tumor is identical to that of the granular cell tumor because the cells have a granular eosinophilic cytoplasm due to the presence of enlarged lysosomes. Certain differences do exist, however. The congenital tumor does not show pseudoepitheliomatous hyperplasia (Figs 9-50a and 9-50b). It is also more vascular. Ultrastructurally, it lacks angulate bod-

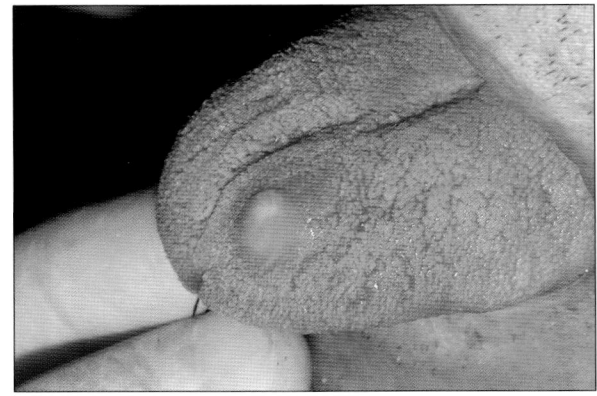

Fig 9-51 Granular cell tumors that occur in the oral cavity are usually located within the tongue or floor of the mouth. They will present as a firm fixed mass and have a thin or smooth surface.

ies but shows smooth muscle features not present in the granular cell tumor. In addition it is negative for S-100 protein.

PROGNOSIS ▶ Excision is curative without recurrence.

Granular Cell Tumor

CLINICAL PRESENTATION AND PATHOGENESIS ▶ The adult granular cell tumor seems to be a type of benign neural tumor with lysosomal alterations producing the granular appearance. The lesion will present most commonly in adults aged 20 to 40 years, although younger and older patients are not excluded. The lesion will present as an asymptomatic mass usually in the submucosa of the tongue or floor of the mouth orally or in the dermal subcutaneous level of the chest, back, or axilla. Lesions will be limited in size; few will become larger than 2 cm. Women are affected twice as frequently as men, and the tongue/floor-of-the-mouth area remains the most common site (Fig 9-51).

Granular cell tumors arise and usually go unnoticed for about 6 months before their size or presence causes the individual to seek attention. They will be firm and fixed within the tissue but not to other structures such as bone or skin. About 10% to 15% of patients will have more than one lesion.

The histogenesis seems to be neural and most likely Schwann cell in origin. The fact that this granular cell tumor reaches a size of 2 cm and then ceases to grow suggests that it may not represent a true neoplasm but is perhaps a reactive process from some unknown stimulation or a hamartoma of Schwann cells (such as a schwannoma) but with a granular cell appearance due to the accumulation of lysosomal vacuoles.

DIFFERENTIAL DIAGNOSIS ▶ Any mass less than 2 cm in the substance of the tongue must be regarded as suggestive of a granular cell tumor. However, its firm nature and lack of encapsulation suggest two other benign tumors, the *rhabdomyoma* and the *lipoma*. *Schwannomas* are also possibilities. In addition, three malignant lesions are serious considerations in the tongue despite the small size of the tumor: *rhabdomyosarcoma* in younger patients; *squamous cell carcinoma* in older patients, particularly smokers; or *adenoid cystic carcinoma* of minor salivary gland origin within the tongue. Minor salivary gland remnants exist in the tongue, and salivary gland neoplasias arising from them are most often small, subtle adenoid cystic carcinomas.

On the chest wall and back, the differential diagnosis changes somewhat. Certainly *neurofibromas, lipomas,* and *schwannomas* remain considerations, but muscle-origin tumors and salivary gland tumors are eliminated. Instead, *sebaceous cysts, dermatofibromas,* and *pilomatricomas* are more likely.

DIAGNOSTIC WORK-UP ▶ The mass lesion should be excised for biopsy and treatment. Frozen sections to rule out a malignancy are advised. If the lesion is benign or confirmed to be a granular cell tumor, excision with 5-mm margins is recommended. Because granular cell tumors are not encapsulated, frozen sections of the re-section margins are recommended.

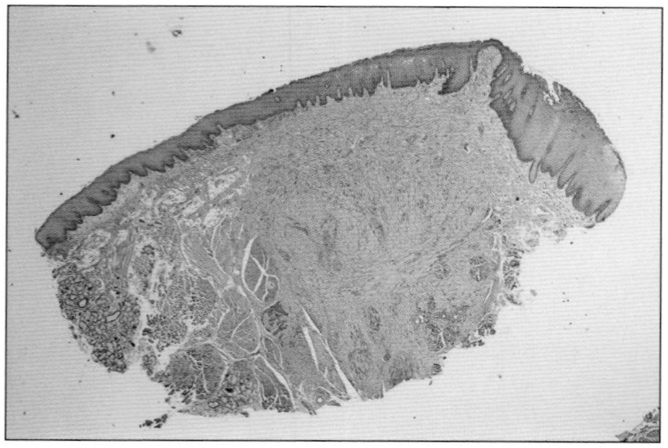

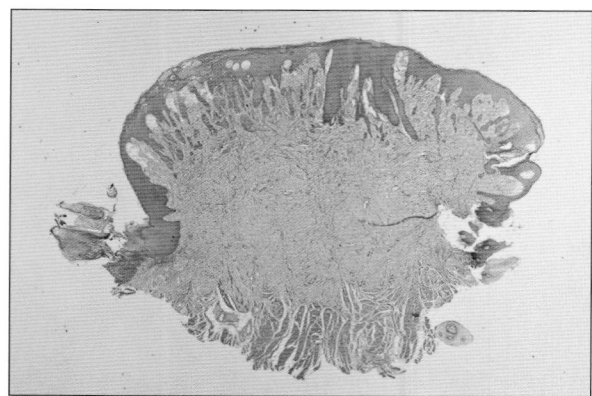

Fig 9-52 A granular cell tumor of the tongue shows that these lesions are ill-defined and unencapsulated. They tend to blend into the surrounding normal stroma. Note also that pseudoepitheliomatous hyperplasia is not present in this particular specimen.

Fig 9-53a This granular cell tumor of the tongue is clearly an exophytic mass. The covering epithelium shows pseudoepitheliomatous hyperplasia.

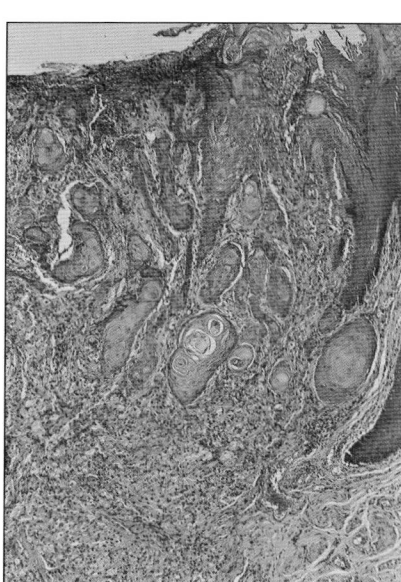

Fig 9-53b High-power view of Fig 9-53a showing a pseudoepitheliomatous reaction of the overlying epithelium, which may be misinterpreted as an invasive carcinoma.

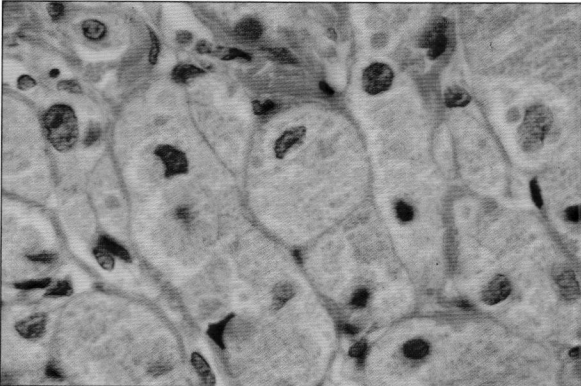

Fig 9-54 High-power view of the granular cells. The granules represent lysosomes.

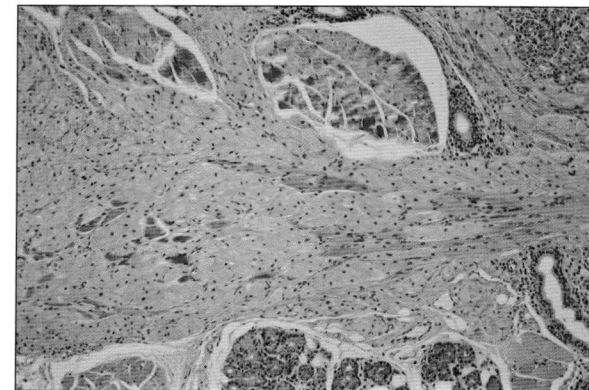

Fig 9-55 This granular cell tumor demonstrates the very intimate relationship it often shares with skeletal muscle.

Excision of lesions in the tongue requires absolute hemostasis and a meticulous closure. It is important to suture corresponding intrinsic and extrinsic muscle edges together so that coordination of the fine muscular movements of the tongue can be regained.

HISTOPATHOLOGY ▶ Granular cell tumors have poorly delineated borders and often appear infiltrative (Fig 9-52). This characteristic together with the tumor's hard consistency will often give the clinical impression of malignancy. Tumors frequently abut the overlying epithelium, in which case a striking pseudoepitheliomatous hyperplasia, which will often mimic an invasive squamous cell carcinoma, may be induced (Figs 9-53a and 9-53b). However, if the apparent epithelial invasion is into granular cells rather than normal tissue such as muscle, it is an associated pseudoepitheliomatus hyperplasia, not a cancer. Therefore, if a granular cell lesion is not considered, this histologic impression of malignancy may lead to a wrong diagnosis.

The tumor itself consists of large polygonal to rounded cells with small nuclei, which are usually centrally located. The cytoplasm is eosinophilic with coarse granules, although sometimes the granules may be quite fine (Fig 9-54). The cells lie in sheets or clusters separated by fibrous septae or skeletal muscle

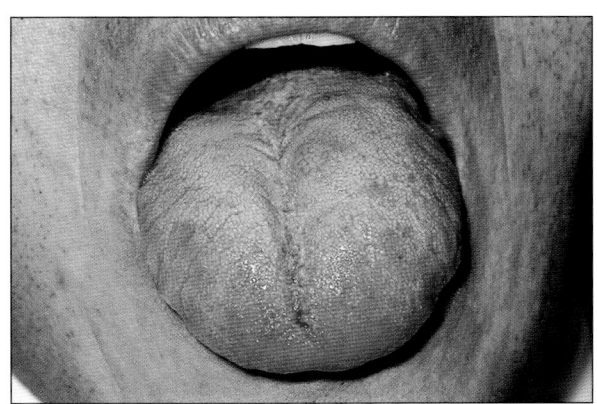

Fig 9-56 Rhabdomyomas are deep-seated benign tumors that are firm and often polypoid. In the tongue they will often give the impression of a diffuse enlargement.

fibers. There is often an intimate relationship with nerve. Because most of these tumors are found in the tongue, there is also proximity to skeletal muscle (Fig 9-55). Smaller interstitial cells with angulated bodies are also present. The granular cells are periodic acid–Schiff (PAS) positive and diastase resistant. Immunohistochemistry suggests a Schwann cell origin for these tumors: the granular cells are positive for S-100 protein, neuron-specific enolase, and myelin protein. Ultrastructural findings also suggest the possibility of pericytes and undifferentiated mesenchymal cells in addition to Schwann cells. The granules represent mainly phagolysosomes and usually contain cellular debris.

PROGNOSIS ▶ Granular cell tumors have a 7% recurrence rate, but many of those may represent new tumors rather than re-emergence of the original tumor. Therefore, local excision should be curative in nearly all cases.

Sporadic cases of spontaneous regression have been reported with the congenital granular cell tumor; however, no such phenomenon has been reported with this granular cell tumor. There is a rare malignant counterpart to this tumor, but it represents only about 1% of cases.

Myogenic Tumors

Rhabdomyoma

CLINICAL PRESENTATION AND ▶ The rhabdomyoma is another benign tumor representing an error in development and is thus a hamartoma rather than a true neoplasm. Two of the three types of rhabdomyomas present in the oral and maxillofacial/head and neck regions, and represent the site of predilection for each.

PATHOGENESIS

Adult Type

The adult type of rhabdomyoma is the most common. It is generally found in older individuals, and men are more frequently affected than are women. It will present as an asymptomatic polypoid or round mass, which displaces or occupies normal structures (Fig 9-56). Its occurrence in the tongue often causes protrusion and at times a tingling sensation. Its occurrence in the pharynx or larynx may lead to obstructive symptoms. It may also be found in the floor of the mouth, soft palate, and strap muscles of the neck, but not in the muscles of the extremities. In some texts, it may also be referred to as the *extracardiac rhabdomyoma* to distinguish it from the ventricular rhabdomyomas seen in children.

Fetal Type

The fetal type is much rarer than the adult type and may be confused with a rhabdomyosarcoma and thus lead to unnecessarily aggressive treatment. This type may be either congenital or arise at any time

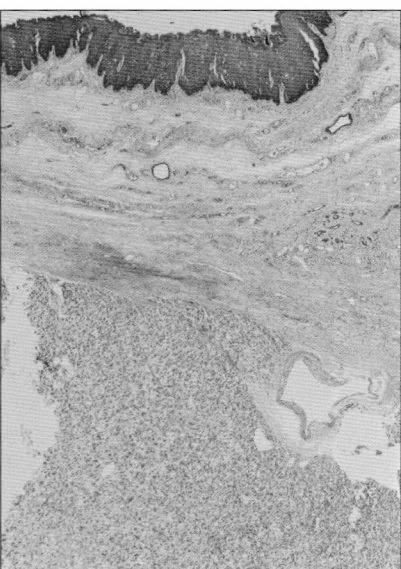

Fig 9-57a Low-power view of a rhabdomyoma showing that it is a well-demarcated but deep unencapsulated mass.

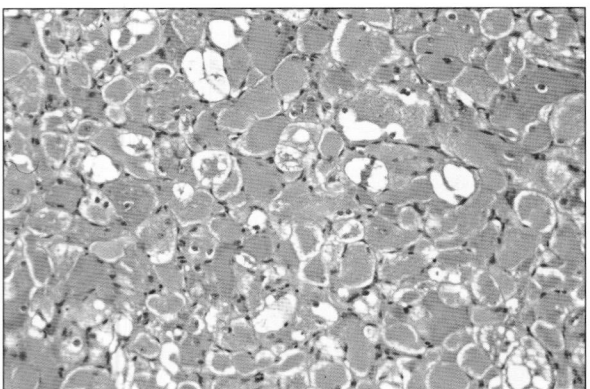

Fig 9-57b High-power view of a rhabdomyoma showing the large eosinophilic, granular cells with peripheral nuclei. Some of these cells have accumulated glycogen and, as the cytoplasm shrinks, the cells take on a spider-like appearance. Ultimately, the cell becomes entirely clear.

before the age of 4 years. The lesion will present as a painless mass, 2 to 5 cm in diameter, within the muscle layer beneath intact skin or mucosa. Most have arisen in the retroauricular area and posterior triangle of the neck. One reported case was associated with basal cell nevus syndrome.

Genital Type

The genital type is the rarest and occurs exclusively in the vagina or vulva in women between 20 and 50 years of age. It is a polypoid mass that is asymptomatic and usually only noticed after mucosal erosion or bleeding. The mass will rarely attain a size greater than 3 cm.

DIFFERENTIAL DIAGNOSIS ▶

The adult-type rhabdomyoma is suggestive of other benign tumors with a polypoid lobulated character, namely *neurofibroma, lipoma,* and *granular cell tumor,* particularly those that occur intraorally. In the neck, the mass may also suggest a *non-Hodgkin lymphoma,* a *branchial cyst,* a *thyroglossal duct cyst,* and several *inflammatory* or *metastatic lymph node diseases.*

The fetal type is so rare and the usual concern about rhabdomyosarcoma so great that the first consideration is almost always that of a *rhabdomyosarcoma.* Other possibilities in young children include *reactive lymph node hyperplasia* and other developmental abnormalities that occur in young children, such as *vascular malformations* and *lymphangiomas.*

DIAGNOSTIC WORK-UP ▶

Small lesions can be explored and excised as a combined diagnostic biopsy and curative excision. Larger lesions often require an incisional biopsy first to confirm the rare diagnosis of a rhabdomyoma and rule out other diseases. Excision requires 2- to 5-mm margins around the clinical lesion.

HISTOPATHOLOGY ▶

The adult rhabdomyoma is a well-defined mass (Fig 9-57a) containing polygonal to rounded, closely packed cells that have deeply eosinophilic, finely granular cytoplasm and peripherally placed nuclei. Many cells appear vacuolated because of the accumulation of glycogen. As this progresses the cytoplasm retracts, creating a so-called spider cell (Fig 9-57b). Cross striations may be seen, a feature that is more clearly delineated with a phosphotungstic acid–hematoxylin stain. The tumor cells are separated by narrow fibrovascular septae.

Distinct from the usually easily recognized adult rhabdomyoma is the fetal rhabdomyoma, which histologically resembles rhabdomyosarcoma. However, it is usually well encapsulated. It consists of spindle cells and muscle fibers in varying stages of differentiation. The degree of differentiation tends to increase toward the periphery. The degree of cellularity is variable. Mitoses are infrequent.

Excision is curative; recurrences are exceedingly uncommon. The paradox of this tumor is that unlike other benign tumors, which are much more common than their malignant counterparts, the rhabdomyoma is much rarer than its malignant counterpart, the rhabdomyosarcoma. Rhabdomyomas account for only 2% of all striated muscle tumors.

Although rhabdomyomas may grow very large, they nonetheless represent hamartomas arising from aberrant tissue development, similar to large odontomas. They are, therefore, expected to reach a certain size and cease growth.

Leiomyoma

Leiomyomas, which are benign tumors of smooth muscle origin, are uncommon in the head and neck regions and oral cavity. Their general distribution correlates with levels of smooth muscle tissue, that is, uterus (95%), gastrointestinal tract, and urinary bladder, in that order.

The sporadic cases in the head and neck region manifest as small, 1- to 2-cm nodules that are characteristically painful. In fact, pain is often severe and will be heightened by palpation or manipulation. In general, three types of leiomyomas are recognized.

Cutaneous Leiomyoma

Cutaneous leiomyomas, the most common, arise from the pilar erector muscle of hair follicles and are significantly painful. They are usually a firm, subcutaneous nodule that is thin and expanded but has an intact overlying skin.

Vascular Leiomyoma

These lesions are almost identical to the cutaneous leiomyomas except that their vessel walls are thick, whereas those of the cutaneous type are thin and indistinct. They have a predilection for women, except in the oral cavity, where they have a predilection for men. This type of leiomyoma is less common than the cutaneous type but tends to occur more frequently in the oral mucosa and head and neck area. These probably arise from smooth muscle around arteriovenous connections. They are no more vascular than are other leiomyomas and do not pose an enhanced bleeding potential. This type is also noted for its pain.

Leiomyoma of Deep Soft Tissue

In leiomyoma of deep soft tissue, the rarest form of leiomyoma, the lesions probably arise from vascular smooth muscle and attain the largest size (Fig 9-58). They are not painful and are usually discovered only as an incidental finding or when their size produces secondary symptoms. Degenerative changes, including calcifications that may be identified radiographically, are found.

The painful nature of leiomyomas, particularly upon palpation, is one of their distinguishing features, but it is not present in every case. Therefore, nonpainful submucosal or skin masses such as a *fibroma, gran-*

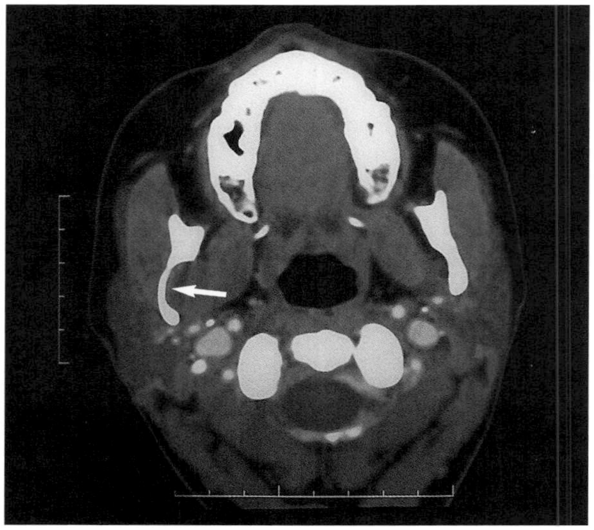

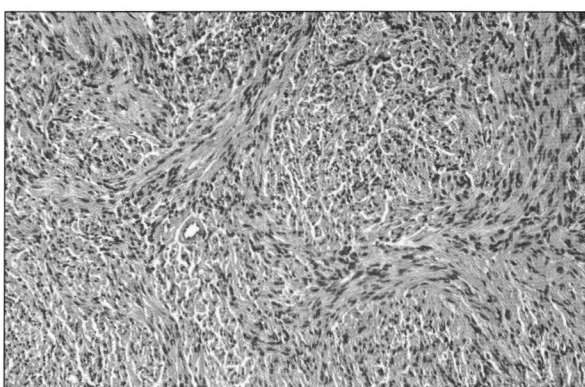

Fig 9-58 A rare deep leiomyoma of the pterygo-mandibular space causing a resorption of the medial surface of the ramus (*arrow*).

Fig 9-59a A leiomyoma showing interlacing bands of spindle cells.

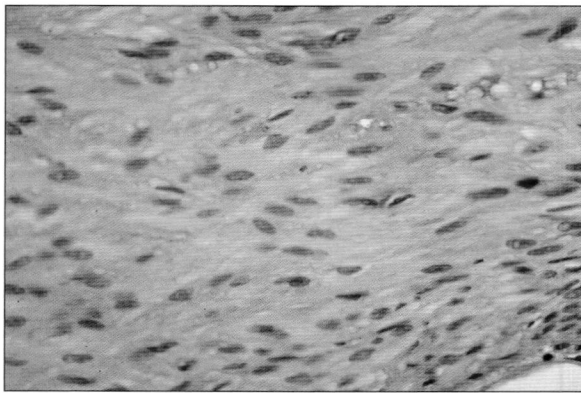

Fig 9-59b A high-power view of Fig 9-59a showing that the nuclei of smooth muscle will often have blunted ends.

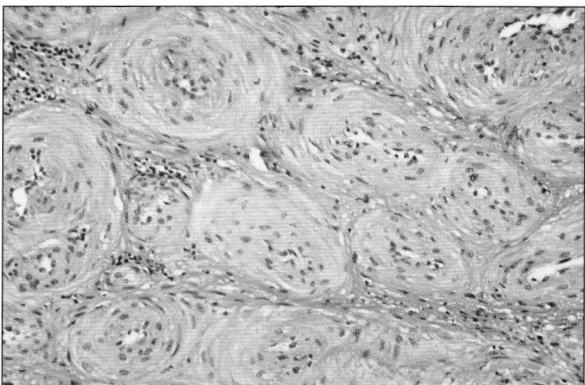

Fig 9-60 A vascular leiomyoma showing the smooth muscle proliferation around the vessels.

ular cell tumor, schwannoma, lipoma, and *minor salivary gland tumor* remain considerations. Other nodular lesions noted to be painful to palpation that can be confused with a leiomyoma are the rare *glomus tumor* (another tumor of arteriovenous smooth muscle origin) and the *C-fiber neuroma.*

DIAGNOSTIC WORK-UP AND TREATMENT HISTOPATHOLOGY

Suspicious lesions require exploration and excision with a 5-mm margin.

Leiomyomas represent true neoplasms with slow but persistent growth. What causes them to be painful is unknown. It is possible that peripheral nerve endings, which richly innervate pilar erector muscles for touch and proprioception, innervate vascular smooth muscle, and register vascular headache pain, also continue to innervate the neoplastic smooth muscle tissue.

Leiomyomas are usually circumscribed masses composed of spindle cells; thus, they bear considerable resemblance to fibrous and neurogenic lesions (Fig 9-59a). The nuclei, however, will frequently have blunted ends (Fig 9-59b). A special stain such as Masson trichrome may be helpful in demonstrating the myofibrils, which will stain red in distinction to the blue staining of collagen. Electron microscopy and immunohistochemistry studies may also be helpful. The former will show myofilaments, the latter positivity for desmin, actin, and myosin.

PROGNOSIS ▶

Vascular leiomyomas are well-demarcated masses of smooth muscle arranged circumferentially around the lumen of blood vessels (Fig 9-60).

Excision is expected to be curative. Recurrent tumors of the cutaneous form usually represent new tumors since multiple tumors of this form characteristically develop in the same general area. Recurrent tumors of deep tissue origin are suggestive of leiomyosarcomas because the deep tissue planes are one of the more common locations of leiomyosarcomas. Malignant transformation of a benign leiomyoma does not occur. Leiomyosarcomas are malignant from their onset.

Lymphatic and Vascular Tumors

Lymphangioma

CLINICAL PRESENTATION AND
PATHOGENESIS ▶

Lymphangiomas represent hamartomas of malformed lymphatics. They are sometimes termed *lymphangiectasias* because they are actually cystic dilations of malformed lymphatic channels that fail to communicate with or drain into other lymphatic channels or veins, and therefore will collect lymph. The fact that a lymphangioma may be seen on ultrasound in utero and that it clinically manifests in early childhood supports the explanation of its origin as an error in embryogenesis. Moreover, its predilection for the head and neck and the axilla, where the embryonic lymph sacs are located, lend further support to this explanation.

The lymphatic system appears alongside the venous drainage of an area at the sixth week of embryo development. Like veins, lymph channels are lined by endothelium, but unlike veins they contain no adventitial support and no basement membrane. This is important to the normal function of the lymphatic system because it allows for direct contact with the interstitial fluid space. The normal lymphatic channels collect the metabolic products and fluid from the interstitial space by direct pinocytosis through the endothelial cell and by means of an opening-closing cycle at the junctions between endothelial cells. Neither process is inhibited by the barrier effect that a basement membrane would pose. This already delicate developmental structure is further weakened by developmental endothelial malformations, which may result in the well-known large cystic hygromas or in multicystic deep and superficial lymphangiomas.

Three types of lymphangiomas have been described: the superficial multicystic type; the deep cavernous type; and the cystic hygroma. However, these actually represent a single type of defect in lymphatic development manifesting different degrees of severity. Generally speaking, lymphangiomas are less common than hemangiomas. Most of those occuring in the head and neck area (50% to 65%) are present at birth, while 90% are clinically apparent by age 3 years; the majority of these are the deep cavernous type.

The most common presentation is that of a painless soft mass that gradually enlarges and then remains static over a long period. Although occasional enlargements and shrinkages occur, a residual mass remains. The superficial multicystic type is the most static of the three types; it will develop slowly in a young adult as a soft enlargement or fullness of the involved area and will usually present with a pebbly surface that may appear to contain fluid-filled vesicles or blood (Figs 9-61 and 9-62).

The deep cavernous type tends to expand outward, creating a generalized enlargement of the area. Individuals will often complain of a swollen face (Fig 9-63) or a swollen tongue. This type is more often reported to undergo episodes of expansion and shrinkage than are the other types.

The cystic hygroma type can reach enormous sizes (Fig 9-64) and lead to the death of the infant. Otherwise, it will remain over a long period of time as a static mass that is either unresectable or can only be incompletely removed.

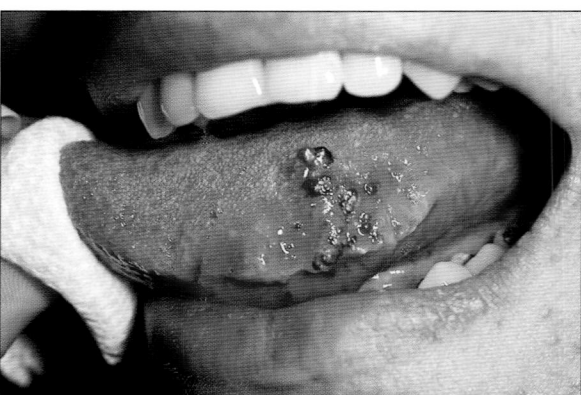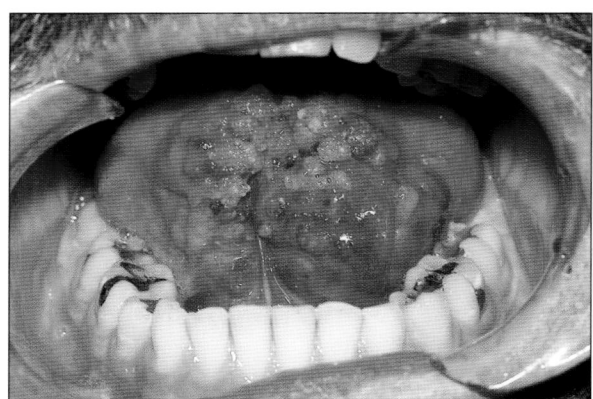

Figs 9-61 and 9-62 Lymphangiomas in the oral cavity are often found on the tongue or floor of the mouth. They will be soft to semisoft, have an irregular surface, and may have blue or red areas where blood has collected in the lymphatic channels. Each of these would represent the superficial multicystic type.

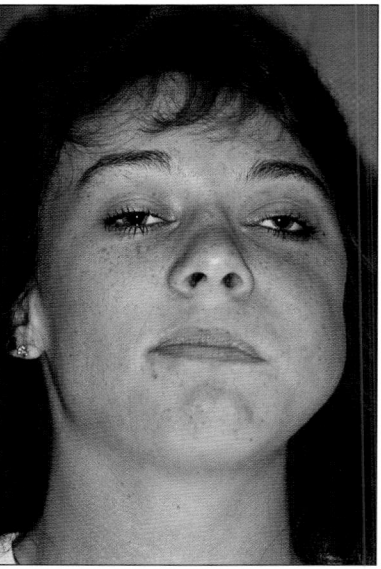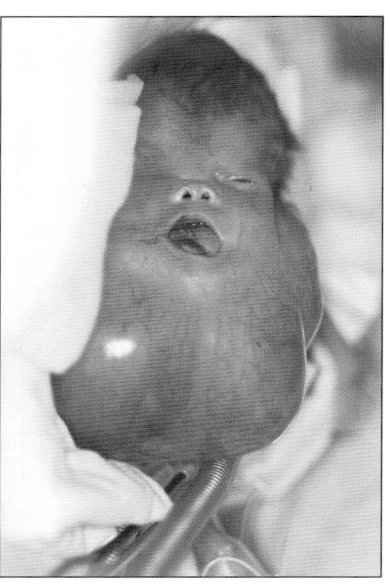

Fig 9-63 A deep cavernous type of lymphangioma in the cheek will present as a diffuse enlargement that may give the clinician a palpable sense of fused nodules, the so-called bag of worms impression.

Fig 9-64 A cystic hygroma is a large lymphangioma that usually appears as a congenital mass. This represents malformed lymphatics, which can obstruct the airway. Some are fatal.

DIFFERENTIAL DIAGNOSIS ▶

Because of their soft quality, lymphangiomas will most closely resemble *lipomas, salivary retention phenomena*, and *hemangiomas*. Since many lymphangiomas actually have some blood in their lymphatic channels, they are most often confused with hemangiomas; thus the term *hemangiolymphangioma* has been applied to such lesions. However, these basically represent lymphangiomas with communications to normal blood vessels.

DIAGNOSTIC WORK-UP ▶

No definitive studies other than an exploration and biopsy will confirm the diagnosis of a lymphangioma. However, ultrasonography will detect the cystic nature and fluid component of a lymphangioma, and angiography will rule out a vascular lesion such as an arteriovenous or cavernous hemangioma. A CT scan will raise suspicions of a lymphangioma if is shows multiple areas or large spaces that are homogeneous and do not enhance with contrast injections.

HISTOPATHOLOGY ▶

Lymphangiomas are unencapsulated lesions consisting of dilated, endothelially lined channels that may contain lymphocytes. The stroma consists of delicate collagen within which lymphoid aggregates are some-

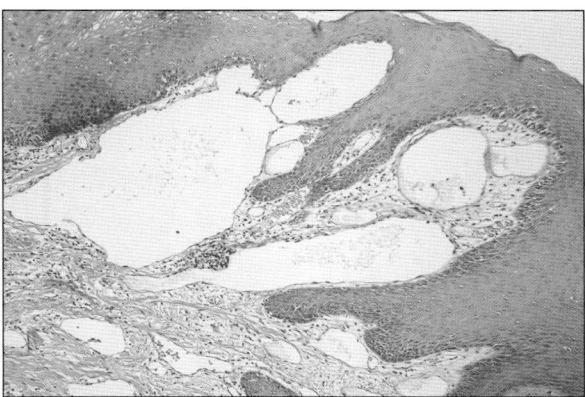

Fig 9-65 A lymphangioma of the tongue with dilated, endothelially lined channels. The lumina may contain lymph and lymphocytes. A lymphoid aggregate is also present.

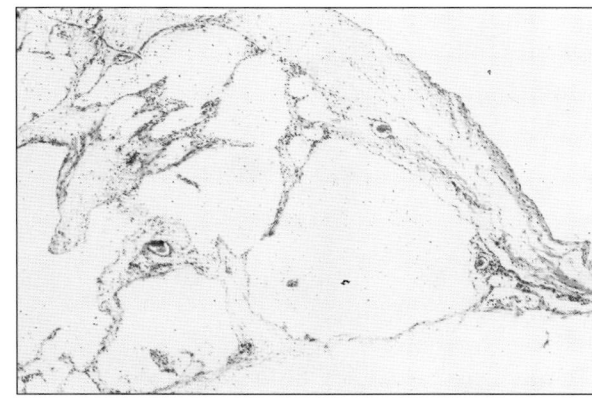

Fig 9-66 A cystic hygroma showing a network of large, endothelially lined sacs. It has formed a circumscribed mass.

times encountered (Fig 9-65). Some lymphangiomas also have a vascular component and may therefore contain some red blood cells. Cystic hygromas differ only in that they are usually composed of very large, interconnecting, endothelially lined, cyst-like spaces (Fig 9-66).

TREATMENT AND PROGNOSIS ▶

Lymphangiomas may be described as benign because they are hamartomas that may become large but will not continue to grow indefinitely and will not metastasize. Nevertheless, they can be life-threatening as a result of their size or secondary infection. Since they do not respond to sclerosing agents, pressure therapy, radiotherapy, or any known chemotherapy, almost all are either tolerated by the patient or treated surgically.

The cystic hygroma that is compatible with life is best removed between the ages of 18 and 24 months. If the cystic hygroma has compromised the airway, a tracheostomy may be required before this time. Cystic hygromas are usually well circumscribed, but they have only a thin connective tissue capsule at best. In such cases, a precise pericapsular excision and removal of any lymph nodes or identifiable lymphatic structures in the neck are recommended. A complete removal of the entire lymphangioma/cystic hygroma may not be possible. However, since it represents a hamartoma rather than a true benign neoplasm, the remaining lymphangioma will not re-proliferate, but what remains may dilate and re-expand.

The localized cavernous types and the superficial multicystic types are either allowed to remain untreated or excised with 5-mm margins. However, since many lymphangiomas extend deeply into the muscle of the lip or tongue, such surgery risks deformity, some functional loss, and possibly nerve injury. It is not uncommon to excise a lymphangioma in one, two, or three stages to minimize these risks.

It is important to emphasize that sclerosing agents, chemotherapy, and radiotherapy are not effective therapies and therefore are not recommended. Moreover, radiotherapy is a known risk for malignant transformation.

Hemangiomas

Hemangiomas are benign proliferations of vessels closely resembling normal vessels. Their similarity to normal vessels is so great that it is unclear whether they represent vessel malformations, true neoplasms, or hamartomatous overgrowths. One school of thought suggests that lesions that have greater numbers of endothelial cells than are required to line their lumen represent neoplasms; the remainder represent hamartomas. Under this definition, hemangioendotheliomas would represent true neoplasms, but so would reactive lesions such as papillary endothelial hyperplasia, while arteriovenous malformations and what are now termed *juvenile capillary hemangiomas* would represent hamartomas.

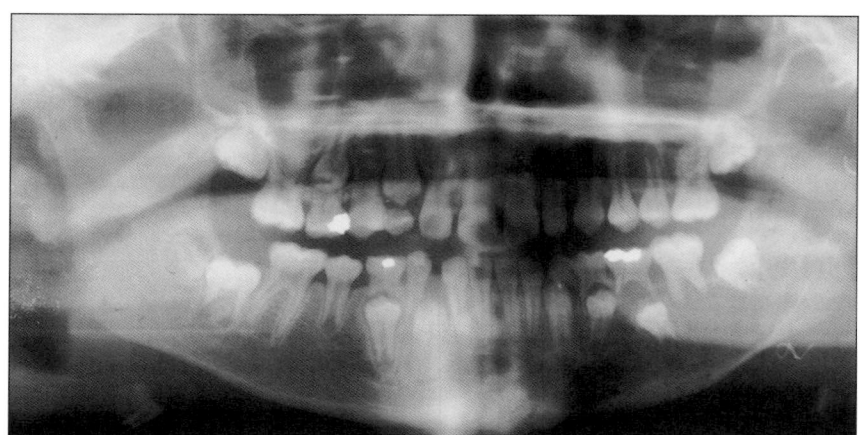

Fig 9-67 Large radiolucency representing a single lumen under arterial pressure. This AVH presented in a 9-year-old girl as a pulsatile expansion of the mandible and mobile teeth.

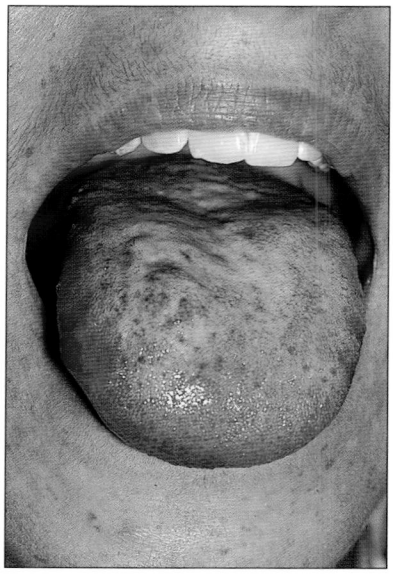

Fig 9-68a An AVH in a 17-year-old girl. It appeared as a subtle, soft-blue mass, but it was pulsatile and an angiogram revealed it as the tip of a large, high-flow vascular network.

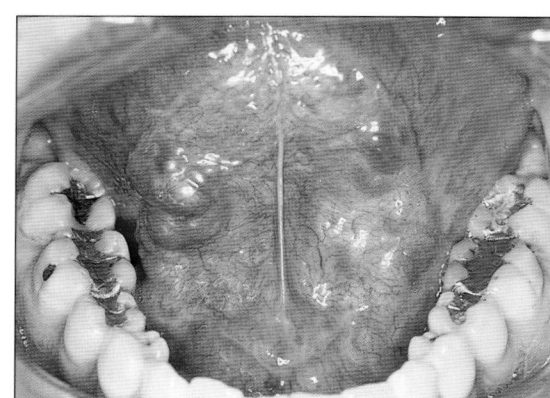

Fig 9-68b Normal draining veins, such as these lingual veins, become enlarged as the result of an AVH.

Another school of thought contends that malformations present at birth or those that appear shortly after birth are all congenital and represent vascular malformations. However, many vascular lesions may be congenital but subclinical at birth, only to appear years later (eg, telangiectasias seen in hereditary hemorrhagic telangiectasia and several facial hemangiomas). Indeed, many arteriovenous hemangiomas that emerge in the late teens and early 20s are associated with other abnormal vessels identified only by angiography.

In the absence of a uniformly accepted classification and in light of the wide range of biologic behaviors, the authors of this text prefer the term *hemangioma* used with the acknowledgment that almost all of these lesions represent vascular malformations that may be expressed at any time from fetal life to old age. They will be distinguished from proliferating cellular entities including hemangioendotheliomas, hemangiopericytomas, and angiosarcomas, which are true neoplasms owing to their continuous cell division without true vessel formation.

Arteriovenous Hemangioma

CLINICAL PRESENTATION AND PATHOGENESIS ▶

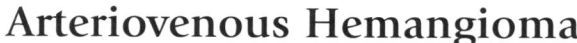

Arteriovenous hemangiomas (AVHs) are the most serious of all the hemangiomas and are life threatening. Those occuring in deep locations or centrally within the bone of the jaws and face are associated with a variable number of direct arteriovenous communications. They may also have a large soft tissue component that is most often located within the overlying skin and the lip. Most will occur within the mandible, the maxilla, or the tongue in the teenage and early adult years (Figs 9-67 and 9-68a). The patient is often able to detect a "whirring sound" or will claim to hear their heartbeat within the lesion. Indeed, some will demonstrate a visible palpation or a palpable thrill, and occasionally some of these will be able to be auscultated with a stethoscope (ie, a bruit). Most can be heard as an increased pulsatile sound with turbulence by Doppler examination. Some AHVs will produce vague paresthesias in the lip, apparently due to pulsatile pressure on the inferior alveolar nerve. In high-flow lesions, jugular venous

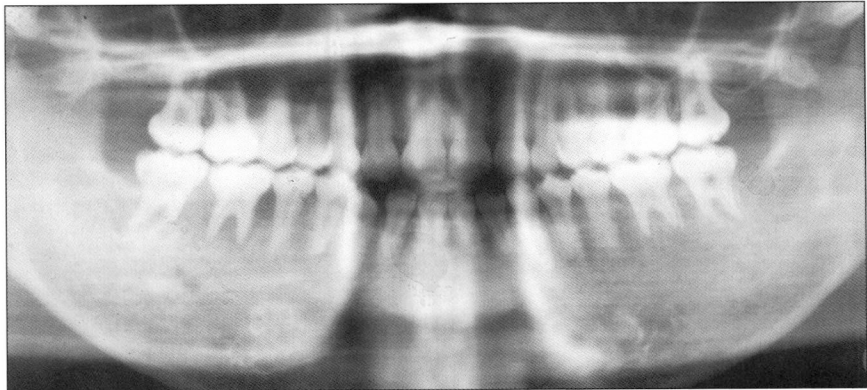

Fig 9-69a An AVH showing a fine trabeculation of bone and a generally enlarged mandible. Note the spiked roots and the radiolucency around the right first molar, which developed a life-threatening bleed from the gingival sulci.

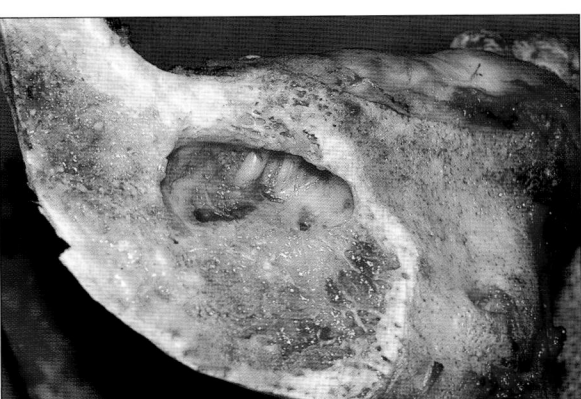

Fig 9-69b AVH resection specimen showing a 1.5 × 3.0–cm vascular space that was under arterial pressure. Note the tooth root in this space. Removal of this tooth would have produced a significant bleeding episode through the socket.

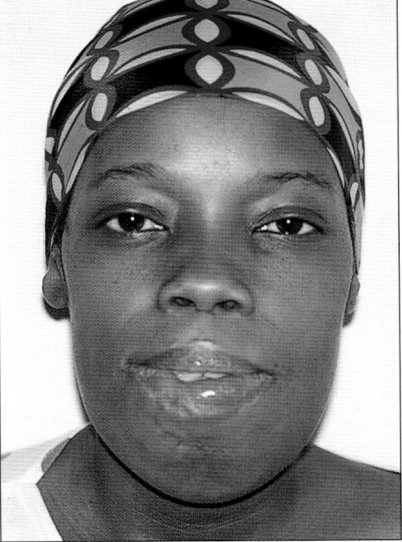

Fig 9-69c A young woman with a large AVH of the mandible shows an enlarged lower lip and a discoloration of the skin and anterior neck.

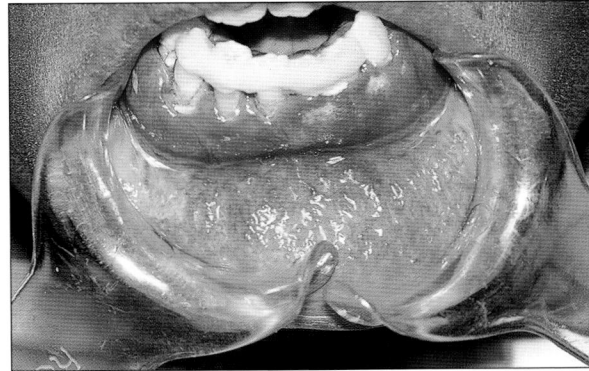

Fig 9-69d The soft tissues of the labial mucosa and lower lip show dilated AVH vessels. Note the blue discoloration of the gingiva and the need for splinting of the mandibular teeth as a result of the AVH within the mandible.

distension can be seen; in those within the tongue, engorgement of the lingual veins on the tongue's ventral aspect becomes apparent (Fig 9-68b).

If this type of hemangioma is located in the mandible or maxilla, the bone will be expanded and a fine multilocular radiolucency will often be present. The radiographic picture will vary from distinctly radiolucent (see Fig 9-67); to a well-defined multilocular appearance, often described as a "soap bubble"; to a fine, mixed radiolucent-radiopaque appearance that resembles fibrous dysplasia (Fig 9-69a). It is also common to see periosteal new bone formation perpendicular to the cortex, which on occlusal radiographs will have the so-called sun-ray appearance more often associated with osteosarcoma. A careful radiographic inspection frequently reveals periodontal bone loss around one or more teeth, which will appear to be elevated in their sockets (see Figs 9-68 and 9-70a). Clinically, these teeth will be mobile and compressible in their sockets. Removal of such teeth has given rise to dramatic high-pressure (arterial) bleeding from traumatic rents in what usually amounts to large arteriovenous dilations (Fig 9-69b).

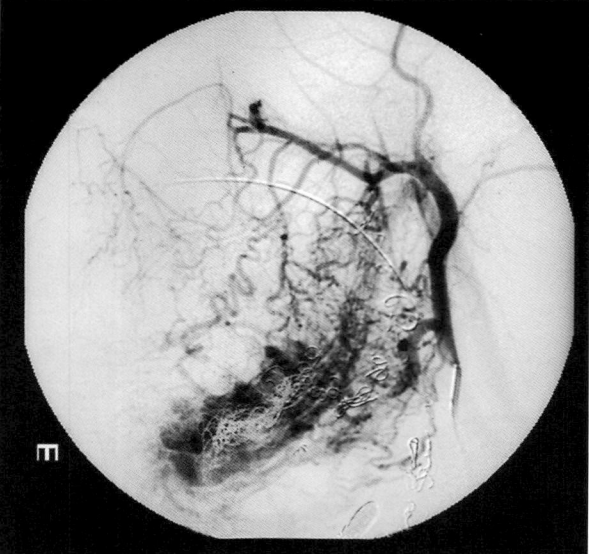

Fig 9-69e An angiogram of an AVH showing serpentine dilated vessels in the mandible and numerous small feeding vessels from the lingual and facial arteries as well as several from the sphenopalatine artery and other branches of the internal maxillary artery.

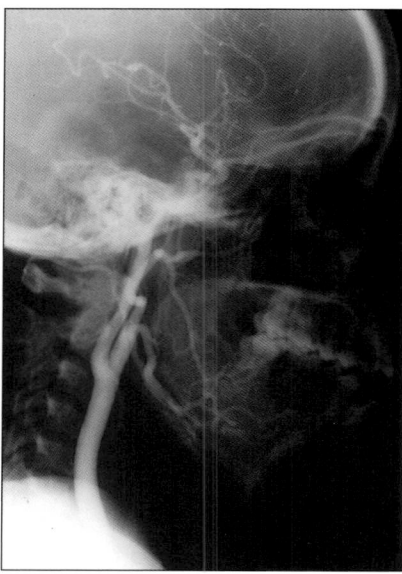

Fig 9-69f Dye has just been injected into this AVH. Although it has not yet entered the venous phase, the AVH filled as rapidly as did the internal carotid, indicating a high flow rate.

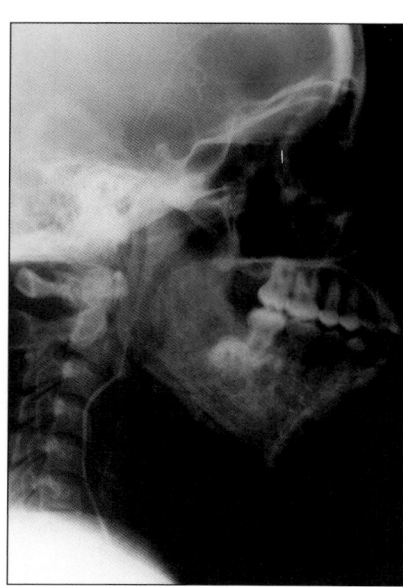

Fig 9-69g A large AVH central nidus retains dye for 5 minutes after all other vessels have cleared, indicating high pressure and turbulence within the AVH.

The soft tissue components of an AVH frequently occur in the skin of the midface and around the lips (Figs 9-69c and 9-69d). Unlike cavernous or capillary hemangiomas, this type is not present in infancy but emerges independently, usually during the teenage years. The lesion will develop into a solitary blue-red nodule located at the submucosal or subcutaneous level. Although arteriovenous communications are apparent in these soft tissues, they do not pose as significant a bleeding risk because the vessels remain small, as does the degree of shunting. Although some will elicit a palpable thrill, they do not present the uncontrollable bleeding potential associated with those in bone.

The pathogenesis of AVHs originates with fetal endothelial cell precursors. During development, one or a few of these cells lose their ability to produce or secrete platelet-derived growth factor (PDGF) and transforming growth factor beta-1 (TGF-β1), which are required to recruit adventitial cells around developing vessels. Consequently, the daughter cells and eventually the vessels that arise from these original cells develop as single cell–lined vessels (arteries, arterioles, veins, and venules). During pre-puberty there is usually insufficient pressure to cause these structurally unsupported vessels to expand and produce symptoms. However, beginning at 10 years of age, the maturity of the cardiovascular system and the increased systemic pressure causes these single cell–lined vessels to expand. As they expand, they create turbulence and a negative pressure that reverses the local flow dynamics to feed blood into these expanded lumen and even recruit new feeder vessels. This process is known as the *black hole phenomenon*.

The black hole phenomenon explains the clinical presentation of patients who are mostly in their early teenage years and the absence of any limitation to a known vascular anatomy. The earlier in fetal development that the loss of these growth factors occurs, the larger the vascular territory that will be involved. Therefore, some will be smaller and some larger in area; most will cross the midline. This pathogenesis also identifies the arteriovenous hemangioma as a developmental malformation rather than a neoplasm. Therefore, its apparent growth during its active phase is not due to a neoplastic process but to either a further manifestation of developmentally unsupported vessels or to recruitment of vessels into its central nidus.

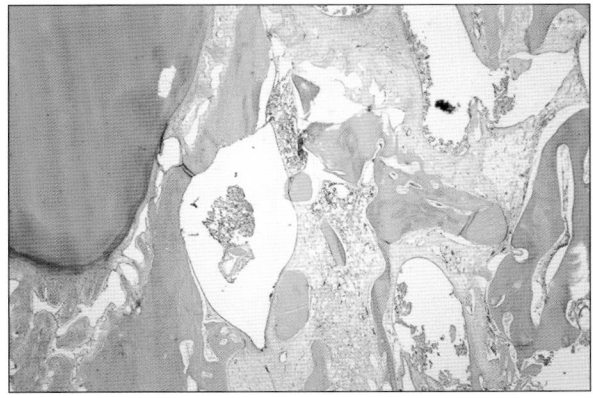

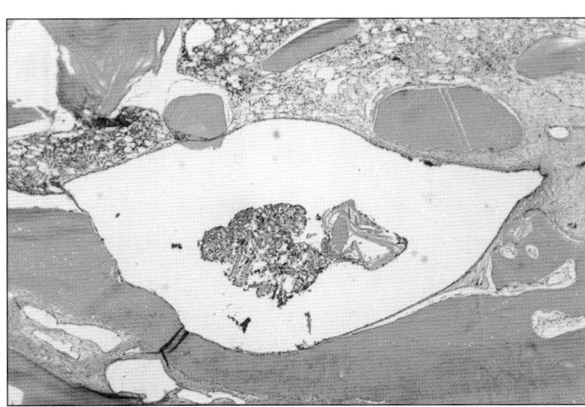

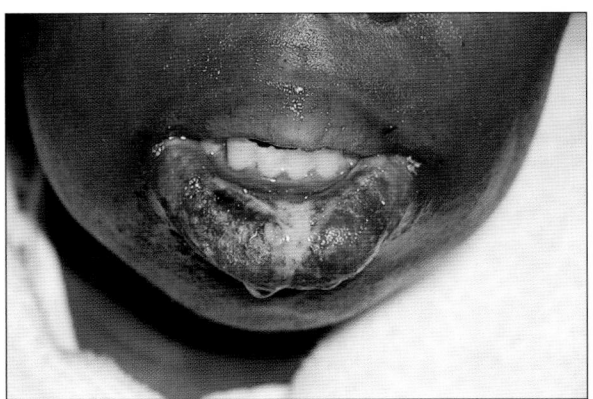

Fig 9-69h AVH showing numerous single cell–lined vessels with no adventitia. Note the proximity to the tooth root and some AVH vessels in the periodontal membrane.

Fig 9-69i High-power view of the AVH shown in Fig 9-69h clearly showing the single-cell layer of the lumen without adventitia.

Fig 9-69j Overaggressive embolizations may lead to ischemic necrosis and tissue loss.

DIFFERENTIAL DIAGNOSIS ▶

Arteriovenous hemangiomas that occur in the jaws may be subclinical (other than a radiolucent expansion). They will resemble odontogenic tumors such as *ameloblastomas, odontogenic myxomas*, and *ameloblastic fibromas*. Those with some fine bone trabeculations may instead resemble fibro-osseous diseases such as *fibrous dysplasia, ossifying fibroma, central giant cell tumors*, or even the infectious disease *chronic sclerosing osteomyelitis*.

DIAGNOSTIC WORK-UP ▶

A lesion that is suggestive of an AVH, whether via clinical examination, radiography, or Doppler sounds, should undergo a CT or MRI scan to determine its extent of involvement and its relationship to other tissues and a diagnostic angiogram of both common carotid systems. A lesion that is not initially thought to be an AVH but returns blood under pressure from aspiration should also undergo scanning and angiography. Both common carotids should undergo angiography separately because possible crossover feeders from the opposite side and/or from the internal carotid circulations need to be assessed. The clinician should be present during the angiography or arrange to review videotapes of the procedure to understand the dynamics of this malformation.

In reviewing the static angiograms, it is important to understand that images are taken one second apart beginning just before dye injection and ending when the dye completely clears from the field. One should, therefore, assess the number of feeders, their size, their location and parent feeding vessels (Fig 9-69e), the time required until the venous phase begins (Fig 9-69f), and the time required for the central lesion to empty (Fig 9-69g). The sooner the venous phase is seen, the greater the arteriovenous shunt and the higher the flow. Prolonged retention of residual dye within the lesion (3 to 5 minutes) is associated with larger lesions, increased flow rates, and turbulence, which creates eddies that retain the dye longer (see Fig 9-69g).

HISTOPATHOLOGY ▶

Histologically, dilated vessels, comprising only a single row of endothelial cells, are present. In close proximity, feeder arteries and veins may be seen (Fig 9-69h). Often there is thickening of the intima of the vein because of increased pressure, but no adventitial cells are present (Fig 9-69i).

TREATMENT ▶

The ideal therapy for these lesions, particularly when located within the jaws, is selective embolization followed by surgeries. The goal is to obstruct or reduce the blood flow to the lesion so that it can be excised with minimal blood loss. This approach is very effective for lesions that are resectable, and little blood loss is the rule. Overaggressive embolization is discouraged because embolization affects the normal as well as the abnormal vessels, and there have been several reports of tissue slough and dehiscences due to skin and other tissue ischemia (Fig 9-69j).

Embolization techniques and materials vary. As of this writing, embolizations are usually achieved with coils, 100% alcohol, or polyvinyl alcohol (PVA) beads. Coil embolizations generally embolize feeder vessels at the small artery level. They are initially effective, but small unembolized and often collapsed feeders enlarge rapidly (within 24 hours) to become dominant feeders, and recanulation of the clot and growth of bypass vessels quickly negate its effects. The surgeon should discourage the invasive radiologist from using coils because their reduction of blood flow is too short and too small. In addition, these coils will block access to these same vessels in future embolizations, which are often required. Absolute alcohol can be injected into the small artery precapillary arteriolar level by what is called "superselective" embolization. The caustic effects of 100% alcohol are, therefore, exerted close to the center of the lesion, which results in fibrosis of many of the lesion's multiple feeders. PVA beads of varying sizes are released in the main feeders and progress downstream to lodge in and embolize at the precapillary arteriolar level or within the lesion itself. Both PVA beads and alcohol are believed to be selectively guided to the more abnormal vessels by the fluid dynamics (higher flow rates than normal) of abnormal vessels.

The timing of surgery following embolization depends on the material used for embolization. If solid or bulky materials, such as coils, fat, muscle, or Gelfoam (Pharmacia) are used, the surgery should follow soon after; that is, the same day or the next day (12 to 24 hours). Because these materials obstruct vessels too proximal in the feeder system, after this time collapsed collateral vessels fill to supply the AVH and restore high-pressure flow. If small PVA beads (250 μm or less) or liquid agents such as 100% alcohol or cyanoacrylate are used, the surgery is best delayed for about 72 hours to gain the maximum reduction of blood flow to the central portion of the AVH. In the case of PVA beads, they will initially lodge at the arteriole level and then flow further downstream toward the center of the AVH, at which level they will clot. Because the clot is closer to the AVH, they encompass more distal feeders in the feeder system. In the case of liquid agents, these flow initially into the distal portions and then hopefully into the central portions of the AVH. However, unlike solid materials, they do not lodge to act as a plug. Instead, they initiate endothelial damage by inducing clotting and eventual fibrosis, which takes time.

Today the standard approach to a serious, life-threatening AVH in bone is resection, which is often large and necessitates later reconstruction (Fig 9-69k). Although it leaves residual AVH in the soft tissues, this approach is effective, and it eliminates the life-threatening bleeds from the bone. An AVH resection requires a wide access via a visor incision in the neck to reduce the blood loss beyond that achieved by preoperative embolization. The external carotids should be isolated and temporarily clamped to reduce the blood flow. As the dissection approaches the mandible, numerous thin, dilated vessels may be encountered in the soft tissue. Each is isolated, clamped, and ligated as it is approached. The approach to either jaw should separate the bone from the attached soft tissue with a supraperiosteal dissection (Fig 9-69l). Attempting a subperiosteal reflection to preserve the periosteum will not promote better healing but will increase the surgical blood loss instead. This is due to multiple high-pressure perforating vessels from the bone to the periosteum that will be opened and difficult to control because they will contract into the cortex. Transsection of these same vessels at the supraperiosteal level makes them more easily controlled with electrocautery. Should bony bleeds occur under high pressure ("pumpers"), the best control measure is bone wax applied to the cortex. Once the mandible or maxilla is circumscribed with a supraperiosteal dissection in the area of resection, the bony resection can be completed with a readiness for electrocoagulation and/or bone wax at each bone end.

In addition to the technical surgical approach described, as part of this type of resection, typed and cross-matched blood (8 units) should be available and hypotensive anesthesia techniques should be used. A tracheostomy will also be necessary because the degree of surgery and the vascular nature of the AVH will predictably create a significant degree of swelling that may compromise the airway (Fig 9-69m). The significant size of most AVHs in the mandible will necessitate reconstruction with a rigid titanium plate (Figs 9-69n and 9-69o). Immediate bone grafting is not recommended because of the time length of most resections and the potential for contamination from oral communications. Instead, the rigid plate will maintain the jaw contours and tissue projection until a well-planned cancellous marrow graft can be accomplished 3 months later (Figs 9-69p to 9-69s).

As of this writing, another surgical approach, one that avoids jaw resection and has shown promising results in several cases, is being tested. This approach exposes the mandible or maxilla with the same soft

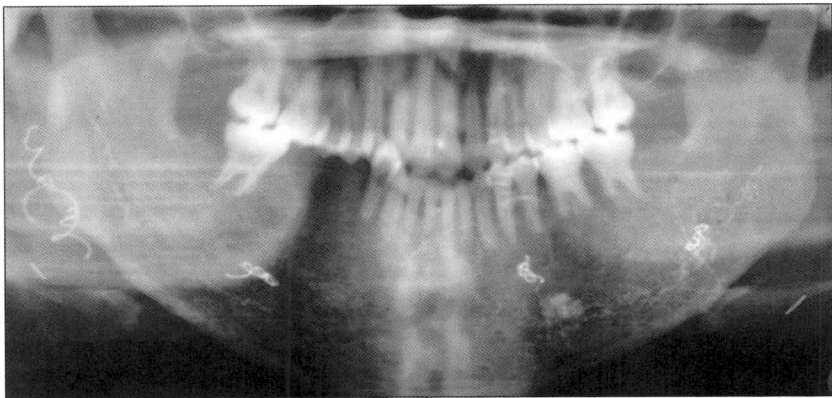

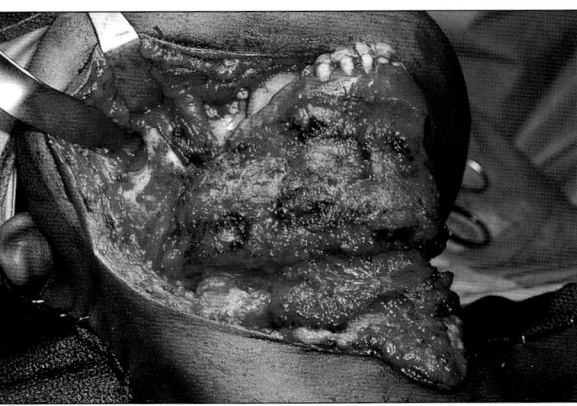

Fig 9-69k This large AVH, originally shown in Fig 9-69a, worsened and enlarged over time in response to a pregnancy, and therefore required a resection as a life-saving measure.

Fig 9-69l The technique of resecting an AVH may require temporary clamping of the external carotids and a supraperiosteal dissection around the bone.

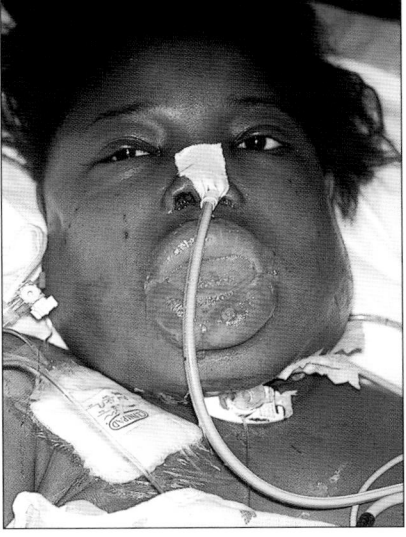

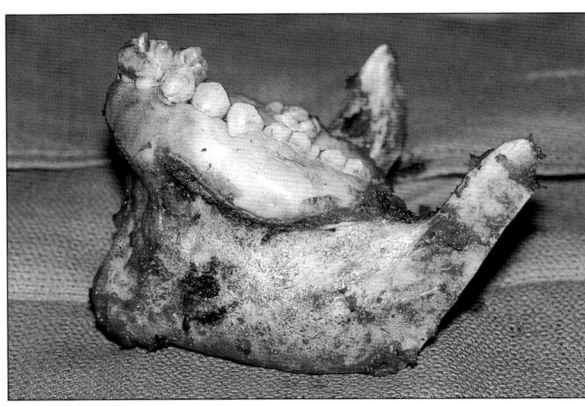

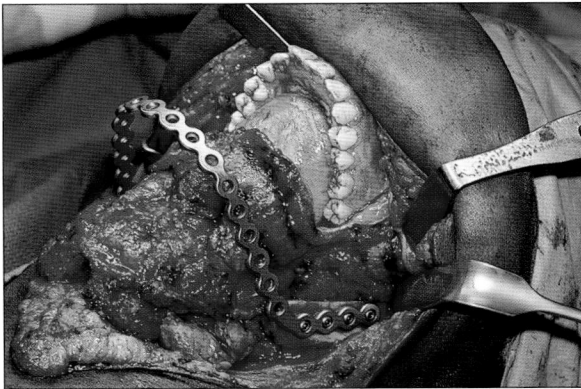

Fig 9-69m AVH surgery produces significant edema. A tracheostomy is usually necessary to secure a reliable postoperative airway.

Fig 9-69n This resection specimen of the AVH shown in Fig 9-69k is noteworthy for its extent, for its multiple feeders (manifested as a pebbly surface), and for the excessive vertical height of the mandible, which was stimulated by the internal perfusion of the jaw over several years.

Fig 9-69o Immediate bone-grafting of an AVH resection is not recommended. Instead, reconstruction with a rigid titanium plate to provide soft tissue support and contours as a preparation for a staged bone graft is advisable.

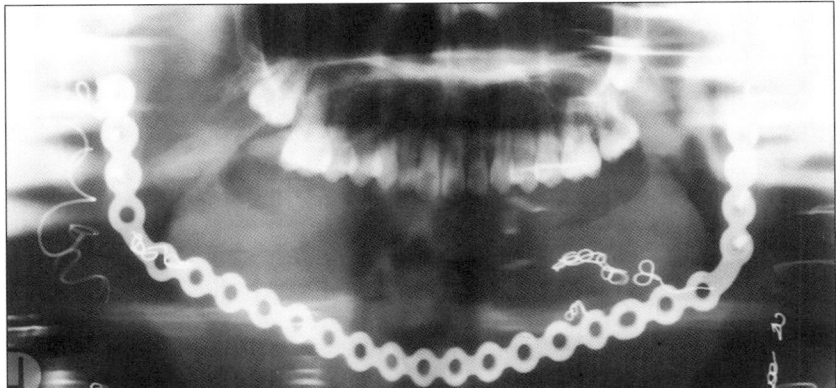

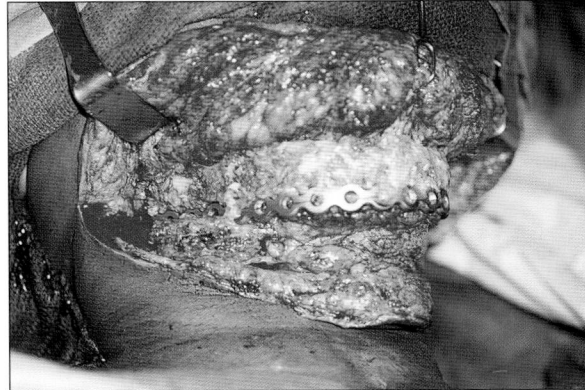

Fig 9-69p The rigid titanium plate can function well until the soft tissues are sufficiently healed for a controlled bone graft. Tissue healing and maturity takes 3 to 4 months.

Fig 9-69q The AVH-related defect is bone grafted with cancellous cellular marrow using the titanium plate as a crib and platelet-rich plasma (PRP) as an accelerator.

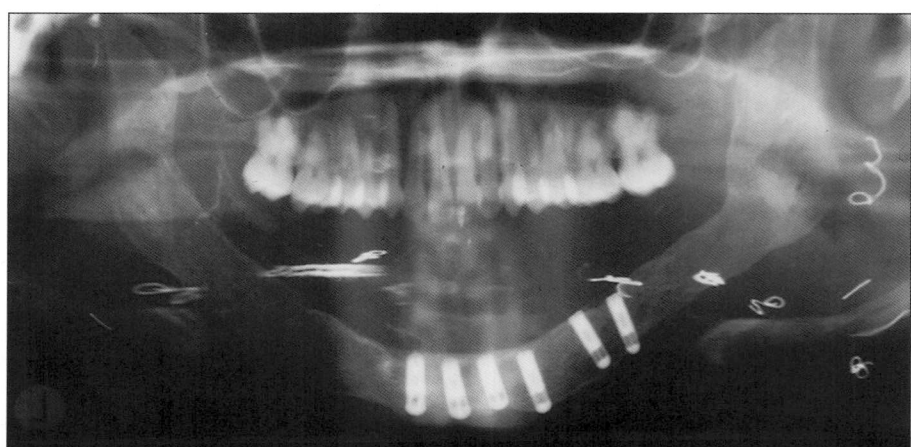

Fig 9-69r Reconstructed mandible after condyle-to-condyle resection of an AVH with mature bone and dental implants.

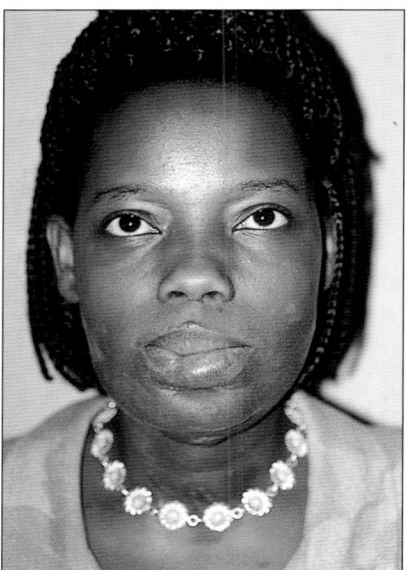

Fig 9-69s Resection and reconstruction of the individual shown in Fig 9-69c has an improved appearance and a cessation of life-threatening bleeds. However, residual AVH in soft tissues of the lower lip and neck remain.

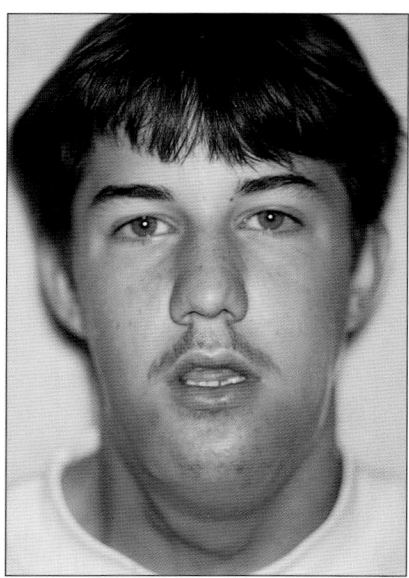

Fig 9-70a This AVH had a large, dilated soft tissue component in the neck and chin in addition to a large central lesion in the mandible.

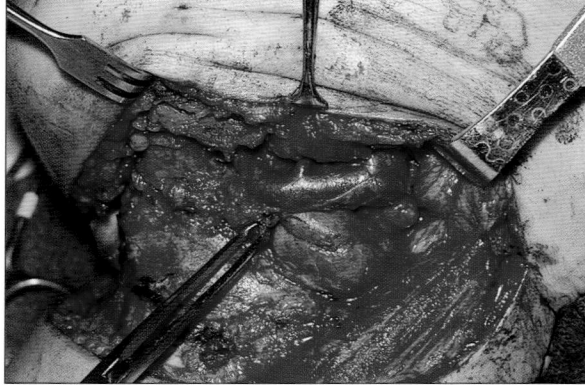

Fig 9-70b These large, dilated AVH vessels in soft tissue can be isolated and ligated like any other large vein.

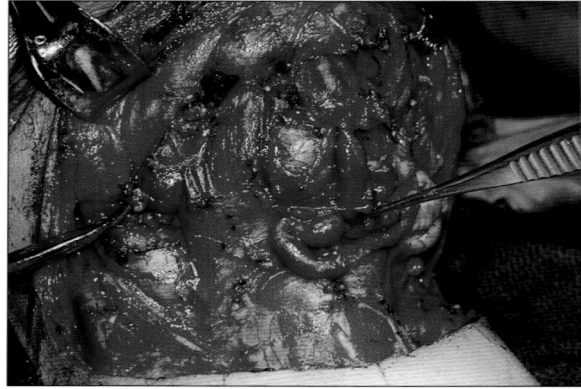

Fig 9-70c The large, dilated AVH vessels in soft tissue can be excised after ligation.

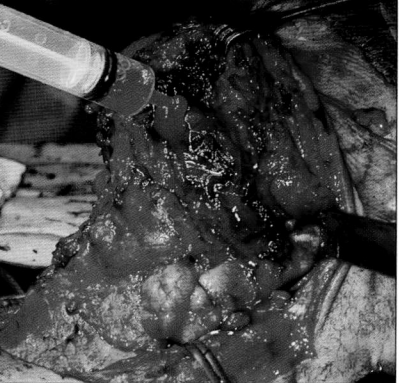

Fig 9-70d The AVH in the mandible was treated by enucleation of the endothelial lining and packed with Surgicel (Ethicon), Avitene (Davon), and PRP.

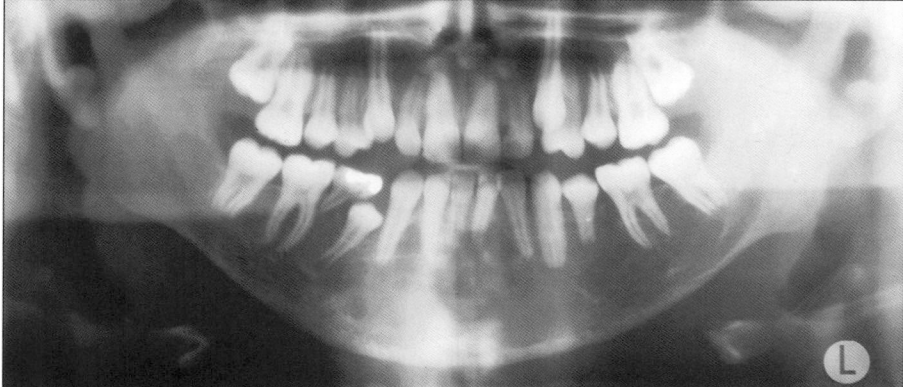

Fig 9-70e Preoperative radiograph showing a large AVH radiolucency extending from the left second molar area to the right canine area.

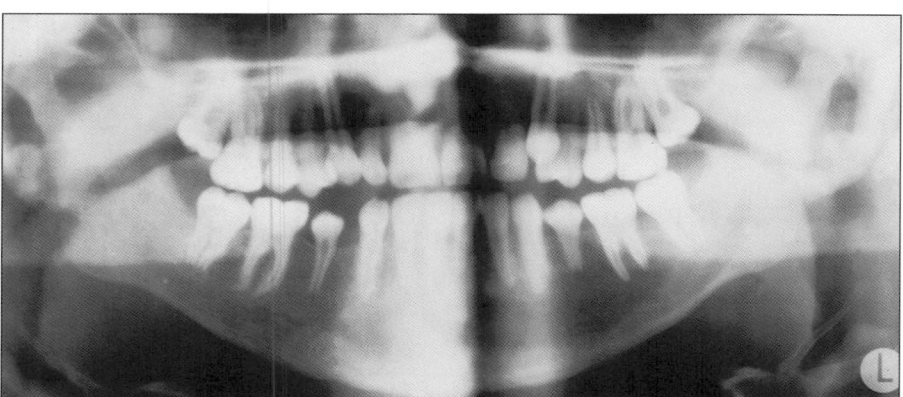

Fig 9-70f Bone regeneration into the defect can be seen within 4 months.

tissue surgical approach to the bone, and, as before, dilated vessels encountered in the soft tissue dissection are isolated and ligated as they appear (Figs 9-70a and 9-70b). This may amount to many vessels, but their removal will further reduce the blood flow to the vessels within bone (Fig 9-70c). In this approach the jaw is not resected, but with the external carotids temporarily clamped and hypotensive anesthesia achieved, the lateral cortex is quickly removed and the endothelial lining of the AVH quickly curetted. The bony cavity is then packed with Surgicel (Ethicon), Avitene (Davol), and platelet-rich plasma (PRP) (Fig 9-70d). A dense compaction of the Surgicel has been effective in stopping any residual AVH bleeding. To date, this approach has shown bone regeneration in the defect without a return of the AVH in bone (Figs 9-70e and 9-70f). However, it is still a relatively new approach that is considered only in cases occuring in bone that have an accessible, single, large radiolucency. The theory supporting the effectiveness of this approach is the removal of the central AVH nidus, which literally sucks in blood from adjacent vessels via its negative pressure and recruits new feeders.

Some lesions in soft tissue may be unresectable. In particular, large lesions of the tongue may require total glossectomy in young adults, creating obvious swallowing, speech, and aspiration difficulties. Such "unresectable lesions" in soft tissue may be managed with serial embolizations, usually performed annually. A few lesions resolve completely after several embolizations; most persist but no longer continue to pose a bleeding threat; and a few others continue to develop new high-pressure vessels, leading to a risky resection or to eventual death.

PROGNOSIS ▶ Arteriovenous hemangiomas that are embolized and resected tend not to recur. Therefore, the focus of management is to embolize and resect those that are resectable and to manage the unresectable AVHs with serial embolizations. Those that undergo serial embolizations have about a 10% chance of resolution, a 60% chance of preventing progression and life-threatening bleeds, and a 30% chance of progressing to uncontrollable disease.

Management of Emergencies and Complications

The two most common AVH-related emergencies that the oral and maxillofacial specialist may need to manage are a life-threatening bleed and a rapid proliferation of the AVH that may obstruct the airway.

The emergency bleed is a time-honored scenario in oral and maxillofacial surgery education. It may start with a single extraction of a tooth that has its roots in an unrecognized AVH. The surprised practitioner is startled to see a rapid high-pressure bleeding (see Fig 9-69b). In the past, the clinician has been taught to replace the tooth in the socket with pressure. However, experience has found this maneuver to be inadequate, as rapid bleeding continues around the tooth. Instead, the socket should be directly packed with Surgicel or plain gauze and digital pressure should be applied until bleeding is stopped; afterward, a tie-over suture maintaining pressure on the packing material is placed using a nonresorbable suture. In the authors' experience, direct packing is universally effective, rendering other more dramatic hemorrhage control measures, such as external carotid ligation and panicked emergency embolizations, unnecessary. This approach is also effective when the patient develops a spontaneous bleed and is brought into the emergency room (Figs 9-71a and 9-71b). In each case, after packing has controlled the rapid bleeding (Fig 9-71c), fluid resuscitation is provided, O Rh negative blood is given, and blood is typed and cross-matched. There should be no reluctance to give O Rh negative blood in such urgent cases. This "universal donor" type of blood has an excellent track record, supported by the use of over a million units during the Vietnam War without a reaction. From this controlled situation, a diagnostic angiogram and initial embolization can be accomplished (Fig 9-71d).

A less common emergency is upper airway obstruction, usually caused by proliferation or expansion of the AVH. In particular, those that occur in the tongue often require emergency intubation or tracheostomy (Fig 9-72a). After an airway is secured, an attempt may be made to manage the AVH by embolization and surgery. However, a total glossectomy is not recommended because of the obvious speech, swallowing, and aspiration difficulties it would create. Therefore, radiotherapy, which would oth-

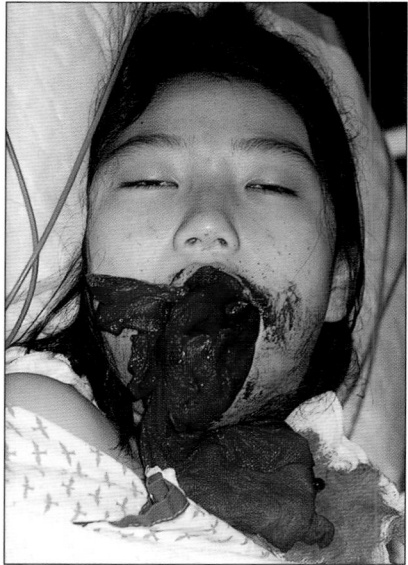

Fig 9-71a This young girl developed a spontaneous bleed at home from an AVH. She presented in hypovolemic shock with a hemoglobin of 6.8 mg/dL and a hematocrit of 17%.

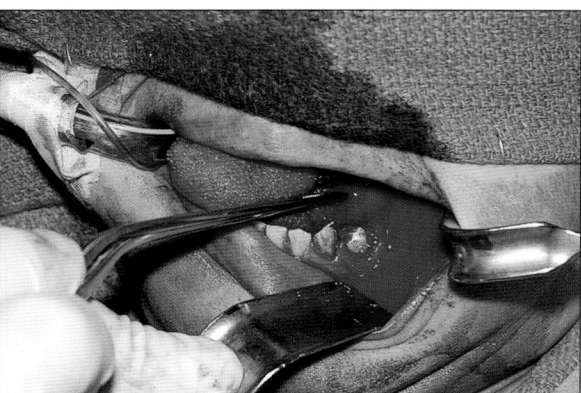

Fig 9-71b The source of the bleeding was an AVH that ruptured through the oral mucosa in the area of an exfoliating primary tooth.

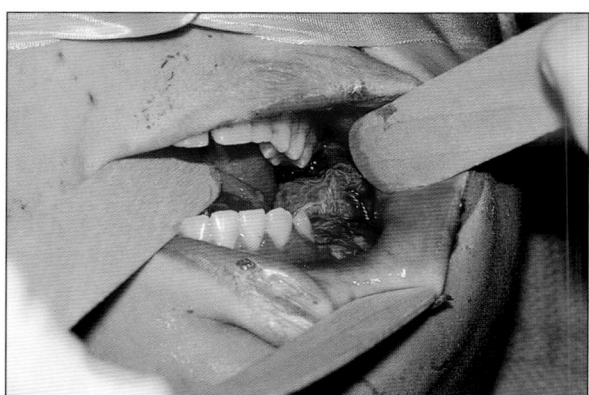

Fig 9-71c Removing the mobile teeth in the AVH and packing the defect stopped the bleeding without the need for external carotid ligations or emergency embolization. Here the pack is being removed after a planned selective embolization.

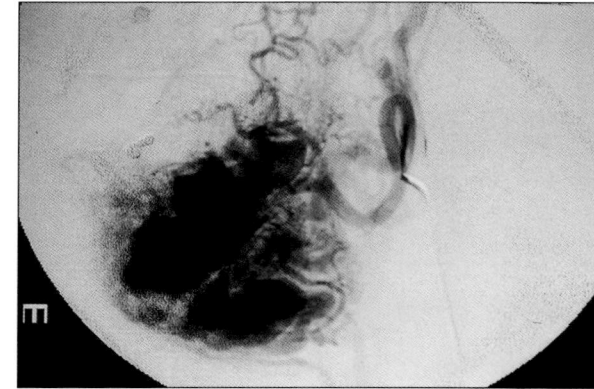

Fig 9-71d Some AVH angiograms, like the one involved in the emergency bleed, will have dramatically large vascular spaces. The bleeding point frequently represents only the "tip of the iceberg."

erwise not be a strong consideration because of the potential for sarcoma transformation, is used in this rare situation. A dose of up to 6,000 cGy will induce a fibrosis and physical shrinkage of the AVH, restoring the airway and allowing discontinuation of the tracheostomy (Figs 9-72b and 9-72c).

Another complication that the oral and maxillofacial specialist must keep in mind is high-output cardiac failure. Even many young patients will have demonstrable cardiomegaly due to the increased blood volume within the AVH (Fig 9-73). This should decrease somewhat with embolization and surgery and is another indication for treating the AVH directly.

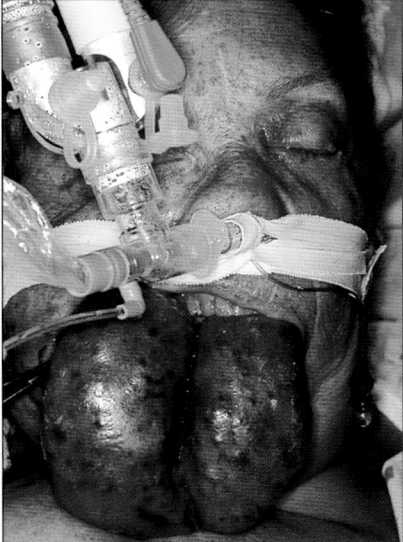

Fig 9-72a This AVH of the tongue proliferated rapidly for no obvious reason and obstructed the airway, necessitating an emergency intubation that was then converted into a tracheostomy. (Courtesy of Dr James Ruskin.)

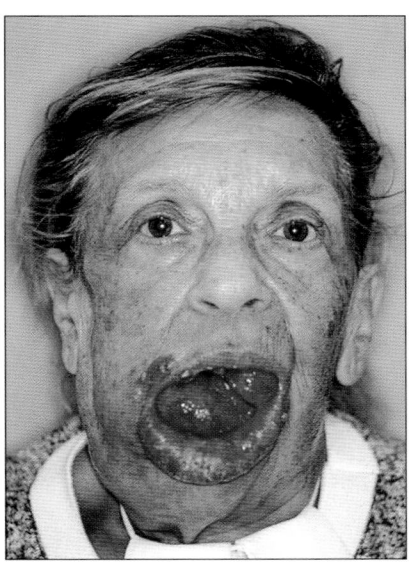

Fig 9-72b After 6 weeks of radiotherapy (6,000 cGy), the tongue and lip have significantly decreased in size and are beginning to become fibrous. (Courtesy of Dr James Ruskin.)

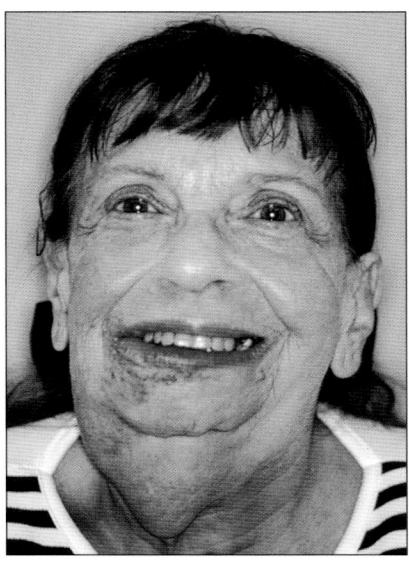

Fig 9-72c After 6 months, the fibrosis induced by the radiotherapy has further reduced the size of the tongue and lower lip, allowing removal of the tracheostomy and a return of contours and tongue position. (Courtesy of Dr James Ruskin.)

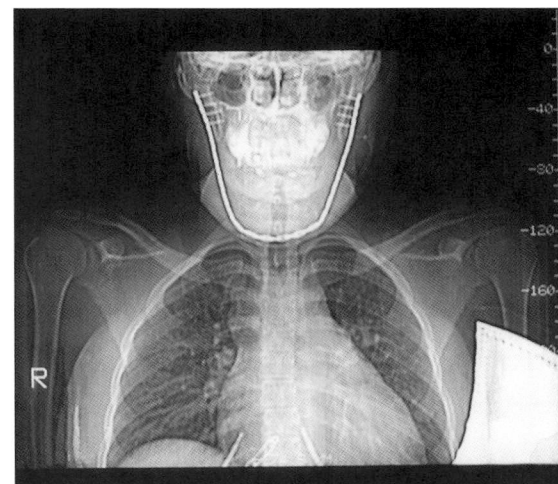

Fig 9-73 A large AVH of the mandible that was present for over 8 years was resected and the mandible replaced with a titanium reconstruction plate. Note the obvious cardiomegaly as a result of the increased vascular volume, which improved after the resection.

Juvenile Capillary Hemangioma

CLINICAL PRESENTATION AND PATHOGENESIS ▶

Juvenile capillary hemangiomas are distinctive lesions that commonly occur in the superficial skin area of the chin (Fig 9-74) and upper neck and slightly less commonly occur in the parotid area. The lesion appears as a red-blue multinodular mass with a thin overlying skin. Although painless, it may ulcerate if the thin overlying skin is ruptured. It is much more common in young girls than in boys, and it is not rare, occurring in 1 of every 200 live births.

The lesion may be described by the parents or obstetrician as congenital, but it usually becomes apparent about 2 to 6 weeks after birth and then rapidly enlarges to its maximum size (usually 4 to 8 cm) by 6 to 9 months of age. Most will then remain static for 2 to 6 months before undergoing a slow but steady involution. As the lesion regresses, it loses its red to violaceous color and takes on a pale appearance. As it involutes it leaves an irregular, almost wrinkled-looking skin surface. By the age of 7 years, 75% to 90% of the lesion will have involuted. Because the involutional process is one of interstitial and vessel fibrosis, it leaves behind a firm, fibrotic, multinodular texture.

This classic appearance and evolution have given this lesion the designation *strawberry nevus*. Nonetheless, this hemangioma is a vascular malformation of a series of abnormal vessels fed by a single normal arteriole and therefore is not under abnormally high pressure and does not pose a bleeding threat.

DIAGNOSTIC WORK-UP ▶

The juvenile capillary hemangioma is a clinically distinctive entity diagnosed by its appearance and history. No known diagnostic studies will add useful information. An angiogram is not indicated.

HISTOPATHOLOGY ▶

Hemangiomas may be classified as either capillary or cavernous; however, both types consist of proliferative vascular channels that are lined by endothelium and lack a muscular coat. Erythrocytes are in the lumen. The arrangement is often lobular, since capillaries proliferate around a feeder vessel. Capillary hemangiomas may initially be extremely cellular lesions composed of endothelial cells and poorly canalized vessels. Mitoses may be present. In early stages, these have been called juvenile hemangiomas (Figs

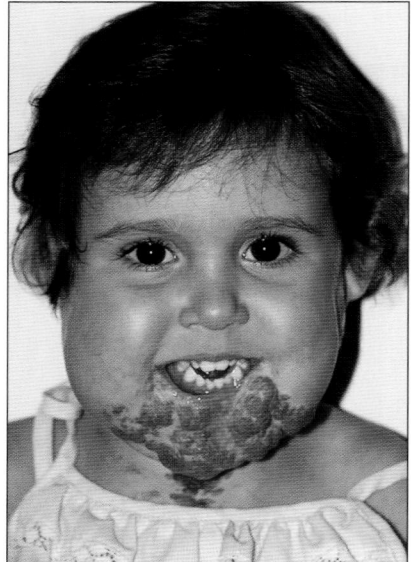

Fig 9-74 Juvenile capillary hemangiomas have a red-blue multinodular appearance. Occurrence in the lower lip-chin area at or shortly after birth is a common presentation.

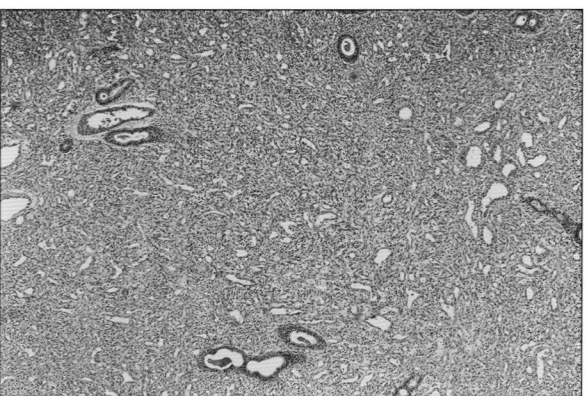

Fig 9-75a Juvenile hemangioma of the parotid. Some residual ducts can be seen within the very cellular hemangioma.

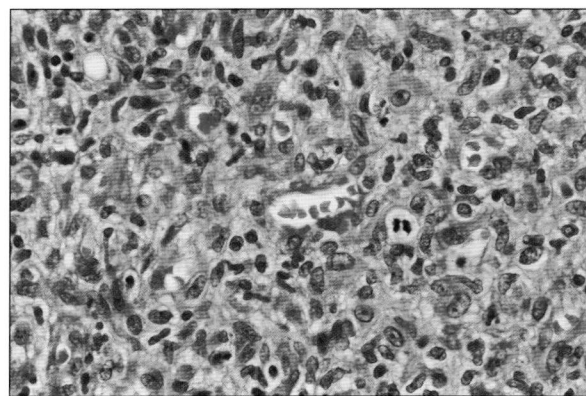

Fig 9-75b High-power view of Fig 9-75a showing the cellularity and rather sparse canalization of these tumors. Mitotic activity also can be seen.

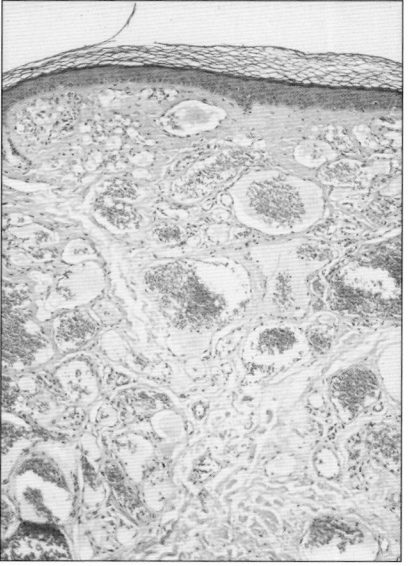

Fig 9-75c Capillary hemangioma consisting of numerous endothelially lined, blood-filled channels supported by scant blood-filled channels.

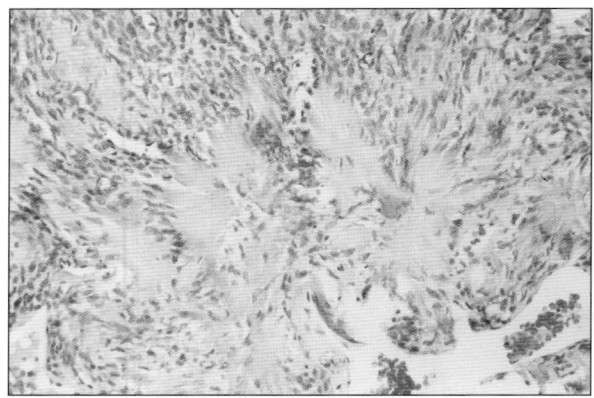

Fig 9-75d Hemangioma showing fibrosis.

9-75a and 9-75b). Mast cells, which may be a source of angiogenic factors, can be seen. As these lesions mature, the vessels are canalized, and the endothelial cells flatten to form the typical capillary hemangioma (Fig 9-75c). When they undergo regression it is through interstitial fibrosis (Fig 9-75d).

TREATMENT AND PROGNOSIS ▶

The best therapy in most cases is time and the avoidance of overaggressive therapy during the hemangioma's active growth phase. Parental education and reassurance about involution are of great value. In addition, it is reasonable to prepare parents for cosmetic/reconstructive surgery, which may be required in later years (ages 8 to 12 years).

Although cryosurgery, sclerosing agents, and surgical excision have all been used, these methods often create more scarring and disfigurement than the lesion itself or its involution. Irradiation also once was used, but today it is not advised because of its possible carcinogenic effects and its scarring and drying effects on skin. Systemic prednisone is a valid and commonly used therapy today. A dose of 1 mg/kg per day at 2-week intervals (interrupted by 2-week intervals) for 3 months at a time will hasten involution and is associated with few side effects or complications.

A more recent alternative therapy for certain juvenile capillary hemangiomas has been developed in the laboratory of Judah Folkman at Boston Children's Hospital. His discovery that interferon alpha 2a is anti-angiogenic has already led to its use in the treatment of Kaposi sarcoma and to ongoing studies of its use in treating hemangiomas. For example, it is used in large and unresponsive hemangiomas, especially in patients who demonstrate increased levels of basic fibroblast growth factor (bFGF) in a 24-hour urine collection. Increased levels of bFGF, which stimulates angiogenesis, is a marker for response to interferon alpha 2a, and the use of interferon alpha 2a, in turn, is predicated on its action to downregulate bFGF, which is overexpressed by certain hemangiomas. Its use in selected hemangiomas is not universal but offers a nonsurgical treatment approach that is less prone to complications. Dosages vary according to the patient and the size of the hemangioma but range from 1 million to 4 million U per day for an indeterminate time.

When natural involution is complete, the residual nodular, irregular skin surface may be improved, requiring only makeup or dermabrasion. However, more severe cases may require excision and advancement of local flaps, which are preferred over distant pedicled or free vascular flaps to match skin thickness and color. If the excised skin surface area is large, it is reasonable to consider placement of a tissue expander adjacent to the area so that the expanded local skin can be rotated or advanced to cover the defect without stretching it or creating tension at the site of closure.

Cavernous Hemangioma

CLINICAL PRESENTATION AND PATHOGENESIS ►

Cavernous hemangiomas are less common than juvenile capillary hemangiomas in all areas of the body except the oral cavity. Like juvenile capillary hemangiomas, they occur most frequently at or just after birth. Cavernous hemangiomas differ from capillary hemangiomas in that they are larger, more diffuse, usually located somewhat deeper, and only partially involute. Therefore, they persist into adult life unchanged or somewhat fibrosed.

The classic presentation is a soft, diffuse, puffy mass in the parotid (Figs 9-76a and 9-76b) and in the skin over the parotid region as well as within bone, mostly in the posterior mandible (Fig 9-77a). They may also present as a large, soft, blue-red, painless blanching mass in the oral mucosa (Fig 9-77b). Soft tissue cavernous hemangiomas will often produce a cupped-out type of resorption of the bony cortex (Figs 9-77c and 9-77d). Although these lesions do not undergo involution, they develop calcifications via phlebolith formation (Fig 9-77e). These dystrophic calcifications in organized thrombi are often first seen on a radiograph. Those that occur in the parotid region are well-known to show multiple small, round radiodensities superimposed over the ramus and posterior body (Fig 9-77f).

Less commonly, cavernous hemangiomas will occur centrally within bone. They will usually cause a painless expansion and a mixed radiolucent-radiopaque appearance due to their stimulation of reactive bone (Fig 9-78). Like their soft tissue counterparts, their blood-filled spaces are not under high pressure and therefore do not pose a significant bleeding threat.

DIFFERENTIAL DIAGNOSIS ►

Because of their deep location, the red-blue vascular nature of cavernous hemangiomas is less apparent and therefore initially may not be correctly recognized. *Lymphangiomas* can bear a strong resemblance to cavernous hemangiomas because they too are soft and diffuse and can impart a red-blue appearance by virtue of their hemangiomatous components, some blood in their abnormal lymphatic spaces, and the bluish color of lymph when viewed through skin. *Neurofibromas* and *lipomas* will also clin-

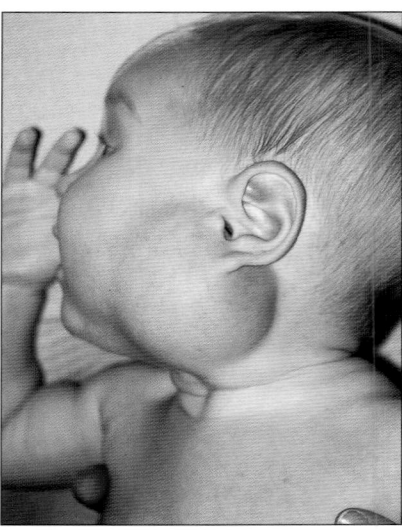

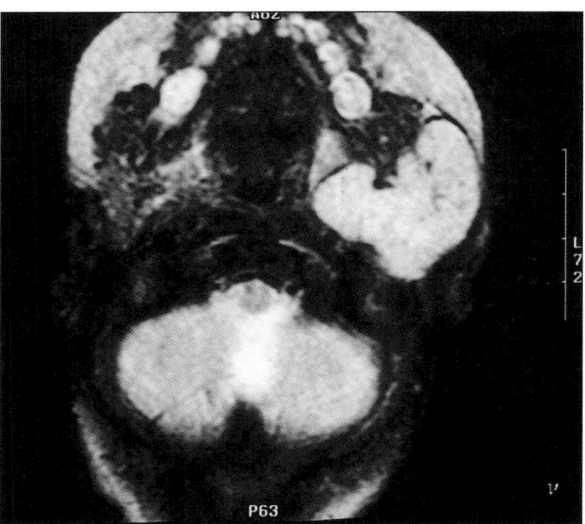

Fig 9-76a One presentation of a cavernous hemangioma is within the parotid in an infant. Here the mass outlines the parotid gland and has a slightly blue color.

Fig 9-76b An MRI scan of the hemangioma shown in Fig 9-76a reveals the distinct outline of the parotid capsule within which it is located.

ically have a soft, diffuse, and irregular quality to their presentation, mimicking that of a soft tissue cavernous hemangioma.

Cavernous hemangiomas centrally located in bone will mostly resemble fibro-osseous disease or bone tumors. They will produce a radiographic appearance most similar to an *ossifying fibroma* or an *osteoblastoma* (see Fig 9-78). In the jaws, some may be confused with a *developing odontoma*, a *calcifying odontogenic cyst*, or a *calcifying epithelial odontogenic tumor*.

DIAGNOSTIC WORK-UP ►

A cavernous hemangioma may require no specific work-up if the lesion is clinically apparent and/or it radiographically demonstrates phleboliths. If there is a suspicion that the lesion represents an arteriovenous hemangioma (also called an arteriovenous malformation), it should be palpated to detect a possible thrill and auscultated for a possible bruit. Although auscultation with a stethoscope is the standard, a more precise auscultation can be accomplished with a Doppler unit and is highly recommended. If bruits are heard by either examination, a diagnostic angiogram is required.

HISTOPATHOLOGY ►

Cavernous hemangiomas are less circumscribed than capillary hemangiomas and have dilated vascular channels with flattened endothelium. Calcifications and formation of phleboliths occur through dystrophic calcification of organizing thrombi, but regression does not occur (Figs 9-79a to 9-79c).

TREATMENT AND PROGNOSIS ►

Cavernous hemangiomas in soft tissue usually require some type of treatment because of their impingement on adjacent structures. Because these lesions are not true neoplasms with continual growth, they do not necessarily require complete removal or wide margins. The goal of therapy is alleviation of their impingement on native structures or their interference with function. Therefore, if they are accessible, soft tissue cavernous hemangiomas should be completely excised if feasible (Fig 9-80). They do not pose a severe bleeding potential and can be managed in many cases by a peripheral resection around their edges (Figs 9-81a to 9-81h; see also Fig 9-78). If the lesion is so large that the excisional wound is unmanageable or major reconstructive surgery would be required, ablation with cryosurgery or laser surgery offers some distinct advantages if performed by experienced practitioners. Sclerosing therapy is less desirable than either excision, cryosurgery, or laser surgery, but it has been used in the past. Sclerosing agents, such as sodium morrhuate, sodium psyllate, or a slurry of 250 mg tetracycline in 5 mL of saline, are useful in inducing fibrosis in most cavernous hemangiomas. However, repeated injections are required, and unpredictable outcomes (from minimal effect on the hemangioma to overfibrosis of the tissues) are common.

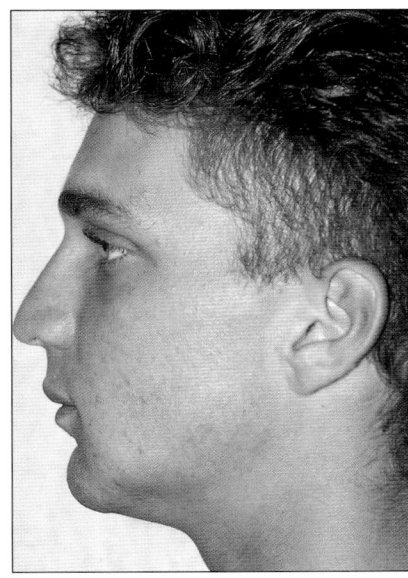

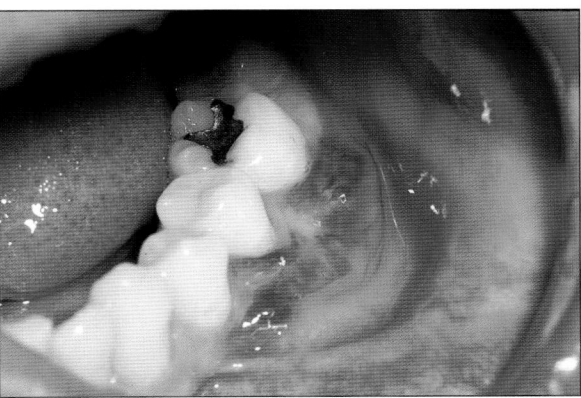

Fig 9-77b A residual cavernous hemangioma in the vestibule and gingiva may create an occasional bleeding episode but will not result in significant blood loss.

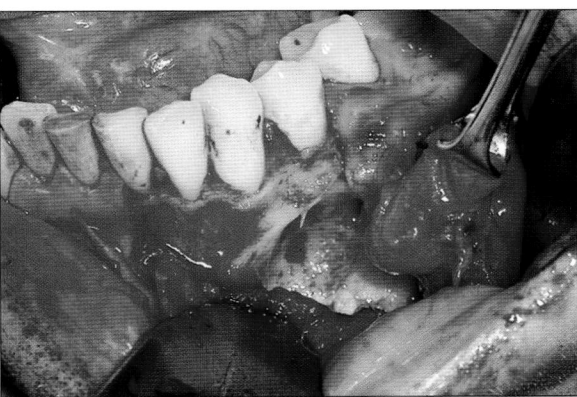

Fig 9-77c Removal of this cavernous hemangioma in the vestibule revealed a cortical defect in the mandible that was caused not by the pressure of the tumor mass but rather by mandibular growth around the mass, which had been present during the growth years.

Fig 9-77a This congenital hemangioma of the parotid and surrounding tissues has undergone significant involution with only a residual increased tissue thickness and bluish color in this 20-year-old individual.

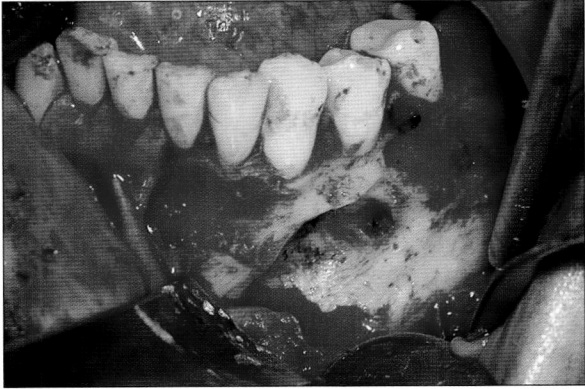

Fig 9-77d Cupped-out resorption of the buccal cortex indicative of the long-standing nature of this hemangioma.

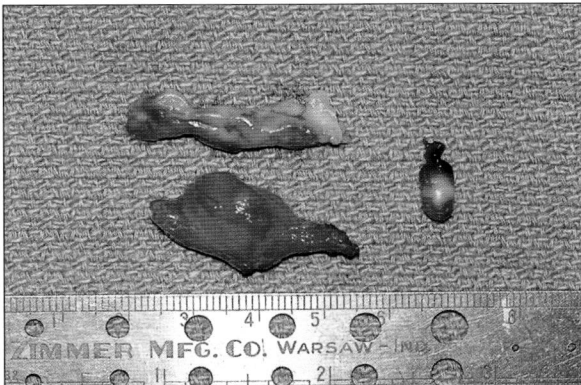

Fig 9-77e Specimens of an excised soft tissue cavernous hemangioma are firm because of fibrosis and may contain an oblong-shaped phlebolith with a smooth surface.

Fig 9-77f Radiopacities over the ramus and below the inferior border in this 20-year-old patient represent phleboliths within a congenital cavernous hemangioma of the parotid and adjacent tissues. The phleboliths develop as calcified thrombi from entrapped blood or within low-flow vessels.

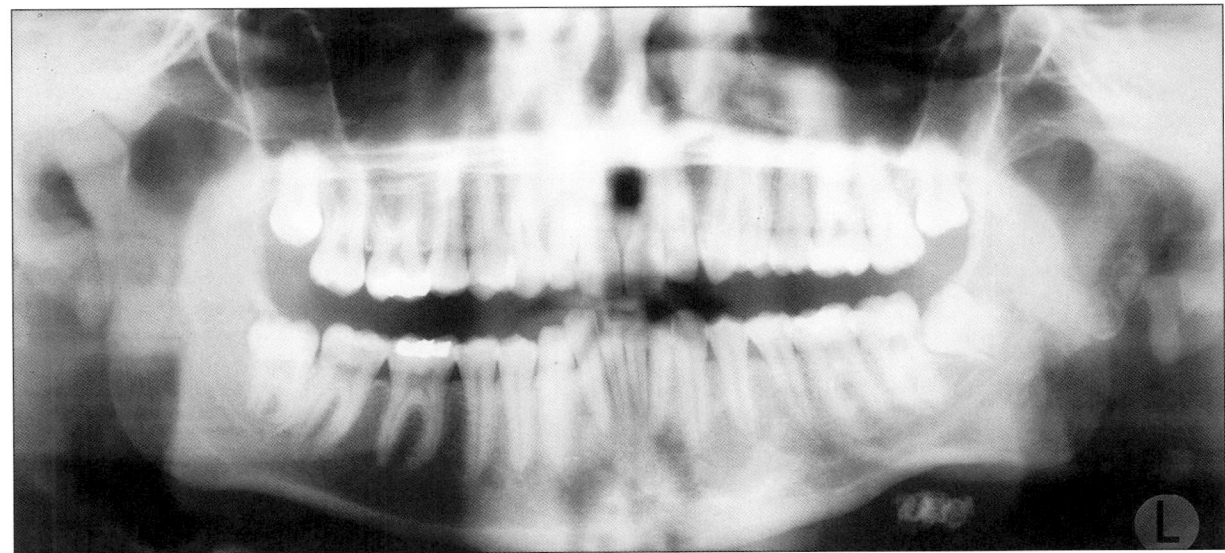

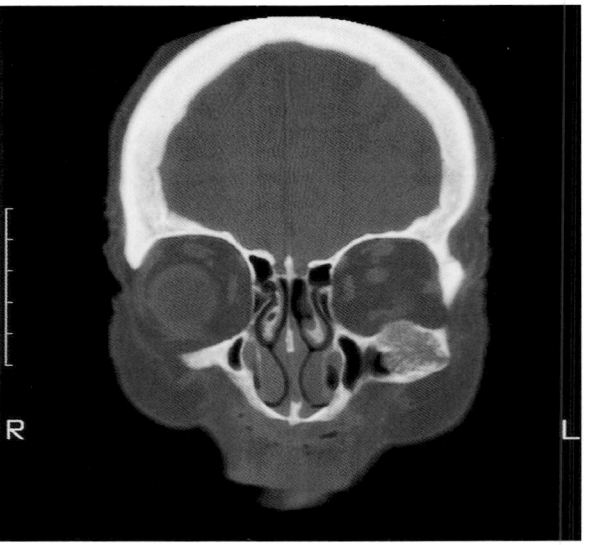

Fig 9-78 A central cavernous hemangioma will stimulate a thickening of its internal trabecular bone and thus will appear as a radiopacity. Consequently, it is often confused with and included with ossifying fibromas and osteoblastomas in differential diagnoses.

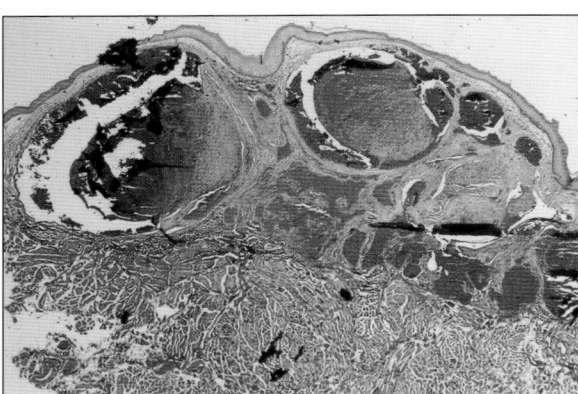

Fig 9-79a Hemangioma showing organizing thrombi within the superficial vessels.

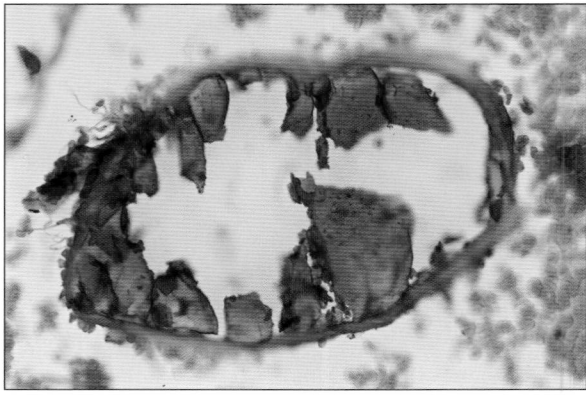

Fig 9-79b If calcification occurs within these areas, a phlebolith is formed. This will show up as a radiopacity within soft tissue.

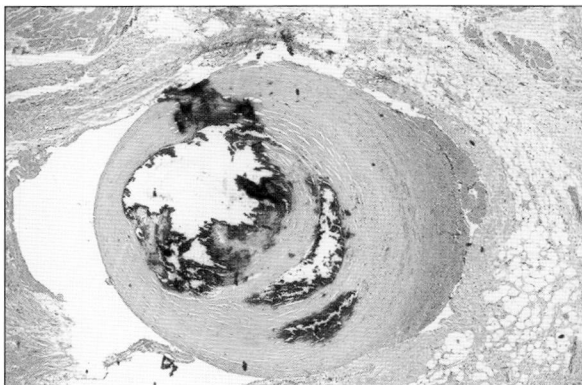

Fig 9-79c Mature phleboliths will show a layering effect due to successive depositions of dystrophic calcifications into concentric rings.

Cavernous hemangiomas in bone will be very well demarcated and somewhat radiopaque. They will resemble the radiographic picture of an ossifying fibroma or an osteoblastoma and are treated in much the same way with a peripheral resection using 2- to 3-mm margins. Since the tumor itself contains lined vessels that are dilated and thinned, the perfusion may produce some extracortical bone formations, giving it a so-called sun ray appearance. The tumor does not pose a significant bleeding threat because of the absence of high-pressure or high-flow rates. Therefore, the resection may be accomplished with saws and osteotomes as needed. When the bone graft can be placed into a contamination-free tissue bed and immobilized, the graft can be done immediately; otherwise the graft should be staged for 3 to 4 months.

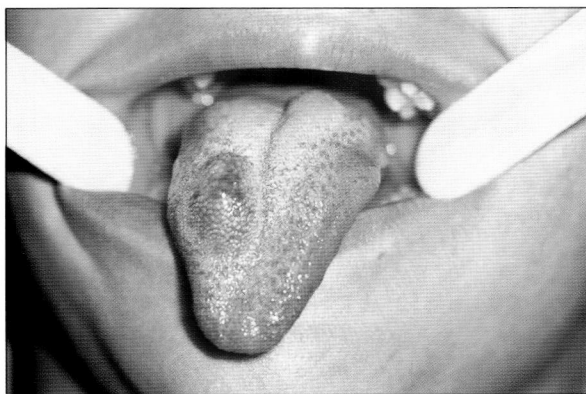

Fig 9-80 A cavernous hemangioma in the tongue is a low-flow hemangioma and therefore not a significant bleeding risk. Before excision, however, the clinician should use a Doppler or angiography to rule out an arteriovenous hemangioma, which is a significant bleeding risk.

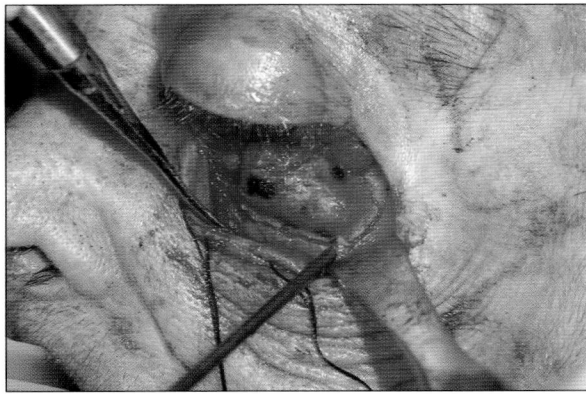

Fig 9-81a Resection of the central cavernous hemangioma of the orbital floor and infra-orbital rim shown in Fig 9-78 needs only 2-mm peripheral margins.

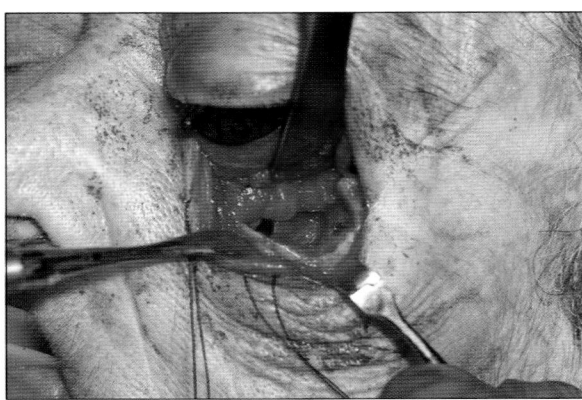

Fig 9-81b Resultant defect of infraorbital rim and orbital floor resection.

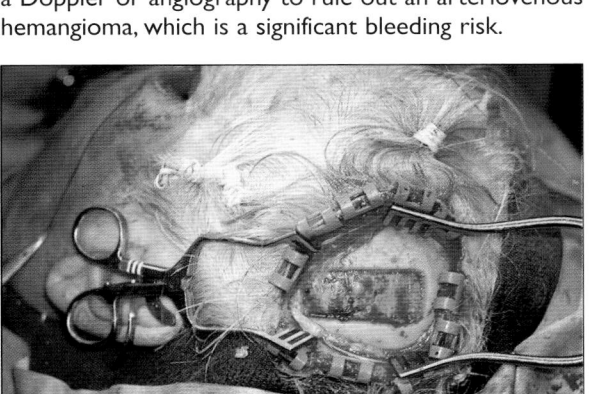

Fig 9-81c Defects of the orbital area are ideally reconstructed with split-thickness cranial bone grafts.

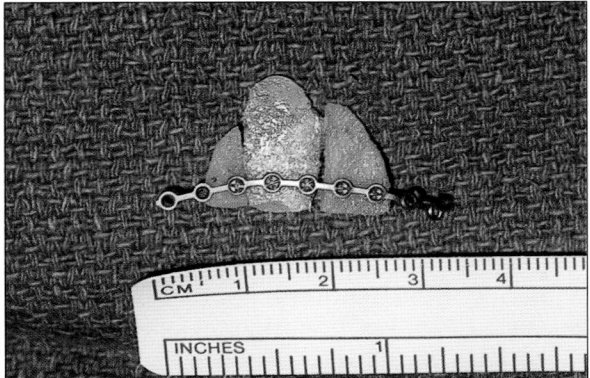

Fig 9-81d Cranial bone graft shaped and fashioned to reconstruct the orbital floor.

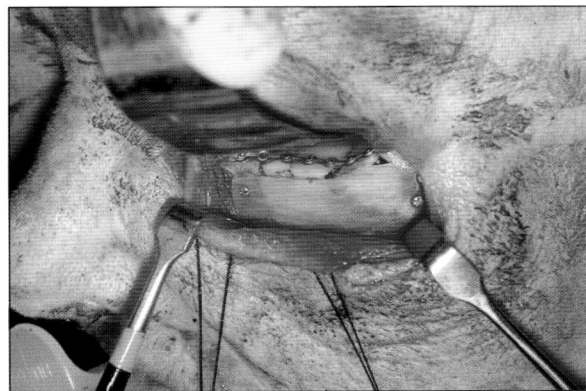

Fig 9-81e Cranial bone graft used to reconstruct the orbital floor here is overlaid with a second cranial bone graft to reconstruct the infraorbital rim and anterior maxillary cortex.

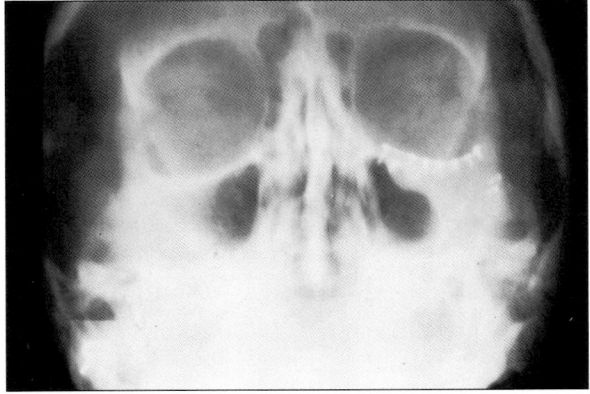

Fig 9-81f Three-year follow-up Waters radiograph shows an excellent orbital size and contour.

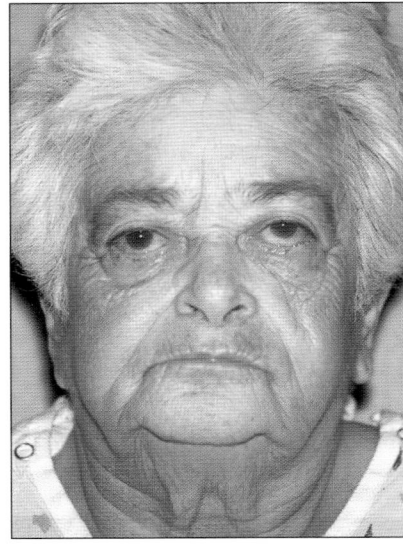

Fig 9-81g Elevation of the left globe by this tumor had produced significant diplopia.

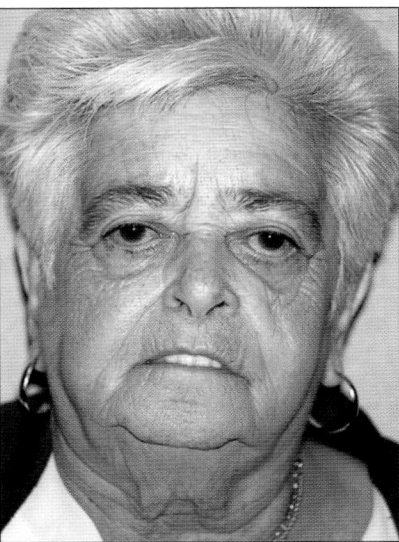

Fig 9-81h After resection of the tumor and immediate orbital floor reconstruction, the globe position returned to normal and the diplopia resolved.

Syndromes Associated with Cavernous Hemangiomas

There is one complication associated with cavernous hemangiomas that is often referred to as a specific syndrome (Kasabach-Merritt syndrome) and two bona fide syndromes (Maffucci and blue rubber bleb nevus syndromes).

Kasabach-Merritt Syndrome

In this syndrome, a large cavernous or arteriovenous hemangioma is complicated by thrombocytopenic purpura. It is believed that the many tortuous and cavernous vascular spaces in some very large hemangiomas undergo intravascular coagulation and, in the process, consume platelets. The result is thrombocytopenia and the development of cutaneous and mucosal petechiae and ecchymosis. The parent hemangioma also increases in size, and internal bleeding may occur.

This syndrome occurs mostly in infants but has been known to occur in adults. In either it will pose a life-threatening situation and is associated with a 30% mortality rate due to exsanguination or secondary infection from attempts to treat the bleeding. In most cases, surgery is impossible because of the size of the hemangioma and the patient's compromised hematologic profile. Therefore, most are treated as a hemorrhagic emergency with anticoagulation (heparin) for what amounts to a type of diffuse intravascular coagulation, along with systemic corticosteroids (methylprednisone [Solu-Medrol], 1.5 mg/kg every 6 hours). Although radiotherapy is not usually advised for uncomplicated hemangiomas, this situation represents such a serious complication that radiotherapy is sometimes used. Radiotherapy will predictably reduce the size of the hemangioma and the extent of the coagulopathy. Such large, unresectable hemangiomas that produce the Kasabach-Merritt syndrome and the uncontrolled expanding arteriovenous hemangiomas are the two rare indications for radiotherapy.

Maffucci Syndrome

Maffucci syndrome is characterized by multiple hemangiomas and enchondromas. The cavernous hemangiomas are present at birth, whereas the enchondromas develop a few years later. Although the hemangiomas do not pose a threat or create significant deformities, the enchondromas usually do. These cartilaginous tumors develop from a defect in endochondral ossification and are the result of a marked but disorganized overgrowth in the cartilage growth plate. They produce a shortened club-shaped bone, usually in the hand. The involved bones, which usually have multiple enchondromas and bony exostoses, undergo frequent pathologic fractures, and one or more of the enchondromas undergoes malignant transformation into a chondrosarcoma in 20% of patients. Histopathologically, these are cavernous hemangiomas with large, irregular, endothelially lined spaces containing erythrocytes. The vascular spaces may be poorly defined.

Blue Rubber Bleb Nevus Syndrome

This rare syndrome, an autosomal-dominant trait, produces a peculiar blue hemangioma that has the appearance and texture of a rubber nipple or rubber skin (Fig 9-82). Identical lesions appear in various locations in the gastrointestinal tract, primarily the small intestines. The skin hemangiomas characteristically respond to pressure, leaving a flat, wrinkled surface that regains its shape and appearance after the removal of pressure. The intestinal lesions are often associated with bleeding and will produce a chronic iron-deficiency anemia. Therefore, therapy is focused on gastroscopic excision of bleeding intestinal lesions. Histopathologically these are cavernous hemangiomas, but they may also have small lumina, and the walls of the superficial vascular spaces may abut the overlying epithelium.

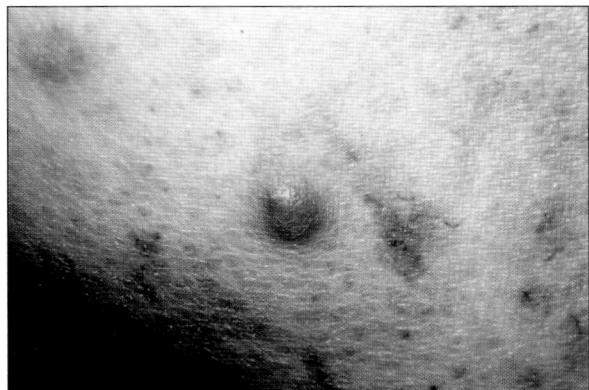

Fig 9-82 This semi-firm blue nodule has the texture of rubber and is part of the rare autosomal-dominant trait of blue rubber bleb nevus syndrome.

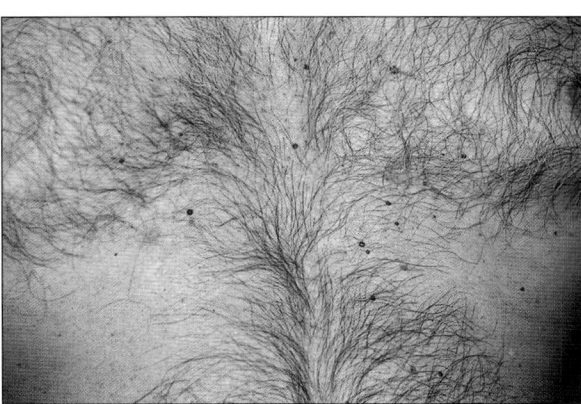

Fig 9-83a Cherry hemangiomas are genetically predetermined, superficial capillary proliferations that first manifest at about the age of 35 to 40 years and become more prominent thereafter.

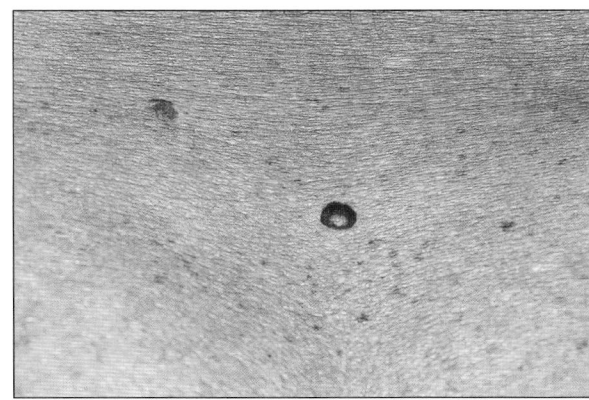

Fig 9-83b Cherry hemangiomas remain small (less than 5 mm in diameter), do not pose a bleeding threat despite their superficial location, and are not known to transform into a malignancy.

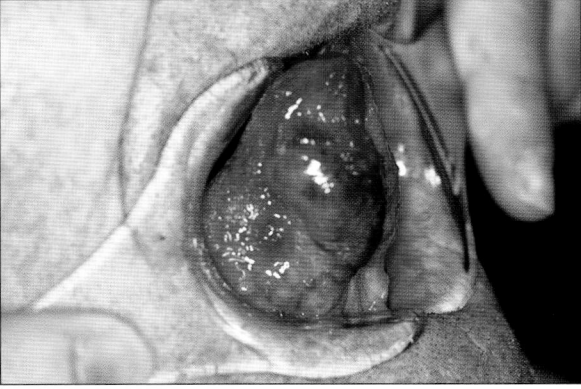

Fig 9-84 Dilated vein on the ventral surface of the tongue represents a varix rather than a true hemangioma.

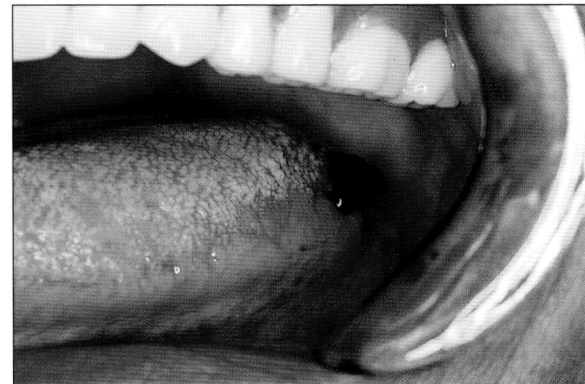

Fig 9-85 This varix of the lingual tonsil merely represents a dilated, blood-filled vein that does not pose a significant bleeding threat.

Cherry Hemangiomas

Cherry hemangiomas, also known as *Campbell de Morgan spots* or "senile" angiomas, are small (0.1 to 1.0 cm), superficial red papules that appear on the skin of the chest, back, and sometimes the extremities (Figs 9-83a and 9-83b). Unlike most capillary hemangiomas, which appear in infancy and childhood, they usually first appear in adults at age 35 to 40 years and reach their maximum number by age 50. They are innocuous, pose no bleeding threat, and have no known transformation into a malignancy.

Histopathologically, these lesions initially are like capillary hemangiomas, with proliferating capillaries that have prominent endothelial lining and small lumina. As the lesions age, however, the capillaries dilate and the endothelial cells flatten. The overlying epithelium is attenuated.

Varix

A varix is merely a dilated vein (Fig 9-84). It is clinically recognizable and may be left as is or ligated and excised if it is symptomatic (Fig 9-85).

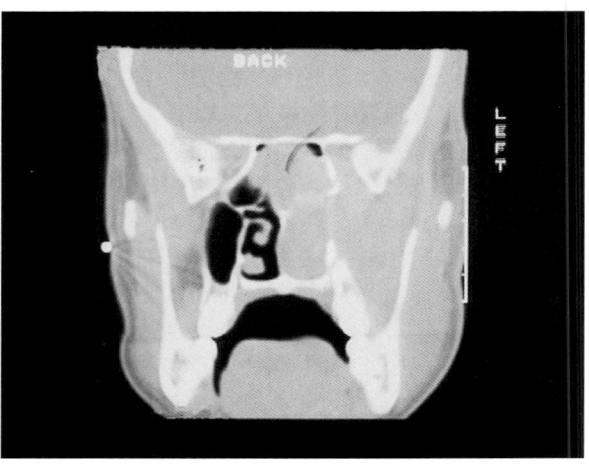

Fig 9-86 Some nasopharyngeal angiofibromas will extend into the maxillary sinus and orbit and may produce diplopia.

Nasopharyngeal Angiofibroma

Nasopharyngeal angiofibromas are benign tumors that are life threatening because of their vascularity and location. The tumor develops almost exclusively in adolescent boys.

It will present with the patient complaining of progressive nasal obstruction over the past 1 to 2 years and episodes of epistaxis. Some of the bouts of epistaxis will be prolonged and severe because the small vessels within the lesion lack vasoconstrictive capacities. A nasal speculum examination or a transoral mirror examination will usually identify a red-blue polypoid mass, which may protrude into the pharynx or into the anterior nasal cavity. The tumor does not cause pain, but its size and erosion into adjacent structures will produce a variety of signs. Orbital invasion will often cause protrusion of the globe and visual changes, particularly diplopia (Fig 9-86). Obstruction of the eustachian tube often creates a secondary otitis media, and obstruction of sinus drainage may cause sinusitis in any of the paranasal sinuses.

The nasopharyngeal angiofibroma represents a benign but true neoplasm as evidenced by its continued growth and recurrence if incompletely excised. Its bleeding nature is due not only to its vascular density, but also to a thin or absent smooth muscle component and the lack of an elastic membrane within the vessel wall. Because of these missing elements, the vessels cannot vasoconstrict or form a platelet plug, which is the first phase of hemostasis.

The clinical presentation of a nasopharyngeal angiofibroma is very distinctive. Occasionally, a *vascular nasal polyp* will produce a mass-related epistaxis, or an *allergic rhinitis* will produce swollen bleeding nasal membranes, which may be mistaken for a nasopharyngeal angiofibroma. *Vascular malformations* and *hemangiomas* are other clinical possibilities.

A CT scan is essential for assessing the extent and location of this tumor. Because the clinical presentation and male predominance are so specific, an incisional biopsy, which may produce profuse bleeding, is often deferred if the CT scan is consistent with a nasopharyngeal angiofibroma. In some cases, a diagnostic angiogram is useful, but usually this procedure is also deferred until just before surgery and includes embolization (Figs 9-87a to 9-87c).

The treatment goal is to accomplish a complete excision with wide access and minimal blood loss. An angiogram is performed 1 to 3 days before surgery. The angiofibroma is embolized, usually with PVA beads, alcohol, or other particulate materials. The surgical access is through a Le Fort I down-fractured maxilla and nasal mucosal incision. The embolized tumor bleeds much less, and the wide access provided by the Le Fort I approach allows for a more complete excision (Figs 9-87d to 9-87f). The down-fractured maxilla is returned to its original position as defined by the dental occlusion and the indexing of rigid fix-

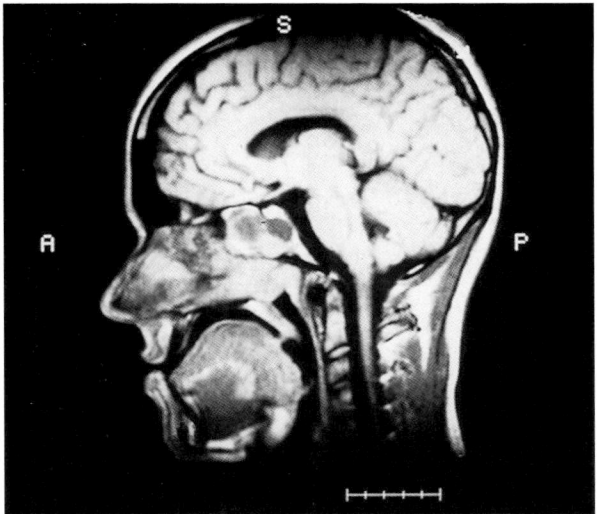

Fig 9-87a Nasopharyngeal angiofibroma extending to the crista gali and base of the skull.

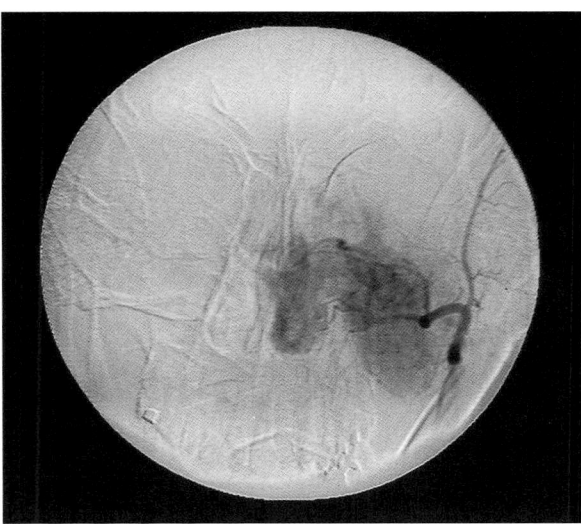

Fig 9-87b A pre-embolization angiogram of a nasopharyngeal angiofibroma will show only one or two discrete normal feeding vessels and an intrinsically vascular tumor.

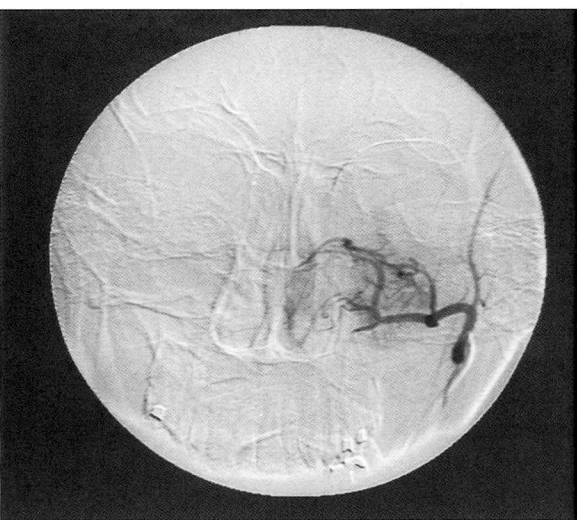

Fig 9-87c A postembolization angiogram of the same nasopharyngeal angiofibroma shows a reduction in the internal vasculature of the tumor and a retention of the larger normal vessels.

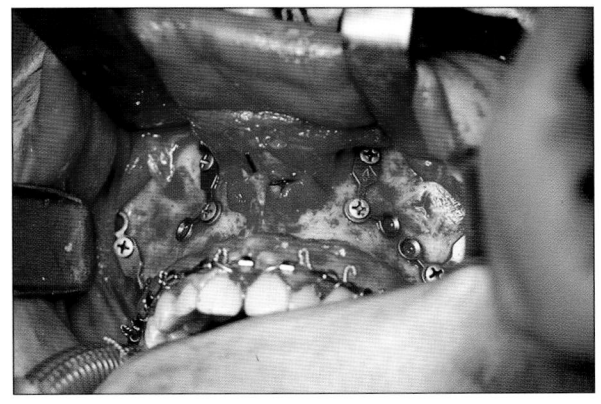

Fig 9-87d The Le Fort I down-fracture access to a nasopharyngeal angiofibroma is preceded by plate placement to index the position of the maxilla.

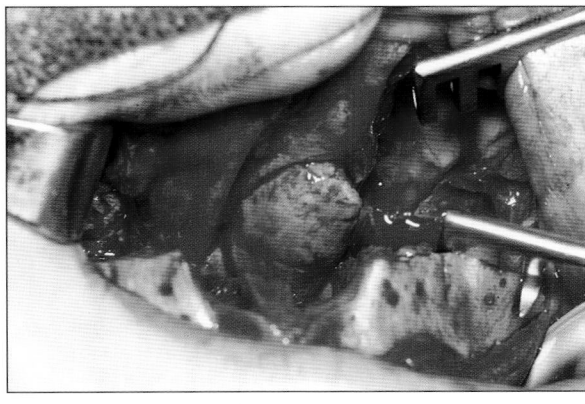

Fig 9-87e The Le Fort I down-fracture provides the most direct access to a nasopharyngeal angiofibroma. Combined with preoperative embolization, the access provided by the Le Fort I approach greatly reduces the blood loss during removal.

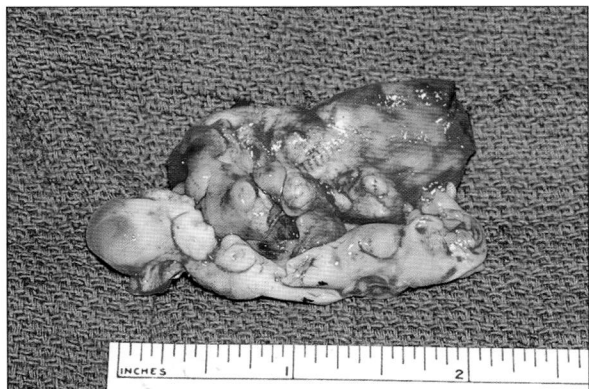

Fig 9-87f A nasopharyngeal angiofibroma is a firm multinodular mass with a thin capsule.

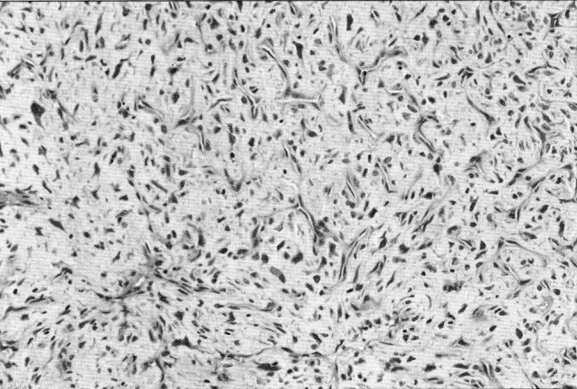

Fig 9-87g A nasopharyngeal angiofibroma with numerous slit-like capillaries.

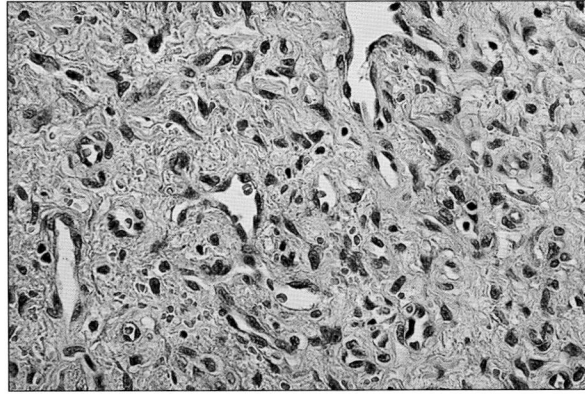

Fig 9-87h This nasopharyngeal angiofibroma shows dilated, angulated capillaries.

HISTOPATHOLOGY ▶

ation plates on the maxillary cortex prior to the Le Fort I osteotomy. It is then rigidly fixated so that the patient can return to function without requiring maxillomandibular fixation.

Histologically, these firm, rubbery, lobulated masses are fibrovascular. The stromal collagen fibers are often in parallel arrangement, and there may be areas of hyalinization and myxoid degeneration. The vessels may be slit-like (Fig 9-87g), but they are characteristically angulated or staghorn in shape (Fig 9-87h). They have a normal endothelial lining but lack elastic fibers, and smooth muscle is sparse or absent. Mast cells are prominent.

PROGNOSIS ▶

Use of the Le Fort I approach has caused a dramatic reduction in the intraoperative blood loss and the recurrence rate of nasopharyngeal angiofibromas. Recurrence rates with the older transnasal approach were around 40% to 60% because of incomplete excision. Recurrence with the Le Fort I approach is 5% to 8% because of higher rates of complete removal.

Because of high recurrence rates in the past, many cases were treated with radiotherapy, which relieved bleeding and nasal obstruction and induced tumor regression. However, a small number of patients developed sarcomas after 10 years or more. Such treatment today is used only as an alternative for cases that cannot be treated surgically.

Hemangiopericytoma

CLINICAL PRESENTATION AND PATHOGENESIS ▶

Benign hemangiopericytomas arise from a vascular supporting cell, the pericyte. They are part of a spectrum of tumors that range from benign to intermediate types to overtly malignant. Those of the intermediate type have features of both the benign and malignant forms and probably represent a low-grade malignancy. However, the overtly benign form is the most common.

It will present as a deep-seated mass within muscle or within deeper fascial spaces (Fig 9-88a). It tends not to occur at superficial levels such as the subcutaneous level or submucosa. Men and women are affected equally. The peak incidence is between the ages of 30 and 50 years. The tumor grows very slowly and will often have a reported duration of several years. Most are of significant size at the time of diagnosis.

The tumor mass is painless but often contains pulsations or audible bruits. This is due to the development of functional vascular spaces and prominent feeding vessels with arteriovenous shunting.

The oral and maxillofacial area is an uncommon location for hemangiopericytomas, accounting for only 16% of cases. Most of these occur within the orbit.

DIFFERENTIAL DIAGNOSIS ▶

The deep-seated location of the mass is strongly suggestive of *salivary gland tumors* such as the pleomorphic adenoma. If pulsations are noted, it may suggest an *arteriovenous hemangioma* or, if the nasal cavity or medial orbit is involved, a *nasopharyngeal angiofibroma*.

DIAGNOSTIC WORK-UP ▶

Despite its vascular nature, the tumor can undergo an incisional biopsy with normal hemostatic controls. The incisional biopsy should be of sufficient size for adequate histopathologic assessment. Determining the cellularity and number of mitotic figures on the basis of examination of 10 to 20 high-power fields (HPFs) is critical in determining whether the tumor is benign or malignant. Because of its deep location, a CT or MRI scan is recommended to determine its size and anatomic relationships. A Doppler examination is also suggested. If the tumor displays audible bruits with the Doppler, an angiogram should follow.

HISTOPATHOLOGY ▶

Hemangiopericytomas have a thin, vascular pseudocapsule. They consist of ovoid to spindle cells, which surround endothelially lined vascular spaces. The vessels may be distended and often have a staghorn contour (Fig 9-88b). A silver stain will stain the basement membrane of the endothelial cells so that the proliferating cells are seen outside the vessel, thus clearly distinguishing these tumors from those of endothelial origin.

TREATMENT ▶

If histopathology confirms a benign hemangiopericytoma, treatment is local excision with margins of 0.5 to 1.0 cm. Because many have feeder vessels and the lesion itself is vascular, ligation of all feeding vessels in the immediate area is advised.

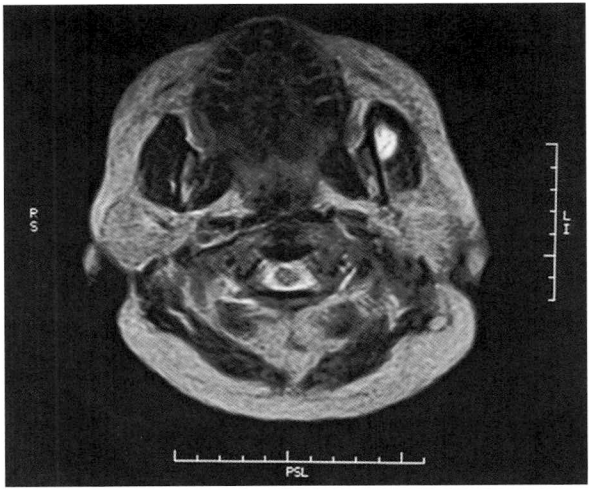

Fig 9-88a A hemangiopericytoma in the oral and maxillofacial area is very rare. When it occurs, it will be deep seated and have an intense signal uptake on a T2-weighted MRI because of its vascular network.

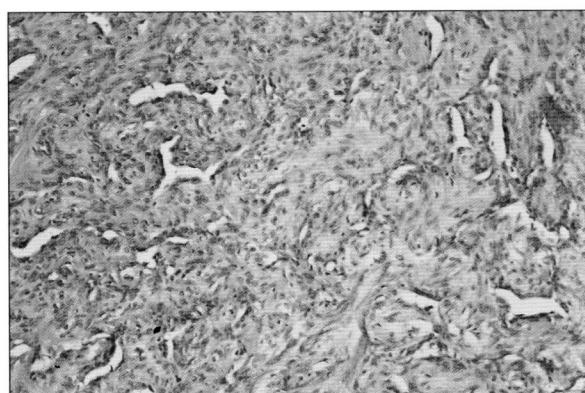

Fig 9-88b Hemangiopericytoma with numerous vessels, many of which have a staghorn appearance.

PROGNOSIS ▶

The prognosis of this tumor is excellent; no recurrences are expected when it is excised with clear margins.

Carotid Body Tumor

CLINICAL PRESENTATION AND PATHOGENESIS ▶

The carotid body tumor is considered one of a group of extra-adrenal paragangliomas; that is, it arises from specialized neural crest cells that develop in association with autonomic ganglia. This group includes the adrenal medulla, which can give rise to an intra-adrenal paraganglioma known as a *pheochromocytoma*; the carotid body tumor; paragangliomas of the aortic and the vagal bodies; as well as smaller paragangliomas in the thorax, abdomen, and retroperitoneal space. The histogenesis of carotid body tumors is the specialized chemoreceptor cells located on the posterior aspect and within the adventitial cell layers of the carotid artery bifurcation. These chemoreceptor cells normally detect small changes in arterial oxygen tensions and pH and in turn regulate each value somewhat by reflexively changing the rate and depth of respiration. The carotid body tumors are very rare, accounting for only 0.012% of all tumors registered in major surgical centers. Nonetheless, it is the most common of the extra-adrenal paragangliomas. The incidence of carotid body tumors increases somewhat in areas of high altitude such as Peru, Mexico City, and Colorado, presumably because of a continuous hypoxic stimulus. Men are reported to be affected more frequently from lower altitudes and women more frequently from higher altitudes. The peak age range is between 40 and 60 years.

The carotid body tumor is a benign tumor that will present as a painless, slowly enlarging, and pulsatile mass in the area of the carotid bifurcation in the neck. It is noted to be movable in the anteroposterior direction but not in the superoinferior direction. A bruit can usually be heard over the mass by means of a stethoscope or, if not, a Doppler sounding. Most carotid body tumors are nonfunctional paragangliomas and therefore will not produce elevated serum or urinary catecholamine levels. The rare ones with catecholamine production may produce systolic hypertension by stress or with surgical manipulations similar to a pheochromocytoma.

DIFFERENTIAL DIAGNOSIS ▶

While the pulsatile quality of a mass in the area of the carotid bifurcation should suggest a carotid body tumor, other unassociated masses in the same area also may seem to be pulsatile because of trans-

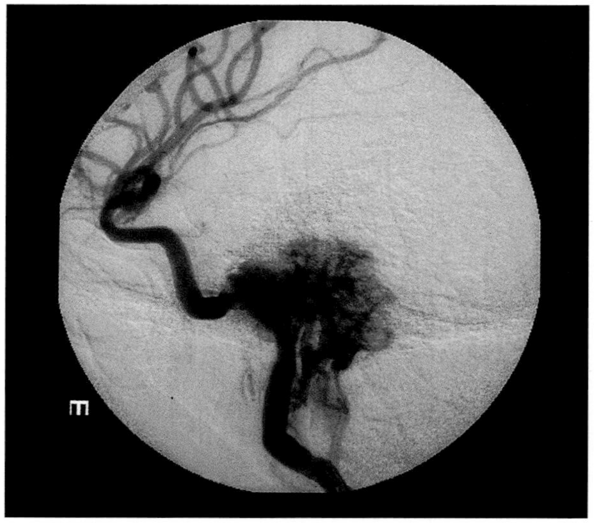

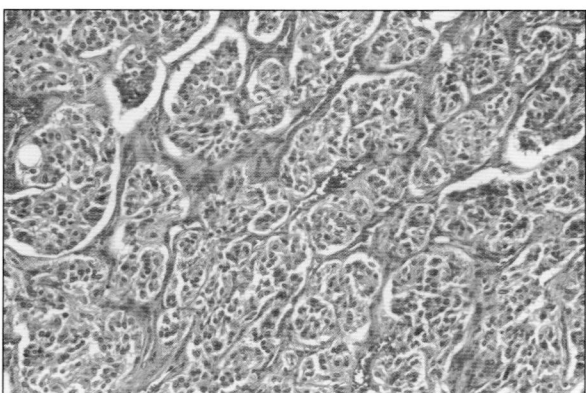

Fig 9-89 An angiogram of a carotid body tumor will show multiple vessels within the tumor.

Fig 9-90a A low-power view of a carotid body tumor showing the nest-like arrangement of cells. These are separated by fibrovascular trabeculae.

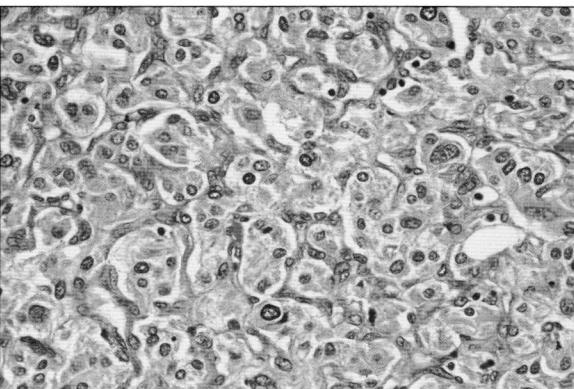

Fig 9-90b A carotid body tumor showing the "zell-ballen" or nests of cells, which have an eosinophilic cytoplasm. Although some of the nuclei are atypical in appearance, this does not necessarily indicate malignancy.

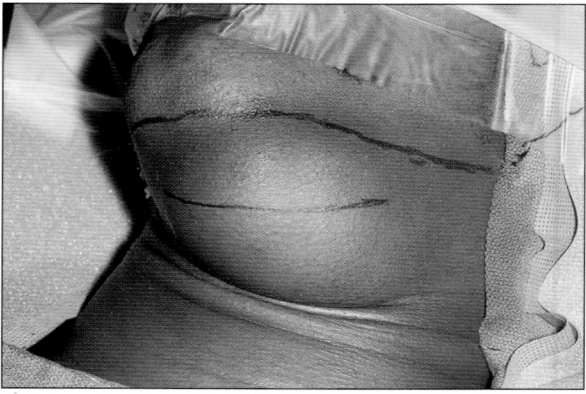

Fig 9-91a The carotid body tumor may attain a large size. It is usually clinically pulsatile and will have harsh arterial Doppler sounds.

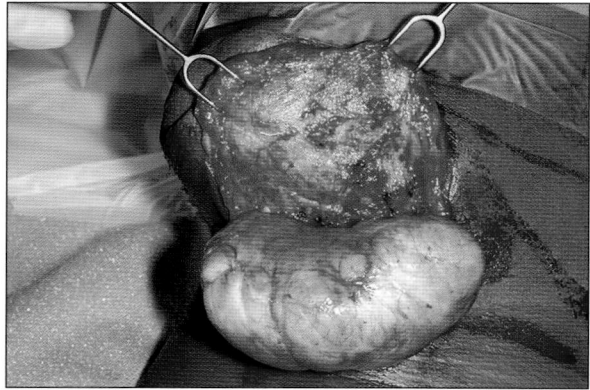

Fig 9-91b Excision of a carotid body tumor is a meticulous dissection because it requires the ligation and cauterization of the numerous vessels entering the tumor.

mission of the pulsatile wave from a normal carotid artery. Therefore, lymph node diseases affecting the jugulodigastric node or other lymph nodes of the upper deep cervical chain are strong considerations: *tuberculosis lymphadenitis* (scrofula), *cat-scratch disease*, *lymphoma*, and *regional lymph node metastasis from a squamous cell carcinoma*. Other diseases that may appear as a mass in this area are the *branchial cyst*, *schwannoma*, and *lipoma*. In addition, an *aneurysm of the carotid artery* itself will be a pulsatile mass.

DIAGNOSTIC WORK-UP ▶

Selective angiography is required of a suspected carotid body tumor. This should be accomplished bilaterally, as carotid body tumors occur bilaterally about 2% of the time and to assess the degree of collateral cerebral blood flow should the carotid circulation become interrupted during surgery. The angiograms of a carotid body tumor will typically show numerous enlarged and tortuous vessels in a round mass engulfing the carotid bifurcation (Fig 9-89). It will also usually show a lateral displacement of the carotid artery system, accounting for its easy clinical palpability and underscoring its origin from the deep surface of the carotid bifurcation. At times, the mass will diverge and separate the internal and external carotid branches. The finding of a pulsatile mass with an angiographic picture is sufficient for diagnosis and is an indication for a neck exploration and local excision.

HISTOPATHOLOGY ▶ Carotid body tumors are lobular tumors that are pale yellow to red-brown. They may envelop the carotid artery or show only partial attachment to it. These tumors are sometimes multifocal, and a thin partial capsule is usually present. The tumor consists of nests of cells separated by delicate fibrovascular tissue (Fig 9-90a). This pattern of the carotid body tumor historically has been described as *zellballen* ("balls of cells"). The cells are large and polygonal with eosinophilic and sometimes granular cytoplasm (Fig 9-90b). Neurosecretory granules containing catecholamines may be identified by Grimelius or another silver stain. Nuclei are rounded. Some may be atypical, but mitoses are rare.

There are no specific criteria for malignancy, and cytologic atypia does not necessarily indicate malignancy. Artifactual changes may sometimes alter the characteristic pattern of this tumor.

TREATMENT ▶ Carotid body tumors are treated with a wide access and slow, painstaking total excision (Fig 9-91a). The intimacy of the tumor to the carotid is the guiding factor in the surgery. Most tumors are attached to the carotid vessel and may be removed using the bipolar electrocautery and scalpel excision with numerous vascular ties. In such cases, the tumor, along with its thin capsule, is literally peeled off the outer surface of the carotid and the surrounding tissues (Fig 9-91b). However, in other cases the carotid is completely encased by the tumor, which therefore cannot be dissected from the carotid. For these situations, complete excision requires a resection of a segment of the carotid and placement of a mesh graft. Therefore, careful study of the preoperative angiograms and CT scans is necessary to assess collateral cerebral blood flow and to try to predict and be prepared for tumors that require a carotid resection.

PROGNOSIS ▶ Although carotid body tumors are thought to be benign and have a first-time surgical cure rate of about 75%, a small number (6% to 9%) metastasize to regional lymph nodes or to lung and/or bone. These seem to be associated with tumors left untreated for long periods of time and with locally recurrent tumors, which identifies a small potential for malignant transformation. Even then, these metastases occur very late, 10 to 30 years after the original excision.

In large and carotid-encased tumors and in those that have been incompletely excised, radiotherapy may be used at 5,000 cGy to 6,000 cGy with a good response.

Malignant Soft Tissue Tumors of Mesenchymal Origin

▶ "If the patient is over 40, think of cancer. If the patient is under 40, think of cancer."
—*Robert E. Marx*

Fibroblastic Malignancies

Fibromatoses

CLINICAL PRESENTATION AND PATHOGENESIS ▶

Fibromatoses found in the oral and maxillofacial region have been categorized as the deep musculo-aponeurotic type. They have been given many terms, including *extra-abdominal desmoids, desmoid tumors, grade 1 fibrosarcomas, nonmetastasizing fibrosarcomas*, and *aggressive fibromatosis*. This abundant nomenclature is indicative of the tumor's vague position in the spectrum of benign to malignant neoplasms. Nonetheless, fibromatoses remain a benign fibrous tissue proliferation with an intermediate biologic behavior between a benign fibroma and a fibrosarcoma; that is, like fibrosarcomas they exhibit destructive infiltrative growth and frequently recur, but like fibromas they do not metastasize.

The oral and maxillofacial region is an uncommon location for a fibromatosis. Most occur in the shoulder (22%), chest and back (17%), thigh (13%), and mesentery (10%). Those that arise in the oral and maxillofacial area (2%) are somewhat unique compared to those that occur in the more common locations around the shoulder girdle and trunk. The oral and maxillofacial locations (mostly the mandible, maxilla, and mastoid area) show a younger peak age range (5 to 20 years compared to 25 to 35 years), more infiltrative and faster growth, and a much greater propensity to invade underlying bone or to arise seemingly from within bone.

The patient is usually a preteen or teenager with a poorly circumscribed, painless fibrous growth apparently arising from the periosteum or from the fascia of muscles attached to the jaws or mastoid (Fig 10-1). The history is one of rapid emergence over a 2- to 6-week period. There is no sex predilection. The mass will seem to be adherent to bone and will extend close to the surface mucosa or skin in most cases.

Radiographs frequently show a poorly demarcated, irregular bony destruction (Fig 10-2). If the lesion is located on the surface of the jaws, it may show an irregular resorption of the adjacent cortex only. If the location is central, it will usually show a destructive pattern in all directions.

Uncommonly, pain or even paresthesia has been reported. The pain seems to be located at the periosteal level during the rapid growth phase or related to jaw motion if the tumor is attached in an area of muscle contraction. Paresthesia is related to the tumor encompassing a sensory nerve but is a slow-to-develop finding and does not occur in all cases.

The pathogenesis of fibromatoses remains unexplained. Both trauma and endocrine influences have been proposed but remain unsatisfactory explanations. Yet, many cases have occurred in an area of previous injury such as that of a surgical scar, radiation, burn scar, or fracture, and a small percentage of lesions have been shown to contain markedly elevated amounts of estrogen-receptor protein.

DIFFERENTIAL DIAGNOSIS ▶

A fibromatosis must be distinguished from a *fibrosarcoma* and a *reactive fibrous proliferation* by means of histopathology and history. A fibromatosis will be distinguished from a fibrosarcoma primarily by its uniform growth pattern, maturity of cells, and paucity of mitotic figures. A fibromatosis is distinguished

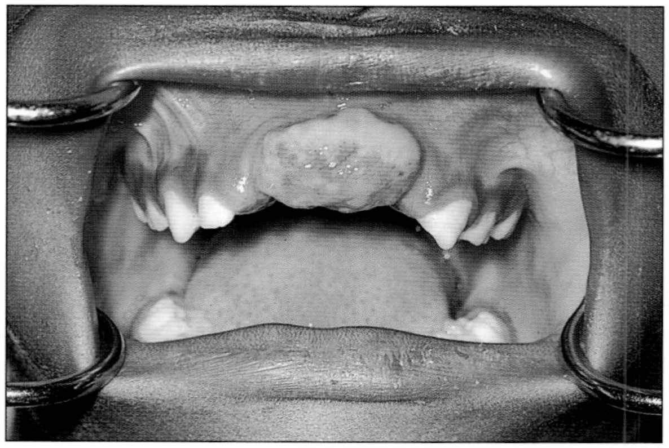

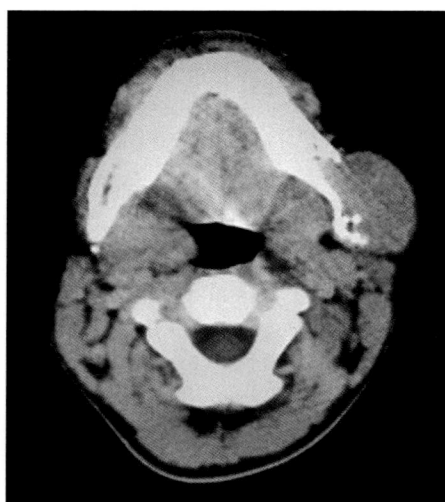

Fig 10-1 Aggressive fibromatosis arising from the periosteum of the anterior maxilla in a preteen. This will behave as a low-grade, nonmetastasizing fibrosarcoma.

Fig 10-2 Aggressive fibromatosis arising from periosteum or fascia may locally invade into the underlying bone and create a cortical resorption.

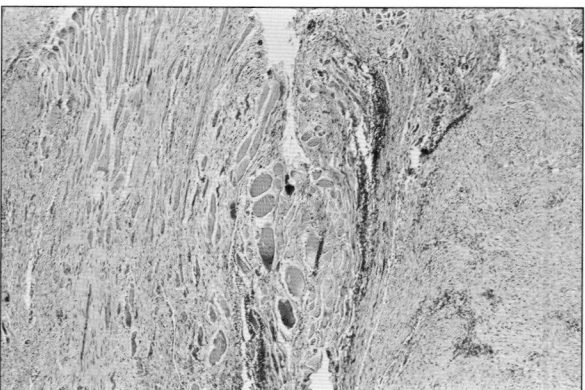

Fig 10-3a Aggressive fibromatosis showing infiltration of skeletal muscle by fibroblasts.

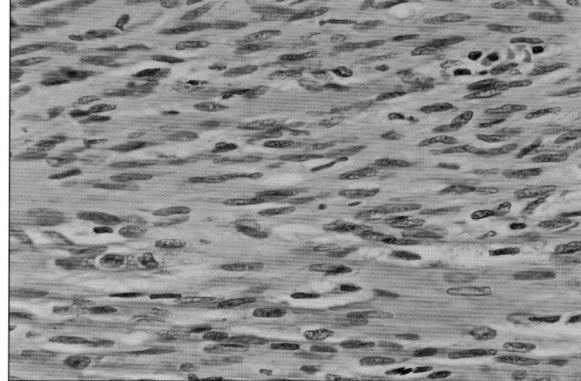

Fig 10-3b High-power view of benign-appearing spindle cells in aggressive fibromatosis.

from a reactive fibrous proliferation by its absence of an apparent stimulus and its lack of inflammatory cells and focal hemorrhages. Clinically, the destructive and infiltrative nature of a fibromatosis will also resemble that of a *neurofibroma* or a *malignant peripheral nerve sheath tumor* as well as that of *nodular fasciitis*. These three entities can be distinguished only by their histopathologic features.

DIAGNOSTIC WORK-UP ▶ The diagnosis requires a deep incisional biopsy in the center of the mass. The biopsy should extend to bone and include periosteum to enable assessment of the infiltrative growth pattern of the mass. It is important not to biopsy the edge of the mass or to take too small a specimen. A biopsy at the edge of the mass will induce scar tissue that is histologically similar to the tumor itself, thereby confusing the margins at the time of excision. If too small a specimen is taken, a subsequent biopsy specimen will contain inflammatory cells and a scar tissue pattern, which may make the mass resemble a reactive fibrous proliferation or nodular fasciitis.

HISTOPATHOLOGY ▶ These are infiltrating tumors composed of fibroblasts and myofibroblasts. They consist of uniform, elongated, slender spindle cells with abundant collagen arranged in broad, elongated fascicles. There is variable cellularity and mitotic activity. Some areas may be hypocellular or hyalinized. At the periphery of the tumor where it infiltrates muscle, there may be atrophy of the skeletal muscle resulting in the for-

Table 10-1 Characteristics of fibromatosis vs fibrosarcoma

	Fibromatosis	**Fibrosarcoma**
Pattern	Fascicular	Herringbone
Mitoses	Few; normal	Few to many; abnormal
Tissue	More collagen; more widely separated nuclei	Less collagen; more closely packed nuclei

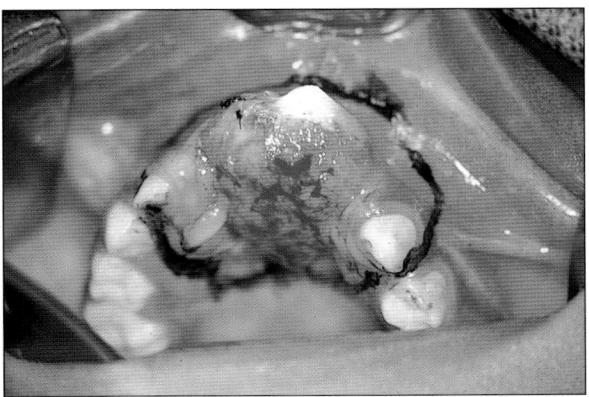

Fig 10-4a Because aggressive fibromatoses are locally infiltrative, they require a wide local resection with 1.0- to 1.5-cm margins.

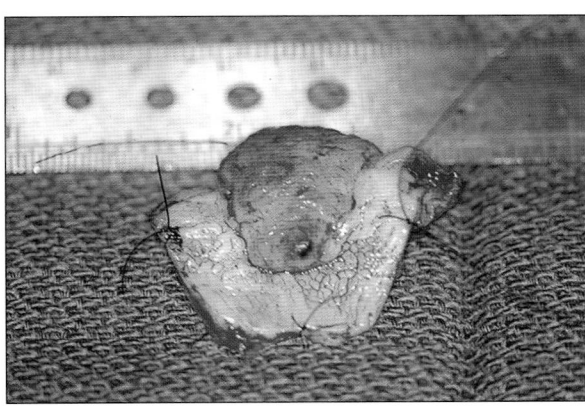

Fig 10-4b The margins of the specimen should be marked and assessed with frozen sections.

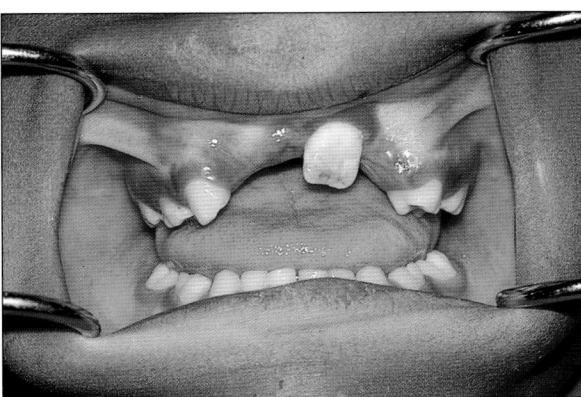

Fig 10-5 Re-epithelialization occurs rapidly in young individuals, minimizing the surgical defect. Recurrence is unlikely if clear tumor margins are obtained. If a recurrence develops, it is usually seen within the first year.

mation of multinucleated giant cells. This may give the impression of malignancy, but this impression is counterbalanced by the fact that the nuclei do not show atypia and there is considerable collagen production. These tumors may appear innocuous on a cellular level even though they are highly infiltrative (Figs 10-3a and 10-3b). These lesions may be difficult to separate from low-grade fibrosarcomas (Table 10-1).

TREATMENT ▶

The focus of treatment is a wide local excision of the tumor and any involved bone. Margins are 1.0 to 1.5 cm with frozen section assessment at the time of surgery (Figs 10-4a and 10-4b). Treatment of regional lymph nodes is not necessary.

Reports from some centers suggest good results with initial chemotherapy protocols using agents often used for sarcomas, such as adriamycin, actinomycin D, cyclophosphamide, and daunorubicin, followed by surgery. This approach may be advantageous in those very large tumors that approach the base of the skull, making complete resection difficult, or those tumors associated with significant functional loss and morbidity. Additionally, radiotherapy may have a role to play in some large unresectable tumors and in recurrent or incompletely excised tumors. Response to radiotherapy in such situations has been documented, but it is slower than it is for epithelial malignancies. Radiation-induced sarcomas have been reported but are very rare.

PROGNOSIS ▶

If a recurrence is to develop, it usually becomes apparent within the first year. The recurrence rate for oral and maxillofacial fibromatoses is unknown because of the paucity of cases, but for fibromatoses in other locations it ranges from 25% to 68%. The recurrence rate is inversely proportional to the attainment of surgically clear margins of clinically uninvolved tissue (Fig 10-5).

Fibrosarcoma

Fibrosarcomas are rare lesions in general and in the oral and maxillofacial area in particular (only 10% of fibrosarcomas occur in the head and neck region). Between 1950 and 1975, they were believed to be the most common soft tissue malignancy. However, the identification and separation of malignant fibrous histiocytomas, fibromatoses, nodular fasciitis, fibrous osteosarcomas, and undifferentiated epithelial malignancies, all of which were previously regarded as fibrosarcomas, has unmasked the rarity of true fibrosarcoma. Fibrosarcoma is less common than liposarcoma, rhabdomyosarcoma, and malignant fibrous histiocytoma. Today, fibrosarcomas are defined as malignant tumors of fibroblasts that show no other evidence of cellular differentiation and are capable of recurrence and metastasis. They are often graded with a grading scale of grade 1 through grade 3. Grade 1 and 2 fibrosarcomas tend to be more differentiated and therefore less clinically aggressive. Grade 3 fibrosarcomas are usually faster growing and very aggressive; they also have a greater tendency to metastasize.

Fibrosarcomas in the oral and maxillofacial area usually arise from bone, periosteum, or muscle fascia (Fig 10-6a). They are usually painless fibrous, fleshy masses that are destructive of bone and will cause mobility of teeth if they are located in alveolar bone. Compared to fibromatoses, they are slower to develop and often somewhat smaller. Fibrosarcomas frequently have a duration of several months to years before presentation and are usually 3 to 5 cm in size. They may occur at any age, but peak incidence in the oral and maxillofacial area is the 20s and early 30s, older than for fibromatoses in this same area (5 to 20 years) and younger than for fibrosarcomas elsewhere (30 to 55 years).

Much has been written about fibrosarcomas arising in sites of previous trauma, and many have indeed been reported to arise from the scar tissue of an old injury site. However, no clear evidence exists to ascribe an etiologic role of trauma. Other than scar tissue being an abundant source of fibroblasts, there is no cause-and-effect relationship. Considering the prevalence of trauma and at least some scar tissue, the simultaneous occurrence of fibrosarcoma and scar is likely only coincidental.

In the oral and maxillofacial area, fibrosarcomas either arise from bone or invade into bone from their deep soft tissue origin. Therefore, *osteosarcomas* are prominent on the differential list, as are *malignant fibrous histiocytomas*, *fibromatoses*, *neurofibromas*, and *malignant peripheral nerve sheath tumors*. Each one must be distinguished by its unique histopathologic features.

Diagnosis of a fibrosarcoma requires a deep incisional biopsy within the lesion's center. Too superficial a biopsy may lead to a diagnosis of a reactive fibrous lesion, since periosteal and fascial reactions to many tumors are manifested by the deposition of collagen. Plain radiographs, computed tomography (CT) scans, or a magnetic resonance imaging (MRI) scan to delineate the extent of the disease is also recommended (Fig 10-6b). Assessment of metastatic activity is best accomplished by a chest radiograph and a technetium-99 methylene diphosphate (^{99}Tc-MDP) bone scan, as metastasis is most frequent to lungs and bone.

Fibrosarcomas are invasive tumors with no distinct margins. The cells are rather uniform and spindle shaped and lie in fascicles, often forming a herringbone pattern (Fig 10-7a). Mitoses are present, but multinucleated and bizarre giant cells are not a feature of this tumor (Fig 10-7b).

Tumors that are poorly differentiated form less collagen and thus have more densely packed nuclei. The pattern is less organized. Mitoses are numerous, but marked cellular pleomorphism is not seen. Tumors that are highly pleomorphic or contain bizarre giant cells are more suggestive of malignant fibrous histiocytoma.

Malignant neoplasms are often given a histologic grade. Parameters between different grading systems may vary, but in general the grade relates to factors such as invasiveness, cellularity, pleomorphism, mitotic rate, atypical mitoses, necrosis, and the quantity of matrix that may be produced. The importance of some of these factors may depend on the tumor type. In the case of fibrosarcomas, grades I and II show the features described above. They are more uniform with distinct fascicles and a herringbone pat-

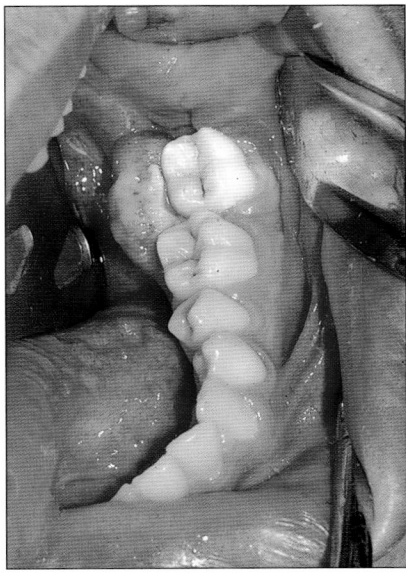

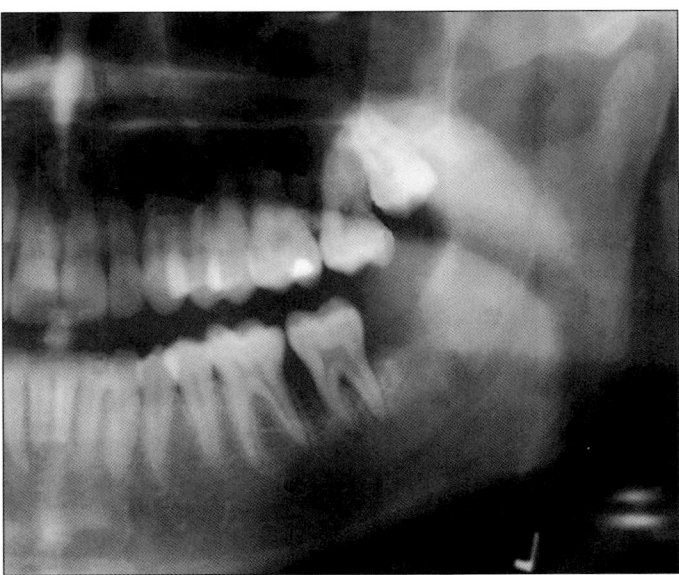

Fig 10-6a Clinical view of a fibrosarcoma emerging as a fleshy to firm mass in the area of the posterior lingual gingiva.

Fig 10-6b Although widening of the periodontal membrane space is often attributed to osteosarcomas, fibrosarcomas and most other sarcomas can produce the same sign.

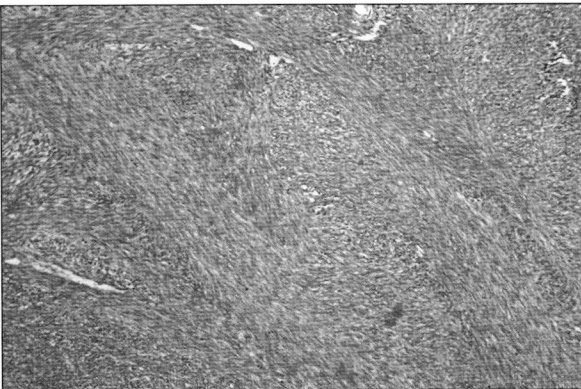

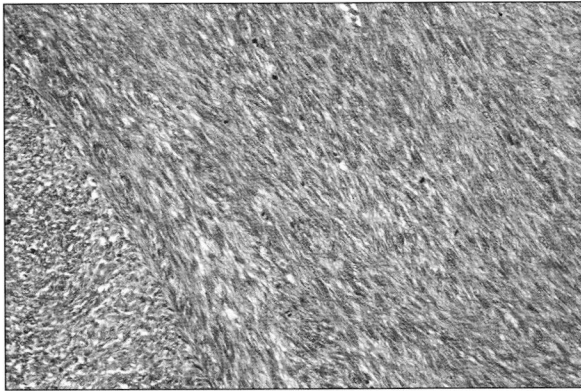

Fig 10-7a Low-power view of a fibrosarcoma showing the herringbone pattern.

Fig 10-7b High-power view of a fibrosarcoma showing plump, closely packed cells with little collagen production and some mitotic activity.

tern. There is a greater production of matrix (collagen). Grade III (high grade) is more cellular, produces less collagen, and has greater mitotic activity. Distinct fascicles and a herringbone pattern are lacking.

TREATMENT ▶

The focus of treatment is very wide local excision using 3-cm clinical margins in soft tissue and bone as well as assessing margins with frozen sections at the time of surgery (Figs 10-8a and 10-8b). Lymph node dissection is not required. In fibrosarcomas that cannot be completely excised because of their location or extreme size, postoperative radiotherapy of 6,000 cGy to 7,000 cGy is appropriate. In grade 3 fibrosarcomas, postoperative adjunctive chemotherapy is recommended, ostensibly to treat potential subclinical or microscopic metastasis. When chemotherapy is employed, agents used successfully for sarcomas are preferred, including adriamycin, actinomycin D, oncovin, cyclophosphamide, prednisone, and daunorubicin.

PROGNOSIS ▶

Like most sarcomas, fibrosarcomas are malignancies for which the prognosis correlates most closely with histologic grade. Conversely, most epithelial malignancies, such as squamous cell carcinoma, correlate better to clinical staging. Using a three-grade system of advancing histologic grade, reported 5-year

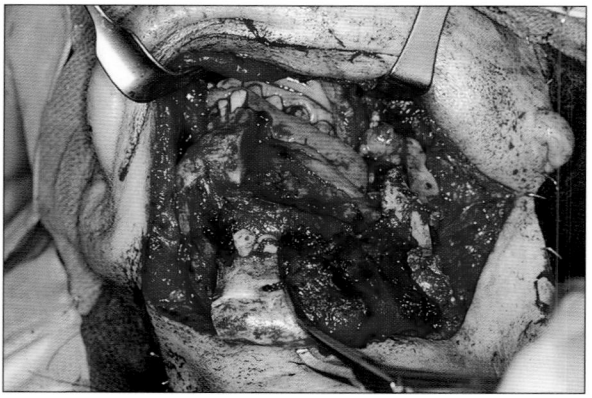

Fig 10-8a Fibrosarcomas require a wide surgical resection with 3-cm soft tissue and bony margins if bone is involved.

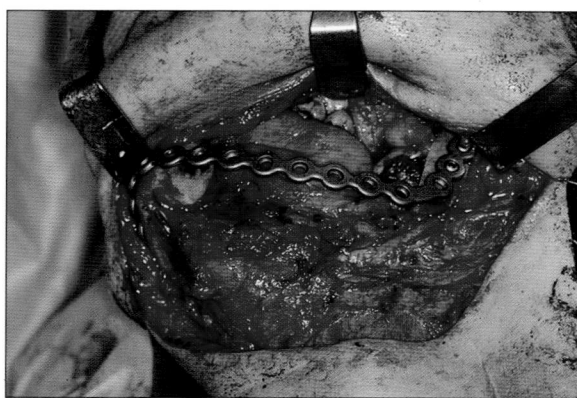

Fig 10-8b Fibrosarcoma resection defects can be immediately reconstructed with titanium reconstruction plates and soft tissue flaps if required.

survival rates are 82% for grade 1, 55% for grade 2, and 36% for grade 3 tumors. In addition, margin integrity and width of excisional margins correlate with recurrence and survival. The simple truth is that the wider the excision, the lower the recurrence rate and the greater the survival rate. Tumor size, duration, and location do not influence recurrence or survival.

Local recurrence (persistence of the original tumor) by incomplete excision is the most common cause of failure to cure. Metastasis is less frequent. When metastasis occurs, it does so via bloodborne routes. Venous tumor emboli most commonly spread to the lungs as they are swept into the right heart chambers by normal venous return and implanted into the lungs via the pulmonary artery system (see Fig 7-7). Other venous tumor emboli spread to bone, especially to the vertebrae and skull, because of their rich venous system of valveless veins (see Fig 18-27).

Malignant Fibrous Histiocytoma

CLINICAL PRESENTATION AND
PATHOGENESIS ▶

The term *malignant fibrous histiocytoma* is relatively new and therefore unfamiliar to many practitioners. Yet it is the most common soft tissue sarcoma of late adult life. Many were previously diagnosed as fibrosarcomas, malignant peripheral nerve sheath tumors, and pleomorphic rhabdomyosarcomas. In particular, its overlap with fibrosarcomas is understandable since both arise from a similar precursor cell within a maturation sequence beginning with the pluripotential mesenchymal stem cell and ending with the mature fibrocyte. In general, malignant fibrous histiocytomas arise from a more immature cell in this sequence and therefore have a more aggressive behavior. Fibrosarcomas arise from a slightly more mature cell in this sequence and therefore are mostly of lower grades. There is some overlap in these tumors, but the histocytic-appearing cells generally represent the more primitive cells in this lineage (Fig 10-9).

Two thirds of those affected are men, and most of those affected are between the ages of 50 and 70 years. The lesion may occur in either soft tissue or bone and is rare in the oral and maxillofacial area; the most common sites are the extremities and retroperitoneum. In the soft tissues it usually presents as a painless firm to fleshy mass. In bone it presents with expansion and an irregular, diffuse radiolucency indicative of a destructive lesion (Figs 10-10a and 10-10b). In the mandible it may produce paresthesia of the lower lip; in the maxilla, paresthesia of the cheek. Its growth rate is intermediate to slow; many will have been present for 3 months to 1 year before the individual seeks medical attention. There is a distinct history of previous radiotherapy in many cases. Radiation-induced malignant fibrous histiocytomas can occur, as do other types of sarcomas, after a postradiation latency period of 20 to 40 years.

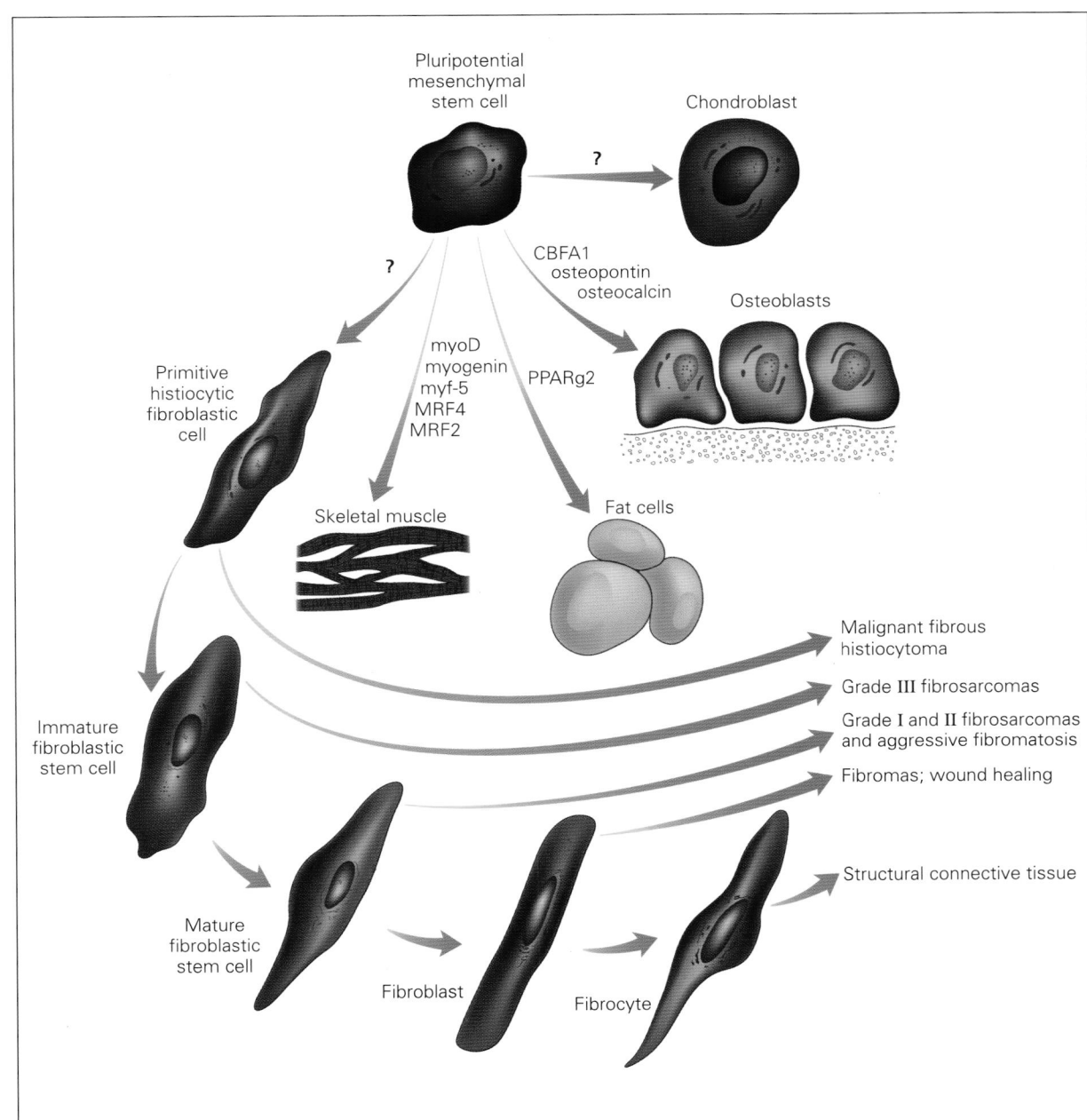

Fig 10-9 All sarcomas arise from the pluripotential mesenchymal stem cell or from one of its early progeny. Each of the multiple stages in this cell maturation sequence can give rise to a neoplasia. The earlier (less differentiated) stages are thought to give rise to the higher-grade and more aggressive malignancies, such as the malignant fibrous histiocytoma and the grade III fibrosarcoma. Cells in the later (more differentiated) stages of the maturation sequence are thought to be the parent cells of the lower-grade sarcomas, the aggressive fibromatoses, and even benign tumors.

Common to those malignant fibrous histiocytomas that occur in the extremities and retroperitoneum but uncommon to those that occur in the oral and maxillofacial area are the clinical signs of fever and leukocytosis with a mature neutrophilia or eosinophilia. This seems to be the result of the tumor's production of eosinophilic and neutrophilic chemotactic and colony-stimulating factors. Both signs regress with surgical removal of the tumor.

There is no evidence that malignant fibrous histiocytomas arise from their benign counterparts. Those that are malignant show malignant features from their outset.

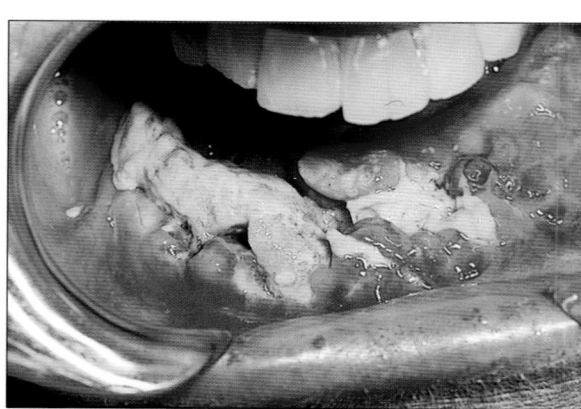

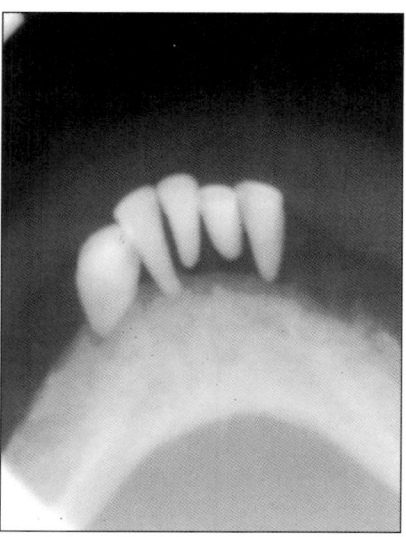

Fig 10-10a Malignant fibrous histiocytomas are aggressive high-grade sarcomas arising from primitive fibroblastic precursors or mesenchymal stem cells.

Fig 10-10b A malignant fibrous histiocytoma will readily invade and resorb bone to produce mobility of teeth in the area.

DIFFERENTIAL DIAGNOSIS ►

Malignant fibrous histiocytomas must be distinguished from the *benign fibrous histiocytoma*, which also may present as a rare radiolucent expansion in the jaws or as a painless soft tissue mass. In addition, it must be distinguished from those entities with which it was historically grouped: *fibrosarcomas, malignant peripheral nerve sheath tumors,* and *rhabdomyosarcomas,* all of which may present in a clinically identical fashion. Although the distinction of these entities is mainly histopathologic, most true fibrosarcomas and rhabdomyosarcomas occur at younger ages.

DIAGNOSTIC WORK-UP ►

The diagnosis should be made by a deep incisional biopsy within the center of the lesion. It is also recommended that plain radiographs, a CT scan, or an MRI scan be performed to ascertain the extent of the tumor and its relationship to adjacent structures. A metastatic work-up should include at the minimum a chest radiograph and liver function tests. It may also include a ^{99}Tc-MDP bone scan in large and high-grade tumors with greater metastatic potential.

HISTOPATHOLOGY ►

Malignant fibrous histiocytomas present a broad histologic spectrum, with fibroblasts, histiocytoid cells, and multinucleated giant cells as common features. Consequently, they are subclassified according to their histologic appearance.

Storiform-Pleomorphic Type

This form, the most common, usually contains short fascicles of plump spindle cells arranged around slit-like vessels in a storiform pattern. In addition, some histiocytic cells are present (Fig 10-11). Numerous mitoses, some of which are atypical, and inflammatory cells may be seen. Other areas of the tumor are pleomorphic and have a less organized pattern. These have more mitoses and numerous multinucleated giant cells (Fig 10-12).

Myxoid Type

In this variant of the storiform-pleomorphic type, loose mesenchymal cells in a myxoid stroma compose at least half of the tumor. This type has a lower metastatic potential.

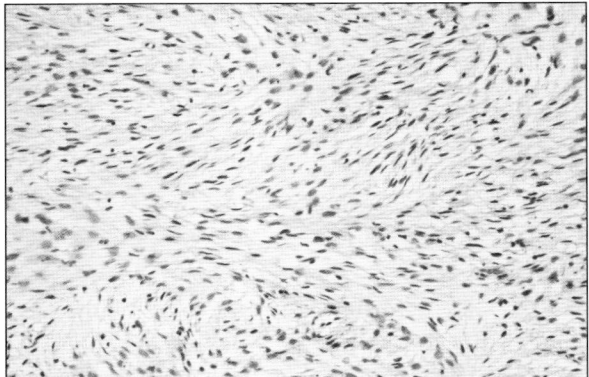

Fig 10-11 Malignant fibrous histiocytoma in which spindle cells form a storiform pattern.

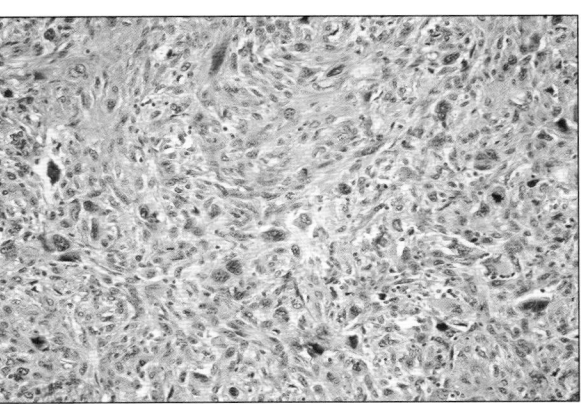

Fig 10-12 Malignant fibrous histiocytoma with a more pleomorphic appearance. Spindle cells, histiocytic cells, multinucleated giant cells, and mitoses as well as some inflammatory cells can all be seen.

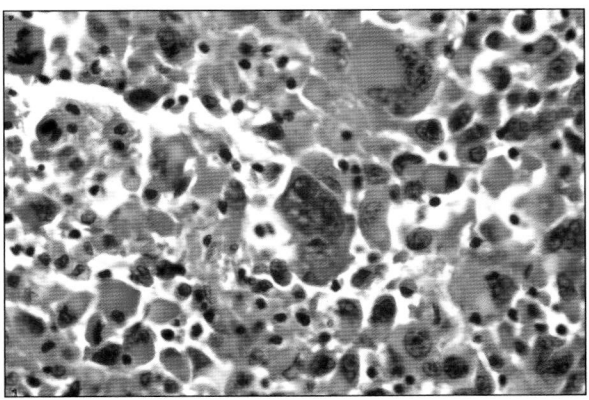

Fig 10-13 The giant cell type of malignant fibrous histiocytoma in which numerous multinucleated giant cells are present.

Giant Cell Type

This type has also been called *malignant giant cell tumor of soft parts*. It consists of fibroblasts and histiocytes showing mitotic activity and pleomorphism, but in addition large numbers of multinucleated giant cells, resembling osteoclasts, are found in association with the histiocytic cells (Fig 10-13). Many tumors contain foci of osteoid or bone.

Inflammatory Type

Sheets of histiocytes, most of them foamy, are seen along with inflammatory cells in a poorly collagenized stroma. The xanthoma cells frequently have malignant features.

Angiomatoid Type

This tumor has areas of hemorrhage with deposition of hemosiderin and fat and a chronic inflammatory component. There is a fibroblastic and histiocytic proliferation, which may show pleomorphism and mitotic activity. The histiocytic component may phagocytose the hemosiderin and fat. This tumor differs from the other types because it tends to occur in children and adults under the age of 40 and is of low grade.

The diagnosis of malignant fibrous histiocytoma has become somewhat of a wastebasket, and care must be employed to exclude other entities such as pleomorphic liposarcomas, pleomorphic rhabdomyosarcomas, and pleomorphic carcinomas. Generally considered to be a high-grade pleomorphic sarcoma, the malignant fibrous histiocytoma is a tumor that shows no differentiation other than collagen production.

As these neoplasms become more clearly defined, some changes may be anticipated. An example of this is the WHO reclassification of the angiomatoid malignant fibrous histiocytoma as an angiomatoid fibrous histiocytoma, thus acknowledging the low-grade behavior of this tumor.

TREATMENT ▶ Malignant fibrous histiocytomas are treated with a very wide excision with 3-cm margins in both soft tissue and bone. All margins need to be assessed with frozen sections, and particular attention must be given to fascial planes, where the tumor seems to have a tendency to proliferate. In the larger or higher-grade tumors (grade III), regional lymph node dissection should be considered. This treatment would be unusual for most sarcomas, which do not metastasize to regional lymph nodes in general, but it is not unusual for malignant fibrous histiocytomas. The overall incidence of regional lymph node metastasis is

12%, but this figure climbs to as much as 35% in the larger tumors, in those with greater depth of invasion (more common in the oral and maxillofacial area), and in those of higher histologic grade.

Chemotherapy and radiotherapy may play adjunctive roles in advanced cases or in those with metastasis, but surgery remains the primary modality for the primary tumor.

PROGNOSIS ▶

The prognosis is directly related to the adequacy of the resection. Widely excised tumors with clear margins show recurrence rates approaching 0%. Tumors excised with less aggressive margins and margins not examined have had recurrence rates ranging from 50% to 80%. Large series in locations other than the maxillofacial area report a 36% overall 5-year survival rate.

Metastasis is mostly by bloodborne routes, but this is one sarcoma that has some tendency to undergo lymphatic spread. Metastasis usually occurs within the first 2 years, mostly to the lung, but bone and regional lymph node metastasis is also possible. Metastatic frequency is related to the depth of the tumor's invasion and to its size. This is especially important in the oral and maxillofacial area, where tumors tend to be more deeply located and a significant percentage occur in bone.

Malignancies of Adipose Differentiation

Liposarcoma

CLINICAL PRESENTATION AND PATHOGENESIS ▶

Liposarcomas are very rare tumors in the oral and maxillofacial area, but they are the second most common sarcoma in adults (after the malignant fibrous histiocytoma) when all areas are considered. Liposarcomas of the head and neck area account for only 5.6% of all liposarcomas, and most occur within the neck proper. They are most common in the thigh and retroperitoneum.

Most liposarcomas present as a slow-growing mass from a deep origin. Liposarcomas originate from primitive mesenchymal cells rather than from mature fat cells; otherwise, they would be common in areas of mature fat stores, particularly subcutaneous fat. Instead, liposarcomas are rare in subcutaneous areas; they most commonly arise in intermuscular fascial planes, which contain populations of residual mesenchymal stem cells. Liposarcomas do not develop from pre-existing benign lipomas. All are malignant from their inception.

Liposarcomas of the head and neck region, as elsewhere, originate from deep tissue planes as a fleshy painless mass in individuals between 40 and 60 years of age. They show a slight preference (60%) for males. Many have been present for several months, and some "well-differentiated" types are present for several years before the individual seeks medical attention (Figs 10-14a to 10-14c). Many attain sizes over 10 cm.

A soft tissue density is seen on plain radiographs. Liposarcomas with less differentiation are more vascular and thus will appear more soft tissue radiodense. The more well-differentiated, and hence more "fatty" liposarcomas, tend to be more radiolucent. In addition, well-differentiated liposarcomas are known to develop focal calcifications and ossifications, which are telling features on plain radiographs.

DIFFERENTIAL DIAGNOSIS ▶

The rarity of a liposarcoma in the oral and maxillofacial area usually precludes its placement on a differential list. Instead, clinicians are most concerned about other neoplasms that can reach large sizes and arise from deep origins, such as a *pleomorphic adenoma*, *carcinoma ex-pleomorphic adenoma*, *neurofibroma*, and *recurrent ameloblastoma* seeded into deep tissue by curettage procedures.

DIAGNOSTIC WORK-UP ▶

A CT scan or an MRI scan is of great value in assessing the size and location of such tumors (Fig 10-14d). The diagnosis requires a deep incisional biopsy from the lesion's center. It is recommended that a sufficiently large specimen be removed so that the pathologist can study enough representative tissue to grade the differentiation of the lesion. A chest radiograph is also required to rule out identifiable lung metastasis.

HISTOPATHOLOGY ▶

The histologic picture is of prime importance because clinical behavior is governed primarily by histologic type. Other factors affecting behavior are the location and the size of the tumor. Liposarcomas

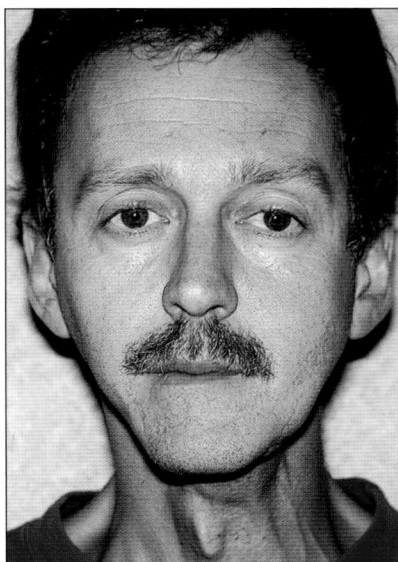

Fig 10-14a Early recurrence of liposarcoma in the left submental submandibular trigone area, which appeared 6 years after the original treatment.

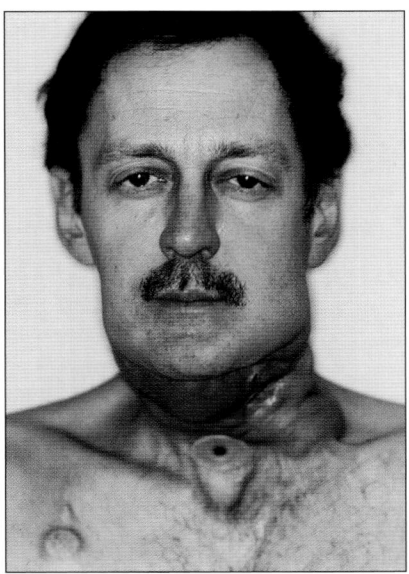

Fig 10-14b This slow-growing tumor took 7 more years to obstruct the airway and pharynx, requiring a tracheostomy and gastrostomy.

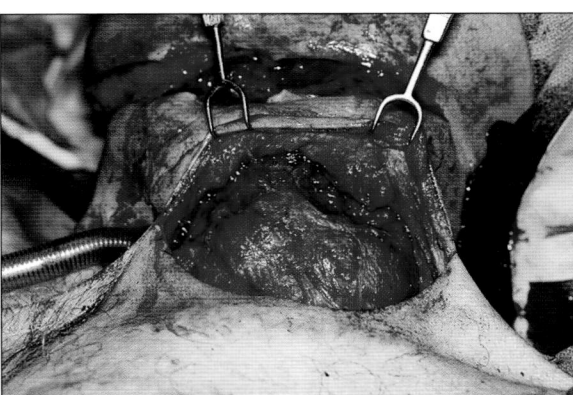

Fig 10-14c Liposarcomas are usually resistant to chemotherapy, radiotherapy, and immune therapy protocols. Repeated surgical debulking to relieve pain and reduce tumor load (cytoreduction surgery) is often performed for palliation.

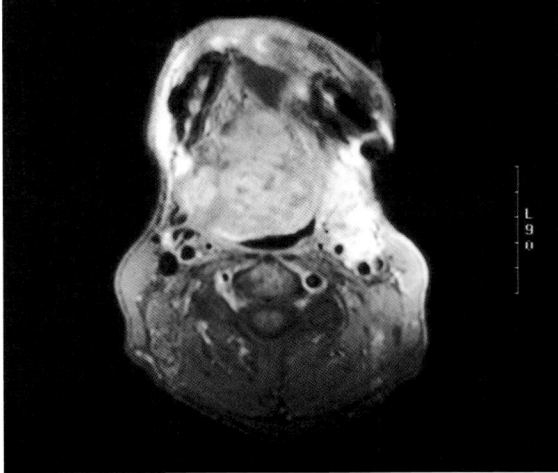

Fig 10-14d This large, recurrent liposarcoma obstructed the airway and the entire pharynx, necessitating a debulking surgery, a tracheostomy, and a gastrostomy feeding tube.

are usually lobulated, circumscribed tumors. The different histologic types are listed below in order of increasingly aggressive behavior.

Well-Differentiated Liposarcoma

Well-differentiated liposarcoma has the appearance of a benign neoplasm with the addition of lipoblasts and some mild nuclear atypism (Fig 10-14e). The behavior depends to a large degree on location. More superficial lesions, such as those in the subcutis, do not metastasize and have also been called *atypical fi-*

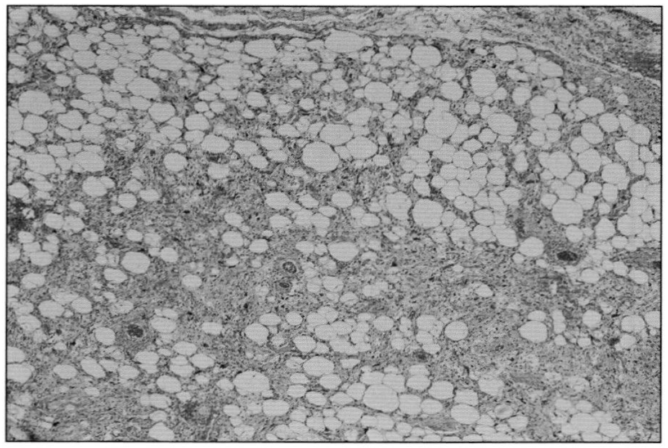

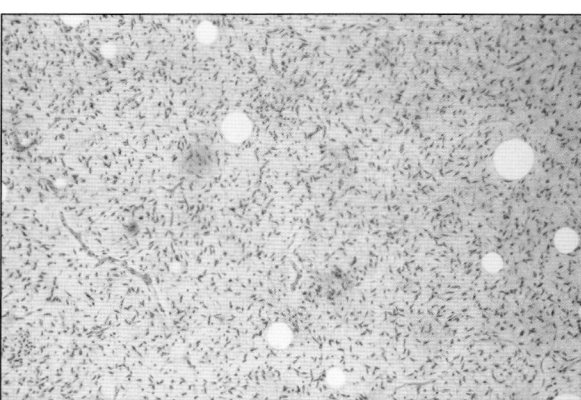

Fig 10-14e A well-differentiated liposarcoma in which normal-appearing fat is dominant. The denser interposed tissue contains some atypical cells with hyperchromatic nuclei.

Fig 10-14f Myxoid liposarcoma showing a rich capillary network and myxoid cells.

bromas. They may undergo repeated recurrences in this area, however. Five-year survival is approximately 100%. Survival drops to 50% at 10 years.

Myxoid Liposarcoma

Myxoid liposarcoma is the most common type of liposarcoma, comprising approximately half the cases. Stellate cells are seen in a mucinous stroma, and there is a prominent network of capillaries (Fig 10-14f). Some tumor cells contain lipid vacuoles within the cytoplasm that may displace the nucleus. Five-year survival approaches 90%.

There is a cytogenic marker for myxoid liposarcomas, a reciprocal chromosomal translocation, t(12;22)(q13;q11–12). This is also present in round cell liposarcomas, which are considered to be a more poorly differentiated form of myxoid liposarcomas. The other types of liposarcoma do not show this marker.

Round Cell Liposarcoma

Round cell liposarcoma is a poorly differentiated form of the myxoid liposarcoma that occurs infrequently. It is separated from the myxoid type because of its much greater aggressiveness and metastatic potential; however, it shows the same chromosomal translocation. Histologically, it resembles other small round cell tumors such as malignant lymphoma. The cells are uniform, and mitoses are uncommon. Lipid formation is not prominent. Five-year survival is approximately 25%.

Pleomorphic Liposarcoma

Pleomorphic liposarcoma occurs only rarely. These highly pleomorphic tumors contain atypical vacuolated giant cells, and mitoses are prominent. As with round cell liposarcomas, prognosis is poor.

Liposarcomas will stain for vimentin and S-100 protein, but poorly differentiated tumors frequently do not. It should be noted that 10-year survival tends to decrease by approximately 15% from the 5-year statistics for all histologic types.

TREATMENT ▶ The primary treatment modality is wide surgical excision with 3- to 5-cm peripheral margins and all margins assessed by frozen section at the time of surgery. Wide margins and frozen section assessments

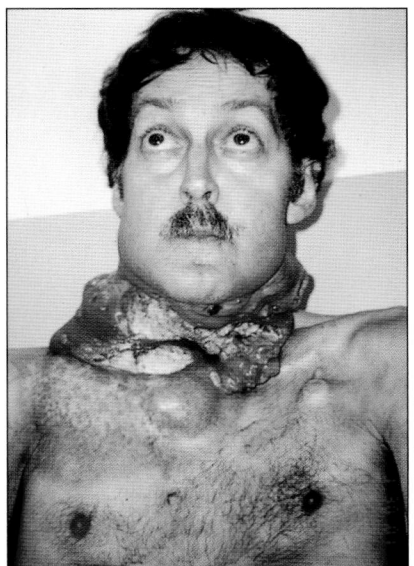

Fig 10-14g Although persistent lipo-sarcomas rarely metastasize, they will slowly and insidiously infiltrate skin and deep fascial planes.

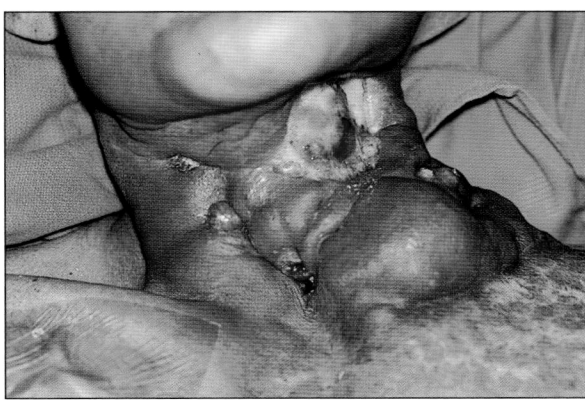

Fig 10-14h Liposarcoma eroding through skin, infil-trating into deeper tissues, and existing as a large mass all at the same time.

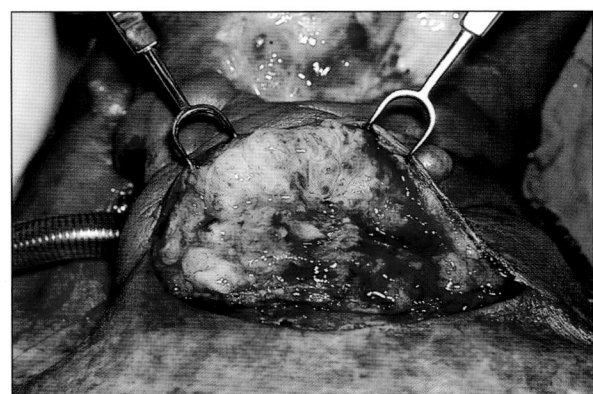

Fig 10-14i Liposarcoma infiltrating the dermis.

are vital because liposarcomas often produce satellite lesions, which are separate from but adjacent to the main body of the tumor. It would be easy to excise the main tumor focus and leave these satellite tumor foci behind. In addition, liposarcomas are well-known to insidiously proliferate along deep fascial planes (Figs 10-14g to 10-14i).

Postoperative radiotherapy is also recommended since these tumors are reasonably responsive to radiation in doses between 5,500 cGy and 7,500 cGy. Lymph node dissections are not required since these tumors usually metastasize only via bloodborne routes to the lungs. Radiation by itself is not ade-quate therapy because the tumor is usually too deep, too large, and not sufficiently radiosensitive for cure by radiotherapy as the sole modality.

PROGNOSIS ▶

Long-term follow-up is important because recurrences may be first observed 5 to 10 years later. Recurrence at the primary site is usually related to the completeness of the resection, which in turn is re-lated to its size, depth, and anatomic location. Recurrence at the primary site overall is about 50%.

Metastasis is directly related to histologic differentiation. The less differentiated, the more cellular, and the more pleomorphic the cells, the more likely the tumor will metastasize mainly to the lungs. The ad-justed 5-year survival rate for liposarcomas in locations other than the oral and maxillofacial area is about 65%. Because late recurrences and late metastases beyond 5 years occur, 10-year survival rates become significant and drop to less than 50%.

Neurogenic Malignancies

Malignant Peripheral Nerve Sheath Tumor (Neurosarcoma)

CLINICAL PRESENTATION AND PATHOGENESIS ▶

Most malignant peripheral nerve sheath tumors arise as isolated malignancies from no known stimulus. Approximately 10% arise from malignant transformation of a neurofibroma in hereditary neuro-fibromatosis with a latency of 15 to 20 years, and about another 10% result from radiation damage with a latency period of 15 to 30 years.

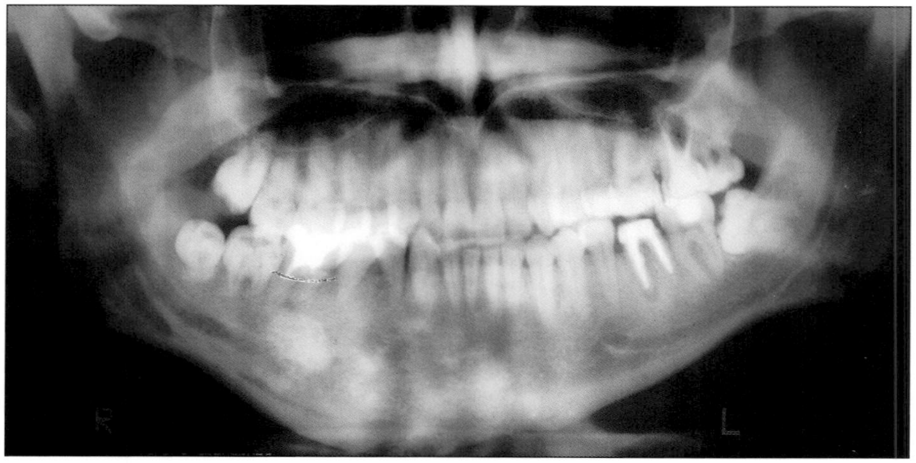

Fig 10-15a Diffuse irregular radiolucency with expansion of the mandibular canal related to a malignant peripheral nerve sheath tumor of the mandible.

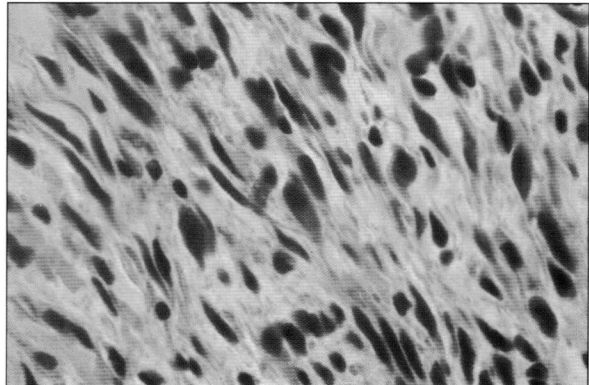

Fig 10-15b Malignant peripheral nerve sheath tumor showing spindle cells and cells with plump, hyperchromatic nuclei.

Malignant peripheral nerve sheath tumors are rare in the oral and maxillofacial area. They may occur centrally within the jaws or as a deep soft tissue malignancy. There is a slight male predilection (3:2) and an average age of 35 years, but a wide age range of 20 to 60 years. When a malignant peripheral nerve sheath tumor occurs within bone, it will produce a diffuse and irregular radiolucency (Fig 10-15a). At times it may demonstrate a widening of the mandibular canal, but mostly it will show a more complete destructive pattern with some bony expansion, erosions, and tooth mobility. It frequently produces a paresthesia or anesthesia of the regional nerve distribution. If it should arise from a motor nerve, which is even more rare, it will produce a paresis.

Soft tissue malignant peripheral nerve sheath tumors are firm to fleshy in consistency and are confluent with adjacent tissues. They usually will not demonstrate surface ulceration.

DIFFERENTIAL DIAGNOSIS ▶

Malignant peripheral nerve sheath tumors in the jaws are sufficiently rare that they are seldom high on a differential list. Instead, *osteosarcoma* is more often considered as are *fibrosarcoma, malignant fibrous histiocytoma,* and even some aggressive odontogenic tumors such as the *odontogenic myxoma* or *ameloblastoma.* Soft tissue malignant peripheral nerve sheath tumors clinically resemble a *fibrosarcoma* and their own benign counterpart, the *neurofibroma.* If the lesion occurs in the paranasal sinuses or the palatal mucosa, malignant salivary gland tumors such as *adenoid cystic carcinoma* and *mucoepidermoid carcinoma* also become realistic considerations.

DIAGNOSTIC WORK-UP ▶

The diagnosis is made from a deep incisional biopsy within the center of the lesion. Plain radiographs, a CT scan, or an MRI scan is recommended to ascertain the extent of the tumor and its involvement with adjacent structures.

HISTOPATHOLOGY ▶

Because they often closely resemble fibrosarcomas, these tumors are difficult to identify histologically. In general they are spindle cell tumors with cells arranged in fascicles. Nuclear pleomorphism and abnormal mitoses are usually present (Fig 10-15b). The nuclei may be wavy or comma shaped. Palisading is sometimes noted. The tumor itself is often hypocellular, and it may also contain myxoid areas.

The spectrum of differentiation can be quite wide, resembling cellular neurofibromas with some pleomorphism and mitoses at one end of the range to highly pleomorphic tumors at the other.

Heterotopic components such as bone and cartilage may be seen. The malignant *Triton tumor,* so named because the tumor cells can be viably transplanted into the Triton salamander, is a highly aggressive variant that also shows rhabdomyoblastic differentiation. In most cases the diagnosis is aided by the recognition that the tumor originates from a nerve trunk or a neurofibroma or is associated with neurofibromatosis. Electron microscopy may be of considerable help, and immunohistochemistry with frequent but not consistent S-100 protein positivity can also be employed.

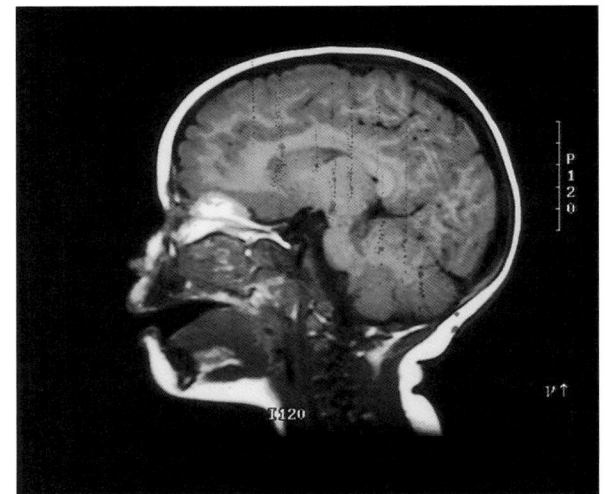

Fig 10-16 Large refractory olfactory neuroblastoma in the ethmoid sinuses and around the cribriform plate. The presenting symptom was loss of smell (anosmia).

TREATMENT

Malignant peripheral nerve sheath tumors are treated with very wide excision using 3-cm peripheral margins in both soft tissue and bone. All margins need to be assessed with frozen sections at the time of surgery. It is especially important to assess the margins along nerve because the tumor will tend to have its leading extension along its nerve of origin. Lymph node dissection is not required since this tumor metastasizes via bloodborne routes rather than via lymphatics. Chemotherapy and radiotherapy do not play a great role in the treatment of malignant peripheral nerve sheath tumors but are reserved for adjunctive care in recurrent, metastatic, or high-grade tumors.

PROGNOSIS

Recurrences represent a persistence of the original tumor and its continual growth after incomplete removal. Head and neck data are sparse, but overall recurrence rates are about 60%, and 5-year survival rates are 50%. The two most important factors related to recurrence and survival are the degree of differentiation of the tumor and the width of the surgical margins.

Metastasis from the oral and maxillofacial area is mostly to lung, skin, and vertebrae. All are related to venous tumor emboli and subsequent seeding into each respective tissue. Generally, malignant peripheral nerve sheath tumors that arise from pre-existing neurofibromas in hereditary neurofibromatosis have a worse prognosis. Recurrence rates are about 80% and metastasis rates about 65%. This is believed to be the result of three factors: later detection, because of their tendency to occur on the trunk and extremities; emergence at a histologically higher grade; and a propensity to develop multiple malignant peripheral nerve sheath tumors. Fortunately, only 4% of individuals with hereditary neurofibromatosis develop malignant peripheral nerve sheath tumors. The very rare Triton tumor has a nearly 0% survival rate.

Olfactory Neuroblastoma (Esthesioneuroblastoma)

CLINICAL PRESENTATION AND PATHOGENESIS

Olfactory neuroblastomas are considered malignant tumors of neuroectodernal cell origin arising from the neuroectodermal cell olfactory placode high in the nasal cavity. They are believed to be of that origin because of their production of norepinephrine and dopamine beta-hydroxylase, which is the enzyme that catalyzes the conversion of dopamine to norepinephrine.

Unlike other neuroblastomas, which occur in infancy up to the age of 3 years and are a common malignancy in children, olfactory neuroblastomas are very rare at any age, and 90% occur after the age of 10 years. The lesions will mainly present with unilateral nasal obstruction and epistaxis. Large lesions that erode into paranasal sinuses or the orbits may obstruct the nasolacrimal duct, causing epiphora, headaches, or anosmia (loss of the sense of smell) (Fig 10-16).

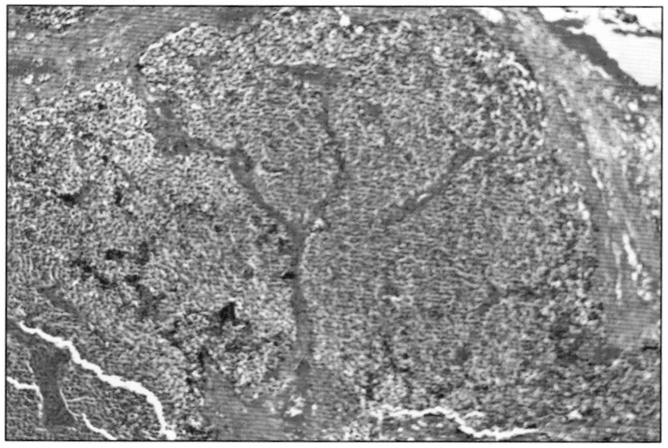

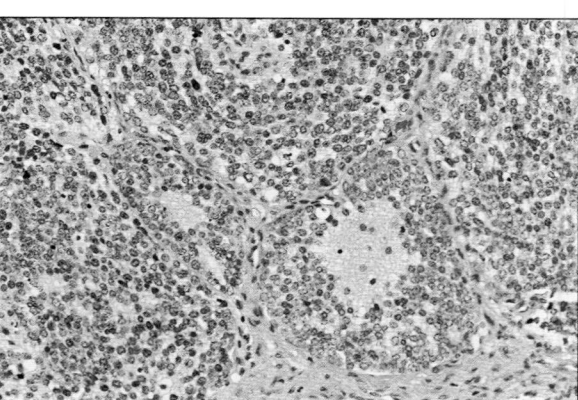

Fig 10-17b A higher-power view of an olfactory neuroblastoma shows the small round cells, which have little cytoplasm. Neurofibrillar material can be seen.

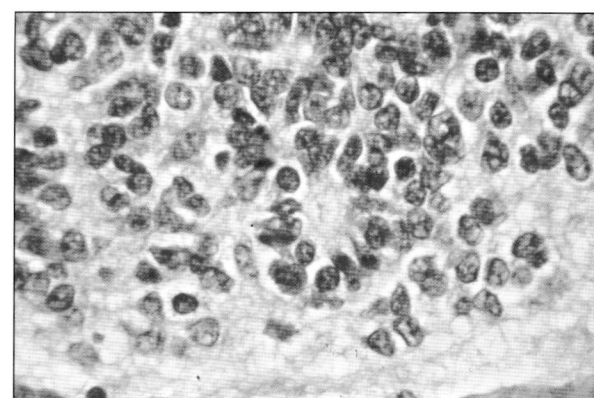

Fig 10-17c A Homer-Wright pseudorosette within an olfactory neuroblastoma.

Fig 10-17a Low-power view of an olfactory neuroblastoma in which fibrovascular trabeculae divide the tumor, which is composed of small dark-staining round cells, into a lobular pattern.

A nasal speculum examination will identify a gray fleshy mass in the superior meatus of the nasal cavity. Radiographs will show bony destruction, expansion, and sometimes focal calcifications within the lesion itself.

DIFFERENTIAL DIAGNOSIS

Nasal obstruction, epistaxis, and periorbital expansion in a teenager or young adult are most suggestive of a *nasopharyngeal angiofibroma* or a *rhabdomyosarcoma*. *Malignant fibrous histiocytoma* or *fibrosarcoma* are other considerations. Rarely, some tissue masses in this area may represent previously undiagnosed *meningioceles* that have perforated the cribriform plate to present in the superior aspect of the nasal cavity.

DIAGNOSTIC WORK-UP

A CT scan or an MRI scan is a necessary part of the work-up to assess size and bony involvement and to rule out a potential meningiocele, which would leak cerebrospinal fluid if it were biopsied. An angiogram may also be required if the epistaxis is prominent or if a nasopharyngeal angiofibroma is strongly suspected. A transnasal incisional biopsy should provide sufficient tissue to establish the diagnosis.

HISTOPATHOLOGY

In general, these tumors have a lobular architecture. The interlobular tissue is fibrovascular, and the tumor cells are small, dark-staining cells with little cytoplasm, resembling those of neuroblastoma (Figs 10-17a and 10-17b). The correlation of histologic grade with behavior has been questioned by some.

Grade I tumors have a large amount of neurofibrillary material. The cells are round and uniform, and mitoses are absent. Homer-Wright pseudorosettes may be seen. (These pseudorosettes are also seen in neuroblastomas.) They consist of tumor cells in a circular arrangement, surrounding a core of eosinophilic neurofibrillar material (Fig 10-17c).

Grade II tumors are more cellular but have less neurofibrillar material. There may be some mitotic activity, and nuclei are more atypical. Homer-Wright pseudorosettes are present, and gland-like structures may be seen.

Grade III tumors show increasing cellularity, mitoses, and anaplasia, along with decreasing neurofibrillar material. Flexner-Wintersteiner rosettes, consisting of a circular arrangement of columnar cells around a central lumen, are present. This type of rosette, also seen in retinoblastomas, is sometimes called a true rosette as opposed to a Homer-Wright pseudorosette.

Grade IV tumors retain their lobular architecture but are anaplastic with numerous mitoses. They resemble lymphomas or poorly differentiated carcinomas.

Electron microscopy is helpful for diagnosis because it identifies the presence of cytoplasmic neurosecretory granules. Immunohistochemically, neurofilament protein and neuron-specific enolase may be positive, and S-100 protein-positive cells surround the neuroblasts.

TREATMENT

Most tumors are treated with surgery and radiotherapy in the dose range of 3,500 cGy to 5,000 cGy. Smaller tumors limited to the nasal cavity are identified as stage A and may be treated by either of these modalities alone. Larger tumors extending from the nasal cavity to involve one or more of the paranasal sinuses are identified as stage B and usually require combination therapy. Tumors extending beyond the nasal cavity and sinuses are termed stage C and also require combination therapy.

Surgical approaches vary with the size of the tumor; smaller tumors are suitable for a transnasal approach or for external ethmoidectomy incisions over the lateral nasal bridges. Such incisions may be connected bilaterally over the nasofrontal suture area; this is termed the *open-sky approach* and is used for increased access. For large tumors, a bicoronal flap approach may be needed together with a Le Fort I downfracture to access the tumor from above and below.

PROGNOSIS ▶ The prognosis is related to the size of the tumor and to the extent to which it was excised. Therefore, early aggressive approaches yield the best results. Stage A patients have a 90% 5-year survival rate; stage B, 71%; and stage C, 47%. Uncontrolled disease will extend into the cranium and eventuate in death with an average survival time of 27 months.

Neuroblastoma

CLINICAL PRESENTATION AND PATHOGENESIS ▶ Neuroblastomas, accounting for about 10% of all childhood malignancies, are the third most common childhood malignancy after leukemias and brain tumors. Neuroblastomas arise from primordial neural crest cells and are, therefore, found mainly in the adrenal glands (50%) and in the paramidline area around the vertebrae. They are rare in the oral and maxillofacial area (2.5%).

Neuroblastomas are the most malignant part of a spectrum of tumors arising from neural crest cells, which originate and migrate from the mantle layer of the developing spinal cord. Proceeding along a scale of further differentiation, neuroblastomas are followed by ganglioneuroblastomas, which are malignant but less aggressive, and ganglioneuromas, which are benign.

Neuroblastomas in the oral and maxillofacial area appear with a variety of presentations, the most common of which is one or more nodular, usually bluish, masses. There may be several areas that are bluish and somewhat flat, resembling ecchymoses and giving the child a battered child appearance, which is characterized by numerous bluish-red cutaneous nodules and has given rise to the term "blueberry muffin baby" (Fig 10-18a). Usually, the child appears wasted, fatigued, and chronically ill. It is not uncommon for the child to have fever, weight loss, and joint pain, a presentation that may mimic that of rheumatic fever.

Whites are more commonly affected than blacks or Asians. About 25% of cases are congenital and 50% are diagnosed by 2 years of age. Almost all (over 90%) are diagnosed by age 5 years. Metastasis is common, and metastatic lesions in the skull, femur, and/or humerus at presentation are not unusual (Fig 10-18b).

DIFFERENTIAL DIAGNOSIS ▶ Depending on location and size, a large mass of darker pigmentation may suggest a *melanotic neuroectodermal tumor of infancy*, particularly in the maxilla and midface area. Similarly, *facial hemangiomas* may resemble a neuroblastoma, and a cluster of several may give rise to a so-called blueberry muffin baby appearance. In addition, other invasive malignancies in this age that may present with a mass and a chronically ill child are *rhabdomyosarcomas* and *Ewing sarcomas*. As stated, internal neuroblastomas, which are not clinically apparent, may produce malaise, fever, and joint pain suggestive of *rheumatic fever*.

DIAGNOSTIC WORK-UP ▶ Incisional biopsy is usually required to establish the diagnosis. Because metastasis is frequent, a radiographic survey or CT scan to assess the most common metastatic sites (skull, femur, humerus, and lung) is necessary. In addition, urine assessment for elevated levels of catecholamines (norepinephrine, epinephrine) and their metabolites (vanillylmandelic acid [VMA], homovanillic acid [HVA], and 3-methoxy-4 hydroxyphenylglycol [MHPG]), which are seen in over 90% of cases, is recommended.

HISTOPATHOLOGY ▶ These are infiltrative lobular tumors composed of round cells that resemble lymphocytes but are usually a little larger. They have deeply staining nuclei and scant cytoplasm. Mitoses are numerous. The cells lie in sheets, separated into lobules by fibrovascular septae (Figs 10-19a and 10-19b). There may be

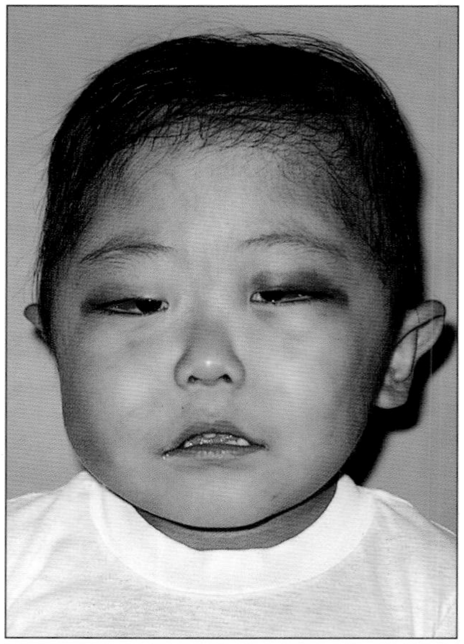

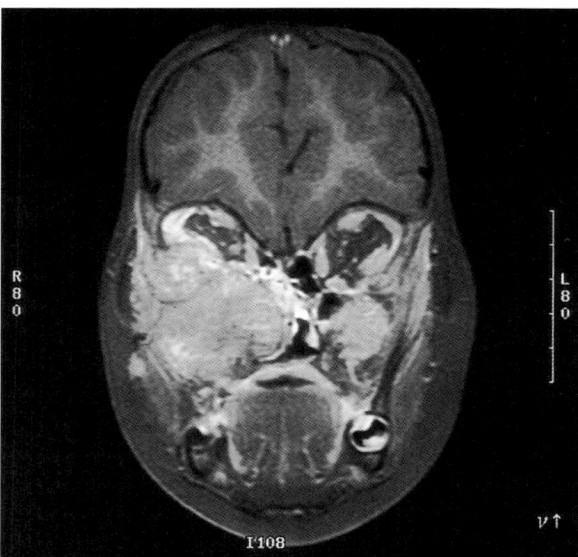

Fig 10-18a Typical presentation of a child with multi-focal neuroblastoma. The appearance resembling that of a battered child is common, as is the resemblance to a blueberry muffin, leading to the term "blueberry muffin baby."

Fig 10-18b Neuroblastomas will often be seen on a CT scan as large masses occupying soft tissue spaces, distorting normal anatomy.

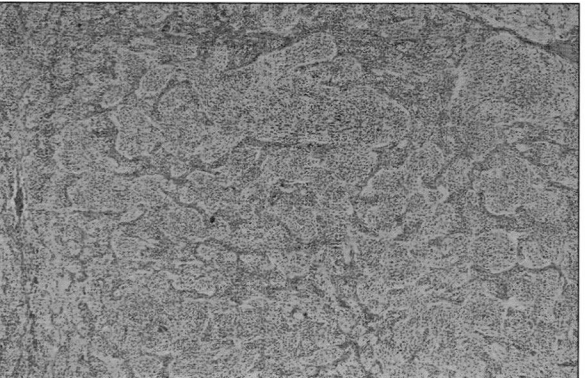

Fig 10-19a Like the olfactory neuroblastoma, this neuroblastoma of the adrenal gland shows the fibrovascular trabeculae dividing the round cell tumor.

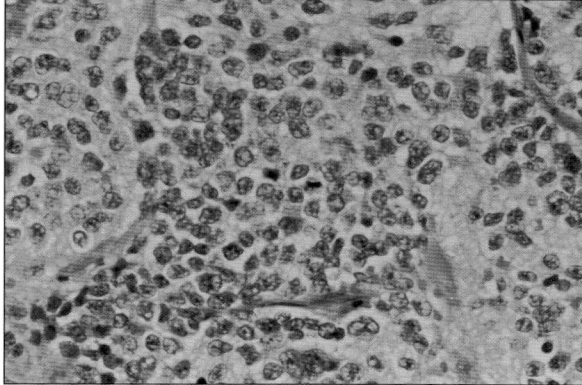

Fig 10-19b Higher-power view of Fig 10-19a shows the small round cells and the many mitoses.

areas of necrosis. When tumors are better differentiated, the cells develop cytoplasmic processes that polarize into a central focus, forming Homer-Wright pseudorosettes (see Fig 10-17c). Some neuroblastomas differentiate further and form ganglion cells. These large cells have eosinophilic cytoplasm and are often binucleated. Such tumors are called *ganglioneuroblastomas*. Further differentiation to ganglion cells and Schwann cells constitutes a *ganglioneuroma*. On rare occasions a neuroblastoma may differentiate into one of these tumors.

The neuroblastoma must be differentiated from embryonal rhabdomyosarcomas, Ewing sarcomas, and malignant lymphomas, which comprise the other major round cell tumors of childhood. In difficult cases, histochemistry and immunohistochemistry may be useful. Ewing sarcomas are glycogen- and neuron-specific enolase–negative, and neuroblastomas are usually neuron-specific enolase–positive. Rhabdomyosarcomas are usually desmin- and glycogen-positive, and lymphomas are leukocyte common antigen–positive.

480

A similar group of tumors, known as *extracranial-primitive neuroectodermal tumors*, are small round cell tumors that arise outside the central and sympathetic nervous systems and are thought to be of neural crest origin. The diagnosis is primarily one of exclusion and demonstration of neural origin through electron micoscopy and immunohistochemistry.

TREATMENT ▶

Surgery and radiation therapy are the focus of treatment for neuroblastomas, although chemotherapy sometimes plays an adjunctive role. Treatment is based on clinical staging. Stage I is a tumor confined to the organ of origin; a stage II tumor extends beyond the organ of origin but not across the midline; stage III is a continuous tumor across the midline; stage IV presents with distant metastasis. There is also a stage IV-S, which is a stage I or stage II neuroblastoma with a single, isolated metastatic deposit in the liver, skin, or bone.

Stage I and stage II neuroblastomas are treated solely with local excision using 2-cm margins. Stage III tumors are treated with local excision and radiotherapy. Stage IV tumors are usually treated with radiotherapy at the primary site as well as at all identified metastatic foci. Stage IV-S tumors are treated with excision of the primary tumor and radiotherapy for the metastatic focus.

PROGNOSIS AND FOLLOW-UP ▶

Although the last two decades have brought great improvement in the prognosis of such childhood sarcomas as leukemia and rhabdomyosarcoma, the same has not been true for neuroblastoma. The two most important clinical factors related to prognosis are age at diagnosis and clinical staging. Children younger than 2 years have a better 2-year survival rate (77%) than those older than 2 years (38%). Similarly, children with stage I or stage II disease have an 88% 2-year survival rate compared to only a 33% 2-year survival rate for patients with stage III or stage IV disease. In general, neuroblastomas in the oral and maxillofacial area are associated with a better prognosis than are those in the adrenal gland, retroperitoneum, or vertebrae, presumably because of earlier recognition. Of prognostic significance is that serum ferritin levels greater than 150 mg/mL and neuron-specific enolase levels greater than 100 mg/mL are associated with an unfavorable prognosis. The serum ferritin protein seems to be a tumor product that coats the surface of T lymphocytes, inhibiting their function. Neuron-specific enolase appears to be a tumor product indicative of the tumor's metabolic activity. These serum parameters, regardless of their initial levels, are useful for assessing recurrent disease, as is the persistence or return of elevated urine catecholamine levels.

Myogenic Malignancies

Rhabdomyosarcomas

CLINICAL PRESENTATION AND PATHOGENESIS ▶

Rhabdomyosarcomas are malignant tumors of primitive mesenchymal cells that undergo partial rhabdomyoblast differentiation. Unlike other soft tissue sarcomas, which generally occur in adults and are more common in sites other than oral and maxillofacial regions, rhabdomyosarcomas are most common in this region (44% of all rhabdomyosarcomas) and occur mostly in children and teenagers. In fact, 2% of rhabdomyosarcomas are present at birth, and 5% occur in individuals younger than 1 year.

There are three basic histologic types: embryonal, alveolar, and pleomorphic, with the embryonal type bearing the best prognosis and being by far the most common type found in the oral and maxillofacial area. Males are affected a little more commonly than females (1.5:1). Tumors have a peak incidence at age 4 years and another at age 17 years.

In the oral and maxillofacial area, the orbit is the most common location, followed by the nasal cavity, mouth, sinuses, cheek, and neck. The tumor presents as a rapidly growing, fleshy mass, which readily invades and destroys bone. In the orbit, the medial upper quadrant is the preferred location with prominent nasal and orbital bone destruction as well as invasion into the eyelids producing marked eyelid edema. Proptosis is another frequent feature of orbital tumors, along with diplopia and epiphora, but vi-

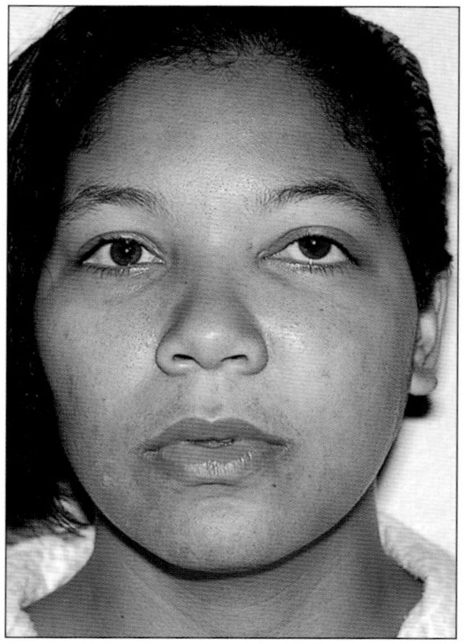

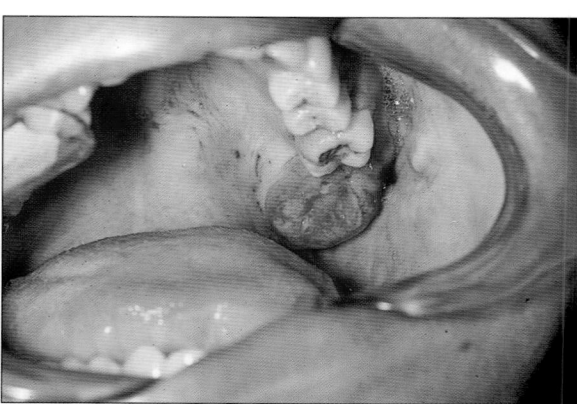

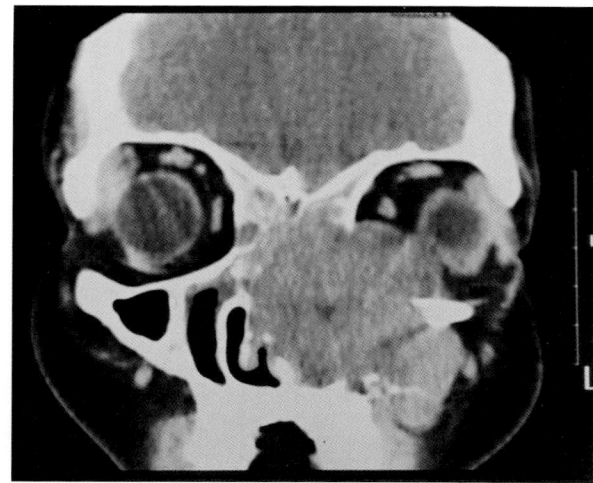

Fig 10-20a Twenty-three-year-old woman who presented with diplopia from an elevation of her left globe due to a rhabdomyosarcoma that expanded into the orbit, the oral cavity, and the naso-ethmoidal area.

Fig 10-20b A common oral presentation of the rare rhabdomyosarcoma is that of a fleshy mass protruding through the posterior maxillary alveolus in a child, teenager, or young adult.

Fig 10-20c The oral presentation of a rhabdomyosarcoma is often the "tip of the iceberg." Examination often reveals an extensive mass in the maxilla, nose, orbit, and ethmoids.

sual acuity usually is not affected (Fig 10-20a). Those that arise in the cheek, maxillary sinus, or masseter area readily invade into adjacent bone and the orbit (Figs 10-20b and 10-20c).

Pain is not a prominent feature of rhabdomyosarcoma despite the tumor's bony destruction and often large size. However, sensory nerve loss (anesthesias and paresthesias) is common, and, if motor nerves are involved, paresis or paralysis may occur.

Rhabdomyosarcomas are not radiographically distinctive but will show primarily the anticipated soft tissue mass and bony destruction.

Although rhabdomyosarcomas are frequently described as tumors of muscle origin or of muscle cells, their histogenesis is, like that of other sarcomas, from primitive mesenchymal cells, which are specific for these tumors and undergo rhabdomyoblast differentiation. They may also arise from residual fetal rhabdomyoblasts, which might explain their predilection for children and their occasional occurrence in fetal life. It is nearly impossible for them to arise from muscle cells proper since these cells do not dedifferentiate, and even injured muscle cells fail to mitose but instead repair via scar tissue formation.

DIFFERENTIAL DIAGNOSIS ▶

A tumor with rapid growth and destructiveness in a child or young adult should suggest a rhabdomyosarcoma. Other rapidly destructive lesions in this age group are *Ewing sarcoma*, *neuroblastoma* (the third most common malignancy in children), an *acute Langerhans cell histiocytosis*, and less commonly, a *malignant peripheral T-cell lymphoma*. All of these are also known to invade bone in a destructive manner.

DIAGNOSTIC WORK-UP ▶

The diagnosis is established by means of a deep incisional biopsy within the center of the tumor. Plain radiographs, a CT scan, or an MRI scan is required to understand the tumor's size, spatial anatomic relationship, and extent of bony destruction. The CT or MRI scan should include detailed cuts of the base of the skull to assess potential invasion into this area and include the entire skull to rule out brain extension or metastasis. A chest radiograph is taken to rule out lung metastasis, and because rhabdomyosarcomas have a propensity to metastasize to bone marrow, a bone marrow aspiration is also a strong consideration.

HISTOPATHOLOGY ▶

Rhabdomyosarcomas are classified according to their histologic appearance into one of three categories.

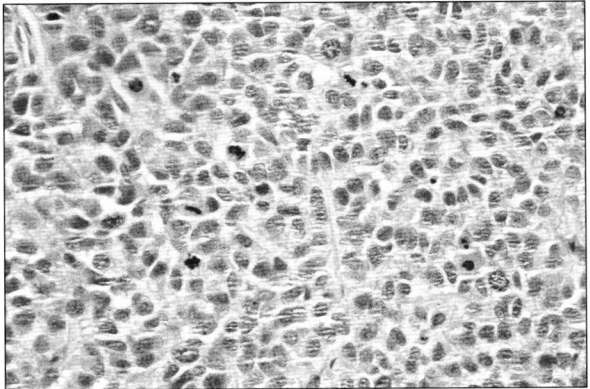

Fig 10-21 An embryonal rhabdomyosarcoma composed predominantly of small round cells. Numerous mitoses can be seen.

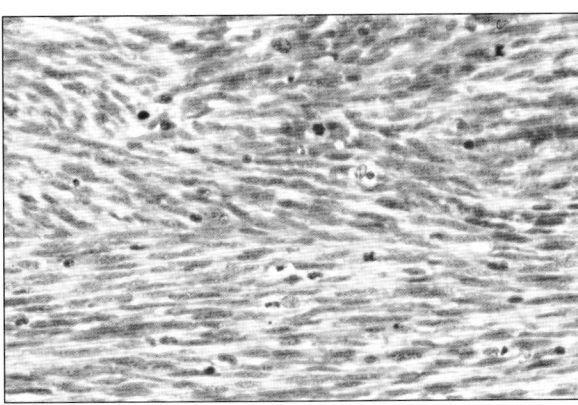

Fig 10-22 A rhabdomyosarcoma with a predominantly spindle cell pattern. Mitoses are present.

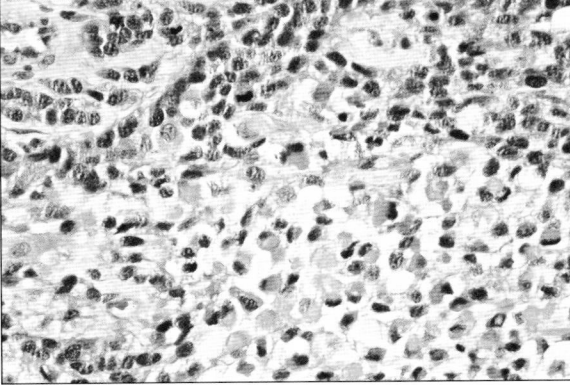

Fig 10-23 In this rhabdomyosarcoma, differentiation to skeletal muscle can be seen. Many cells have intense eosinophilic cytoplasm and peripherally placed nuclei.

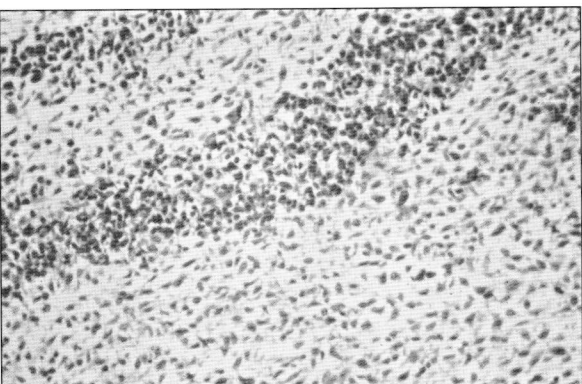

Fig 10-24 An embryonal rhabdomyosarcoma with closely packed, poorly differentiated round cells within a more myxoid arrangement.

Embryonal Rhabdomyosarcoma

The embryonal rhabdomyosarcoma develops from undifferentiated mesenchymal stem cells, which can resemble different stages in the development of skeletal muscle. Thus, the histologic picture can be quite varied. In many instances the tumors may contain small round cells, but they may also contain spindle cells (Figs 10-21 and 10-22). Depending on their differentiation, the cytoplasm may be scant and indistinct or more abundant and strongly eosinophilic (Fig 10-23). The cytoplasm may be vacuolated because of the deposition of glycogen. Tadpole-shaped cells may be present, and cross striations can sometimes be identified in more well-differentiated tumors. Nuclei are usually hyperchromatic and on occasion may be eccentrically situated (see Fig 10-23). Mitoses may be numerous. Stromal collagen is scant. A characteristic pattern shows areas of hypercellularity with densely packed cells alternating with less cellular myxoid areas (Fig 10-24). These tumors are infiltrative. They may be difficult to distinguish from other round cell tumors of childhood, such as neuroblastoma, Ewing sarcoma, and malignant lymphoma.

A variant of embryonal rhabdomyosarcoma is the botryoid type, which is usually seen within mucosa-lined cavities such as the nasopharynx and nasal and oral cavities. Because of their unrestricted growth, these polypoid tumors have a mucoid stroma and myxoid appearance with relatively few cells. Below the covering epithelium, a dense zone of undifferentiated cells, which has been termed the *cambium layer of Nicholson*, is often found.

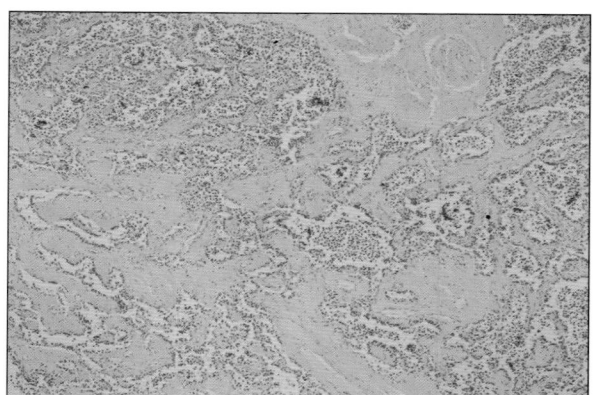

Fig 10-25a A low-power view of an alveolar rhabdomyosarcoma shows the alveolar spaces.

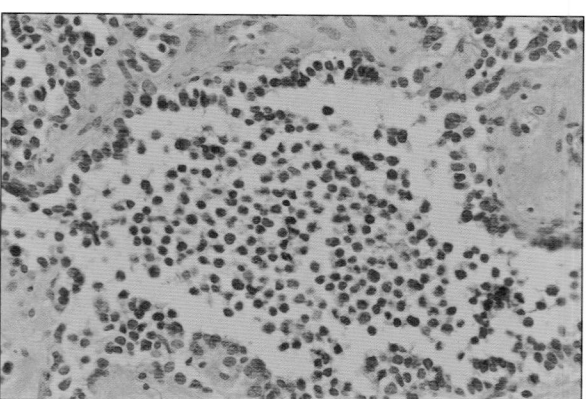

Fig 10-25b A higher-power view of Fig 10-25a shows the small round cells composing the tumor.

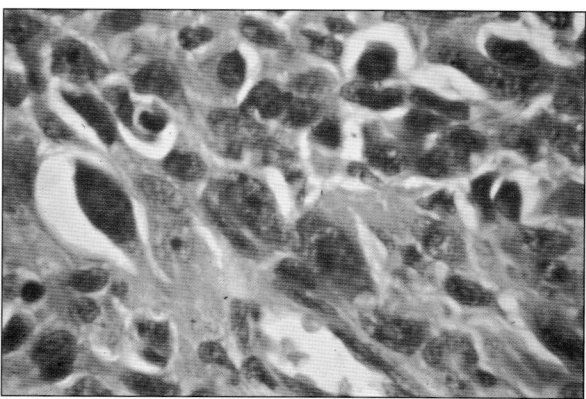

Fig 10-26 A pleomorphic rhabdomyosarcoma showing a tadpole-shaped cell with the nucleus at the dilated head and cytoplasm forming the tail.

Alveolar Rhabdomyosarcoma

The alveolar rhabdomyosarcoma is characterized by the presence of clefts or alveolar spaces, which are formed through loss of cohesion within the tumor cell aggregates. The spaces are lined by a single layer of tumor cells, which are attached to fibrous septae (Figs 10-25a and 10-25b). Some of the cells may protrude into the space in pseudopod-like fashion. Most of the tumor cells are rounded. Multinucleated giant cells and mitoses are common. Cross striations may sometimes be identified.

Pleomorphic Rhabdomyosarcoma

Pleomorphic rhabdomyosarcoma may be difficult to separate from other pleomorphic sarcomas such as malignant fibrous histiocytoma. There is great variation in the size and shape of the cells. Racquet-shaped cells, tadpole-shaped cells, strap cells, and giant cells may be present, and bizarre mitoses are not uncommon (Fig 10-26). Cross striations are not usually observed.

The histologic diagnosis of rhabdomyosarcoma is often difficult and usually requires ultrastructural examination and immunohistochemistry. Immunohistochemistry in particular is of considerable help. While there are many markers available, myoglobin and desmin are probably the most useful. Cytogenetic studies can be diagnostic for alveolar rhabdomyosarcoma, which typically shows a chromosomal translocation, t(2;13)(q35;q14) or rarely t(1;13)(p36;q14).

TREATMENT ▶ The treatment of rhabdomyosarcoma has been a great success story dating back to 1960, when the Intergroup Rhabdomyosarcoma Study (IRS) created staging and combination treatment protocols. Until that time, rhabdomyosarcoma survival rates were dismal. For oral and maxillofacial tumors, the 5-year survival rate was only 6% and the average survival time was only 16 months. Today, the outcome is vastly improved.

The IRS clinical staging parameters are presented in Table 10-2. The staging is based on local excision rather than on radical surgery and takes into account tumor size as it relates to the degree of excision. Therefore, the initial therapy is local excision without radical ablation of normal tissues. This is a decided deviation from normal oncologic surgical principles, but one that is acceptable in these cases because of the responsiveness of residual tumor cells at the margins to chemotherapy and radiotherapy. Examination of the resected specimen for residual disease at the margins then becomes critical because tumor staging will depend on this assessment.

Table 10-2 Rhabdomyosarcoma staging (after local excision)

Group I:	Localized disease
Group II:	Residual microscopic disease
Group III:	Residual gross disease
Group IV:	Metastasis present at diagnosis

Table 10-3 Multimodal therapy for rhabdomyosarcoma

1. Local excision
2. 4,000-cGy to 6,000-cGy radiation
3. Vincristine-adriamycin-cytoxan (VAC) chemotherapy for 1 to 2 years; add actinomycin-D (VACA) for groups III and IV

The surgeon's assessment of visible disease remaining after surgery as well as the identification of any distant metastasis will dictate the staging. From this information alone, the choice and degree of additional therapy is made. Group I refers to localized disease and microscopic margins free of tumor. Group II indicates grossly negative but microscopically positive margins. Group III indicates grossly visible disease left at the time of surgery. Group IV indicates identification of distant metastasis irrespective of the tumor resection margins (see Table 10-2). In general, group I and group II tumors are treated with three chemotherapeutic agents: vincristine, adriamycin, and cyclophosphamide (Cytoxan) (VAC). Group II tumors receive, in addition, radiotherapy of 4,000 cGy to 6,000 cGy over 6 weeks. Group III and group IV tumors receive the same chemotherapy, but with the addition of actinomycin D (VACA) and radiotherapy of the same dose to the primary site and to any metastatic focus (Table 10-3).

For tumors of the oral and maxillofacial area, surgery does not include regional lymph node dissection. Chemotherapy is continued for 1 year, or up to 2 years if there remains a suspicion of residual disease.

PROGNOSIS ▶ The strict protocol of the IRS staging has allowed for reliable survival statistics. The 5-year survival rate is 83% for group I tumors, 70% for group II tumors, 52% for group III tumors, and 20% for group IV tumors. Inherent in these data is the conclusion that the size of the tumor and its resectability are the most important prognostic factors. Therefore, a speedy diagnosis and work-up are recommended; prompt surgery followed by clinical staging with follow-on therapy is the challenge.

When cure is not obtained, it is usually because of uncontrollable disease at the primary site. Metastasis, when it occurs, is to lung or bone marrow and will frequently be associated with a local recurrence as well.

Because the therapy advanced by the IRS group is very effective, many children live into adult life. However, they must accept and at times be treated for the long-term complications of their therapy. Complications possibly related to early life chemotherapy are leukemia, neutropenia, anemia, and chronic diarrhea. Those seemingly related to radiotherapy are xerophthalmia, xerostomia, hypoplastic facial bones and mandible, hypoplastic dentition (Fig 10-27a), dysphasia with a propensity for aspiration, radiation fibrosis limiting jaw opening (Figs 10-27b and 10-27c), and osteoradionecrosis. In fact, the ongoing damage of radiation cellular injury has caused a significant number of patients to develop osteoradionecrosis of the mandible 20 to 30 years later.

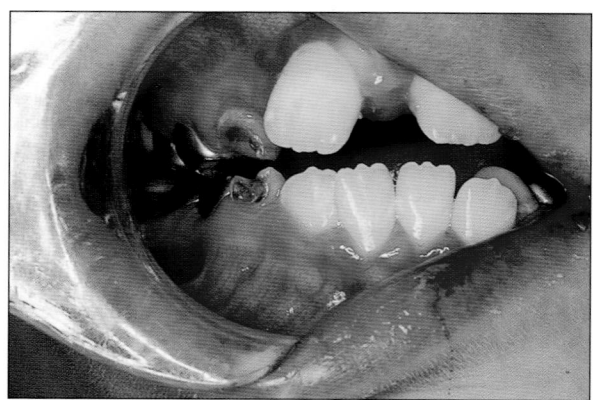

Fig 10-27a Radiation caries, hypoplasia of teeth, and a limited jaw opening in a 10-year-old child who received radiotherapy for a rhabdomyosarcoma at the age of 2 months. (See also Fig 8-10b.)

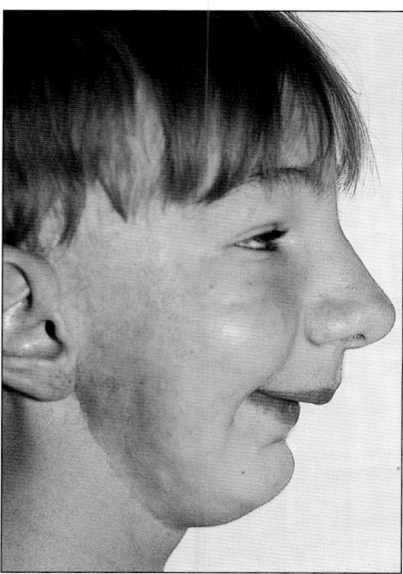

Fig 10-27b Radiation-induced hypoplasia of the mandible and restricted opening secondary to radiotherapy to the masseter and ramus area for a rhabdomyosarcoma at the age of 2 months.

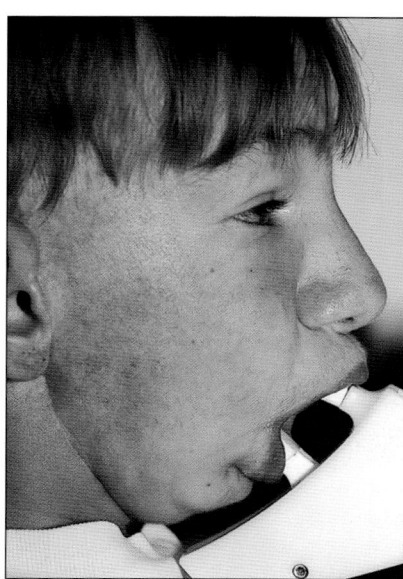

Fig 10-27c Early-life radiotherapy to the area of the pterygomasseteric sling creates a lifelong problem of limited opening. Here, after a surgery to release radiation fibrosis, a Therabite device is used at frequent daily intervals to maintain the opening.

Leiomyosarcoma

CLINICAL PRESENTATION AND PATHOGENESIS ▶

Leiomyosarcomas are a relatively uncommon type of sarcoma, accounting for only 7% of all soft tissue sarcomas. Most occur in the retroperitoneum and within the abdomen; others are associated with large blood vessels, such as the inferior vena cava and pulmonary artery, and are often referred to as *leiomyosarcomas of vascular origin*. Intraoral leiomyosarcomas are extremely rare because of the paucity of smooth muscle in oral tissues; the palate (Fig 10-28) and tongue are their most common locations. Similarly, cutaneous leiomyosarcomas in the facial skin and skin of the neck also are rare, accounting for only about 2% of sarcomas involving skin. Both oral mucosal and facial skin leiomyosarcomas are presumed to arise from the smooth muscles around arteries and arterioles.

Leiomyosarcomas are malignancies that occur in adults, most of whom are older than 50 years. The tumors are generally small (2 cm or less). Those that occur in the dermis often produce a discoloration, a corrugated appearance, or an ulceration of the skin. Those that occur at the subcutaneous level cause an elevation of the skin but no surface changes and may attain a larger size.

Leiomyosarcomas are solid tumors. Although they often arise from the smooth muscle cells of blood vessels, they do not form blood vessels and do not contain blood. They also arise de novo and are not known to transform from a benign leiomyoma. Each tumor is usually fixed within the submucosa or the subcutaneous layer of the skin and may infiltrate the underlying bone or muscle.

DIFFERENTIAL DIAGNOSIS ▶

The presentation of a small, usually nonnucleated fixed mass would suggest malignancies that are more common than a leiomyosarcoma. When a leiomyosarcoma is diagnosed, it is usually a surprise finding. In the oral cavity, a fixed palatal mass would be more suggestive of minor salivary gland malignancies such as *adenoid cystic carcinoma, mucoepidermoid carcinoma*, and a *polymorphous low-grade adenocarcinoma*. If it occurs within the tongue, a concern about a *squamous cell carcinoma* from an unseen surface ulceration or a *granular cell tumor* would be appropriate.

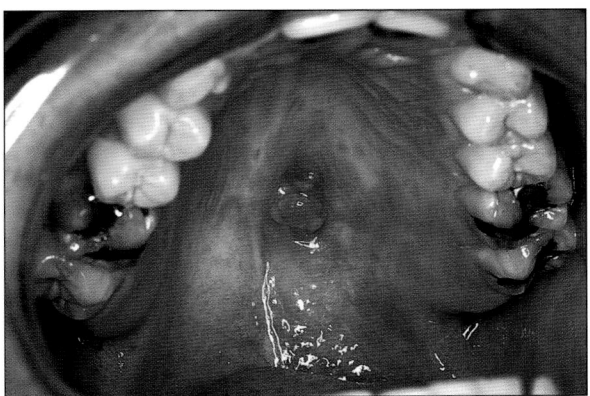

Fig 10-28 A leiomyosarcoma of the palate presenting as a soft tissue mass.

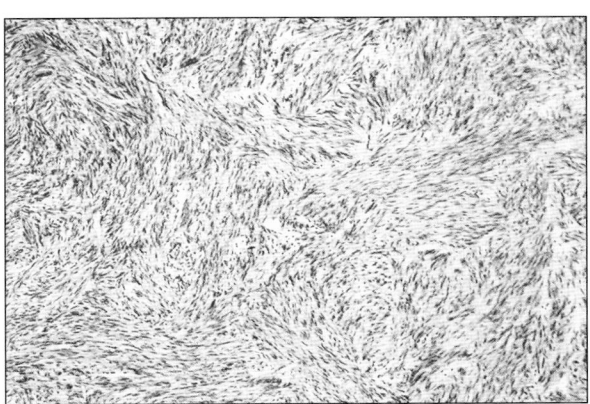

Fig 10-29a Low-power view of a leiomyosarcoma showing fascicles of spindle cells.

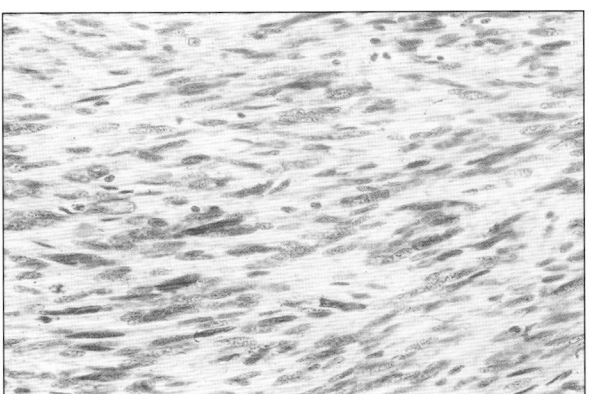

Fig 10-29b High-power view of the tumor shown in Fig 10-29a demonstrating the often blunt-ended nuclei.

DIAGNOSTIC WORK-UP ▶

HISTOPATHOLOGY ▶

On facial skin a leiomyosarcoma would mimic several of the malignant skin appendage tumors such as a *pilomatric carcinoma*, a *microcystic adnexal carcinoma*, and a *ductal eccrine carcinoma*.

A CT scan or an MRI is recommended to more precisely assess the size of the tumor, its infiltration, and its relationship to normal structures. An exploration and biopsy usually follows.

These tumors are usually composed of fascicles of spindle cells with eosinophilic cytoplasm and centrally placed nuclei, which are blunt ended and cigar shaped (Figs 10-29a and 10-29b). Multinucleated giant cells are frequently present. Sometimes the cells are more epithelioid and rounded with eosinophilic or clear cytoplasm. Pleomorphism is a variable feature. It may be difficult to separate the malignant from the benign tumors. One widely used criterion for malignancy is the presence of 5 or more mitoses per 10 high-power fields.

A trichrome stain will color the longitudinal parallel myofibrils red, and PAS stain will indicate the presence of glycogen, which can be helpful in separating the tumor from other spindle-cell neoplasms that it might resemble. These include fibrosarcomas and neurogenic tumors, the latter particularly when there is a palisading pattern. Leiomyosarcomas sometimes also may demonstrate myxoid changes.

TREATMENT AND PROGNOSIS ▶

Leiomyosarcomas of the oral cavity and facial skin area are usually low-grade malignancies. They are best treated with an excision using 2-cm margins and supported with frozen sections at the time of surgery. Although recurrence rates are between 25% and 40%, metastases and tumor-related deaths are very uncommon. Recurrences are associated with the more deeply infiltrating tumors, underscoring the particular importance of attaining a tumor-free margin at the deep surface. Recurrences are treated with re-excision. Adjunctive radiotherapy or chemotherapy is ineffective.

Vascular Malignancies

Angiosarcoma

CLINICAL PRESENTATION AND PATHOGENESIS ▶

Angiosarcomas are malignant tumors that arise from either vascular or lymphatic endothelium; thus, the term *angiosarcoma* here includes malignancies that would otherwise be termed *malignant hemangioendotheliomas* or *lymphangiosarcomas*. Even as a group, angiosarcomas are the rarest form of soft tissue sarcomas, accounting for less than 1% of all sarcomas. However, one of their common sites is the skin of the maxillofacial area and the scalp (52%). They may occur at any age but are more common with advancing age, with most occurring in the elderly. Men are affected twice as frequently as women.

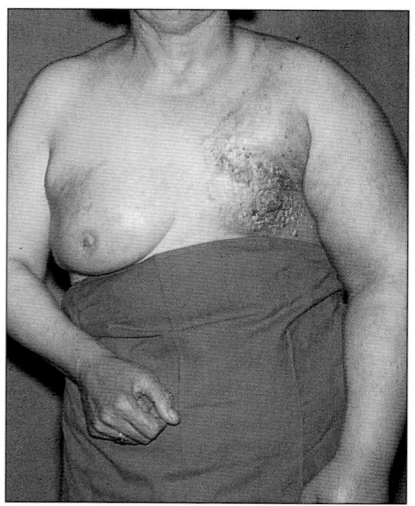

Fig 10-30 Chronic lymphedema from a radical mastectomy and an axillary lymph node dissection is a predisposing factor to the development of an angiosarcoma.

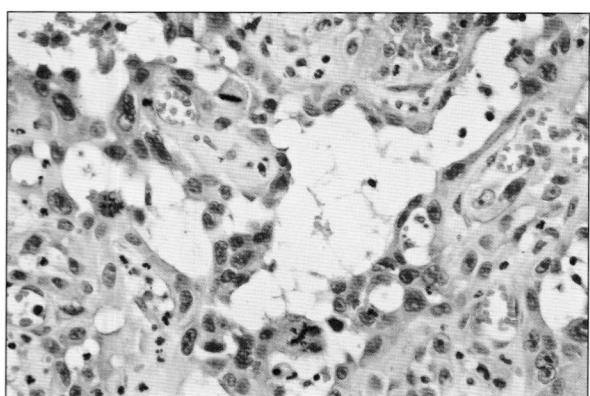

Fig 10-31 An angiosarcoma showing intercommunicating vascular channels lined by atypical cells with plump nuclei, many of which project into the lumen. Mitotic figures are apparent.

The tumor usually begins as a flat, ecchymotic-looking area with a firm, indurated edge. Many are associated with facial edema and are presumably of lymphatic endothelial origin. As the lesions mature, they become nodular and fleshy and will ulcerate. Most are painless, but secondary infection of ulcerated lesions may produce pain. They are not vascular lesions, per se, and therefore do not pose a bleeding risk. Instead, they are of vascular cellular origin.

Angiosarcomas in sites other than the oral and maxillofacial area and scalp are more closely associated with chronic lymphedema, not as a manifestation of the tumor but as an etiologic agent. It is believed that chronic lymphedema from past surgeries such as mastectomies or injuries is a predisposing factor. About 10% of angiosarcomas develop in chronic lymphedematous tissues (Fig 10-30). Another 10% are believed to be late effects of radiotherapy for previous malignancies of other types.

DIFFERENTIAL DIAGNOSIS

Induration and ulceration of angiosarcomas lead to a suspicion of malignancy. However, their rarity makes them an unusual consideration on a differential list. Instead, more common ulcerating malignant lesions that can occur on facial and forehead skin as well as scalp are considered, primarily *basal cell carcinoma, melanoma, skin squamous cell carcinoma,* and *eccrine tumors of sweat gland origin.* If the tumor is nodular and bulky, a so-called turban tumor or, more appropriately, *cylindroma of the scalp,* is another possibility.

DIAGNOSTIC WORK-UP

A deep incisional biopsy within the lesion's center is diagnostic.

HISTOPATHOLOGY

Angiosarcomas are infiltrating tumors that usually form irregular vascular channels that often intercommunicate to form a network. The endothelial cells lining the channels are plump and hyperchromatic and may proliferate to form papillary projections. Nuclear irregularities and atypical mitoses are usually present (Fig 10-31). There is a range of differentiation in these tumors, from lesions resembling hemangiomas at one end to those so anaplastic that they resemble melanoma or carcinoma. A reticulin stain can be useful to demarcate the lumen and show the tumor cells within it. Immunohistochemical staining for factor VIII antigen, which is a marker of vascular differentiation, is variably present in almost all tissues and is therefore not reliable.

TREATMENT

Radical excision with 5-cm margins and/or radical electron-beam radiotherapy of 7,000 cGy or more are the treatments associated with the best outcomes. Because this tumor is known to spread peripherally along the dermis and microscopically appears at a distance from the clinical borders, wide excision

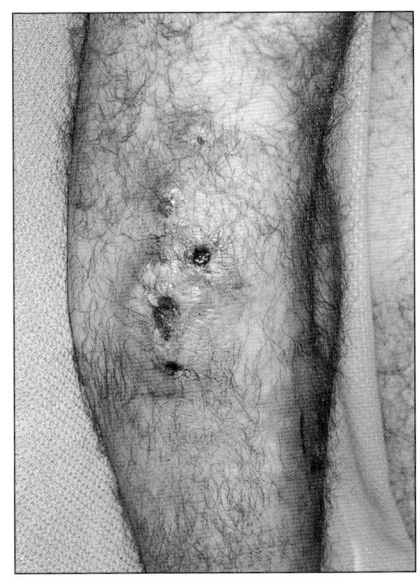

Fig 10-32a Multiple chronic classic Kaposi sarcoma lesions of the leg. Some are present as patch lesions, some as plaque lesions, and others as nodules.

or wide-field radiotherapy is important. In addition, lymph node metastasis is common, necessitating surgical lymphadenectomy or requiring that radiotherapy fields include the neck.

PROGNOSIS ▶

The biologic behavior of angiosarcomas runs the spectrum of low grade to very high grade. Some of the low-grade types are singled out and called malignant hemangioendotheliomas, but this is arbitrary and misleading. However, most are high-grade malignancies with a poor prognosis. Most studies have shown a 10% to 15% 5-year survival rate due to late diagnosis, complications with elderly patients, and aggressive tumor behavior. One half of patients die within 15 months of the diagnosis. The tumor's size at the time of treatment is the factor most affecting prognosis. Patients who were cured were treated early; a lesion size of 5 cm is the critical size over which survival percentage falls precipitously. Death occurs equally from complications related to recurrence and from metastasis. Metastasis is mostly to cervical lymph nodes regionally and to lung distantly.

Kaposi Sarcoma

CLINICAL PRESENTATION AND PATHOGENESIS ▶

Kaposi sarcoma is a vascular neoplasm that was rarely seen in the US before the emergence of HIV/AIDS in 1980. It is now thought to be a multifocal viral-induced tumor that occurs as a result of a genetic predisposition. This theory is based on the high incidence of HLA-DR5 antigens in individuals with any of the five types of Kaposi sarcoma, which are described below.

Classic Kaposi Sarcoma

Moritz Kaposi first described this form in five individuals in 1872. It principally affects elderly men in their 60s and 70s who are usually of Jewish, Greek, or Italian ethnicity. It forms violaceous macules, papules, and nodules often symmetrically on the skin of the lower extremities. It is chronic and slowly progresses through an early patch stage and into plaque and nodular stages (Fig 10-32a). The lesions increase slowly in size and number, spreading proximally and emerging into plaques or vascular nodules. Characteristically, individuals live with these lesions and die of unrelated causes years later. About 35% develop a second malignancy, usually lymphoma, leukemia, multiple myeloma, or colon cancer.

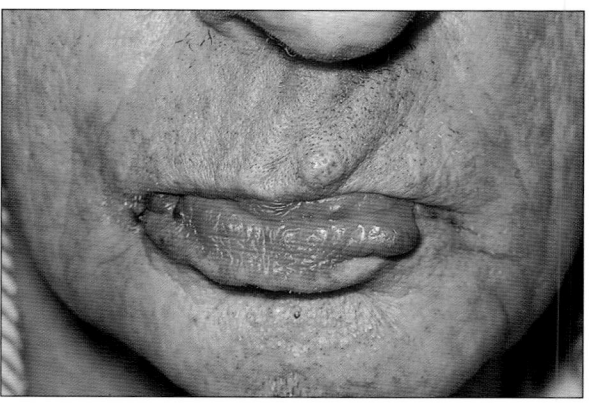

Fig 10-32b Chronic classic Kaposi sarcoma nodule of the lower lip resembling a varix or a small hemangioma.

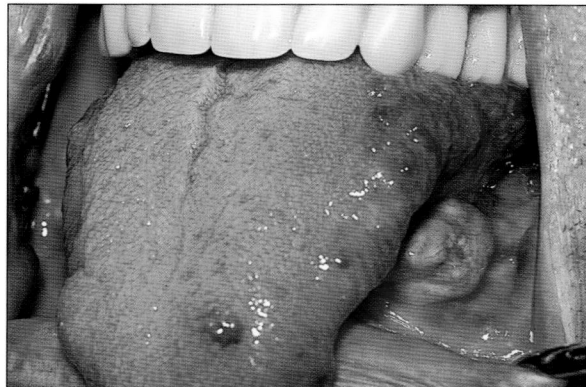

Fig 10-32c Multiple classic Kaposi sarcoma lesions on the tongue and floor of the mouth.

African Cutaneous Kaposi Sarcoma

One of two African types, the cutaneous form of African Kaposi sarcoma is endemic and parallels the course of classic Kaposi sarcoma but in a more infiltrating and aggressive manner. It typically occurs in men, but the average age is 35 years as compared to an average of 68 years for classic Kaposi sarcoma. This form does not usually involve lymph nodes, but the lesions spread proximally more rapidly and infiltrate more extensively.

African Lymphadenopathic Kaposi Sarcoma

This form is also endemic and occurs specifically in African children, who present with prominent generalized lymphadenopathy of most lymphatic systems and with only sparse skin lesions. The salivary glands are frequently involved as well. The course is fulminant, with internal organ Kaposi sarcomas developing in several organs, and rapidly leads to death. Despite the well-documented high rate of HIV/AIDS in Africa, these African forms of Kaposi sarcoma are not associated with HIV infections.

AIDS-Related Kaposi Sarcoma

The emergence of AIDS brought renewed interest in and attention to Kaposi sarcoma. Initially, Kaposi sarcoma was seen in 30% to 50% of homosexual men infected with AIDS as opposed to only 4% in heterosexual IV drug users and others who had AIDS. Today, however, Kaposi sarcoma is also rare in homosexual men with AIDS. The incidence has dropped to 5%. The leading theory for this decline is the control of secondary viral infections, which are cofactors in the oncogenic stimulus of Kaposi sarcoma. Homosexual men are known to have a higher incidence of coviral infection, explaining the initial high incidence of Kaposi sarcoma in this group and its reversal with today's broad-based anti-viral therapies.

Kaposi Sarcoma in Immunosuppressed Individuals

Approximately 0.4% of renal transplant patients develop Kaposi sarcoma, representing a 200-fold increase over that of the general population. About 30% of these patients die of multifocal pulmonary or gastrointestinal Kaposi sarcoma or of a second malignancy, usually a lymphoma. Transplant-associated Kaposi sarcoma has been associated with all of the immunosuppressive drugs that are currently used to reduce the risk of rejection: azathioprine, cyclophosphamide, prednisone, and cyclosporine, either alone or in combination. The Kaposi lesions usually develop 18 months after the transplant and emerge with

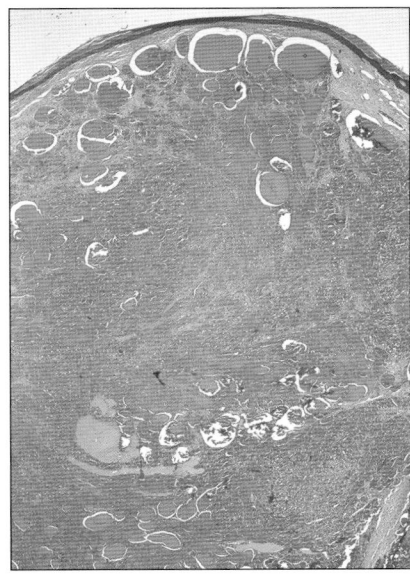

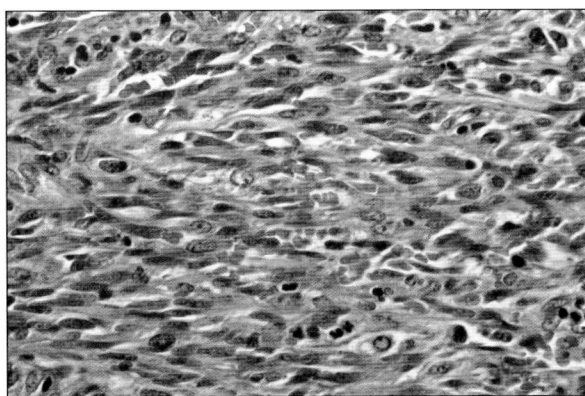

Fig 10-33a The tumor stage of Kaposi sarcoma. Low-power view shows the rounded, exophytic contour of the mass. Numerous dilated blood-filled channels can be seen, but in addition more solid areas compose the major portion of the tumor.

Fig 10-33b High-power view shows the spindle cell proliferation, with erythrocytes lying between the cells, that is typical of Kaposi sarcoma.

the loss of cellular immunity as diagnosed by skin testing with phytohemagglutinin (PHA) and dinitrochlorobenzene (DNCB).

DIFFERENTIAL DIAGNOSIS ▶

Because of its vascular nature, Kaposi sarcoma strongly resembles other vascular lesions. Lesions in the oral cavity, as well as those on the maxillofacial skin, may initially resemble *bruising* (ecchymosis) or a deeply located *low-grade mucoepidermoid carcinoma*. As they become more papular and nodular (Figs 10-32b and 10-32c) they appear more like *hemangiomas, lymphangiomas,* and *arteriovenous hemangiomas*. Even though it is uncommon, *bacillary epithelioid angiomatosis* may appear as multifocal Kaposi sarcoma lesions. On the alveolar ridge, they may resemble a *pyogenic granuloma*, or a *peripheral giant cell proliferation*.

DIAGNOSTIC WORK-UP ▶

Distinguishing a Kaposi sarcoma from similar lesions and confirming the diagnosis can be accomplished only via biopsy. If the biopsy confirms a Kaposi sarcoma, a CT scan of the abdomen and pelvis is recommended to assess for internal lesions. If the individual has not been tested previously for HIV antibodies, written consent must be obtained and blood drawn for HIV testing.

HISTOPATHOLOGY ▶

The histologic appearance of Kaposi sarcoma is determined not by the background in which the disease has arisen but by the maturity of the lesion. As the tumor develops from patch through plaque and nodular stages, the histologic picture changes.

In the early patch stage, changes may be extremely subtle and show only a proliferation of both small and dilated vessels. Subsequently, anastomosing, jagged, thin-walled vessels may develop superficially. The lining cells are unremarkable. A mild infiltrate of lymphocytes and plasma cells may be seen at the periphery. The presence of extravasated erythrocytes and hemosiderin should arouse suspicion.

Vascular proliferation continues in the plaque stage, and foci of spindle cells, typically related to the vascular component, develop.

In the nodular stage, the spindle cell component dominates, encroaching on the previously obvious vascular spaces (Fig 10-33a). Intersecting bands of spindle cells are seen. The rather bland nuclei are densely packed. Some mitoses may be seen, but they are not prominent. The picture resembles fibrosarcoma, but Kaposi sarcoma will show the presence of slit-like spaces between the spindle cells, which contain varying numbers of erythrocytes and some hemosiderin (Fig 10-33b). Hyaline globules may be seen within the cytoplasm of the spindle cells, but they are not unique to Kaposi sarcoma and may represent degenerated membranes of phagocytosed erythrocytes. They are periodic acid–Schiff (PAS) positive and diastase resistant. At the periphery of the nodules, dilated vessels, lymphocytes, and plasma cells are usually noted.

The vascular nature of Kaposi sarcoma is supported by positive CD_{31} and CD_{34} immunostaining. There is some evidence that it may arise from lymphatic endothelium. Electron microscopy and immunostaining have produced conflicting results that may simply be related to the maturity of the lesion.

It is still not clear if Kaposi sarcoma is a true neoplasm or a diffuse reactive hyperplasia. Some cases have been shown to be a clonal process (implying neoplasia). There is a consistent association in all types of Kaposi sarcoma with human herpesvirus 8 (HHV8), a gamma herpesvirus, also known as *Kaposi sarcoma–related virus*. Immunostaining for this virus can also be helpful diagnostically.

Within the histopathologic differential diagnosis of Kaposi sarcoma is bacillary epithelioid angiomatosis. This multifocal proliferative vascular disease found predominantly in HIV-positive patients typically affects the skin, although lymph nodes, oral mucosa, and even alveolar bone may be involved. Clinically, it frequently resembles Kaposi sarcoma. However, like cat-scratch disease, it seems to be caused by *Bartonella henselae* and responds to treatment with erythromycin.

Bacillary epithelioid angiomatosis may be distinguished from Kaposi sarcoma histologically because of their well-formed vascular channels lined by protuberant endothelial cells. In addition, there is an inflammatory component usually consisting of neutrophils as well as aggregates of bacterial colonies that can be identified by means of Warthin-Starry silver stain. Immunohistochemically, factor VIII–related antigen positivity is usually demonstrated.

TREATMENT AND PROGNOSIS ▶

The overall management of all types of Kaposi sarcoma is usually handled by a medical oncologist. Isolated lesions can be treated with intralesional injections of vinblastine, 0.1 to 0.5 mg/mL, or with focal radiotherapy of 1,800 cGy to 2,400 cGy. Widespread lesions usually require systemic chemotherapy. Effective drugs include vinblastine, etoposide, doxorubicin (Adriamycin), and bleomycin. In addition, alpha-2 interferon has been used but only a 20% response has been noted.

The prognosis for individuals with the classic and the African cutaneous forms is considered to be good. Nevertheless 10% to 20% die of these forms of Kaposi sarcoma and another 35% die of a second malignancy. The African lymphadenopathic form has a nearly uniformly fatal prognosis. The AIDS-related form has a prognosis that is improving each year as fewer AIDS patients develop Kaposi sarcoma or develop fewer and smaller lesions. In addition, combination anti-retroviral drug therapies have improved the control and prognosis of AIDS sufficiently that today concomitant therapies for secondary viral infections are included in their overall management, resulting in a lower incidence of Kaposi sarcomas in this group.

The prognosis for individuals with transplant-associated Kaposi sarcoma is related to the patient's degree of immunosuppression and his or her ability to discontinue the immunosuppressive drugs without rejection of the transplanted organ. If the immunosuppressive drugs are discontinued, the Kaposi lesions often regress without further treatment. However, the overall mortality rate is 30%.

Malignant Hemangiopericytoma

CLINICAL PRESENTATION ▶

Although some hemangiopericytomas are obviously benign and others are obviously malignant, there are also a number that are intermediate; these are included in the malignant hemangiopericytoma category to avoid the possibility of undertreatment. Nevertheless, benign hemangiopericytomas far outnumber the rare malignant ones, and the oral and maxillofacial area is an uncommon site, accounting for only 16% of all types of hemangiopericytomas.

Truly malignant hemangiopericytomas are diagnosed and graded by their cellular nature and mitotic figures per high-power field (HPF). Clinically, both benign and malignant hemangiopericytomas present as painless, deep-seated tumors (often arising within muscle or deep fascia). Males and females are affected

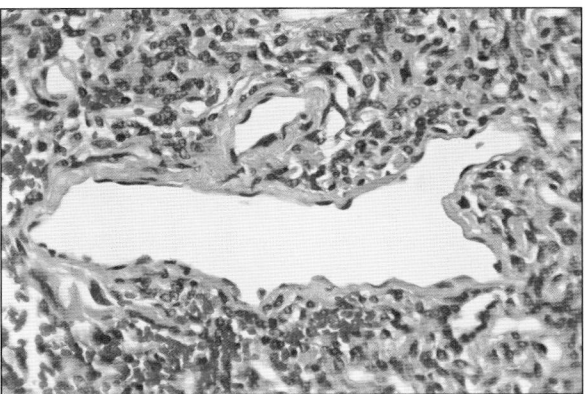

Fig 10-34 The staghorn shape of the vascular channels typically seen in malignant hemangiopericytomas.

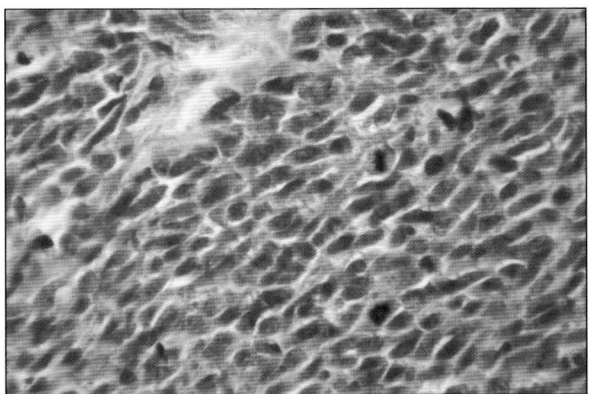

Fig 10-35 This malignant hemangiopericytoma is very cellular and shows several mitotic figures. These features help distinguish benign from aggressive lesions.

equally. The lesions are richly vascular with functional vessels that may produce a pulsatile thrill or an audible bruit.

The incidence increases with advancing age up to a peak in the 30- to 50-year age range. However, a separate infantile form occurs more commonly in the superficial subcutaneous fat rather than deep within muscle as does the adult type, and it grows in a rapid infiltrative pattern, forming satellite lesions. By contrast, the adult type is slower growing and develops into a lobulated mass, sometimes reaching large sizes. Most adult types are present for several months or even years before the individual seeks medical attention.

DIFFERENTIAL DIAGNOSIS ▶

Because of its rarity, a malignant hemangiopericytoma is usually not an initial consideration. Deep-seated tissue masses in the oral and maxillofacial area in mid-adult life may suggest several salivary gland neoplasms, particularly the more common ones such as the *pleomorphic adenoma*, *adenoid cystic carcinoma*, and *mucoepidermoid carcinoma*. The deep location and large size are also consistent with *benign* and *malignant fibrous histiocytomas*. If pulsations are present or a bleeding history is elicited, an *arteriovenous hemangioma* is appropriate, and if it is located in the nasal area, a *nasopharyngeal angiofibroma* should be considered.

DIAGNOSTIC WORK-UP ▶

The tumor's deep location requires a CT or MRI scan to delineate its true size and anatomic relationships. It is also recommended that angiography be performed because many tumors have a rapid circulation pattern with feeders and considerable arteriovenous shunting. The diagnosis requires an incisional biopsy of sufficient size to take several sections for histopathology. Because the differentiation between benign and malignant (and thus the treatment approach) is based on the mitotic figures and the cellular pattern, the biopsy is exceedingly important.

HISTOPATHOLOGY ▶

These circumscribed tumors arise from pericytes. They consist of closely packed cells arranged around ramifying, thin-walled, endothelially lined, vascular channels of greatly varying size. Small vessels may be obscured by tumor cell proliferation and compression. The cells have round to oval nuclei and may sometimes be spindled. They can resemble endothelial cells, fibroblasts, and histiocytes. The vessels often have a "staghorn" configuration (Fig 10-34). Because it acts as an arteriovenous shunt, the periphery of the tumor tends to be under increased venous pressure with resultant vascular dilation, so that there is the potential for considerable hemorrhage during surgical removal.

The behavior of the malignant hemangiopericytoma can be difficult to predict, but it is most closely associated with mitotic activity. Fewer than 2 per 10 HPFs indicates a favorable prognosis, whereas 4 or more per 10 HPFs correlates with recurrent disease and metastasis. Greater aggression may also be seen with tumors that show increased cellularity, pleomorphism, and/or necrosis and hemorrhage (Fig 10-35).

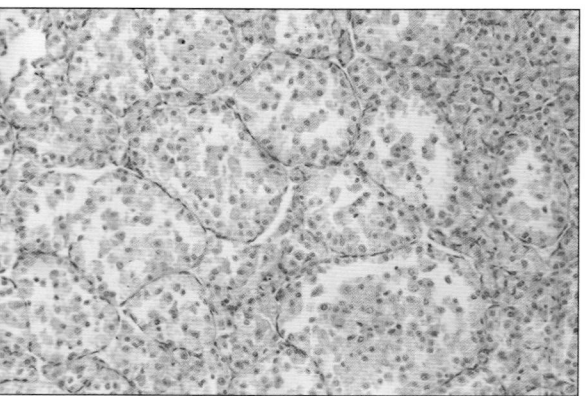

Fig 10-36a Low-power view of an alveolar soft part sarcoma showing the striking nest-like arrangement and the pseudoalveolar pattern.

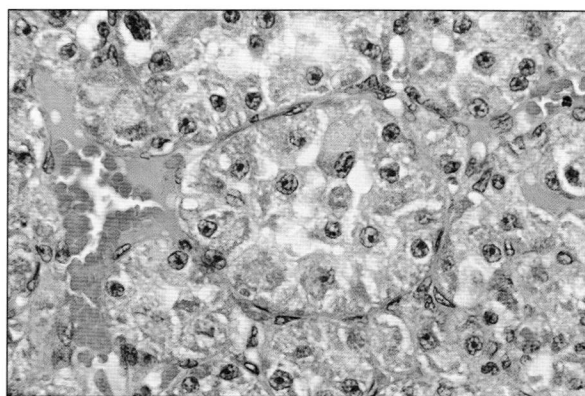

Fig 10-36b High-power view of an alveolar soft part sarcoma showing the abundant granular eosinophilic cytoplasm, pseudoalveolar arrangement, and dilated, thin-walled blood vessel.

Malignant hemangiopericytomas occurring in the upper aerodigestive tract typically lack these aggressive histologic features and metastatic potential.

The diagnosis depends on the architecture of the lesion. Immunocytochemistry is nonspecific.

TREATMENT ▶

Truly malignant hemangiopericytomas are usually treated with preoperative embolization and surgical excision followed by postoperative radiotherapy in doses between 3,500 cGy and 5,500 cGy. Even with preoperative embolization, it is wise to approach the lesion with identification and ligation of the known feeding vessels as identified by the angiogram.

PROGNOSIS ▶

The prognosis of malignant hemangiopericytomas depends on the tumor's size and the number of mitotic figures per HPF. Metastasis, usually to lungs or bone, can occur as much as 10 years after initial therapy. Metastasis incidence is difficult to ascertain because of this tumor's rarity, but it ranges from 20% to 50%. Five-year survival rates for those with fewer than 4 mitotic figures per 10 HPFs is about 85%; for those tumors with more than 4 mitotic figures per 10 HPFs, the 5-year survival rate is 45%.

Malignancies of Uncertain Histogenesis

Alveolar Soft Part Sarcoma

CLINICAL PRESENTATION AND PATHOGENESIS ▶

The alveolar soft part sarcoma is an uncommon tumor of uncertain histogenesis. The most prevalent location is the thigh and buttocks, but the head and neck, particularly the tongue and orbit, are often the involved sites in children. The usual age range is 15 to 35 years, and there is a female preponderance. These tumors are typically asymptomatic. An important characteristic is the marked vascularity with the potential for severe hemorrhage at surgery.

HISTOPATHOLOGY ▶

The alveolar soft part sarcoma is a poorly circumscribed, friable tumor, typically with a uniform histology in which the tumor cells have a nest-like arrangement (Fig 10-36a). The cell clusters are divided by thin-walled blood vessels. The cells are large, usually polygonal, with single or multiple nuclei. The abundant cytoplasm is eosinophilic and granular. Mitoses are rare. In the center of the nests there is frequently necrosis with loss of cell adhesion, giving a pseudoalveolar pattern (Fig 10-36b). A characteristic feature is the presence of PAS-positive, diastase-resistant crystals that are rhomboid- or rod-shaped and are visible ultrastructurally. Dilated veins, often showing tumor invasion, are seen at the periphery. Occasionally, but particularly in children, the tumors have a more uniform appearance and lack the nesting arrangement. These often have a better prognosis.

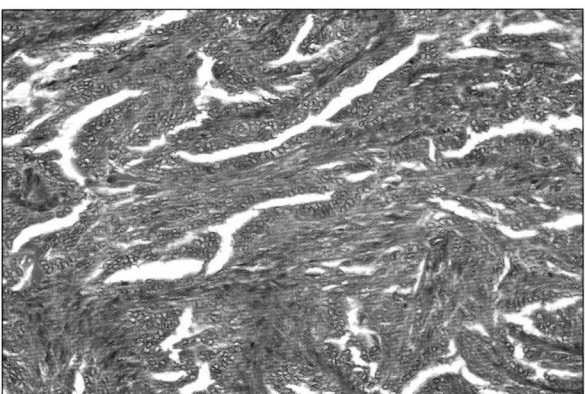 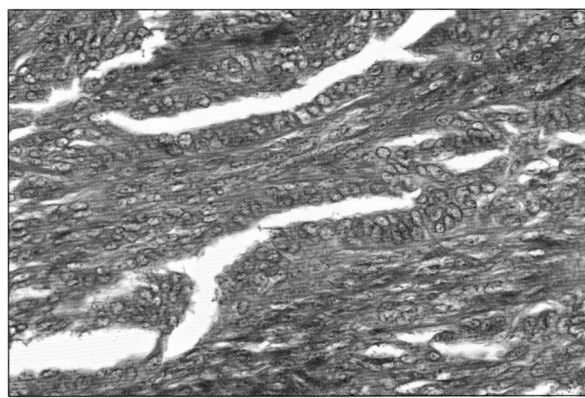

Fig 10-37a The cleft-like pattern frequently seen in synovial sarcomas is readily apparent.

Fig 10-37b A higher-power view of Fig 10-37a shows the biphasic pattern of this synovial sarcoma. The epithelial-like cells line the clefts, beneath which spindle cells are seen.

Synovial Sarcoma

CLINICAL PRESENTATION AND PATHOGENESIS ▶ Although it shows a histologic resemblance to developing synovium, there is no evidence that the synovial sarcoma originates from synovial tissue. It is seen predominantly in the 15- to 40-year age range with a slight male predilection. It presents as a painful but slow-growing mass, often evolving over many years. Most are found in the lower extremity, particularly around the knee. Ten percent of cases are seen in the head and neck, particularly in the paravertebral area. They may present as a retro- or parapharyngeal mass, but they also can occur in the tongue, soft palate, and parotid. Radiographically, small calcifications may be present; this feature can be helpful diagnostically.

HISTOPATHOLOGY ▶ The histology of the synovial sarcoma embraces a broad spectrum of features. The classic form is a biphasic tumor consisting of plump but uniform spindle-shaped cells that resemble a fibrosarcoma but are devoid of a herringbone pattern. These are accompanied by cuboidal- to columnar-shaped epithelial-like cells that line spaces or clefts or form nests (Figs 10-37a and 10-37b). There can be a pseudoglandular appearance. Mitoses are infrequent but may be seen in both cell types. Calcifications may be present in about 20% of cases. Vascularity varies from dominant to scant. There may be replacement of the cellular component by collagen or myxoid tissue.

A variant of this form is a monophasic fibrous type. The majority of spindle cells are positive for cytokeratin and epithelial membrane antigen, confirming its relationship to the biphasic form in which both cell types are positive.

A monophasic epithelial form also exists but is very uncommon, and there can be considerable difficulty in separating this from metastatic carcinoma and malignant melanoma.

The poorly differentiated synovial sarcoma consists of closely packed cells that are often intermediate in form between epithelial and spindle cells. There may be a rich vascular background, in which case it may resemble hemangiopericytoma. Synovial sarcomas are associated with the chromosomal translocation t(X;18)(p11.2;q11.2).

TREATMENT ▶ Malignancies of uncertain histogenesis are also malignancies of uncertain treatment. The alveolar soft part sarcoma and synovial sarcoma are so rare that they are almost always an unexpected and surprise finding and therefore will not be included in any differential diagnosis. There are also too few reported cases to have any meaningful data related to treatment outcomes. Most will present similar to a fibrosarcoma or a rhabdomyosarcoma as an infiltrative soft tissue mass. It is suggested that they be treated in similar fashion to an osteosarcoma, with presurgical chemotherapy followed by a resection with 2- to

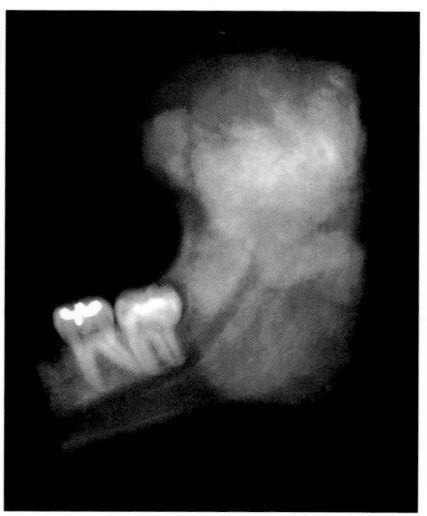

Fig 10-38a Resection of a synovial sarcoma arising from the temporomandibular joint requires 3-cm margins in soft tissue and bone.

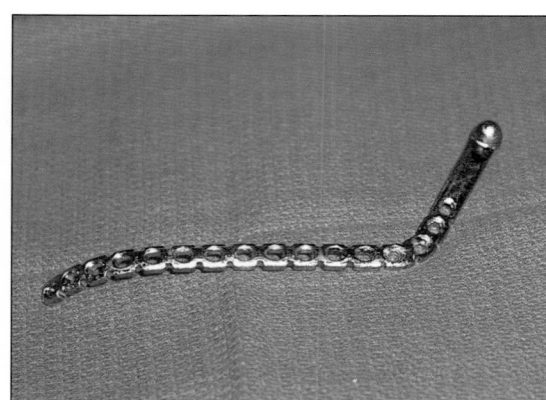

Fig 10-38b Invasion of the ramus due to a synovial sarcoma.

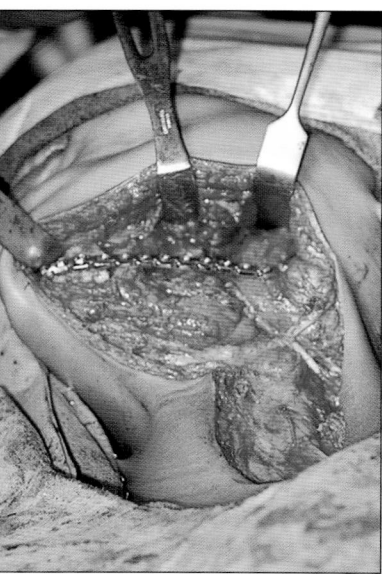

Fig 10-38c Effective immediate reconstructions of mandibular resections can be accomplished with rigid titanium reconstruction plates that include a condylar replacement.

Fig 10-38d Reconstruction plate in place along with a sternocleidomastoid muscle flap, which eliminated dead space and provided an articulating surface for the condylar replacement via the sternal tendinous insertion.

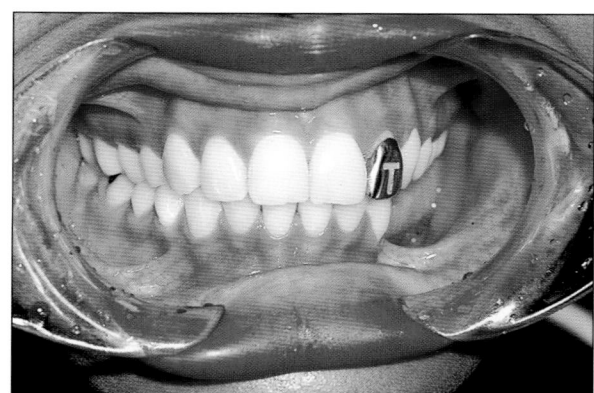

Fig 10-38e Eleven-year follow-up with no recurrent disease and a long-term stability of the occlusion achieved solely by the reconstruction plate.

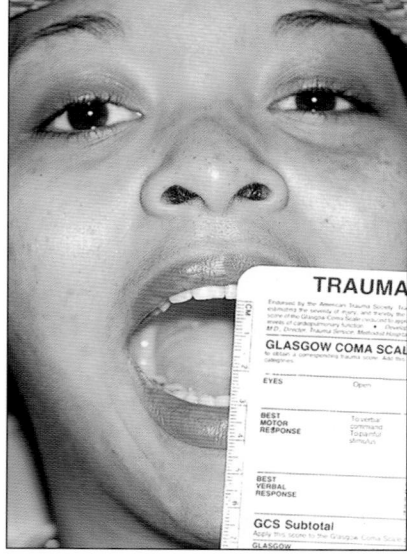

Fig 10-38f Full rotational jaw opening with minimal deviation achieved with the reconstruction plate and its condylar replacement.

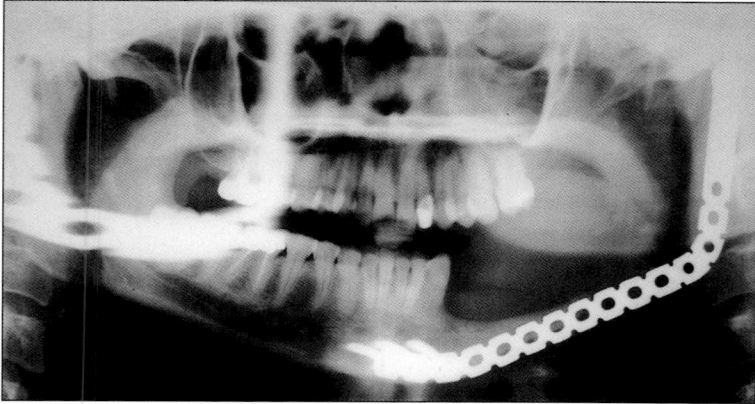

Fig 10-38g An 11-year follow-up demonstrates maintenance of the condylar replacement in the temporal fossa and stability of the plate. Note the small amount of spontaneous bone regeneration arising from the distal segment and coursing along the plate.

3-cm margins (Figs 10-38a and 10-38b). The rationale for initial chemotherapy is to select agents to which the tumor is responsive and to treat any microscopic metastatic deposits at distant sites. As with any sarcoma, the surgical defect may be significant and will require initial rigid titanium plate stabilization if the mandible is involved (Figs 10-38c to 10-38g), a maxillary obturator if the maxilla is involved, and a soft tissue myocutaneous free vascular flap if sufficient soft tissue is extirpated. Use of postoperative chemotherapy would be expected.

Non-neoplastic Salivary Gland Diseases

CHAPTER 11

▶ The Three Stages of a Scientific Theory:
First, it is thought to be preposterous and ridiculous.
Second, it is admitted to be true but insignificant.
Third, it is embraced as true and even revolutionary.
Those who criticized it most now claim they were the ones who discovered it first.

—Author unknown

Mumps

CLINICAL PRESENTATION ▶

Mumps, the most common salivary gland disease, is a paramyxovirus infection usually of both parotid glands and to some extent the submandibular and sublingual glands. The usual case involves a child who is not immunized (Fig 11-1a), while a more severe involvement with more complications occurs in adults (Fig 11-1b). Transmission occurs via infected saliva droplets, which require a 14- to 21-day incubation period before the onset of symptoms.

The child usually will develop low-grade fever and malaise. High-grade fevers are suggestive of metastatic orchitis (in males) or meningitis. Both parotid glands become enlarged in 75% of cases, but not always at the same time; therefore, unilateral parotid gland enlargement is frequently observed (see Fig 11-1b). The enlarged parotid glands are tender to the touch and will be uncomfortable during jaw movements. Submandibular glands are frequently tender and enlarged as well.

Most cases run a course of slightly less than 2 weeks. When the infection resolves, a permanent immunity is incurred. However, in rare cases in children and more commonly in adults, involvement of other organs complicates the usual benign, self-limiting course. Orchitis occurs in 25% of adult men and is heralded by testicular swelling and pain. Less frequently, mumps pancreatitis develops, which will produce upper abdominal pain, nausea, and vomiting. In females, oophoritis parotidea uncommonly develops and is heralded by lower abdominal pain and cramping. The most severe complication is meningitis, which may eventuate in encephalitis and death in rare cases. Early signs of meningitis are headaches and neck stiffness.

DIFFERENTIAL DIAGNOSIS ▶

A child with swollen, tender parotid glands is considered to have mumps until proven otherwise. Other diseases that can cause swollen, tender parotid glands include *bacterial parotitis*, other viral parotitis (*coxsackie A virus*, *cytomegalovirus*, *echovirus*, and *parainfluenza viruses*), and *obstructive parotitis*, usually from mucus plugs in Stensen duct. Other conditions, such as sialosis, sarcoidosis, Sjögren syndrome, bulimia, and lymphomas, among others, produce parotid gland enlargement, but none of these will be associated with marked tenderness and fever.

DIAGNOSTIC WORK-UP ▶

The diagnosis of mumps is confirmed by isolating paramyxovirus from saliva or by paired serum studies that show a fourfold rise in mumps antibody titers. Other laboratory tests will show an absolute lymphocytosis, but the overall white blood cell count usually will be normal. Serum amylase levels are usually increased; this is not indicative of pancreatitis because most of the amylase is derived from the parotid gland.

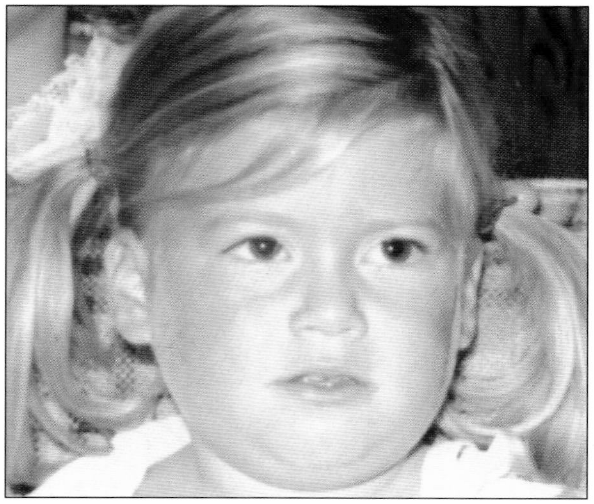

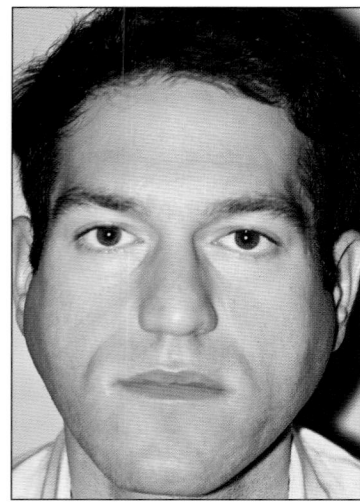

Fig 11-1a Mumps typically occurs in children and will mostly exhibit bilateral parotid gland enlargements, low-grade fever, and malaise. (Courtesy of Dr Irwin Stolzenberg.)

Fig 11-1b Mumps may create unilateral or bilateral tender parotid enlargements. It also uncommonly occurs in adults.

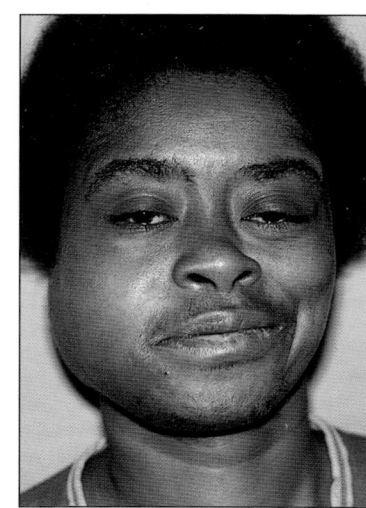

Fig 11-2 A swollen and painful parotid gland is suggestive of a bacterial parotitis.

HISTOPATHOLOGY ▶

Biopsy is not customarily used to diagnose mumps. However, the parotid gland will show swelling of acinar cells with vacuolation of the cytoplasm and considerable interstitial edema with infiltration by lymphocytes and plasma cells. Ductal dilation occurs, and desquamated epithelium may be found within the lumen.

TREATMENT ▶

Mumps, including complications involving other organs, is self-limiting. No specific therapy is given other than supportive care, which usually consists of bed rest, antipyretics, analgesics, and hydration.

Orchitis, if it develops, is treated with testicular elevation and ice. Meningitis, if it develops, may require corticosteroids, elevation of the head, and induced hyperventilation to combat cerebral edema.

PROGNOSIS ▶

Mumps is self-limiting and mostly resolves without residua. Rare deaths occur from meningitis progressing to encephalitis. Cases that progress to orchitis also resolve completely, and the patients rarely become sterile. Mumps, unlike rubella, is not teratogenic and is not associated with fetal death.

Mumps vaccine, a live attenuated virus preparation, is completely safe. It is usually administered to children as part of the MMR (mumps-measles-rubella) preparation first at age 15 months and then at age 4 to 6 years. Repeat vaccinations are not harmful in the already immunized individual. However, neither the MMR nor isolated mumps vaccine should be given to immunocompromised individuals or those allergic to eggs or neomycin, both of which are used in the preparations.

Bacterial Parotitis

CLINICAL PRESENTATION AND PATHOGENESIS ▶

Bacterial parotitis occurs both in a childhood form (recurrent) and in an adult form. The recurrent childhood form seems to be unrelated to any predisposing factors or underlying pathology. The adult form occurs more commonly with advancing age and is often related to dehydration secondary to debilitation, decreased parotid flow secondary to parasympatholytic drugs (atropine, propantheline bromide, etc), inspissated mucous plugs producing static salivary flow, or decreased salivary flow related to Sjögren syndrome.

In either form, the gland becomes swollen and painful (Fig 11-2). In the infection's early stages, the gland will become more swollen and painful with eating, and salivary production further distends the parotid capsule. The patient is often febrile, but mild cases may not be accompanied by fever. The opening of Stensen

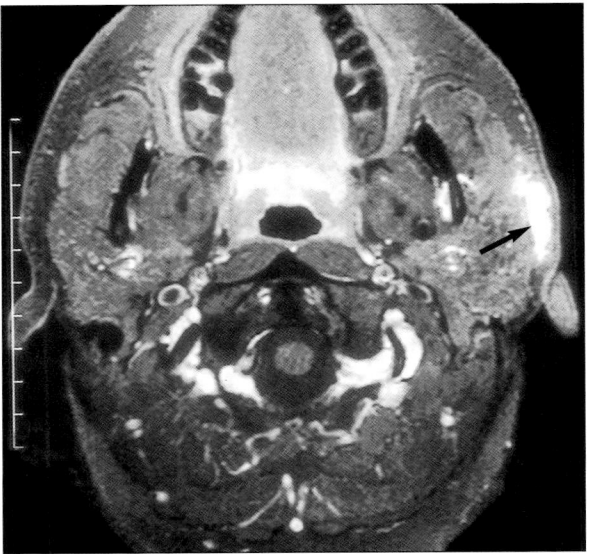

Fig 11-3a Inflammation, edema, and suppuration from bacterial parotitis are usually well illustrated by an MRI scan of the parotid glands. Note the increased T-2 signal uptake (*arrow*) indicating a parotid abscess.

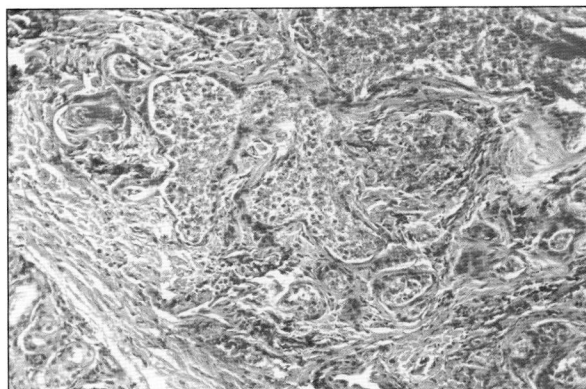

Fig 11-3b Accumulation of neutrophils within salivary ducts.

duct is often erythematous, and a suppurative exudate or saliva-diluted suppurative exudate, which will appear as a milky exudate, may be expressed. The most common causative organism is *Staphylococcus aureus*, which is usually the methicillin-resistant strain (MRSA). However, the infection usually is not caused by MRSA alone, but is accompanied by several species of streptococci.

Severe infections will extend beyond the parotid capsule and may result in a salivary-cutaneous fistula, a pharyngeal space infection, or an external or middle ear infection.

Bacterial parotitis is much less common than bacterial submandibular gland sialadenitis, probably because of the downward tract of the parotid duct, which makes stasis less likely, and the more proteinaceous parotid secretion. Unlike the mucoprotein secretions of the submandibular gland, parotid secretions are less viscous and do not support bacterial growth as well.

DIFFERENTIAL DIAGNOSIS ▶ Most cases of infectious parotitis are evident by the clinical signs and symptoms of an enlarged, painful parotid gland with an altered salivary flow. However, in adults, an underlying pathosis should be considered. In the absence of debilitation or drug-induced xerostomia, one must consider a *sialolith* or early *Sjögren syndrome*, particularly in women, and a *benign lymphoepithelial lesion* in either sex. *HIV parotitis* also produces a painful parotid enlargement, although it is caused not by bacteria but by multiple lymphoepithelial cysts. In addition, *sarcoidosis* and *sialosis* cause parotid enlargement; however, the pain associated with these conditions is mild and pus is not produced.

DIAGNOSTIC WORK-UP ▶ The most important aspect of the work-up is culture and sensitivity testing of the exudate. It is important to establish the presence of *S aureus* and to determine whether it is true MRSA or only penicillin-resistant via the elaboration of β-lactamase. Sialography has been superceded by computed tomography (CT) and magnetic resonance imaging (MRI) because of the more detailed information they offer (Fig 11-3a). In addition, sialography may force some infection beyond the parotid capsule, causing extension and spread. Sialography may be accomplished once the acute infection is under control and if a sialolith is strongly suspected. A blood count will usually show a slight leukocytosis with a shift to the left indicative of immature neutrophils.

HISTOPATHOLOGY ▶ Purulent exudate within the ducts may erode into the adjacent parenchyma, causing formation of small abscesses and focal areas of necrosis (Fig 11-3b).

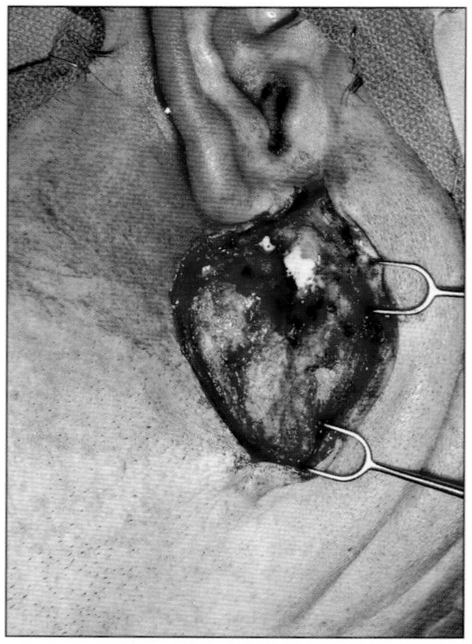

Fig 11-3c Pus and fibrosis in a bacterial parotitis refractory to antibiotic therapy. Surgical debridement was required in the form of a superficial parotidectomy.

Histologic differences between recurrent parotitis in children and that found in adults have been reported. In children, the inflammatory component primarily affects the supporting connective tissue, whereas in adults the infiltrate is ductal and parenchymal.

Initial treatment includes hydration, which may require intravenous fluids and antibiotics. If cultures identify *S aureus* that is not MRSA and the usual streptococci, then antibiotics such as ampicillin with sulbactam (Unasym, Pfizer), 1.5 g every 6 hours intravenously, is a good choice, as is ciprofloxacin (Cipro, Bayer), 400 mg every 12 hours intravenously. For outpatient therapy, amoxicillin with clavulanate (Augmentin, GlaxoSmithKline), 875 mg orally twice daily, or ciprofloxacin (Cipro), 500 mg orally twice daily, are good choices. If the cultures identify MRSA, the best therapy is 500 mg vancomycin administered intravenously every 12 hours. As an outpatient drug for follow-up care, 100 mg vibramycin orally twice a day is effective against MRSA.

If the parotitis is refractory to culture-specific antibiotics or if a defined abscess is in evidence, then incision and drainage and a reculturing of a drainage specimen must be performed. If a parasympatholytic drug is part of the patient's medications, its use should be discontinued if possible. On rare occasions, a persistent bacterial parotitis will require a superficial or total parotidectomy (Fig 11-3c).

Specific antibiotics and hydration therapy are very effective. Persistent infection should alert the clinician to look for several possibilities: a parotid mucous plug or sialolith; immunosuppression; resistant bacteria; incorrect initial interpretation of cultures; an undiagnosed abscess; or an unrecognized underlying pathology such as Sjögren syndrome.

Sialosis

Sialosis will produce a bilateral, diffuse, soft-textured enlargement of both parotid glands. Most cases are painless, but a small number have been associated with chronic pain. Two general types have been identified. One type, sometimes called *idiopathic sialosis*, arises unassociated with any specific nutritional abnormality or related to unrecognized bulimia and its nutritional deficit or to an unrecognized reflex sympathetic dystrophy (RSD). This type forms enlarged parotid glands caused by acinar cell hypertrophy. Acinar cells are enlarged to 2 to 5 times their normal size. The other type is associated with theoretic nutritional imbalances related to chronic disease states such as diabetes, cirrhosis, alcoholism, and chronic obesity. This form shows a smaller degree of acinar hypertrophy, but a more prominent fatty infiltration into the

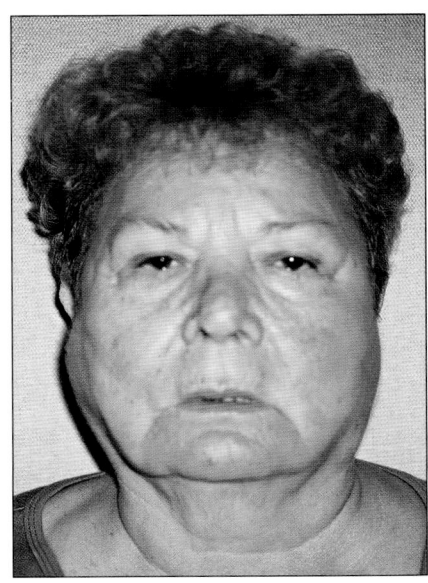

Fig 11-4a Diffuse parotid enlargements related to nutritional sialosis secondary to diabetes.

gland. It is primarily this fatty infiltration that accounts for the enlargement because fat cells (adipocytes) are larger than parotid acinar cells (Fig 11-4a).

The idiopathic-bulimic or RSD-related group fits the profile of bulimic patients: young (20 to 40 years), white, middle- to upper-class women. The chronic disease–related group tends to be older (50 years or more) and of either sex.

The nutritional abnormality is not defined and remains speculative. In bulimic patients, serum electrolyte changes may be the causative factor.

DIFFERENTIAL DIAGNOSIS ▶

Sialosis is only one of a specific subset of diseases that cause painless or mildly painful soft enlargement of both parotid glands. The others are *sarcoidosis*, *Sjögren syndrome*, a *lymphoma* developing in Sjögren syndrome, *benign lymphoepithelial lesions*, and a case of *mumps* later in life. Parotid tumors other than lymphomatous processes are ruled out by the diffuse, soft-textured bilateral nature of sialosis, which is different from the discrete, firm mass and unilateral location of parotid tumors. Even Warthin tumors that occur bilaterally are not likely because of their discrete feel and their circumscribed location in the superficial lobe.

DIAGNOSTIC WORK-UP ▶

Soft, diffuse parotid enlargements require an incisional parotid biopsy. The approach is via the skin under the earlobe, which will enable access to the posterior aspect of the superficial lobe. This approach is effective in distinguishing sarcoidosis, sialosis, Sjögren syndrome, and other diffuse parotid enlargements without risking facial nerve damage. (In this location the facial nerve is 3.2 cm below the skin surface, whereas the parotid is 1.0 to 1.3 cm.)

In those patients in whom bulimia is suspected, it is useful to look for other signs of this disease, such as incisal or cusp tip caries, lingual erosion of mandibular teeth, pharyngitis, and hemorrhoids.

HISTOPATHOLOGY ▶

The glandular changes are characterized by hypertrophy of the acini. The cells may enlarge to 2 to 3 times their normal size, which causes compression of the ducts. The cytoplasm is packed with zymogen granules in its early involvement, but becomes gradually degranulated to become almost clear over the course of the disease. The nuclei are displaced to the base of the cell. Interstitial fatty infiltrates may develop (Figs 11-4b to 11-4d).

TREATMENT ▶

Reassuring patients that the enlarged parotid glands do not represent neoplastic or preneoplastic disease is important. Patients with bulimia require behavioral modification programs and sometimes antidepressants, of which fluoxetine and other selective seratonin reuptake inhibitors are reported to be preferred. Patients whose sialosis is related to chronic disease usually require no treatment other than

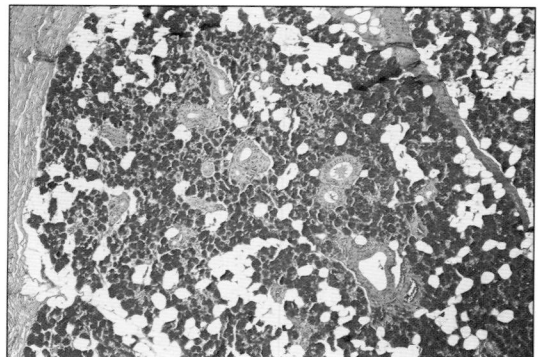

Fig 11-4b To assess a sialosis histopathology, it should be compared to a normal parotid histology. The normal parotid gland acinar cells are smaller than the cuboidal cells of the ducts, as shown here.

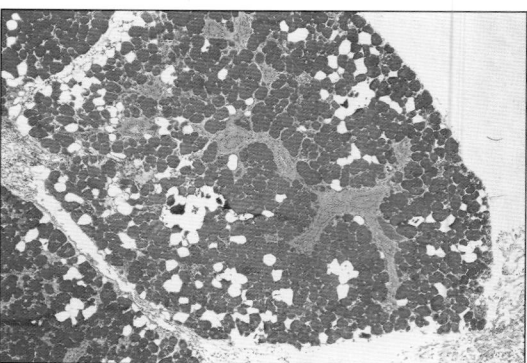

Fig 11-4c In early sialosis, the acinar cells are hypertrophied and will be larger than the cuboidal cells of the ducts.

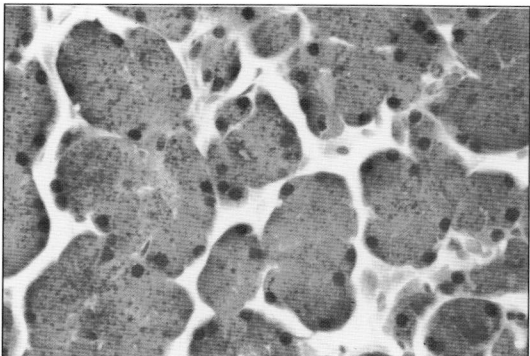

Fig 11-4d A high-power view of sialosis will show large ballooned acinar cells and a degranulation of zymogen granules with only a few remaining.

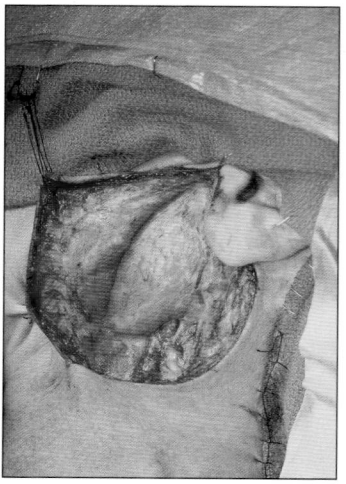

Fig 11-4e An even and homogeneous enlargement of the parotid due to sialosis. A superficial parotidectomy may be used to contour the sialosis enlargement and alleviate the discomfort of parotid expansion.

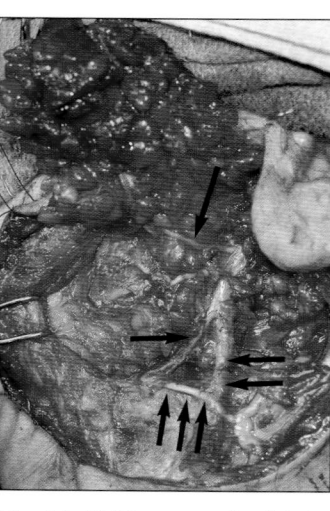

Fig 11-4f The superficial lobe is removed using the landmarks of the facial nerve branches (*single arrow*), the retromandibular/external jugular vein (*double arrows*), and the anterior branch of the greater auricular nerve (*triple arrows*) as dissection guides.

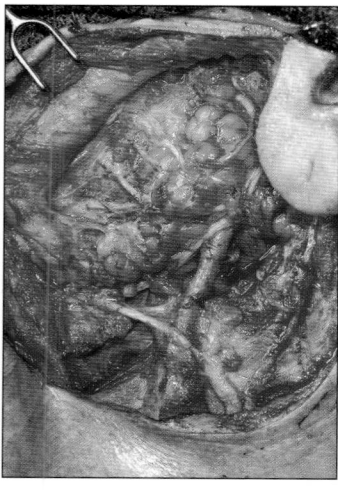

Fig 11-4g The intact branches of the facial nerve remain within the substance of the parotid's deep lobe after the superficial parotidectomy.

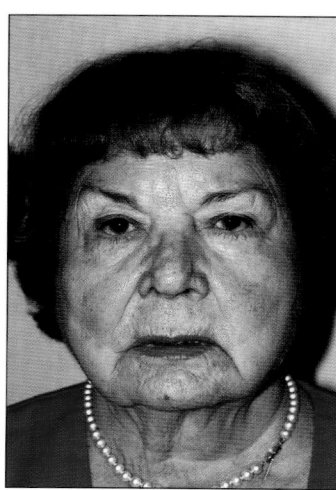

Fig 11-4h An improvement in contour as well as relief of discomfort are gained by the patient shown in Fig 11-4a when treated by a superficial parotidectomy.

PROGNOSIS ▶

reassurance. In selected cases in which the underlying nutritional disorder is controlled, superficial parotidectomies will alleviate facial expansion and the pain in painful cases (Figs 11-4e to 11-4h).

Sialosis is neither life threatening nor debilitating. It is merely a clinical sign of a specific pathology.

Benign Lymphoepithelial Lesion

CLINICAL PRESENTATION AND PATHOGENESIS ▶

The benign lymphoepithelial lesion (BLEL) can be conceptualized as a Sjögren-like infiltration and enlargement of the parotid glands without the mucosal dryness (sicca syndrome) and without the rheumatoid manifestations. Sjögren syndrome occurs in middle-aged women as a painless enlargement of one or both parotid glands. Benign lymphoepithelial lesions occur in adults of either sex (Fig 11-5a). As the disease progresses, both parotid glands become involved in nearly all cases. The parotid gland enlargements are diffuse and soft at first, becoming more firm throughout the years. Secondary bacterial parotitis frequently occurs because of stasis of salivary flow and ductal obstruction. Lymphoepithelial lesions may include a single lymphoepithelial cyst. However, in HIV infection, multiple cysts are the rule.

The pathogenesis is unknown but is suggestive of age-related or viral-related alterations of surface antigens on the acinar cells of the gland. This antigenicity stimulates and attracts both T and B lymphocytes (mostly the latter) into the gland, where they mediate the devitalization of acinar cells. As a result, the acinar cells are replaced by lymphocytes while the myoepithelial cells, which are not antigenic, remain within the tissue among the lymphocytes. Constant antigenic stimulation is thought to occasionally promote the uncontrolled proliferation of a single line of B cells, resulting in the few cases of lymphoma that develop from a BLEL.

DIFFERENTIAL DIAGNOSIS ▶

The bilateral and diffuse presentation rules out discrete parotid neoplasms other than *lymphomas*, which may be the result of a BLEL. Other diseases that can cause bilateral parotid enlargement include *sarcoidosis*, *nutritional sialosis*, *HIV parotitis*, and *mumps*. In addition, because it is histologically indistinguishable from BLEL, *Sjögren syndrome* must be ruled out by means of clinical and laboratory testing.

DIAGNOSTIC WORK-UP ▶

The lymphoepithelial nature of the lesion must be confirmed by an incisional parotid biopsy accomplished beneath the earlobe. If a lymphoepithelial lesion is identified, Sjögren syndrome must be ruled out by assessing mouth dryness empirically or by a timed collection of parotid flow, which is time-consuming and inaccurate because of unknown normal values and daily flow variations. Xerophthalmia can be measured more accurately by a Schirmer tear function test (see page 507). Other conditions found in laboratory testing that indicate Sjögren syndrome include anemia, leukopenia, sometimes eosinophilia, and hypergammaglobulinemia. Additionally, positive antinuclear antibodies (ANAs), rheumatoid factor (RF), and anti-Sjögren syndrome antibodies (either anti-Sjögren syndrome antibody-A [SS-A] or anti-Sjögren syndrome antibody-B [SS-B]) may be required. Sjögren syndrome itself may be secondary (secondary Sjögren syndrome) to another disease. Therefore, the clinical examination and work-up may need to pursue possible systemic lupus erythematosus, progressive systemic sclerosis, scleroderma, and biliary cirrhosis, among others. The histopathologic specimen should also be assessed for a developing lymphoma by immunohistochemistry or gene probe analysis. A lymphoma is identified if the lymphocytes show a monoclonal origin. A polyclonal origin implies a benign process.

HISTOPATHOLOGY ▶

Initially, lymphocytic infiltrates are seen in a periductal location with resultant acinar atrophy. Hyperplastic and metaplastic changes occur within the duct, such that the epithelium encroaches on the lumen. These are the epimyoepithelial islands that are characteristic of this lesion (Fig 11-5b). There may be eosinophilic hyaline material, representing excess basement membrane material, within or surrounding the islands. Ultrastructural studies of epimyoepithelial islands have not produced uniform results, but when coupled with immunohistochemistry, these studies suggest a structural composition of ductal epithelium and myoepithelium. The lymphocytic infiltration is a progressive process with increasing loss of functional acini. They are polyclonal and predominantly of the CD4 type. The final picture is of a background of lymphocytes within which are scattered epimyoepithelial islands still contained within the capsule of the gland (Fig 11-5c). Lymphoid follicles with germinal centers may be seen. Studies have indicated that the distribution of the cells in benign lymphoepithelial lesions is similar to that in reactive lymph nodes. Monoclonality of the lymphocytes, which may be demonstrated by immunohistochemistry or molecular techniques, would indicate development of low-grade B-cell lymphoma (Figs 11-6a and 11-6b).

In HIV, the cysts are lined with squamous or cuboidal epithelium. The lymphocytic infiltrate is predominantly of the CD8 type, and epimyoepithelial islands are seen. Follicular hyperplasia, sometimes with granulomatous inflammation, is usually prominent (Figs 11-7a and 11-7b).

TREATMENT ▶

A benign lymphoepithelial lesion requires no specific treatment if the lymphocytic infiltrate is a polyclonal infiltrate. Such lesions are followed up for signs of monoclonal proliferation indicated by an increase in size, a greater firmness, or a darkening of color. If this occurs or if the original biopsy specimen was identified as a monoclonal lymphoproliferative infiltration (usually indicating a B-cell lymphoma), bi-

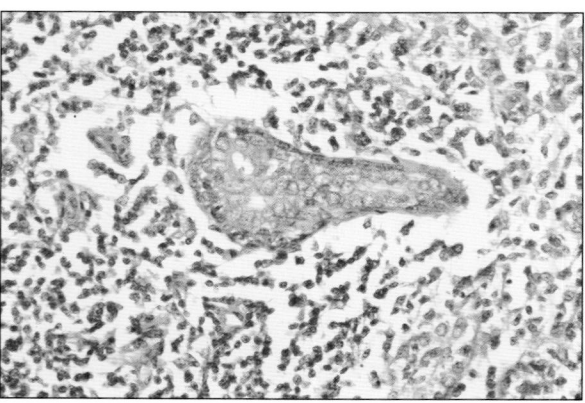

Fig 11-5a Benign lymphoepithelial lesions occur equally in men and women, unlike Sjögren syndrome, and present without signs of xerostomia or xerophthalmia.

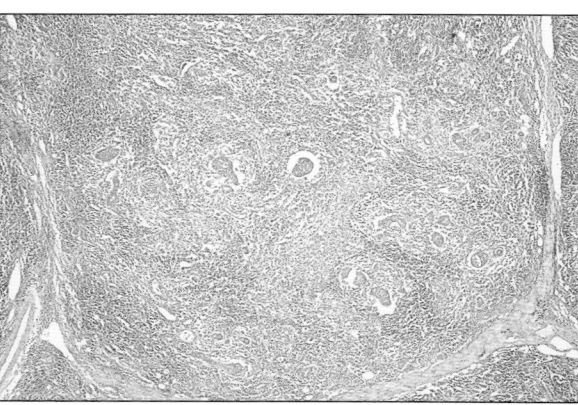

Fig 11-5b A benign lymphoepithelial lesion in the parotid gland demonstrating an epimyoepithelial island surrounded by lymphocytes.

Fig 11-5c Low-power view of the benign lymphoepithelial lesion shown in Fig 11-5b. Scattered epimyoepithelial islands can be seen in a sea of lymphocytes.

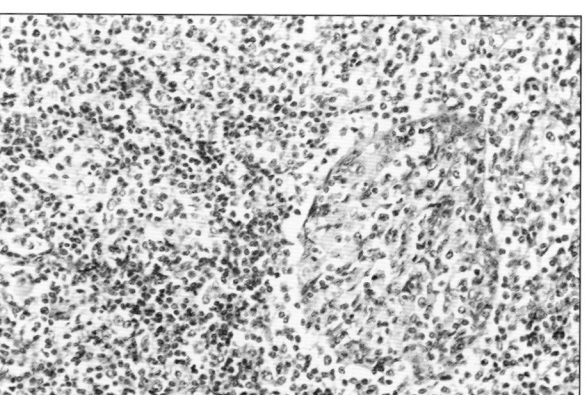

Fig 11-6a Development of a lymphoma in a lymphoepithelial lesion in a patient with Sjögren syndrome. The neoplastic lymphocytes here are infiltrating the epimyoepithelial island.

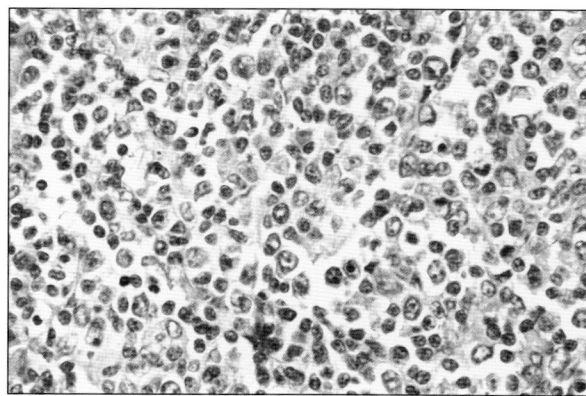

Fig 11-6b The same lesion shown in Fig 11-6a revealing neoplastic lymphocytes.

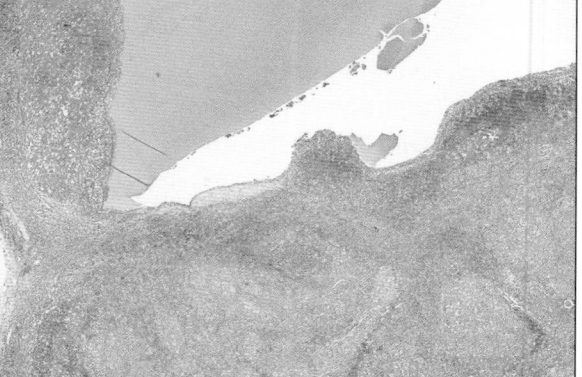

Fig 11-7a Lymphoepithelial cyst of the parotid gland.

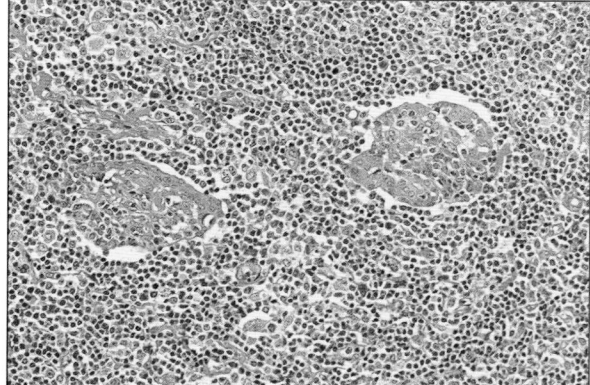

Fig 11-7b The same case shown in Fig 11-7a. The tissue adjacent to the cyst reveals a lymphoepithelial lesion with epimyoepithelial islands and surrounding lymphocytes.

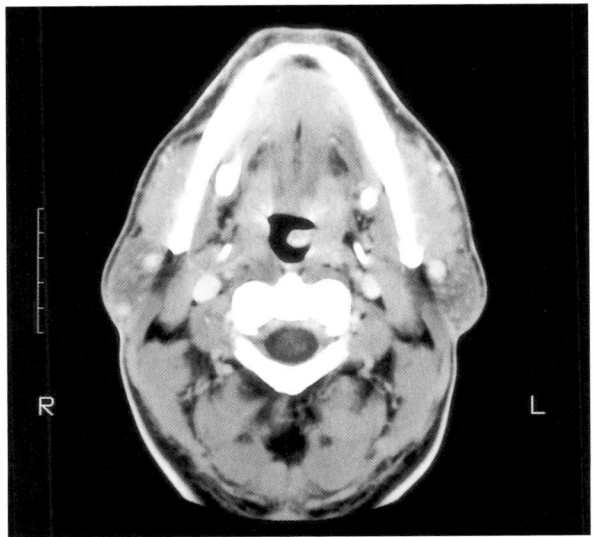

Fig 11-8 Diffuse enlargement of both parotid glands due to benign lymphoepithelial lesion infiltration. There is no evidence of loculations suggesting a lymphoepithelial cyst.

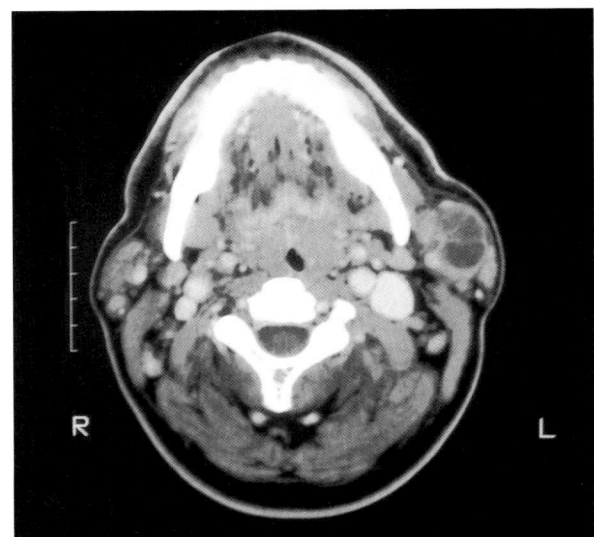

Fig 11-9 A multilocular fluid-filled cyst in the parotid gland is part of the presentation of this benign lymphoepithelial lesion.

lateral port radiotherapy in the range of 5,000 cGy to 6,800 cGy is indicated. If a benign lymphoepithelial cyst develops in the parotid gland, it will be noted by a more discrete mass and a CT scan finding of loculated fluid-filled spaces (Figs 11-8 and 11-9). In such cases, a superficial parotidectomy is indicated.

PROGNOSIS ▶ Most BLELs remain benign. Only 5% to 10% progress to a lymphoma, most of which are B-cell lymphomas.

Sjögren Syndrome

CLINICAL PRESENTATION AND PATHOGENESIS ▶ A syndrome is defined as a clinical symptom complex. Sjögren syndrome is an autoimmune destruction of exocrine glands (primarily salivary and lacrimal) that produces the clinical manifestations of dry mouth (xerostomia), dry eyes (xerophthalmia or keratoconjunctivitis sicca), and, in more than 50% of cases, parotid gland enlargement. Primary Sjögren syndrome is diagnosed when the syndrome is limited to this pattern of involvement. However, this pattern of involvement may be a manifestation of another well-defined autoimmune disease such as rheumatoid arthritis, systemic lupus erythematosis, or primary biliary cirrhosis. In this context, it is referred to as secondary Sjögren syndrome. This is an important distinction because lymphoma development is mostly seen in the primary type of Sjögren syndrome.

Sjögren syndrome primarily affects women older than 40 years (Figs 11-10a to 11-10c). However, newer diagnostic techniques such as parotid biopsies and antibody identifications have shown that many children and teenagers with dry mouth conditions actually have Sjögren syndrome. Caries at the cervical tooth margins and mucosal candidiasis are frequent (Fig 11-10d). An absence of flow from Stensen duct or a thick, mucoid secretion is common. The parotid enlargements are usually asymmetric and painless. Those larger than 6 cm, irregular by palpation, or darkened in color should be considered suggestive of lymphoma, particularly if the Sjögren syndrome is of the primary type (see Fig 11-10c). The dry eyes will often become secondarily infected and may have a suppurative collection in the lacrimal lake area and a reddened conjunctiva. Some patients will present with fatigue and mild arthralgia, but most will be active and tolerant of their disease. Many patients will have tooth loss secondary to caries, but they usually tolerate dentures well despite their dryness.

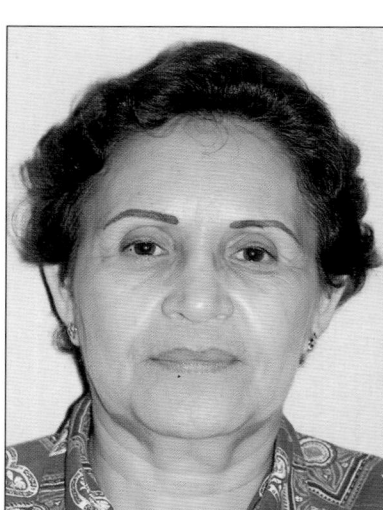

Fig 11-10a Some Sjögren syndrome patients will present with xerophthalmia and xerostomia but no parotid enlargement.

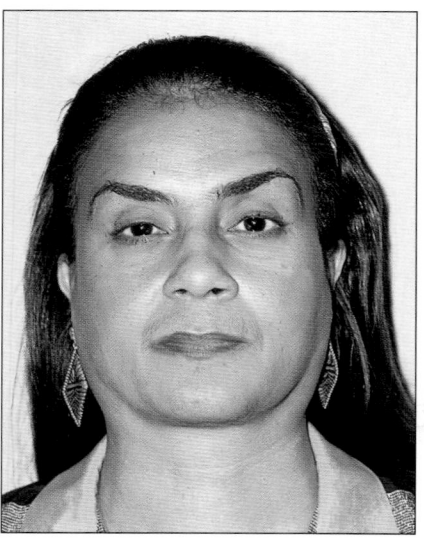

Fig 11-10b Other Sjögren syndrome patients will present with parotid enlargement with or without clinical xerophthalmia or xerostomia. This presentation, with both parotids enlarged but one more so than the other, is typical.

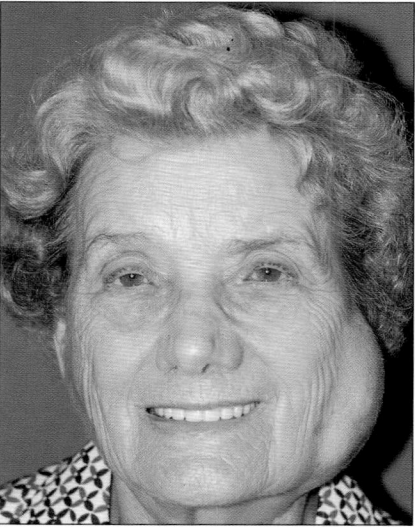

Fig 11-10c Still other Sjögren syndrome patients will present with overt parotid enlargement and clinically obvious xerophthalmia (note the conjunctivitis) and xerostomia (see Fig 11-10d). The clinician should be suspicious of lymphoma when the parotid enlarges to this degree, if it is firm, or if the skin color darkens.

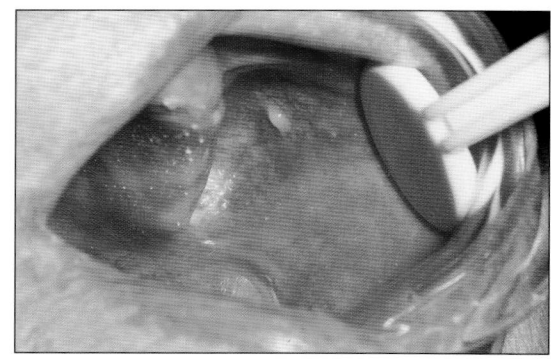

Fig 11-10d Severe xerostomia in Sjögren syndrome. Note the thick mucoid secretion of altered saliva from the parotid duct and the white tufts of candidiasis on the dry mucosa. The patient's edentulism was the end result of cervical caries that was contributed to by the xerostomia.

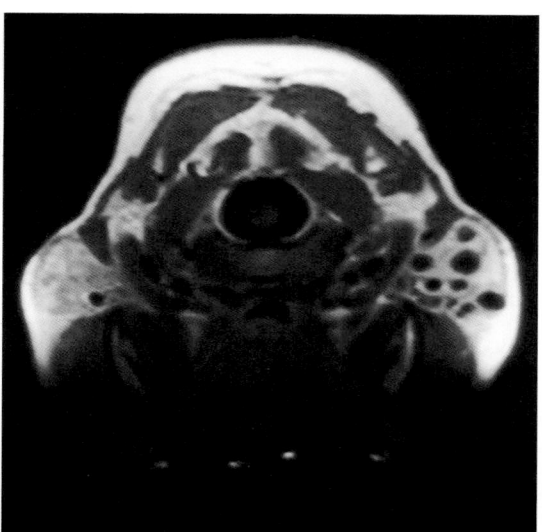

Fig 11-10e Multiple loculations within the parotid gland representing ductal ectasia in Sjögren syndrome.

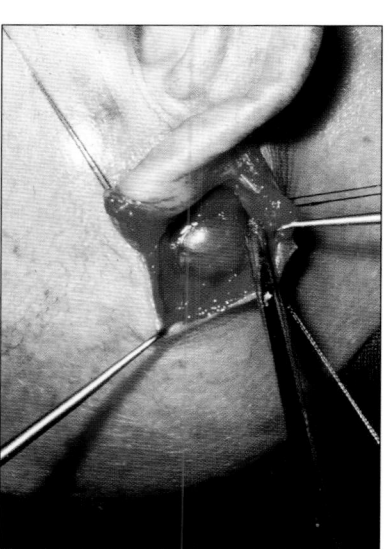

Fig 11-10f The incisional parotid biopsy is the most direct and effective method of confirming Sjögren syndrome. These dilated, mucous-filled portions of the parotid gland are consistent with Sjögren syndrome.

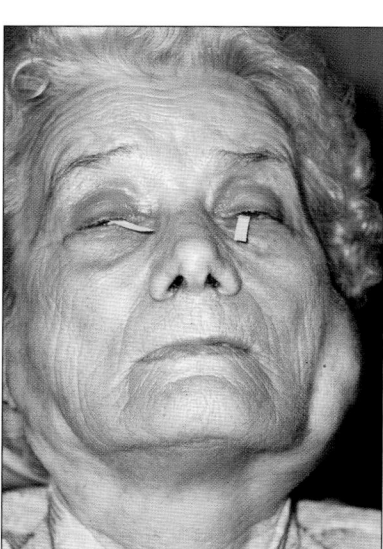

Fig 11-10g The Schirmer tear function test is simple to perform and will provide an index of tear production.

The pathogenesis of Sjögren syndrome is complex and uncertain, but thought to be similar to that of the benign lymphoepithelial lesion. It is suspected that age or viral changes in exocrine acinar cells result in an antigenicity on the cell surface. This, in turn, creates a stimulation and intense activity of mainly B cells, which infiltrate these glands and destroy the glandular acini. The myoepithelium and ductal elements lack the antigen and are thus spared. The result is dryness of the affected area and enlargement of the gland if sufficient numbers of lymphocytes have accumulated in it. In the 6% to 10% of cases that undergo transformation to a lymphoma (over a period of 5 to 15 years), the constant polyclonal B-cell overactivity selects a single clone (usually of B cells) that overtakes the population, resulting in a lymphoma.

Sjögren syndrome, like many autoimmune diseases, is associated with certain human lymphocyte–associated (HLA) or histocompatability antigens, indicative of a genetic vulnerability. HLA-DR4 antigen is found in patients who develop secondary Sjögren syndrome. HLA-B8 and HLA-DR3 antigens are found in patients with primary Sjögren syndrome.

DIFFERENTIAL DIAGNOSIS ▶

The dry eyes and dry mouth are defining features of Sjögren syndrome and distinguish it from other entities that cause parotid enlargement but are not associated with overt dry mouth and dry eyes (*sarcoidosis, sialosis, mumps,* and *benign lymphoepithelial lesions*). Some medications such as atropine, nifedipine, and antidepressants can produce a subjective dry mouth, but objectively saliva is more plentiful, and dry eyes usually is not a complaint.

DIAGNOSTIC WORK-UP ▶

A Sjögren syndrome work-up can include a host of studies, such as nuclear imaging and injection sialography, that add little to the diagnosis but provide information about the degree of ductal and acinar destruction. The same information can be obtained from a CT or MRI scan, which will often show internal hypodense areas indicative of ductal ectasia and salivary pooling (Fig 11-10e).

A more focused work-up should seek to establish histopathologic confirmation. For this purpose, an incisional parotid biopsy beneath the earlobe for each parotid gland is preferred over labial gland biopsies because the parotid is more yielding, the major salivary glands are affected earlier and more severely than the minor glands, and lymphoma can be ruled out at the same time (Fig 11-10f). Lymphomas associated with Sjögren syndrome develop only in the parotid gland and systemic lymphatics and are not associated with minor salivary glands. Moreover, labial salivary gland biopsies require regimented biopsy techniques and histopathologic assessment, which are more prone to error.

A Schirmer tear function test is recommended to assess the degree of xerophthalmia. It is not worth the effort, however, to measure parotid salivary flow. Therefore, only a clinical judgment as to the degree of xerostomia is recommended. The Schirmer test is conducted by placing Schirmer porous paper in the inferior fornix of each unanesthetized eye for 10 minutes (Fig 11-10g). The wetting of the paper indicates tear production; less than 10 mm is dry, 10 to 15 mm is borderline, and greater than 15 mm is considered normal.

Laboratory tests should include a complete blood count to assess for anemia, leukopenia, or eosinophilia; serum immunoglobulins to assess for hypergammaglobulinemia consistent with Sjögren syndrome or hypergammaglobulinemia related to a lymphoma developing in a Sjögren syndrome; and the following autoantibody assessments: ANA, RF, SS-A, and SS-B. A positive ANA or RF indicates a possible secondary Sjögren syndrome. A positive SS-A or SS-B is consistent with Sjögren syndrome and may be seen with either the primary or the secondary form, although SS-B is more strongly associated with secondary Sjögren syndrome.

HISTOPATHOLOGY ▶

Lymphocytic infiltration of exocrine glands is the hallmark of Sjögren syndrome. In major salivary glands, the previously described benign lymphoepithelial lesion is considered typical. However, it is not consistently seen in minor salivary glands. Marx et al identified this process in only 65 (57%) of 114 known Sjögren patients who underwent minor salivary gland biopsies. The parotid gland will show an early lymphocytic infiltration, acinar atrophy, and epimyoepithelial islands.

Within minor salivary glands, the formation of epimyoepithelial islands is uncommon. The usual picture is of a focal lymphocytic sialadenitis (Fig 11-11a). To distinguish this from a nonspecific chronic

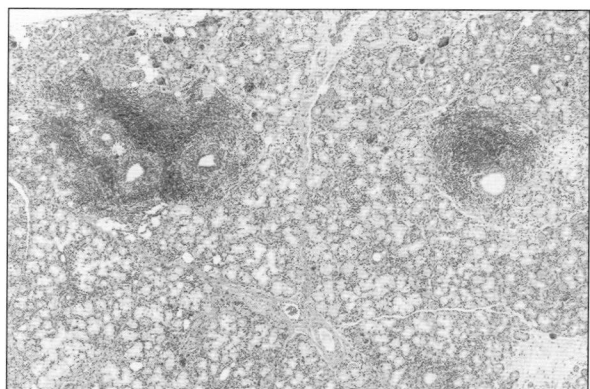

Fig 11-11a Tissue from a lip biopsy specimen of a patient with Sjögren syndrome showing focal aggregates of lymphocytes in a periductal distribution.

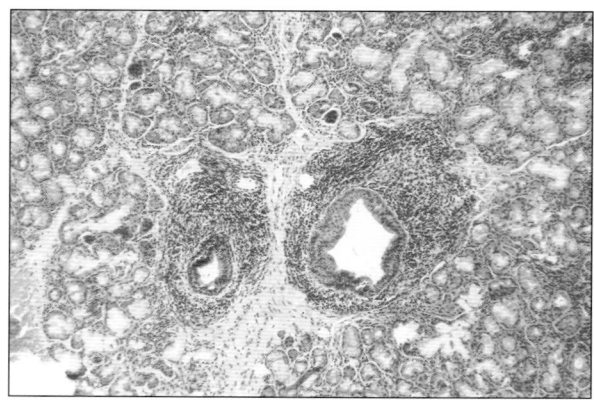

Fig 11-11b Periductal lymphocytes in a patient with Sjögren syndrome. The adjacent acini are normal in appearance.

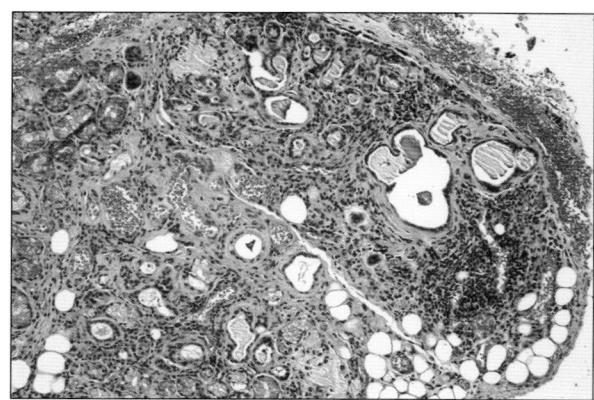

Fig 11-11c A nonspecific chronic sialadenitis in which the ducts are prominent and often dilated. This pattern is not seen in focal lymphocytic sialadenitis associated with Sjögren syndrome.

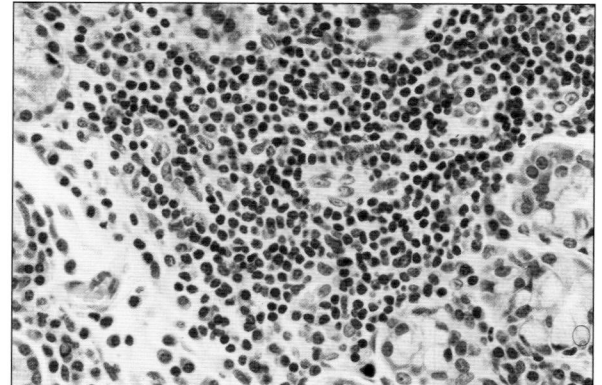

Fig 11-11d A focus of normal-appearing lymphocytes in Sjögren syndrome.

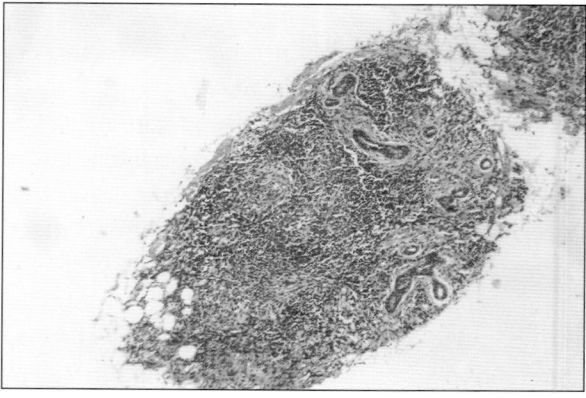

Fig 11-11e As the lymphocytic infiltrates become confluent, the acini are lost in a patient with long-standing secondary Sjögren syndrome.

sialadenitis, a certain set of cumbersome criteria must be met. The lymphocytic foci must be observed in otherwise normal glands that do not demonstrate the diffuse atrophy, ductal dilation, and interstitial fibrosis of nonspecific sialadenitis (Figs 11-11b and 11-11c). The biopsy specimens should be taken from beneath a clinically normal mucosa, and it is recommended that 5 to 10 individual glands be removed for examination. In such a specimen, aggregates of 50 or more lymphocytes (ie, a "focus") are sought adjacent to normal acini (Fig 11-11d). The presence of more than 1 focus per 4 mm^2 in most of the specimen supports the diagnosis of Sjögren syndrome. Because of this involved biopsy protocol, a reliable diagnosis is less likely. Therefore, tissue from an incisional parotid biopsy is preferred. While plasma cells may be seen, they are usually peripheral to the lymphocytic focus. As time passes, the extent of lymphocytic infiltration increases with consequent loss of acini and a resultant clinical xerostomia (Fig 11-11e).

TREATMENT ▶

Like any autoimmune disease, Sjögren syndrome is incurable. However, its symptoms and complications often require management. The symptom of dry eyes is best managed with a slowly dissolving methylcellulose (Lacrisert, Merck) preparation on a daily basis. The eyes also often require topical antibiotics such as sulfacetamide or ophthalmologic gentamycin. The oral dryness may be managed with oral pilocarpine (Salagen), 5 mg three times daily; atomized water spray (Evian, Evian); or sips of water. Caries controls and topical fluoride carriers, which are used in irradiated patients, also are useful. Frequently, nystatin oral suspensions, 100,000 units/mL used as a 1-tsp oral swish and swallow, is needed to control *Candida* colonization.

For the 6% to 10% of cases in which Sjögren syndrome progresses to lymphoma, a complete work-up for lymphoma in other locations and staging are required. Most are B-cell lymphomas. The parotid focus of lymphoma is most often treated with radiotherapy of 5,000 cGy to 6,000 cGy, although chemotherapy for stage II or stage IV lymphoma is also used.

PROGNOSIS ▶ Sjögren syndrome is compatible with long-term survival. A repeat parotid biopsy is indicated if the gland increases in size, darkens, or becomes irregular. In this manner, lymphomatous transformation can be detected early and treated, resulting in a good prognosis.

Necrotizing Sialometaplasia

CLINICAL PRESENTATION AND PATHOGENESIS ▶ Necrotizing sialometaplasia will most commonly present as an inflammatory ulcer on the mucosa of the posterior hard or soft palate. The ulcer will have indurated edges that are often raised, features strongly suggestive of a carcinoma (Fig 11-12a). The ulcer is usually deep with a gray to yellow fibrinous base. The ulcer is tender but not as overtly painful as its appearance might suggest. Frequently, the immediate surrounding mucosa will show red dots that represent inflamed openings of minor salivary gland ducts. The ulcer will be of short duration, usually a few days to a few weeks. It rarely gets larger than 3 cm, and although it may occur bilaterally, it neither crosses the midline nor occurs as a single lesion in the midline.

Occasionally, an early necrotizing sialometaplasia is seen prior to ulceration, which is produced by the onset of necrosis. In such situations, the lesion will appear as an indurated firm elevation. Its slight tenderness and possibly darkened color are the only features differentiating it from a minor salivary gland neoplasm.

Some patients will report a history of trauma or a palatal anesthetic injection 3 or more weeks earlier, but most cannot identify a particular inciting agent.

The pathogenesis of this lesion has frequently been attributed to ischemic necrosis related to palatal injections, trauma, or smoking. This is based on the occasional patient history report of such antecedent events and the observation of pale, devitalized mucous salivary glands among the inflammatory cells and around the metaplastic ductal epithelium. This, however, does not explain the majority of cases, and considering the vast numbers of palatal injections dentists give each year, one would expect a much higher incidence of this disease if this lesion were related to injections or trauma. Because necrotizing sialometaplasia occurs in both smokers and nonsmokers, it also cannot be directly linked to smoking.

DIFFERENTIAL DIAGNOSIS ▶ Palatal ulcers with induration are strongly suggestive of malignant tumors known to occur in this area. Of these, *squamous cell carcinoma* is a strong consideration, as are the salivary gland malignancies, *adenoid cystic carcinoma* and *mucoepidermoid carcinoma*. However, all of these tumors should have a longer duration than that of necrotizing sialometaplasia. A common problem is that a long-standing lesion may not have been noticed for some time and then is reported as a recent happening; alternatively, an unrelated trauma may focus attention on the lesion, and as a result a traumatic cause is falsely attributed. Additionally, the palate is a preferred site for extranodal *non-Hodgkin lymphoma*. However, such lesions tend to be fleshy masses without ulceration.

DIAGNOSTIC WORK-UP ▶ Because a patient's history may be confused and even misleading, all such lesions should be biopsied. An incisional biopsy of the base of the ulcer and the edge that is most indurated and raised will yield the most representative specimen. It is important to take a large specimen and to include the deep base of the lesion because a necrotizing sialometaplasia may occur over a true neoplasm. While many lesions of necrotizing sialometaplasia in the past were overdiagnosed as invasive malignancies, the opposite can also occur, that is, a necrotizing sialometaplasia can obscure a malignancy.

HISTOPATHOLOGY ▶ Necrotizing sialometaplasia is characterized by lobular necrosis and associated squamous metaplasia of ducts and acini. At low power, the preservation of lobular architecture is apparent. The areas of necrosis consist of small pools of mucin rimmed by neutrophils. Within or adjacent to these areas are metaplastic ducts. These may be seen as ducts with a thickened squamous epithelial lining, or as solid,

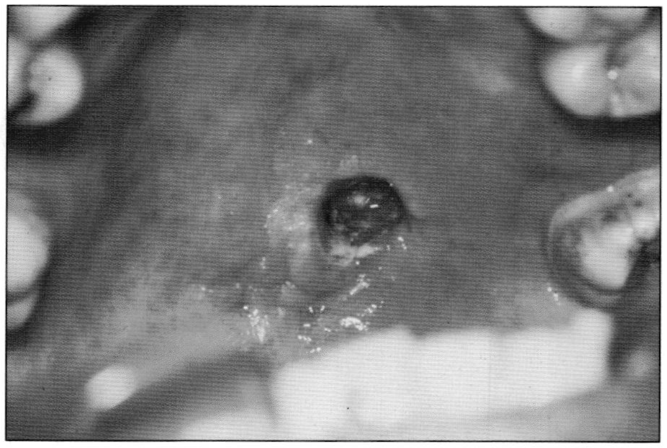

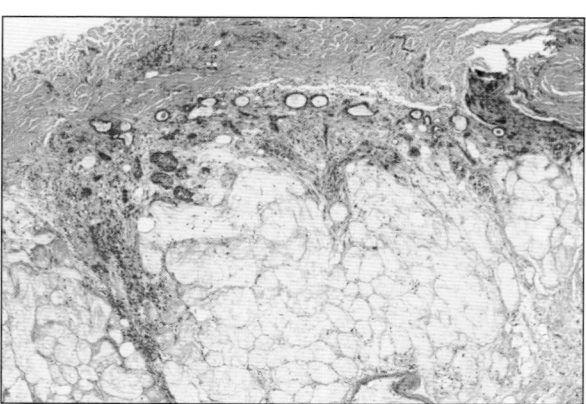

Fig 11-12a Sialometaplasia ulcers often have ragged raised edges and will be indurated because of inflammation, giving the clinical impression of a carcinoma.

Fig 11-12b Necrotizing sialometaplasia of the palate showing the reactive process immediately overlying the necrotic mucous glands.

Fig 11-12c A higher-power view of Fig 11-12b revealing some inflammatory cells within the necrotic glands. The associated ducts and acini have undergone squamous metaplasia.

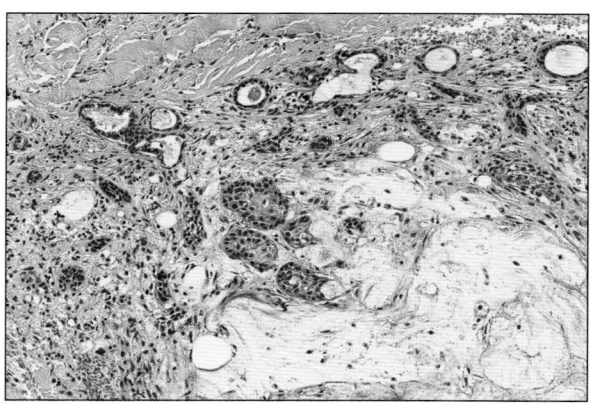

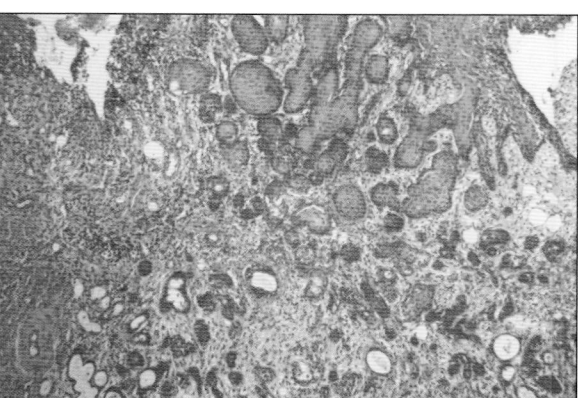

Fig 11-12d Necrotizing sialometaplasia. Pseudoepitheliomatous hyperplasia can be seen above, and some metaplastic ducts and acini can be seen below.

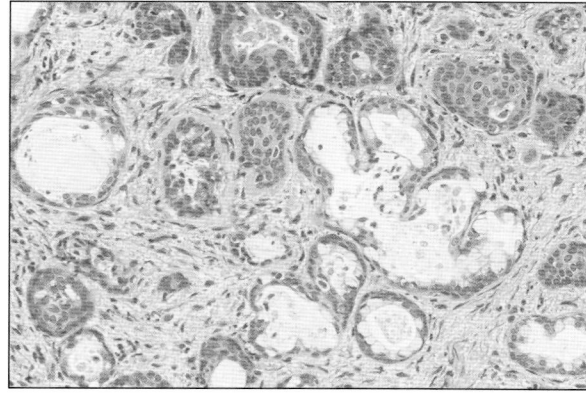

Fig 11-12e Necrotizing sialometaplasia in which some residual mucous cells, together with the squamous metaplasia, can mimic a mucoepidermoid carcinoma.

compact, rounded nests of epithelium. An inflammatory background is typically present (Figs 11-12b and 11-12c). The mucosal surface is often ulcerated, and pseudoepitheliomatous hyperplasia is seen as a result of squamous metaplasia of the excretory ducts. The epithelial cells are usually bland but may be hyperchromatic (Fig 11-12d). The pseudoepitheliomatous hyperplasia as well as the deeply seated islands of metaplastic squamous epithelium can lead to an erroneous diagnosis of squamous cell carcinoma. In addition, the squamous metaplasia of the ducts and acini juxtaposed with residual mucous cells may suggest a mucoepidermoid carcinoma (Fig 11-12e). In most cases, however, the lobular architecture, areas of necrosis, and mixed inflammatory background, together with the distinctive epithelial nests, distinguish necrotizing sialometaplasia.

TREATMENT AND PROGNOSIS ▶

A true necrotizing sialometaplasia requires no specific treatment other than follow-up. However, follow-up over the subsequent 3 months is extremely important because a necrotizing sialometaplasia should resolve in that time. The clinician should remember that incorrect diagnoses can go both ways. Just as diagnosing a necrotizing sialometaplasia as a mucoepidermoid carcinoma or a squamous cell carcinoma is possible, so is diagnosing each of these malignancies as a necrotizing sialometaplasia. Lesions that worsen over the first 2 months or show no evidence of resolving require re-biopsy and a second review of the original histopathologic features.

Necrotizing sialometaplasia fills in with granulation tissue and completely epithelializes its surface within 3 months.

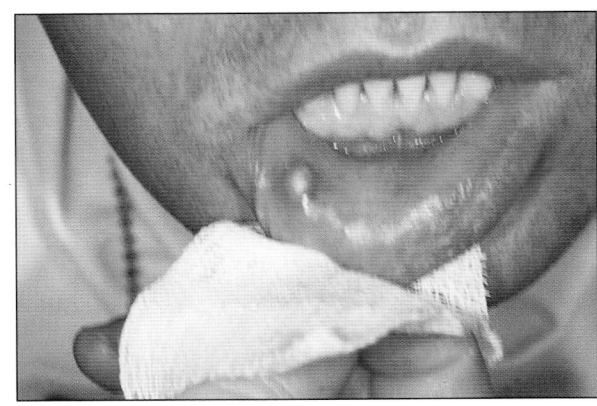

Fig 11-13 Mucoceles will usually appear on the lower lip as thin-walled, fluid-filled, blue vesicles.

Salivary Retention Phenomena

Mucoceles are mucous extravasation phenomena resulting from traumatic severance of salivary excretory ducts or, occasionally, their spontaneous rupture. The extravasated mucin elicits an inflammatory reaction and some fibrosis, resulting in what is recognized as a mucocele. Mucoceles can occur almost anywhere minor salivary glands exist but are most common in the lower lip. They also occur related to the sublingual gland (called a ranula) and even the parotid gland (called a sialocele). In each location, it is important to note that ductal injury, rather than glandular injury, is the cause of mucoceles. This explains why most lip surgeries do not cause mucoceles and parotid gland surgeries do not cause sialoceles.

As stated earlier, the three clinical types of mucous extravasation have a similar pathogenesis and development. They differ only in their glands (ie, ducts) of origin.

Mucoceles

Mucoceles of minor salivary gland origin will present as painless or only mildly uncomfortable, soft, fluid-filled vesicles (Fig 11-13). Those that occur on the lower lip are usually located paramidline, measure 1 cm or less, and appear bluish because of the mucin. Deeper mucoceles, which often occur on the ventral surface of the tongue or the floor of the mouth unassociated with the sublingual gland, are frequently gray or yellowish in color. Most occur in children, teenagers, and young adults.

A separate type of minor salivary gland mucocele, known as a *superficial mucocele*, is formed after a duct rupture in the subepithelial location. Preferred sites are the palate and retromolar areas. The mucoceles will appear as small (1- to 5-mm) yellow to gray vesicles.

Ranulas

Ranulas result from extravasation of saliva from any one of the 20 ducts that arise from the sublingual gland and empty into the floor of the mouth or into the anterior portion of Wharton duct. Some, therefore, are initiated by ductal injury or inflammation created by sialoliths of Wharton duct. Ranulas are characteristically large (3 to 6 cm) and form a blue, tense vesicle in the floor of the mouth (Fig 11-14). The typical size of a ranula and the firmness of the floor of the oral mucosa together resemble a frog's belly, hence the name "ranula," which refers to the frog's genus, *Rana*.

Some ranulas will attain sufficient fluid pressure as to herniate through the mylohyoid muscle and present in the submental triangle as a soft mass (Figs 11-15a and 11-15b). These are called *plunging ranulas*. Some become so large that they compromise swallowing or breathing and extend as far as the mediastinum.

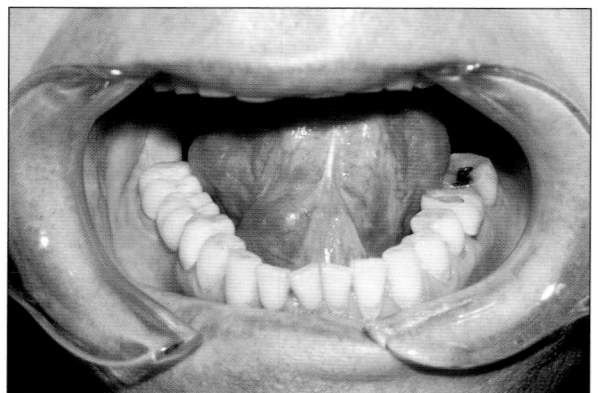

Fig 11-14 A ranula is a mucocele in the floor of the mouth usually arising from the sublingual gland. It will therefore also present as a thin-walled, fluid-filled, blue vesicle.

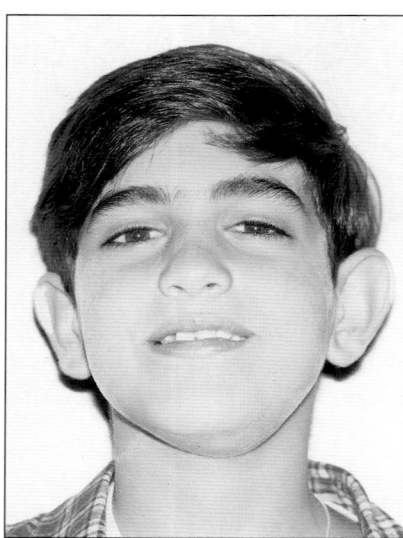

Fig 11-15a Some ranulas will protrude through the mylohyoid muscle to present in the submandibular triangle as a plunging ranula.

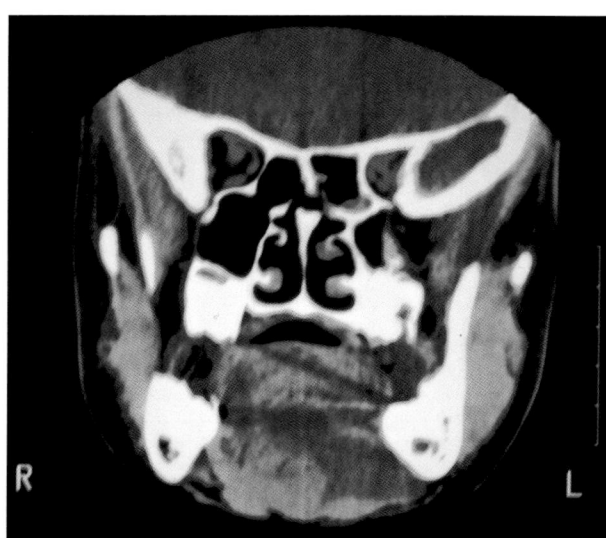

Fig 11-15b This CT scan of a plunging ranula shows fluid in the floor of the mouth and in the left side of the submental triangle.

Sialoceles

Sialoceles of the submandibular gland and parotid gland (Fig 11-16a) are uncommon. When they do occur, they are more often related to penetrating injuries rather than to surgery. In either situation, the ductal injury is found in the main duct or in one of the large interlobar ducts (Figs 11-16b and 11-16c). Sialoceles of the parotid gland are more common than those of the submandibular gland. In the parotid gland, the extravasation of saliva forms a cutaneous collection, which thins the overlying skin, frequently to the point of rupture, or communicates to an area of penetrating injury to form a salivary cutaneous fistula.

DIFFERENTIAL DIAGNOSIS ▶

Mucoceles

Because mucoceles of minor salivary gland origin are bluish and the history of trauma may be vague, other lesions that may appear blue must be considered. Of these, *low-grade mucoepidermoid carcinomas* are the most significant. They will also produce mucin in vacuolated spaces within the tumor, imparting the blue color. *Cavernous hemangiomas*, *small lymphangiomas*, and a *venous varix* will give a similar appearance. Although rare, a *vascular leiomyoma* appears blue and has a predilection for the lip.

Ranulas

Because of its denseness, the ranula will palpate as a firm mass, and because it is sufficiently deep that a blue coloration often is not seen, it may resemble a *dermoid cyst*, which is known to occur in the floor-of-the-mouth area. Other developmental cysts, including *epidermoid cysts*, *teratoid cysts*, and the *gastrointestinal heterotopic cyst*, occur more rarely in this area as well. The firmness and doughy quality of a ranula also may suggest a *salivary gland tumor of the sublingual gland*, a *lymphangioma*, or a lymph node enlargement that may represent a *lymphoma*, *sarcoidosis*, or *HIV-related lymphadenopathy*, among other conditions.

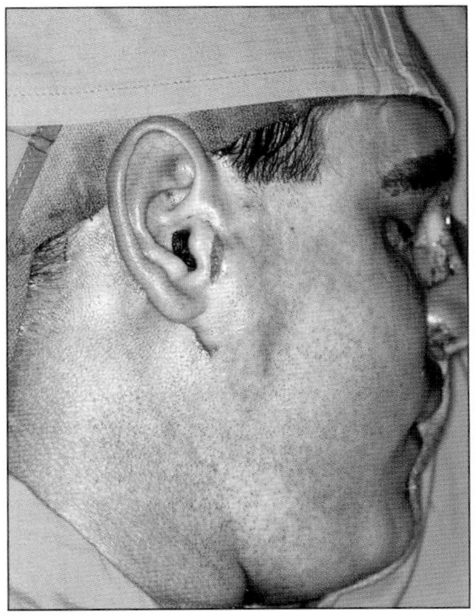

Fig 11-16a A parotid sialocele presents with thinning of the overlying skin and a saliva collection usually associated with eating or other salivary stimulations.

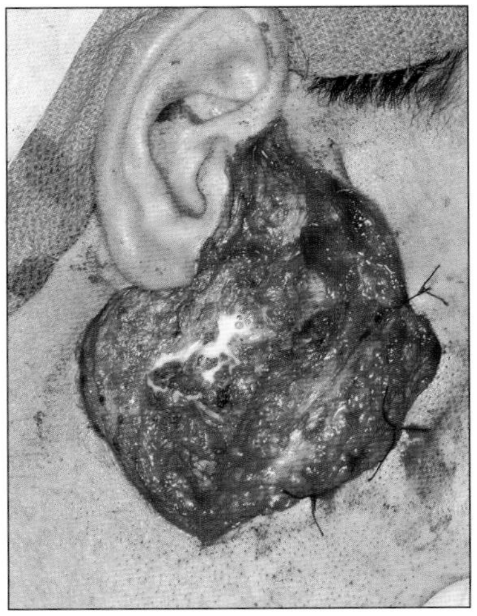

Fig 11-16b Injection of sterile milk will locate and identify a tear or laceration in the main parotid duct and/or one of the major interlobar ducts.

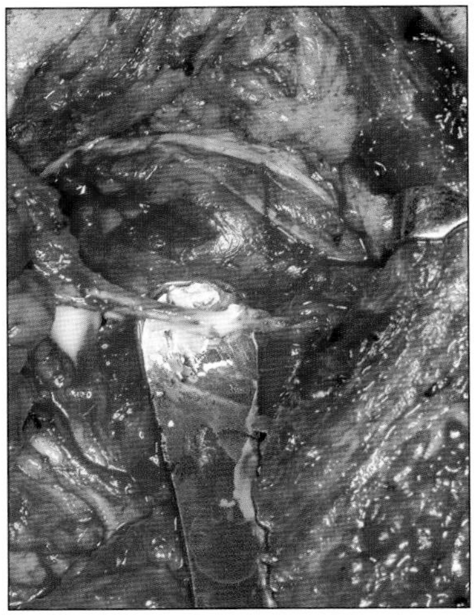

Fig 11-16c Injection of sterile milk will guide the dissection to isolate the parotid duct injury so that magnification-assisted repair or a ligation can be accomplished.

Sialoceles

Sialoceles are somewhat distinctive because of their history of more obvious trauma. Their main challenge is the identification of the actual injured duct producing the phenomenon.

Diagnostic Work-Up, Treatment, and Prognosis

Mucoceles

Minor salivary gland mucoceles are managed by local excision, including excision of the tense overlying epithelium. This will establish the diagnosis and resolve the condition with little chance of recurrence of the original lesion or generation of a new lesion. However, it is important to be sure the surgery does not create another partially transsected minor salivary gland, which can produce a recurrent mucocele.

Ranulas

The most predictable approach to a ranula is excision of the fibrous capsule and the entire sublingual gland from which it arises (Figs 11-17a and 11-17b). Transoral approaches to a ranula/sublingual gland excision should attempt to minimize the risk of damage to small branches of the lingual nerve. A common approach is to incise the mucosa over the submandibular duct in which a lacrimal probe has been placed for identification. The ranula and the sublingual gland are then bluntly dissected from the submandibular duct and the lingual nerve. The lingual nerve is known to "double cross" the submandibular duct; that is, in the posterior lingual vestibule (second premolar–first molar region), the lingual nerve will cross the duct from its medial to lateral aspects and will course superficial to the duct. It is, therefore, at greatest risk for damage in this location. The nerve will then cross under the duct from the lateral to the medial aspects in the first premolar region and ramify into numerous branches into the tongue musculature from its deep surface. The ranula can be separated from these branches using blunt dissection parallel to the branches (Figs 11-17c and 11-17d).

Because the sublingual gland is positioned adjacent to the lingual cortex, it is anterior to the lingual nerve entering the tongue. Therefore, another approach to the sublingual gland is a lingual gingival incision via reflection of lingual periosteum. An incision through the periosteum will enable assessment

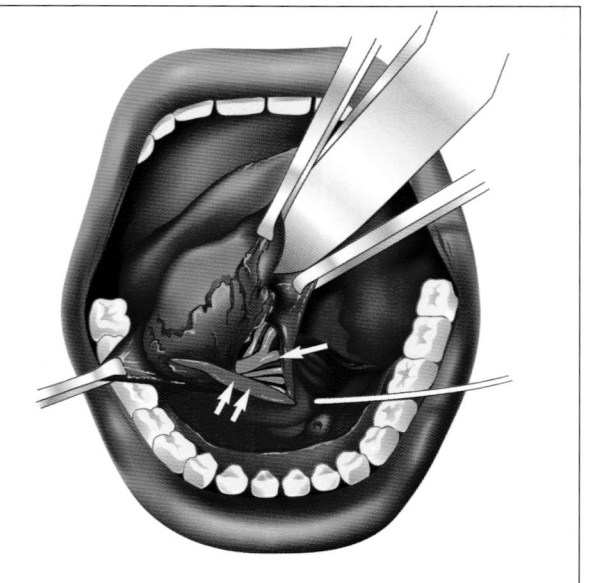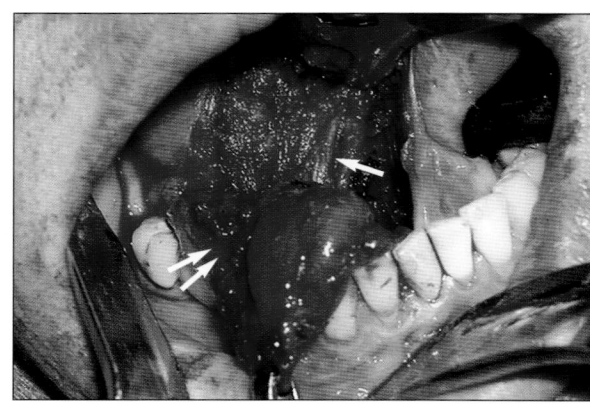

Figs 11-17a and 11-17b The best method for assuring resolution of a ranula is via excision of the entire mucous-filled capsule and the sublingual gland of origin. Noted here are the preserved branches of the lingual nerve posterior to the ranula (*single arrow*, lingual nerve; *double arrows*, submandibular duct).

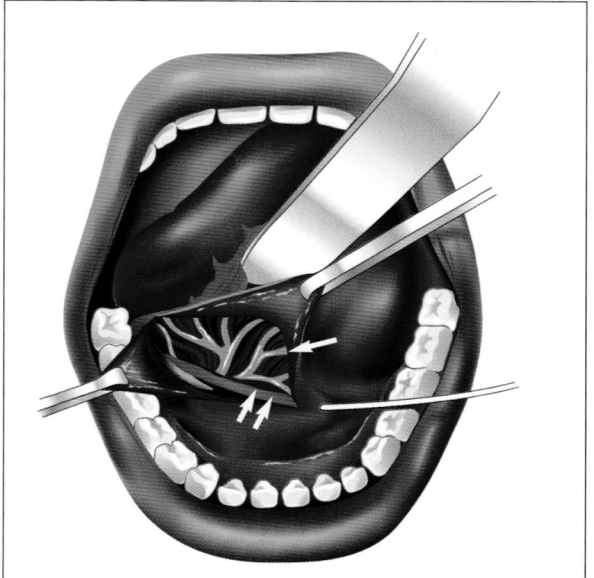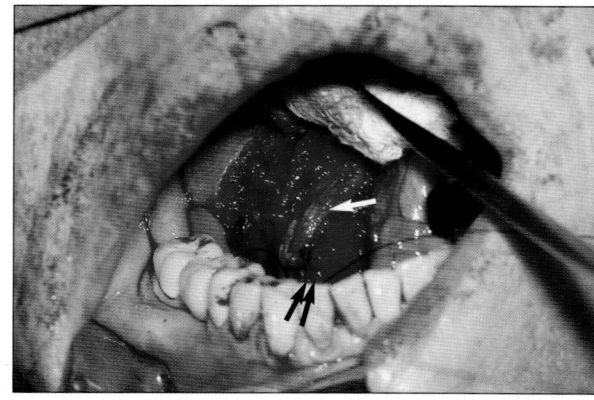

Figs 11-17c and 11-17d The wound defect after a ranula excision should allow visualization of the lingual nerve entering the tongue. The wound is usually left to granulate and epithelialize. It may also be skin grafted or closed primarily, but these maneuvers are not necessary (*single arrow*, lingual nerve; *double arrows*, submandibular duct).

of the sublingual glands at the point most distant from the lingual nerve. This approach avoids the need for incisions through the floor of the oral mucosa in which lingual nerve branches course and may have been displaced by the ranula.

Marsupialization procedures have been used to temporarily decompress a large ranula. Marsupialization may also occasionally resolve a ranula, but several procedures are often required and even then often do not resolve the ranula.

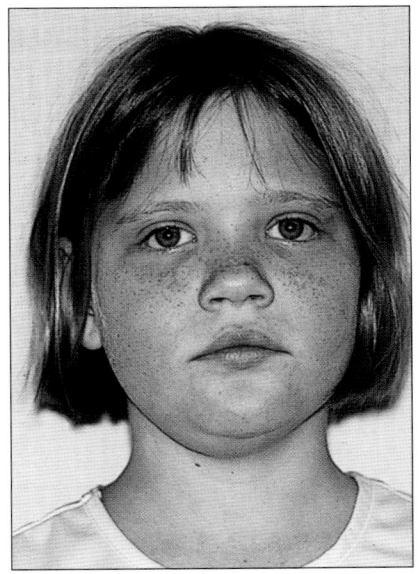

Fig 11-18a Expansion in the submental triangle to the right of the midline related to a plunging ranula.

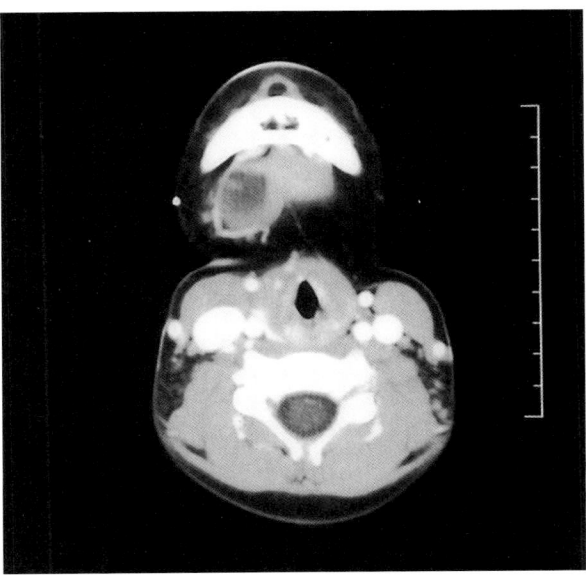

Fig 11-18b A CT scan of this plunging ranula shows a hypodense space indicative of a fluid-filled lesion and suggesting its origin from the right sublingual gland.

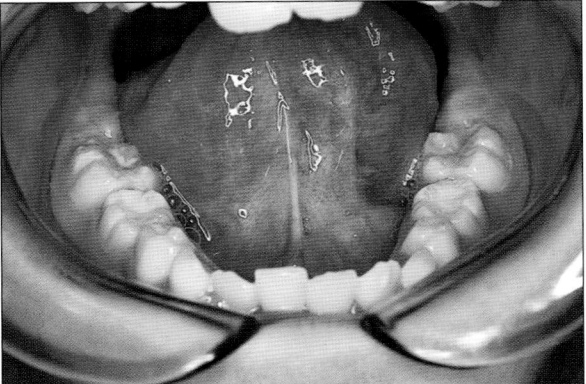

Fig 11-18c A plunging ranula may have only a slight presentation in the floor of the mouth.

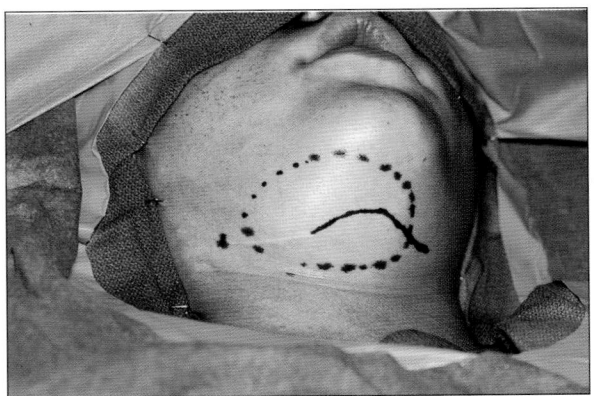

Fig 11-18d Access to a plunging ranula is made through a symmetric incision in the submental triangle.

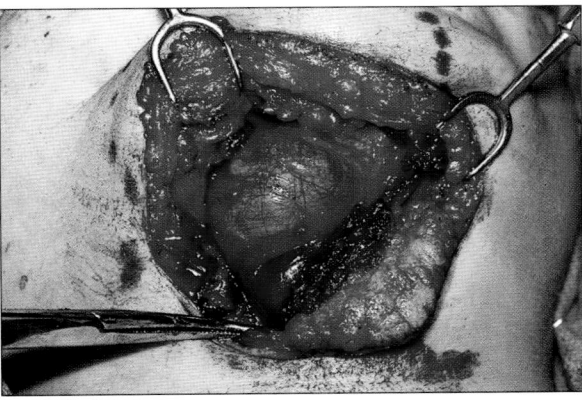

Fig 11-18e A plunging ranula is exposed through a cutaneous incision in the submental triangle. Here, the tense fluid-filled ranula is distending and herniating through the mylohyoid muscle.

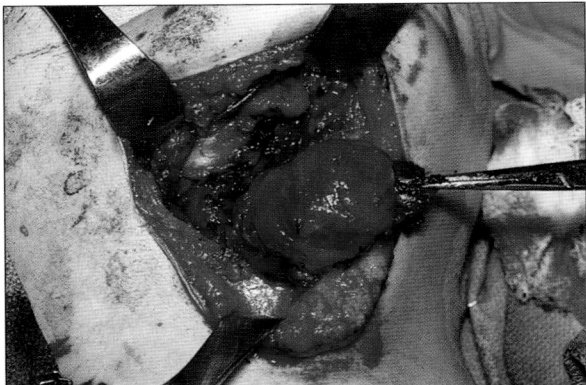

Fig 11-18f Ranulas may become very large. The entire connective tissue lining and the offending sublingual gland must be removed to prevent recurrences. In some cases, removal of both sublingual glands may be necessary.

Plunging ranulas are best approached through a transcutaneous incision in the submental triangle. This access will allow removal of the ranula directly and permit repair of the mylohyoid muscle. With this approach, a symmetric incision is made across the midline within the submental triangle. The distended ranula may be just deep to the surface and can be accessed by reflecting the two portions of the mylohyoid muscle created by the rent in this muscle from the pressure of the plunging ranula. The ranula and the offending gland are then excised with a pericapsular blunt dissection and separated from the lingual nerve, which will be positioned on the oral side of the ranula (Figs 11-18a to 11-18f).

Sialoceles

Sialoceles of the parotid gland may be treated with repair assisted by loop magnification or the operating microscope if the main parotid duct is severed and is identifiable. To locate the injured duct, it is help-

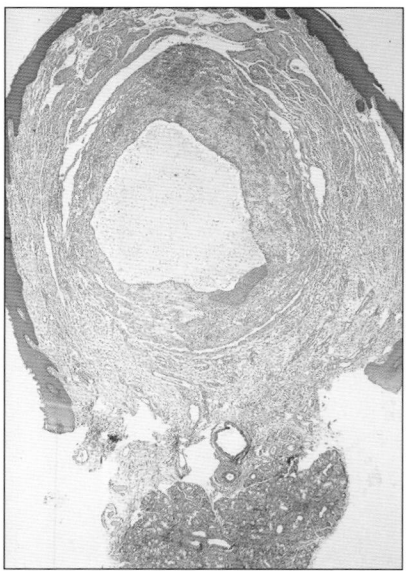

Fig 11-19a A mucocele with a fragment of the ruptured duct at the base and the liberated mucin walled off by inflammatory tissue.

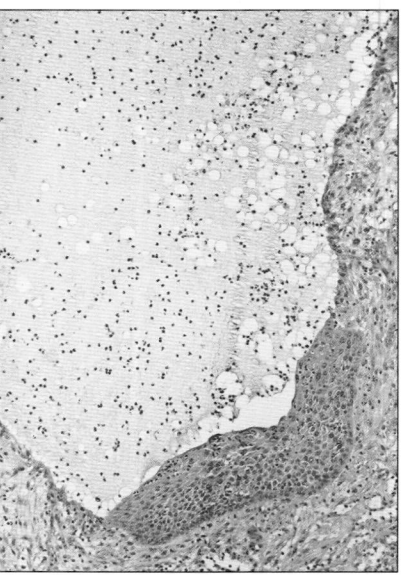

Fig 11-19b A higher-power view of Fig 11-19a showing the epithelium of the ruptured duct.

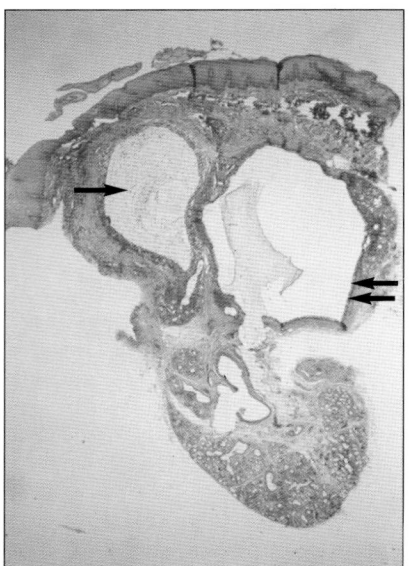

Fig 11-20 A mucocele (*single arrow*) with a dense inflammatory lining and a mucus retention cyst (*double arrows*) with the ductal epithelial lining. The feeder duct and mucous glands, showing chronic sialadenitis, are at the base.

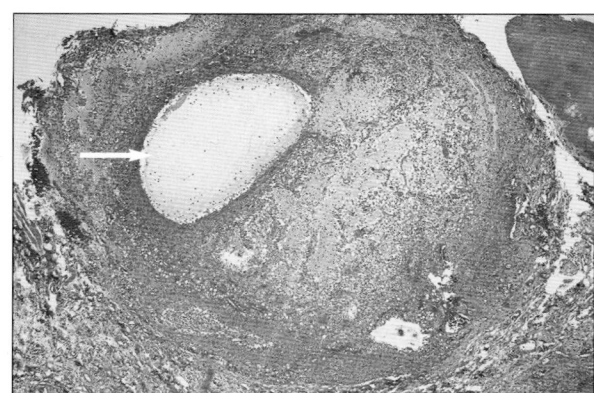

Fig 11-21a Mucin has been liberated into the tissues. The mucin has pooled and is walled off by inflammatory tissue (*arrow*).

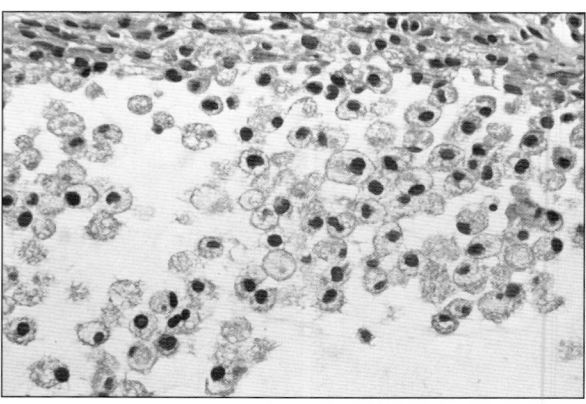

Fig 11-21b In mucoceles, macrophages associated with the mucin may be found in large numbers. The cytoplasm contains mucin.

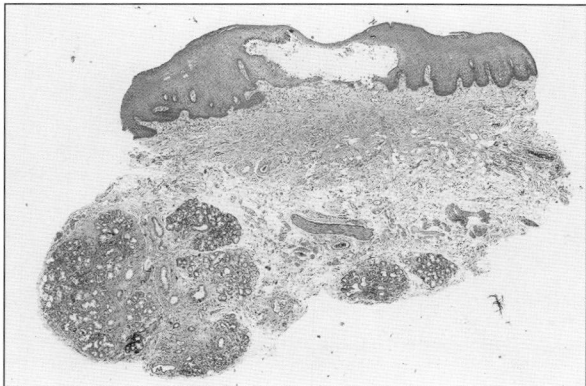

Fig 11-22 A superficial mucocele can simulate a vesiculobullous lesion.

ful to cannulate and inject sterile milk into Stensen duct (see Figs 11-16a to 11-16c). If the duct is repairable, it is sutured and retested with another injection of sterile milk. Postoperatively, the patient must be well hydrated and maintained on sialagogues to prevent ductal collapse and fibrosis. Most injuries causing sialoceles are located deep within the gland so that a cannula or stent cannot be retrieved.

If the ductal system is macerated and there is no chance of individual ductal repair, a superficial parotidectomy is very effective. Prolonged occlusive dressings, ligation of Stensen duct, and even radiation therapy have been used, but each is less ideal than either ductal repair or superficial parotidectomy

HISTOPATHOLOGY ▶

The histologic picture is characterized by the liberation of mucin from an injured duct into connective tissue, accompanied by an inflammatory reaction that includes neutrophils, plasma cells, lymphocytes, and macrophages (Figs 11-19a, 11-19b, and 11-20). The mucin collects in pools and is walled off by a compressed fibrovascular tissue, which usually contains inflammatory cells (Fig 11-21a). This gives the impression of a cystic structure, but no epithelial lining is present. The pooled mucin often contains neu-

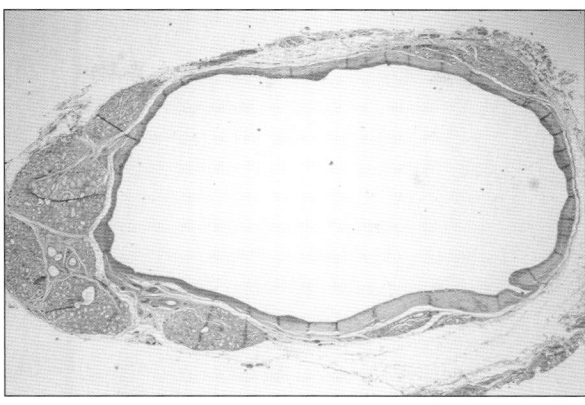

Fig 11-23a A mucus retention cyst with an epithelial lining. The inflammatory features that accompany a mucocele typically are not seen.

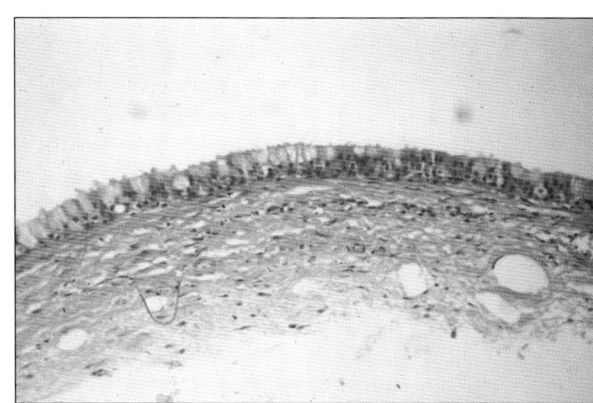

Fig 11-23b The lining of a mucus retention cyst with mucous-secreting cells. This is a variable finding.

trophils and large numbers of active macrophages with a vacuolated cytoplasm (Fig 11-21b). As the lesion ages, reparative features may become apparent with formation of granulation tissue and ultimately fibrosis. Some lesions may show prominent vascularity. Adjacent mucous glands usually show features of a sialadenitis with inflammatory infiltrates, ductal dilation, and acinar atrophy. The surface epithelium is frequently attenuated. In some instances, the mucocele may be extremely superficial with mucin collecting within or immediately below the epithelium (Fig 11-22), giving the impression of a vesiculobullous process.

Mucus Retention Cyst

CLINICAL PRESENTATION AND PATHOGENESIS ▶

Mucus retention cysts are distinguished from mucous extravasation phenomena by the histopathologic identification of an epithelial lining rather than a lining of granulation tissue. Mucus retention cysts therefore are often clinically referred to as mucoceles. Unlike true mucoceles, however, they rarely form in the lower lip (3% of lower lip mucoceles are mucus retention cysts). Instead, they are more commonly located in the floor of the mouth, buccal mucosa, posterior palate, and upper lip. Because they arise from ductal obstruction by calculi, mucous plugs, or fibrosis, they also differ from true mucoceles by their absence of traumatic duct injury or rupture.

Mucus retention cysts will present as a 0.3- to 1.0-cm painless mass within the mucosa. The distended overlying epithelium will be of normal color. Unlike mucoceles, the cysts will not appear bluish, and there is usually no history of an inciting event or other pathology. The mass will be freely movable without induration.

DIFFERENTIAL DIAGNOSIS ▶

The firm, freely movable mass characteristic of a mucus retention cyst is suggestive of a small or developing benign salivary gland tumor. Therefore, *pleomorphic adenoma* is a strong consideration, as is a *canalicular adenoma* and a *basal cell adenoma*. In addition, their very development makes them akin to mucoceles of the mucous extravasation type, particularly an older, mature mucocele often referred to as a *fibrosed mucocele*.

DIAGNOSTIC WORK-UP AND TREATMENT ▶

Mucus retention cysts require excision for diagnosis and definitive treatment. Only a "shelling out" type of a dissection is required, but the cyst is often removed with 0.5-cm margins because of the possibility that the mass may represent a benign salivary gland tumor.

HISTOPATHOLOGY ▶

Because these lesions develop as a consequence of retention within a salivary duct, an epithelial lining is present (Figs 11-23a and 11-23b). The cells are often cuboidal to columnar with eosinophilic cytoplasm and resemble striated ducts. Mucous-secreting cells may be present, and squamous epithelium is

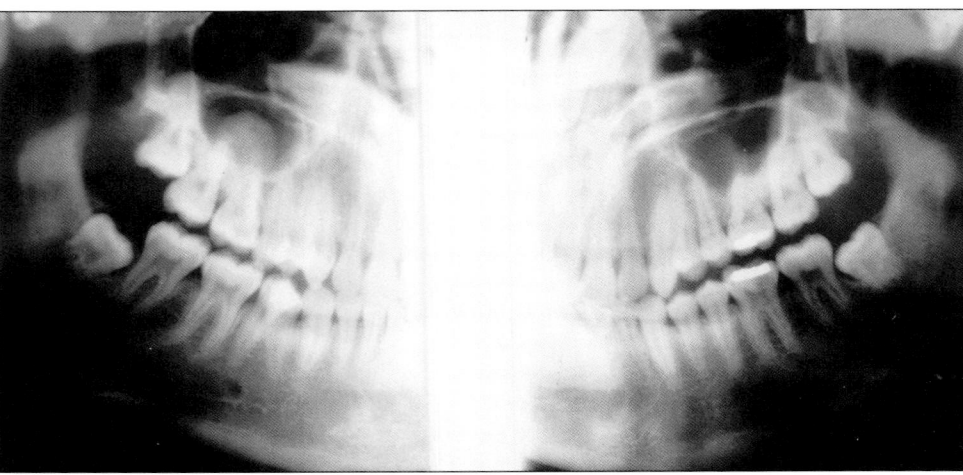

Fig 11-24 Mucoceles in the maxillary sinus are frequently seen as rounded or dome-shaped soft tissue masses arising from the sinus lining.

not unusual. The lumen contains mucin. An inflammatory component, usually prominent in the mucocele, is typically absent except within the adjacent salivary glands.

PROGNOSIS ▶ Excision is curative. A true mucus retention cyst will be limited in size compared to large mucous extravasations, such as the ranula, because the cystic pressure created behind the obstructed and dilated duct will compress the gland of origin, eventually causing it to atrophy and cease salivary production. Therefore, mucus retention cysts tend to be small, isolated, and uncommon.

Mucoceles and Mucous Cysts of the Sinuses

CLINICAL PRESENTATION AND PATHOGENESIS ▶ Both mucoceles and mucous cysts occur in the paranasal sinuses. Most are incidental radiographic findings of a dome-shaped soft tissue mass seen radiographically or on a CT scan. They are most commonly seen in one or both maxillary sinuses on a panoramic radiograph (Fig 11-24). They are primarily seen in young adults and are associated with airborne allergens or chronic sinusitis. The mucoceles or, more rarely, the cysts that they may represent are asymptomatic in themselves, but their presence usually indicates an inflammatory sinus condition.

Sinus mucous extravasations are mostly induced by allergens and/or chronic inflammatory sinus disease. The goblet cells of the schneiderian membrane hypertrophy, secrete additional mucous, and undergo hyperplasia. A collection of mucin accumulates between the bony sinus floor and the distended sinus membrane to create the classic dome-shaped soft tissue density. Rarely, part of the schneiderian membrane may proliferate and prolapse over another part, forming a mucous cyst lined by a sinus membrane.

DIFFERENTIAL DIAGNOSIS ▶ The main entity on the differential list of a sinus mucocele is a *sinus polyp*. However, sinus polyps have a greater soft tissue density because they are solid cells rather than mucous extravasations or cysts, which are fluid filled. Sinus polyps also tend to erode bone and emanate from the sinus roof and upper portions of the walls, whereas mucoceles arise from the sinus floor. While some would place certain tumors on the same differential—in particular, *adenoid cystic carcinoma*, which is well-known to arise within the sinus, and a *squamous cell carcinoma of sinus origin*—these would each be more radiodense with soft tissue, erode bone, and have an irregular outline. Mucoceles of the sinus have a smooth, dome-shaped outline.

DIAGNOSTIC WORK-UP AND TREATMENT ▶ A careful review of the radiograph should be sufficient to distinguish the sinus mucocele from other entities. If doubt remains, a CT scan, which will give a clearer picture of the shape, location, and density of the lesion, should be performed. No specific treatment is required.

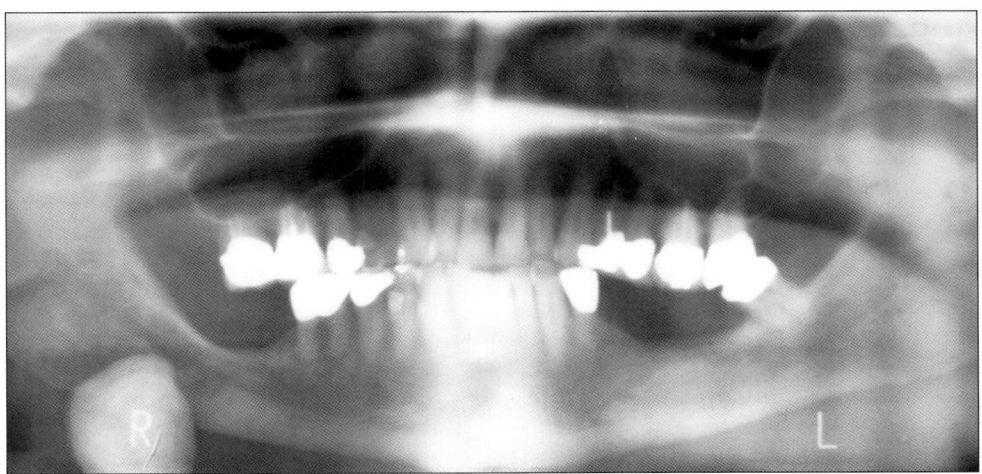

Fig 11-25 Because they are composed of calcium carbonate and calcium phosphate, sialoliths in the submandibular gland are most always visible on a panoramic radiograph. They may be located in the proximal duct or within the gland parenchyma.

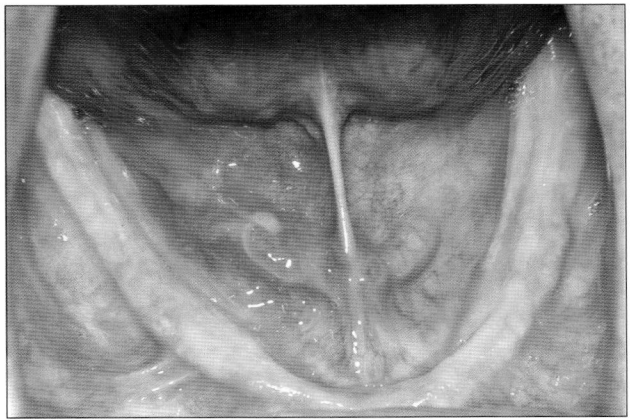

Fig 11-26 Sialoliths may produce a sialadenitis with pain and suppuration, which will be characterized either by pus emanating from the duct, as seen here, or by a submandibular space abscess.

HISTOPATHOLOGY ▶

The true sinus mucous cyst is an epithelially lined, mucin-filled structure that may arise either from a blocked sinus ostium or from sinus lining displaced during surgery or following trauma. More commonly, it results as a reaction to allergens or as part of a chronic sinusitis. The epithelium may be mucous secreting or cuboidal. The mucous may escape into the adjacent tissue and cause an inflammatory reaction. Hemorrhage may occur and result in hemosiderin and cholesterol deposition.

Mucus retention cysts arise from obstruction of a duct within the sinus lining. They are typically lined by pseudostratified columnar epithelium. Some mucous-secreting cells may also be present.

The true sinus mucocele has no epithelial lining. It consists of a mucoid or serous fluid that collects under the mucosa of the sinus, causing compression of the adjacent connective tissue.

Sialolithiasis

CLINICAL PRESENTATION AND PATHOGENESIS ▶

Sialolithiasis (calculi, salivary stones) can form in all of the salivary glands, including minor salivary glands, but the gland that most commonly produces such stones is the submandibular gland. The so-called stones that form in the parotid duct system are rarely calcified and are actually mucous plugs that do not appear on radiographs. Stones that form in the submandibular duct system are almost always radiopaque because they are composed of calcium carbonate and calcium phosphate (Fig 11-25). Stones are believed to be more common in the submandibular duct system because of the more viscous glycoprotein consistency of the secretions and the upward course of the duct, which makes it more prone to stasis and retrograde bacterial invasion. The parotid gland secretion is much less viscous because of its higher protein levels and because the course of Stensen duct is downward. There is no association in either gland with altered serum calcium levels or renal stones.

Sialoliths form around a nidus in concentric layers, suggesting that some event (eg, inflammation, bacterial colonization, a foreign body, or sloughed cells) precedes their formation. They can occur along any part of the duct and are most frequent at anatomic bends. In the submandibular duct, stones are often found at the duct's bend around the posterior edge of the mylohyoid muscle.

When sialoliths form, they will obstruct the duct either partially or completely. Therefore, individuals present with a painful swelling of the gland and usually with signs of secondary infection, including a suppurative exudate from the duct, fever, and mild to moderate leukocytosis (Fig 11-26). Individuals will

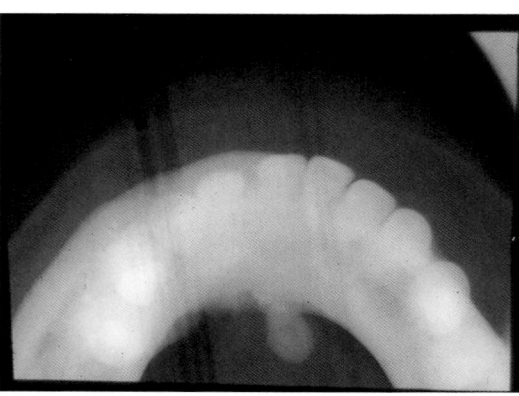

Fig 11-27 The location of a suspected sialolith in the distal portion of the submandibular duct may be confirmed by direct clinical examination or by a simple occlusal radiograph.

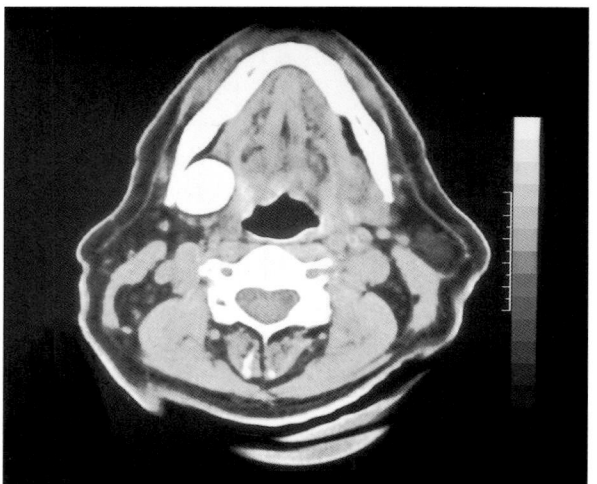

Fig 11-28 The location of a suspected sialolith within the submandibular gland can be confirmed by a CT scan, as seen here.

report an increase in pain and swelling upon eating. The gland will be palpably firm and anywhere from mildly tender to very painful.

Radiographs may identify one or more stones in the submandibular duct. However, to identify stones that may also have formed within the gland itself, a CT scan is recommended as the most unequivocal study to accomplish.

DIFFERENTIAL DIAGNOSIS ▶ The diagnosis may seem apparent with the identification of sialolithiasis and apparent sialadenitis. However, the clinician must confront two subtle difficulties. The first is whether the radiographic stone is indeed in the submandibular duct. Stones in the anterior portion of the duct can often be palpated or seen on an occlusal radiograph; these can hardly be in any place other than the duct. Those more posterior, within the hilum of the gland or at the posterior edge of the mylohyoid, may be confused with calcifications from other sources, such as *calcified lymph nodes* from previously resolved tuberculosis, *phleboliths* (particularly if an old cavernous hemangioma were present), *tonsoliths*, and even *calcifications of the carotid bifurcation*.

The second difficulty is determining whether the stone is related to a sialadenitis, which is most likely, or whether it is one of about 10% of cases associated with a tumor within the gland.

DIAGNOSTIC WORK-UP ▶ A critical part of the work-up is a CT scan with 2- to 3-mm cuts (Figs 11-27 and 11-28) to identify the location of the stone. In most cases, this will eliminate the need for sialography. Computed tomography cannot diagnose a tumor in the gland, but its pattern can identify glands suspicious for a concomitant tumor. Most obstructed submandibular glands will have both inflammation and fibrosis in a homogeneous pattern throughout the gland. If a tumor is present, the CT scan will usually reveal it with a heterogeneous pattern whereby the soft tissue windows will show a different density in the tumor than in the remainder of the gland.

TREATMENT ▶ Stones that are accessible in the floor of the mouth are removed via a direct approach, and the damaged duct is sutured to the mucosa of the floor of the mouth (sialodochoplasty). With this approach there is always concern about the course of the lingual nerve in the floor of the mouth. The lingual nerve will begin lateral and superficial to the submandibular duct in the second premolar–molar region. It will curve beneath the duct at the first premolar region to course deep and medial to the duct anterior to the premolars, where it sends branches to innervate the floor of the mouth and tongue proper. Therefore, the incision for stone removal in the anterior floor of the mouth is best placed somewhat lateral to the duct. In the molar region and posterior, it is best to place it medial to the duct. As the

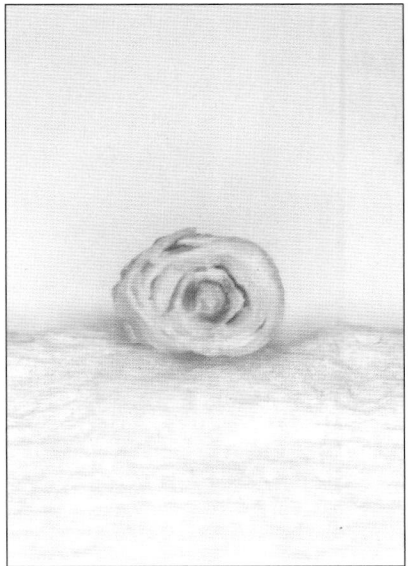

Fig 11-29a Cross section of a sialolith. Note the yellow color and the appearance of a central nidus surrounded by concentric layers.

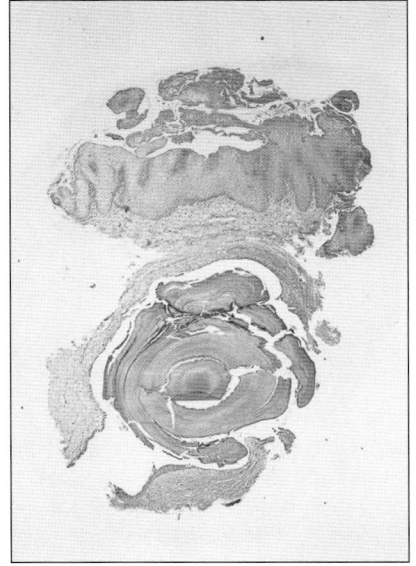

Fig 11-29b A sialolith associated with a minor salivary gland. It lies within the dilated duct and has a lamellar pattern.

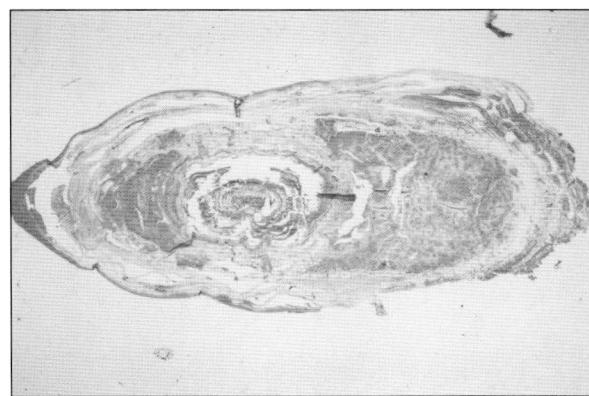

Fig 11-29c A section of a submandibular gland sialolith with a central nidus. This specimen was decalcified.

Fig 11-29d Sialoliths associated with minor salivary glands showing the marked inflammatory response in the surrounding tissue.

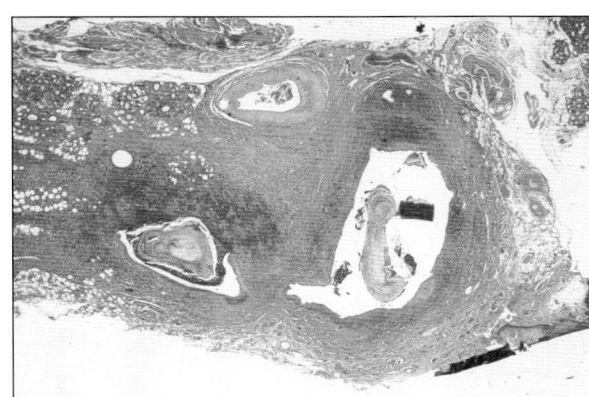

stone and duct are identified, a holding suture should be placed around the duct posterior to the stone to prevent forcing the stone proximally. Postoperatively, patients should be placed on hydration and sialagogues as well as culture-specific antibiotics based on cultures of the removed stones. At times, it is helpful to suture a polyethylene tube into the duct opening in an effort to prevent constriction of the new opening.

There are three indications for excision of the submandibular gland related to sialoliths: (*1*) when sialadenitis persists after removal of stones from the floor of the mouth; (*2*) when the stones are at the mylohyoid bend or the hilum of the gland and duct; or (*3*) when clinical suspicion or scan evidence suggests a tumor.

Parotid stones usually do not produce a long-term clinical problem. Most are passed with parotid flow, and a few require removal from the duct with either a repair or duct transposition. Parotid stones or plugs are not associated with tumors, which are sometimes seen in the submandibular gland.

HISTOPATHOLOGY ▶ Sialoliths may be off-white to yellow or orange in color and have smooth or rough surfaces (Fig 11-29a). Examined microscopically, they are seen to consist of calcified material arranged in a concentric, lamellar pattern (Fig 11-29b), often around a central nidus (Fig 11-29c). Admixed organic material is usually present. The surrounding ductal epithelium may undergo metaplastic change, and adjacent glands will usually show varying degrees and stages of sialadenitis, atrophy, and fibrosis (Fig 11-29d).

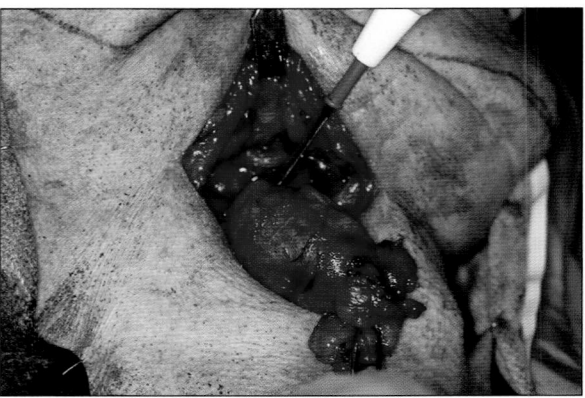

Fig 11-30a Submandibular gland excision is often required to resolve symptoms and eradicate infections associated with sialoliths and sialadenitis. Here, the preservation of the lingual nerve is gained by direct visualization from downward traction on the gland and transsection of the submandibular ganglion connecting fibers.

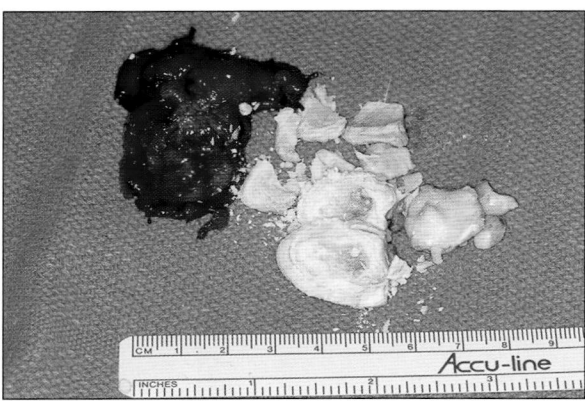

Fig 11-30b Sialoliths will be chalky in consistency and will break apart upon manipulation. Note the concentric rings indicative of sequential layers in their formation.

Sialoliths themselves damage submandibular glands by their obstruction of salivary flow. The back-pressure, inflammation, and subsequent fibrosis develop within the gland parenchyma. Therefore, if the sialolith has been present for a short time, the gland may recover after sialolith removal. However, if the sialolith is of long standing, the gland may harbor irreversible inflammation and fibrosis, so that it cannot recover even if the sialolith is removed. These glands will often have persistent pain after an initial sialolith removal. The ratio is close to 1:1. Glands in which recovery does not occur are usually those with longer histories of obstruction and more clinically apparent infection. In addition, the presence of tumors can initiate stone formation. Firm, hard glands, those with radiographic heterogeneity, and those with persistent symptoms should be removed. If there is any doubt in the clinician's mind, the gland should be removed (Figs 11-30a and 11-30b). The absence of a single damaged submandibular gland results in no functional loss, but the presence of a tumor with a 40% malignant potential can be life threatening.

Submandibular Gland Sialadenitis

Submandibular gland sialadenitis may occur in association with sialolithiasis or a tumor in the gland, or unassociated with either as a direct bacterial infection. Clinically, the gland will be enlarged, tender, and painful to the touch or exhibit pain upon swallowing. Most patients will present with a history of recurrent episodes. If the process has persisted for more than 1 year, the gland will be palpably firm, presumably related to fibrosis. The floor of the mouth will often be elevated because of inflammation within the duct and/or a suppurative exudate emerging from the opening of Wharton duct. There is usually no association with systemic disease processes or with medication. There is also no known association with diet, dental pathology, or periodontal disease.

Depending on the acuteness and the degree of the infection, patients will show varying degrees of leukocytosis and a shift to the left (toward immature forms). Most cases of submandibular gland sialadenitis undergo periodic acute exacerbations from a baseline of chronic disease. During the acute episodes, fever, leukocytosis, and pain are more prominent. The organisms most commonly associated with submandibular gland sialadenitis are the same penicillin-resistant *S aureus* (often methicillin-resistant) and streptococci species that are associated with bacterial parotitis.

DIFFERENTIAL DIAGNOSIS ▶

With submandibular gland sialadenitis, it is important to determine whether it is a straightforward gland infection or if it is associated with *sialolithiasis* or a *salivary gland tumor*. It is also important to rule out a *submandibular space abscess from an odontogenic infection*.

DIAGNOSTIC WORK-UP ▶

Initially, the exudate should be cultured and the patient placed on empiric antibiotics covering streptococci and most penicillin-resistant organisms. Oral therapy such as amoxicillin with clavulanate (Augmentin, SmithKlineBeecham), 875 mg twice daily, dicloxacillin, 500 mg four times daily, or erythromycin ethyl succinate, 400 mg four times daily, are reasonable choices.

A panoramic radiograph and occlusal radiographs to assess for sialoliths are required, as is a thorough dental examination to rule out an odontogenic infection. A CT or MRI scan should be performed to assess for sialoliths within the proximal duct system and for a tumor within the gland.

TREATMENT ▶

Patients with a history of only one or two acute episodes may be treated with an intense, 1-month course of culture-specific antibiotics, hydration, and sialagogues. In cases that are refractory to this regimen, submandibular gland excision should be performed. Additionally, submandibular glands with a history of recurrent episodes or scan evidence suggestive of a tumor should also undergo excision.

Surgical excision of submandibular glands with a history of chronic sialadenitis will exhibit fibrosis of the gland and adherence to surrounding structures. The approach to the gland is best made by an incision at the gland's inferior edge placed in a curvilinear fashion in a natural neck crease or resting skin tension line. The gland is approached at its inferior edge because the dissection will proceed through the subcutaneous layer, platysma, and the superficial layers of deep cervical fascia. The facial vein will require ligation in two locations, as will the facial artery. The first ligation of the facial vein will occur as it courses over the gland at its inferior edge. The first ligation of the facial artery will occur as it enters the gland at its deep inferior-lateral edge. The submandibular gland can then be dissected in a pericapsular fashion from the inferior to superior aspect. The facial nerve branches will remain superior and superficial to this dissection. As the gland is dissected from its deep boundaries of the intermediate tendon and the hyoglossus muscles, the lingual nerve will come into view in the superior aspect of the dissection medial to the mandible's inferior border. Visualization of the lingual nerve, which is a 4- to 7-mm–wide, flat, ribbon-like structure, will be facilitated by downward traction of the gland (see Fig 11-30a). Surgery of glands with significant inflammation and fibrosis may find the lingual nerve to be adherent to and resemble the submandibular duct. Separation of these two structures can be facilitated by inserting a lacrimal probe into the duct through its oral opening. The rigid probe will be palpable in the wound, identifying the duct and permitting a more straightforward dissection around it. Once the gland is separated from the small parasympathetic fibers entering the gland from the submandibular ganglion, the lingual nerve will retract superiorly. The duct is then transsected and ligated, and the gland delivered by ligating and transsecting the facial vein as it passes superior to the gland and by ligating the facial artery as it emerges from the gland at its superior edge. The resultant wound contains dead space and should, therefore, be drained and a pressure dressing applied. Patients should continue on culture-specific antibiotics for a 10-day course after surgery.

HISTOPATHOLOGY ▶

The histologic features are variable as they follow the spectrum of inflammation and repair. An inflammatory infiltrate consisting predominantly of lymphocytes and plasma cells is present and may be focal or diffuse. Consequently, there is ductal dilation and acinar atrophy (Fig 11-31a). Metaplastic changes may occur within the ducts, which can be manifested by a mucous-secreting epithelium (Fig 11-31b). Over time, fibrosis occurs, resulting in a fibrosed, nonfunctional gland.

PROGNOSIS ▶

About 50% of submandibular glands recover with antibiotics, hydration, and sialagogue therapy. Cases that undergo excision resolve without recurrence. About 10% of submandibular sialadenitis cases are related to a tumor, most of which are determined to be malignant. In such cases, further therapy is required. If the tumor is benign, gland removal should be sufficient. However, malignant disease warrants additional surgery of either a supraomohyoid or functional neck dissection followed by radiotherapy.

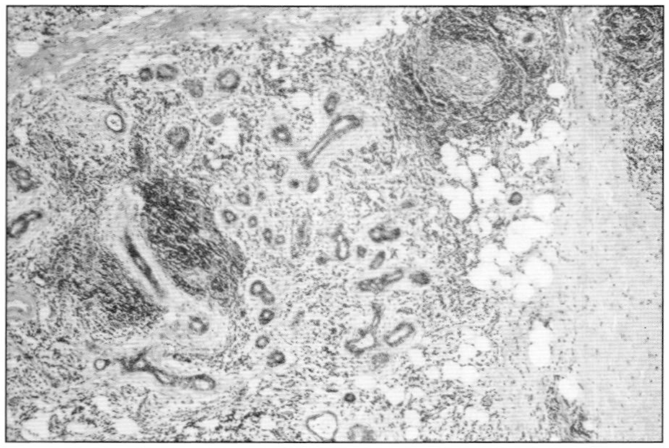

Fig 11-31a Sialadenitis of the submandibular gland. The histologic picture varies depending on the stage of the lesion. Here, the inflammatory component is both focal and diffuse. Acini are not evident, and numerous ducts can be seen. Ultimately, fibrosis will take place.

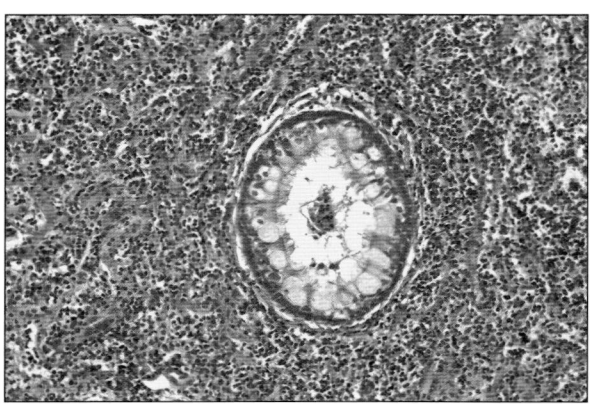

Fig 11-31b Mucous metaplasia of ductal epithelium is frequently seen secondary to marked inflammation.

HIV Parotitis

CLINICAL PRESENTATION ▶ In a small number (less than 3%) of HIV-infected patients, multiple lymphoepithelial cysts proliferate in the parotid glands, resulting in a painful enlargement of one, or more commonly both, glands. The enlargements can become significant and result in a presentation suggestive of bilateral tumors (Fig 11-32a). Most patients have not progressed to advanced AIDS and therefore have CD4 counts greater than 200 cells/mL.

The enlarged parotids are mildly tender to palpation. Although they may be tense because of fluid accumulation in the multiple cysts, the lesions are not firm. Since this disease involves the entire parotid parenchyma, the lesions do not present as a discrete mass and are not moveable.

DIFFERENTIAL DIAGNOSIS ▶ If the HIV status is known to be positive, HIV parotitis should be the first consideration. However, like Sjögren patients, HIV-infected patients may also develop *lymphomas* in the parotid gland. In addition, tuberculosis is more common in HIV patients and thus may exist as a *TB parotitis* or a *TB adenitis* within the parotid lymph nodes. *Kaposi sarcoma* or *sarcoidosis* can also develop in the parotid of an HIV-infected individual.

If the HIV status is unknown, HIV parotitis remains a consideration, but the subset of systemic diseases that cause parotid enlargements must be included on the differential list. These are *sarcoidosis, Sjögren syndrome, sialosis,* and *lymphoma of the parotid,* as well as *benign lymphoepithelial lesions of the parotid* unassociated with Sjögren syndrome or sialosis.

DIAGNOSTIC WORK-UP ▶ If the HIV status of the patient is unknown, it should be tested. HIV testing should be accomplished after requesting the patient's consent. A CD$_4$ count should also be conducted. A CT scan of the parotid is nearly pathognomonic and will show multiple discrete hypodense areas indicating fluid-filled cysts within the parotids. Although lymphoepithelial cysts can develop in the HIV-negative individual, these are usually single cysts in only one gland.

If the individual is HIV positive and a CT scan shows multiple hypodense areas, this constitutes sufficient evidence to accept a working diagnosis of HIV parotitis and to proceed to treatment (Fig 11-32b). However, if the HIV status is negative, either an incisional parotid biopsy or a superficial parotidectomy is recommended for diagnostic purposes. The incisional parotid biopsy is recommended if the parotid is diffusely enlarged and no defined mass can be seen on the CT scan. A superficial parotidectomy is recommended if the clinical examination or CT scan suggests a defined mass in the parotid.

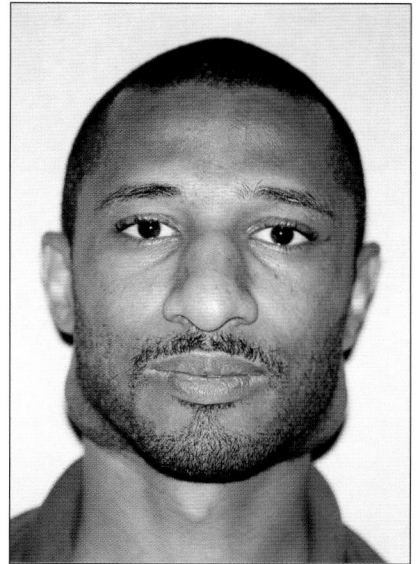

Fig 11-32a Bilateral parotid enlargements due to multiple lymphoepithelial cysts in an HIV patient.

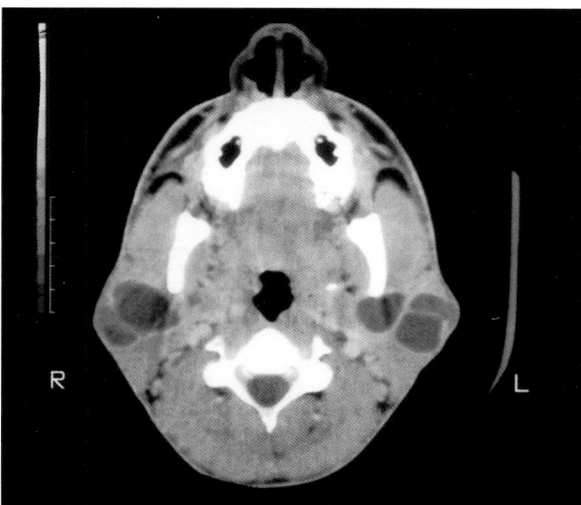

Fig 11-32b CT scan showing multiple hypodense loculations in each parotid consistent with HIV parotitis.

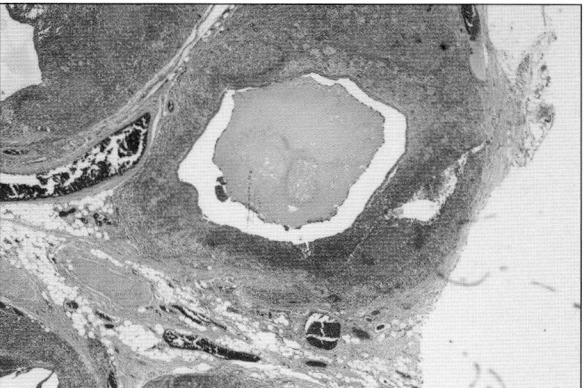

Fig 11-32c Lymphoepithelial cyst showing a fluid-filled space with a thin epithelial lining and surrounded by a dense lymphocytic infiltrate and a hyperemic vascular stroma. An HIV parotitis will have multiple lymphoepithelial cysts.

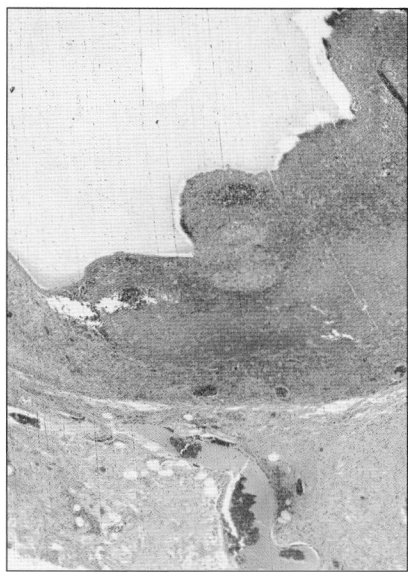

Fig 11-32d The lymphocytic infiltrate in an HIV parotitis may organize to form a recognizable germinal center similar to those seen within a lymph node.

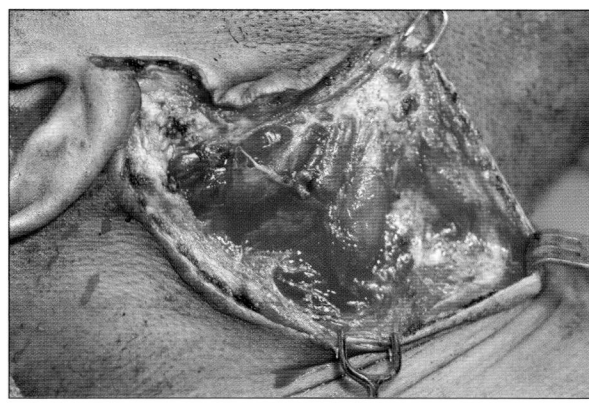

Fig 11-32e A superficial parotidectomy in HIV parotitis is difficult because of the enhanced vascular nature of the diseased tissue and its multiple fluid-filled cysts.

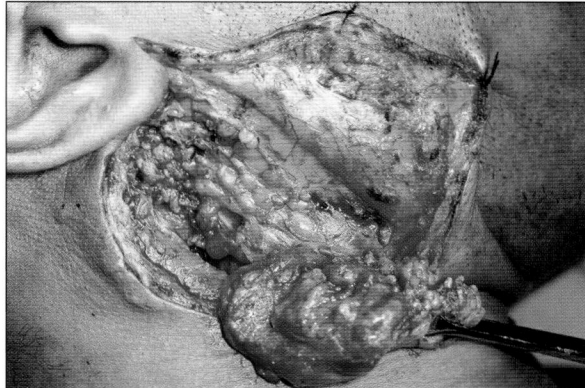

Fig 11-32f A superficial parotidectomy in HIV parotitis will remove about 75% of the diseased tissue. The remaining disease in the deep lobe of the parotid does not seem to produce symptoms or cause a recurrent enlargement of the area.

HISTOPATHOLOGY

The parotid gland will show multiple fluid-filled cysts (Fig 11-32c). These are lymphoepithelial cysts with a squamous or cuboidal epithelial lining and lymphocytes in the wall that may form germinal centers (Fig 11-32d). Connective tissue septae contain numerous dilated and engorged veins. Parotid tissue is replaced by the cysts and lymphocytic infiltrate. The latter are predominantly CD8 cells. Epimyoepithelial islands may be present (see Fig 11-7b), and follicular hyperplasia, sometimes with granulomatous inflammation, is usually prominent. The picture is essentially that of a benign lymphoepithelial lesion with prominent cyst formation.

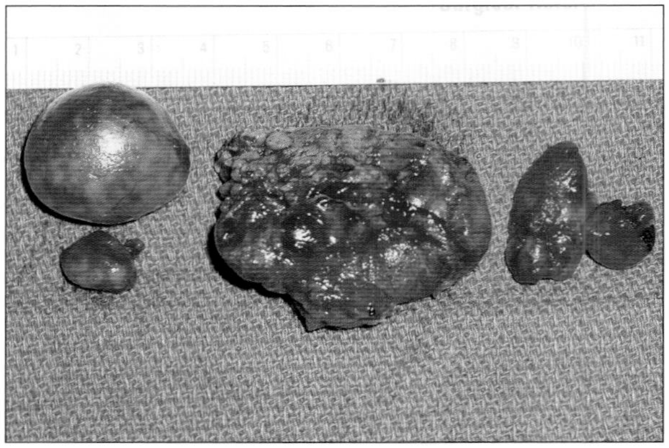

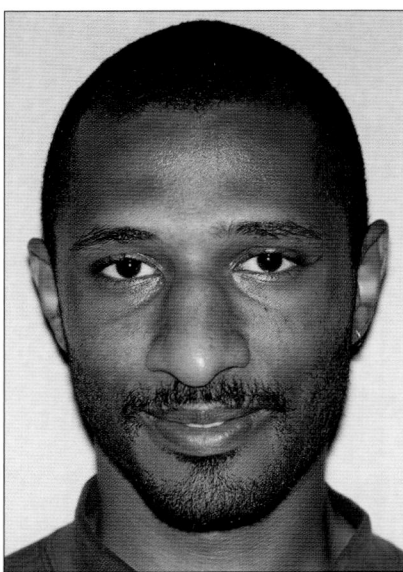

Fig 11-32g Fluid-filled cysts of all sizes, together with a diffuse inflammation, make up HIV parotitis.

Fig 11-32h Superficial parotidectomies are effective in correcting the parotid enlargements as well as reducing pain.

TREATMENT ▶

Superficial parotidectomy and radiotherapy can be used to control and resolve clinical disease. Surgery is preferred by these authors because of its predictability and because it provides tissue sufficient for a definitive diagnosis. A standard superficial parotidectomy resolves the pain and enlargement and, despite leaving residual HIV parotitis in the deep lobe of the gland, achieves a permanent resolution of symptoms and a return to normal contours. Recurrence of clinical disease does not seem to occur. Although the superficial parotidectomy is approached in the standard fashion, in this disease it is much more technically difficult. The gland is highly vascularized and the cysts contain fluid under pressure, which causes a spray of HIV-containing fluid (Figs 11-32e to 11-32g). Therefore, absolute barrier techniques and HIV precautions should be undertaken.

As an alternative to surgery, external beam radiotherapy may be used. Doses of 2,000 cGy to 4,000 cGy are effective in reducing the size of the parotid glands and inducing a fibrosis of the lymphoepithelial cysts. However, given the increased longevity of HIV-infected patients now achieved through multidrug therapy, a concern about radiation-induced lymphoma must be considered.

PROGNOSIS ▶

Both surgery and radiotherapy have proven to be effective as a long-term treatment (Fig 11-32h). Regardless of the control or progression of the HIV disease spectrum, recurrence is uncommon, presumably because of the physical removal of the superficial lobe of the parotid or to the complete atrophy of the gland induced by radiotherapy.

Salivary Gland Neoplasms

▶ *"Special stains are wonderful. They allow us to see what we still don't recognize in a different color."*

—*Anonymous*

While the clinical presentation of a salivary gland neoplasm is usually an asymptomatic mass that may occasionally be ulcerated or cause pain, the histologic presentation is far more complex. The tumor spectrum is vast, and yet repetitive features may be seen in a variety of neoplasms with differing biologic behavior.

Developing salivary glands arise from the stomodeum as ectodermal buds that proliferate as cords into the underlying mesenchyme. The ends thicken to form terminal bulbs. These undergo branching, followed by continued advancement into the mesenchyme. This process repeats itself, all the while maintaining continuity with the oral epithelium. This branching process gives rise to the lobular architecture of the gland. The terminal tubular elements differentiate into acinar cells, and between the acinar cells and basal lamina myoepithelial cells form. These are strap-shaped and stellate cells, which may appear as clear cells prior to the development of myofilaments. Intercalated and smaller striated ducts also differentiate from this area. The original cords and their branches become the excretory ducts (Fig 12-1).

The histogenesis of salivary gland tumors has been controversial. Some suggest acinar cells, since these have been shown to have a regenerative capacity. Others however, propose a stem or reserve cell in the salivary duct system. The complexity of salivary gland tumors is due in part to the fact that in most instances more than one cell type is involved. These may be acinar, luminal, myoepithelial, basal, or squamous. Adding to this diversity, extracellular secretory products are a striking component of many tumors. These products include basal lamina, collagen fibers, elastic fibers, and glycosaminoglycans. It is believed that these substances are probably secreted by the neoplastic myoepithelial cells.

Salivary gland tumors may involve major or minor glands. The largest number of cases are found within the parotid. While most types of tumors may be found in both sites, relative frequency can vary. Thus approximately 80% of parotid tumors are benign. In minor salivary glands, however, the benign-malignant ratio is closer to 1:1, while in the sublingual gland, an uncommon site for neoplasms, the majority are malignant.

The pleomorphic adenoma is the most common tumor both in major and in minor salivary glands. Warthin tumors, basal cell adenomas, oncocytomas, acinic cell carcinomas, and sebaceous tumors have a strong predilection for the major glands, but the polymorphous low-grade adenocarcinoma has a marked predilection for the minor glands. While most intraoral salivary gland tumors favor the palate, the canalicular adenoma favors the upper lip.

Tumors occurring within salivary glands are predominantly of epithelial origin. However, it should be appreciated that nonepithelial neoplasms also may arise within the gland that are not actually of salivary

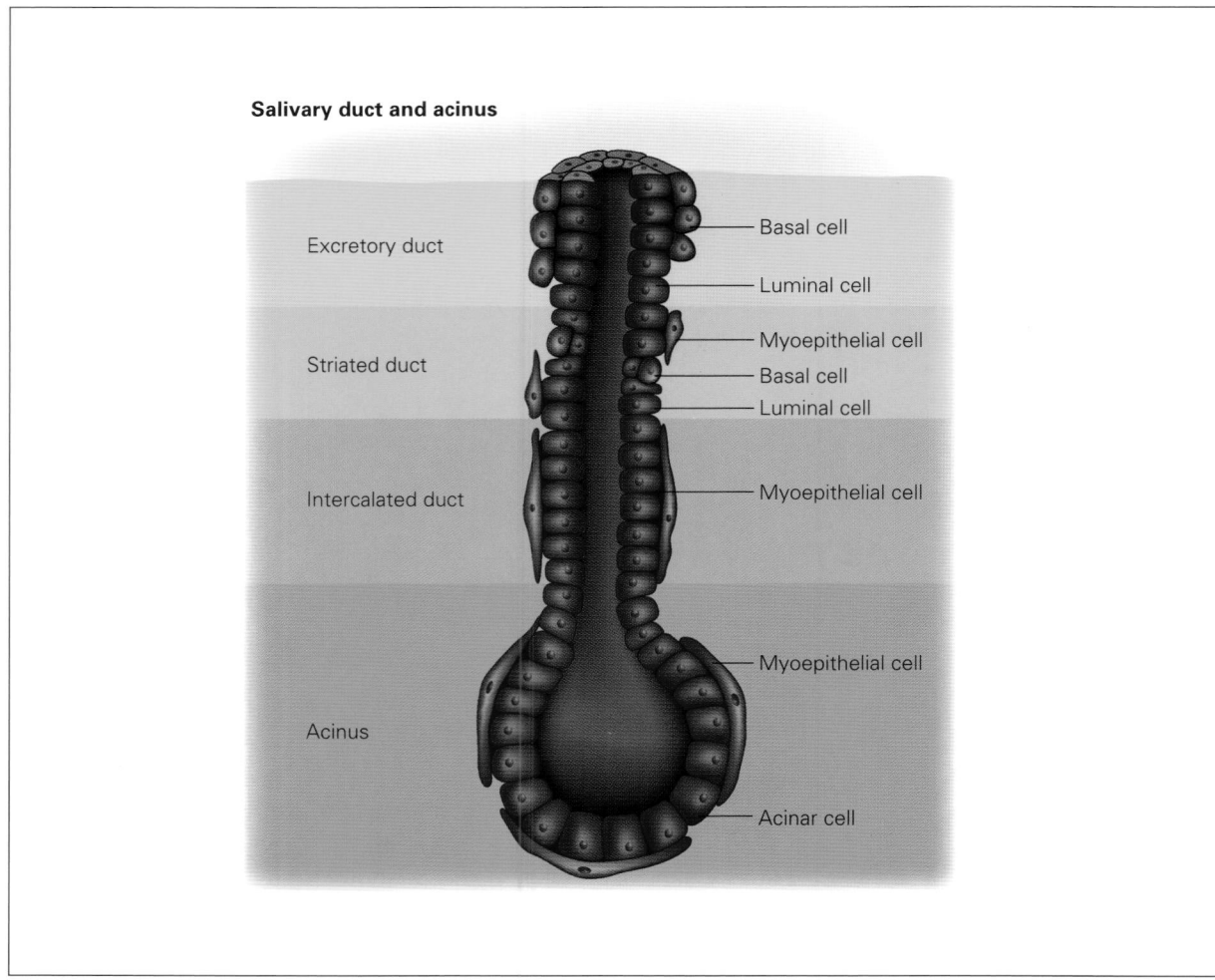

Salivary duct and acinus

Excretory duct — Basal cell, Luminal cell

Striated duct — Myoepithelial cell, Basal cell, Luminal cell

Intercalated duct — Myoepithelial cell

Acinus — Myoepithelial cell, Acinar cell

Fig 12-1 Development of salivary glands arises from ectodermal ingrowth, resulting in specialized ducts and terminating in the functional acinus.

gland or ductal origin. Most of these are found in the parotid gland. Among the more common benign tumors is the hemangioma, which is the most frequently occurring tumor in the parotid gland in children. Lipomas and neurogenic tumors also may be seen. Hodgkin and non-Hodgkin lymphomas and, most infrequently, soft tissue sarcomas may develop. Metastatic tumors such as renal cell carcinoma and melanoma may also occur.

Pleomorphic Adenoma

CLINICAL PRESENTATION ▶

The pleomorphic adenoma is the prototypical benign yet true neoplasm; that is, it will continue to grow—or regrow if not completely removed—but it is incapable of metastasis. It occurs at different statistical incidences in all salivary glands. Eighty percent of tumors that occur in the parotid gland are benign: of these, 75% are pleomorphic adenomas and 5% are Warthin tumors (papillary cystadenoma lymphomatosum). Pleomorphic adenomas, and salivary gland tumors in general, are not commonly found in the submandibular and sublingual glands. Nevertheless, they account for about 20% to 30% of all tumors

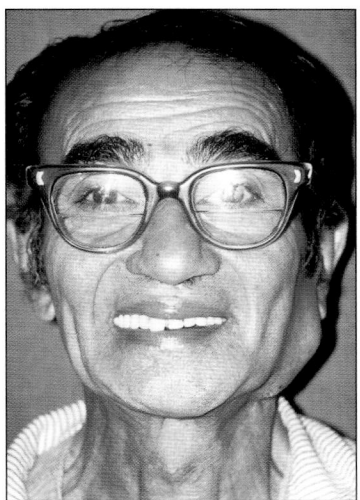

Fig 12-2 Pleomorphic adenoma of the parotid superficial lobe, which typically presents as a freely movable, nontender but firm mass.

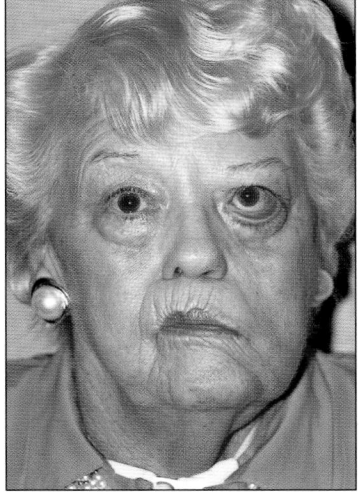

Fig 12-3a Left facial nerve palsy resulting from a large untreated pleomorphic adenoma that transformed into a malignancy. The facial nerve palsy developed with the malignancy.

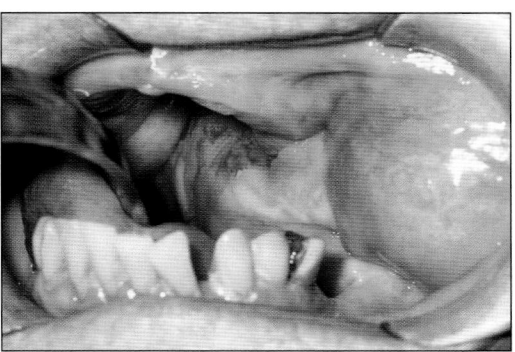

Fig 12-3b A pleomorphic adenoma that arises from the deep lobe of the parotid gland may present as a firm nontender mass in the tonsillar fossa or buccopharyngeal raphe area.

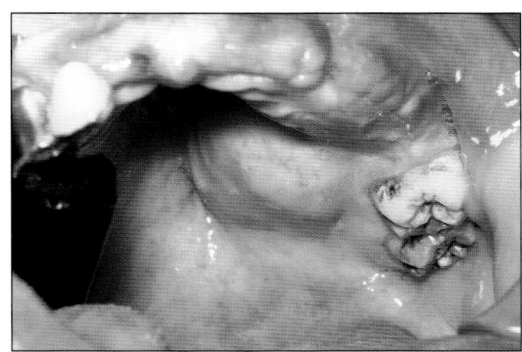

Fig 12-4 The most common presentation for an oral mucosal pleomorphic adenoma is a firm nontender mass with an intact mucosa at the junction of the hard and soft palates.

in these glands. Oral pleomorphic adenomas are somewhat common, accounting for about 45% of all oral minor salivary gland tumors. When they arise in the oral mucosa, the site of predilection is the mucosa over the posterior hard palate and anterior soft palate; otherwise, pleomorphic adenomas can occur in any location where minor salivary glands exist. Consequently, the two most common clinical presentations are a painless firm mass in the superficial lobe of the parotid gland and a painless firm mass in the posterior palatal mucosa.

Eighty percent of all pleomorphic adenomas in the parotid gland develop in the superficial lobe, which constitutes 80% of the parotid gland (Fig 12-2). It presents as a freely movable, firm mass. Peculiarly and rarely, these can fluctuate in size or be painful. Pleomorphic adenomas do not induce facial nerve paresis. Any facial nerve weakness not attributable to previous surgery should be considered a malignancy until proven otherwise (Fig 12-3a). When a pleomorphic adenoma arises from the deep lobe of the parotid gland, it usually goes unrecognized for a number of years until its size creates symptoms of dysphagia or gagging. These present orally as a bulge arising from the tonsillar fossa area (Fig 12-3b).

When a pleomorphic adenoma presents in the mucosa of the hard palate–soft palate junction, it will be a firm, painless mass with intact overlying mucosa (Fig 12-4). If the mucosa is ulcerated and the ulceration is not attributable to trauma or a biopsy, the mass should be considered a malignancy. In the palatal mucosa, the mass will seem to be fixed to the palate. Since the pleomorphic adenoma cannot invade bone, this is not caused by bony invasion but rather by the inelasticity of the palatal mucosa, which becomes distended by the tumor mass and may eventuate in a cupped-out resorption of bone. In other oral mucosal sites, the pleomorphic adenoma presents as a freely movable, circumscribed mass.

Pleomorphic adenomas can arise at any age but are somewhat more common between the ages of 30 and 50 years and are slightly more common in women.

DIFFERENTIAL DIAGNOSIS ▶

The differential diagnosis of a firm mass in the parotid gland must include a *Warthin tumor* (papillary cystadenoma lymphomatosum), which is particularly likely in men, and *basal cell adenoma*, which preferentially develops in the parotid gland. In addition, malignant salivary gland tumors that must be considered include *mucoepidermoid*, *adenoid cystic*, and *acinic cell carcinomas*. Nonsalivary gland neoplasms that

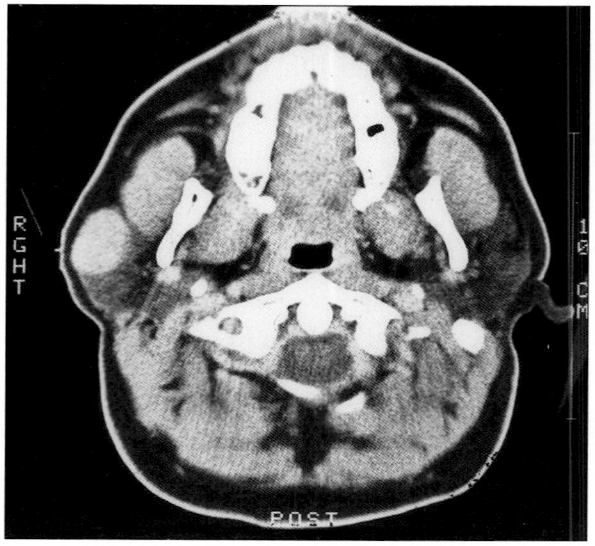

Fig 12-5 A CT scan will confirm the location of the tumor, seen here in the superficial lobe. The soft tissue density of the tumor, its homogeneity, and any areas of extension should be noted.

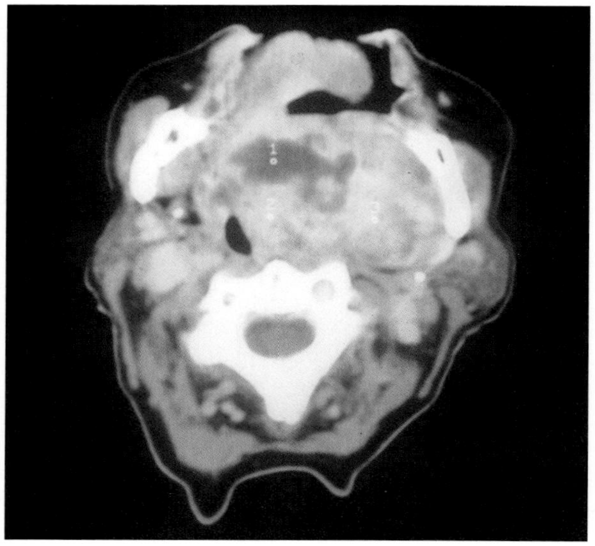

Fig 12-6 CT scan showing a large mass (pleomorphic adenoma) arising from the deep lobe of the parotid. It is obstructing the airway and appears heterogeneous, a typical feature of pleomorphic adenomas.

are known to occur in the parotid gland—ie, *hemangiomas, lymphangiomas, lipomas*, and *lymphomas* within parotid lymph nodes—may also present in a similar fashion. The clinician must also be aware that skin nodules such as *sebaceous cysts* can form a subcutaneous mass in the area that may give an impression of being located in the parotid gland.

The differential diagnosis of a firm mass in the palatal mucosa with intact overlying epithelium is primarily a subset of other salivary gland neoplasms. In order of statistical likelihood, they are *adenoid cystic, mucoepidermoid*, and *polymorphous low-grade adenocarcinomas*. Another benign tumor that requires some consideration is the *canalicular adenoma*. In addition, several nonsalivary gland tumors may present with a similar appearance, such as *non-Hodgkin lymphoma* and *neurofibroma*.

Diagnostic Work-Up and Treatment

For a mass in the parotid gland, a computed tomography (CT) scan or magnetic resonance imaging (MRI) scan is valuable to confirm its location in the parotid, specifically in the superficial lobe (Figs 12-5 and 12-6). This should be followed by a superficial parotidectomy, which represents both the diagnostic biopsy and the definitive treatment (see pages 567 to 569). In such a presentation, an incisional parotid biopsy would be contraindicated because seeding of tumor cells throughout the biopsy site is a concern.

For a mass in the palatal mucosa, a CT scan, particularly coronal views, also is recommended to determine its extent and the degree of any resorption of the palate. A deep incisional biopsy of the mass is recommended in its center to establish a firm permanent-section diagnosis prior to planning definitive surgery. This is different from the parotid gland approach, in which biopsy and definitive surgery are one and the same, because an oral incisional biopsy can be accomplished without seeding tumor cells.

If a pleomorphic adenoma is confirmed, it is excised with 1-cm clinical margins at its periphery and includes the overlying surface epithelium and the periosteum of the palate (see page 560). Excision or scraping of the palatal bone is not required because the periosteum is an effective anatomic barrier and pleomorphic adenomas do not elaborate osteoclast-activating factor to invade bone. If the tumor extends to the area of the soft palate, the excision includes the fascia over the soft palate musculature. The muscles of the soft palate need not be excised unless frozen sections indicate tumor at this margin.

For pleomorphic adenomas in other mucosal sites, a peripheral excision with 1-cm margins is recommended. This will include overlying mucosa but should not include overlying skin if the mass is located in the lip or buccal mucosa. In these instances, the muscle fascia of the orbicularis oris or buccinator is an effective anatomic barrier.

In any site, enucleation, or a "shelling out" of a pleomorphic adenoma, is contraindicated. The pseudo-capsule of a pleomorphic adenoma will certainly give the clinical impression of a complete removal of an "encapsulated nodule or mass" with these approaches, but the extracapsular tumor projections left behind may lead not only to recurrence but to multicentric recurrences caused by the remaining tumor projections and foci within the tissue at the circumference of the resections.

HISTOPATHOLOGY ▶

From a therapeutic standpoint, the most significant histologic features relate to the capsule of the tumor. While not all pleomorphic adenomas, particularly those affecting minor salivary glands, will have a well-developed capsule, these are well-demarcated masses. Unfortunately, this characteristic, coupled with the fact that these tumors are clinically freely moveable, particularly when palpated in such areas as the lip, belies the fact that tumor cells are found within the capsule and as extensions through and beyond it (Figs 12-7a to 12-7c). Thus a "conservative" enucleation would almost ensure residual tumor cells and set the patient up for multifocal recurrences (Figs 12-7d and 12-7e). Grossly, these tumors have a smooth, sometimes bosselated surface. The cut surface is typically white and resembles a cut potato (Fig 12-8). Bluish areas representing cartilage-like material may be seen, and a gelatinous component may be present. Older tumors often show cyst formation.

The microscopic picture is typically diverse (Fig 12-9). Essentially, there is a proliferation of both ductal epithelium and a myoepithelial component. This gives rise to cellular, epithelial areas as well as mesenchymal-like tissue that usually has a myxochondroid appearance (Fig 12-10). The relative quantities of these two types can vary considerably. In general, the minor salivary gland tumors are more cellular than those of the major glands. The cellular portion of the tumor may form a variety of patterns such as islands, sheets, ribbons, or ductal configurations (Fig 12-11). Squamous cells and keratin pearls may be present (Fig 2-12). Occasionally, there may be cribriform areas, suggesting the pattern of adenoid cystic carcinoma. However, such areas usually compose only a small portion of the tumor, and the infiltrative nature of the carcinoma is not evident. Aggregates of oncocytic cells may be seen, but this can occur in a variety of salivary gland tumors. Plasmacytoid (hyaline) cells (Fig 12-13) and spindle cells (Fig 12-14) may also be seen. Both of these have been identified as myoepithelial cells. In some tumors, one or both of these cell types constitute practically the entire lesion. If the ductal and glandular component constitutes less than 5% of the tumor, these would be classified as myoepitheliomas. Basal lamina produced by myoepithelial cells appears to be responsible for the eosinophilic hyalinized material that can form a striking component of many tumors (see Fig 12-12). The myoepithelium also deposits the basophilic, mucoid material, which then separates the cells so that the tissue appears myxoid. Degeneration of cells with vacuolation produces the chondroid pattern. Crystalline material may sometimes be seen.

Malignant degeneration is possible within pleomorphic adenomas, and the incidence increases with tumor duration and size. Histologic features suggestive of malignant transformation include extensive hyalinization, cellular atypism, necrosis, calcification, and invasion.

PROGNOSIS ▶

Excision with controlled frozen sections and clear intraoral margins and excision via superficial parotidectomy are associated with a cure rate of more than 95%. Incomplete removals uniformly result in tumor recurrence. Clinically, recurrence is first manifested about 4 to 6 years postoperatively and is often unknown to the original surgeon, which has given false credence to enucleation procedures.

Pleomorphic adenomas are benign tumors with a well-documented transformation to malignancy (carcinoma ex pleomorphic adenoma). It is estimated that up to 25% of untreated pleomorphic adenomas undergo malignant transformation, a process that is size- and time-related. Therefore, early definitive treatment is strongly recommended. Although malignant transformation requires histopathologic confirmation, clinical clues of such transformation may be readily apparent. They include ulceration, fluctuance, pain, neural deficits, or a change from a single circumscribed mass to a lobulated mass (Figs 12-15 and 12-16).

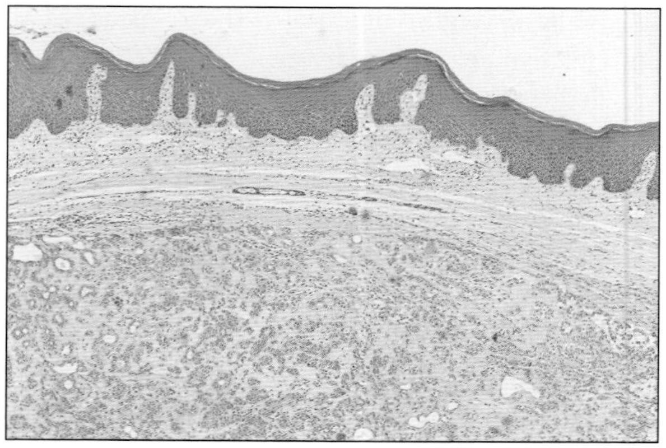

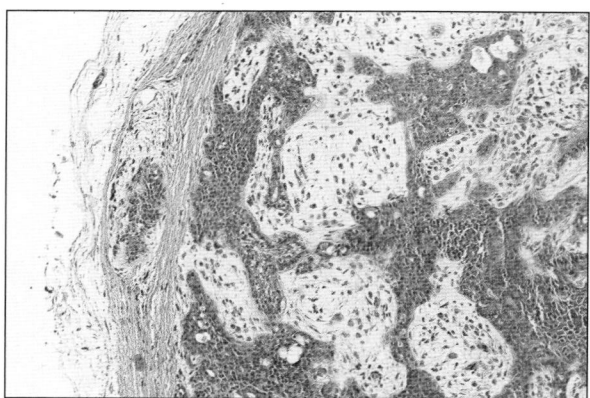

Fig 12-7a Pleomorphic adenoma of the palate showing tumor islands lying beyond the tumor capsule.

Fig 12-7b Pleomorphic adenoma with an island of tumor in the capsule.

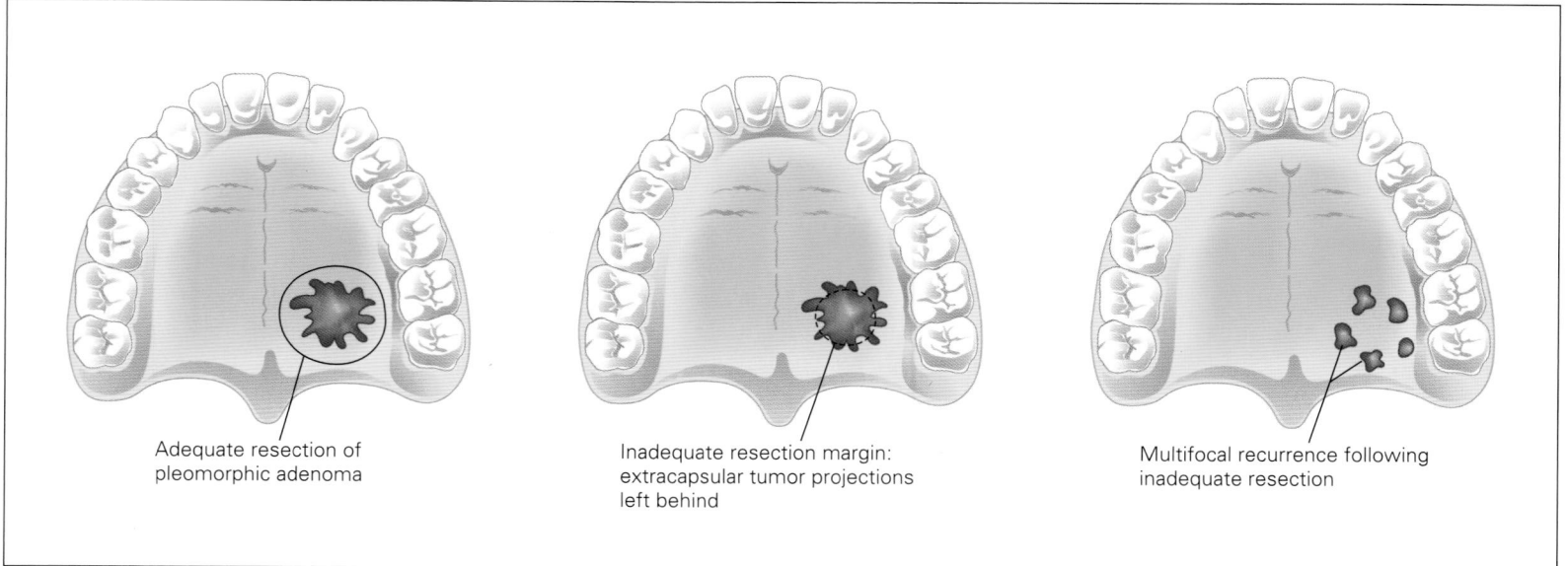

Adequate resection of pleomorphic adenoma

Inadequate resection margin: extracapsular tumor projections left behind

Multifocal recurrence following inadequate resection

Fig 12-7c Diagrammatic representation of the growth pattern of pleomorphic adenoma. There may be a well-developed capsule, but the tumor has extensions that exceed it.

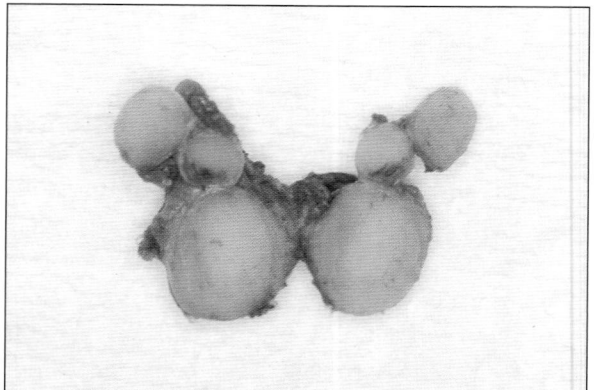

Fig 12-7d A formalin-fixed specimen from the upper lip showing a pleomorphic adenoma that recurred 8 years after initial presentation. Note the multiple, discrete tumor nodules.

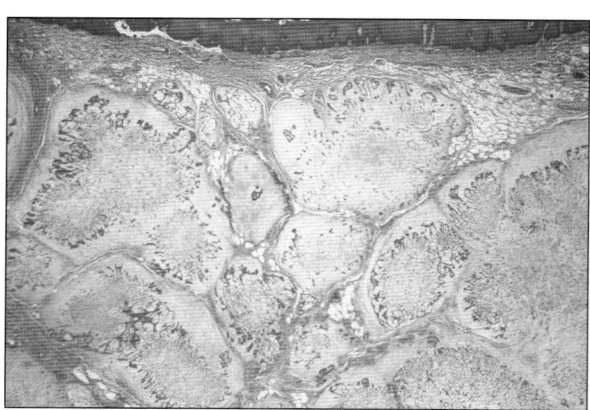

Fig 12-7e Pleomorphic adenoma recurring in the upper lip 10 years after the first presentation. Multiple nodules have coalesced into a single mass.

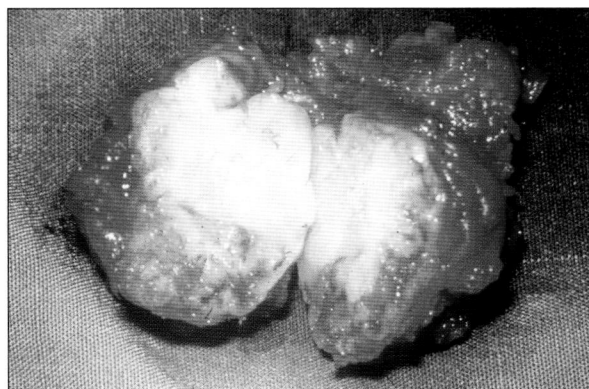

Fig 12-8 Gross specimen of a pleomorphic adenoma of the parotid gland showing the so-called cut-potato surface.

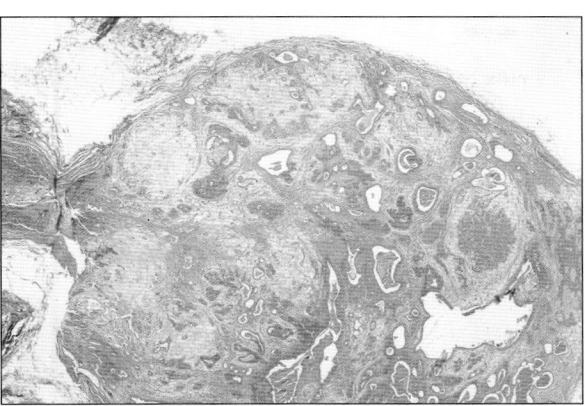

Fig 12-9 Pleomorphic adenoma showing a well-defined mass with a varied pattern. There are areas of cellularity with solid, ductal, and cystic patterns. Myxochondroid areas appear sparsely cellular.

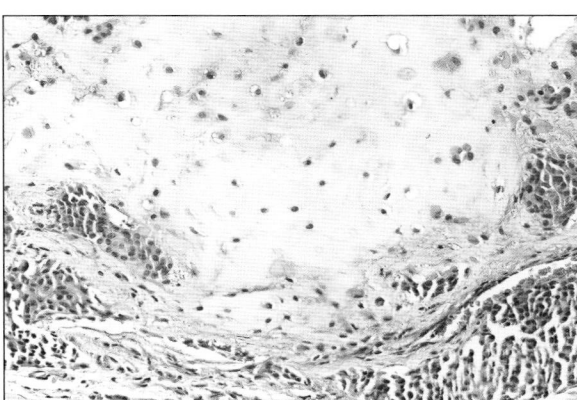

Fig 12-10 Myxochondroid area with epithelial islands, the classic appearance of a pleomorphic adenoma.

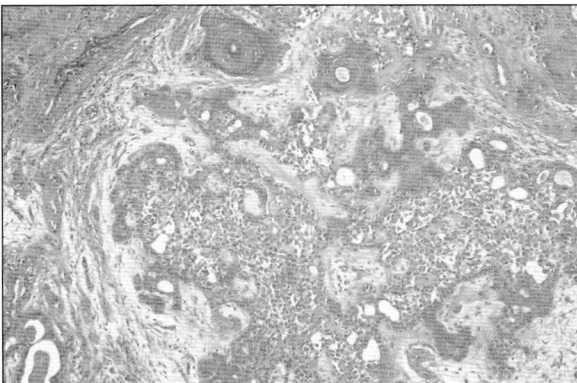

Fig 12-11 A cellular area of a pleomorphic adenoma showing the epithelium in sheets, ductal configurations, and squamous differentiation.

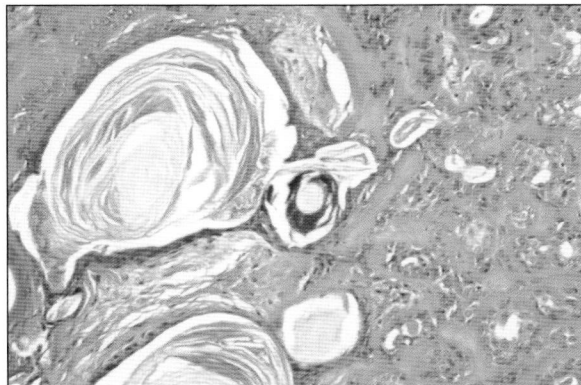

Fig 12-12 An area of a pleomorphic adenoma with a more hyalinized stroma and keratin formation.

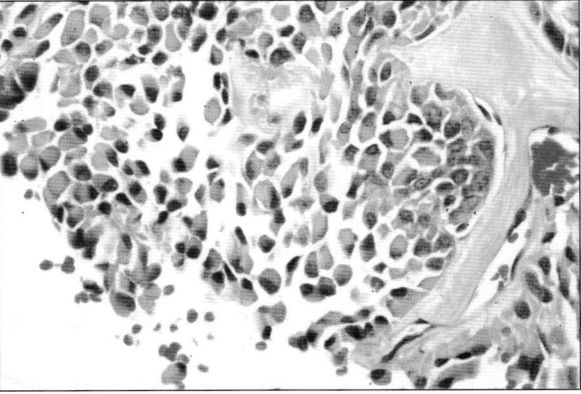

Fig 12-13 Plasmacytoid cells will often lose their cohesiveness, creating a stronger resemblance to plasma cells. Areas such as this are often seen in pleomorphic adenomas.

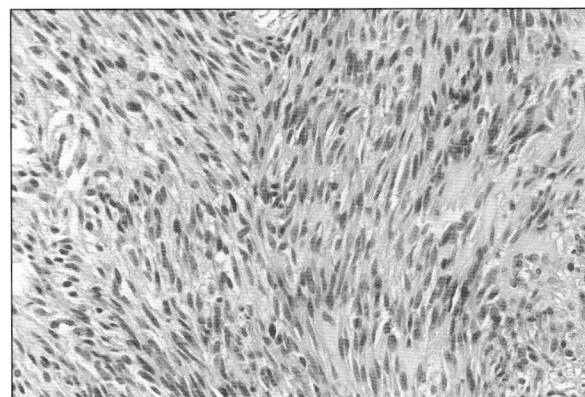

Fig 12-14 Myoepithelioma with spindle cells arranged in fascicles. Spindled myoepithelial cells can also be seen in pleomorphic adenomas.

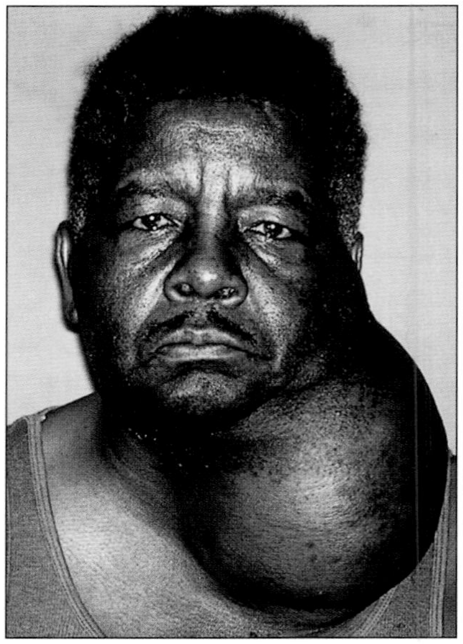

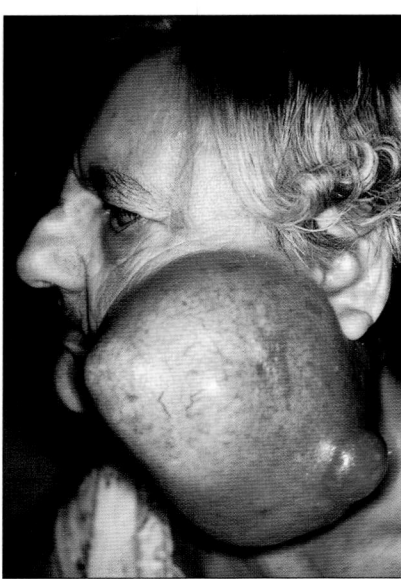

Fig 12-15 Untreated pleomorphic adenomas may attain a very large size. The transformation to a carcinoma ex pleomorphic adenoma is related to the size and longevity of the mass. This one is still benign.

Fig 12-16 This large pleomorphic adenoma has transformed into a malignancy. Clinical signs of malignancy may include fluctuance, irregularity of texture, ulceration, and facial nerve palsy.

Myoepithelioma

CLINICAL PRESENTATION AND PATHOGENESIS

The myoepithelioma is a rare, benign salivary gland neoplasm with a biologic behavior similar to that of the canalicular and basal cell adenomas. It is rare in any site but will occur more frequently in the parotid gland's superficial lobe than in other major salivary glands or in oral mucosal sites. It will present as a firm, circumscribed, painless mass with an intact overlying epithelium. In sites other than the palatal mucosa, it will be freely movable. It occurs equally among men and women, mainly during the mid-adult years.

This neoplasm seems to result from a monoclonal proliferation of myoepithelial cells, which may partially differentiate into spindle-shaped or plasmacytoid cells. Their histogenesis from myoepithelial cells is reflected in their most frequent location, that is, the parotid gland, where myoepithelial cells are more common.

DIFFERENTIAL DIAGNOSIS

The rarity of myoepithelioma makes it a surprise diagnosis identifiable only histopathologically. Its clinical differential diagnosis usually consists of the more common salivary gland tumors. In the parotid gland, a *pleomorphic adenoma*, *Warthin tumor* (papillary cystadenoma lymphomatosum), *basal cell adenoma*, *adenoid cystic carcinoma*, or *mucoepidermoid carcinoma* would be appropriate. In oral sites, the same differential would generally prevail except that a Warthin tumor would not be included and the *canalicular adenoma* would be substituted for the basal cell adenoma.

DIAGNOSTIC WORK-UP AND TREATMENT

In the parotid gland, this lesion would require a superficial parotidectomy for diagnosis and definitive treatment. In an oral mucosal site, the tumor requires excision with 0.5-cm margins peripherally and deep margins of periosteum or muscle fascia as appropriate.

HISTOPATHOLOGY

A myoepithelioma may occur in one of three histologic forms. The most common is the spindle-cell form (70%), which is found most frequently in the parotid gland (see Fig 12-14). The cells have eosinophilic cytoplasm and may form fascicles or have a more diffuse pattern. There is little supporting

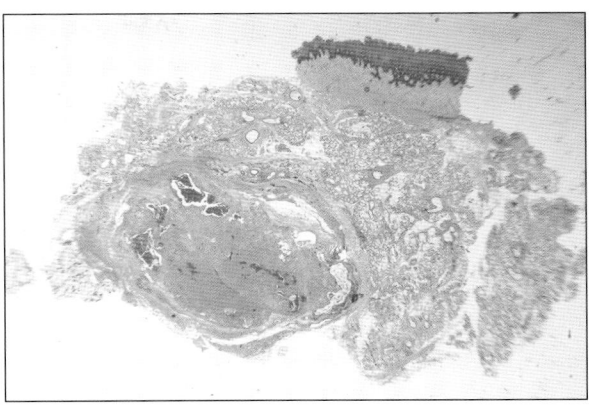

Fig 12-17a A myoepithelioma of the palate showing a well-defined mass.

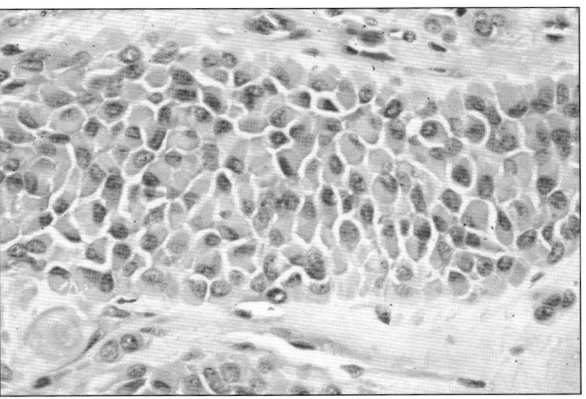

Fig 12-17b This myoepithelioma is composed of plasmacytoid cells, here seen lying in sheets.

stroma. The plasmacytoid form (17%), which has a predilection for the palate, consists of rounded to polyhedral cells with eosinophilic cytoplasm and eccentric nuclei (Figs 12-17a and 12-17b; see also Fig 12-13). A myxoid stromal component may be present. The third form is a mixture of plasmacytoid and spindle cells (13%).

Myoepitheliomas are best conceptualized as part of a spectrum that includes pleomorphic adenomas. Many pleomorphic adenomas have numerous myoepithelial cells. A criterion that may be used to separate the two lesions is that if the tumor contains less than a 5% component of ducts and glands, it should be called a myoepithelioma.

Plasmacytoid myoepitheliomas are methyl green–pyronin negative, which distinguishes them from plasmacytomas. Spindle-cell myoepitheliomas mimic other spindle cell tumors such as schwannomas and leiomyomas but may be distinguished from them immunohistochemically because the other spindle-cell tumors are negative for cytokeratin but myoepithelial cells are positive for both epithelial and mesenchymal markers.

PROGNOSIS ▶ Excision is curative and carries little chance of recurrence. In fact, a recurrence should be considered a potential unrecognized malignancy.

Warthin Tumor (Papillary Cystadenoma Lymphomatosum)

CLINICAL PRESENTATION AND PATHOGENESIS ▶ Papillary cystadenoma lymphomatosum is a benign hamartomatous or reactive proliferation of ductal salivary gland cells and lymphoid elements that is commonly referred to as a *Warthin tumor*.

The tumor will present almost exclusively in the superficial lobe of the parotid gland as a firm to doughy painless mass of several months' duration (Fig 12-18a). It is said to occur most frequently in the "tail" of the parotid gland, which is the most inferior and posterior portion of the gland below the ear and the angle of the mandible. Men are affected more frequently than women by a 3:1 ratio, and it affects those between 30 and 70 years of age.

Warthin tumors are known to occur bilaterally (synchronous tumors) in about 4% to 6% of cases, or two or more tumors are known to occur simultaneously in the same gland (also synchronous tumors). This is less than the overall bilateral development of about 10% because second and even third lesions may develop years later (metachronous tumors) in the same or opposite gland or may even recur as a new tumor in residual elements of a treated gland. Overall, Warthin tumors account for about 5% to 6% of parotid gland tumors.

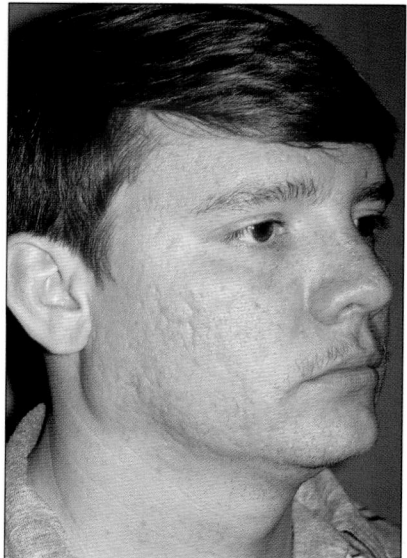

Fig 12-18a A Warthin tumor will be seen more commonly in men. Like a pleomorphic adenoma, it will present as a firm, nontender, freely movable mass in the superficial lobe of the parotid gland. A Warthin tumor will not present in the deep lobe of the parotid gland or in an oral site.

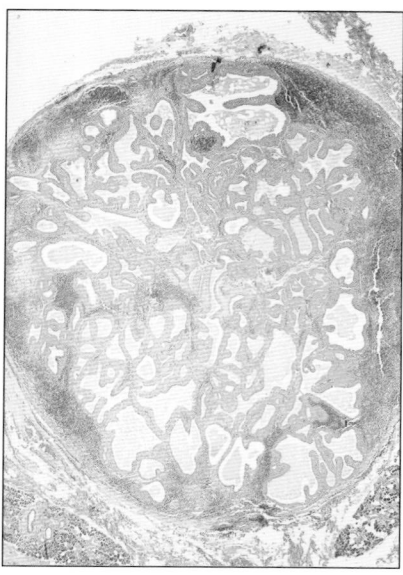

Fig 12-18b A Warthin tumor showing an encapsulated mass within the parotid gland. The cystic nature of the tumor is apparent, with papillary projections extending into the lumina. The lymphoid stroma can also be seen.

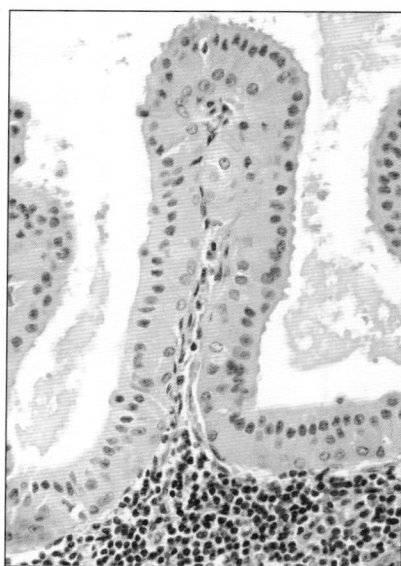

Fig 12-18c A portion of the tumor shown in Fig 12-18b reveals a papillary projection lined by two layers of oncocytic cells. The basal cells are cuboidal and the luminal cells are columnar with an orderly arrangement of nuclei.

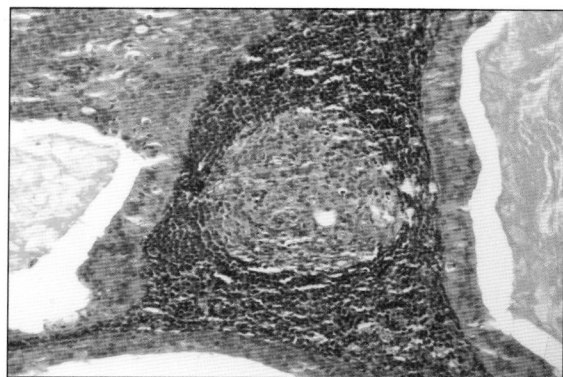

Fig 12-18d Lymphoid stroma with a germinal center in a Warthin tumor. Adjacent cysts lined by the oncocytic cells and containing a typical eosinophilic coagulum are also visible.

A Warthin tumor is believed to arise from the incorporation of salivary gland cells into lymph nodes during their development; these later become reactive and induce a proliferation of both salivary and lymph node elements. The fact that Warthin tumors reach a certain size and remain static and that multiple or bilateral tumors occur indicates that they are not true neoplasms but hamartomas or reactive hyperplasias of salivary gland and lymphoid elements.

Reports of rare oral Warthin tumors may reflect a similar histogenesis. In most cases, reactive lesions such as a reactive epulis fissuratum may induce a proliferation of oncocytically changed minor salivary glands and lymphoid follicles, thus bearing a resemblance to a Warthin tumor and representing a stimulated oncocytic hyperplasia (see Fig 2-5).

DIFFERENTIAL DIAGNOSIS ▶

Statistically, a firm mass in the tail of the parotid gland would most likely represent a *pleomorphic adenoma*. Less commonly, the *basal cell adenoma* should also be considered, as should several malignant parotid tumors such as *adenoid cystic, mucoepidermoid*, and *acinic cell carcinomas*. Other lymph node–related diseases within the parotid gland, such as *lymphoma, HIV-related parotitis, lymphadenopathy*, and *tuberculosis-related lymphadenitis* (which is increasing in incidence secondary to HIV-related immunosuppression) may also be seen. In addition, a mass in this location may actually originate in the dermis rather than the parotid gland. Lesions such as *sebaceous cysts* require some consideration, particularly if the individual's complexion suggests it.

DIAGNOSTIC WORK-UP AND TREATMENT ▶

A clinician can easily get carried away with a work-up for this tumor. No doubt the lymphoid elements within the tumor will cause an increased uptake of ^{99}technetium pertechnetate, but this will not affect treatment. A CT scan may also be performed to document the tumor's location in the parotid gland, but an experienced clinician can determine the same by examination. A fine-needle aspirate is quick and straightforward and may be the most yielding study. It will identify the lesion as a Warthin tumor or at least rule out a malignancy, which would require a more aggressive surgery. Barring any suspicion of a malignancy, a Warthin tumor or a mass in this location suspected of being either a pleomorphic adenoma or a Warthin tumor is excised with a superficial parotidectomy, representing both a diagnostic biopsy and the definitive treatment for this tumor. The cut gross specimen will often reveal the characteristic finding of a soft, sponge-like multicystic lesion containing a thin brown fluid.

HISTOPATHOLOGY ▶

This lesion is encapsulated and discrete; its name, papillary cystadenoma lymphomatosum, is its histologic description (Fig 12-18b). Grossly, the specimen is usually multicystic with projections in the wall of the cysts. The lumina may contain clear, mucoid, or semisolid often brownish material. The solid components of the tumor are gray-white.

Just as the gross appearance is virtually pathognomonic, so is the microscopic picture. It is a multicystic structure lined by a double row of oncocytic cells. The inner layer is columnar and rests on a layer of cuboidal cells. The cytoplasm in both layers is eosinophilic and somewhat granular because of the presence of numerous mitochondria. Papillary projections extend into the lumen, which may contain eosinophilic periodic acid–Schiff (PAS)–positive material (Fig 12-18c). The subjacent tissue is separated from the lining epithelium by a basement membrane. The supporting tissue consists of lymphoid tissue, which appears reactive and usually contains germinal centers (Fig 12-18d).

PROGNOSIS ▶

A superficial parotidectomy is curative for a Warthin tumor. In rare instances, an apparent recurrence is noted, but such phenomena probably represent new tumors arising from residual gland elements.

Basal Cell Adenoma

CLINICAL PRESENTATION ▶

Basal cell adenomas are benign neoplasms of salivary gland origin with a less infiltrative growth behavior than that of a pleomorphic adenoma. They are more common in the parotid gland (70%) than in oral mucosal sites. When they do occur in oral mucosa, they have a predilection for the upper lip and rarely occur in the palatal mucosa, in contrast to the pleomorphic adenoma, which frequently occurs within palatal mucosa and uncommonly in the upper lip. The lesions are painless, well-circumscribed masses that tend to be smaller (1 to 3 cm) than most pleomorphic adenomas. Most occur in men and in older adults (average age, 60 years).

DIFFERENTIAL DIAGNOSIS ▶

In its most common location in the parotid gland, basal cell adenoma is similar to a small or recently developed *pleomorphic adenoma* or *Warthin tumor* (papillary cystadenoma lymphomatosum). Its superficial location may make it appear to be a *sebaceous cyst of skin* or an *enlarged lymph node*, which may be related to *lymphoma, HIV-related parotitis, lymphadenopathy,* or *tuberculosis-related lymphadenitis.* In addition, a variety of *malignant salivary gland tumors* may also be small and appear as a similar mass.

DIAGNOSTIC WORK-UP AND TREATMENT ▶

When the mass is located in the parotid gland, a fine-needle aspiration should be performed to rule out malignancy. If malignancy is ruled out, a superficial parotidectomy should be undertaken. In an oral mucosal site, an excision with 0.5-cm margins is adequate.

HISTOPATHOLOGY ▶

These tumors are usually well-circumscribed or encapsulated masses whose cut surface is homogeneous but often interrupted by cystic spaces containing brownish material. They may be multifocal.

The tumors consist of uniform cells with eosinophilic cytoplasm and oval nuclei. The cells may be arranged in several patterns. In the solid pattern, there are large islands with peripheral cells that may be more hyperchromatic and palisading. Occasionally, the central cells are squamous and form keratin pearls. The stroma is usually scanty (Fig 12-19). The trabecular-tubular pattern forms cords and ductal structures. The membranous pattern has a jigsaw arrangement of epithelial islands in a multilobulated and often unencapsulated tumor. The islands are surrounded by eosinophilic, PAS-positive, hyalinized material representing replicated basal lamina. The islands may also contain small intercellular hyaline masses that may coalesce. This pattern strongly resembles that of dermal cylindroma.

Rarely, basal cell adenomas may develop invasive properties; in such cases, they are classified as basal cell adenocarcinomas.

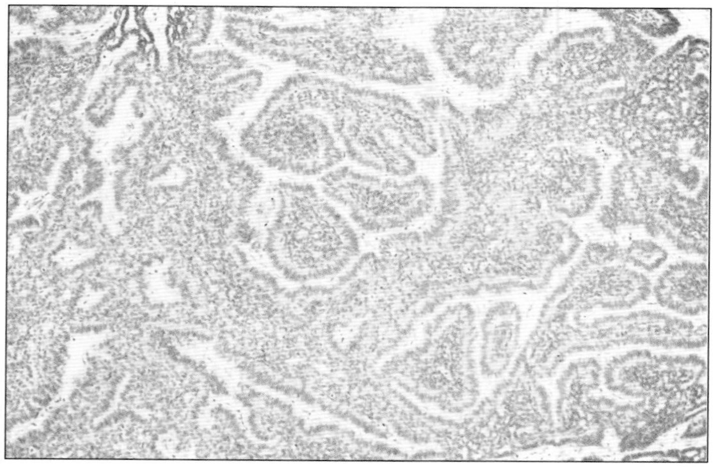

Fig 12-19 A basal cell adenoma with tumor islands consisting of basaloid cells with columnar, palisading cells at the periphery.

PROGNOSIS ▶ Excisions are curative, leaving little chance of recurrence. When a rare clinical recurrence develops, it is usually a second tumor rather than a persistence of the original tumor. Some have reported significant recurrence rates with the membranous variant because of its multilobular and multifocal nature. However, these are the result of "conservative" excisions without frozen section–assessed margins. Superficial parotidectomy of parotid lesions reduces such recurrences.

Canalicular Adenoma

CLINICAL PRESENTATION ▶ Canalicular adenomas are benign neoplasms that arise exclusively from oral mucosal minor salivary glands. About 80% occur in the upper lip, their site of predilection; the rest occur in other oral mucosal sites. They have a distinct female predilection and occur in those older than 50 years of age, which is usually older than patients with basal cell adenomas. The tumor will usually present as a single, firm, painless, freely movable mass in the upper lip submucosa. About 20% will occur multifocally, requiring a complete examination of the entire lip for smaller, developing tumors. Most will be small, ranging in size from 0.5 cm to no larger than 3 cm. The overlying epithelium will be intact (Fig 12-20a).

DIFFERENTIAL DIAGNOSIS ▶ A freely movable mass in the upper lip will suggest a *mucocele* or a true *mucus retention cyst*, although mucoceles are uncommon in the upper lip compared to the lower lip. It may represent a *basal cell adenoma*, which can occur in the upper lip but occurs most commonly in the parotid gland. A *pleomorphic adenoma* may be considered, but it is uncommon in the upper lip.

DIAGNOSTIC WORK-UP AND TREATMENT ▶ Diagnosis and definitive treatment are accomplished by an excision of the mass with 0.5-cm margins, including the overlying epithelium and the muscle fascia usually of the orbicularis oris muscle. Frozen sections should be used to assess margins at the time of excision.

HISTOPATHOLOGY ▶ These tumors are discrete and may have a capsule (Fig 12-20b). They are sometimes multifocal. The cut surface of the tumor can have cystic spaces and gelatinous areas. The cells are uniform, cuboidal to columnar in shape, with regular nuclei. They are often arranged in double rows with duct-like separations, resembling links in a chain (Fig 12-20c). There may be single rows arranged as parallel, canalicular structures or as cysts. The stroma is striking for its poorly defined, wispy quality and lack of collagen. Capillaries are prominent, however.

PROGNOSIS ▶ Excision is curative, leaving little chance for recurrence. However, because these tumors may occur as multifocal tumors, a second tumor may arise in the local area or elsewhere.

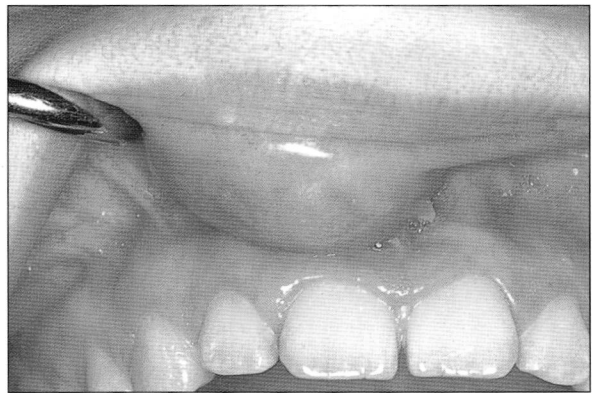

Fig 12-20a Canalicular adenoma has a predilection for the upper lip, where it will present as a small, firm, non-tender, and freely movable submucosal mass on the oral side of the orbicularis oris muscle. (Reprinted from Strassburg M and Knolle G, *Diseases of the Oral Mucosa: A Color Atlas*, with permission from Quintessence Publishing Co.)

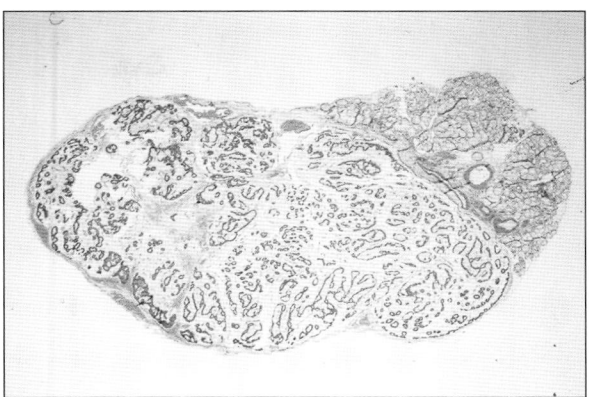

Fig 12-20b A canalicular adenoma showing a tumor mass that is well defined, vascular, uniform, and seemingly without stroma.

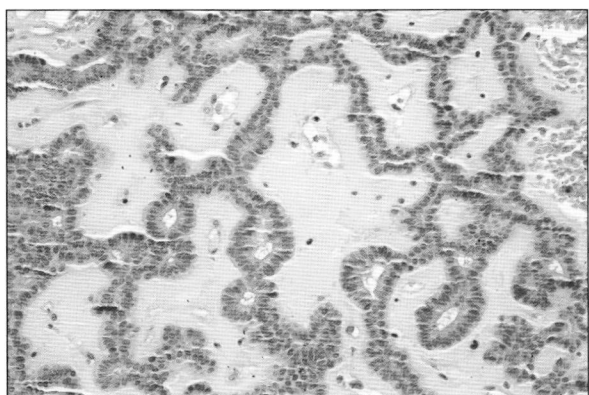

Fig 12-20c The same tumor as shown in Fig 12-20b showing a sparsely cellular stroma that contains numerous capillaries. The cells are uniform and often arranged in double rows with ductal configurations. These double rows have a canalicular appearance when the two layers are more widely separated.

Oncocytoma

CLINICAL PRESENTATION AND PATHOGENESIS ▶

The oncocytoma is a very rare, benign salivary gland tumor that may represent a reactive proliferation of activated oncocytes. It is found mostly as a small tumor of less than 5 cm in size in the parotid gland. Rarely, it will also occur in an oral mucosal site. The tumor presents as a slow-growing, painless, firm mass that is freely movable in the parotid gland's superficial lobe. In rare instances, multiple masses composed of onco-cytes arise in the same location; this condition is called *oncocytosis*. Most occur in individuals older than 50 years, and because of its rarity no gender predilection is known.

Because these tumors rarely exceed 5 cm and oncocytes are normally found as age-related changes in the intralobular ducts of the parotid gland, it is suspected that they represent a limited proliferation of striated duct origin, essentially an oncocytic hamartoma rather than a true neoplasm such as a pleo-morphic adenoma.

DIFFERENTIAL DIAGNOSIS ▶

In the parotid gland, the neoplasm will mimic the more common parotid tumors, such as a *pleomorphic adenoma*, *Warthin tumor* (papillary cystadenoma lymphomatosum), and *adenoid cystic*, *mucoepidermoid*, and *acinic cell carcinomas*, among others. It may also present as a lymph node enlargement in the parotid gland, as would a *lymphoma, HIV-related lymphadenopathy*, and *tuberculosis-related lymphadenitis*.

DIAGNOSTIC WORK-UP AND TREATMENT ▶

In the parotid gland, most masses of this nature should undergo a fine-needle aspiration to rule out malignancy. If the results rule out a malignancy or suggest an oncocytoma, a superficial parotidectomy is the treatment of choice. In an oral mucosal site, excision with 0.5-cm margins assessed by frozen sections is recommended.

HISTOPATHOLOGY ▶

These are usually encapsulated tumors that may be multinodular (Fig 12-21a). They consist of large polyhedral or rounded cells with a granular eosinophilic cytoplasm and a dense nucleus (Fig 12-21b). The granularity of the cytoplasm is caused by the large numbers of densely packed mitochondria, which can be identified by electron microscopy. Histochemistry is less reliable, but phosphotungstic acid–hema-toxylin stain will usually identify mitochondria. The cells tend to be arranged in sheets, cords, or nests. There may be an alveolar pattern with delicate fibrovascular septae. Rarely, cystic structures may be formed. Clear cells sometimes may be prominent (Fig 12-21c). Ultrastructurally and histochemically, they are identified as oncocytes. Their changed appearance is probably the result of processing artifact.

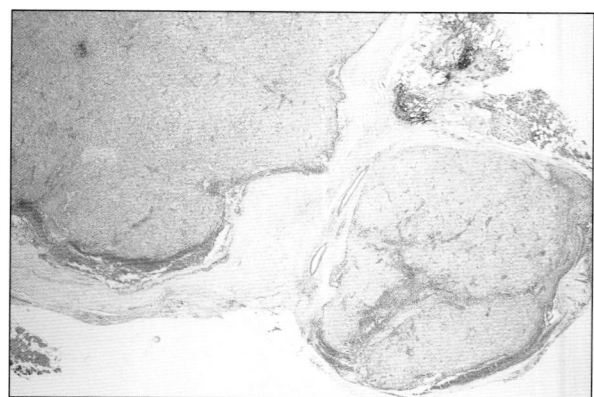

Fig 12-21a An oncocytoma showing multinodularity.

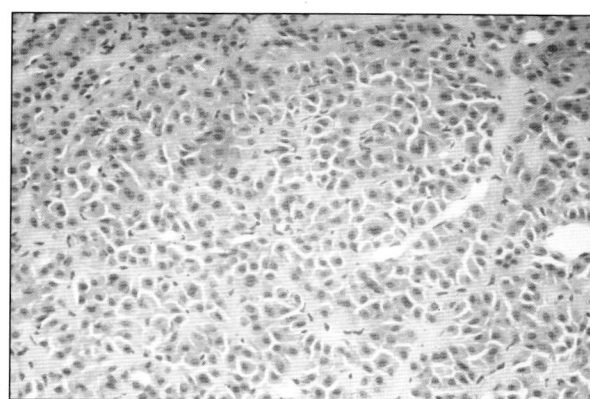

Fig 12-21b Oncocytic cells with granular cytoplasm.

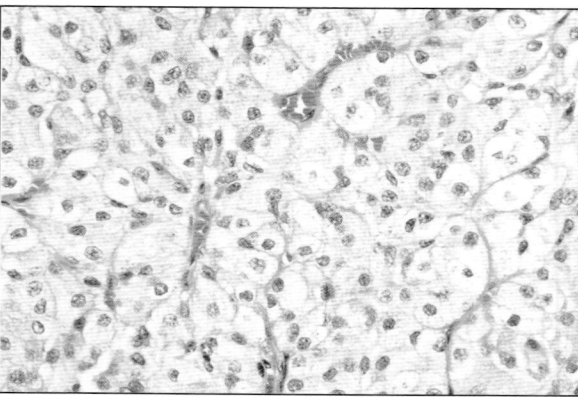

Fig 12-21c Oncocytic cells, many of which have a clear cytoplasm.

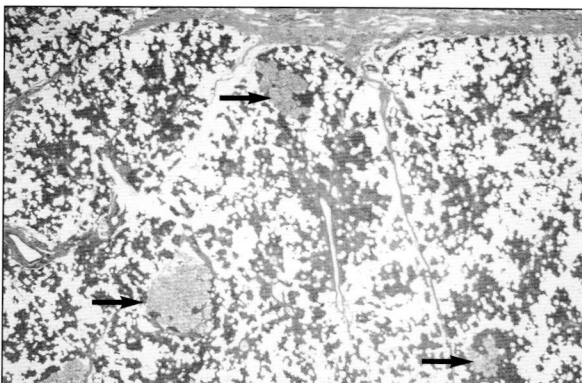

Fig 12-21d Oncocytosis of the parotid gland showing scattered clusters of oncocytes (*arrows*).

Oncocytosis, which may represent a hyperplastic or metaplastic process, consists of focal aggregates of oncocytes that may be multiple or solitary. This is seen most frequently in the parotid gland (Fig 12-21d). A rare malignant counterpart of the oncocytoma does occur.

PROGNOSIS

Excision via a superficial parotidectomy or local excision is generally curative with little chance for recurrence.

Inverted Ductal Papilloma

CLINICAL PRESENTATION AND PATHOGENESIS

The inverted ductal papilloma is a submucosal proliferation of ductal epithelium of the excretory duct that produces a small (0.5 to 2.0 cm), raised nodular mass in the submucosa. The mass will be connected to the surface but will be otherwise movable. The surface may have a small indented pit from the ductal opening; otherwise, the surface is intact. Like the sialadenoma papilliferum, this entity occurs mostly in older men.

The inverted ductal papilloma is a limited hyperplasia of ductal epithelium of a minor salivary gland. It produces a nodule by its increase in cell numbers, but it is neither a truly invasive lesion nor a true neoplasm.

DIFFERENTIAL DIAGNOSIS

The diagnosis of an inverted ductal papilloma is always an unexpected diagnosis discovered upon histopathologic examination. Most are removed with a working diagnosis of a *mucocele, mucus retention cyst*, or *fibroma*, or a *canalicular adenoma* if located in the upper lip.

DIAGNOSTIC WORK-UP AND TREATMENT

Excision with minimal margins is diagnostic and represents a definitive treatment.

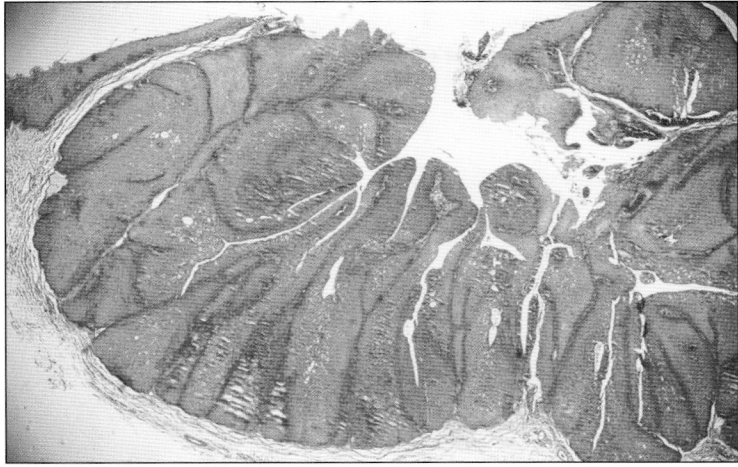

Fig 12-22 An inverted ductal papilloma shows the downward proliferation of the epithelium. The lesion does not project above the surface of the mucosa, a portion of which can be seen here.

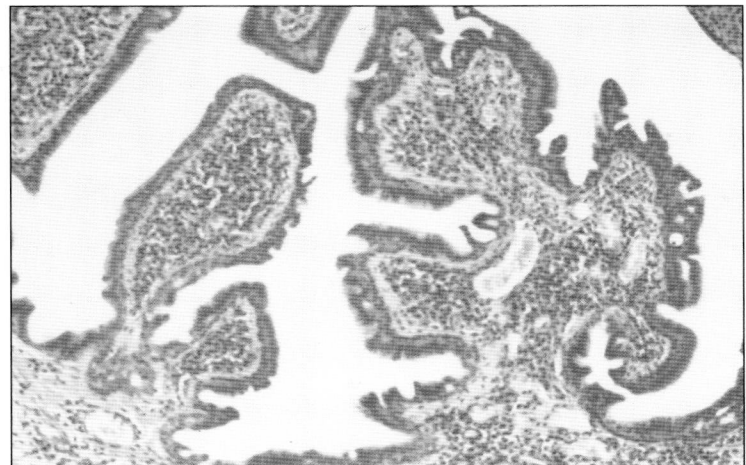

Fig 12-23 An intraductal papilloma in which the papillary projections can be seen within a dilated duct lumen.

HISTOPATHOLOGY ▶

Although this lesion originates from the distal component of the excretory duct, it does not protrude above the mucosal surface. Also, unlike the sialadenoma papilliferum, it is circumscribed. The ductal epithelium proliferates into the stroma with a pushing border and forms broad folds within the lumen (Fig 12-22). The cells are often basaloid, but the surface may be covered by columnar or cuboidal cells with eosinophilic cytoplasm. Mucous cells and even microcysts may be present.

PROGNOSIS ▶

Recurrence is not seen after excision.

Intraductal Papilloma

CLINICAL PRESENTATION AND PATHOGENESIS ▶

The intraductal papilloma is similar to the inverted ductal papilloma because it is a limited submucosal proliferation of ductal epithelium. It will tend to produce a small (0.5- to 2.0-cm) mass somewhat deeper in the submucosa because of its deeper origin. It will be a freely movable, painless mass seemingly without a surface connection. In some glands, particularly larger glands, it may produce an obstruction and result in mucus retention cysts. Most occur in older men.

The intraductal proliferation may be age- or inflammation-related, but it does not represent a true neoplasm with unlimited growth. Its intraductal location often causes cystic degeneration of the parent gland or the duct more proximal to its location.

DIFFERENTIAL DIAGNOSIS ▶

The diagnosis of an intraductal papilloma, like the diagnosis of an inverted ductal papilloma, is a specific histopathologic interpretation rarely anticipated clinically. Instead, the lesion usually has been excised with a working diagnosis of a *mucocele, mucus retention cyst,* or *fibroma,* or a *canalicular adenoma* if located in the upper lip.

DIAGNOSTIC WORK-UP AND TREATMENT ▶

Excision with minimal margins is diagnostic and represents a definitive treatment.

HISTOPATHOLOGY ▶

This papilloma appears to arise from a more proximal portion of the duct than the preceding lesions. It is unicystic and lined by one or two layers of cuboidal to columnar epithelium, which form papillary projections into the lumen (Fig 12-23). Mucous cells may be present.

PROGNOSIS ▶

Recurrence is not seen after excision.

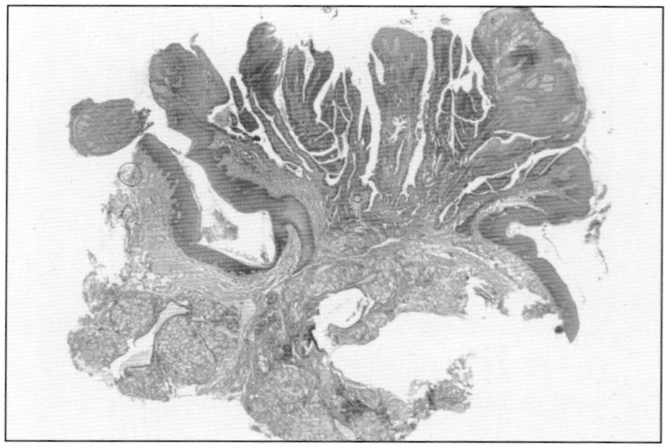

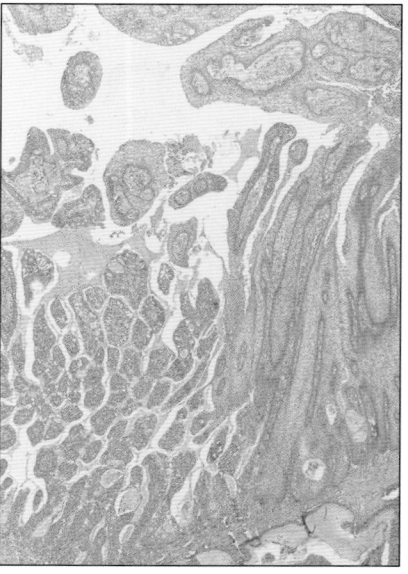

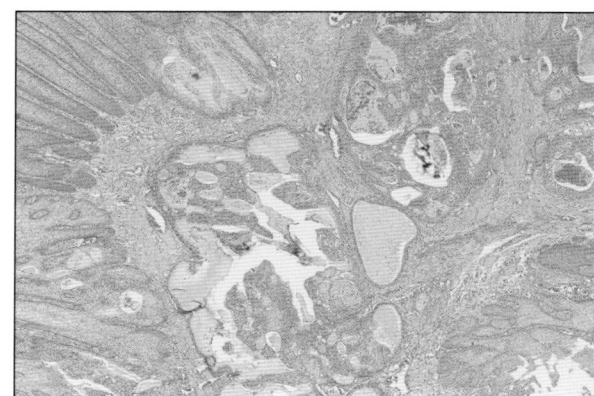

Fig 12-24a Sialadenoma papilliferum with an exophytic papillary appearance.

Fig 12-24b Sialadenoma papilliferum showing the continuity of the surface squamous epithelium with the ductal epithelium.

Fig 12-24c Dilated ductal spaces can be seen at the base of the sialadenoma papilliferum.

Sialadenoma Papilliferum

CLINICAL PRESENTATION AND PATHOGENESIS

Sialadenoma papilliferum is an exophytic benign proliferation of the superficial portion of an excretory duct. Because most arise from minor salivary glands, particularly of the buccal mucosa and palate, it will present as a small, verrucous-like lesion of the oral mucosa. It is more common in men and tends to occur in later life (in those older than 50 years). It is slow growing and will usually not exceed 2 cm.

The sialadenoma papilliferum also represents a limited hyperplasia of ductal epithelium that, because of its superficial location, fuses to the surface epithelium to develop its verrucous appearance. Its growth potential is limited.

DIFFERENTIAL DIAGNOSIS

The papillary nature of the lesion will make it appear like a *squamous papilloma*, a *verruciform xanthoma*, or a *verrucous carcinoma* rather than a salivary gland lesion. It may also resemble a small *squamous cell carcinoma*.

DIAGNOSTIC WORK-UP AND TREATMENT

Excision with minimal margins is all that is required both to establish a diagnosis and to eradicate the lesion.

HISTOPATHOLOGY

These are papillary lesions with an exoendophytic growth pattern that appears to arise from the distal portion of a salivary excretory duct. The exophytic component resembles a squamous papilloma with fibrovascular cores covered by acanthotic, parakeratinized, stratified squamous epithelium (Fig 12-24a). This merges into a glandular component with pseudostratified columnar epithelium or a double row of columnar and cuboidal cells (Fig 12-24b). At the base, there may be a proliferation of ducts and glandular structures that are not encapsulated, which can give the false impression of invasion (Fig 12-24c).

PROGNOSIS

Recurrence is not seen after excision.

Sebaceous Adenoma and Sebaceous Lymphadenoma

CLINICAL PRESENTATION AND PATHOGENESIS

Sebaceous cells are normally present in major salivary gland tissue and occur ectopically as so-called Fordyce granules in oral mucosa. Only rarely do they become neoplastic or proliferate as a tumorous

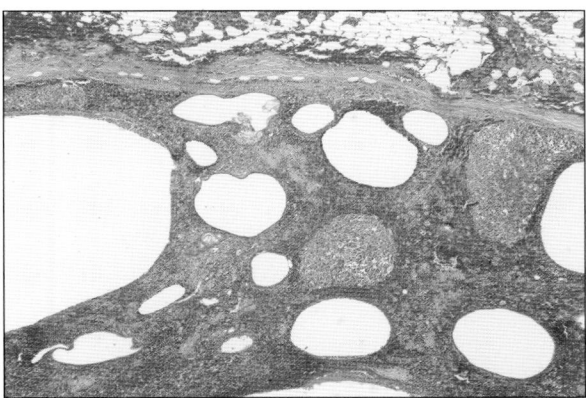

Fig 12-25a Sebaceous lymphadenoma showing abundant lymphoid tissue with germinal centers. There are dilated ducts and sebaceous glands.

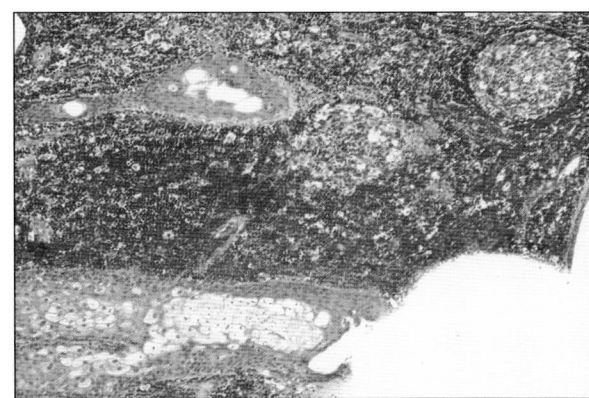

Fig 12-25b Higher-power view of Fig 12-25a with germinal centers, epithelially lined cystic spaces, and sebaceous glands.

mass. Two sebaceous tumors, sebaceous adenoma and sebaceous lymphadenoma, arise mainly in the parotid gland. Each is a rare finding.

Like the pleomorphic adenoma, the sebaceous adenoma and sebaceous lymphadenoma will each present as a slow-growing mass in the parotid gland. They are painless, soft to doughy in consistency, and movable because they tend to be encapsulated and well circumscribed. The reported cases to date indicate that they most commonly occur in women 50 years or older.

The pathogenesis of the sebaceous lymphadenoma is similar to that of the Warthin tumor (papillary cystadenoma lymphomatosum). Both arise from salivary gland ducts entrapped within lymph nodes. The sebaceous lymphadenoma probably arises from the intralobular ducts, unlike the Warthin tumor, which arises from striated ducts. Both, therefore, have similar biologic behavior. The sebaceous adenoma probably arises from the interlobular ducts or from sebaceous cells not entrapped within lymph nodes.

DIFFERENTIAL DIAGNOSIS ▶
The more common parotid tumors are the major considerations: *pleomorphic adenoma, Warthin tumor, basal cell adenoma*, and, less likely, some malignant *salivary gland tumors* or a *lymph node enlargement*.

DIAGNOSTIC WORK-UP AND TREATMENT ▶
Diagnosis and treatment are achieved with a superficial parotidectomy. For the rare tumor that occurs outside the parotid gland (fewer than 20 reported to date), a local excision with 0.5-cm margins is adequate.

HISTOPATHOLOGY ▶
Sebaceous adenomas are well-demarcated, often encapsulated tumors consisting of nests of sebaceous cells in a fibrous stroma. Frequently, cysts develop.

Sebaceous lymphadenomas are usually encapsulated and may be cystic or solid. They consist of sebaceous glands and salivary ducts in a lymphoid stroma, which may contain germinal centers (Figs 12-25a and 12-25b). Liberation of sebum can induce a stromal reaction of inflammatory cells, macrophages, and foreign-body giant cells.

PROGNOSIS ▶
The prognosis is excellent. Recurrence is not seen after adequate excision.

Mucoepidermoid Carcinoma

CLINICAL PRESENTATION AND PATHOGENESIS ▶
Mucoepidermoid carcinoma is the most common malignant salivary gland tumor. Statistical data indicate that it is the most common parotid malignancy (89%) and that it is the most common malignant salivary gland tumor in children. About 70% of these tumors are found in the parotid gland, 15% to 20% in the oral cavity, and 6% to 10% in the submandibular gland. A few are also found centrally within the mandible. In most large series, it has a distinct female predilection of about 3:1.

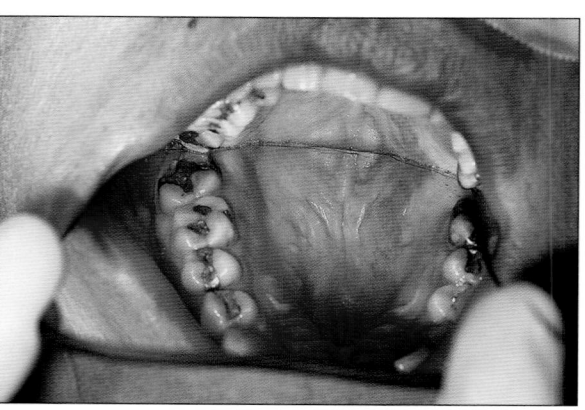

Fig 12-26 Low-grade mucoepidermoid carcinoma may be long-standing but usually is less than 3 cm in diameter. The surface may or may not be ulcerated.

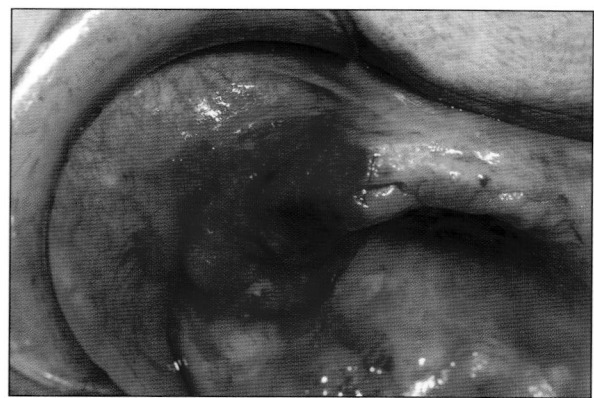

Fig 12-27 High-grade mucoepidermoid carcinoma closely resembles a squamous cell carcinoma by its larger size, faster infiltrative growth, invasion of bone, and greater likelihood to be ulcerated.

Mucoepidermoid tumors are the one malignancy in which histologic grading and clinical behavior characteristics correlate and are somewhat predictive of biologic behavior. Treatment decisions are, therefore, based on histologic grading. The tumors will span a wide range, from low grade to very high grade and with different gradations in between subtly blending from one form into another. Low-grade mucoepidermoid carcinomas will possess an infiltrative growth pattern and a very slow growth rate similar to that of a pleomorphic adenoma. They metastasize infrequently and only late in their course. Conversely, high-grade mucoepidermoid carcinomas behave like poorly differentiated squamous cell carcinomas with rapid infiltrative growth and metastasis.

Determination of the grade (low, intermediate, or high) is not limited to histopathologic criteria alone. The clinical features of each differ and are important in the final determination of grade. Low-grade tumors are characteristically less than 3.0 cm and grow very slowly (Fig 12-26). Patients frequently will have been aware of their presence for 3 to 6 years. Most tumors will not be ulcerated or will have only recently ulcerated after many years, prompting the patient to seek treatment. Many tumors will appear bluish because their well-differentiated character creates mucin-filled spaces that appear blue through the mucosal cover. Most will not invade bone until late in their course. Intermediate- and high-grade mucoepidermoid carcinomas are faster growing, more diffuse, and ulcerate early. Many are obviously destructive to underlying bone, and some are painful. Because they are not sufficiently differentiated to produce mucin, they will not appear blue or vacuolated. They will present as solid masses with a normal color of the overlying epithelium or with an ulcerated surface.

A parotid mucoepidermoid carcinoma will present as a parotid mass, which may be freely movable, like the more common benign parotid tumors, but may also be diffuse and less circumscribed. If the facial nerve is infiltrated by tumor, facial muscle paresis may be evident.

Mucoepidermoid carcinomas arise from reserve cells in the salivary duct system. Therefore, they can partially differentiate into mucin-producing cells or duct-like epidermoid cells. Both cell types are altered neoplastic cells. Because the reserve cell can become neoplastic at any stage of its maturation, the resultant tumor may emerge with variable biologic behavior and histologic grading as is typical of the mucoepidermoid carcinomas.

DIFFERENTIAL DIAGNOSIS ▶ A low-grade mucoepidermoid carcinoma in the mucosa of the palate may or may not be ulcerated. If it has an intact overlying mucosa, the most likely lesion would be a *pleomorphic adenoma* followed by an *adenoid cystic carcinoma* and a *polymorphous low-grade adenocarcinoma*. If the surface is ulcerated unattributable to trauma, the likelihood of pleomorphic adenoma is remote. Therefore, because of its slow growth rate and malignant nature, which can ulcerate the surface mucosa, *adenoid cystic carcinoma* becomes the primary differential lesion, followed by *polymorphous low-grade adenocarcinoma* and perhaps a *carcinoma ex pleomorphic adenoma.*

A high-grade mucoepidermoid carcinoma of the palate will be infiltrative, ulcerated, and destructive of bone (Fig 12-27). Therefore, *squamous cell carcinoma* is the most important differential lesion in this location. Other considerations are *sinus* or *nasal carcinomas* that have extended down through the palate and perhaps a *carcinoma ex pleomorphic adenoma* as well. An adenoid cystic carcinoma would not appear clinically like a high-grade mucoepidermoid carcinoma despite its malignant nature. Adenoid cystic carcinomas tend to be slower in growth and develop more of a mass than a diffuse growth pattern. Although extranodal non-Hodgkin lymphomas occur in the palatal mucosa as a preferred site, their presentation is more that of a nonulcerated fleshy mass.

A low-grade mucoepidermoid carcinoma in the parotid gland would present as the more common benign parotid tumors (*pleomorphic adenoma, Warthin tumor,* and *basal cell adenoma*) as well as some malignant tumors, mainly *adenoid cystic carcinoma* and *acinic cell carcinoma.*

A high-grade mucoepidermoid carcinoma in the parotid gland usually has a presentation suggestive of an aggressive malignancy, including rapid growth, large size, possible facial muscle paresis, and induration. Its differential would include *adenoid cystic carcinoma* (though this lesion tends to be a small primary), *salivary duct carcinoma, carcinoma ex pleomorphic adenoma,* and possibly seeding of a *regional metastasis from an oral or a nasopharyngeal squamous cell carcinoma.*

DIAGNOSTIC WORK-UP ▶

If the mass is in a location other than the parotid gland, a representative incisional biopsy is required. It should be in the lesion's center and include overlying mucosa. If the tumor is in the palate, a CT scan or MRI scan with coronal views is needed to assess for sinus, nasal, or palatal bone invasion. If the tumor is in the parotid gland, the same type of scan is required to assess its location and size.

HISTOPATHOLOGY ▶

The biologic behavior of these tumors, which ranges from extremely low grade to highly aggressive, depends primarily on the histology. In general, these masses are unencapsulated, although the low-grade tumors are usually well circumscribed (Fig 12-28a) while the high-grade tumors show considerable infiltration.

Several cell types are seen, including:

1. Mucous-secreting cells, which are usually large cells with pale foamy cytoplasm. They may occur in clusters or single cells, or they may line cystic spaces. They elaborate epithelial mucin, which can be identified by mucicarmine or PAS stain; the latter is resistant to diastase digestion. Particularly when the mucous component is scant, special stains may be necessary for identification.

2. Epidermoid cells, which lie in sheets or line cystic spaces. They may show interlacing patterns with intercellular bridges. Occasionally, keratin pearls are seen.

3. Intermediate cells, which are basaloid cells that vary from small, dark-staining cells to larger, more epidermoid-like cells. They may lie in sheets or line cystic spaces. They tend to blend into epidermoid cells. These cells are believed to differentiate into epidermoid, mucous, and clear cells.

4. Clear cells that may form broad sheets or occur as single cells or clusters within epidermoid cells. Although these cells are usually negative on mucin staining, some mucin may occasionally be identified.

The grading of mucoepidermoid carcinoma depends primarily on the relative mix of cell types, although growth pattern and cellular atypia also play significant roles.

Low-grade mucoepidermoid carcinomas are characterized by well-formed cysts that may be quite large. These cysts frequently contain mucin and are lined by a mixture of mucous, intermediate, and epidermoid cells (Figs 12-28a to 12-28c). These cells may also form more solid foci between the cysts. The cells are mature and do not show atypia or mitotic activity. The cysts may rupture, liberating mucin and causing an inflammatory reaction within adjacent tissue (Fig 12-28d). Rupture also facilitates the spread of tumor cells. In relation to other grades, low-grade tumors have a more prominent mucous cell component. Clinically, the mucin-filled cysts appear similar to mucus retention phenomena. A potential

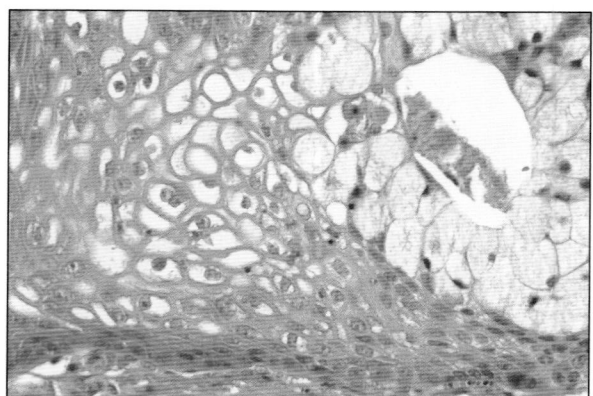

Fig 12-28a A mucoepidermoid carcinoma of the lower lip showing a circumscribed but unencapsulated mass with numerous cystic spaces. This indicates a low-grade tumor.

Fig 12-28b From the tumor shown in Fig 12-28a. Numerous mucous cells are seen with some adjacent clear cells and intermediate cells.

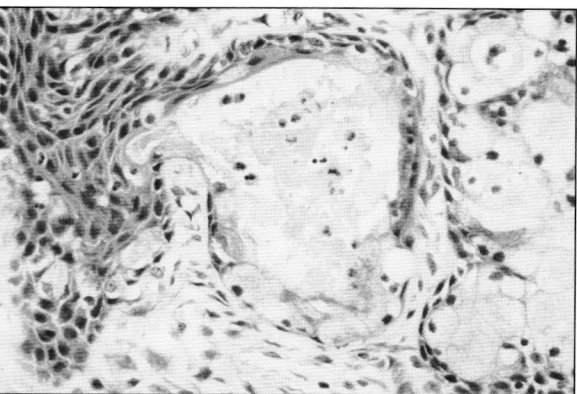

Fig 12-28c A low-grade mucoepidermoid carcinoma showing cystic spaces that are lined by mucous cells and epidermoid cells.

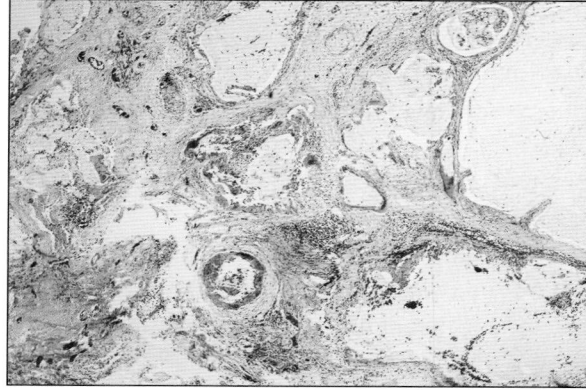

Fig 12-28d Low-grade mucoepidermoid carcinoma in which some cysts have ruptured, releasing mucin and inducing a foreign-body reaction.

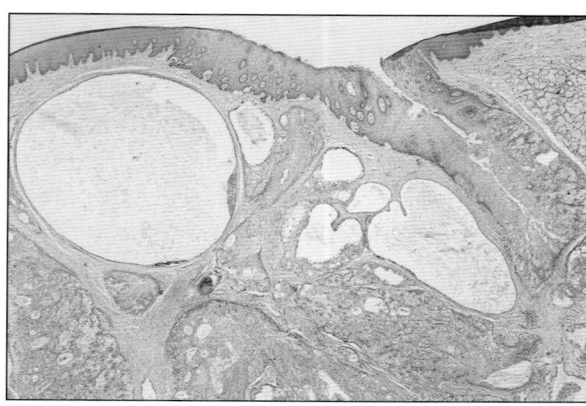

Fig 12-28e Low-grade mucoepidermoid carcinoma in which several large cysts are seen at the surface of the tumor. A biopsy specimen with insufficient depth may show only an innocuous cyst.

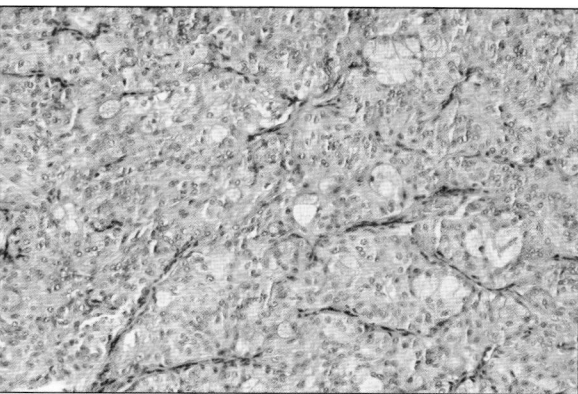

Fig 12-29 Intermediate-grade mucoepidermoid carcinoma with a more solid pattern. Fewer mucous cells are present. Intermediate cells and some epidermoid cells are seen.

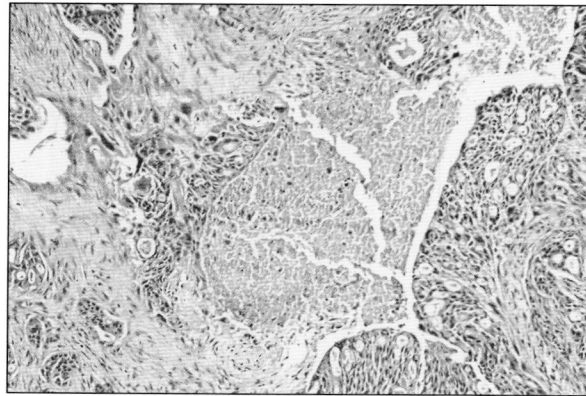

Fig 12-30a A high-grade mucoepidermoid carcinoma showing necrosis.

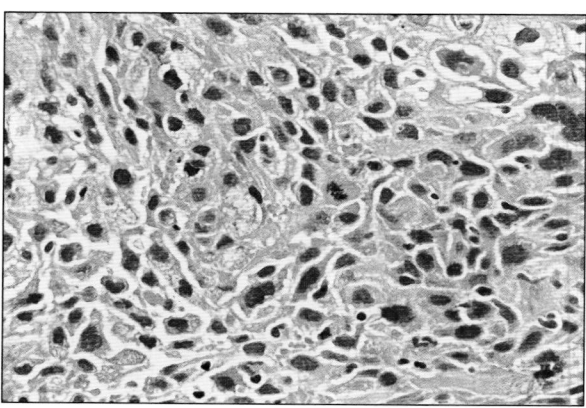

Fig 12-30b A high-grade mucoepidermoid carcinoma with pleomorphic cells, large hyperchromatic nuclei, and a mitotic figure in the center of the field.

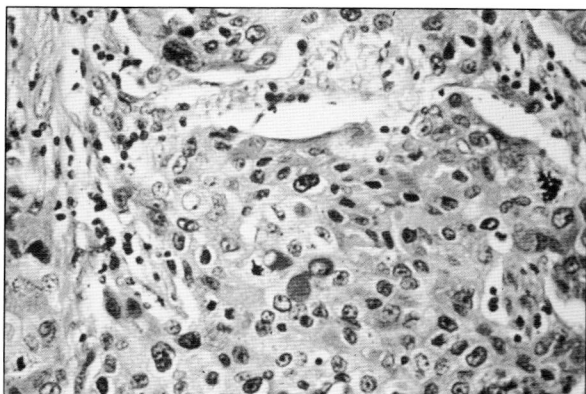

Fig 12-30c A high-grade mucoepidermoid carcinoma showing pleomorphic and atypical epithelial cells. A PAS stain demonstrates the sparse mucous cells.

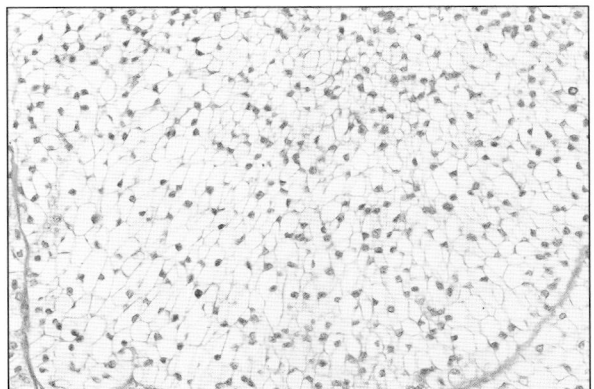

Fig 12-31 Sheets of clear cells within a mucoepidermoid carcinoma.

problem with low-grade tumors is that large cysts may sometimes develop in the superficial aspect of the tumor (Fig 12-28e). In these cases, an insufficiently deep incisional biopsy may miss the diagnostic portion of the tumor.

Intermediate-grade tumors contain smaller and fewer cysts and have a more solid appearance. The solid areas consist of intermediate cells, epidermoid cells, and some mucous cells (Fig 12-29). Mitoses are not usually present, but nuclear atypism may be seen. Compared to low-grade tumors, intermediate and epidermoid cells are more prominent and mucous cells are sparser.

High-grade tumors are solid and consist of intermediate and epidermoid cells, which show considerable atypia. Mitotic activity also is present. Mucous cells may be readily noted, but in many tumors they are so sparse that there is a marked resemblance to squamous cell carcinoma. In these cases, special stains, such as mucicarmine or PAS, are necessary to demonstrate their presence and clarify the diagnosis. These are infiltrative, unencapsulated tumors (Figs 12-30a to 12-30c).

Clear cells may be seen in all grades of mucoepidermoid carcinoma. Occasionally, they can represent the majority of the tumor. In these instances, they must be differentiated from other clear cell neoplasms, including metastatic renal cell carcinoma (Fig 12-31).

TREATMENT AND PROGNOSIS ▶

Low-grade mucoepidermoid carcinomas of the palate require a soft tissue palatal excision with 1-cm peripheral margins and anatomic barrier margins. The palatal bone does not require excision unless radiographs, scans, or direct observation indicate tumor extension into it. Postoperative radiotherapy or prophylactic neck dissection is not indicated. The same lesion in other oral mucosal sites requires a local excision with 1-cm margins and anatomic barrier margins. The 5-year survival rate for individuals with low-grade mucoepidermoid carcinoma of the oral mucosa treated in this fashion is about 95%.

Low-grade mucoepidermoid carcinomas of the parotid gland are treated with superficial parotidectomy unless they originate from or extend into the deep lobe or involve the facial nerve, in which case a total parotidectomy is required. The 5-year survival rate is about 90% to 95%.

Intermediate- and high-grade mucoepidermoid carcinomas of the palate require a hemimaxillectomy-type excision with postoperative radiotherapy in the dose range of 5,000 cGy to 7,000 cGy. The bilateral necks should be treated prophylactically with either surgery or radiotherapy. If nodal disease presents in the neck, then surgical neck dissection is accomplished in addition to radiotherapy of the primary tumor site and the neck. The 5-year survival rate for such high-grade tumors is about 35%; at 10 years, the survival rate drops to about 25%. Metastasis to regional lymph nodes and uncontrolled tumor at the primary site with cranial invasion are a prime cause of death. Distant metastasis to the lungs is also seen.

Intermediate- and high-grade mucoepidermoid carcinomas of the parotid gland require a total parotidectomy and ipsilateral neck dissection followed by postoperative radiotherapy in the dose range of 5,000 cGy to 7,000 cGy. The 5-year survival rate is about 40%; the 10-year rate is approximately 25%.

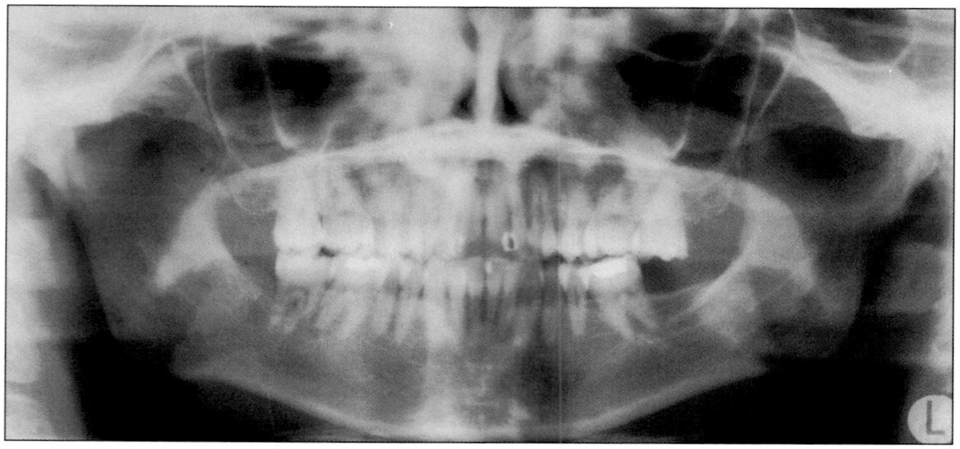

Fig 12-32 Radiolucency in the right third molar area, where a biopsy identified a low-grade central mucoepidermoid carcinoma.

Central Mucoepidermoid Carcinoma

CLINICAL PRESENTATION AND PATHOGENESIS ►

Central mucoepidermoid carcinomas are almost always low grade in terms of both histology and behavior. They occur in the mandible but are difficult to discern in the maxilla because central mucoepidermoid carcinomas in this location soon become indistinguishable from those arising in the sinus or palatal mucosa. In fact, when they occur in the mandible, they must be confined to bone with no soft tissue extension to qualify as a true central mucoepidermoid carcinoma. They can occur in all tooth-bearing areas of the mandible but seem to be more frequent in the third molar and premolar regions.

These carcinomas will often be an incidental finding on a panoramic radiograph or present with a painless bony expansion (Fig 12-32). The inferior alveolar nerve is usually unaltered in its lip sensation but can develop paresthesia in large lesions of long standing. Radiographically, about one half will appear as a well circumscribed unilocular radiolucency unassociated with an impacted tooth crown. Another one half will appear as a multilocular radiolucency. They occur more frequently in the 30- to 50-year age range.

The pathogenesis of a central salivary gland tumor remains obscure. One theory suggests embryologically entrapped salivary gland elements in the mandible, which later become neoplastic. However, this theory does not answer the question of why these are almost exclusively mucoepidermoid tumors and not other types. The other theory is based on neoplastic transformation of the mucous cells found within some odontogenic cysts. This theory would explain why these tumors are primarily mucoepidermoid carcinomas and occur almost exclusively in the tooth-bearing areas of the jaws.

DIFFERENTIAL DIAGNOSIS ►

A central mucoepidermoid carcinoma is usually not part of a differential diagnostic list concerning a radiolucent expansion of the mandible. Instead, this presentation is more common to odontogenic cysts and tumors. Therefore, lesions such as *ameloblastomas, odontogenic keratocysts, odontogenic myxomas*, and *dentigerous cysts* are more to be anticipated, as is the more radiolucent bone tumor, the *central giant cell tumor*.

DIAGNOSTIC WORK-UP ►

Most central mucoepidermoid carcinomas are diagnosed by an exploration and incisional biopsy or by enucleation. A CT scan is recommended to assess the bony extent and any soft tissue extension of the tumor.

HISTOPATHOLOGY ►

Central mucoepidermoid carcinomas do not differ histologically from their soft tissue counterparts. Most reported cases have been low-grade tumors.

TREATMENT ►

Central mucoepidermoid carcinomas should not be left to follow-up if they were diagnosed by enucleation. The recurrence rate is over 60%, and there is risk of the lesion extending out of the bone into adjacent structures and the neck. These tumors are low-grade malignancies that may be completely

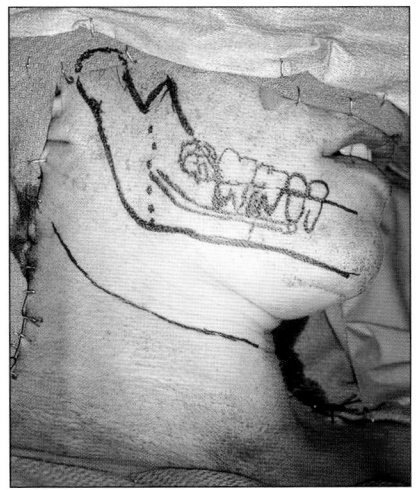

Fig 12-33a A central mucoepidermoid carcinoma of the mandible is best treated with 1.5-cm resection margins.

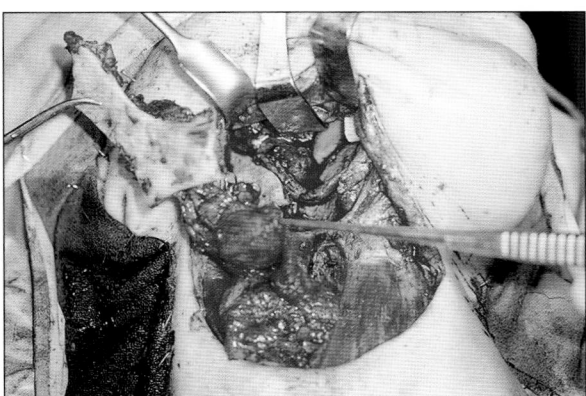

Fig 12-33b Unless 1 cm of the inferior border can be preserved while maintaining 1.5-cm bony margins, a continuity resection is needed.

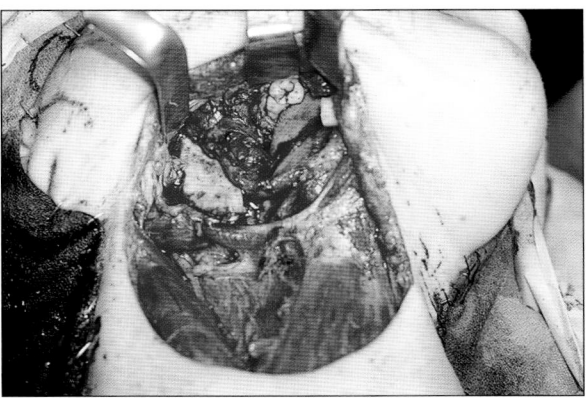

Fig 12-33c Resections for a central mucoepidermoid carcinoma should not attempt to preserve the inferior alveolar nerve.

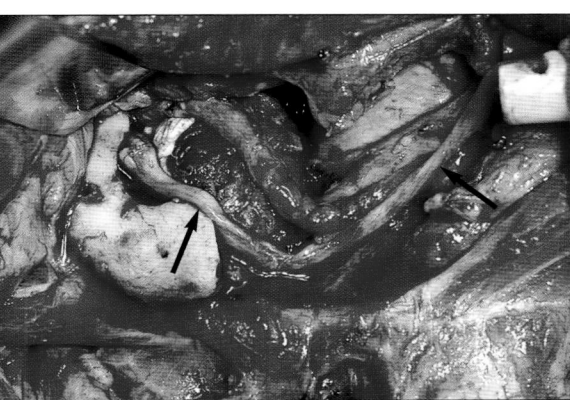

Fig 12-33d Because central mucoepidermoid carcinomas rarely require postoperative radiotherapy, nerve grafts to reconstruct the inferior alveolar nerve are a consideration. Here a sural nerve graft was cabled between the proximal and distal nerve ends (*arrows*).

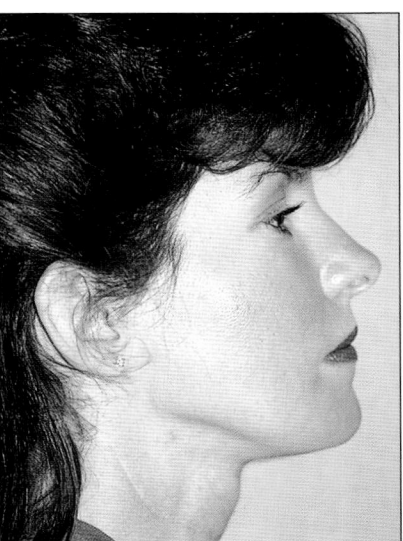

Fig 12-33e Resections of a central mucoepidermoid carcinoma that are reconstructed with just a rigid titanium reconstruction plate result in a stable mandible and retention of facial contours.

cured with definitive surgery. They are best treated with a resection of bone with 1.0- to 1.5-cm bony margins (Fig 12-33a). In some cases this allows for a peripheral resection, which preserves mandibular continuity, but mostly it requires a continuity resection. Unless the inferior alveolar nerve is more than 1 cm from the tumor, the nerve should be included in the resection (Fig 12-33b). Although central mucoepidermoid carcinomas are low grade, they exhibit perineural invasion. In most resections, preservation of the nerve invites recurrence (Fig 12-33c). However, nerve grafting may be accomplished in selected cases (Fig 12-33d). Postoperative radiotherapy and/or neck dissection is not required unless the clinical behavior or histologic grading is more advanced than low grade.

The resultant continuity defect is best treated with a reconstruction plate initially (Fig 12-33e), followed by a definitive bony reconstruction at least 3 months later. This approach will avoid the higher in-

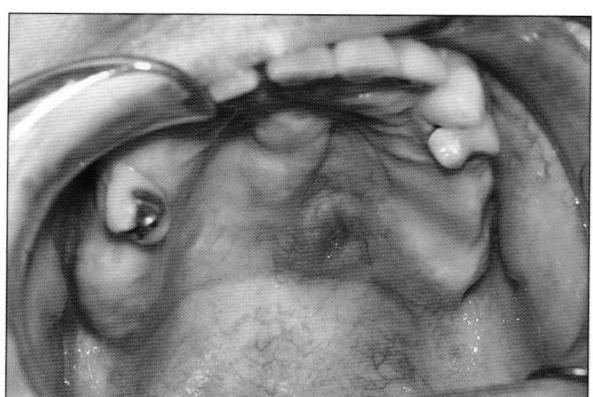

Fig 12-34 Like many adenoid cystic carcinomas, this one presented as a small tumor mass of several years' duration. Undiagnosed for 5 years despite numerous dental visits, the tumor had already undergone metastasis to the lung at the time of diagnosis.

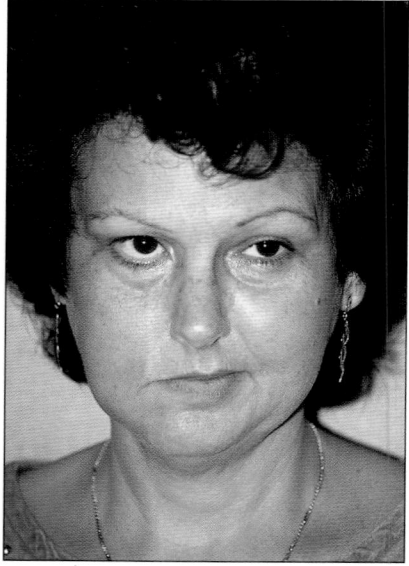

Fig 12-35 Adenoid cystic carcinoma in the parotid has a marked propensity to infiltrate nerves. It may initially present with facial nerve palsy with no obvious mass because of its small size.

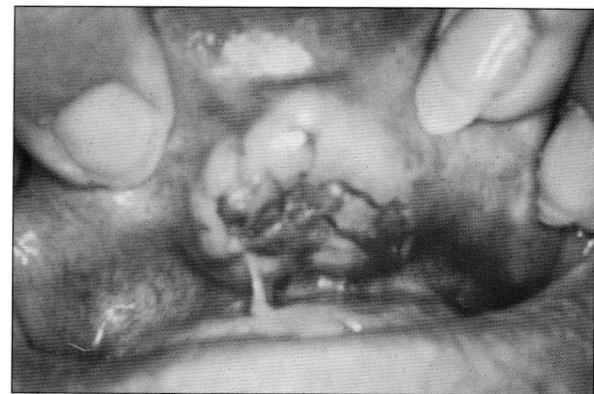

Fig 12-36 Some adenoid cystic carcinomas attain a large size in addition to prominent neural invasion and vascular spread.

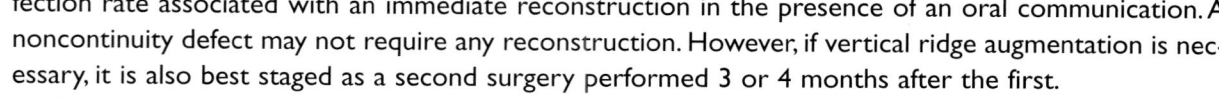

PROGNOSIS ▶

fection rate associated with an immediate reconstruction in the presence of an oral communication. A noncontinuity defect may not require any reconstruction. However, if vertical ridge augmentation is necessary, it is also best staged as a second surgery performed 3 or 4 months after the first.

Central mucoepidermoid carcinomas have a 90% cure rate with prompt, definitive surgery. Otherwise local recurrences may occur, becoming uncontrolled and metastasizing to regional lymph nodes and to the lungs, leading to death.

Adenoid Cystic Carcinoma

CLINICAL PRESENTATION ▶

Adenoid cystic carcinoma is a clinically deceptive and histologically specific malignancy of salivary gland origin. It is clinically deceptive by virtue of its small size and slow growth, which belie its extensive subclinical invasion and marked ability for early metastasis (Fig 12-34). It is a malignancy that reinforces the point that tumor growth rate and metastatic capability are independent tumor properties.

Adenoid cystic carcinoma is the most common oral minor salivary gland malignancy. However, it also occurs in all the major salivary glands with an equal male-female distribution, except in the submandibular gland, where it occurs almost exclusively in women. Peculiar to adenoid cystic carcinoma, the tumor is occasionally found deep within the substance of the tongue, presenting a diagnostic problem. Other salivary gland tumors rarely occur in the tongue.

Wherever it arises, it presents as a single, solid tumor mass that is usually less than 4 cm in size. In the oral mucosa of the palate, the mucosa will be ulcerated 50% to 60% of the time. The palate may have objectively testable decreased sensation, but most patients are subjectively unaware of it. In the parotid gland, it will frequently occur deeper in the superficial lobe and cause facial nerve paresis or paralysis (Fig 12-35). In the submandibular gland, it presents as a mass usually associated with obstructive sialadenitis unassociated with any specific nerve dysfunction. In other mucosal sites, it will present as a firm, indurated mass with fixation either to bone or to adjacent structures, unless it is a very early tumor (Fig

12-36). When it occurs in the tongue, it may be asymptomatic for a long period and then identified by the patient as a "lump in the tongue." Other times, it will present as a deep pain in the tongue or, rarely, with paresis of one side. Such symptoms should alert the clinician to consider this tumor on a differential diagnosis of unexplained deep tongue pain in adults.

DIFFERENTIAL DIAGNOSIS ▶

The differential diagnosis in each site is usually a composite of primarily malignant and some benign salivary gland tumors, depending on the presence or absence of certain findings. In the palatal mucosa, if the epithelium is intact, statistically *pleomorphic adenoma* would be the most likely entity, followed by *mucoepidermoid carcinoma* (usually low grade) and *polymorphous low-grade adenocarcinoma*. If an ulceration is present, only malignant tumors would be a consideration, of which *mucoepidermoid carcinoma* (usually low grade) would be the most likely, followed by *polymorphous low-grade adenocarcinoma* and a *carcinoma ex pleomorphic adenoma*.

In the parotid gland, a deep palpable mass without facial nerve paresis would most likely represent a *pleomorphic adenoma*, a *Warthin tumor* (papillary cystadenoma lymphomatosum), or a *mucoepidermoid carcinoma*. However, if there is a detectable weakness of facial muscles, the differential diagnosis would change. Benign tumors would be removed from consideration, and malignancies that can produce functional neurologic loss would be considered. These include *mucoepidermoid carcinoma* (usually high grade) as the most likely because of its propensity to appear in the parotid gland, followed by the less common *salivary duct carcinoma*, and a *carcinoma ex pleomorphic adenoma*. Although it is known for its perineural invasion, the polymorphous low-grade adenocarcinoma would not be a consideration because it does not occur in the parotid gland. It remains primarily a tumor of minor salivary gland origin.

DIAGNOSTIC WORK-UP ▶

In each oral site, a deep incisional biopsy in the lesion's center that recovers sufficient tissue to take several sections is important. In the parotid gland, a fine-needle aspiration is indicated. In all sites, a CT scan or MRI scan is necessary to assess depth of invasion and identifiable extent.

HISTOPATHOLOGY ▶

These tumors are typically unencapsulated and infiltrative. Occasionally, however, they may show a degree of demarcation. The proliferating cell is a small cuboidal cell with a round, hyperchromatic nucleus and scant cytoplasm. Mitotic activity, pleomorphism, and cellular atypia are not usually seen. The cells may be arranged in various patterns that have been described as tubular, cribriform, and solid. These patterns may coexist in the same tumor, but one pattern usually predominates. This is of clinical significance since adenoid cystic carcinomas that are predominantly solid are found to be more aggressive and associated with a worse prognosis than those that are predominantly tubular or cribriform.

The cribriform pattern, classic for this tumor, occurs most frequently. Islands of cells form pseudocystic spaces, which yield a honeycomb, "cylindromatous," or "Swiss-cheese" appearance (Figs 12-37a to 12-37c). The spaces may contain basophilic, mucinous material or hyaline eosinophilic material that ultrastructurally is replicated basal lamina. The hyalinized material may also surround the islands, and continuity between the two can be seen.

The tubular pattern shows the cells in ductal arrangement with a single lumen (Fig 12-37d). The solid pattern has broad sheets and solid islands of the small, dark-staining cells. Sometimes a mature ductal structure can be seen within the islands (Fig 12-37e). Areas of necrosis may occur.

The stroma is fibrous and lacks the myxoid feature of a pleomorphic adenoma. Extensive hyalinization can take place. When this occurs, the epithelial component will often form small cords (Fig 12-37f).

A significant feature of adenoid cystic carcinoma is its ability to show perineural and even intraneural invasion (Fig 12-37g). Thus, paresthesia and facial paralysis can develop. This tumor will also readily invade bone (Fig 12-37h).

TREATMENT ▶

The underlying principles in all adenoid cystic carcinoma therapy are that tumor cells extend well beyond the clinical or radiographic margins and that this tumor undergoes not only perineural invasion but perineural spread. Therefore, it generally requires excision with the widest margins possible and postoperative radiotherapy of 6,000 cGy to 7,500 cGy. In the palate, this will require a hemimaxillectomy with at least 3-cm margins and a complete extirpation of tissue contents of the pterygomaxillary space to the base of the skull. Frozen sections are, of course, required for the peripheral margins, but a neg-

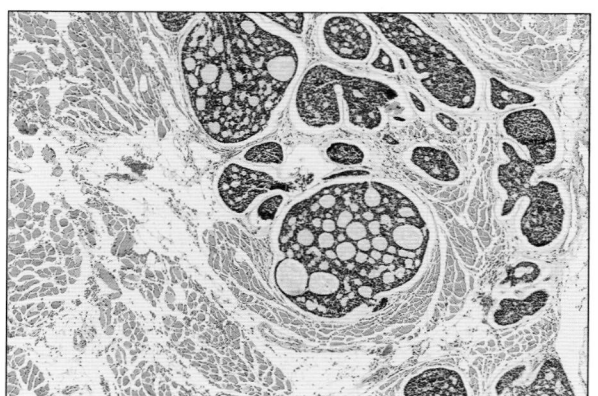

Fig 12-37a Adenoid cystic carcinoma showing its infiltrative character. Note the cribriform pattern.

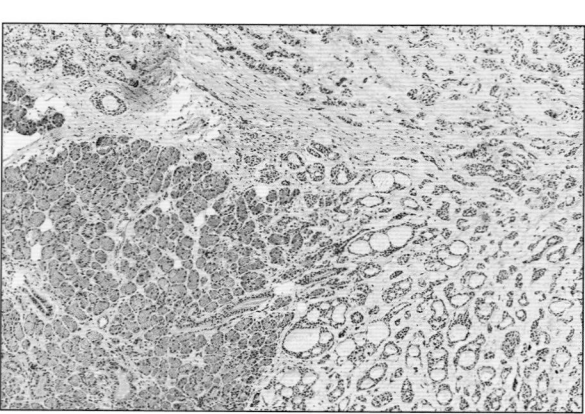

Fig 12-37b Adenoid cystic carcinoma of the submandibular gland. This patient had a 2-year history of a condition that had been interpreted clinically as a chronic obstructive sialadenitis. This is not an unusual presentation for this neoplasm.

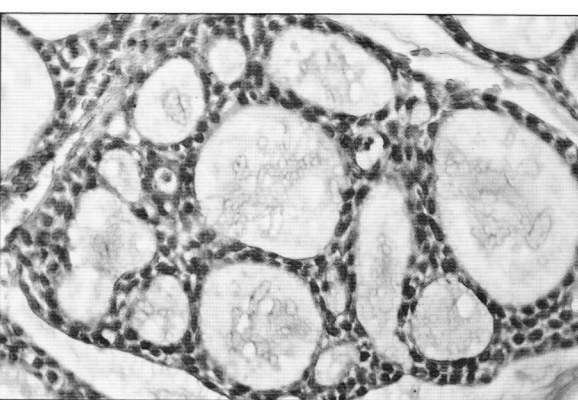

Fig 12-37c The classic cribriform pattern of adenoid cystic carcinoma showing small, cuboidal cells with hyperchromatic nuclei. The cells are uniform. The spaces contain a basophilic, often mucoid material.

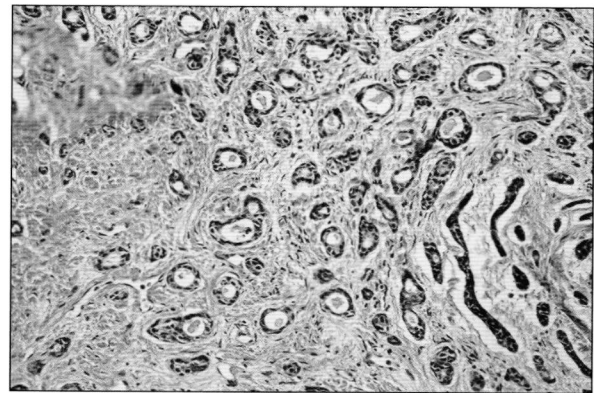

Fig 12-37d A tubular pattern within the same tumor shown in Fig 12-37c. The same cells as formed the cribriform pattern form single ductal structures here.

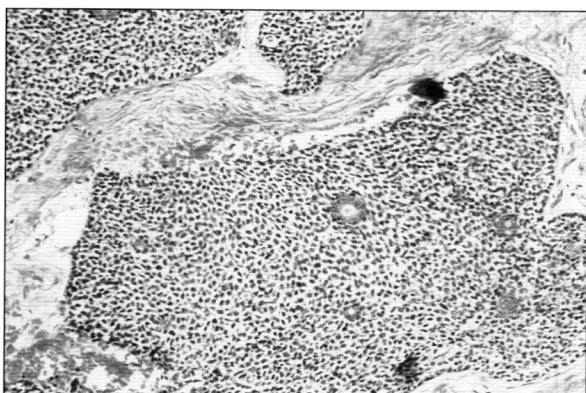

Fig 12-37e A solid pattern within the adenoid cystic carcinoma shown in Figs 12-37c and 12-37d. The cells are the same but the pattern differs; here they form solid sheets. A normal duct is seen within the island.

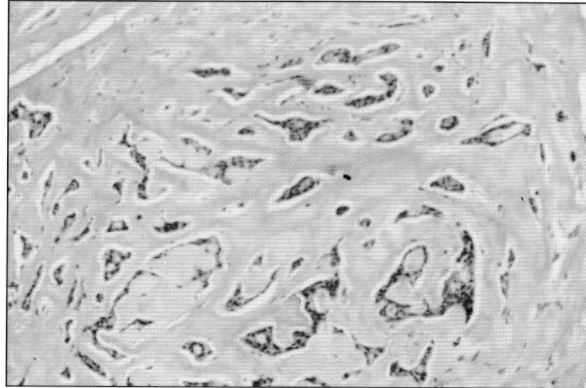

Fig 12-37f An area of extensive hyalinization with the tumor cells, forming small cords in an adenoid cystic carcinoma that shows a predominant cribriform pattern.

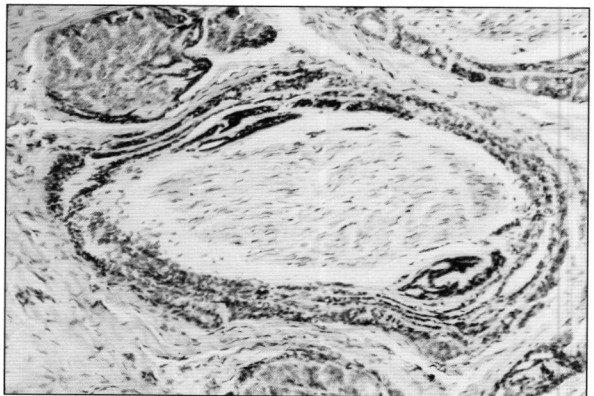

Fig 12-37g Neural invasion by an adenoid cystic carcinoma.

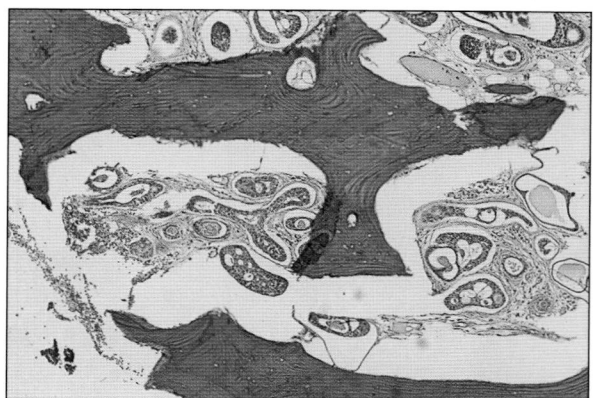

Fig 12-37h Adenoid cystic carcinoma invading bone.

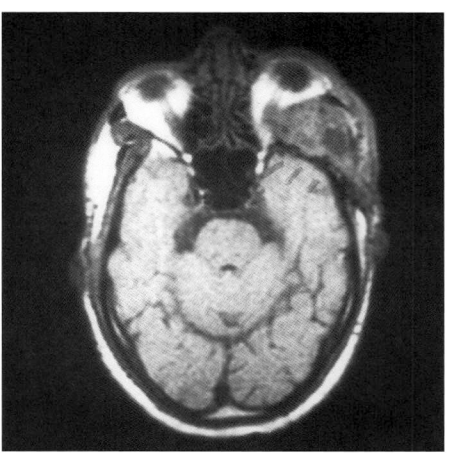

Fig 12-38 Some adenoid cystic carcinomas from the maxilla extend into the orbit via perineural and intraneural spread through the infraorbital fissure.

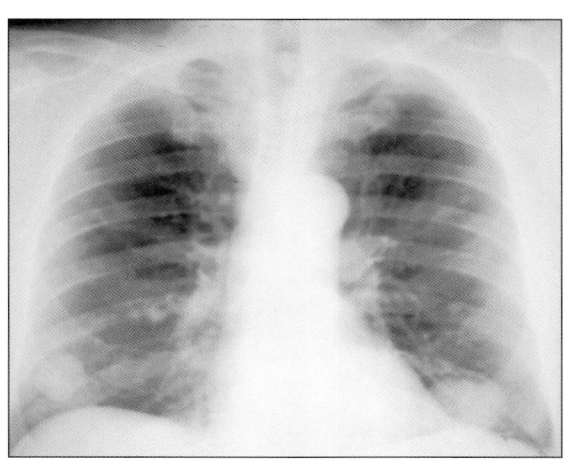

Fig 12-39 The most common metastasis of adenoid cystic carcinoma is to the lungs via bloodborne routes. Here several soft tissue masses in the lungs, known as *cannonball lesions*, originated from a maxillary adenoid cystic carcinoma.

ative margin at the midlevel of the greater palatine neurovascular bundle should not dissuade the surgeon from a complete extirpation to the skull base; perineural spread is not a solid cord of tumor cells migrating proximally up a nerve. Breaks in their continuum, called *skip lesions,* make a complete extirpation necessary.

In the parotid gland, a total parotidectomy is required. If the facial nerve is not involved, a preservation of the nerve is possible if radiotherapy follows. If the facial nerve shows involvement by facial muscle paresis or by direct observation at surgery, excision of a section of the nerve and nerve grafting, followed by radiotherapy, are usually required.

For those lesions discovered unexpectedly when a submandibular gland is removed because of sialadenitis or sialolithiasis, further surgery to accomplish a supraomohyoid neck dissection, in which the lingual nerve and portions of the hyoglossus and mylohyoid muscle are also removed, is recommended. Postsurgical radiotherapy also is recommended.

For lesions in the tongue, there is a greater reliance on radiotherapy. Usually, a local excision of accessible tumor is followed by high-dose radiotherapy (7,000 cGy to 8,000 cGy). This is because of the morbidity and near unresectability of what are mostly base-of-tongue locations.

PROGNOSIS ▶ Adenoid cystic carcinomas have a well-known prognosis profile. The 5-year survival rate is 75%, but the 10-year survival rate is only 20%, and survival at 15 years is about 10%. However, this tumor, which was once thought to be radioresistant, has been shown to be at least somewhat radiosensitive. Postoperative radiotherapy, combined with more aggressive surgeries, is showing signs of increasing long-term survivals into the 30% to 40% range.

Adenoid cystic carcinoma rarely metastasizes to lymph nodes, and then only late in the course of recurrent or uncontrolled disease. Failure occurs with local recurrence that extends proximally into the retro-orbital tissue and/or into the brain or with distant metastasis into the lungs via blood-borne routes (Fig 12-38). In the lungs, metastatic foci will appear as round, soft tissue densities called *cannonball* or *cotton ball* lesions (Fig 12-39). These, like the original primary tumor, are slow growing, and patients may live many years after their appearance.

The overall prognosis relates to several factors. Histologically, solid patterns bode worse than cribriform patterns. Clinical size greater than 4 cm indicates an even greater subclinical spread and, therefore, is associated with a worse prognosis. Delayed diagnosis and/or delayed treatment also worsens the prognosis. Surgical margins that are not clear or are "close" despite postoperative radiotherapy are also associated with a worse prognosis; this is the single most important factor associated with local recurrence.

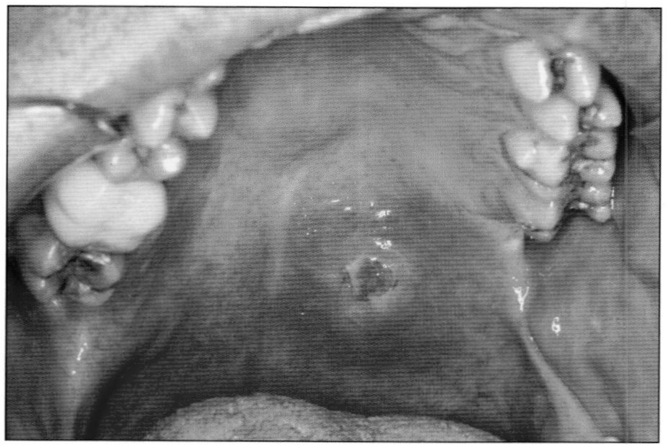

Fig 12-40a Like many other salivary gland tumors, a polymorphous low-grade adenocarcinoma usually presents as a firm, nontender mass at the junction of the hard and soft palates. The surface may or may not be ulcerated. (Courtesy of Dr Eric Carlson.)

Polymorphous Low-Grade Adenocarcinoma

CLINICAL PRESENTATION ►

The polymorphous low-grade adenocarcinoma is a malignancy associated with slow growth, a small size (usually less than 4 cm), and almost no metastatic potential. It arises from the oral mucosal minor salivary glands and does not occur as a primary tumor in any of the major salivary glands. The palate is the preferred site (Fig 12-40a), where about 65% of tumors occur, followed by the buccal mucosa (13%) and upper lip (10%). Like most mucosal salivary gland tumors, it will present as a firm, painless mass and will only rarely develop surface ulceration. The tumor has a female sex predilection, and it occurs in patients 50 years or older. This tumor, like the adenoid cystic carcinoma, will occasionally develop in the base of the tongue.

DIFFERENTIAL DIAGNOSIS ►

Because it typically presents as a slow-growing palatal mass with an intact surface, the tumor is most consistent with a *pleomorphic adenoma*. Otherwise, *adenoid cystic carcinoma*, *low-grade mucoepidermoid carcinoma*, or *canalicular adenoma* (especially if the site is the upper lip) should be considered.

DIAGNOSTIC WORK-UP ►

The mass should undergo incisional biopsy deep in the lesion's center. A sufficient specimen should be taken to enable viewing of several sections. Histologically, this tumor may resemble adenoid cystic carcinoma, particularly because both show perineural invasion. Several sections may need to be reviewed to distinguish them because the extent of the surgical excision required differs greatly between the two. In addition, a CT scan or an MRI scan is recommended to ascertain the size and extent of the tumor. If evidence of palatal or other bony invasion is present, it may suggest another diagnosis, because this finding would be rare for a polymorphous low-grade adenocarcinoma. A reassessment of the histopathologic features would be in order.

HISTOPATHOLOGY ►

These unencapsulated tumors often appear circumscribed but demonstrate infiltration (Figs 12-40b and 12-40c). Cytologically they are uniform, but morphologically they are diverse. The tumor cells typically have bland, pale nuclei with scant, ill-defined cytoplasm (Fig 12-40d). Occasionally, the nuclei are more hyperchromatic. Mitoses are rare. The stroma may be fibrous, myxoid, or hyalinized. The growth pattern may vary considerably from tumor to tumor or within the same tumor. Solid nests, strands, ducts, cysts, concentric whorls, and cribriform patterns may all be seen (Figs 12-40e to 12-40g), but concentric whorls or a targetoid pattern is characteristic of this tumor because of the perineural arrangement of the cells (Fig 12-40h). In a given section, the nerve may not always be apparent (Fig 12-40i). Single-file arrangement is common, occurring most often at the periphery (Fig 12-40j). The tumor may demonstrate an alarming degree of infiltration with invasion of small nerves, vessel walls, surface epithelium, and bone, which belies its low-grade behavior. Necrosis is not seen. Pseudoepitheliomatous hyperplasia may occur in the overlying epithelium. The particular histologic pattern of the tumor does not appear to relate to behavior.

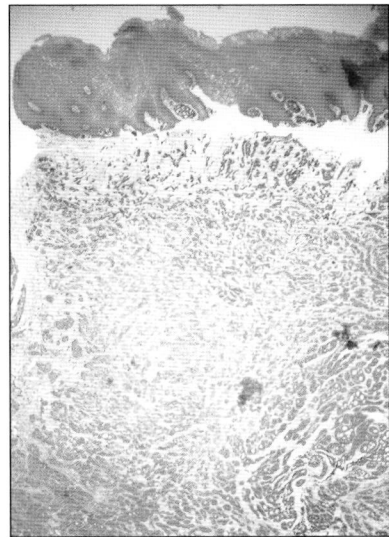

Fig 12-40b Polymorphous low-grade adenocarcinoma showing infiltration up to the surface epithelium and no encapsulation.

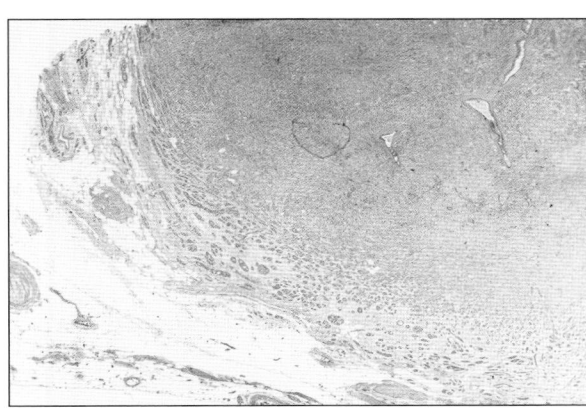

Fig 12-40c Polymorphous adenocarcinoma showing tumor islands that are infiltrative, which is particularly apparent within the fat.

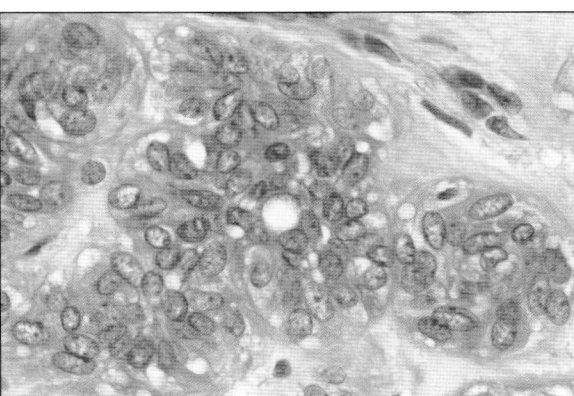

Fig 12-40d Polymorphous low-grade adenocarcinoma showing cells uniform in appearance with bland nuclei.

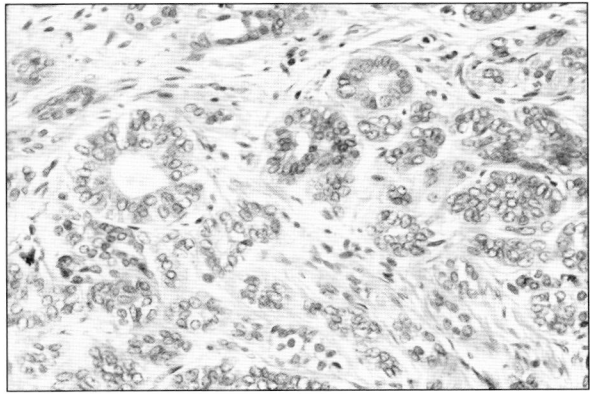

Fig 12-40e The uniform cells of polymorphous low-grade adenocarcinomas forming ductal arrangements.

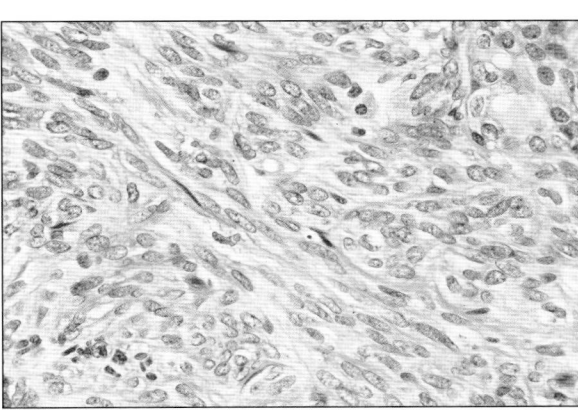

Fig 12-40f An area of haphazardly arranged cells in the polymorphous low-grade adenocarcinoma.

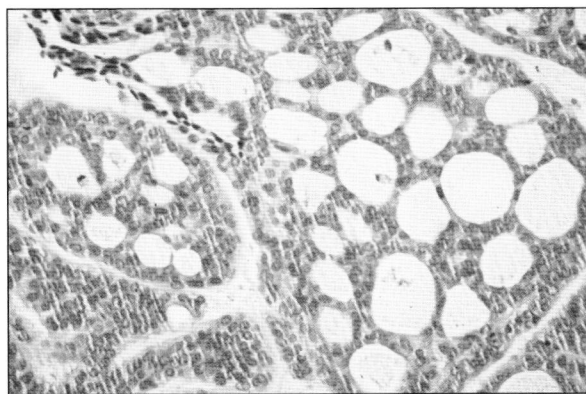

Fig 12-40g Areas showing a cribriform pattern in a polymorphous low-grade adenocarcinoma.

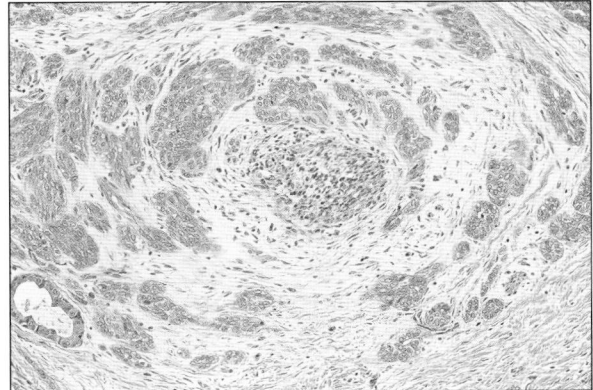

Fig 12-40h Polymorphous low-grade adenocarcinoma showing the characteristic whorled arrangement of tumor cells.

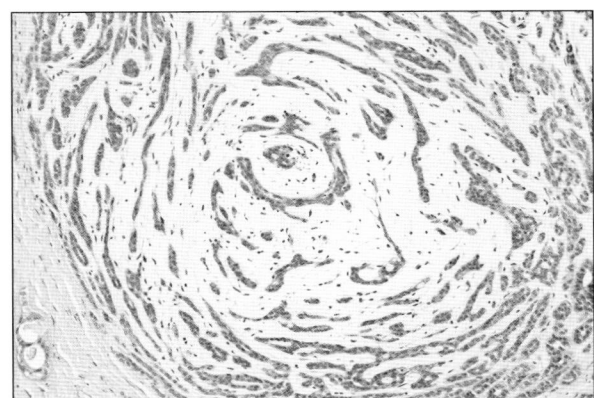

Fig 12-40i The whorled or targetoid arrangement of a polymorphous low-grade adenocarcinoma showing no apparent nerve.

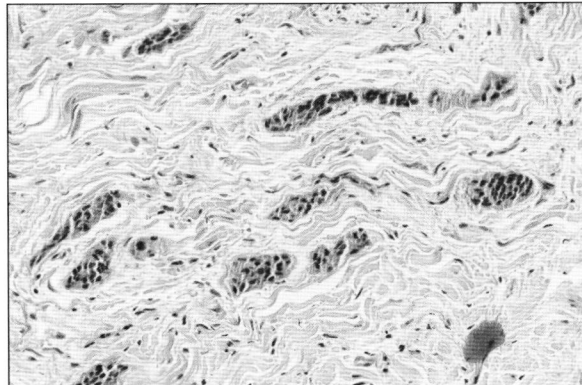

Fig 12-40j A single-file arrangement of tumor cells seen at the periphery of a polymorphous low-grade adenocarcinoma.

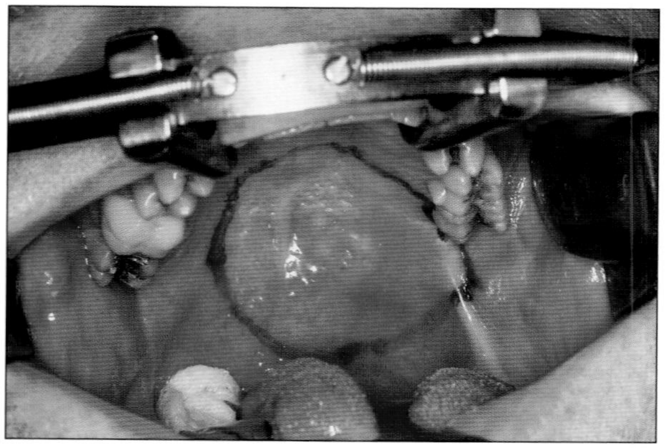

Fig 12-40k A palatectomy excision is outlined with 1.5-cm peripheral margins. A Dingman-Dot (Walter Lorenz) mouth prop device, as seen here, will facilitate access. (Courtesy of Dr Eric Carlson.)

Before the recognition of this entity, most of these tumors had been diagnosed as pleomorphic adenomas or adenoid cystic carcinomas. Pleomorphic adenomas, however, do not show this type of infiltration or invasion. There may be more difficulty with adenoid cystic carcinoma, but usually the cells of this tumor are more hyperchromatic. Probably the most striking feature of the polymorphous low-grade adenocarcinoma is that at one level it demonstrates aggressiveness by its ability to invade, yet cytologically it appears to be bland and innocuous.

TREATMENT ▶

Despite this tumor's perineural invasion and lack of a capsule, it is treated with either a soft tissue excision with 1.5-cm peripheral margins assessed by frozen sections or a palatectomy if located on the palate (Fig 12-40k). The palatal bone may not require excision unless radiographic or observational evidence indicates its involvement. Radiotherapy is not required.

PROGNOSIS ▶

Recurrences are rare and parallel the incidence observed with pleomorphic adenoma or low-grade mucoepidermoid carcinoma. The few long-term follow-up reports available suggest a 10-year survival rate of over 80%.

The good prognosis and lack of recurrence seen with this tumor are not what would be expected based on its histologic invasiveness and prominent perineural invasiveness. This is probably because of its slow growth and slow rate of invasion. Additionally, perineural invasion is not associated with a poorer prognosis unless accompanied by perineural spread, which apparently does not occur with this tumor. Perineural spread is, however, part of the biologic behavior spectrum of adenoid cystic carcinoma.

Acinic Cell Carcinoma

CLINICAL PRESENTATION AND PATHOGENESIS ▶

Acinic cell carcinomas are uncommon low-grade adenocarcinomas, of which 99% are found in the superficial parotid lobe. Accounting for about 2% to 4% of all parotid tumors, they will usually present as a painful mass within the parotid gland; this is unusual for both benign and malignant salivary gland tumors. Another unusual aspect of the acinic cell carcinoma is that 3% are found bilaterally, which means that it ranks second only to Warthin tumors (papillary cystadenoma lymphomatosum) in bilateral occurrence. The masses are characteristically small and usually freely movable. They have been reported in children but are otherwise usually found in adults. There is a slight increased incidence in women. Despite their malignant nature, they are not noted to induce facial muscle paresis and are slow-growing tumors that are often present for up to 5 years before the patient seeks medical attention.

Acinic cell carcinomas may arise from direct neoplastic transformation of parotid acinar cells, but it is more likely that such mature and differentiated cells do not undergo dedifferentiation. Instead, it is suspected that these tumors arise from reserve cells at the most proximal end of the intercalated duct and partially differentiate to develop acinar cell cytomorphologic features.

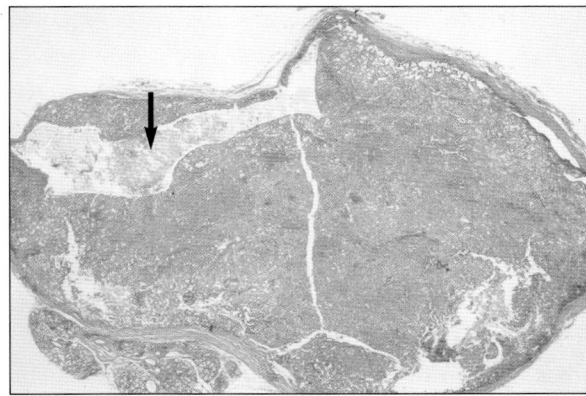

Fig 12-41a An acinic cell adenocarcinoma of the upper lip showing a mass with a thin capsule. An area of necrosis *(arrow)* can be seen.

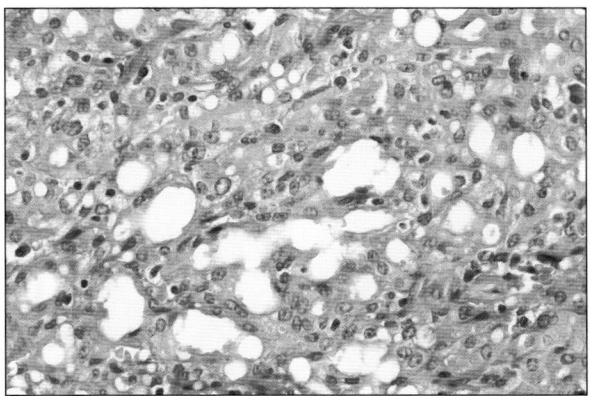

Fig 12-41b The microcystic pattern in an acinic cell adenocarcinoma in a background of glandular cells.

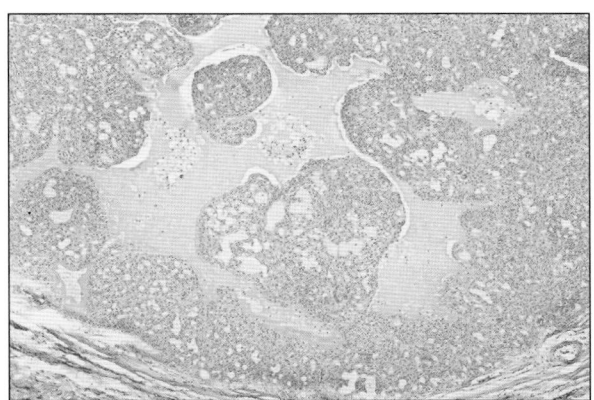

Fig 12-41c A papillary cystic pattern of an acinic cell adenocarcinoma.

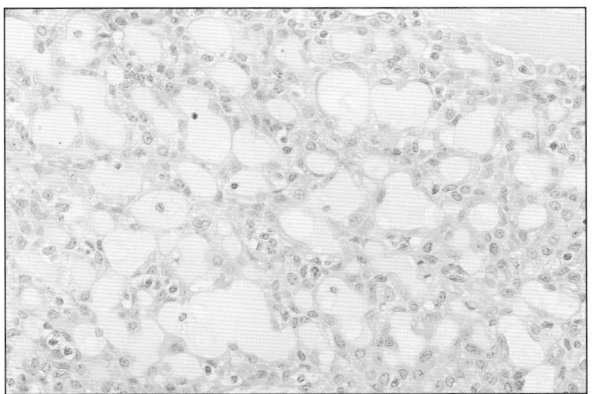

Fig 12-41d The follicular pattern of an acinic cell adenocarcinoma with eosinophilic material in the lumina.

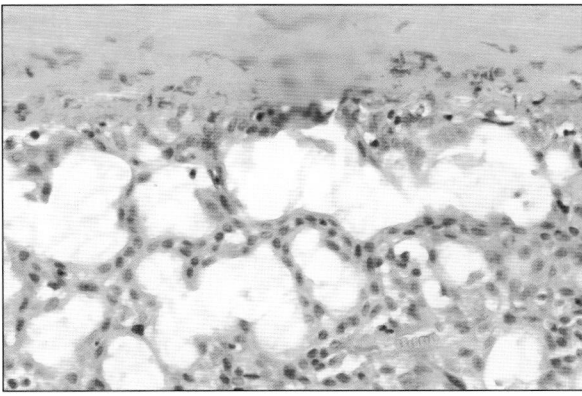

Fig 12-41e Intercalated duct-type cells in an acinic cell adenocarcinoma.

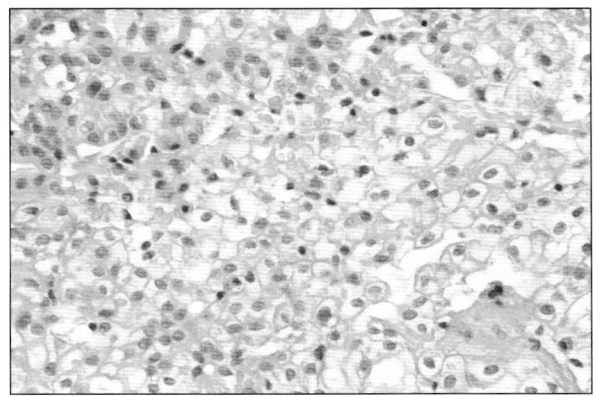

Fig 12-41f Acinic cells and some clear cells in an acinic cell adenocarcinoma.

DIFFERENTIAL DIAGNOSIS ▶

The solitary mass's location in the superficial lobe of the parotid gland without clinical signs of malignancy suggests the more common benign parotid tumors, *pleomorphic adenoma*, *Warthin tumor* (papillary cystadenoma lymphomatosum), and *basal cell adenoma*. Its presentation is also consistent with some *adenoid cystic carcinomas, mucoepidermoid carcinomas*, and lymph node enlargements within the parotid gland, such as *lymphoma, HIV-related lymphadenopathy*, and *tuberculosis-related lymphadenitis*.

DIAGNOSTIC WORK-UP AND TREATMENT ▶

With a mass in the parotid gland, the primary diagnostic work-up and definitive treatment is a superficial parotidectomy without regional neck dissection. However, a fine-needle aspiration cytologic study is recommended first to rule out other malignancies. A CT scan or an MRI scan is also useful to assess the tumor's location in the gland and its proximity to the facial nerve.

HISTOPATHOLOGY ▶

Acinic cell carcinomas are often well circumscribed and may show some encapsulation, particularly when they arise in minor salivary glands (Fig 12-41a). Occasionally they are multinodular. A variety of patterns may be seen, including a solid pattern within which organoid areas formed by intervening fibrovascular trabeculae may be visible. A microcystic pattern is characteristic and probably results from coalescence of intracellular vacuoles or ruptured cells. Papillary-cystic and follicular patterns are less common (Figs 12-41b to 12-41d). The latter can resemble a thyroid carcinoma with a central eosinophilic coagulum and a cuboidal epithelial lining. These varying patterns may coexist in the same tumor.

Morphologically, there are several cell types. Acinar cells are rounded or polygonal and have deeply staining, uniform, eccentric nuclei and a variable number of PAS-positive cytoplasmic granules. Intercalated duct-like cells are smaller and cuboidal with centrally placed nuclei and eosinophilic cytoplasm. They often line ductal spaces. Vacuolated cells have an eccentric nucleus. The nonspecific glandular cells tend to form a syncytium and lack the features of the other cells. Atypia may be present, but mitoses are infrequent and are usually found in glandular cells (Figs 12-41e and 12-41f; see also Fig 12-41b).

The stroma is usually fibrovascular but may be hyalinized. On occasion, there may be considerable vascularity. A striking feature is the frequent presence of a lymphoid infiltrate, which can be quite prominent and contain germinal centers.

Despite the circumscription, histologic evidence of infiltration is often seen. There does not appear to be a correlation between behavior and pattern or cell type. However, multinodularity, hyalinization, and infiltration are often seen in recurrent and metastasizing tumors.

PROGNOSIS ▶ Typical of low-grade carcinomas, acinic cell carcinomas tend to recur locally but seldom metastasize. Recurrences may not appear for 5 to 10 years. Five-year survival rates are about 75%, 10-year survival rates are about 60%, and 15-year survival rates are about 50%.

Carcinoma Ex Pleomorphic Adenoma and Malignant Pleomorphic Adenoma

CLINICAL PRESENTATION AND PATHOGENESIS ▶ There is a confusing set of terms involving these rare entities. The most common, most straightforward, and most important of these is *carcinoma ex pleomorphic adenoma*. This term denotes a malignant transformation of a benign pleomorphic adenoma. Only one cell component becomes malignant, usually the epithelial component, but it can form any one of several types of malignancies. Such malignant transformations are time- and size-dependent. The average age of occurrence is in the 60s, which is 20 years older than the average age for those with a benign pleomorphic adenoma. It will present in a large, long-standing pleomorphic adenoma or in one that was previously treated but has recurred (Fig 12-42a). The transformation of a large, untreated pleomorphic adenoma is clinically suggested if the mass is not uniform and singular, if it is fluctuant in parts (tumor necrosis), if it is fixed to other tissues, or if it is ulcerated (see Figs 12-15 and 12-16).

Another malignant tumor has been termed *malignant pleomorphic adenoma*. This primary malignant tumor has both epithelial and mesenchymal components that are malignant. It is sometimes called a *carcinosarcoma*. It will grow rapidly and metastasize quickly like a high-grade malignancy. Its true diagnosis is discovered only on histopathologic examination. Yet a third malignant pleomorphic adenoma has been described. It is a histologically benign pleomorphic adenoma called the *metastasizing pleomorphic adenoma*. It undergoes metastasis, where the metastatic deposits remain histologically benign pleomorphic adenoma.

The carcinoma ex pleomorphic adenoma occurs in 20% to 25% of untreated benign pleomorphic adenomas and accounts for up to 10% of all malignant salivary gland tumors. Therefore, it occurs frequently enough to warrant early and definitive surgery for all benign pleomorphic adenomas and should be a consideration in any long-standing mass involving salivary gland tissue. Most (75%) occur in the parotid gland, while about 20% occur in the minor glands of the oral mucosa.

Malignant pleomorphic adenomas, carcinosarcomas, and the metastasizing pleomorphic adenoma are too rare to enable much understanding about their sites of occurrence.

Spontaneous or induced malignant transformation of a single cell line in a benign tumor is noted in only a few other lesions: neurofibroma to neurosarcoma, especially that seen in hereditary neurofibromatosis; Paget disease to osteosarcoma; and radiation sarcomas arising from irradiated fibro-osseous disease. The carcinoma ex pleomorphic adenoma transformation is more common than any other. It is suggested that the already altered genome within the cells of a benign pleomorphic adenoma develops further alterations within one cell that express new oncogenes. These oncogenes add the properties of

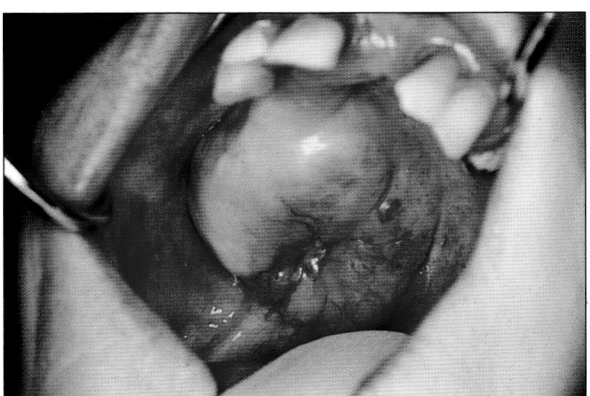

Fig 12-42a This large palatal pleomorphic adenoma developed into a carcinoma ex pleomorphic adenoma, as evidenced by its surface ulceration. It had been present for 18 years.

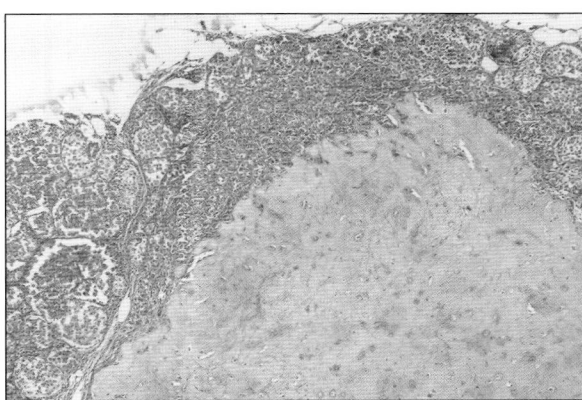

Fig 12-42b An area of myxochondroid tissue representing a pleomorphic adenoma surrounded by a poorly differentiated, cellular epithelial component in this carcinoma ex pleomorphic adenoma.

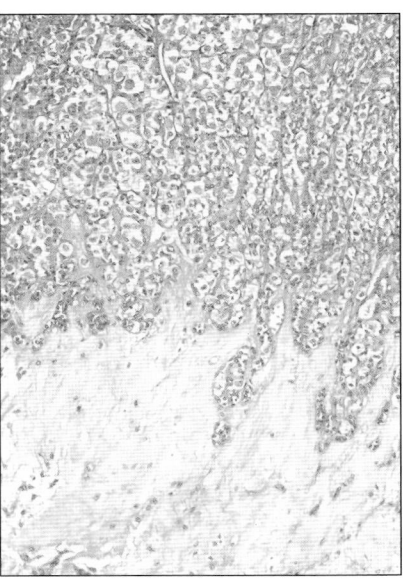

Fig 12-42c A higher-power view of Fig 12-42b showing the malignant cellular component and some of the myxochondroid tissue.

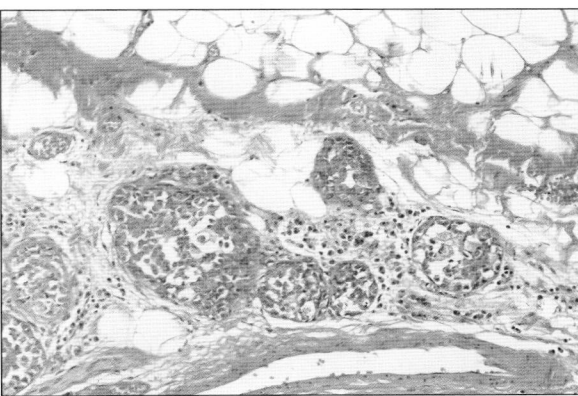

Fig 12-42d The same neoplasm as shown in Figs 12-42b and 12-42c demonstrating infiltration into fat.

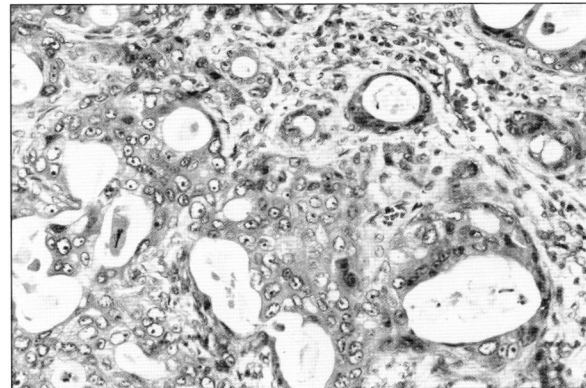

Fig 12-42e A carcinoma ex pleomorphic adenoma showing hyperchromatism and pleomorphism.

faster growth, greater tissue infiltration, invasion of bone (perhaps by the elaboration of osteoclast-activating factor), and metastasis—that is, the properties of a malignant tumor.

DIAGNOSTIC WORK-UP ▶

A differential diagnosis is not germane to a carcinoma ex pleomorphic adenoma because of its origin in a pre-existing pleomorphic adenoma. Clinically, the tumor will show evidence of malignancy of a type that can be confirmed by an incisional biopsy. Before definitive therapy, a CT scan or an MRI scan is performed to assess the size and extension of the primary tumor. A chest radiograph is required to assess potential lung metastasis.

HISTOPATHOLOGY ▶

The feature that these tumors have in common is the presence of some residual benign pleomorphic adenoma (Fig 12-42b). The malignant component can be quite variable. Most frequently, they are poorly differentiated adenocarcinomas or undifferentiated carcinomas. Less often the malignant component may be another specific salivary gland neoplasm, such as acinic cell carcinoma or adenoid cystic carcinoma. The overall features associated with these neoplasms are infiltration and cellular atypia, including an increase in nuclear/cytoplasmic ratio and mitoses (Figs 12-42c to 12-42e). Necrosis and calcifications may be present. There may also be an abundant, hyalinized stroma. Because these tumors typically develop from a focus within the benign tumor, careful inspection of the entire specimen is necessary. Carcinoma ex pleomorphic adenomas are to be distinguished from metastasizing pleomorphic adenomas, which are histologically benign, and from carcinosarcomas, in which there are both epithelial and mesenchymal malignant components.

TREATMENT ▶ Invasive carcinomas that begin in a pleomorphic adenoma and primary malignant pleomorphic adenomas are both highly aggressive malignancies that readily metastasize. Each is ideally treated with an extensive resection of 3- to 5-cm margins, a neck dissection, and postoperative radiotherapy in the dose range of 6,000 cGy to 7,500 cGy. In the parotid gland, the surgery would be a total parotidectomy.

PROGNOSIS ▶ The recurrence rate of this tumor is about 60%. The metastasis rate to regional lymph nodes is about 25%, and to distant organs (such as a lung) about 33%. Therefore, the prognosis is poor despite aggressive therapy. The 5-year survival rates are 40%, 10-year survival rates are 24%, and 15-year survival rates are 17%.

Transoral Minor Salivary Gland Tumor Surgery

Soft Tissue Palatal Excision

INDICATIONS ▶ Benign and low-grade malignant tumors of the palatal mucosa such as pleomorphic adenomas and low-grade mucoepidermoid carcinoma require a soft tissue excision with documented clear margins.

PROCEDURE ▶ The tumor is excised with a 1-cm margin of clinically uninvolved tissue around its periphery to and including the palatal periosteum. The specimen is delivered by reflecting palatal periosteum from the anterior to posterior aspect (Fig 12-43a). As the tumor becomes pedicled off the greater palatine vessels, the vessels are double clamped and incised between each clamp (Fig 12-43b). The proximal vessels are ligated or cauterized, and the reflection of palatal periosteum is continued posteriorly. If the tumor extends into the soft palate mucosa, the periosteal plane of dissection is continued onto the subfascial plane of the soft palate musculature. This dissection is continued for 1 cm posterior to the clinical tumor. It will preserve the integrity of the soft palate unless tumor extension requires extending the excision into the nasal cavity. The specimen is then oriented with a clock-face orientation (Fig 12-43c), the anterior edge representing 12 o'clock and the posterior edge 6 o'clock. Each division in between can then be precisely referenced to the wound to pinpoint a close or tumor-positive margin.

In this dissection, the periosteum serves as an effective anatomic barrier so that the palatal bone does not require excision, burring, or scraping, even if a "cupped out" pressure resorption has taken place.

The exposed palatal bone will granulate completely in 3 to 6 weeks (Figs 12-43d and 12-43e). At the time of surgery, a palatal splint lined with a soft denture liner or placed over a packing material of iodoform gauze lightly sprayed with benzoin and coated with bacitracin ointment is very useful. The benzoin provides a medicinal taste and reduces the odor of decaying fibrin and blood over the 10 to 14 days the splint is in place. The bacitracin is an excellent bacteriocidal lubricant, reducing bacterial colonization and preventing the gauze from adhering to the wound.

Palatectomy

INDICATIONS ▶ A palatectomy is indicated in the treatment of low-grade and some intermediate-grade malignant tumors. The polymorphous low-grade adenocarcinoma in particular will exhibit perineural invasion but not perineural spread and will otherwise show infiltrative behavior. Therefore, when located on the palate, this tumor is often removed by palatectomy rather than soft tissue palatal excision.

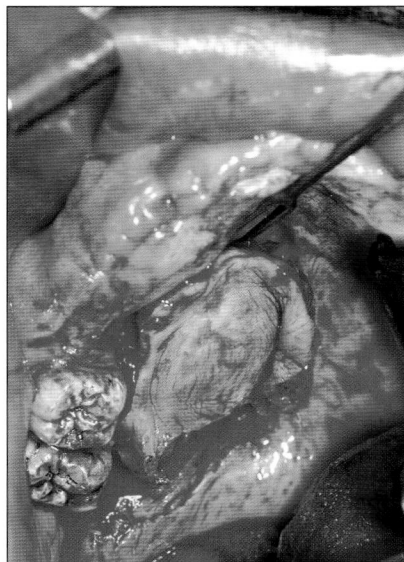

Fig 12-43a Benign and low-grade malignant tumors are excised with clinical margins of 1.0 to 1.5 cm, including the full thickness of palatal mucosa and periosteum.

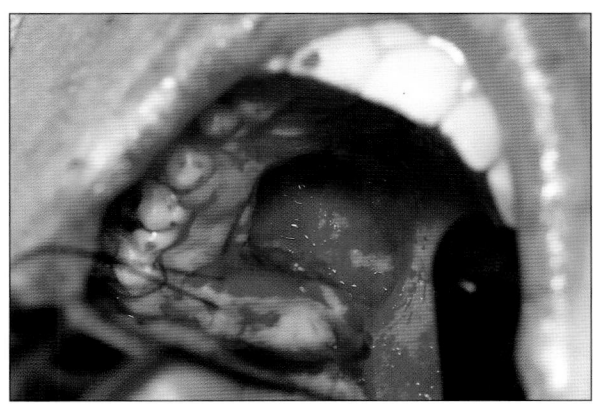

Fig 12-43b Palatal mass excisions are best approached anterior to posterior. The greater palatine vessels can be clamped and either ligated or cauterized under direct vision.

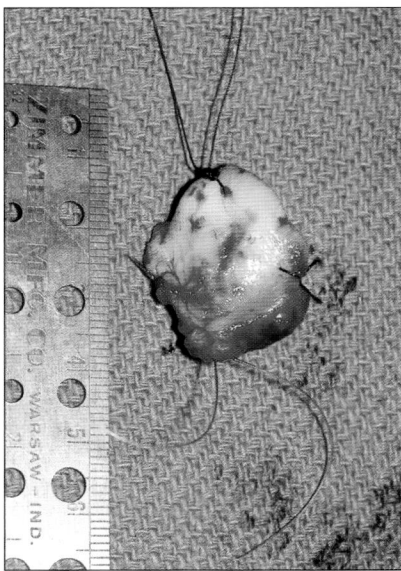

Fig 12-43c Excised specimens should be sent for frozen sections with the edges marked by sutures, preferably using a clock-face orientation (ie, 3 o'clock, 6 o'clock, 9 o'clock, etc).

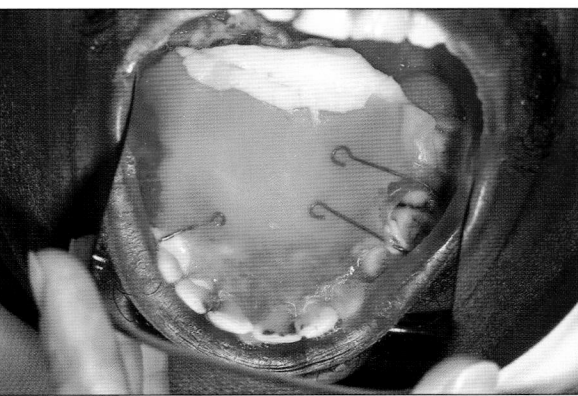

Fig 12-43d A palatal acrylic splint will protect the wound and increase the patient's comfort. It may be retained with single clasps, wires, or screws and is removed after approximately 2 weeks.

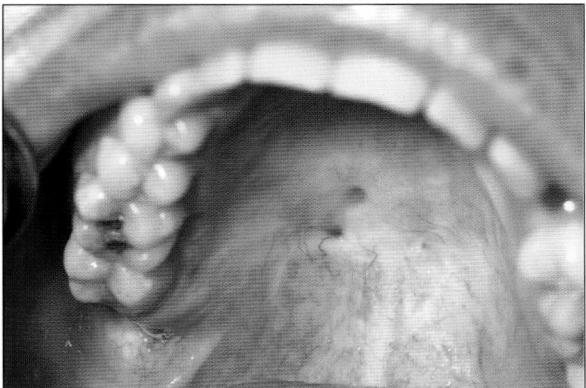

Fig 12-43e Palatal wounds will granulate over exposed palatal bone and completely epithelialize.

PROCEDURE ▶

These tumors are excised with 1.5- to 2.0-cm clinical margins (Fig 12-44a). The incision is made to the palatal periosteum, which is then reflected from the native bone for a short distance rather than from the tumor-bearing specimen. A reciprocating saw is then used to follow the soft tissue peripheral incision. In fact, the saw tip needs to protrude into both the nasal cavity and the maxillary sinus. The specimen is then down-fractured as in a Le Fort I surgery so that the greater palatine neurovascular bundle can be accessed. This neurovascular bundle is clamped as superiorly as possible and transsected on the tumor side of the clamp. The parent vessels are then ligated or cauterized after the tumor specimen is delivered.

The composite soft tissue–bony palate specimen is marked with the same clock-face orientation for frozen section analysis (Fig 12-44b). The resultant wound, an oral-antral-nasal communication, is managed with a similar oral palatal splint as is recommended for a soft tissue palatal excision (Figs 12-44c and 12-44d).

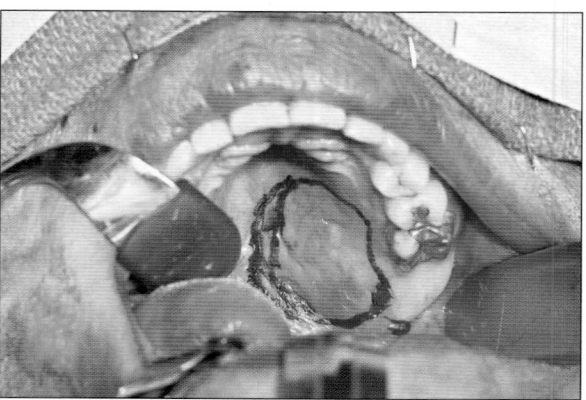

Fig 12-44a A palatectomy is performed only for malignant tumors and usually for low- to intermediate-grade tumors. The alveolar bone and teeth are preserved.

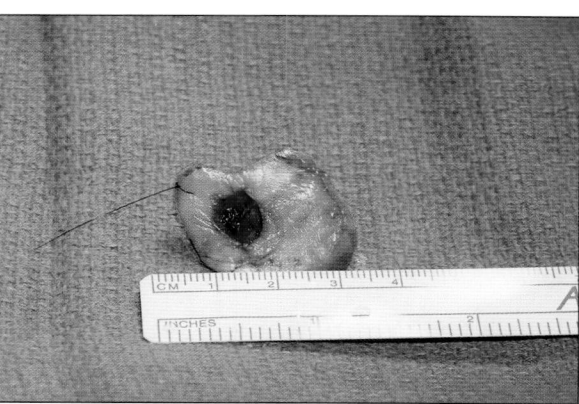

Fig 12-44b A palatectomy specimen also should be sent for frozen sections to assess the soft tissue margins. The bone edges can also be assessed during surgery using a touch preparation for cytology (see Chapter 1).

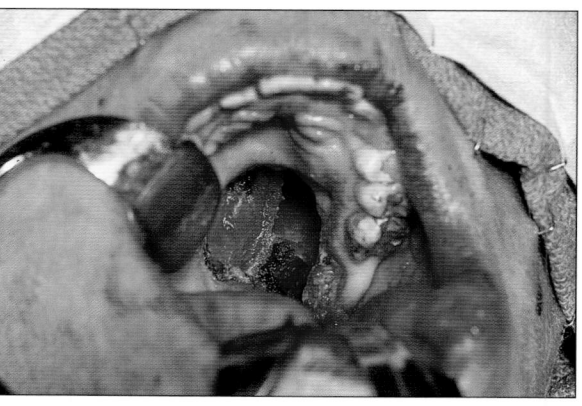

Fig 12-44c The palatectomy defect will naturally communicate into the nose and maxillary sinus.

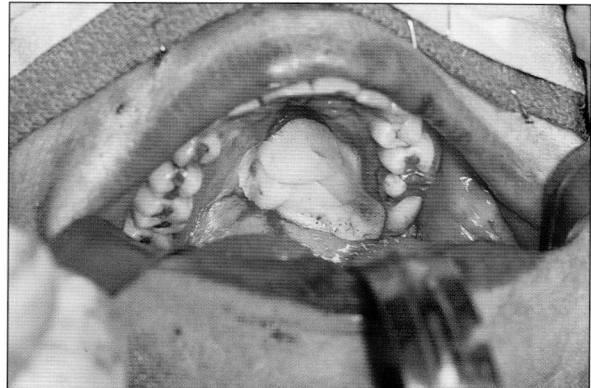

Fig 12-44d The palatectomy defect also is covered and "obturated" with an oral splint to prevent hypernasal speech and to protect the wound.

The splint can be fixated with premade clasps if the individual is dentate. Otherwise, palatal screw fixation, zygoma drop wires, or circumzygomatic wires can be used. This larger defect also is managed with a soft tissue liner or a lubricated packing material.

Hemimaxillectomy

INDICATIONS ▶ A hemimaxillectomy is indicated in the treatment of malignant tumors of the palatal mucosa. Tumors such as intermediate and high-grade mucoepidermoid carcinomas, adenoid cystic carcinoma, and most squamous cell carcinomas of the palate and similar tumors generally require this procedure.

PROCEDURE ▶ The term for this procedure, transoral "hemimaxillectomy," is a small misnomer because the maxilla is not transsected at the midline or between the maxillary incisor teeth. The maxilla is resected, including its overlying mucosa, through an alveolar area other than that of a central incisor 2 to 3 cm from the clinical tumor margin (Fig 12-45a). A periphery of 1.5 to 3.0 cm of mucosa and bone is excised around the lesion. Soft tissue incisions are made to the level of bone. Periosteum attached to bone that is not part of the tumor is reflected to enable use of a reciprocating saw. The maxilla is separated from the pterygoid plates, the nasal septum, and the lateral nasal wall as in a Le Fort I osteotomy. As the tumor is pedicled from the greater palatine vessels above, it is transsected through the neurovascular bundle at

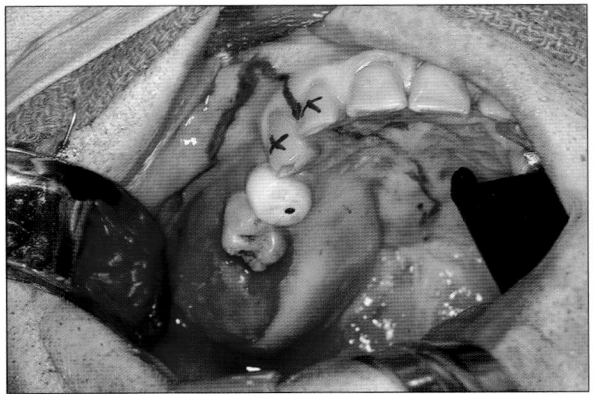

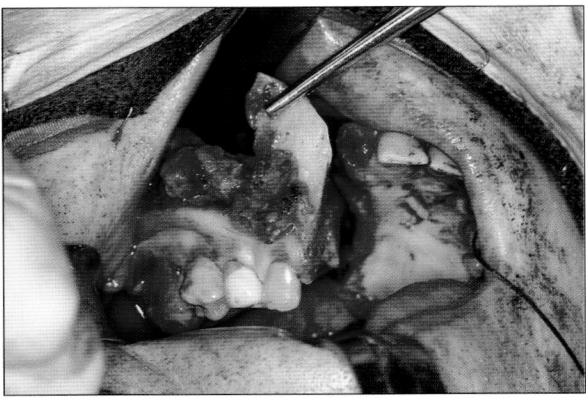

Fig 12-45a A transoral hemimaxillectomy includes bone, teeth, and mucosa. The anterior resection will proceed through a tooth socket to provide an appropriate margin and edge for a prospective prosthesis.

Fig 12-45b This hemimaxillectomy specimen proceeded through the lateral incisor socket, the left paramidline palate, and the pterygoid plates. The specimen is delivered as an en-bloc unit.

the foramen rotundrum (Fig 12-45b). The tumor's margins are marked with sutures for orientation, and each margin, particularly the neurovascular bundle, is checked for tumor by frozen sections. The patient's existing denture or a premade acrylic splint is then lined with a resilient material and fixated with wires or screws. The surgical splint is removed after 2 weeks, cleaned, relined, and modified into a removable provisional prosthesis.

Occasionally an external approach of the Weber-Ferguson type is needed to remove a salivary gland tumor in the maxilla or in the maxillary sinus. The tumor type (benign versus malignant) does not influence the choice of approach so much as does the tumor location, regardless of its histopathology. The standard findings that recommend serious consideration for a Weber-Ferguson approach are (*1*) tumor invading the orbit; (*2*) tumor invading the ethmoid bone or sinus; or (*3*) tumor extending into the retromaxillary or pterygomaxillary space. In these situations the added access gained via the Weber-Ferguson approach permits a more assured complete removal of the tumor than could be gained from a transoral approach.

The Weber-Ferguson incision is a lip-split incisional approach. The incision begins in a convenient crease beneath the lower eyelid with a lateral crow's foot extension. It is extended to the nasomaxillary area medially, where a rounded turn is made. The incision then courses inferiorly paralleling the curvature of the nose and alar crease while staying 1 to 2 mm lateral to the alar crease (an incision placed in the alar crease will produce an inward retraction of the alar crease, resulting in significant asymmetry). The incision continues around the alar crease subnasally to the ipsilateral philtrum. It then courses inferiorly through the crest of the philtrum to the uppermost edge of cupid's bow of the upper lip. The incision then follows the vermilion-skin line to the midline, where the lip is split through the vermilion. The incision turns in the subnasal-philtrum–cupid's bow–midline of the lip are all at 90 degrees. The resultant Z-shaped lip split acts as Z-plasties do elsewhere to break up the line of scar retraction and will thus work to prevent a snarl-like retraction of the upper lip (Fig 12-46a).

The oral areas of the Weber-Ferguson incision will either correspond to the location of the skin incision or be dictated by the margin gained around the tumor (Fig 12-46b). The result should be a posteriorly based hemifacial flap that can provide direct access to the tumor and then be repositioned over an obturator splint to regain facial contours (Figs 12-46c, 12-47a, and 12-47b).

The wound is obturated with a palatal obturator splint with soft liner or packing of the defect as described for a soft tissue palatal excision. The obturator splint may require screw fixation or wire suspension to maintain its position for the 7 to 10 days it is in place (Figs 12-47c and 12-47d).

Hemimaxillectomies that include the orbital floor and preserve the globe will result in enophthalmos and significant diplopia if not prevented by some type of immediate reconstruction. The surgical obtura-

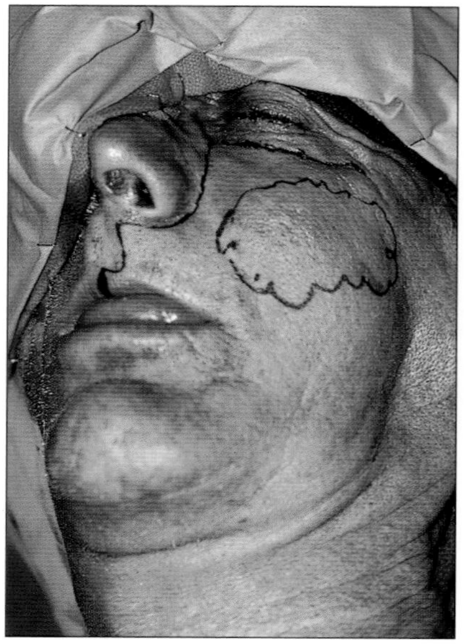

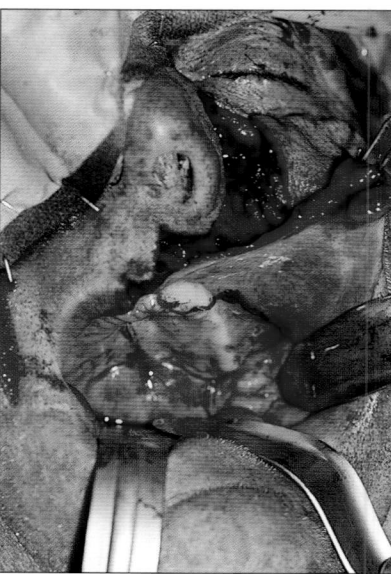

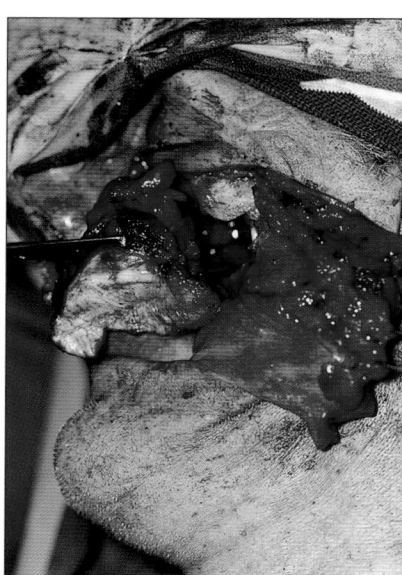

Fig 12-46a Weber-Ferguson incision outlined with a stepped lip-split design, which will prevent an upward lip retraction once healed. This approach was required to access an adenoid cystic carcinoma that had invaded the orbital floor.

Fig 12-46b The Weber-Ferguson access is carried orally through the stepped lip-split incision and continues with a vestibular incision.

Fig 12-46c The Weber-Ferguson approach is a posterior-based cheek flap that provides wide access. Here the tumor is being removed en-bloc with the orbital floor.

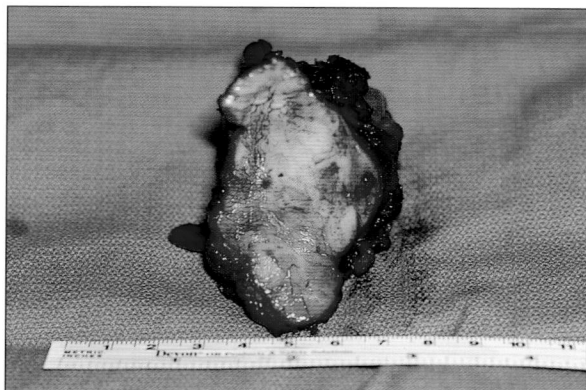

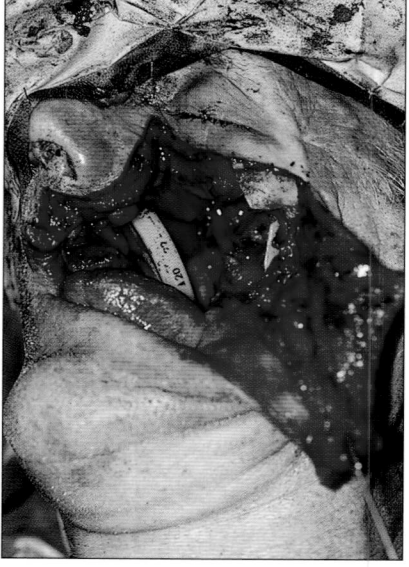

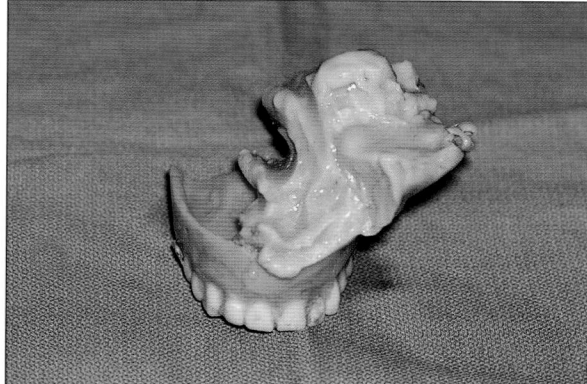

Fig 12-47a Excision of this adenoid cystic carcinoma included not only the orbital floor, but also the pterygoid plates and soft palate of the involved side, which is indicative of the infiltration and perineural spread of this tumor.

Fig 12-47b Excisions of large tumors will leave a large dead space and unsupported structures. The left eye and cheek have lost their support.

Fig 12-47c The surgical obturator splint or modified denture will require significant relining and buildup to support the cheek flap and to obturate the oral-antral-nasal communication.

tor splint cannot be expected to support the globe. A more straightforward approach is to use the temporalis tendon–muscle complex to position and support the eye. The surgical defect itself provides access to the coronoid process of the mandible and the temporalis tendons via either a Weber-Ferguson or even a transoral approach. The temporalis muscle's tendonous attachment to the mandible is reflected so that it can be medially rotated toward the medial canthus and nasal bone areas (Fig 12-47e). In doing

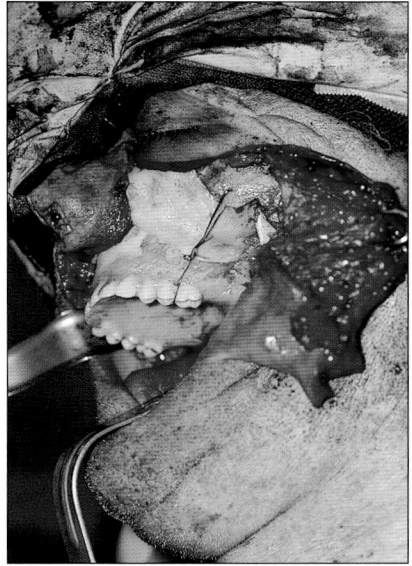

Fig 12-47d In large defects, surgical obturator splints will have little native tissue remaining for retention and will have added weight from the relining material. Therefore, they will require either direct screw fixation or suspension wire fixation, as shown here.

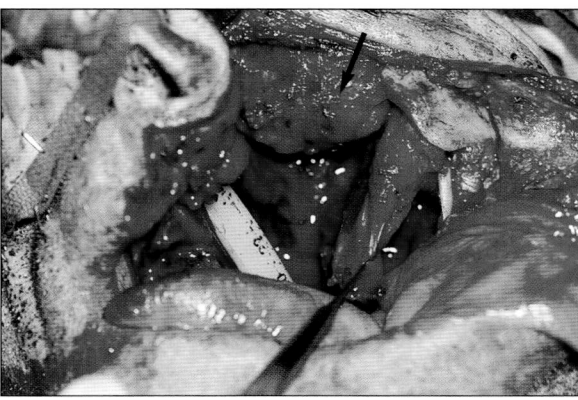

Fig 12-47e To prevent enophthalmos when the orbital floor is removed, the temporalis tendon is detached and rotated medially to uplift and suspend the globe from beneath. The tendon is sutured to the nasal bone through a bur hole once the position matching the unaffected eye is attained. In this view, the globe (*arrow*) has prolapsed into the defect. The temporalis muscle has been detached to develop the flap.

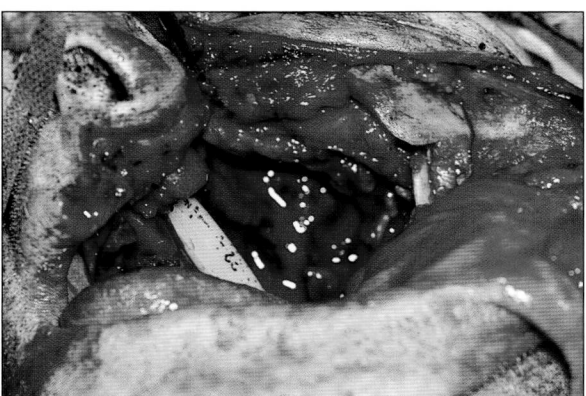

Fig 12-47f The temporalis tendon is sutured to the nasal bones. The eye is now suspended and supported by the temporalis muscle.

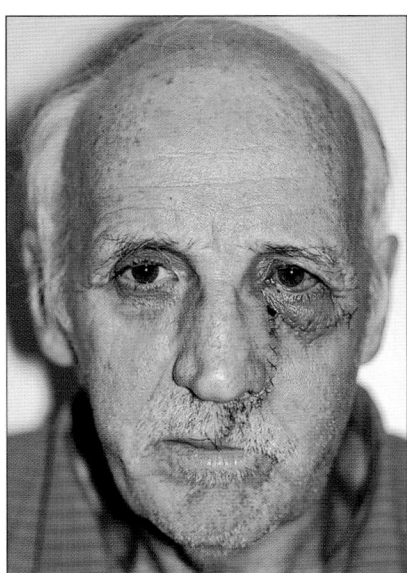

Fig 12-47g Early postoperative view of the position of the involved eye to match that of the uninvolved eye. This patient did not experience diplopia. The cheek is well supported by an obturator prosthesis.

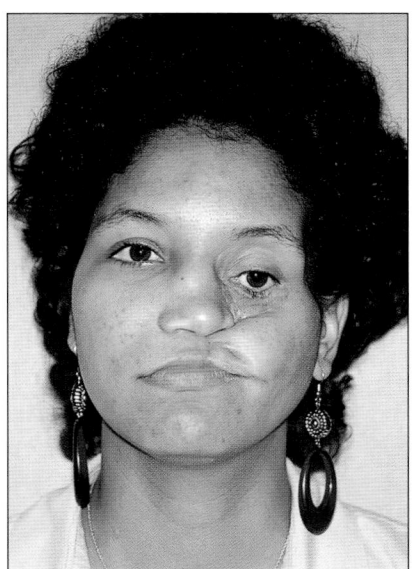

Fig 12-48a A temporalis muscle-tendon flap was not used to support the eye, resulting in severe enophthalmos and diplopia.

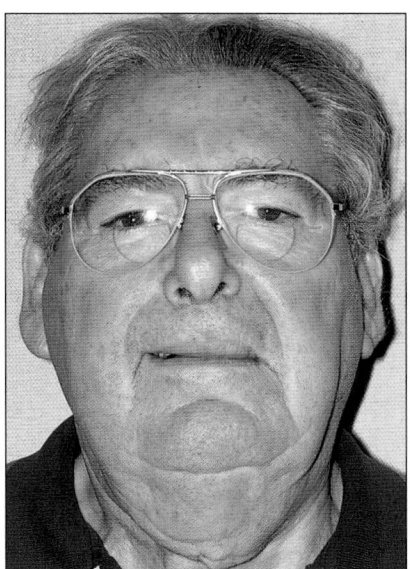

Fig 12-48b Once healed, the combined use of a temporalis tendon–muscle flap, a denture-obturator prosthesis, and a well-designed Weber-Ferguson incision with a stepped lip-split incision to prevent upward lip retraction will provide good tissue support and normal contours while preventing lip incompetence, enophthalmos, and diplopia.

so, the muscle will lift the eye and assume a position beneath and in support of it. The tendon is then sutured to a drill hole placed in the nasal bone, and the tension of the temporalis muscle is adjusted so that the level of the involved eye matches that of the uninvolved eye (Fig 12-47f). By this means, permanent support will be provided for the involved eye, thus preventing enophthalmos and diplopia. In addition, a vascular soft tissue will be available for bony reconstruction of the orbital floor (Figs 12-47g, 12-48a, and 12-48b).

Soft Tissue Excision

INDICATIONS ▶ Soft tissue excisions are indicated in the treatment of benign tumors and mucus retention phenomena. Pleomorphic adenomas, canalicular adenomas, and basal cell adenomas of the lip, buccal mucosa, or other sites are treated in this manner.

PROCEDURE ▶ This surgery often follows a subtotal removal of a pleomorphic adenoma from a small nodule enucleation for what was thought to be a mucocele or mucus cyst. It should closely follow the first procedure as if it were an incisional biopsy so that healing does not distort its location. The surgical area or, if it is the primary procedure, the tumor itself is excised with 1-cm margins. Because a pleomorphic adenoma in these locations arises from minor salivary glands within the submucosa, the overlying mucosal epithelium and underlying muscle fascia are included in the excision. The underlying muscle and even the skin closest to the lesion need not be included in the excision unless frozen sections indicate tumor infiltration. Once frozen sections are clear, a primary wound closure is performed.

Surgeries of the Parotid Gland

Parotid surgery for all conditions comprises six definitive basic procedures: (*1*) fine needle aspirations for diagnostic cytology; (*2*) incisional parotid biopsy; (*3*) superficial parotidectomy; (*4*) total parotidectomy with nerve preservation; (*5*) total parotidectomy with nerve transsection and nerve grafting; and (*6*) excision of the deep lobe of the parotid gland. Each is discussed with reference to its indications and surgical technique.

Fine Needle Aspiration for Diagnostic Cytology

INDICATIONS ▶ Fine needle aspirations (FNAs) are indicated in the treatment of solitary parotid masses suspected to represent a tumor. The purpose of an FNA cytology is to gain a diagnosis prior to definitive parotid surgery without risking the seeding of tumor cells by performing an incisional parotid biopsy. Because of the limited number of cells obtained, it is often impossible to gain a definitive diagnosis. However, the clinician is well served if the pathologist can distinguish the specimen as either benign or malignant. This presurgical knowledge, along with a CT or MRI scan, allows the surgeon to plan the necessary type of parotid surgery (ie, superficial parotidectomy versus total parotidectomy with nerve preservation versus total parotidectomy with nerve transsection and grafting, etc). This also allows the surgeon to better advise the patient and elicit more definitive informed consent.

PROCEDURE ▶ The FNA technique for a parotid mass is identical to an FNA for cervical lymph nodes. The skin is prepared with a surgical scrub and draped. It is anesthetized with local anesthesia. With the parotid mass stabilized between two fingers, a 21-gauge or smaller needle attached to a 10-mL syringe is inserted. The clinician should be able to discern the needle entering the tumor mass by an increase in resistance as it enters it. To confirm the needle's presence in the mass, it is toggled back and forth by the fingers used to stabilize it. If the needle is within the mass, the syringe will move with it. The syringe plunger is drawn back forcibly to dislodge cells into the needle lumen. Negative pressure should be maintained as the needle is withdrawn.

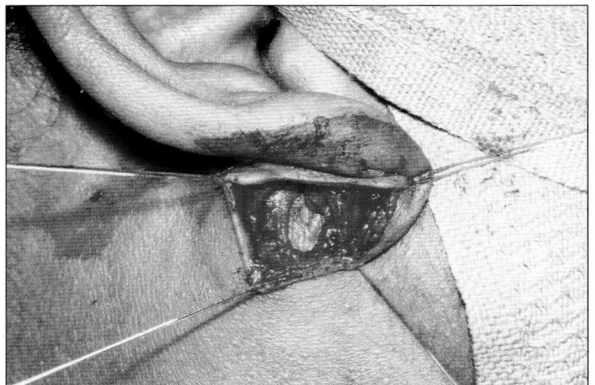

Fig 12-49a The incisional parotid biopsy is accomplished through a 1.5-cm incision under the lobule of the ear, which provides access to the superficial lobe of the parotid.

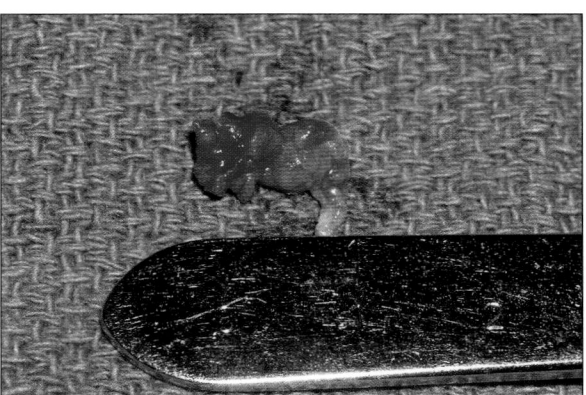

Fig 12-49b The incisional parotid biopsy provides major salivary gland tissue in greater quantities than oral minor salivary gland biopsies.

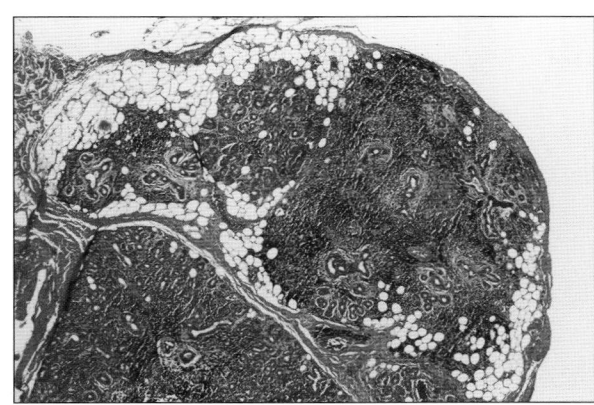

Fig 12-49c A clinically normal-looking parotid shows some fatty replacement as well as complete parenchymal effacement with a dense lymphocytic infiltrate indicative of Sjögren syndrome.

The cells within the needle lumen are forcibly expressed onto a dry glass slide and quickly smeared as thin as possible with the needle itself. The specimen slide is then immediately placed into the fixative (it is best to use 95% alcohol, although formalin will also suffice). This process should take less than 10 seconds.

Incisional Parotid Biopsy

INDICATIONS ▶ Incisional parotid biopsies are indicated when it is necessary to confirm or rule out autoimmune or systemic diseases that involve salivary gland tissue. They are particularly indicated to confirm Sjögren syndrome, benign lymphoepithelial lesions, sarcoidosis, sialosis, and lymphoma in the parotid gland. They are contraindicated in firm, circumscribed masses in the parotid or known neoplasms.

PROCEDURE ▶ Incisional parotid biopsy may be accomplished as an office procedure under local anesthesia. An incision is placed at the inferior margin of the pinna beneath the earlobe for cosmetic reasons (Fig 12-49a). A 1.5-cm incision is made through skin and subcutaneous tissue to expose and identify the thicker white parotid-masseteric fascia (see Fig 12-49a). This fascia and the thin parotid capsule, which are usually fused together, are incised to expose a small portion of the parotid (Fig 12-49b). The gray lobulations of the parotid confirm the location, which is distinguishable from yellow subcutaneous fat (12-49c). Several lobules are then taken and placed in formalin (parotid tissue, which will sink, can again be distinguished from fat, which will float, once the container has been shaken). The parotid-masseteric fascia is closed, as are the subcutaneous and skin layers; no drain is required. Sialoceles do not result as a complication of this procedure because no major ducts are transsected. Facial nerve injury is also not a complication of this procedure because this surgical site is in an area where the facial nerve is much deeper (2.3 cm) than the biopsy level.

Superficial Parotidectomy

INDICATIONS ▶ A superficial parotidectomy is indicated in cases of benign tumors in the superficial lobe and some low-grade malignant tumors (if frozen sections document clear margins). It is also indicated in selected cases

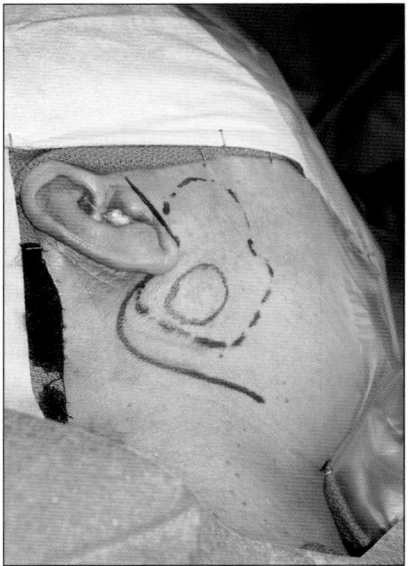

Fig 12-50a The superficial parotidectomy incision combines a pre-auricular incision with a classic Risdon incision to develop a skin flap that will access the parotid.

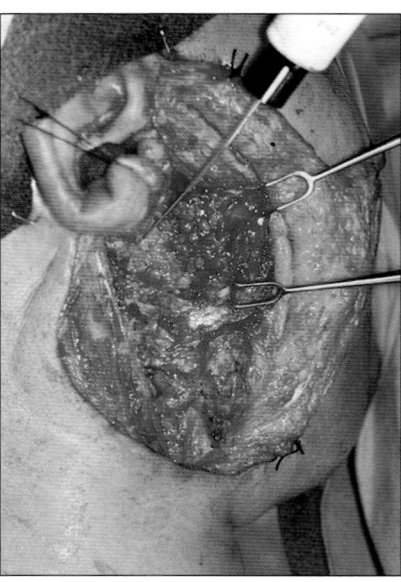

Fig 12-50b A nerve tester is used during a superficial parotidectomy to identify the facial nerve. The glandular tissue superficial to the five branches of the facial nerve is removed, containing the tumor within it.

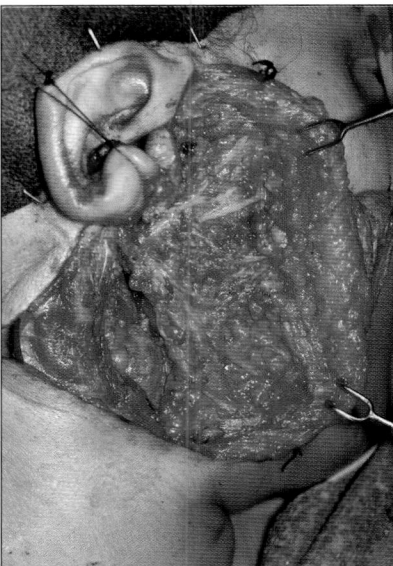

Fig 12-50c A superficial parotidectomy should leave a cuff of parotid parenchyma around the nerve to maintain the blood supply so as to promote fast and optimal nerve recovery.

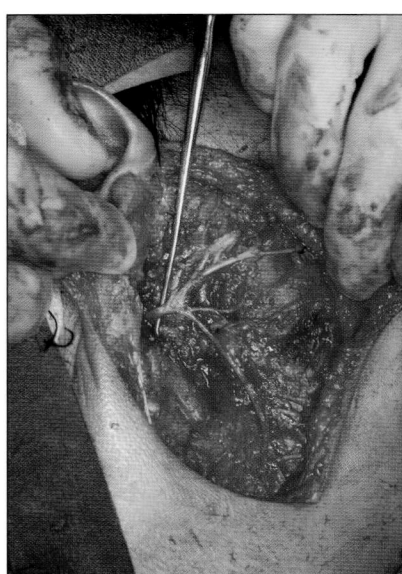

Fig 12-50d A completely "skeletonized" nerve in a superficial parotidectomy will often result in slight facial paresis due to interruption of the nerve's blood supply.

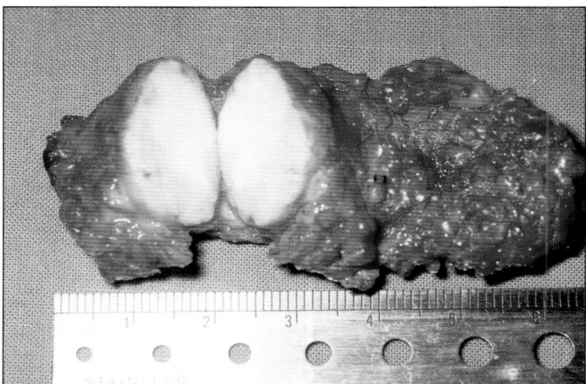

Fig 12-50e A pleomorphic adenoma excised en-bloc within the superficial lobe of the parotid. A pleomorphic adenoma is said to have a "cut potato" look when bisected.

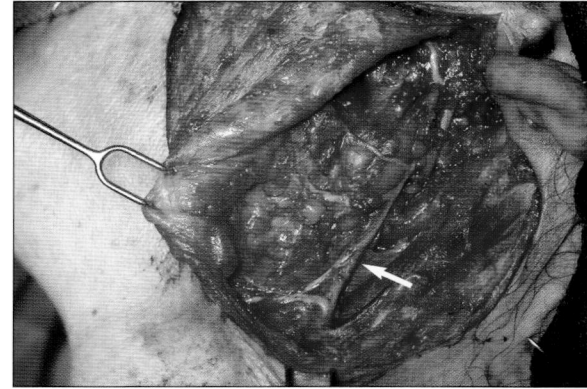

Fig 12-50f An alternative approach to a superficial parotidectomy is to find the cervical branch of the facial nerve outside the gland as it courses alongside the external jugular vein (*arrow*). This branch is then followed into the gland to identify the main trunk of the facial nerve.

of symptomatic sialosis, Sjögren syndrome, HIV parotitis, lymphoepithelial cysts, and parotid injuries with refractory sialocele or salivary-cutaneous fistulae.

PROCEDURE ▶

The standard superficial parotidectomy, called the "central approach," is accomplished with a continuous incision that begins in the preauricular area and continues around the earlobe and gently curves to parallel the angle and posterior body of the mandible about 2 to 3 cm below the inferior border (Fig 12-50a). The first part of the dissection is the development of a skin flap at the level of the parotid capsule, exposing the entire gland. The edge of the skin flap is usually sutured to the skin anteriorly for retraction.

The gland dissection is begun with blunt dissection at its posterior edge to identify the main trunk of the facial nerve. A nerve tester set at 2 mA and an unparalyzed patient are required (Fig 12-50b). The trunk of the facial nerve is deep in this location (average 3.0 to 3.5 cm beneath the skin surface) and requires considerable dissection. It consistently emerges from the stylomastoid foramen between four well-known landmarks: (1) the palpable bony transverse process of the atlas inferiorly; (2) the palpable external cartilaginous meatus superiorly; (3) the palpable bony posterior border of the ramus anteriorly; and (4) the mastoid tip posteriorly. The surgeon can easily pinpoint its anticipated location by advancing a finger anteriorly along the mastoid tip until it falls into a hollow below the cartilaginous meatus just posterior to the ramus of the mandible. Once the trunk of the facial nerve is identified, it is used as the main anatomic guide in the dissection. The parotid tissue is bluntly dissected off the nerve from the posterior to anterior aspect as the nerve bifurcates first into its two major divisions and then into its five terminal branches. As the dissection progresses from anterior to posterior, the nerve will course more superficially. The dissection continues anteriorly until gland tissue ends, which is usually along the buccal branch of the facial nerve and the parotid duct. The parotid duct arises deep and is not excised with the tumor; in fact, it is not even visible in this surgery. The superficial lobe and deep lobe distinction is arbitrary. There is no fascia separating them. The facial nerve is only a convenient anatomic guide that has created a conceptual separation of the parotid gland into two lobes. Therefore, completely skeletonizing the facial nerve branches is not necessary and actually may result in a small amount of unnecessary paresis caused by disruption of the epineurial blood supply (Figs 12-50c and 12-50d). Instead, it is better to leave a small amount of glandular tissue on the nerve unless the tumor's location does not allow it (Fig 12-50e). The resultant wound is closed in layers, and a suction drain and pressure dressing are used.

A modified approach to the superficial parotidectomy, called the "peripheral approach," is preferred by some, especially those familiar with the surgical approaches to the mandible. The incision and initial skin flap are the same as in the standard approach. However, the facial nerve is located at its cervical branch rather than at its trunk (Fig 12-50f). The cervical branch is anatomically consistent in its course just deep to the platysma and along the external jugular vein. The nerve is identified by nerve testing and in this dissection is found at the point where the greater auricular nerve courses superficially across the external jugular vein. The cervical branch in this location is outside the parotid gland. It is followed into the parotid gland, which is separated first from the marginal mandibular branch and then from each succeeding branch as the inferior division is traced superiorly to the nerve trunk and beyond to the upper division. The gland-tumor complex is then dissected off these nerve branches until the gland ends and the specimen is delivered, as is done in the central approach. This approach accomplishes the same superficial lobe excision but avoids the initial deep dissection in the preauricular area in search of the facial nerve trunk. It also uses landmarks more familiar to most oral and maxillofacial surgeons. The surgeon should anticipate and be prepared for the natural vascularity of the parotid gland. The surgeon will find numerous small vessels and capillaries within the gland, especially coursing with the facial nerve branches. A bipolar electrocautery is recommended when performing this surgery.

Total Parotidectomy with Nerve Preservation

INDICATIONS ▶ A total parotidectomy with nerve preservation is indicated in cases of benign and low-grade malignant tumors that encroach upon or extend into the deep lobe (Fig 12-51a).

PROCEDURE ▶ The surgery is identical to the standard or modified superficial parotidectomy except that access to the deep lobe is gained between the upper and lower divisions of the facial nerve. In this approach, each division, including the buccal branch, must be dissected completely. The upper division, along with the buccal branch, is retracted superiorly, and the lower division is retracted inferiorly. A portion or, in some cases, all of the deep lobe may be removed through this access (Figs 12-51b to 12-51d).

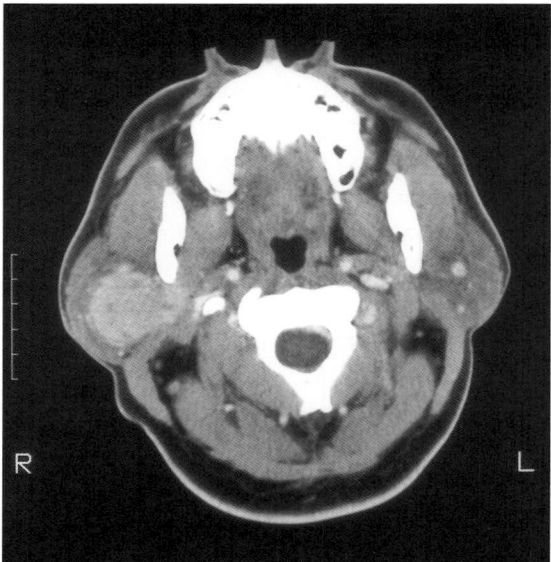

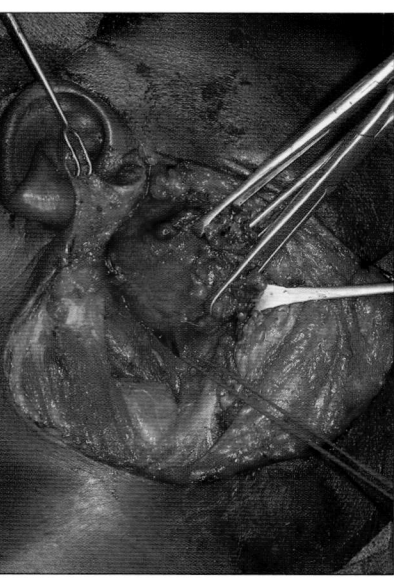

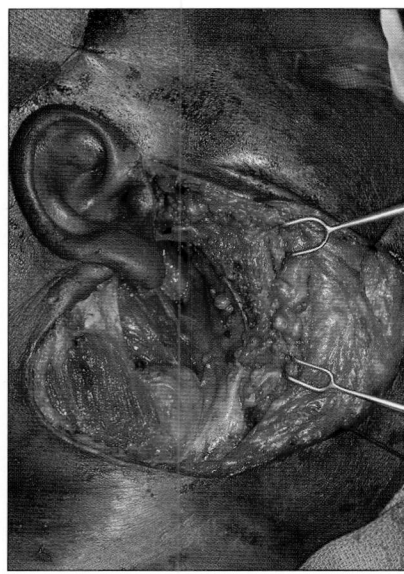

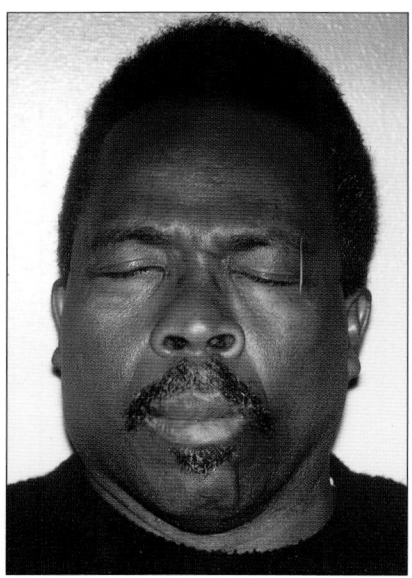

Fig 12-51a Pleomorphic adenoma extending from the superficial lobe into the deep lobe of the parotid, the so-called dumbbell tumor.

Fig 12-51b Tumor removed with a total parotidectomy, accessing the deep lobe between the zygomatic frontal division and the cervico-mandibular division of the facial nerve.

Fig 12-51c The retromandibular vein and the intact facial nerve following removal of the superficial and deep lobes.

Fig 12-51d With this type of total parotidectomy, facial nerve function is preserved.

Total Parotidectomy with Nerve Transsection and Nerve Grafting

INDICATIONS ▶ A total parotidectomy with nerve transsection and nerve grafting is indicated in cases of malignant tumors of the superficial lobe that require aggressive resection and diffuse benign tumors that involve both lobes.

PROCEDURE ▶ This surgery is identical to the standard or modified superficial parotidectomy except that access to the deep lobe is gained through transsection of all five branches of the facial nerve and a nerve graft is accomplished after the tumor is removed (Fig 12-52). As each branch of the facial nerve is transsected, each end is tagged and allowed to retract. The mandible is dislocated forward and each portion of the facial nerve ends is retracted to excise a deep lobe tumor extension. At the same time, a 6- to 8-cm length of the greater auricular nerve is harvested and separated into five fascicles. Each fascicle is grafted to the proximal and distal ends of the transsected nerve, usually via an epineurial closure with 8-0 nylon suture on a BV130-5 needle with the aid of a microscope. Direct re-anastomosis may be accomplished, but nerve retraction will place tension on the anastomosis and may compromise nerve regeneration.

Excision of the Deep Lobe of the Parotid Gland

INDICATIONS ▶ Excision of the deep lobe of the parotid gland is indicated in cases of benign or low-grade malignant tumors located in and limited to the deep lobe of the parotid gland (Fig 12-53).

PROCEDURE ▶ Access to the deep lobe of the parotid gland is blocked by the mandible and the superficial lobe. An access approach developed for parapharyngeal space tumors (Attia approach) also provides access to the deep lobe of the parotid gland. The incision resembles a posteriorly extended Risdon approach to the mandible (Fig 12-54a). A preauricular or superficial parotidectomy incision is not needed. As the

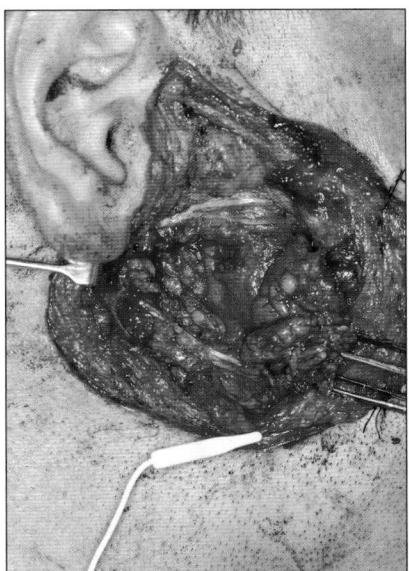

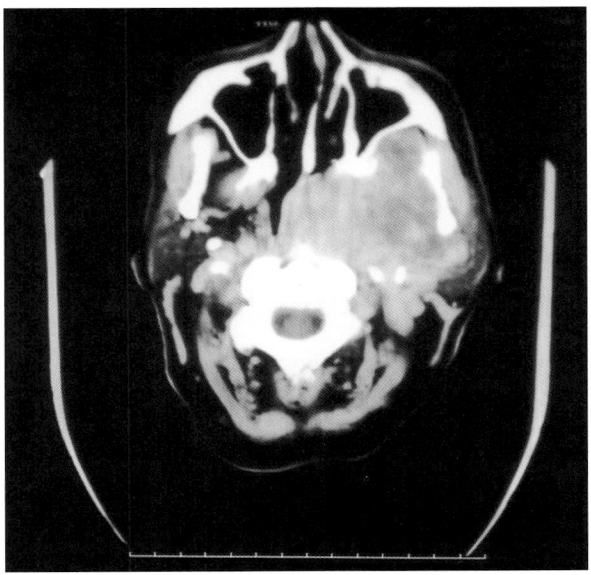

Fig 12-52 When a total parotidectomy requires extensive access, the facial nerve must be selectively transsected. It is then re-anastamosed or nerve-grafted under magnification so as to return as much facial muscle activity as possible.

Fig 12-53 A deep lobe of the parotid tumor will be located medial to the mandibular ramus and will encroach on the airway, the parapharyngeal spaces, the maxilla, and the cervical vertebrae.

mandible is approached, the masseter attachments and the lateral periosteum are not reflected, except just anterior to the mental foramen and just above the lingual aspect, in anticipation of osteotomies in each area. The ramus access is gained by incising the periosteum at the posterior ramus border and reflecting the upper fibers of the masseter anteriorly. Reconstruction plates of 2.4 or 2.7 mm are adapted to the mandible in the areas of the anticipated osteotomies (Fig 12-54b). Fixation screws are placed into tapped sites and then removed and marked to enable replacement in the same positions. A vertical osteotomy is made either between the first premolar roots or through the first premolar alveolus (after a planned removal of this tooth). A second osteotomy is made horizontally above the lingula. The segment of the mandible between these osteotomies can now be reflected laterally, along with the masseter and superficial lobe of the parotid (Fig 12-54c). The mandible is thus pedicled on its lateral attachments and receives additional blood supply through the intact inferior alveolar neurovascular bundle. The deep lobe of the parotid gland and any tumor within it, as well as the parapharyngeal space, will be directly in view. The tumor can be excised along with the entire deep lobe (Fig 12-54d).

The mandible is replaced after the tumor is excised and the plates are refixated into position. Maxillomandibular fixation is not usually required (Figs 12-54e and 12-54f). This approach provides excellent access while maintaining mandibular viability and contour, and it preserves the inferior alveolar and facial nerves.

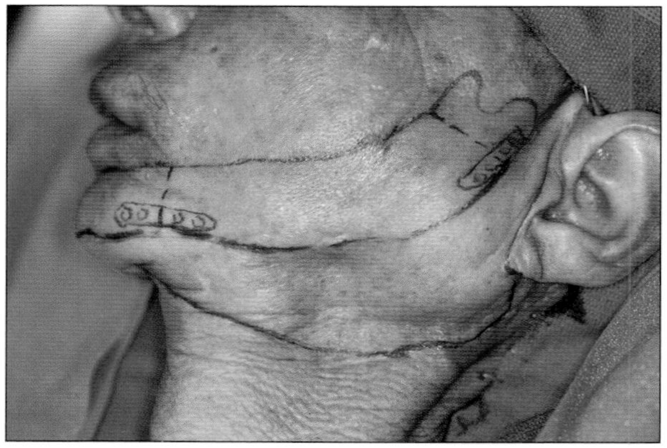

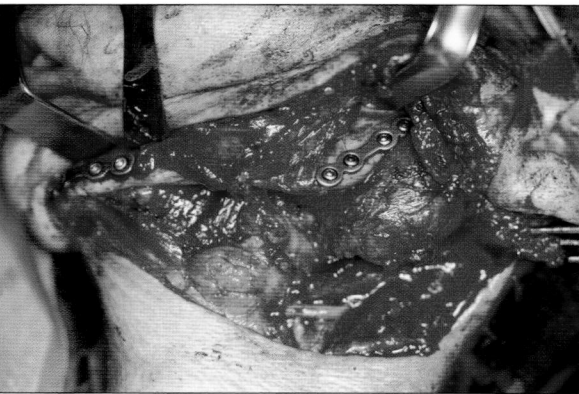

Fig 12-54a Outline of the incision and strategy of the Attia approach to a deep lobe of the parotid tumor.

Fig 12-54b The Attia approach places rigid plates before the osteotomies and maintains the buccal soft tissue attachments.

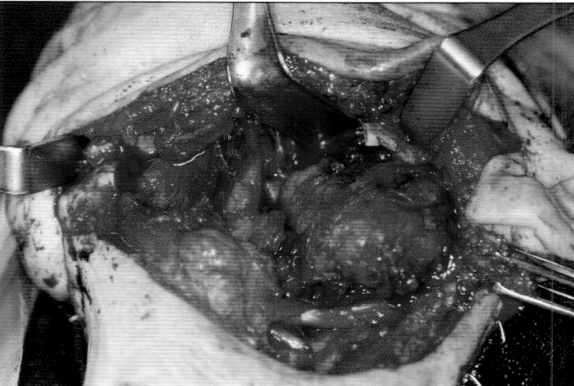

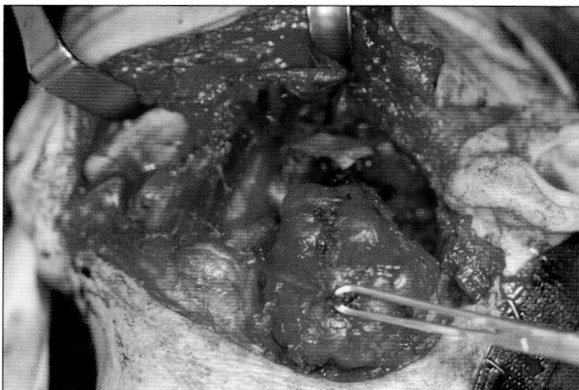

Fig 12-54c Osteotomies above the lingula of the ramus and anterior to the mental foramen allow the resultant mandibular pedicled segment to be reflected superiorly to expose this large, deep lobe tumor.

Fig 12-54d Removal of a large tumor in the deep lobe with the improved access provided by the Attia approach.

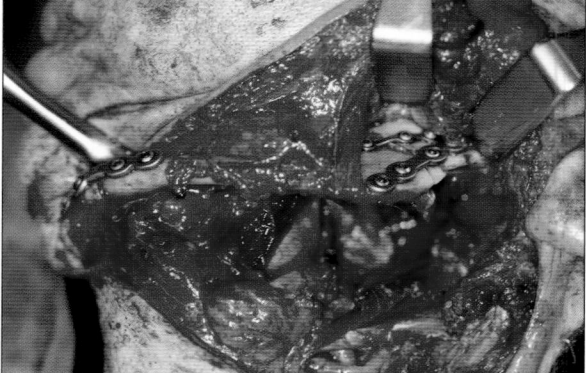

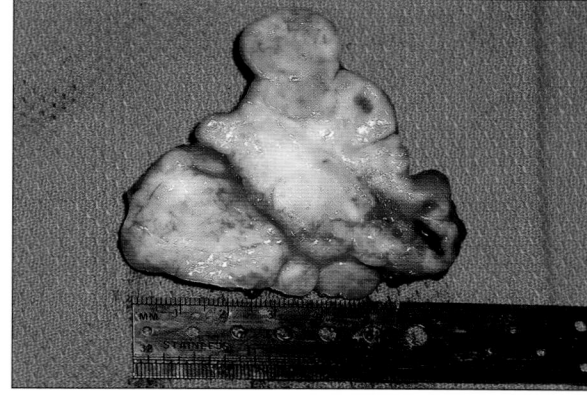

Fig 12-54e After the tumor is removed, the viable mandibular segment is returned to its original position as indexed by the same rigid plates.

Fig 12-54f The large pleomorphic adenoma of the parotid's deep lobe excised through the access provided by the Attia approach.

Odontogenic and Nonodontogenic Cysts

CHAPTER 13

▶ *"A surgeon must be a pathologist who does operations."*
—*Eric Carlson*

A cyst is defined as a pathologic cavity lined by epithelium. All cysts described in this chapter arise from epithelial remnants related to some embryologic development and are therefore referred to as *developmental cysts*. Some arise from epithelial cells left over from tooth development (eg, odontogenic keratocysts), from embryonic ducts (eg, nasopalatine duct cysts), or from organ or facial unit development and fusion (eg, thyroglossal duct cysts, nasolabial cysts, and branchial cysts). Some, such as the common radicular cyst, are said to be inflammatory cysts; however, this categorization is somewhat artificial. In such radicular cysts, inflammation may indeed produce cytokines and growth factors that stimulate epithelial rests to proliferate into a cyst, but the epithelial rests are from tooth root development (rests of Malassez). This chapter will also show that both the branchial cyst and the thyroglossal duct cyst arise rapidly after a pharyngitis, again seemingly because of the stimulatory effects of inflammatory cytokines on dormant epithelium in these areas. Yet these are still best conceptualized as developmental cysts because the source of their epithelium is from the development of specific structures.

The so-called noninflammatory cysts also arise from stimulated epithelial rests or developmental tracts. The primordial origin keratocyst and the dentigerous cyst arise from rests and from reduced enamel epithelium, respectively. Some are stimulated and arise from growth-related cytokines, hence the common finding of cysts in teenagers and young adults. Some arise from genetically stimulated growth factors, hence the multiple keratocysts seen in the basal cell nevus syndrome. And some still presumably result from loss of cell replication inhibitors, hence the potential for a cyst to develop at any age.

The so-called traumatic bone cyst, which is actually a cavity in bone, is not included in this chapter because it is not lined by epithelium and therefore is not a cyst, nor is it related to trauma. Instead, it is now termed an *idiopathic bone cavity,* reflecting both its obscure etiology and its true nature as a cavity in bone without any lining. Similarly, the so-called aneurysmal bone cyst also is not included in this chapter, since it is now recognized as a variant of the giant cell tumor of bone. Its cavities or spaces are lined with young fibroblasts rather than epithelium. Conversely, what has in the past been referred to as the adenomatoid odontogenic tumor (AOT) is now recognized to consistently represent a lumen lined with a specific type of epithelial proliferation arising from Hertwig epithelial root sheath, and is therefore identified in this chapter as an *adenomatoid odontogenic cyst* (AOC), not a true neoplasm or hamartoma.

Development of a Cyst

The common behavioral feature of all cysts is the stimulation of residual developmental epithelial cells, leading to proliferation but not invasion of adjacent tissues. The epithelial rests proliferate into a solid mass of epithelial cells. As the mass enlarges, the epithelial cells in the center become positioned further from the blood supply at the periphery of the mass. At some point, usually 180 to 200 μm (0.18 to 0.20 mm), the cells at the center become too far removed from the nearest blood vessel to survive by nutritional diffusion. They die, creating a lumen. Their intracellular products make the lumen hypertonic, which transudates fluid into the lumen. This in turn creates a hydrostatic pressure, producing bone re-

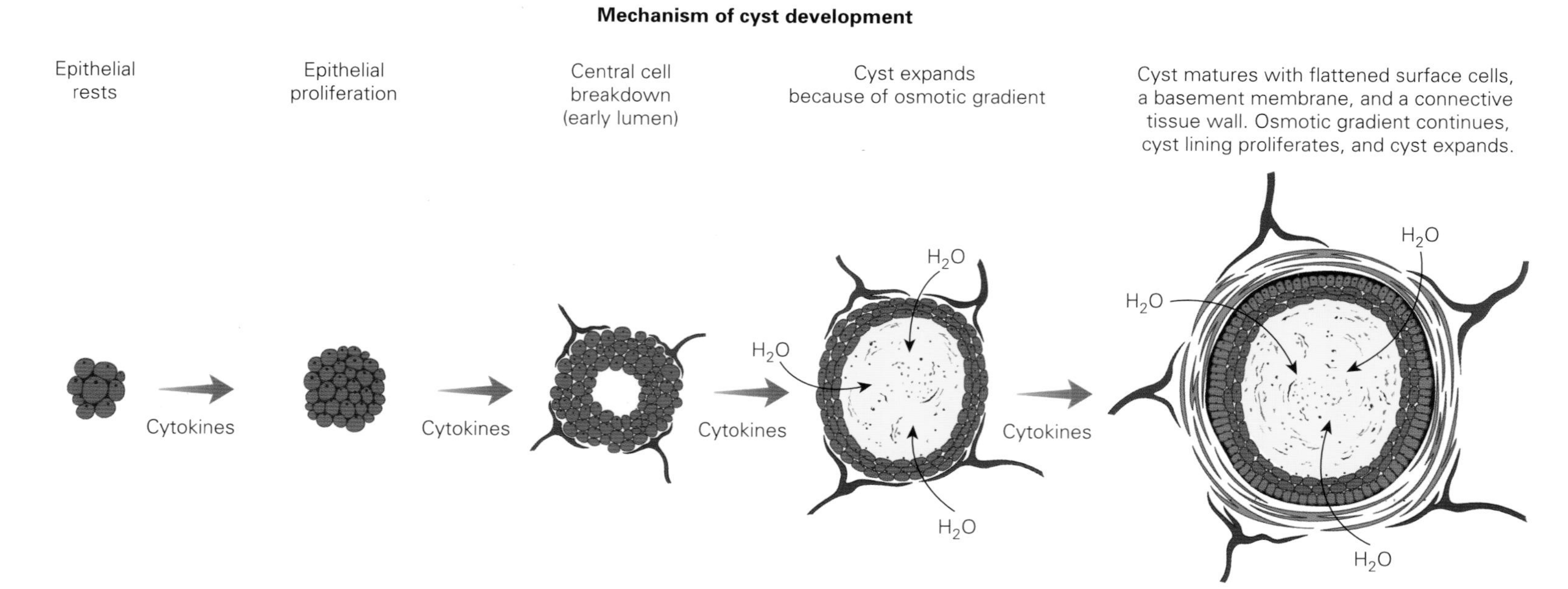

Mechanism of cyst development

Fig 13-1 Cyst development begins and continues by cytokine stimulation of epithelial rests and is added to by the central cellular breakdown products, which create a hypertonic intraluminal solution that transudates fluid for further cyst expansion.

sorption, clinical expansion, and sometimes mild paresthesia or pain. As additional epithelial cells die off and are sloughed into the lumen, their contents perpetuate the hypertonic state and the hydrostatic pressure. The cell membranes and nuclear membranes of these sloughed cells are high in cholesterol, hence the common finding of cholesterol clefts in the lumen or even in the walls of many cysts. As the cyst enlarges, it compresses surrounding connective tissue into a connective tissue wall. The epithelial lining matures and develops a basement membrane. The cyst lining continues to proliferate, thus causing the cyst to enlarge until (*1*) it is removed (enucleation), (*2*) the proliferating cells are communicated into the oral cavity or an external surface so as to break the proliferation–hydrostatic pressure cycle (marsupialization), or (*3*) the inciting cytokines are removed (via tooth removal or root canal therapy in radicular cysts) (Fig 13-1).

Odontogenic Cysts

Radicular Cyst

CLINICAL PRESENTATION AND PATHOGENESIS ▶

The radicular cyst (Fig 13-2a) is an inflammatory cyst associated with the root apex of a nonvital tooth. Because of the high incidence of pulpal pathology, it is the most common cyst of the oral and maxillofacial region. Radicular cysts can occur at any age, but curiously they are seldom seen in children despite the high incidence of pulpal and periapical pathology in this group, which implies that there are few if any epithelial rests that result from the development of primary teeth.

Clinically, these cysts are associated with a tooth that is carious, has undergone previous restorative care, has sustained trauma, or is an apparent failure of root canal therapy (Fig 13-2b). Radiographically, an apical radiolucency will be noted, but rarely will there be bony expansion unless there is secondary infection.

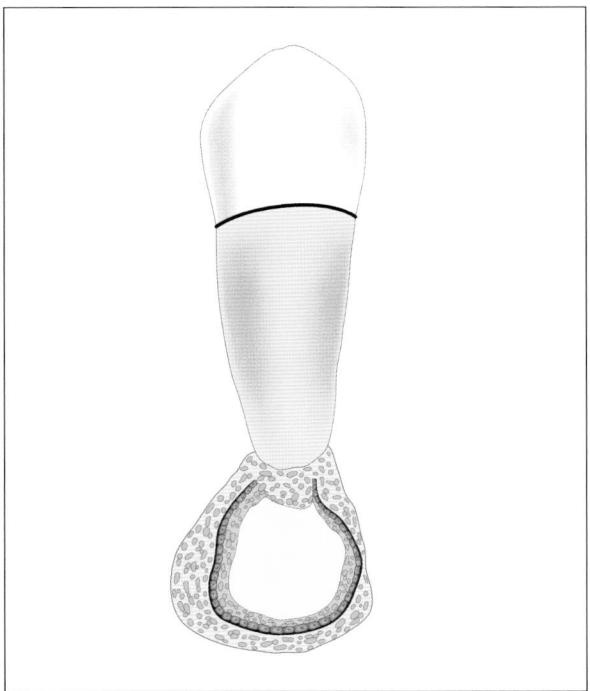

Fig 13-2a Illustration of a radicular cyst showing a lumen and a wall that is attached to the tooth and is confluent with the periodontal membrane. Note that the root surface is not confluent with the lumen of the cyst.

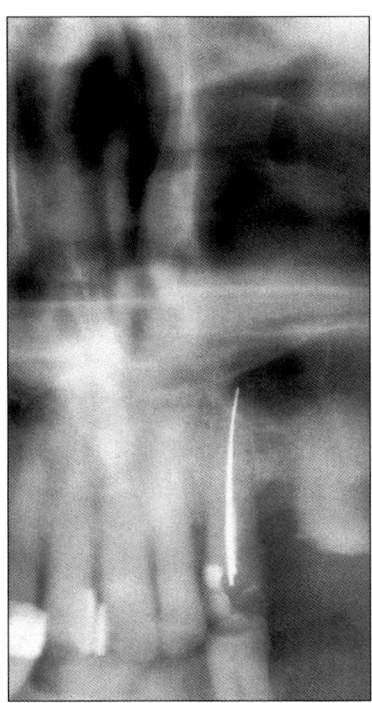

Fig 13-2b Failing root canal treatment with apical radiolucency, which was determined to be caused by a radicular cyst upon removal of the tooth.

Much has been written about the radiographic distinction between periapical granulomas and radicular cysts, and yet there is no real distinction. The presence of a thin rim of sclerotic bone around the radiolucency is as indicative of a periapical granuloma as it is of a cyst.

Most radicular cysts are small, in the range of 0.5 to 1.5 cm, but they can exceed 5 cm. Some will also cause a regular smooth resorption of adjacent tooth roots, or they may have an irregular resorption of their roots of origin, presumably because of infection or osteoclastic factors elaborated by the cyst.

The radicular cyst is the model pathogenesis of an inflammation-stimulated cyst and has been extensively studied. The origin of the cyst epithelium lies with rests of Malassez, which are epithelial remnants of Hertwig epithelial root sheath that lie dormant within the periodontal ligament. The products of pulpal infection and necrosis spill out into the periapical tissues, inciting an inflammatory response. The inflammatory cells secrete a host of lymphokines to neutralize, immobilize, and degrade bacteria. They also induce bone resorption through the elaboration of interleukin-1 and osteoclast-activating factors. These same cells are thought to elaborate many other factors that either directly or indirectly act as epithelial growth factors, stimulating the proliferation of the rests of Malassez in the periapical granuloma. As the epithelial cell mass enlarges, the central cells become distant from their blood supply and break down, thereby forming a cyst. The cyst continues to enlarge by epithelial proliferation in the lining and by hydrostatic pressure generated in the cyst lumen from the hyperosmolarity created by cellular breakdown and sloughing of cells into the lumen. Therefore, the osmotic gradient favors transudation of fluid into the lumen, which maintains its hydrostatic pressure and causes further resorption of the surrounding bone (see Fig 13-1). This cycle can be broken and reversed in most situations if the inflammatory focus is removed (ie, root canal therapy or tooth removal). However, if the tooth is removed, the apical lesion should be removed as well.

DIFFERENTIAL DIAGNOSIS ▶ A *periapical granuloma* is radiographically and clinically indistinguishable from a radicular cyst. In the anterior mandible, the early osteolytic phase of *periapical cemento-osseous dysplasia* is a consideration, as is

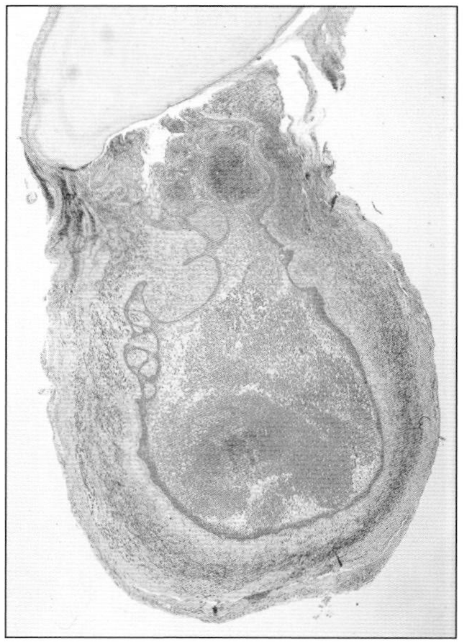

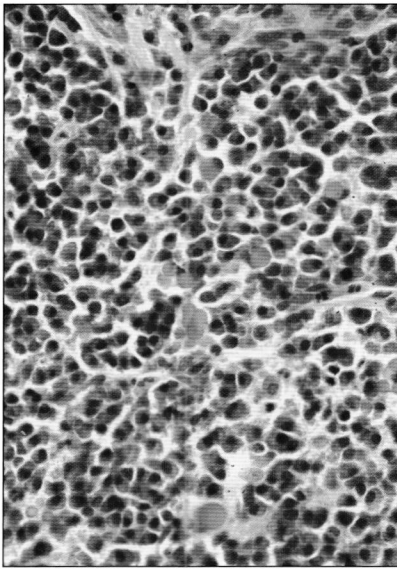

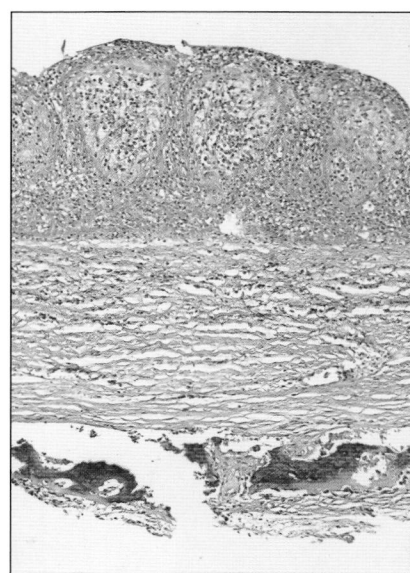

Fig 13-2c Radicular cyst attached to the apex of the tooth root. The periodontal membrane is continuous with the wall of the cyst, which is densely inflamed. The lining is stratified squamous epithelium and the lumen contains erythrocytes, inflammatory cells, and debris.

Fig 13-2d A dense, chronic inflammatory infiltrate, predominantly plasma cells, with rounded eosinophilic globules. These are Russell bodies, which consist of immunoglobulin.

Fig 13-2e The wall of a radicular cyst with a stratified squamous epithelial lining and prominent rete ridges. A dense, chronic inflammatory infiltrate invades the epithelium. The wall is fibrous, and some reactive bone can be seen at the periphery.

the uncommon *sublingual salivary gland depression.* In the posterior mandible, a *submandibular salivary gland depression* is a possibility as are *idiopathic bone cavities.* It is important to remember that throughout both jaws, a wide array of *odontogenic cysts* and *tumors,* plus *central mucoepidermoid carcinoma* and certain *fibro-osseous diseases,* can begin or develop radiolucencies that may appear periapically.

DIAGNOSTIC WORK-UP AND TREATMENT

Periapical radiographs and pulp tests are the most reliable diagnostic aids. If the tooth is nonvital and has a periapical radiolucency, the working diagnosis remains the more common periapical granuloma, followed by a radicular cyst. Because a radicular cyst is derived from the stimulated epithelium of a periapical granuloma, the treatment implications are the same. Treatment is then dictated mostly by the restorability of the tooth. Treatment for nonrestorable teeth involves tooth removal and surgical curettage of the apical area. The apical soft tissue lesion should be evaluated histopathologically, not to distinguish cyst versus granuloma but to rule out unexpected neoplasms or more aggressive cysts. Restorable teeth are treated with endodontic therapy followed by full occlusal coverage restorations.

HISTOPATHOLOGY

Grossly, the contents of radicular cysts are usually a soft brown material, often with glistening, oily, yellow flecks. Nodules of opaque yellow material, representing cholesterol, may be seen protruding into the lumen or within the wall.

The radicular cyst is typically lined by a nonkeratinizing stratified squamous epithelium of varying thickness. The epithelium may be quite proliferative and demonstrate a plexiform arrangement. Mucous-secreting cells occur but are uncommon. As an inflammatory-based cyst, its wall usually contains a dense, mixed inflammatory infiltrate, rich in plasma cells and lymphocytes (Fig 13-2c). Russell bodies (round eosinophilic globules) can be seen within or outside the plasma cell and are the result of very active immunoglobulin synthesis (Fig 13-2d). Immunofluorescence staining confirms the presence of immunoglobulin. The epithelial lining is also frequently infiltrated by inflammatory cells (Fig 13-2e), predominantly neutrophils. The infiltrate may be so dense as to mask the epithelium, and there may be considerable intercellular edema. Ulceration of the lining often occurs, and on occasion the entire epithelium may be

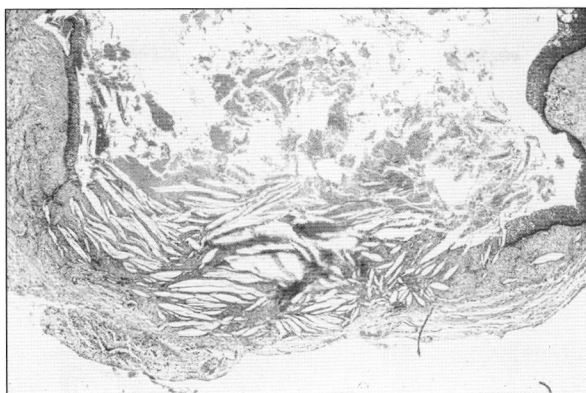

Fig 13-2f A radicular cyst with focal cholesterol slits. The epithelial lining has been disrupted.

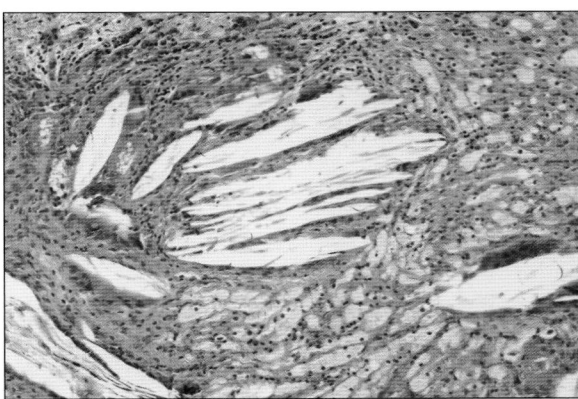

Fig 13-2g Cholesterol may be found in needle-like clefts surrounded by multinucleated giant cells or within the foamy macrophages. The clefts appear clear because the cholesterol is lost during tissue processing.

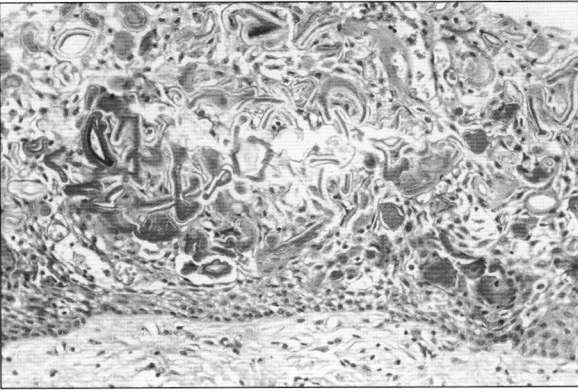

Fig 13-2h Rushton bodies within the epithelial lining of a radicular cyst. These hyaline structures may be linear, curved, hairpin, or rounded in shape.

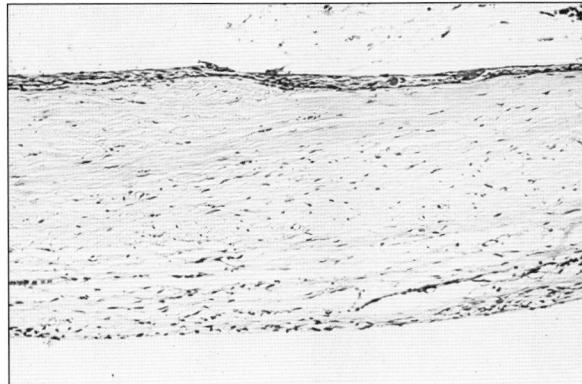

Fig 13-2i This radicular cyst was lined by a thin, flat, squamous epithelium, and the inflammatory process has resolved. Histology alone can be deceptive in diagnosing many cysts.

virtually destroyed (Fig 13-2f). As a consequence of cellular destruction, cholesterol is liberated and may be found within macrophages as foamy histiocytes, singly or more often in sheets, or as clefts within the connective tissue wall, epithelial lining, or lumen (Fig 13-2g). These usually provoke a foreign-body reaction with multinucleated giant cells contorted around the clefts. Such areas are typically associated with hemorrhage and hemosiderin deposition.

Other changes within the epithelium include the formation of Rushton bodies, which are hyaline structures that are eosinophilic and brittle in consistency. They may be linear, curved, hairpin, or round shaped (Fig 13-2h). Their exact nature has been controversial, and studies have produced conflicting results. Possibilities include odontogenic and hematogenous origins. Their presence, however, does appear to be limited to odontogenic cysts. Rushton bodies may sometimes become basophilic as calcium salts are deposited.

The wall itself, in addition to its inflammatory component, is fibrous and will often contain numerous capillaries, particularly in areas adjacent to the epithelial lining. Dystrophic calcifications may also be seen, and at the periphery, reactive osteophytic bone is often noted.

There is nothing pathognomonic about these features; most odontogenic cysts that become significantly inflamed can show similar changes. There are also radicular cysts in which the inflammatory component is absent and the fibrous wall supports a thin, flattened epithelium (Fig 13-2i).

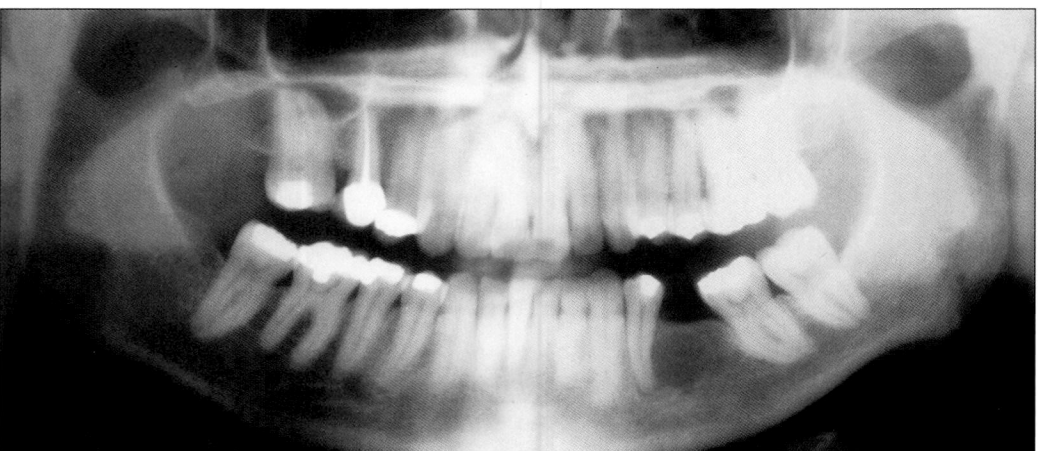

Fig 13-3a Clinical expansion from a residual cyst continued and enlarged after removal of the left mandibular second premolar.

It should be understood that a histologic spectrum exists, ranging from a periapical granuloma, which is a focal aggregate of chronic inflammatory tissue, to an "epitheliated granuloma," in which proliferating epithelium may be seen within the inflammatory focus. This may further progress to a lesion with a central lumen, lined by stratified squamous epithelium with an inflammatory component in the surrounding wall—a radicular cyst.

PROGNOSIS ▶ Radicular cysts are definitively resolved if the tooth and the apical lesion are removed. If the tooth is removed and the cyst is not, most cysts will involute because of the removal of the inflammatory focus. A few rare cases will retain their cystic stimulation independent of the tooth, probably by ongoing inflammation in the wall of the cyst. This is termed a *residual cyst*. Endodontically treated teeth will resolve radicular cysts as they do periapical granulomas as long as they have a successful pulp canal debridement and fill. In cases of endodontic failure due to incomplete fills or other pulpal leakage, the apical radiolucency will darken and enlarge, indicating a continuation of the granuloma-radicular cyst spectrum. In such cases, performing endodontic therapy again, often with assisted magnification techniques, will enable the treatment of accessory untreated canals. These accessory canals must be instrumented and filled and the previously treated canals re-treated to larger sizes and filled. Apicoectomies with a retrofill of the apical area and curettage of the residual lesion or tooth removal is indicated if this re-treatment fails.

Residual Cyst

CLINICAL PRESENTATION ▶ The term residual cyst refers to an inflammatory cyst of the jaws that fails to involute after root canal therapy or tooth removal. It is therefore not a recurrent cyst because it has not yet been removed. It is usually conceptualized as resulting from a tooth extraction that did not include removal of an associated radicular cyst (Fig 13-3a). However, a residual cyst more frequently occurs after endodontic therapy that either failed to eliminate the inflammatory focus or had undiagnosed accessory canals. It may even occur with a successful seal in a case where residual inflammation in the periapical tissue led to cyst progression.

Radiographically, residual cysts will be evident on postoperative radiographs by an enlarging and darkening radiolucency. Like radicular cysts, even large residual cysts will not show much bony expansion. Most are small, in the range of 1 to 3 cm, but sizes in excess of 6 cm are possible.

DIFFERENTIAL DIAGNOSIS ▶ A residual cyst rarely occurs after tooth removal. The fact that it did not resolve a radiolucency should elicit concern that the radiolucency may not have represented a radicular cyst; it may have represented a more aggressive lesion, such as a *primordial odontogenic keratocyst,* or an odontogenic tumor such as an *ameloblastoma* or a *myxoma,* particularly if the radiolucency has enlarged. If the radiolucency has remained

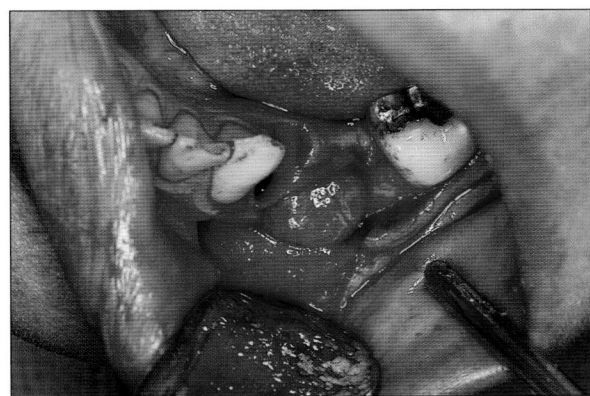

Fig 13-3b Removal of the lesion shown in Fig 13-3a confirmed it to be a residual cyst and resolved it.

static or enlarged only slowly, it may represent an *idiopathic bone cavity* or, if in the posterior mandible, a *submandibular salivary gland depression*. A *periapical cemento-osseous dysplasia* or a *sublingual salivary gland depression* are considerations if the lesion is in the anterior mandible. It may also simply represent a radicular cyst from another tooth that has not been recognized as nonvital.

A residual cyst is more commonly seen after root canal therapy. However, a persistent or enlarging radiolucency after root canal therapy should not be assumed to be a treatment failure. It may also represent these same differential lesions.

DIAGNOSTIC WORK-UP AND TREATMENT ▶

Pulp testing of adjacent teeth to rule out the possibility of a source for another radicular cyst is recommended. After this, an exploration and enucleation of the residual cyst is required and should resolve the lesion. In addition, an exploration and removal of any inflammatory focus, such as residual roots or root canal filling materials, etc, should be accomplished (Fig 13-3b).

HISTOPATHOLOGY ▶

Since these lesions represent radicular cysts (see above), the same histologic picture applies.

PROGNOSIS ▶

Removal of the residual cyst is curative. Recurrence does not occur. The enlargement of this cyst after tooth removal presupposes that it can act independently of its initial inflammatory stimulation or that a residual inflammatory stimulation apart from the tooth remains. Because this is a complicated and uncommon biology, such residual cysts are very rare entities. Residual cysts from failing root canal treatments are not rare entities. These residual cysts require re-instrumentation and root canal fills, an apicoectomy, or removal of the tooth and associated cyst.

Dentigerous Cyst

CLINICAL PRESENTATION AND PATHOGENESIS ▶

The dentigerous cyst (Fig 13-4a) arises from the dental follicle of an unerupted or developing tooth. It is the second most common odontogenic cyst after the radicular cyst. These cysts occur most commonly in the posterior mandible or maxilla and are usually associated with third molars. The second most frequent location is the maxillary canine region (Fig 13-4b) associated with the maxillary canine. Peak incidence is in the teenage years and in the 20s. There is a male predilection of 1.6:1. However, dentigerous cysts have been associated with every tooth and may occur at any age.

A dentigerous cyst may be discovered as an incidental radiographic finding or by examination of a clinical expansion. Because this cyst can attain a very large size (10 to 15 cm), some present with bony expansion and facial fullness. The cysts are not painful unless secondarily infected or unless their size has created a pathologic fracture. Some expand sufficiently to resorb one or both cortices. In such cases, the cyst appears translucent and may be compressible. The tooth from which it arises is clinically absent. Regardless of the degree of resorption or the cyst's size, inferior alveolar nerve sensation in the mandible or superior alveolar nerve plexus sensation in the maxilla is not altered unless a pathologic fracture, or more rarely an infection, causes paresthesia.

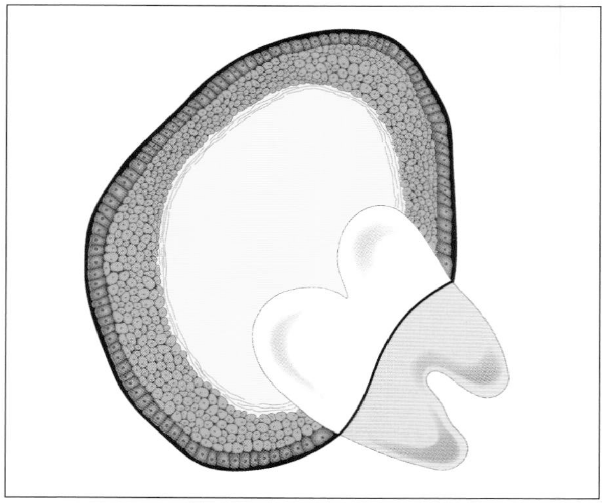

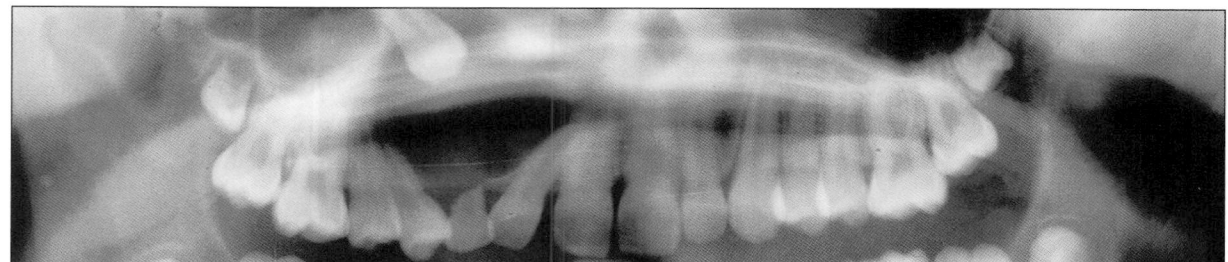

Fig 13-4a Illustration of a dentigerous cyst. Note its attachment at the cementoenamel junction.

Fig 13-4b Displacement of roots of erupted teeth and displacement of the canine into the maxillary sinus region by a dentigerous cyst. The maxillary canine region is the second most common site for a dentigerous cyst.

There are two leading theories about the formation of dentigerous cysts. The first begins with fluid accumulation between the reduced enamel epithelium and the crown of the tooth. The fluid pressure incites a proliferation of the reduced enamel epithelium into a cyst, which is attached at the cementoenamel junction and includes the tooth crown as one of its boundaries. The other theory begins with a breakdown of the stellate reticulum, which forms a fluid between the inner and outer enamel epithelium. The fluid's pressure incites a proliferation of the outer enamel epithelium, which remains attached to the tooth at the cementoenamel junction; the inner enamel epithelium is then pressed onto the crown surface. In each theory, the fluid generates the cystic proliferation by its hyperosmolar content created by cellular breakdown and cell products, causing an osmotic gradient to pump fluid into the cyst lumen.

RADIOGRAPHIC FINDINGS ▶

Radiographically, a dentigerous cyst is a well-demarcated, unilocular radiolucency associated with the crown of an unerupted tooth. The tooth may be displaced: it is not surprising to see teeth displaced to the condylar neck, the nasal floor, or high in the maxillary sinus approaching the orbit. Frequently, teeth are displaced to the inferior border of the mandible and in some cases partially through it. The cyst will displace the radiographic outline of the mandibular canal usually toward the inferior border. It may also displace roots of erupted teeth or create a smooth, regular resorption of their roots (Fig 13-5a). The incidence of root resorption of adjacent teeth has been reported to be as high as 50%.

DIFFERENTIAL DIAGNOSIS ▶

A unilocular radiolucency associated with the crown of a tooth is a classic differential diagnosis in which a dentigerous cyst is the most likely entity. The other specific diseases on the differential list have more troubling biologies and include an *odontogenic keratocyst,* an *ameloblastoma in situ* or a *microinvasive ameloblastoma within a dentigerous cyst,* an *invasive ameloblastoma,* and an *ameloblastic fibroma* in younger

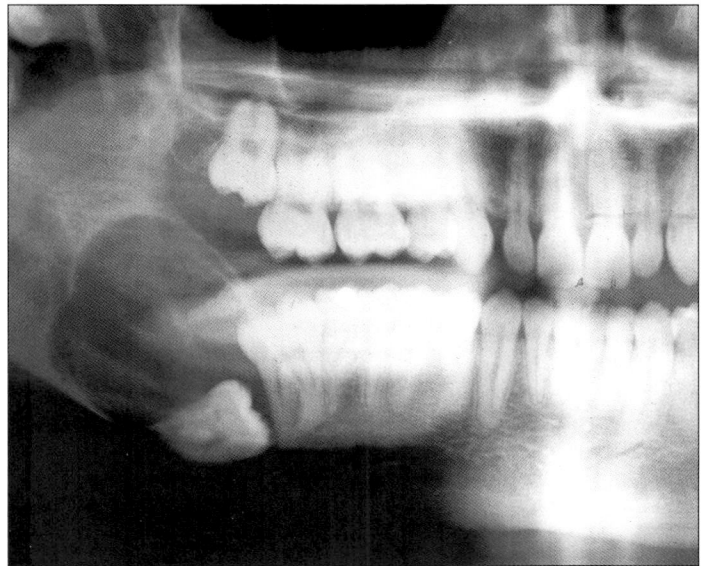

Fig 13-5a Panoramic radiograph of a large dentigerous cyst showing displacement of the tooth of origin (a third molar) and of the mandibular canal.

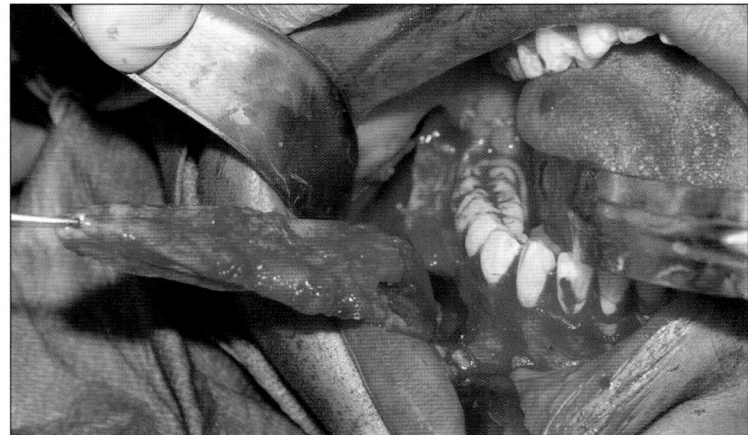

Fig 13-5b Large dentigerous cyst enucleated from the mandible with preservation of erupted teeth and the neurovascular bundle. The lining of a dentigerous cyst will be noticeably thicker than that of a keratocyst unless the keratocyst has undergone a previous entry or infection.

DIAGNOSTIC WORK-UP AND TREATMENT ▶

teenagers and children. If the dentigerous cyst occurs in the anterior maxilla, an *adenomatoid odontogenic cyst* would also be a prime consideration, especially in a young person.

An aspiration of the lesion is recommended. If it returns a straw-colored fluid, this finding together with the radiographic appearance provides a sufficient index of suspicion to indicate an exploration with an intention to remove the cyst via an enucleation procedure. If the aspiration fails to return any fluid, the implication is one of a solid lesion, in which case it would be better to perform an incisional biopsy. If the lesion unexpectedly returns blood, one should not immediately consider performing an angiogram as the needle introduction may have caused the bleeding. If a second aspiration a few days later also returns blood and blood spurts from the needle with the syringe barrel disconnected or a Doppler sounding is positive for vascular sounds, an angiogram is required. A computed tomography (CT) scan or a magnetic resonance imaging (MRI) scan, if necessary, may distinguish between a fluid-filled cyst and a solid tumor. However, the densities of cystic fluid vary greatly, as do the consistencies of solid tumors of many possible types, making this comparison unreliable.

The preferred treatment is a complete removal of the lesion from the bony cavity by enucleation, with preservation of the inferior alveolar neurovascular bundle in the mandible and adjacent erupted teeth. This is best accomplished by using an extended, broad-based full-thickness mucoperiosteal flap to expose the entire expanded cortex over the cyst. It is further facilitated by a complete removal of overlying and usually thinned cortex so as to access the entire cyst. The cyst can then be carefully separated from the bony cavity using the back edge of a curette. When the neurovascular bundle is encountered, it can be lifted with a nerve hook so that either the curette or blunt dissection with a hemostat will separate it from the connective tissue wall of the cyst. Traction can then be applied to the cyst with an Alice clamp, which will further facilitate separation of the cyst from adjacent normal tissues (Fig 13-5b). Marsupialization is less ideal; it runs the risk of allowing an ameloblastoma in situ or a microinvasive ameloblastoma or other neoplastic transformations of the cyst lining to develop into a more invasive disease. It also commits the wound to a slower healing process, a more laborious postoperative course, and a reduction in the final bone regeneration. Marsupialization is indicated in only two situations: (*1*) when it will allow a tooth to spontaneously erupt or to be orthodontically guided into a functional position in

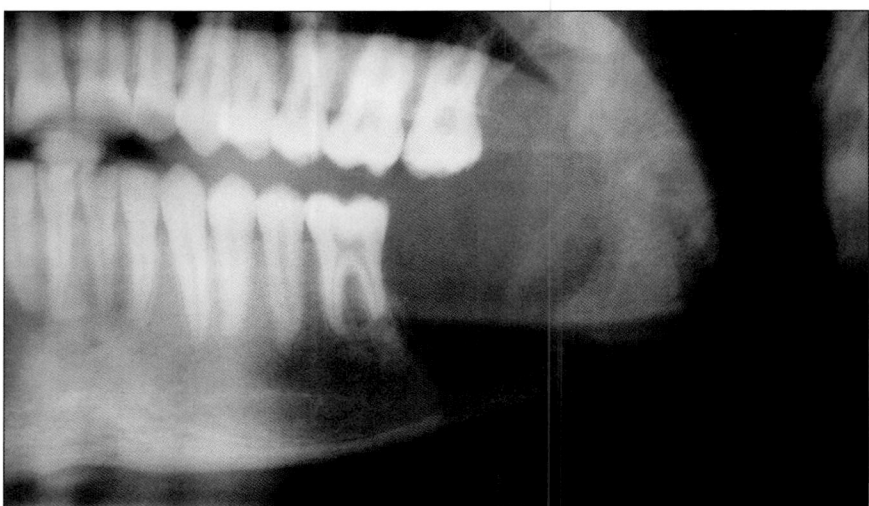

Fig 13-6 This postsurgical fracture in the center of the defect occurred 3 weeks after removal of a cyst. This is the most likely time and location for this complication.

the arch, or (2) when the surgeon identifies a realistic risk of damaging developing teeth or neurovascular bundles during the enucleation. Marsupialization will not reduce the risk of pathologic fracture or infection. The choice of procedures, therefore, depends on the surgeon's experience and training and on the facilities available.

Large dentigerous cysts with resorption of bone close to a pathologic fracture may be treated with postoperative maxillomandibular fixation. This is a valid concept but requires a full 6 to 8 weeks of fixation to actually prevent a fracture. Pathologic fracture related to a dentigerous cyst removal most commonly occurs either at the time of removal, ostensibly because of forces placed on the structurally weakened bone, or 2 to 3 weeks after removal because of revascularization and resorption-remodeling of the bone after surgery. The bone from which the periosteum was reflected, once stripped of its blood supply, will undergo a process by which new blood vessels enter the inferior border and resorb bone before adding new osteoid. This creates resorption cavities in the inferior border, which weaken the bone structurally. These resorption cavities are at their maximum size at 2 to 3 weeks postoperatively in adults, after which new bone apposition progressively remodels the area and fills in some of the defect enough to support jaw function on a soft diet (Fig 13-6).

HISTOPATHOLOGY

Grossly, the dentigerous cyst surrounds the crown and is attached to the tooth at the cementoenamel junction (Fig 13-7a). In the uninflamed cyst, the lining resembles the reduced enamel epithelium from which it is derived and consists of two to three rows of cuboidal or flattened epithelium (Figs 13-7b and 13-7c). Mucous cells may be present and sometimes are quite prominent. Some are ciliated (Fig 13-7d). The wall is fibrous, and the stroma contains abundant mucopolysaccharides so that it may appear basophilic and myxoid. Often rests of odontogenic epithelium are present, and dystrophic calcifications may be seen (Fig 13-7e). As in radicular cysts, Rushton bodies can be found within the lining. Many dentigerous cysts are inflamed, and consequently proliferative changes may occur within the epithelium with the formation of rete ridges. Cholesterol clefts may also be seen. These inflammatory changes can result in a picture indistinguishable from a radicular cyst.

PROGNOSIS

Enucleation of a dentigerous cyst is curative and recurrences are almost unheard of, unlike the odontogenic keratocyst, which has a recurrence rate ranging from 5% to 70%. The difference seems to be that if a portion of a dentigerous cyst lining remains, it will lie dormant and not retain its stimulation to form another cyst. Because the cells seem to be more independent in their proliferation and more active, an odontogenic keratocyst seems to recur if the slightest portion of cyst lining remains. In addition, many recurrent odontogenic keratocysts are actually new primary keratocysts arising from other epithelial

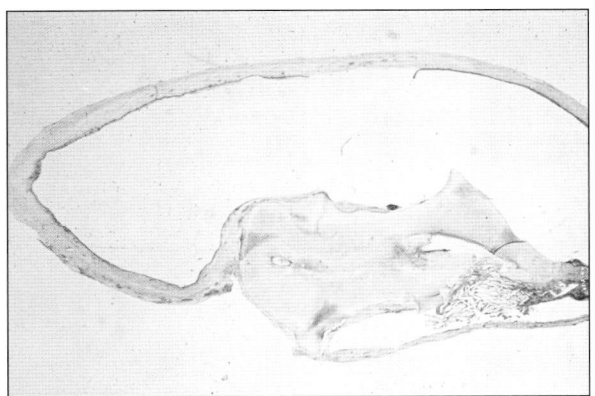

Fig 13-7a This decalcified specimen shows a dentigerous cyst attached to the crown of the tooth.

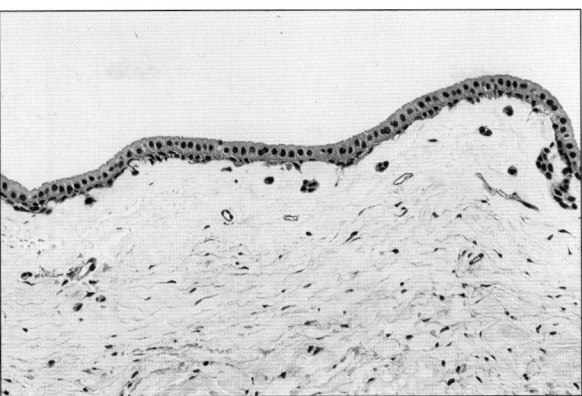

Fig 13-7b Dentigerous cyst lined by simple reduced enamel epithelium.

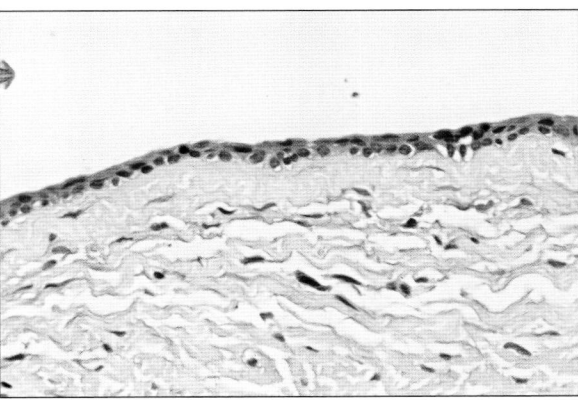

Fig 13-7c Dentigerous cyst lined by a thin stratified squamous epithelium.

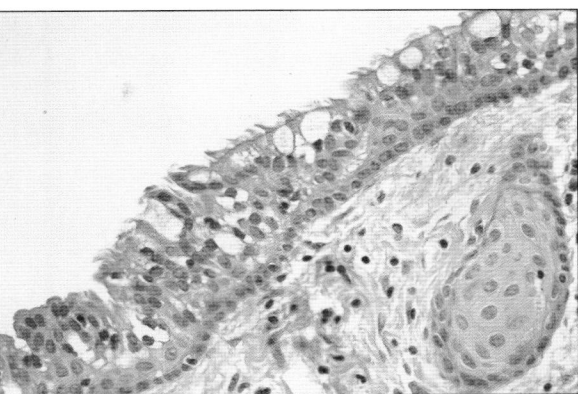

Fig 13-7d Dentigerous cyst with mucous glands and cilia in the lining.

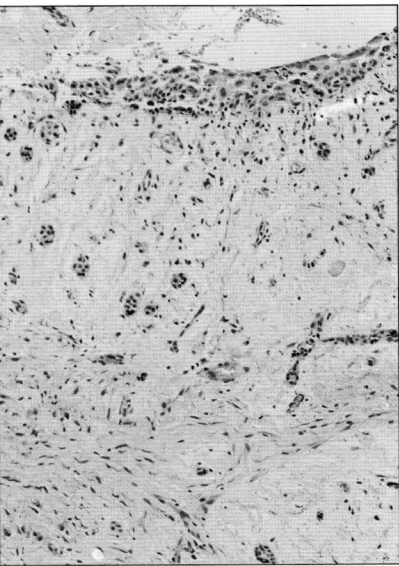

Fig 13-7e The wall of a dentigerous cyst will frequently have areas of myxoid tissue and rests of odontogenic epithelium, which may be numerous.

rests. The low recurrence potential of a dentigerous cyst is also related to the exhausted nature of the reduced enamel epithelium, which has differentiated and formed tooth crown enamel before becoming a cyst. In contrast, the odontogenic keratocyst of primordial origin arises from reactivated dental lamina cells that have not differentiated or formed enamel. Therefore, these cells are more primitive and retain a more active biologic potential. This may also explain to some degree the reduced biologic activity and reduced recurrence rate of odontogenic keratocysts of dentigerous origin.

Paradental Cyst

The paradental cyst is a clinical variant of the dentigerous cyst. It is actually a dentigerous cyst arising from a third molar (or, rarely, other teeth) that is partially erupted. It often arises as an inflammatory process. The partially erupted tooth displaces the cyst buccally so that it lies against the buccal roots or bifurcation of these teeth. It will produce a unilocular radiolucency superimposed over the roots of the involved tooth or an adjacent tooth. Its treatment and prognosis are the same as with any other dentigerous cyst.

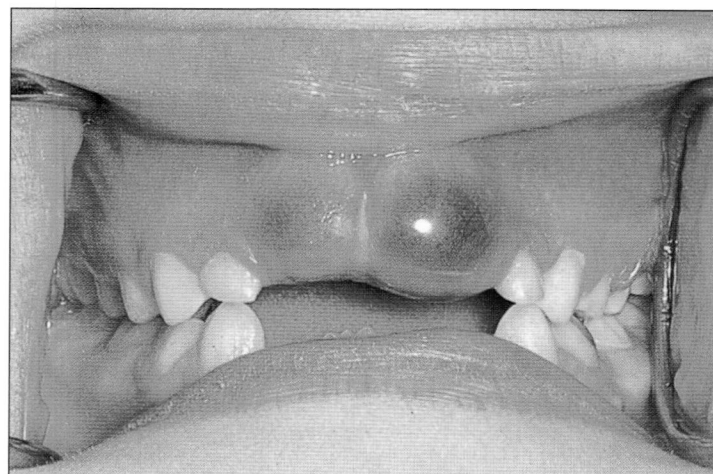

Fig 13-8a Illustration of an eruption cyst. Note that the cyst lining is attached at the cementoenamel junction of the tooth but is separate from the crestal mucosa at this time.

Fig 13-8b Thinned and expanded oral mucosa in the area of an anticipated tooth eruption. The mucosa may be tense and sometimes blue because of the fluid within the eruption cyst. (Reprinted from Strassburg M and Knolle G, *Diseases of the Oral Mucosa: A Color Atlas*, with permission from Quintessence Publishing Co.)

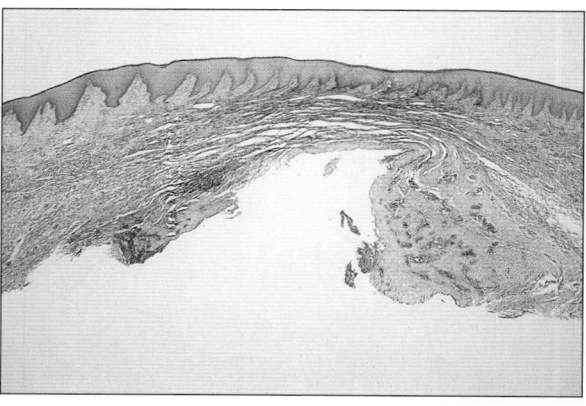

Fig 13-8c Fragments of a thin epithelium can be seen lining the fibrous tissue, which has become compressed by the eruption cyst.

HISTOPATHOLOGY ▶ Paradental cysts are frequently inflammatory cysts and have the same histologic appearance as the radicular cyst, despite the fact that they probably arise from reduced enamel epithelium.

Eruption Cyst

An eruption cyst (Fig 13-8a) is another type of dentigerous cyst. Its pathogenetic theories are the same, but the cyst occurs just as the tooth is erupting. It is mostly seen in children with eruption of their primary teeth or permanent incisors and molars. It will present as a compressible expansion of the soft tissue ridge, where a radiograph shows signs of eruption. Because the cyst is not in bone, there is no discernible radiolucency, but a soft tissue thickness can be appreciated (Fig 13-8b). The cyst will often thin the overlying mucosa so that the fluid inside, viewed through the ridge mucosa, may appear blue. This appearance, together with occasions when actual bleeding occurs in the cyst, has led to the term *eruption hematoma*.

No treatment is usually necessary since eruption of the tooth will naturally marsupialize the cyst lining to the ridge mucosa as it does with normal dental follicles. At times it may be necessary to uncover the erupting tooth. The excision of a small amount of crestal gingiva marsupializes the cyst so that the cyst epithelium becomes confluent with the gingival epithelium, enabling cyst resolution and continued tooth eruption.

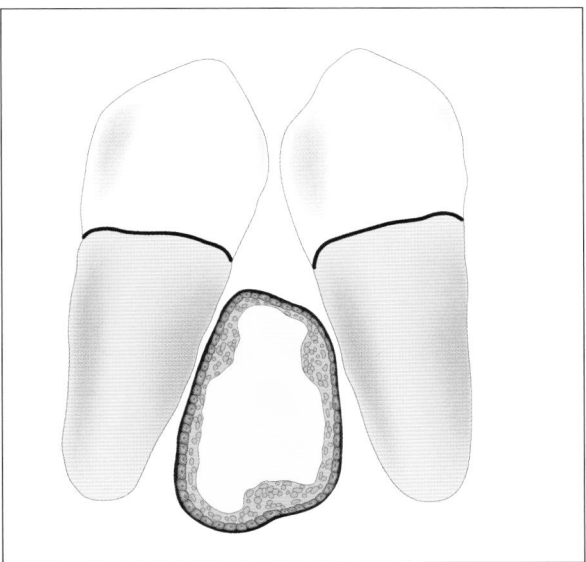

Fig 13-9a Illustration of a lateral periodontal cyst. Note the generally thin lining with focal thickened areas.

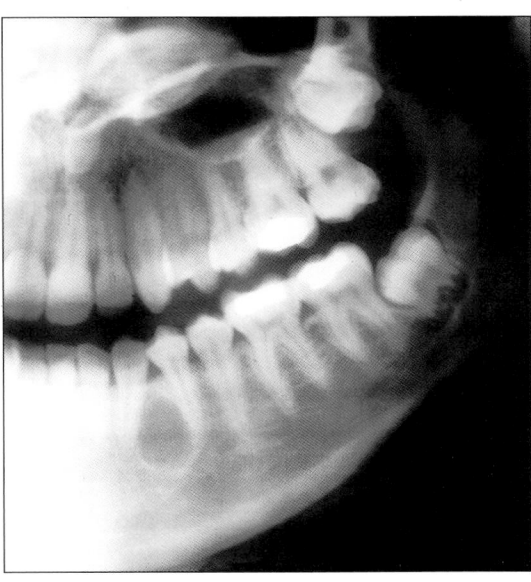

Fig 13-9b A lateral periodontal cyst often appears as an oval or teardrop-shaped radiolucency around and between the premolar or canine teeth.

HISTOPATHOLOGY ▶

Eruption cysts are essentially dentigerous cysts in an extraosseous location. The cyst envelops the crown of the developing tooth and is lined by reduced enamel epithelium as in the dentigerous cyst. The overlying mucosa is compressed and thinned by the cyst (Fig 13-8c).

Lateral Periodontal Cyst

CLINICAL PRESENTATION AND PATHOGENESIS ▶

The lateral periodontal cyst (Fig 13-9a) is a primordial cyst that arises from dental lamina rests that lie within the interradicular crestal or midroot-level bone. Therefore, it develops between teeth. In the mandible as well as the maxilla it develops around the premolars and the canine areas. It occurs mostly in adults older than 21 years and has a male predilection.

The lateral periodontal cyst will usually present as an incidental radiographic finding of a round or teardrop-shaped unilocular radiolucency between teeth. The teeth will be vital and nonmobile and may show root divergence. There is usually no soft tissue swelling associated with the cyst and no root resorption (Fig 13-9b).

It would be reasonable to assume that a cyst arising between teeth would arise from the seemingly ubiquitous rests of Malassez. However, the evidence points toward dental lamina rests, which are usually found in the ridge mucosa (rests of Serres) but can also be found in the interradicular bone. The lateral periodontal cyst is then akin to the gingival cysts of the newborn and the adult as well as the odontogenic keratocyst, all of which arise from dental lamina rests.

DIFFERENTIAL DIAGNOSIS ▶

Because the lateral periodontal cyst forms an interradicular radiolucency, its differential list includes other lesions that can do the same. The *botryoid odontogenic cyst,* the main differential lesion, represents a variant of the lateral periodontal cyst. Its unique histologic features and slightly greater potential to recur warrant its distinction on a differential list. Another differential lesion noted to occur in this fashion is the *odontogenic keratocyst,* which is still another primordial cyst that arises from dental lamina rests. In addition, odontogenic tumors such as an early *ameloblastoma* or *odontogenic myxoma* are prime considerations. Although a rare lesion, the *squamous odontogenic tumor* bears some consideration because of its propensity to occur between premolars. Idiopathic bone cavities can also occur in this location.

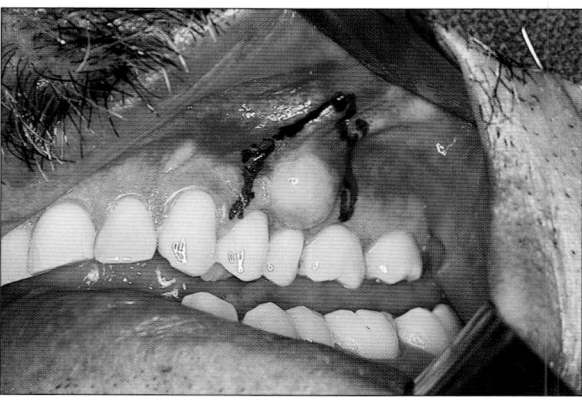

Fig 13-10a The lateral periodontal cyst is usually located between premolars and may significantly thin the overlying attached gingiva.

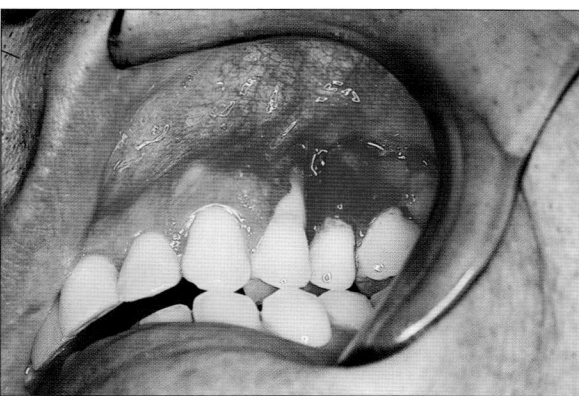

Fig 13-10b Excision of the overlying mucosa along with the cyst will result in a periodontal defect, gingival loss, and root exposures.

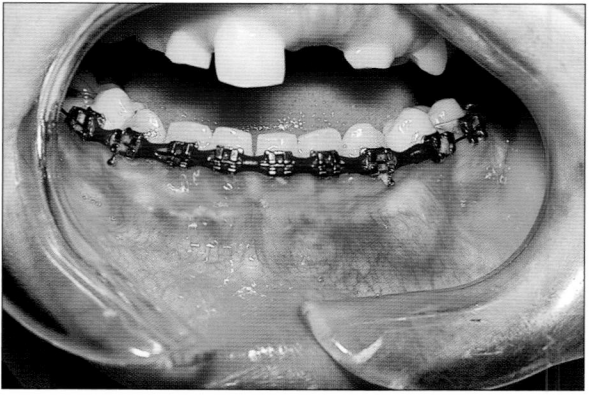

Fig 13-10c A lateral periodontal cyst (or similarly located cysts) should be removed with an attempt to separate the labial gingiva/mucosa from the cyst.

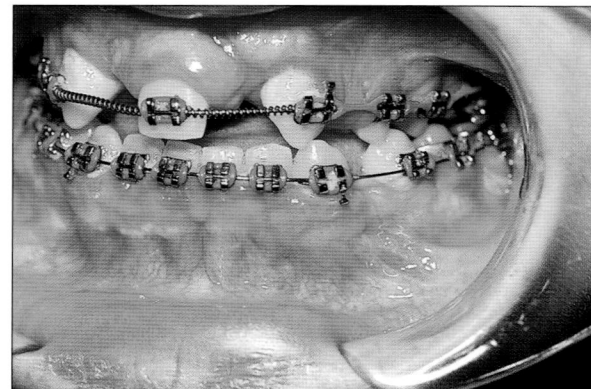

Fig 13-10d Preservation of the labial gingiva/mucosa will prevent interradicular bone loss and root exposures.

DIAGNOSTIC WORK-UP AND TREATMENT

Periapical radiographs and a panoramic radiograph are best suited to reveal the details of this lesion and to enable assessment of the jaws for other lesions. The cyst is enucleated by a labial mucoperiosteal flap, since most cysts lie toward the lateral cortex of the interradicular bone (Figs 13-10a and 13-10b). To avoid damage to adjacent root surfaces, a broad-based flap for direct access and complete coverage of the resultant defect is recommended. Due to the usually large buccal wall defect, long-term resorbable membrane techniques or permanent membranes that require removal later will enhance bone regeneration and prevent collapse and ingrowth of soft tissue into the defect (Figs 13-10c and 13-10d).

HISTOPATHOLOGY

Lateral periodontal cysts are lined by a thin epithelium of two to three cell layers that resembles reduced enamel epithelium (Fig 13-11a). Within this lining, thickenings or "plaques" may be seen, which either protrude into the lumen or push into the wall. In these areas, the cells tend to be flattened and may form whorls (Fig 13-11b). Clear cells may be present within the plaques or elsewhere in the lining (Fig 13-11c). Their nuclei are pyknotic, and many of these cells contain glycogen. In some areas, the thin epithelial lining may be squamous. The attachment of the epithelium to the fibrous wall is often tenuous, so that artifactual separation may be observed. The wall is usually uninflamed, and there may be hyalinized areas subjacent to the epithelium.

PROGNOSIS

Enucleation of a lateral periodontal cyst should resolve the cyst without recurrence, and bone will likely be regenerated in the bony defect over 6 months to 1 year. Root divergence, if present, will be reduced or become normalized even without orthodontic tooth movement (Figs 13-12a and 13-12b).

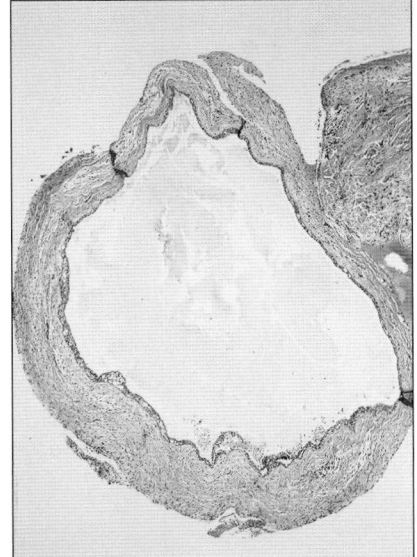

Fig 13-11a Lateral periodontal cyst showing a thin lining with some plaque-like thickenings.

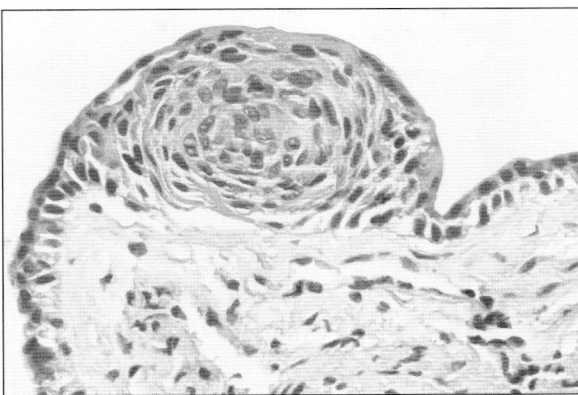

Fig 13-11b The wall of this lateral periodontal cyst shows a lining two cells thick with this area of thickening. Here the epithelial cells have a whorled arrangement.

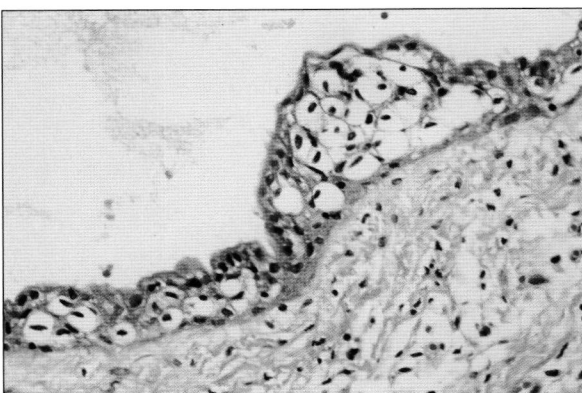

Fig 13-11c The thickened area of this lateral periodontal cyst consists of glycogen-containing clear cells.

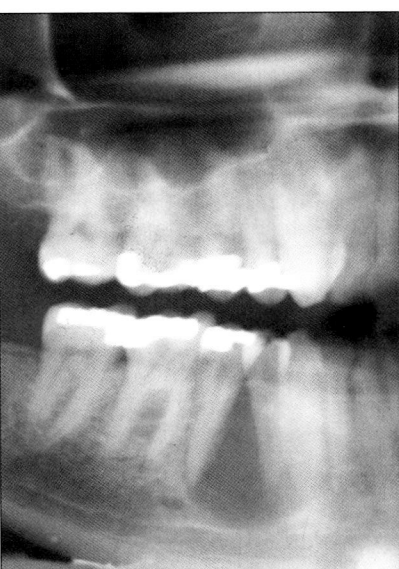

Fig 13-12a Bony defect and root divergence as a result of a lateral periodontal cyst.

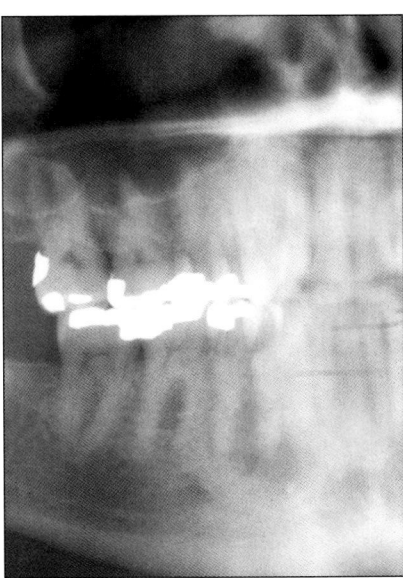

Fig 13-12b Bone fill of the defect shown in Fig 13-12a is evident 1 year later, as is correction of the root divergence.

Botryoid Odontogenic Cyst

The botryoid odontogenic cyst (Fig 13-13a) is a separate variant of the lateral periodontal cyst. Although its histogenesis, locations, and sex and age distribution are identical, it differs from the lateral periodontal cyst radiographically, histologically, and prognostically (Fig 13-13b). It creates a multilocular radiolucency between teeth that will resemble a grape cluster (botryoid), which corresponds to a cyst lining

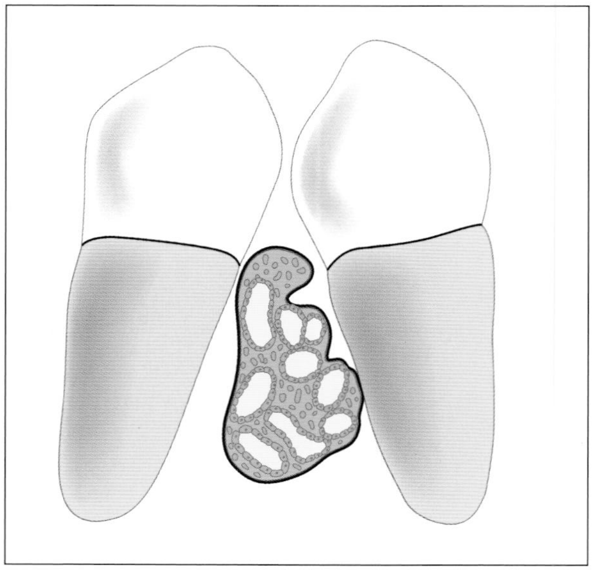

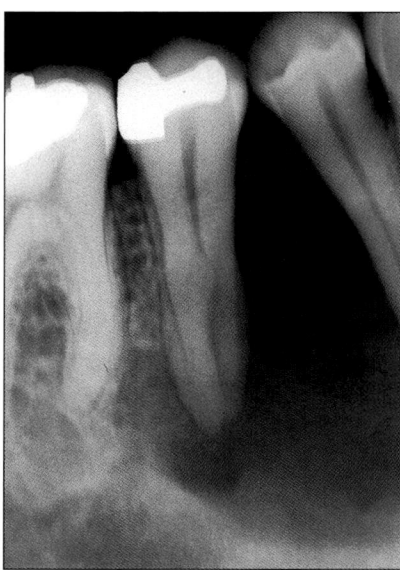

Fig 13-13a Illustration of a botryoid odontogenic cyst. Note the thin epithelial lining, which is 1 to 3 cells thick, and its multilocularity.

Fig 13-13b An interradicular multilocular radiolucency between premolars caused by a botryoid odontogenic cyst, resulting in root divergence. Ameloblastomas, keratocysts, myxomas, and hemangiomas, among others, can produce an identical radiographic picture.

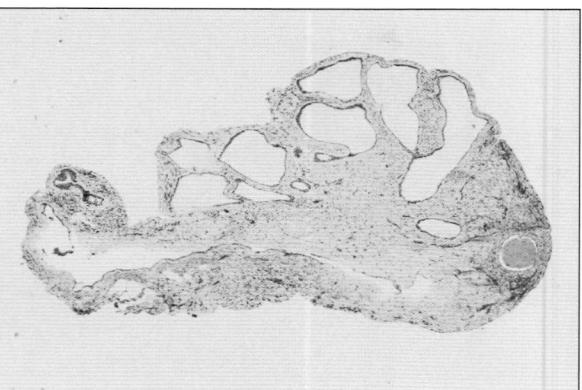

Fig 13-13c Botryoid odontogenic cyst showing its multilocularity.

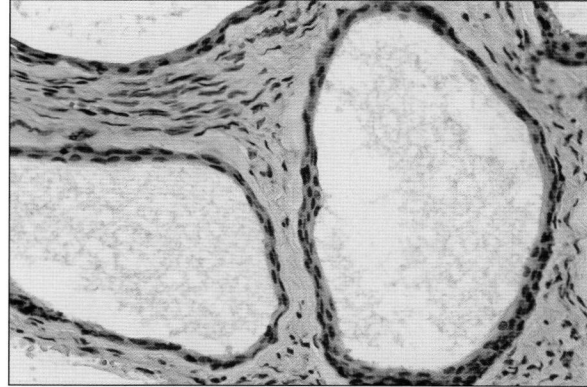

Fig 13-13d The botryoid odontogenic cyst is lined by a thin stratified squamous epithelium.

with numerous lobulations and thickened epithelial tufts again resembling a grape cluster. These numerous loculations impart an added degree of difficulty in the removal of a botryoid odontogenic cyst. Therefore, the probability of an incomplete removal is greater, causing a higher recurrence potential.

HISTOPATHOLOGY ▶ The botryoid odontogenic cyst appears to be a multilocular variant of the lateral periodontal cyst. The thin epithelial lining may be cuboidal or squamous. Plaque-like thickenings may occur. The locules are separated by thin fibrous septae (Figs 13-13c and 13-13d).

Gingival Cyst of the Adult

The gingival cyst of the adult (Fig 13-14a) is the soft tissue counterpart to the lateral periodontal cyst. It arises from the same dental lamina rests, those that came to be located in the ridge mucosa rather than in the bone (Fig 13-14b). Like the lateral periodontal cyst, it occurs in the adult mandibular pre-

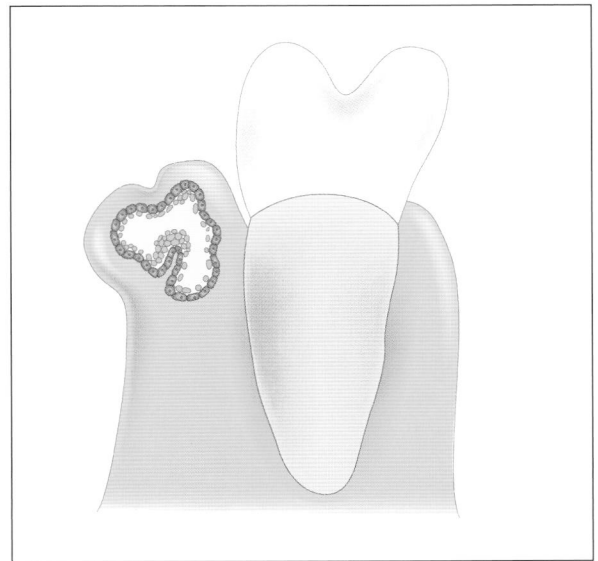

Fig 13-14a Illustration of a gingival cyst of the adult. Note its thin folded lining and its position strictly within soft tissue.

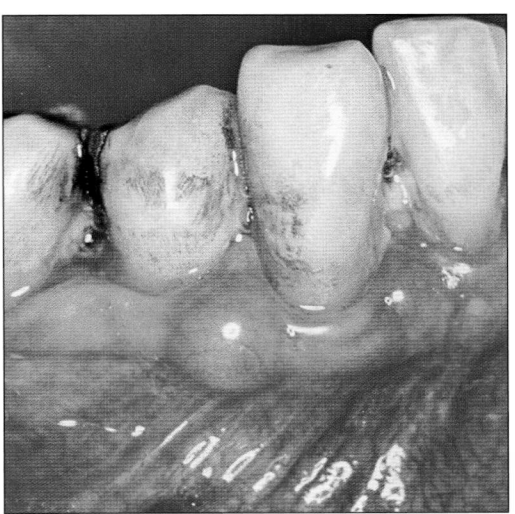

Fig 13-14b A gingival cyst is restricted to the gingiva and has no presence in bone. Unlike the lateral periodontal cyst or botryoid odontogenic cyst, it probably arises from more crestally positioned rests of Serres in the gingiva.

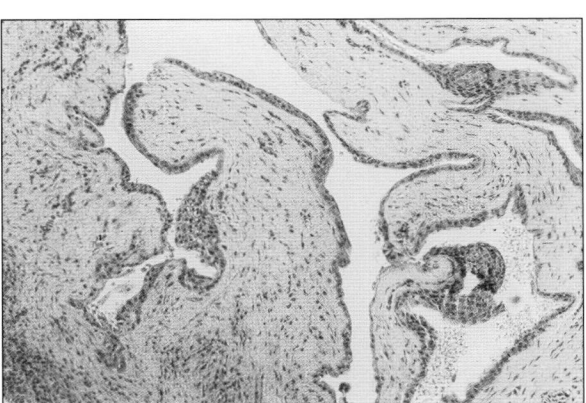

Fig 13-14c Gingival cyst of the adult with a thin lining showing plaque-like thickenings, as in the lateral periodontal cyst.

molar areas and in the maxillary incisor and canine areas. Unlike the lateral periodontal cyst, it shows no male predilection, but the wide age range is identical.

The gingival cyst of the adult clinically presents as a small soft tissue swelling, 1 cm in diameter or less, within the dental papilla or in the midcrestal area in edentulous ridges. Its thinning of the overlying mucosa imparts a bluish color. There is no radiographic evidence of bone resorption, and only a reduced KVP potential exposed periapical radiograph will show its soft tissue density. It is treated by simple excision and a primary closure. Recurrence is not seen.

HISTOPATHOLOGY ▶

The gingival cyst of the adult is similar to the lateral periodontal cyst histologically; the lining is usually thin, resembling reduced enamel epithelium, and may have plaque-like thickenings (Fig 13-14c). Clear cells may also be present. Sometimes the lining may be a stratified squamous epithelium without rete ridges, and occasionally it is keratinized. Termed *gingival cysts* because of their location, these may more appropriately be considered dental lamina cysts.

Gingival Cyst of the Newborn

The gingival cyst of the newborn, which appears clinically as multiple nodules along the edentulous ridges of newborns, is a curiosity (Fig 13-15a). Formerly called *Bohn's nodules*, they represent small dental lamina cysts that produce keratin to form firm white gingival nodules. They require no specific treatment other than reassurance to the newborn's parents. Their natural history will be one of involution or rupture into the oral cavity, where their lining becomes marsupialized and then normalized into the oral mucosa before 3 months of age.

A similar phenomenon may occur in the palatal midline, where small epithelial inclusion cysts arise in newborns related to the fusion of the palatal and nasal process. These are often termed *Epstein's pearls* or *palatine cysts of the newborn*. Their natural history is also one of involution or oral rupture and fusion to the palatal mucosa within just a few months.

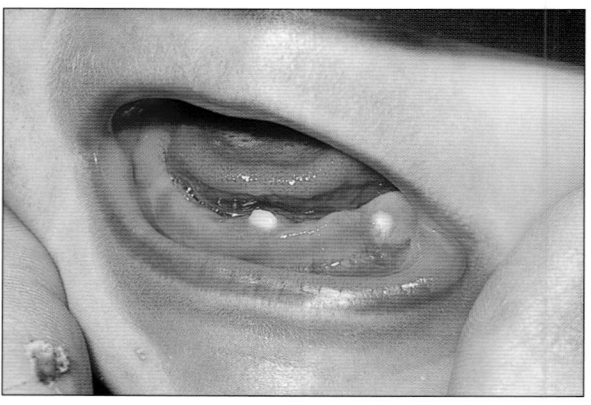

Fig 13-15a Gingival cysts of the newborn will appear as small nodules and will be white because of keratin in the lumen.

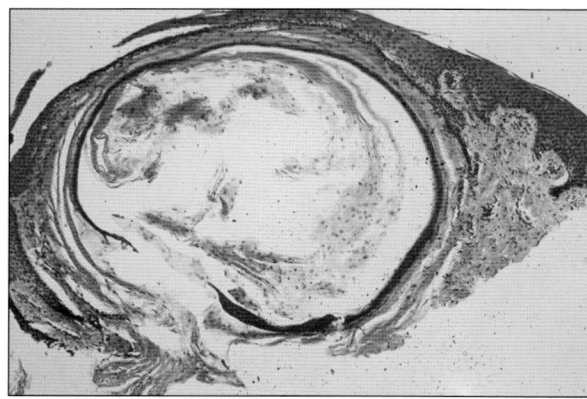

Fig 13-15b A gingival cyst of the newborn is lined by a keratinizing stratified squamous epithelium with keratin in the lumen.

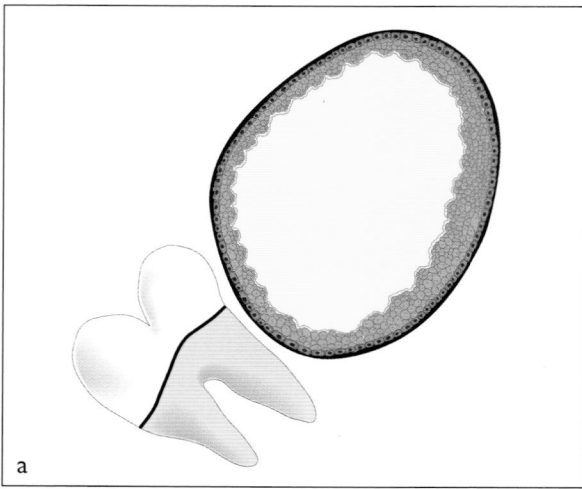

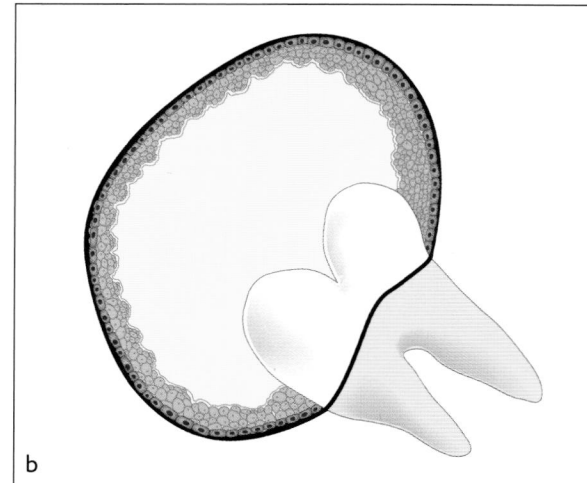

Figs 13-16a and 13-16b There are two basic types of odontogenic keratocysts: (*a*) the primordial-origin keratocyst and (*b*) the dentigerous-origin keratocyst. Note that the thickness and the details of the cyst lining are the same. They differ only in their origin.

HISTOPATHOLOGY ▶

Gingival cysts of the newborn are small and round. They are lined by a thin, stratified, squamous epithelium that is parakeratinized but has a flat basal cell layer. The lumen is filled with keratin (Fig 13-15b).

Odontogenic Keratocyst

CLINICAL PRESENTATION AND PATHOGENESIS ▶

The odontogenic keratocyst is a histopathologically and behaviorally unique, specific entity. It is the most aggressive and recurrent of all the odontogenic cysts and shows characteristics resembling both a cyst and a benign tumor. Most (60%) arise from dental lamina rests or from the basal cells of oral epithelium and are thus primordial-origin odontogenic keratocysts (Fig 13-16a). The remaining 40% arise from the reduced enamel epithelium of the dental follicle and are thus dentigerous-origin odontogenic keratocysts (Fig 13-16b). This clinical identification is of some importance because recurrences are more frequently seen after treatment of the primordial origin type.

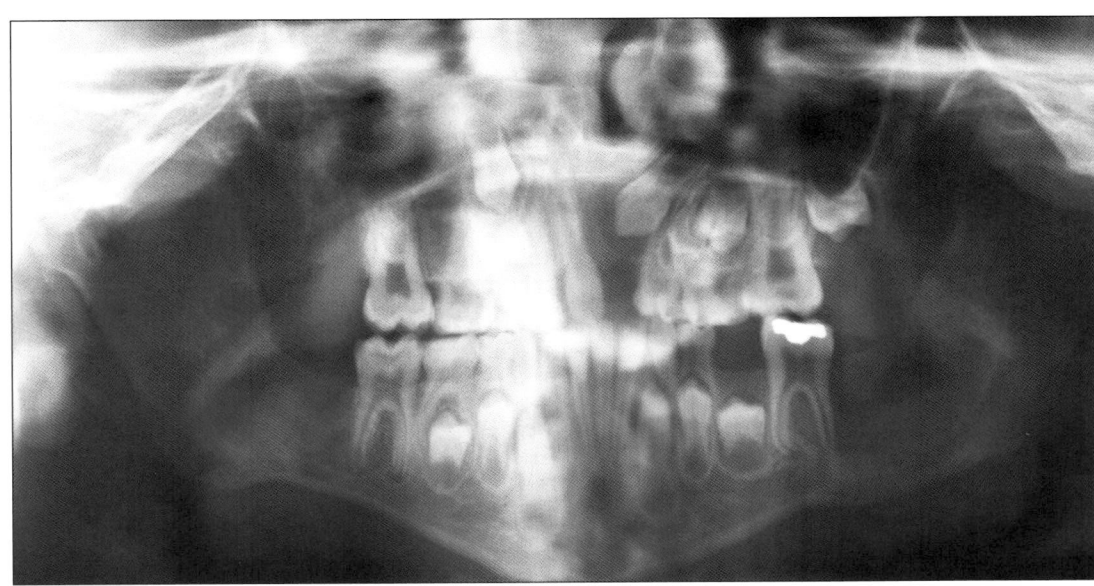

Fig 13-16c Several synchronous odontogenic keratocysts in an individual with basal cell nevus syndrome.

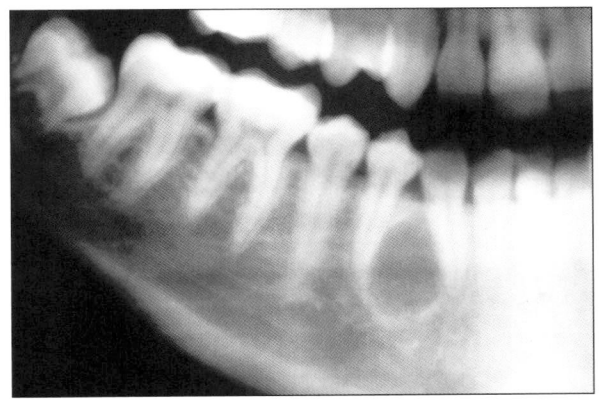

Fig 13-17 An odontogenic keratocyst may also present as a small, unilocular radiolucency. The premolar area is a well-known location and may be identical to the presentation of a lateral periodontal cyst.

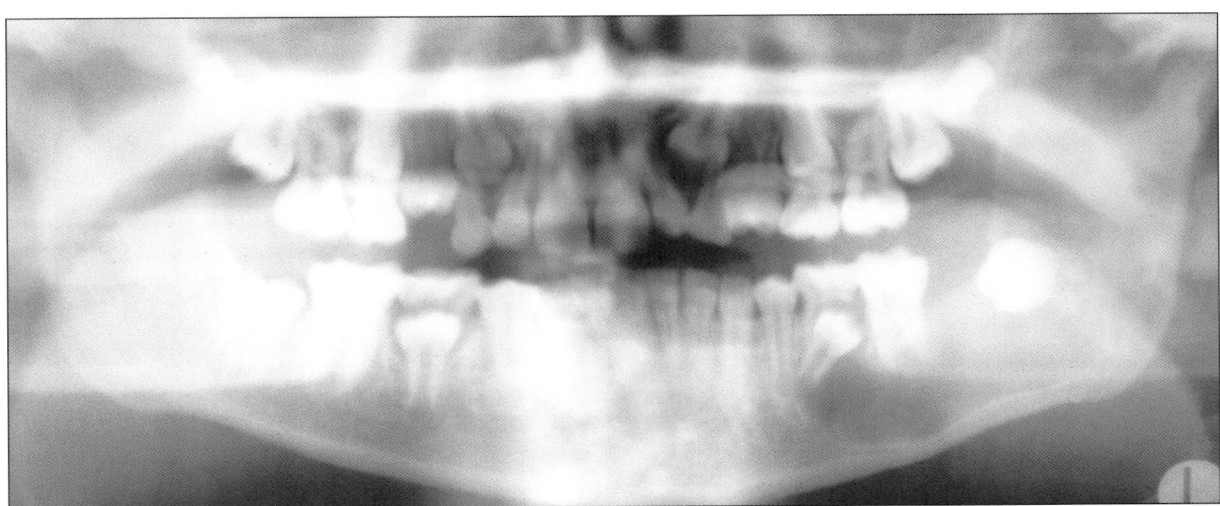

Fig 13-18 A large, unilocular keratocyst may displace teeth and the mandibular canal. The radiolucency is usually asymmetric because of the cyst's faster and more advanced progression through the medullary bone compared to the cortices.

While odontogenic keratocysts have a peak incidence in the teenage years and 20s, they occur at all ages. They occur in children as part of the basal cell nevus syndrome and have the propensity for several to occur at one time or for several new primary cysts to occur over several years (Fig 13-16c). Twice as many odontogenic keratocysts form in the mandible as in the maxilla, and as anticipated most are in the third molar region. In the maxilla, the third molar and canine areas have a high incidence.

An odontogenic keratocyst may present in a variety of sizes and situations. Some are small and unilocular (Fig 13-17), others large and unilocular (Fig 13-18), and still others multilocular (Fig 13-19). Most will be asymptomatic. The larger cysts will cause expansion and may cause tooth mobility. Some will rupture and leak keratin into the surrounding tissue, provoking an intense inflammatory response

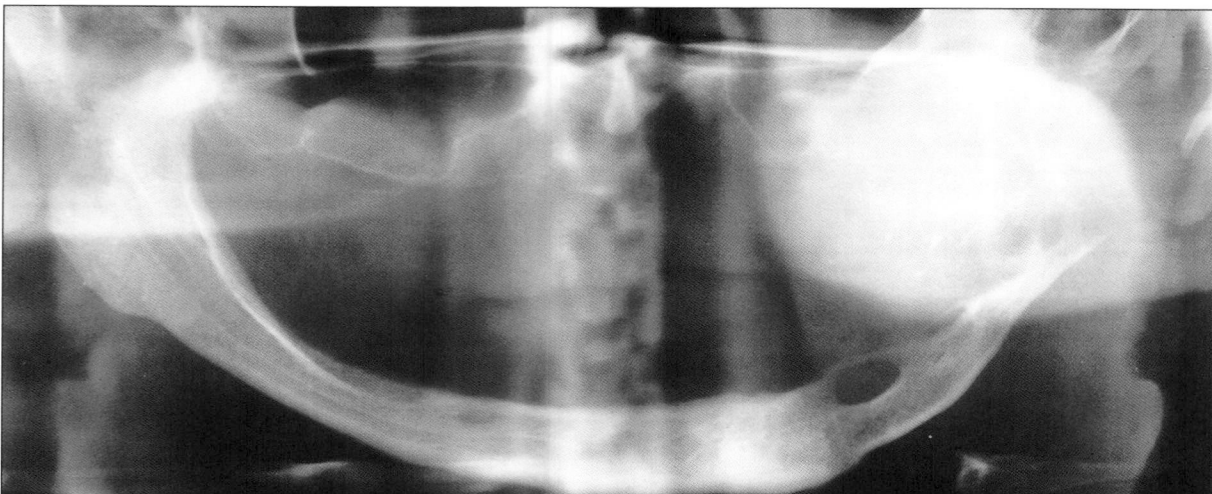

Fig 13-19 Large, multilocular keratocysts will be suggestive of benign tumors and may even produce a pathologic fracture, as this one did.

that causes pain and swelling. The cysts will not affect nerve sensation, although they will frequently displace the inferior alveolar neurovascular bundle to the inferior border. Their resorption of bone will include cortex and inferior border, but at a slower rate than the intermedullary trabecular bone, which is less dense. Therefore, they extend further anteroposteriorly than buccolingually (see Fig 13-18). This principle of further extension through bone that is less dense also explains the finding of greater buccal expansion than palatal expansion in the maxilla. The cysts also frequently resorb the roots of adjacent teeth in a smooth and regular pattern.

DIFFERENTIAL DIAGNOSIS ▶

The odontogenic keratocyst essentially includes three separate differential lists, depending on its general presentation: a dentigerous-origin keratocyst presents a picture that is statistically most likely to be the more common *dentigerous cyst.* If the cyst is located in the anterior region of the jaws, an *adenomatoid odontogenic cyst* becomes a serious consideration. The *ameloblastoma* and *ameloblastic fibroma* would follow.

The unilocular, primordial-origin keratocyst often resembles a *lateral periodontal cyst* if it is located between premolar teeth, a *residual cyst* if it occurs in an area of a previous cyst removal or endodontic therapy, and an *idiopathic bone cavity* if it interdigitates between teeth, as can an odontogenic keratocyst. In the anterior region of the jaws, the cyst resembles an *adenomatoid odontogenic cyst* because approximately one third of adenomatoid odontogenic cysts are of primordial origin and unassociated with an impacted tooth. This presentation may also be compatible with that of an *ameloblastoma* or an *ameloblastic fibroma.*

The multilocular, primordial origin keratocyst does not resemble most cystic lesions. Therefore, entities such as dentigerous cysts, adenomatoid odontogenic cysts, and idiopathic bone cavities are inappropriate with this presentation. Instead, this presentation is much more suggestive of tumors. Three entities well-known to cause mandibular expansion with a multilocular presence are the *ameloblastoma,* the *odontogenic myxoma,* and the *central giant cell tumor.* Less common, but well-known to be multilocular, is a *central arteriovenous hemangioma* of the jaws. In addition, if the lesion is a small, multilocular lesion between premolar or canine teeth, a *botryoid odontogenic cyst* is a strong consideration.

DIAGNOSTIC WORK-UP ▶

Small, unilocular lesions can be diagnosed and treated based on periapical and panoramic radiographs with an enucleation and curettage procedure. Large lesions and those that are multilocular should undergo an incisional biopsy to rule out a neoplasm and a CT scan to define lesion extent and to plan surgical removal (Fig 13-20a).

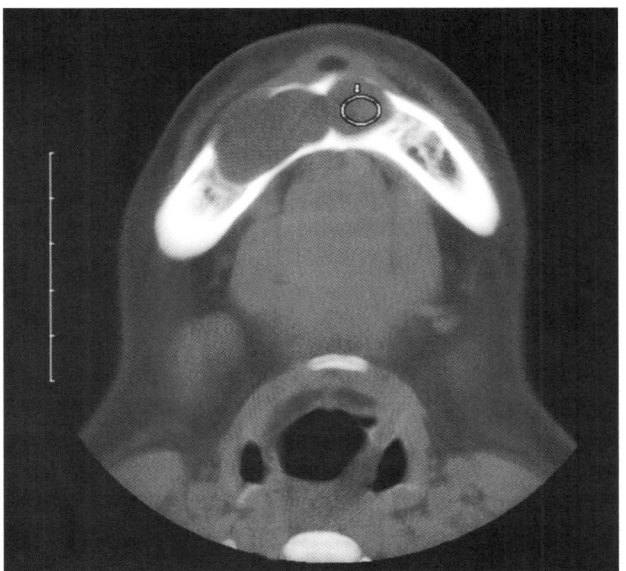

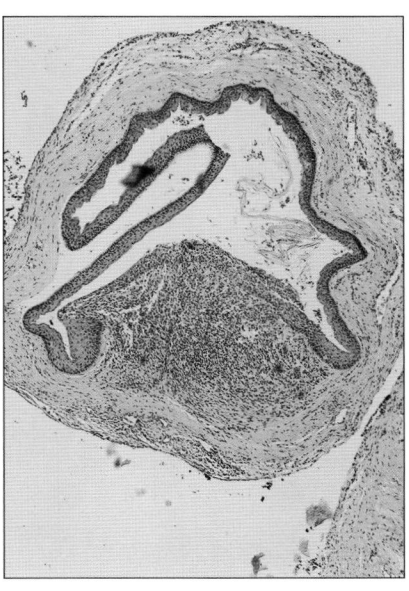

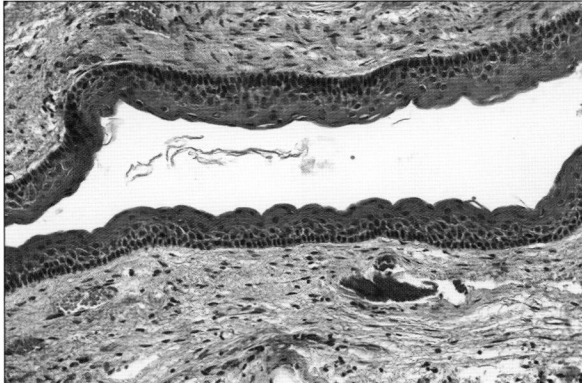

Fig 13-20a Since large, multilocular odontogenic keratocysts will radiographically appear similar to benign tumors,
an incisional biopsy to establish a conclusive diagnosis is
preferred in this situation.

Fig 13-20b Odontogenic keratocyst
with foldings in the lining.

Fig 13-20c Typical odontogenic keratocyst lining
showing a flat epithelial–connective tissue interface, a
parakeratinized corrugated surface, and hyperchromatic
palisaded basal cells. The wall is fibrous with no apparent inflammation.

HISTOPATHOLOGY ▶

While the diagnosis of many odontogenic cysts depends primarily on history, clinical presentation, and radiographic appearance, the diagnosis of the odontogenic keratocyst is made purely on its histologic features. In most cases, this is straightforward. The typical odontogenic keratocyst is lined by stratified squamous epithelium that lacks rete ridges so that the epithelial-connective tissue interface is flat. The lining tends to separate readily from the wall and may be considerably folded (Fig 13-20b). Both of these features make it more difficult to obtain a total removal of the cyst. The epithelial surface is parakera-tinized and often corrugated. Most significantly, the basal cells are hyperchromatic and cuboidal to colum-nar in shape and have palisaded nuclei (Fig 13-20c).

The fibrous wall may contain epithelial islands, which show central keratinization and cyst formation (Fig 13-20d). These are known as "daughter" or "satellite" cysts. Sometimes the keratinization of these islands is such that it may suggest squamous cell carcinoma. The cyst lining will occasionally show small basal extensions (Fig 13-20e). These do not appear to be the source of the daughter cysts but instead represent additional dental lamina rests.

The cystic lumen contains keratin in varying quantities, but it is usually quite sparse, and sometimes only a clear fluid will be found. Because the development of an odontogenic keratocyst is not mediated by an inflammatory process, typically the wall is not inflamed. However, secondary inflammation is not uncommon. If this is sufficiently severe, the epithelium can lose its distinctive features and revert to a nonspecific, nonkeratinizing stratified squamous epithelium (Figs 13-20f and 13-20g). Usually, some areas of the lining retain their diagnostic features.

The odontogenic keratocysts associated with basal cell nevus syndrome are histologically the same as the solitary cysts. However, a higher incidence of basal budding and satellite cysts has been consistently re-ported in these cases.

Odontogenic cysts that exhibit keratinization are not necessarily odontogenic keratocysts. Areas of squamous metaplasia may occur within radicular or residual cysts, although this is not common. Cysts that are orthokeratinized often have the radiographic appearance of dentigerous cysts. Histologically,

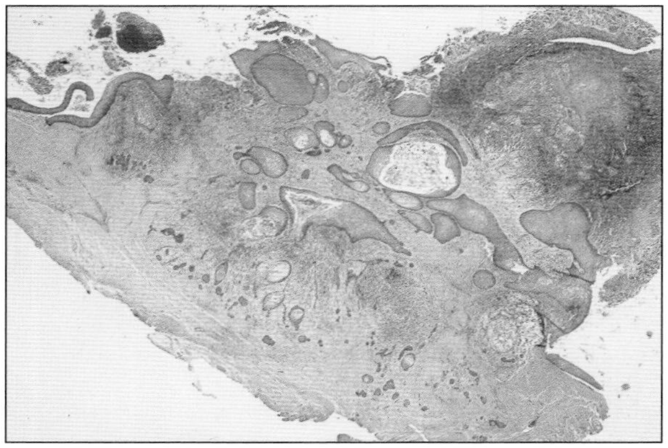

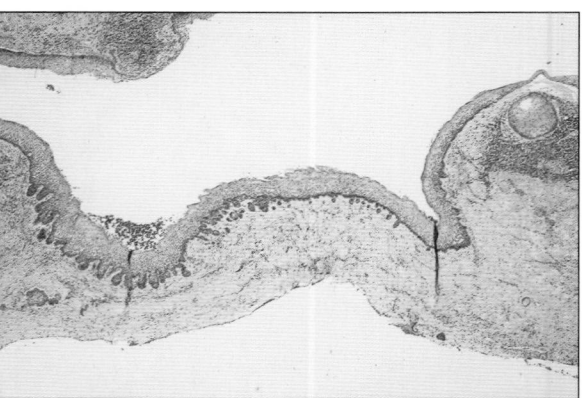

Fig 13-20d Odontogenic keratocyst with daughter cysts in the wall.

Fig 13-20e Odontogenic keratocyst showing bud-like proliferations in the basal area.

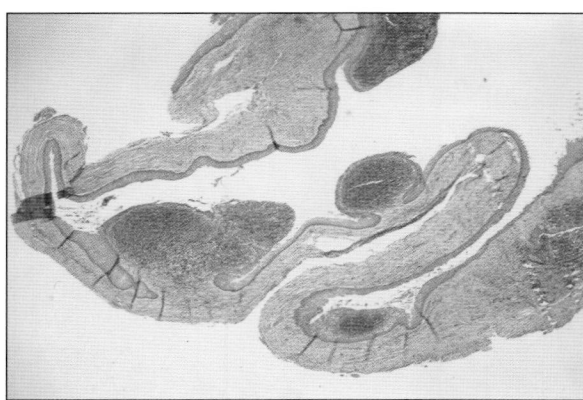

Fig 13-20f Odontogenic keratocyst with foci of chronic inflammation.

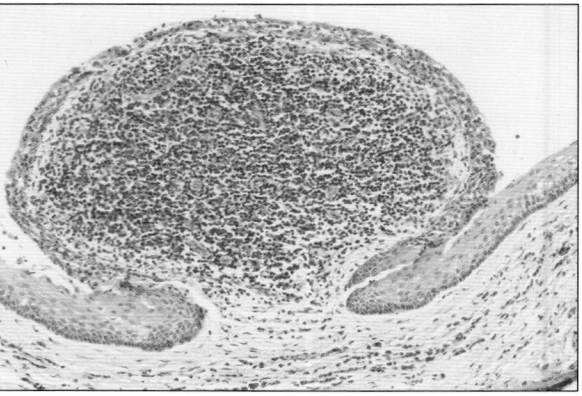

Fig 13-20g Higher-power view of Fig 13-20f showing the change in the epithelium overlying the area of inflammation. The pathognomonic features of the odontogenic keratocyst are no longer present.

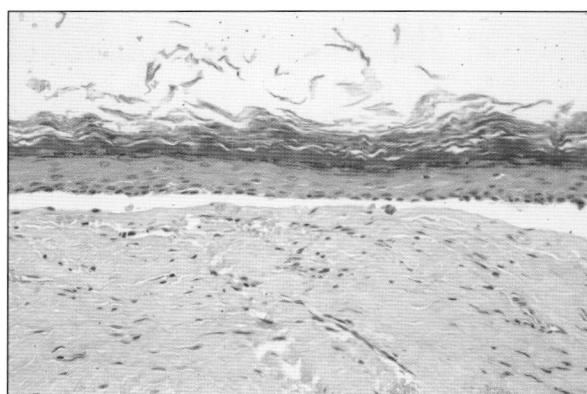

Fig 13-20h Keratinizing odontogenic cyst showing orthokeratin, a granular cell layer, and flattened basal cells.

they have a thin lining with a flat orthokeratinized surface, a prominent granular cell layer, and a flat epithelial–connective tissue interface. Most significantly, the basal cells are flat or low cuboidal and are not hyperchromatic or palisaded (Fig 13-20h). In addition, satellite cysts are not seen. It is well recognized that these cysts do not have the propensity for recurrence as seen in the true odontogenic keratocyst. We therefore prefer to call these cysts *keratinizing odontogenic cysts* to reflect their true origin and to distinguish them from true odontogenic keratocysts.

Occasionally, a cyst will demonstrate features of both the odontogenic keratocyst and keratinizing odontogenic cyst. In this situation, it is best to treat them as odontogenic keratocysts.

TREATMENT ▶

The general approach to treating odontogenic keratocysts is enucleation and curettage. The alternative therapies of marsupialization and resection are also valid but have specific limited indications. One specific indication for marsupialization relates to dentigerous-origin keratocysts, which, through marsupialization, can bring their associated tooth into a functional position in the arch. Another indication applicable to either a dentigerous-origin keratocyst or a primordial-origin keratocyst is when the surgeon's abilities and available facilities pose a risk to developing tooth buds or neurovascular structures (Figs 13-21a to 13-21c). Resection of odontogenic keratocysts is specifically indicated in two instances: (*1*) when there have been multiple (two or more) recurrences after enucleation and curettage procedures, or (*2*) in the case of large multilocular keratocysts in which an enucleation and curettage procedure would result in a near continuity loss by itself (Fig 13-22; see also Fig 13-19).

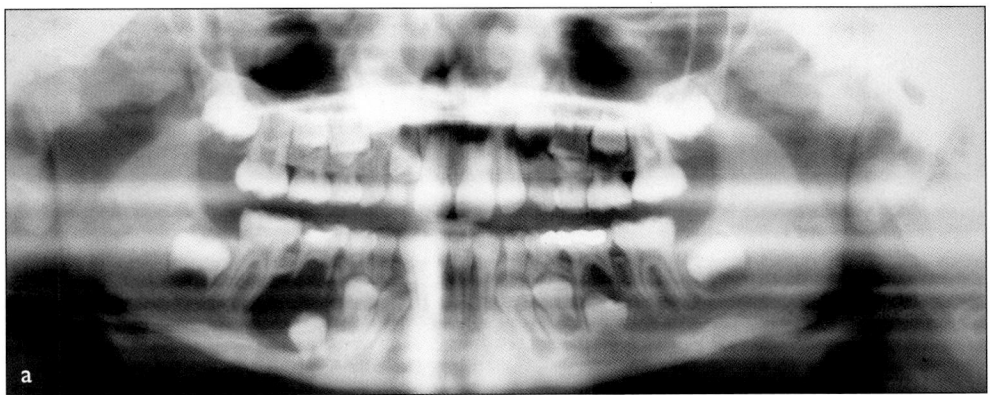

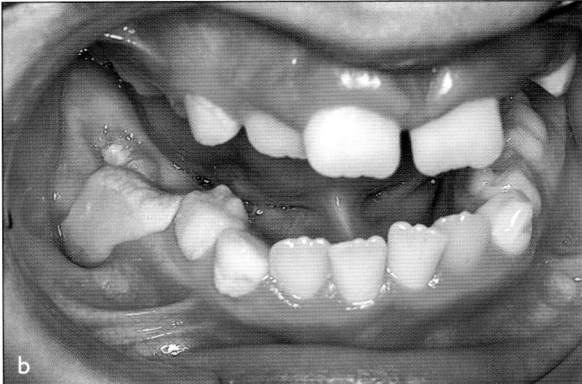
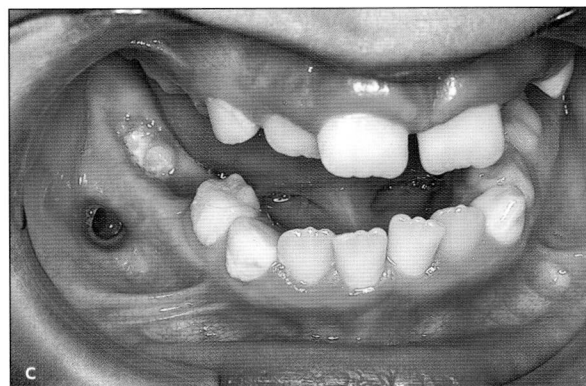

Figs 13-21a to 13-21c Marsupialization is valid in odontogenic keratocyst treatment in selected areas. Here an unerupted tooth that is associated with the cyst is being guided into the arch.

Because recurrence is the major concern in odontogenic keratocyst treatment, specific enucleation and curettage procedures must be followed to minimize the recurrence potential. The two most common reasons for recurrence are failure to remove all of the original cyst lining within bone and new primary cyst formations from additional activated rests or oral basal epithelium. Therefore, the key to reducing recurrence is wide-access enucleation and curettage for all odontogenic keratocysts and the excision of overly keratinized ridge mucosa for those of primordial origin.

The wide access frequently requires a complete lateral decortication so that all of the cyst can be directly visualized during its removal and can be removed in one unit (Fig 13-23). Curetting blindly in a bony pocket invites recurrences. At times, a transcutaneous approach to enucleation and curettage may be necessary, primarily when a large lesion involves the ramus and the condyle area. Because odontogenic keratocysts do not invade epineurium, the inferior alveolar nerve can be separated from the cyst and preserved. In those areas of cortical perforation, the odontogenic keratocyst will herniate out of bone, but it will not infiltrate into the soft tissue as would an ameloblastoma or odontogenic myxoma (Fig 13-24). Therefore, there is no indication to excise a margin of soft tissue in these areas as there is to excise the keratinized ridge mucosa in primordial-origin keratocysts, which is accomplished for the different purpose of eliminating residual activated epithelial rests that have the potential to form new cysts. If the cyst is enucleated as a single, intact unit, curettage of the bony cavity is not necessary as was previously believed. If the entire cyst is enucleated intact, it has by definition been completely removed. "Recurrences" would then only arise from dental lamina rests in the overlying keratinized tissue rather than from the bony cavity. Therefore, curettage of the bony cavity walls, which was previously performed

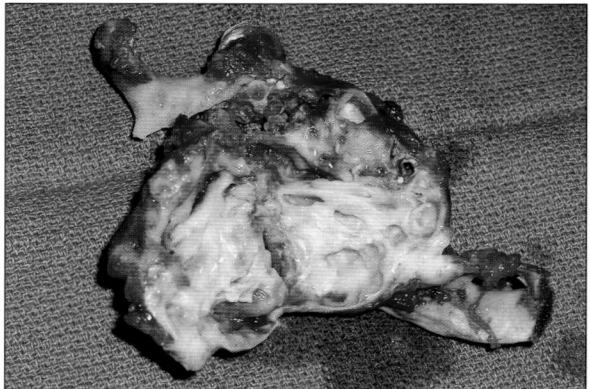

Fig 13-22 This resected keratocyst was multilocular and, as can be seen, multicystic. It caused a pathologic fracture of the mandible, providing no opportunity to curette this lesion for cure while maintaining continuity.

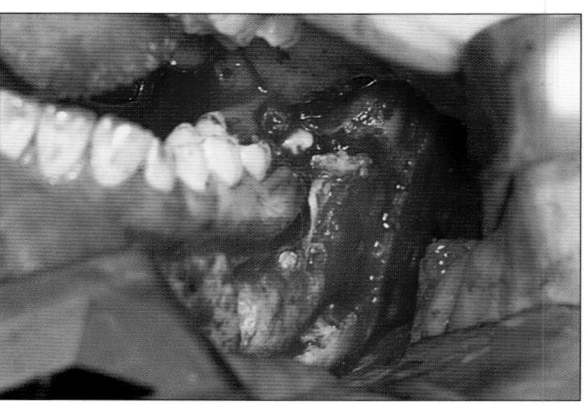

Fig 13-23 Complete lateral decortication, allowing unrestricted access for the removal of a keratocyst in a single unit. This is the most effective means of preventing recurrences from redevelopment of the original cyst.

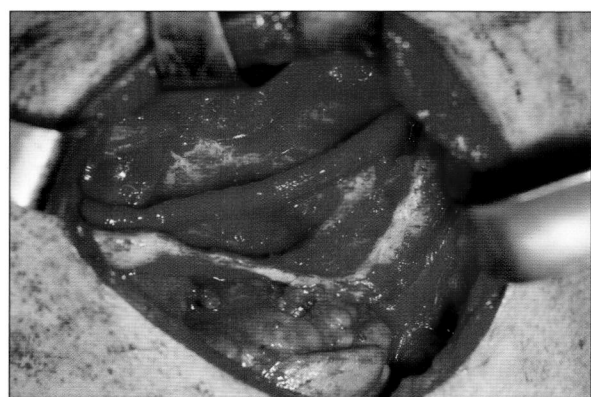

Fig 13-24 A transcutaneous (extraoral) approach to enucleation and curettage of a keratocyst is indicated when much of the ramus and condyle are involved. The neurovascular bundle is preserved and the lingual cortex has been perforated. The keratocyst does not infiltrate the soft tissues adjacent to the mandible. This defect was reinforced with a reconstruction bone plate to prevent fracture (see also Figs 13-26a and 13-26b).

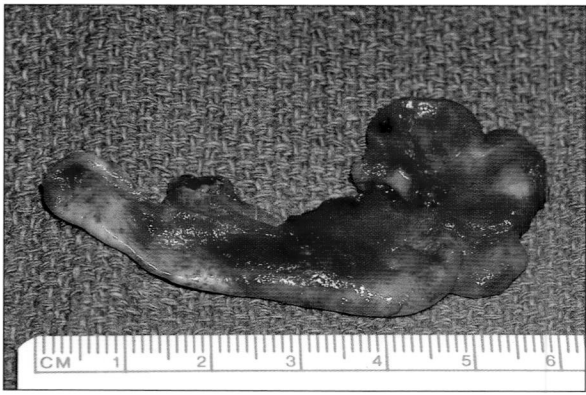

Fig 13-25a An odontogenic keratocyst should be removed in a single unit, as shown here. Note the outpouchings and elongated nature of the keratocyst. The notchings and outpouchings make removal more difficult because they increase the risk of shredding the lining and thus promote recurrence.

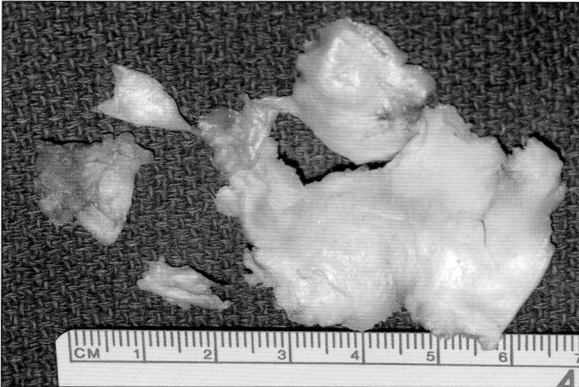

Fig 13-25b An odontogenic keratocyst removed in several pieces, as shown here, will have a much higher recurrence potential regardless of the curettage technique or chemical agents used on the wall of the bony cavity.

to remove residual cyst buds or residual lining in the bony walls, is unnecessary if the cyst was completely removed as a single unit (Fig 13-25a). However, if the thin lining of the cyst is torn or shredded, curettage of the bony wall in an effort to remove the remaining lining is warranted (Fig 13-25b). This is best and most simply achieved with sharp curettes. Other curettage mechanisms have been used, including physical curettage with a rotary bur, thermal curettage with cryotherapy, and chemical curettage with Carnoy's solution; however, they all lack control of precise depth of effect, and none has shown any greater ability to prevent recurrence. In fact, when these modalities are used, there is a risk of justifying less-than-complete cyst removal.

In some cases, the remaining bony integrity is at risk for pathologic fracture. As with dentigerous cysts, this may be managed with 6 to 8 weeks of maxillomandibular fixation or with a rigid fixation plate that can be removed after 6 months or left in place in the adult (Figs 13-26a and 13-26b). In individuals

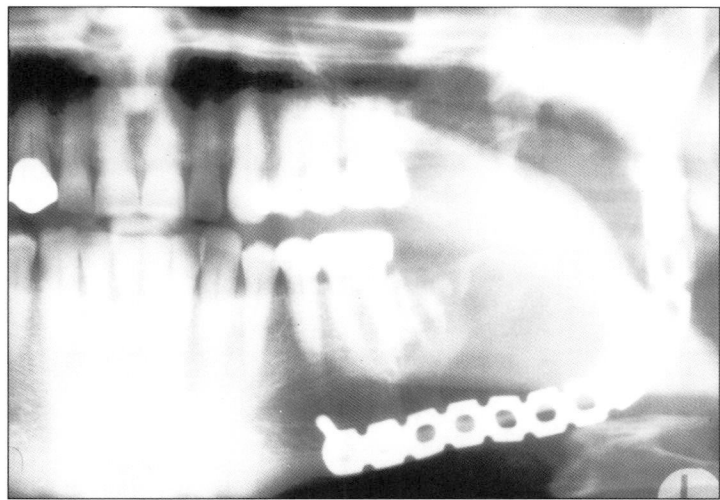

Fig 13-26a Resultant bony defect from the keratocyst removal and plate placement (shown in Fig 13-24) in a 60-year-old man.

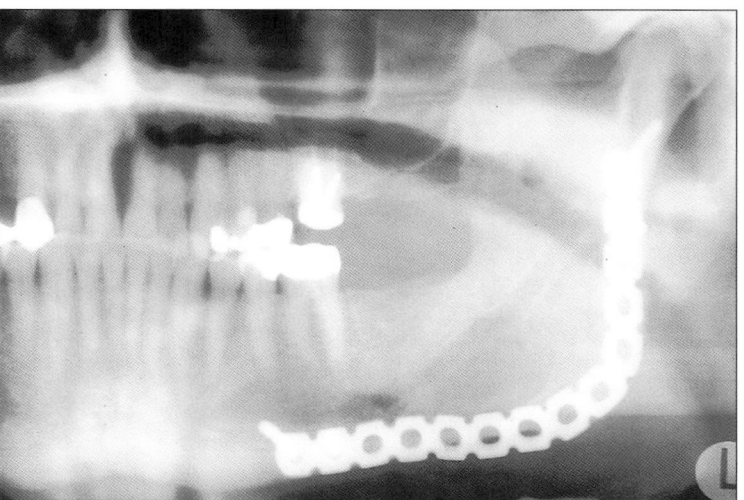

Fig 13-26b Ten-year postoperative radiograph showing complete bone regeneration and mandibular outline with no recurrence. The bone regeneration was complete within 6 to 9 months without grafting.

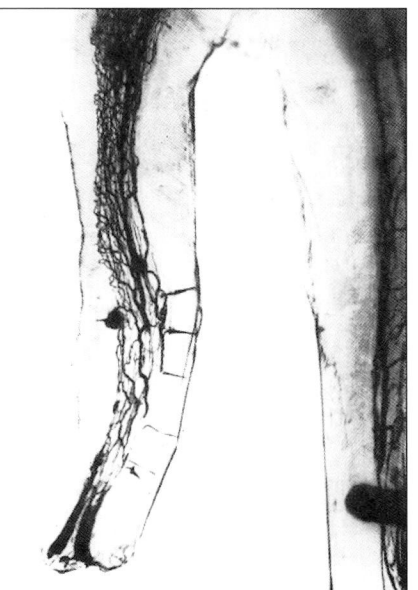

Fig 13-27 Histologic evaluation of combined pulpal-periodontal vasculature using india ink perfusion in the buccal root of a maxillary first molar. Note six groups of blood vessels connecting the root canal with the periodontal ligament. Such nonapical vascular supply maintains pulp vitality even when the apical area is curetted. (Reprinted from Kramer IRH, Vascular architecture of human dental pulp. Arch Oral Biol 1960;2:177, with permission from Elsevier Science.)

younger than 18 years, it is advisable to remove the plate to prevent its becoming enveloped by the growing mandible.

Odontogenic keratocysts that interdigitate around and between the roots of teeth may be removed from the root surfaces and curetted without a commitment to root canal therapy. In fact, root canal therapy is ill-advised because it does not improve access for curettage and commits otherwise sound teeth to extensive restorative work and the potential complications of root canal therapy and occlusal coverage. Teeth that are curetted apically in this fashion become de-innervated, but not devitalized (a blood supply is maintained through pulpal connections through the periodontal ligament) (Fig 13-27). Most will regain responsiveness to pulp testing in 6 months to 1 year, and those that do not remain asymptomatic because the pulp is actually still vital owing to these periodontal membrane collateral vessels.

Odontogenic keratocysts that occur in the maxilla often displace or become adherent to the sinus membrane. Enucleation and curettage in this area often causes a sinus communication, which will read-

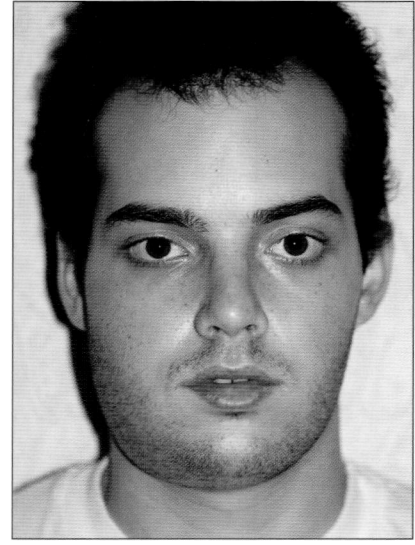

Fig 13-28a This young man experienced four recurrences of an odontogenic keratocyst after an initial enucleation and curettage that shredded the cyst lining. Note the expansion, which was accompanied by pain due either to keratin leaking into the soft tissues and provoking inflammation or to secondary infection.

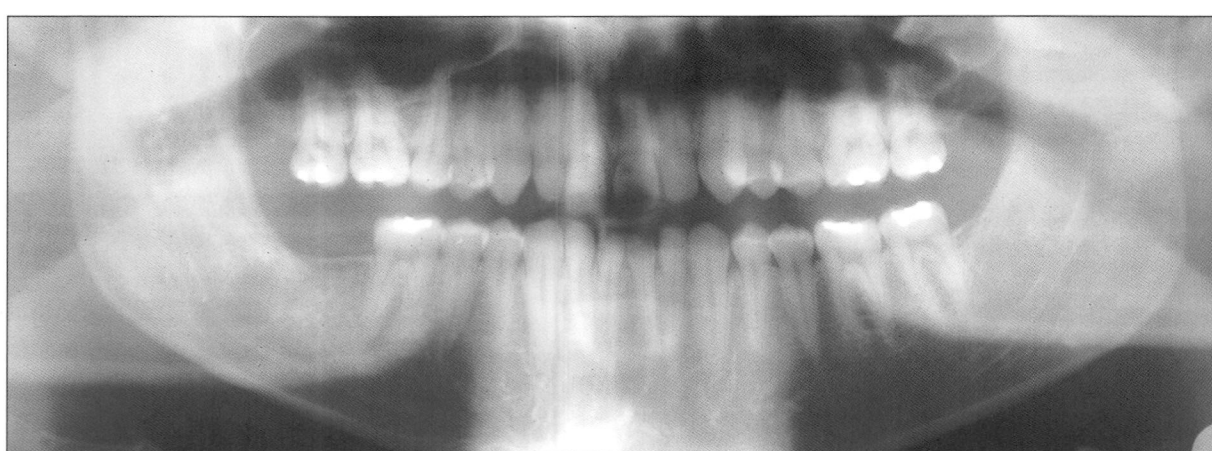

Fig 13-28b Panoramic radiograph of the patient shown in Fig 13-28a. A multilocular radiolucency is visible in the second and third molar areas.

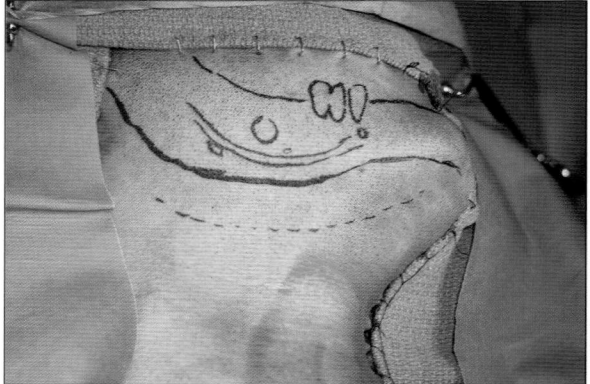

Fig 13-28c The multiple recurrences of this keratocyst are an indication for a curative resection. Here a submucosal resection, nerve preservation, and immediate bony reconstruction are planned.

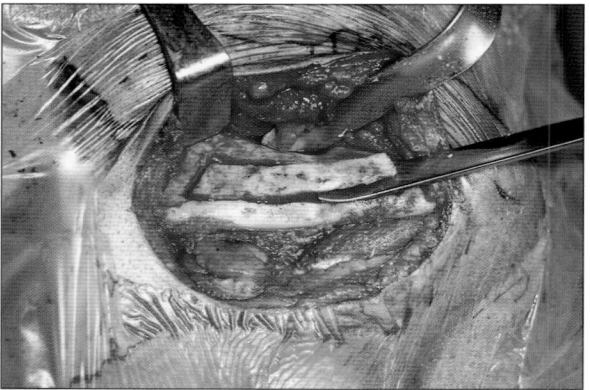

Fig 13-28d Since a keratocyst does not have the ability to truly invade into soft tissues, an en-bloc resection, as is indicated for an ameloblastoma or a myxoma, is not required. Here a lateral decortication to preserve the mandibular neurovascular bundle is accomplished.

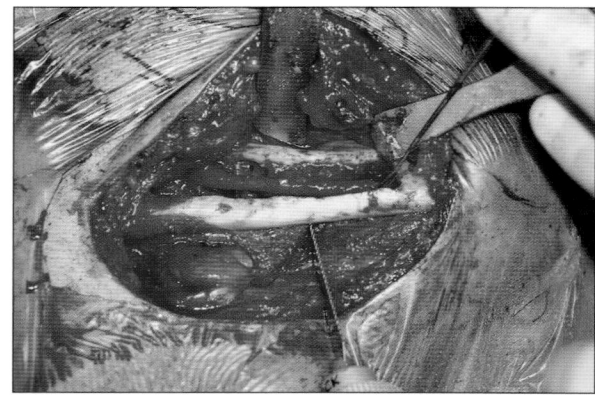

Fig 13-28e With the neurovascular bundle lifted with a nerve hook, a resection of the bone, containing multiple keratocysts within it, can be accomplished without injury to this structure.

ily heal after a primary oral closure without resulting in oro-antral communications or residual sinus disease. The presence of the maxillary sinus should not intimidate the clinician into being less thorough in this location and thereby invite recurrence.

When resection of an odontogenic keratocyst is indicated, it may be accomplished in a fashion similar to the resection of a benign tumor such as an ameloblastoma or a myxoma. However, because an odontogenic keratocyst does not possess the enzymes to infiltrate the soft tissues outside the jaws, it may be resected with modifications to preserve the inferior alveolar neurovascular bundle. Moreover, since the odontogenic keratocyst only protrudes through the cortex without infiltrating into the periosteum, the resection can usually be accomplished in the subperiosteal plane. Figures 13-28a through

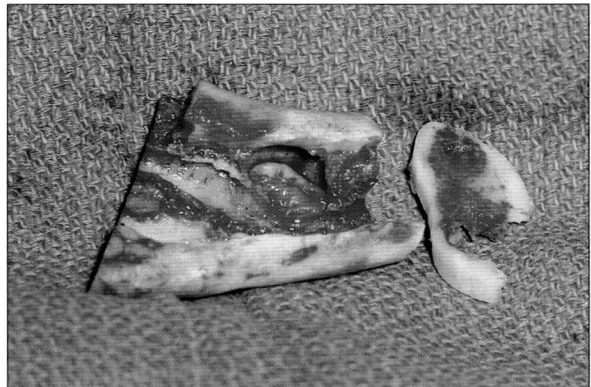

Fig 13-28f Specimen containing four separate keratocysts, an indication of the wide field of recurrence in some recurrent keratocysts. The posterior margin goes through two keratocysts and therefore requires a further resection at this margin.

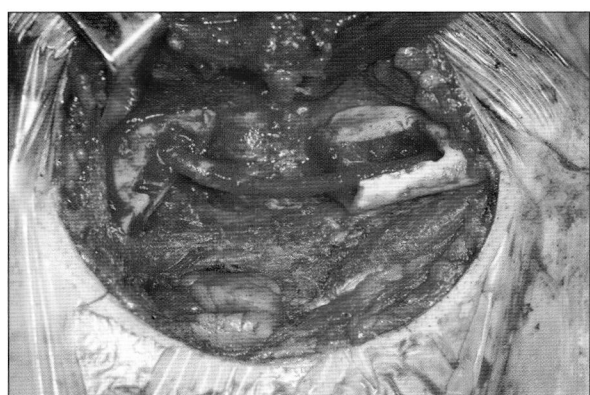

Fig 13-28g Once clear bone margins are obtained, the tissue bed is prepared for a bone graft. Here the patient is placed in maxillomandibular fixation and the recipient tissue bed is dissected without entry into the oral cavity.

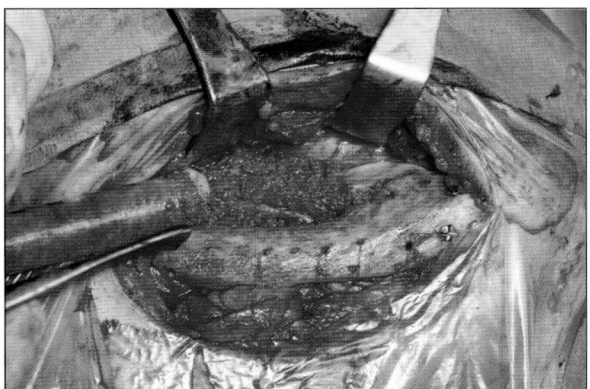

Fig 13-28h An allogeneic bone crib is used to contain an autogenous cancellous marrow graft. The cancellous marrow is condensed around the neurovascular bundle, which is left in its original position.

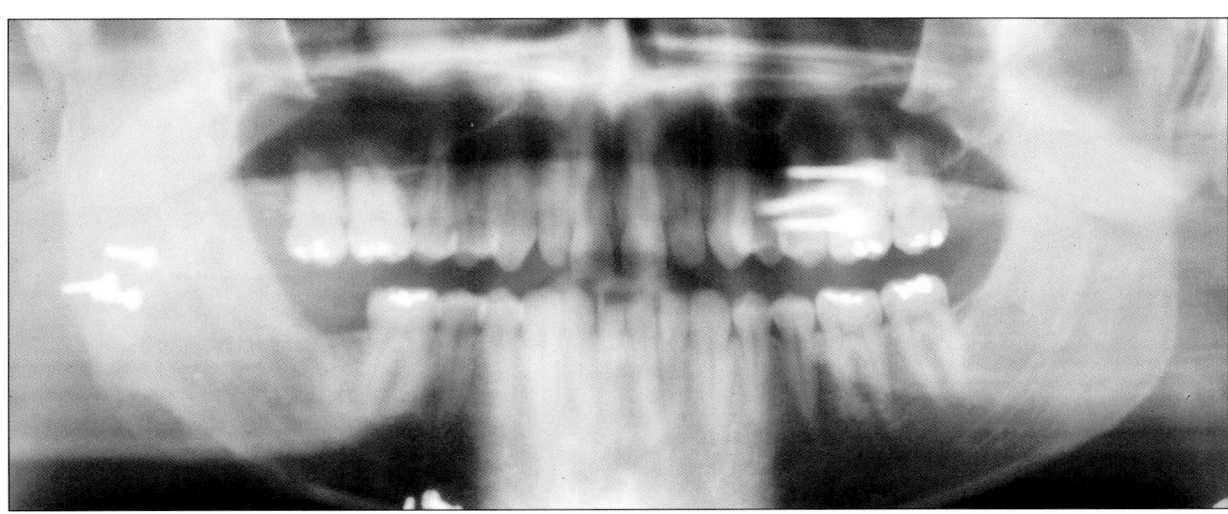

Fig 13-28i Eight-year postoperative radiograph documents an end to this young man's yearly recurrences, regeneration of bone, remodeling of the graft, and the development of a new mandibular canal.

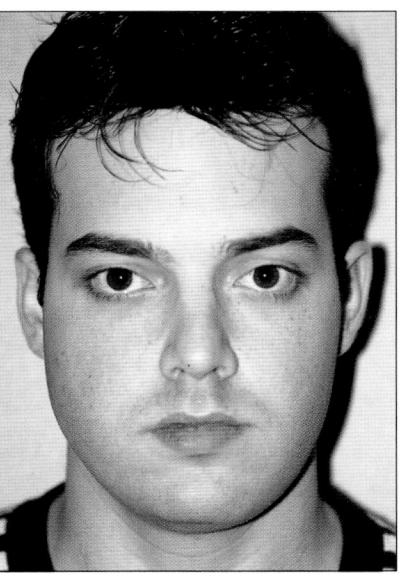

Fig 13-28j Facial photograph showing a return to normal contours. His lip sensation was retained and reported as "completely normal."

13-28j illustrate a single case with multiple recurrences that required a resection based on these principles. In this case, the neurovascular bundle was preserved and an immediate bone graft was made possible by the avoidance of an oral communication. The resection must include the entire field of recurrence, where multiple cysts will be dispersed. Initial margins can be 1 cm based on panoramic radiographs or CT scans. However, the margins may need to be widened if cysts are found at or close to the initial margins by direct gross specimen inspection or by frozen sections from the marrow space. In the case presented here, two of four separate cysts were found at the posterior margin, necessitating a further resection of 0.5 to 1.0 cm.

PROGNOSIS ▶

Published recurrence rates for odontogenic keratocysts range from 5% to about 70%. This wide range is due to the nature of the reports, which are retrospective chart reviews of cysts removed using dif-

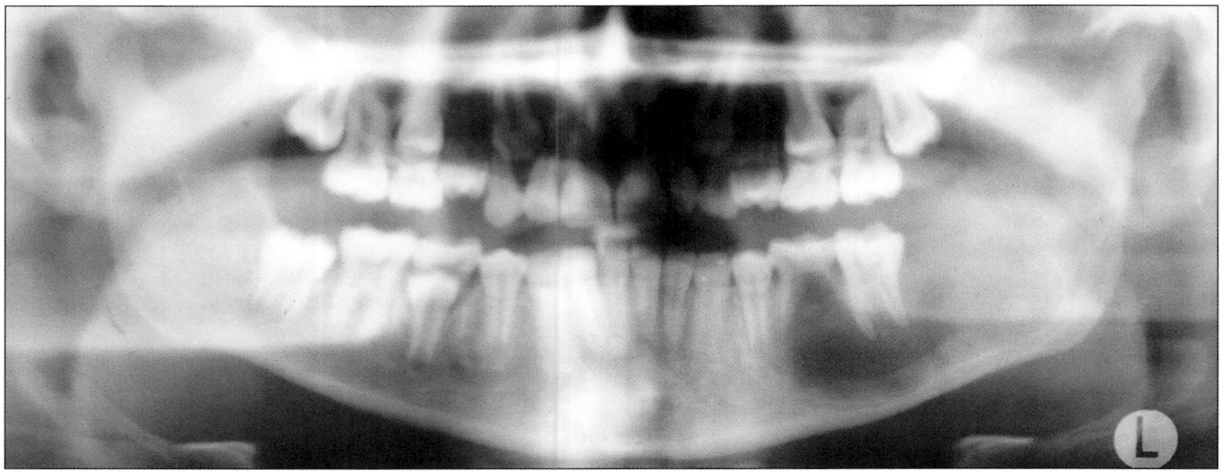

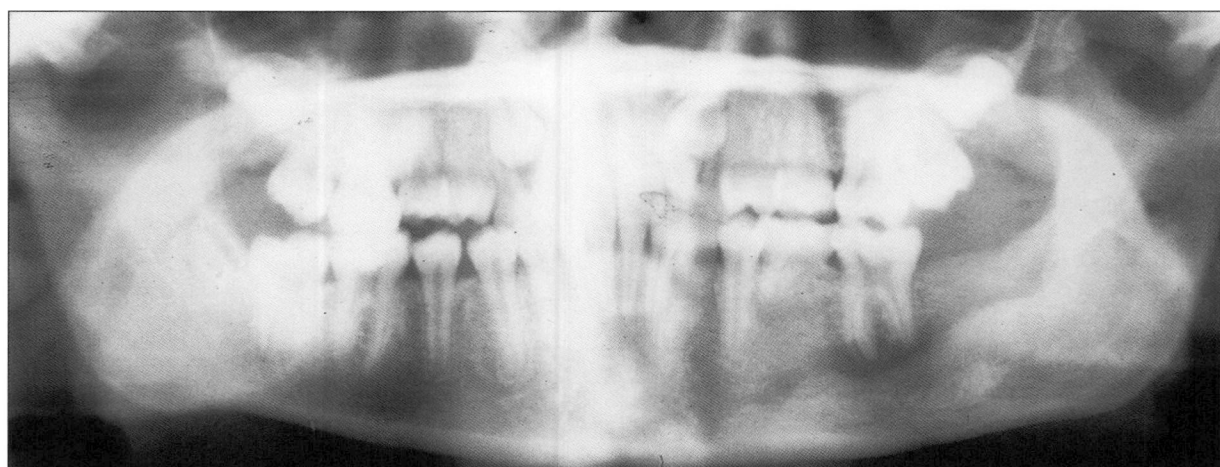

Fig 13-29a Postoperative panoramic radiograph of the remaining defect after the transoral removal of the keratocyst shown in Figs 13-23 and 13-25a.

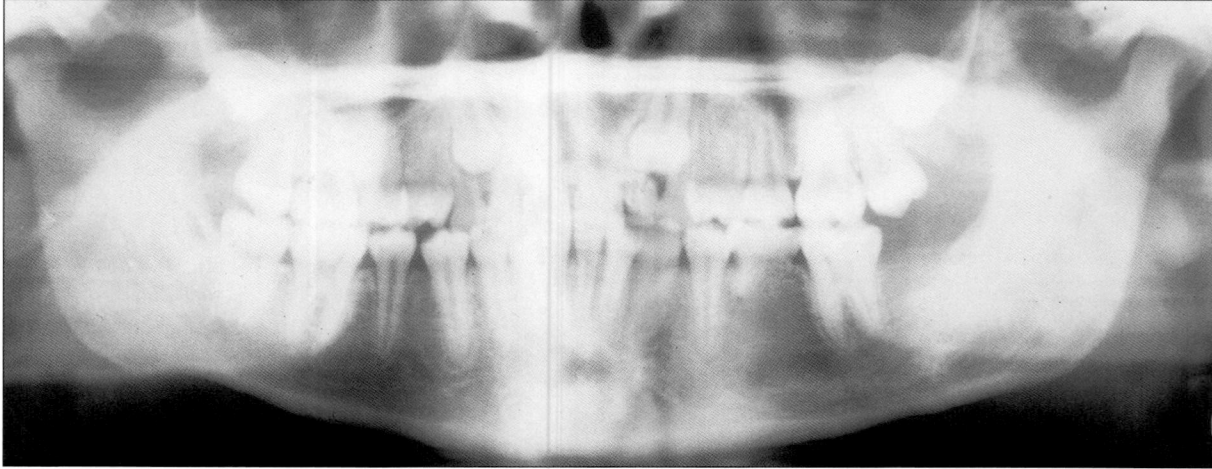

Fig 13-29b At 6 months, the patient shown in Fig 13-29a, a 12-year-old girl, has spontaneously regenerated the entire defect with the exception of a radiolucency around the first molar apices. The first molar is unresponsive to pulp testing. Does this represent an apical granuloma from a nonvital tooth, an area yet to fill in with regenerative bone, or a recurrent keratocyst?

Fig 13-29c The 1-year panoramic radiograph answers the question raised by Fig 13-29b. An apical granuloma would have maintained its size, whereas a recurrent keratocyst would have enlarged and become more radiolucent. The complete regeneration of bone discounts both. The first molar became responsive to pulp testing at 1 year.

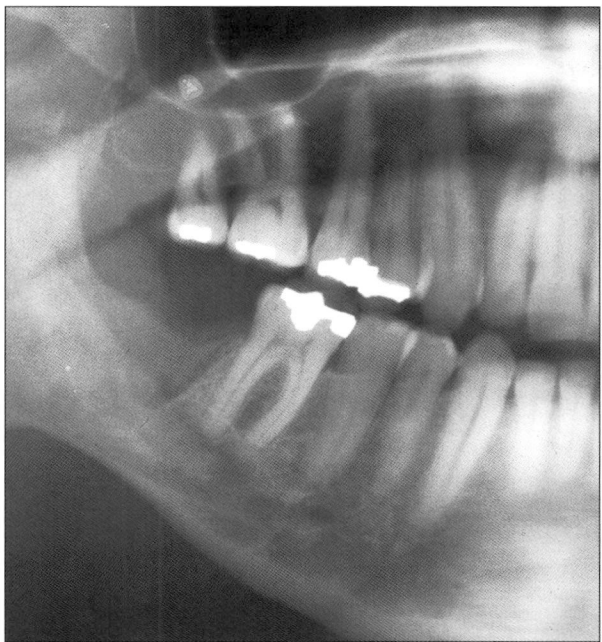

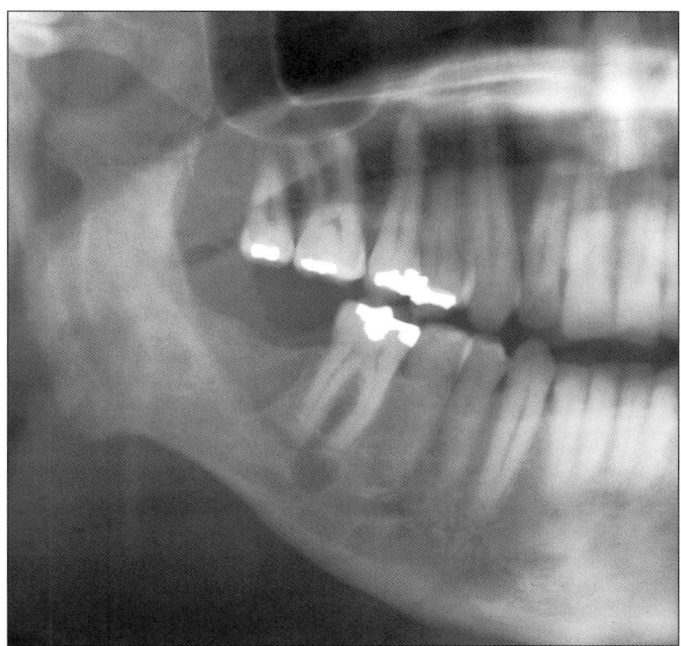

Fig 13-30a Healed keratocyst defect after an incomplete enucleation and curettage.

Fig 13-30b A recurrent keratocyst (redevelopment from remaining cyst lining) becomes apparent when an enlarging and darkening radiolucency appears.

ferent techniques, different surgeons, different patient anesthesias, and no stratification accounting for size, location, or origin. They are, therefore, nearly meaningless, identifying only a marked biologic potential for recurrence.

There are many theories about why odontogenic keratocysts recur, including collagenase production, daughter cysts, budding, and others; however, only two methods of recurrence are supported by data. One is related to incomplete cyst removal. In this sense, odontogenic keratocysts behave like tumors because they can continue to grow and recur without a stimulus. These recurrences, somewhat related to the surgical approach, represent *persistence of original disease.* The other method of recurrence relates to new primary keratocysts where other activated dental lamina rests or activated oral basal epithelium develop into a second cyst. Therefore, recurrences are more common when associated with certain factors, including cysts enucleated in several pieces, primordial-origin keratocysts, cysts of larger size, multilocular cysts, and cysts complicated with perforation and keratin leakage into soft tissues or complicated by infection.

When recurrences develop, those associated with the surgeon *leaving residual cyst lining in bone* become radiographically apparent within 18 months. At first it may be difficult to distinguish between a postsurgical bone lucency that has not undergone complete bone regeneration and a recurrent cyst. However, within a short time the distinction will become apparent. An uncomplicated postsurgical bony cavity will continue to regenerate bone. The radiolucency will appear to become smaller and lighter on the film (Figs 13-29a to 13-29c). In contrast, a recurrent keratocyst will radiographically appear to become larger and darker with time (Figs 13-30a and 13-30b). Those that seem to arise as new *primary cysts* can occur (recur) at any time. Some have been observed to develop 10 years after original treatment, and some even in bone grafts, documenting their origin (Figs 13-31a to 13-31c) from other dental lamina rests or from other rests of Malassez that become activated sometime after the original treatment.

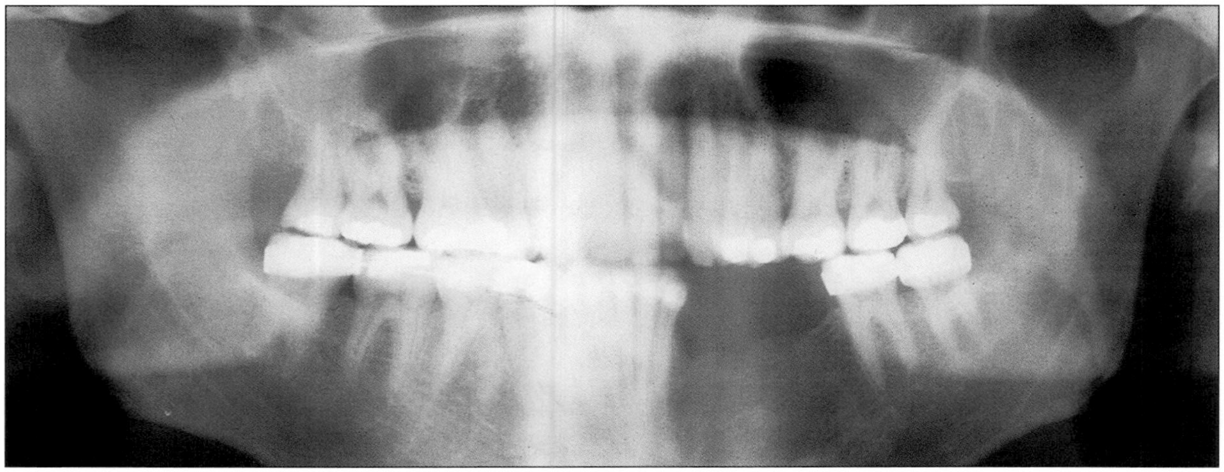

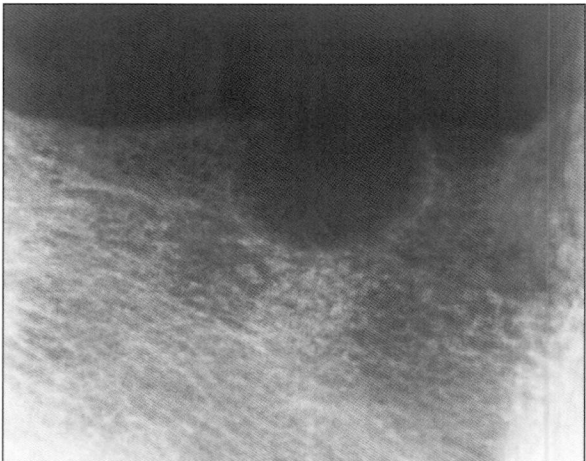

Fig 13-31a Bone graft in the area of a resected primordial origin keratocyst, which did not excise overlying attached gingiva. A suspicious crestal radiolucency appeared at 9 months.

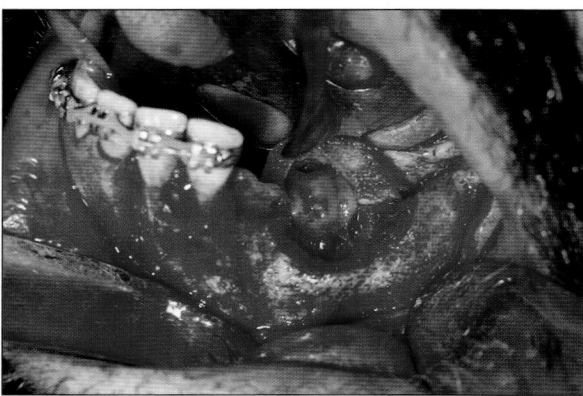

Fig 13-31b Confirmation of the suspicious radiolucency shown in Fig 13-31a in the center of the crestal surface of the graft.

Fig 13-31c On exploration, this radiolucency is identified as a recurrent (new primary) keratocyst arising from residual dental lamina rests in the overlying attached gingiva, which invaded into the graft.

Basal Cell Nevus Syndrome

CLINICAL PRESENTATION AND PATHOGENESIS ▶

The basal cell nevus syndrome is very familiar to the oral and maxillofacial specialist. A fully expressed case will present with several of the many possible abnormalities involving the jaws, skin, craniofacial area, axial skeleton, or central nervous system. A subtle case will present with only one or two abnormalities that may not even be very obvious. The clinician is usually alerted to the possibility of basal cell nevus syndrome when more than one odontogenic keratocyst is found in the jaws, when sequential new primary keratocysts are identified, or when a young individual (10 to 30 years of age) develops basal cell carcinomas.

Because of the need to identify and diagnose patients with basal cell nevus syndrome, it is important for clinicians to know the specific components of this syndrome and their relative frequencies (Table 13-1). Without question, the two most common physical findings are multiple odontogenic keratocysts and

Table 13-1 Components of basal cell nevus syndrome and their frequency

I. Jaw and skull	
1. Odontogenic keratocysts	> 85%
2. Calcified falx cerebri	> 85%
3. Large calvaria	> 60%
4. Large paranasal sinuses	> 60%
5. Hypertelorism	> 50%
6. Bridging of the sella turcica	> 70%
7. Cleft lip and palate	< 15%
II. Skin and internal organs	
1. Basal cell carcinomas	> 70%
2. Milia/epidermoid cysts	> 50%
3. Palmar-plantar pits	> 50%
4. Calcified ovarian fibromas	> 50%
5. Subcutaneous calcifications	< 15%
6. Fetal rhabdomyomas	< 15%
7. Ovarian fibrosarcomas	< 15%
III. Axial skeletal abnormalities	
1. Rib abnormalities	> 60%
2. Spina bifida	> 50%
3. Kyphoscoliosis	> 40%
4. Short fourth metacarpal	> 25%
5. Lumbarization of sacrum	> 40%
6. Pseudocysts of phalanges	> 30%
IV. Central nervous system	
1. Medulloblastomas	< 2%
2. Congenital hydrocephalus	< 3%
3. Mental deficiency	< 3%
4. Craniopharyngiomas	< 1%
5. Meningioma	< 1%

basal cell carcinomas. Multiple odontogenic keratocysts are seen in 85% of cases, nearly all of which develop between the ages of 7 and 40 years. The peak age of development is between 12 and 25 years. Odontogenic keratocysts develop three times more frequently in the mandible than in the maxilla. The growth rate and aggressiveness of odontogenic keratocysts associated with basal cell nevus syndrome are no different than those associated with isolated odontogenic keratocysts. However, the emergence of odontogenic keratocysts from odontogenic rests and dental follicles is much more likely (Fig 13-32a).

The basal cell carcinomas associated with basal cell nevus syndrome are noted to be much less aggressive than sun damage–related basal cell carcinomas except in a few rare cases. The basal cell carcinomas of this syndrome will be multiple and will often resemble acne or milia or will appear as small red-brown lesions (Figs 13-32b and 13-32c). They will appear on areas not usually exposed to the sun, such as the back and trunk, as well as on the sun-exposed areas of the face and neck. They will also appear at much earlier ages (less than 30 years) than do sun damage–related basal cell carcinomas (over 40 years of age).

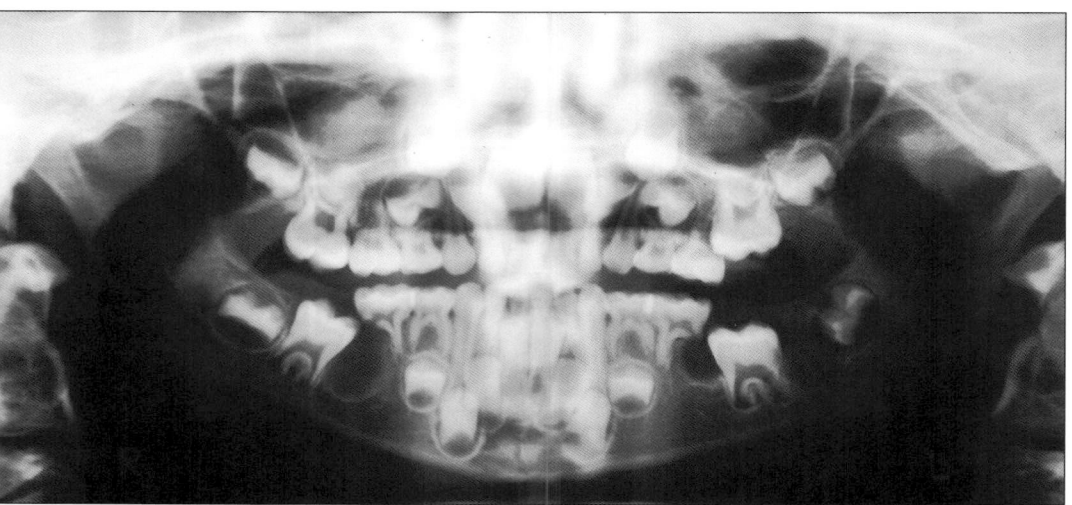

Fig 13-32a Multiple odontogenic keratocysts developed early in this young individual with basal cell nevus syndrome.

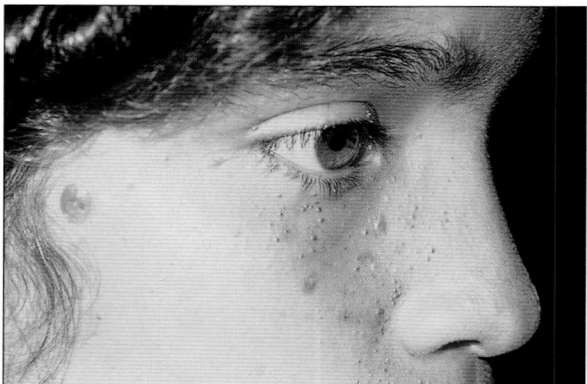

Fig 13-32b The basal cell carcinomas of basal cell nevus syndrome appear as small, reddish-brown, acne-like lesions. The infraorbital skin is a common site.

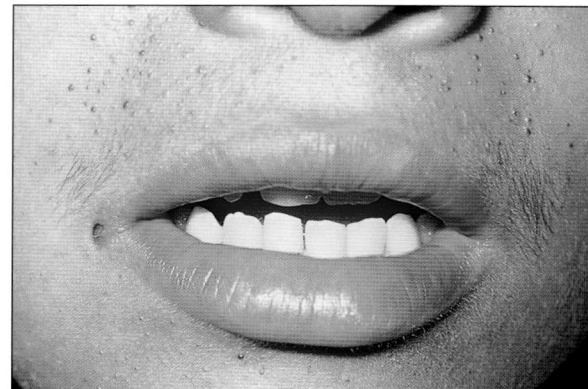

Fig 13-32c Numerous small basal cell carcinomas, a large basal cell carcinoma at the right commissure, and lip pits at the commissures are all components of the basal cell nevus syndrome.

Other likely findings the clinician should look for are increased calvarial size; hypertelorism and frontal bossing (Figs 13-32d and 13-32e); palmar and plantar pits (Fig 13-32f); calcified falx cerebri (Fig 13-32g); rib abnormalities (bifid, absent, fused, hypoplastic ribs or cervical ribs) (Figs 13-32h to 13-32j); spina bifida (Fig 13-32k); multiple epidermoid cysts of the skin; pectus excavatum (Fig 13-32l); kyphoscoliosis; and hyperpneumatized sinuses.

DIFFERENTIAL DIAGNOSIS ▶ The diagnosis of basal cell nevus syndrome is mostly straightforward. However, because *odontogenic keratocysts unrelated to this syndrome* may occur together or closely spaced in time, and because they may recur, multiple odontogenic keratocysts by themselves do not establish the diagnosis. Similarly, *sun damage–related basal cell carcinomas* or basal carcinomas related to other syndromes (*Bazex syndrome* and *Rombo syndrome*) without at least two other features of basal cell nevus syndrome also does not establish the diagnosis. In addition, rare syndromes associated with similar-looking skin lesions like *Rasmussen syndrome*, which has tricoepitheliomas and milia, and the *multiple keratoacanthoma syndromes* of the Ferguson-Smith or Grybowski types may give the impression of a basal cell nevus syndrome.

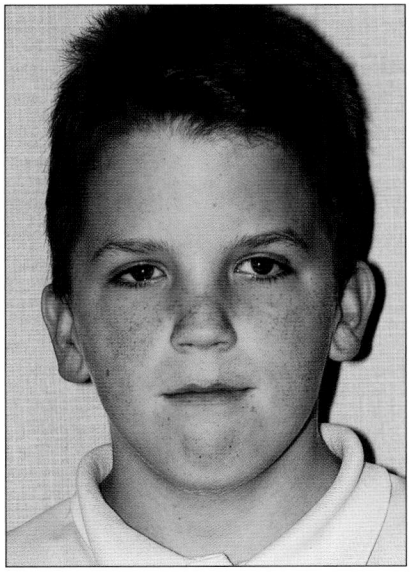

Fig 13-32d Mild hypertelorism and an increased calvarial size in an individual with basal cell nevus syndrome.

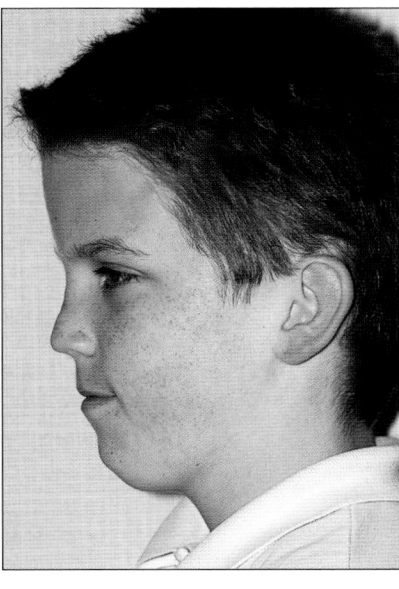

Fig 13-32e Frontal bossing in an individual with basal cell nevus syndrome.

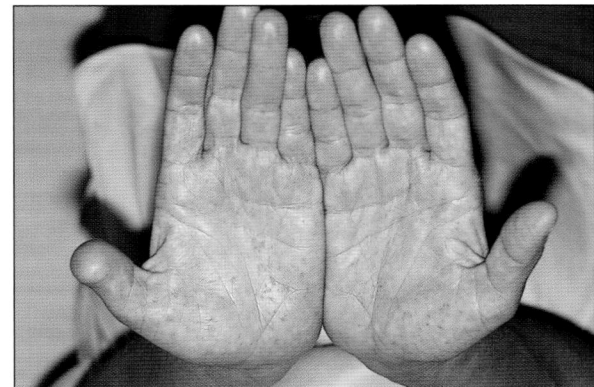

Fig 13-32f Palmar pits in an individual with basal cell nevus syndrome.

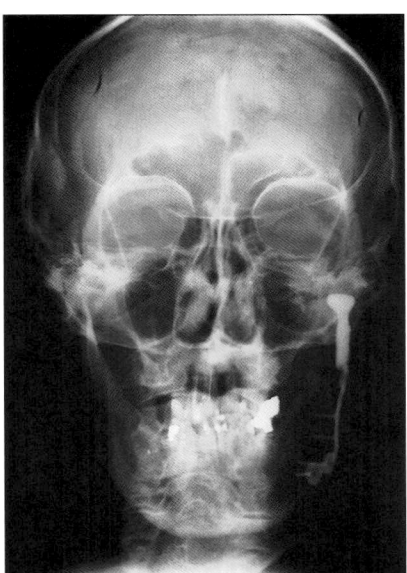

Fig 13-32g Calcification of the falx cerebri seen as a midline linear calcification in a patient with basal cell nevus syndrome.

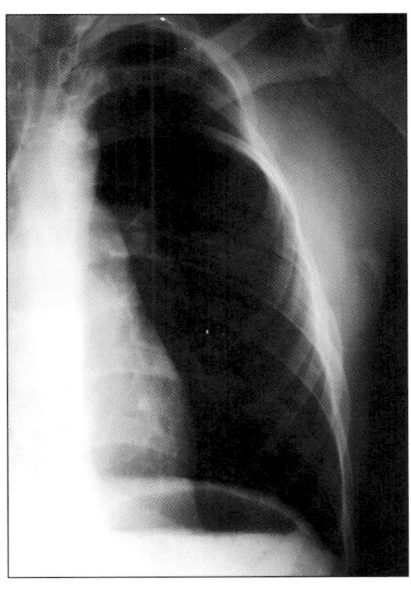

Fig 13-32h Chest radiograph showing a bifid third rib in a patient with basal cell nevus syndrome.

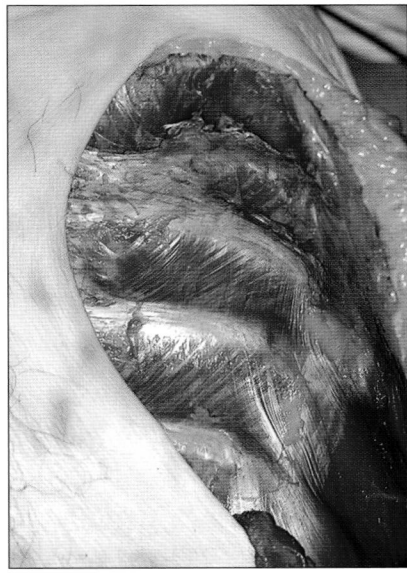

Fig 13-32i Anatomic postmortem dissection specimen with a fused second and third rib. This individual also had basal cell nevus syndrome.

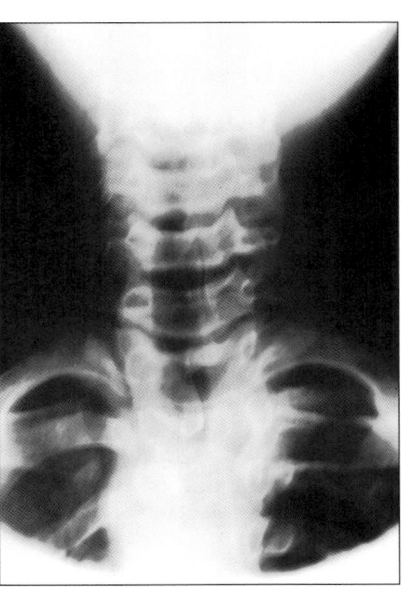

Fig 13-32j Cervical ribs in an individual with basal nevus syndrome.

DIAGNOSTIC WORK-UP ▶

It is impossible for the clinician to explore every possible abnormality associated with this syndrome. However, several quick, straightforward, and yielding tests can be performed. Of course, a panoramic radiograph is essential with removal and documentation of keratocyst formation, as is a thorough topographic skin examination with biopsy of any suspicious lesions. Simple measurements of the occipitofrontal circumference (those greater than 55 cm are significant) and the intercanthal distance (those greater than 36 mm are significant) can be easily accomplished. An anteroposterior skull radiograph, a

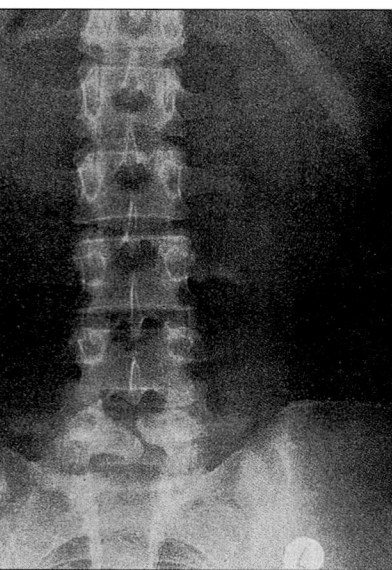

Fig 13-32k Lumbosacral discontinuity in an individual with spina bifida from basal cell nevus syndrome.

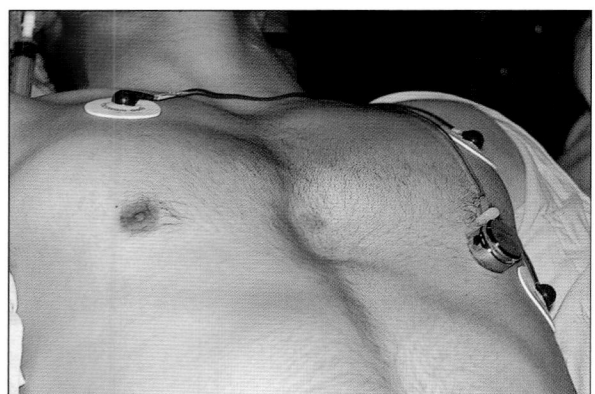

Fig 13-32l Pectus excavatum in an individual with basal cell nevus syndrome.

chest radiograph, and a lumbosacral radiograph will assess for intracranial calcifications, rib abnormalities, and spina bifida, respectively. Palmar and plantar pits, and less commonly lip pits, may be highlighted by coating the area with a Betadine povidone iodine "paint solution" and then wiping the area with a moist cloth. The brown Betadine solution will remain in the pits to highlight their presence.

TREATMENT ▶
The oral and maxillofacial specialist should treat the odontogenic keratocysts associated with this syndrome in the same manner as any isolated keratocyst (see pages 594–599). Enucleation, the most common therapy, is very effective. Because of the relatively young age of individuals who develop basal cell nevus syndrome, the odontogenic keratocysts are often associated with the follicle of a potentially functional tooth. Therefore, marsupialization and orthodontic eruption guidance might be considered if feasible. In addition, because keratocyst surgeries are often required between the ages of 8 and 16 years and because the risk of odontogenic keratocyst development from the third molar follicles is great, removal of third molars at an early age is recommended.

Surgical removal of skin lesions suspected to be basal cell carcinomas should be selective. Since the basal cell carcinomas in this syndrome are much more quiescent than are those related to sun damage, an observation period is advised before removal. Only those with signs of ulceration, enlargement, crusting, and bleeding indicative of transformation to a more aggressive behavior are recommended for removal.

Many of the other syndrome-related abnormalities, such as plantar pits, lip pits, and pectus excavatum, are pertinent only to the diagnosis and do not require therapy. Identification of specific abnormalities that may be correctable or pose a further risk to the individual, such as spina bifida, central nervous system tumors, and kyphoscoliosis, need to be referred to other specialists. In addition, genetic counseling is recommended for each individual and family, who should be made aware that the basal cell nevus syndrome is an autosomal-dominant inheritance. However, 40% of cases result from new mutations and therefore have no familial involvement. Such situations can create guilt, suspicion, and even resentment that can be alleviated or prevented with genetic information and counseling.

PROGNOSIS ▶
The prognosis is excellent. Although most individuals will require more than one surgery related to odontogenic keratocyst removal or another syndrome-related procedure, the syndrome is compatible with a full life span. In rare cases, however, fulminant multiple basal cell carcinomas have produced disfigurement and disability, and in fewer cases central medulloblastomas have caused death.

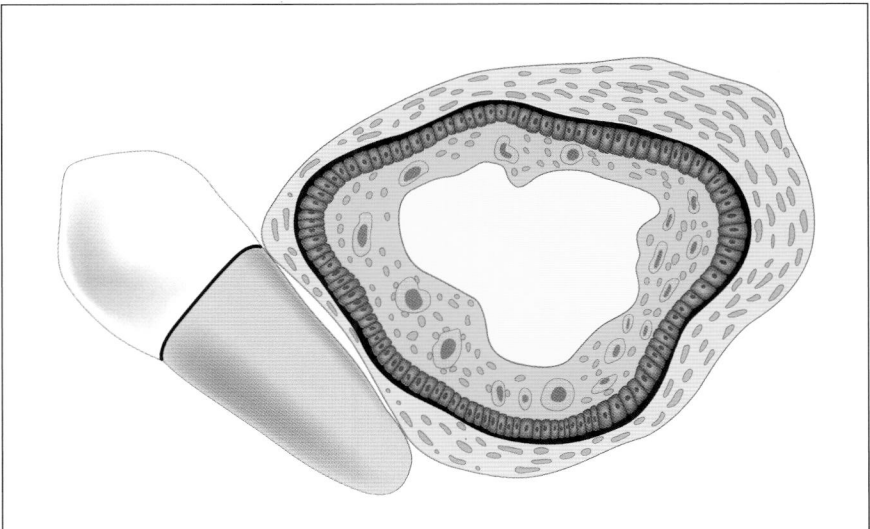

Fig 13-33a Illustration of a calcifying odontogenic cyst. Note the intraluminal proliferation with ghost cells, keratinized areas, and calcified areas.

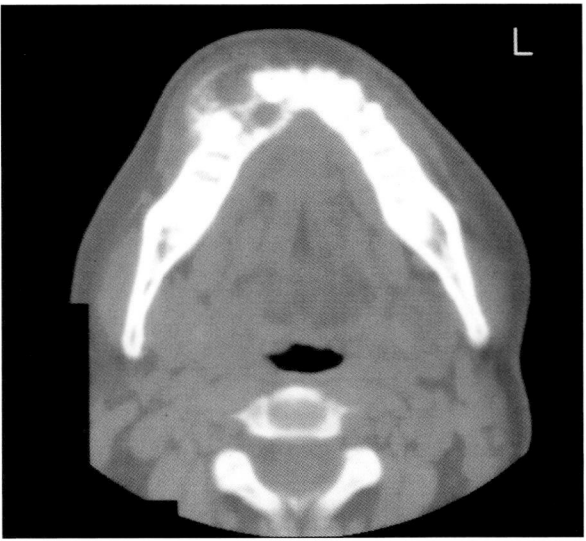

Fig 13-33b A calcifying odontogenic cyst will present as a mixed radiolucent, radiopaque, and asymptomatic expansile lesion.

Calcifying Odontogenic Cyst

CLINICAL PRESENTATION AND PATHOGENESIS ▶

The calcifying odontogenic cyst (Fig 13-33a), like the odontogenic keratocyst, is a histopathologically, radiographically, and clinically unique, specific cyst. Unlike the odontogenic keratocyst, however, it has a much less aggressive behavior. That is, it behaves like any other cyst with little recurrence potential.

Calcifying odontogenic cysts may occur at any age but are more common in the teenage years. They have a marked predilection for females and for occurrence in the maxilla. The cysts are usually discovered as an incidental radiographic finding. Early in their development, they will appear completely radiolucent. As they mature, they develop calcifications that produce a well-circumscribed, mixed radiolucent-radiopaque appearance. Three general patterns of radiopacity are seen. One is a salt-and-pepper pattern of flecks, the second is a fluffy cloud–like pattern throughout, and the third is a crescent-shaped pattern on one side of the radiolucency in a "new moon"–like configuration (Fig 13-33b). The cyst creates mild expansion if it gets reasonably large but is otherwise asymptomatic. Average size is about 3 cm, with a range of 1 to 8 cm.

An extraosseous calcifying odontogenic cyst accounts for 25% of all calcifying odontogenic cysts. It occurs anterior to the first molar and mostly in individuals older than 50 years. It presents on the alveolar ridge or interdental papilla as a firm, soft tissue mass in which calcifications may be seen radiographically.

The cells responsible for the calcifying odontogenic cyst are dental lamina rests (rests of Serres) within either the soft tissue or bone. Therefore, calcifying odontogenic cysts are cysts of primordial origin and are not associated with the crown of an impacted tooth (see Fig 13-33a).

DIFFERENTIAL DIAGNOSIS ▶

Because calcifying odontogenic cysts have three possible clinical-radiographic presentations, there are three differential lists. When a calcifying odontogenic cyst presents as a unilocular radiolucency unassociated with calcifications or an impacted tooth, it will suggest an *odontogenic keratocyst,* an *ameloblastoma,* an *adenomatoid odontogenic cyst* if it is in the anterior jaws, or an *ameloblastic fibroma.* When it presents as a mixed radiolucent-radiopaque lesion, all of these except the *adenomatoid odontogenic cyst* become inappropriate because they do not produce a calcified product. The adenomatoid odontogenic cyst remains a serious consideration because about two thirds produce a salt-and-pepper, flecked radiopaque

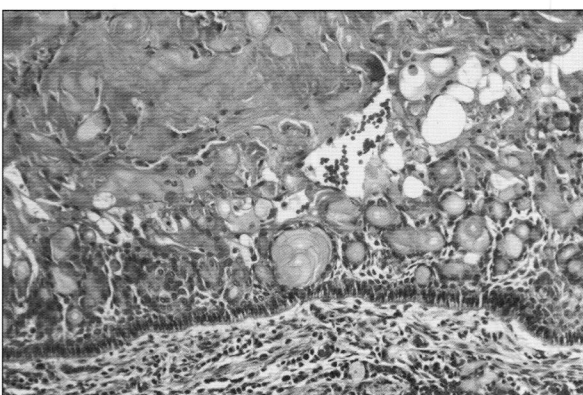

Fig 13-33c Calcifying odontogenic cyst with the characteristic lining of columnar cells in which the nuclei are polarized away from the basement membrane. Above this are ghost cells and extensive keratinization.

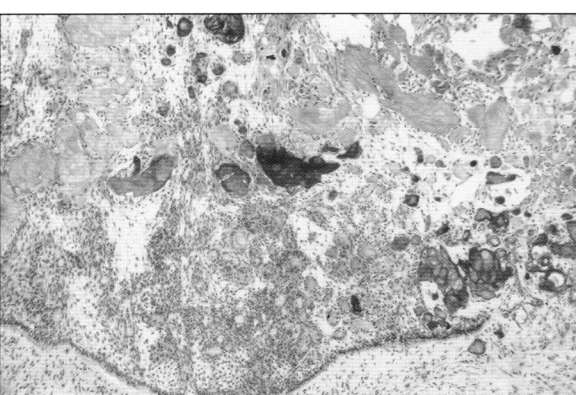

Fig 13-33d Calcifying odontogenic cyst showing the extensive intraluminal proliferation and variation within the lining. Also visible are stellate reticulum–like areas, areas that are more cellular, ghost cells, and calcifications. The latter are essentially dystrophic calcifications involving ghost cells.

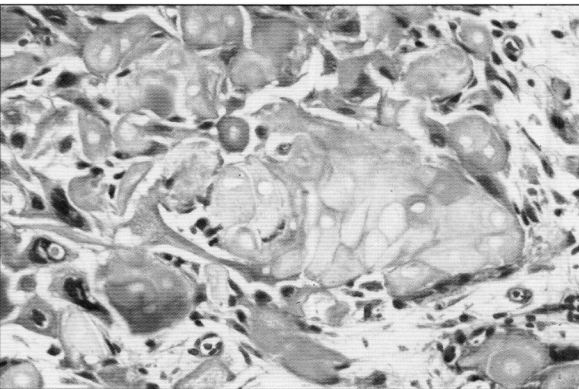

Fig 13-33e Higher-power view of ghost cells showing distinct cell outlines and clear spaces representing the nucleus. Some multinucleated giant cells are present.

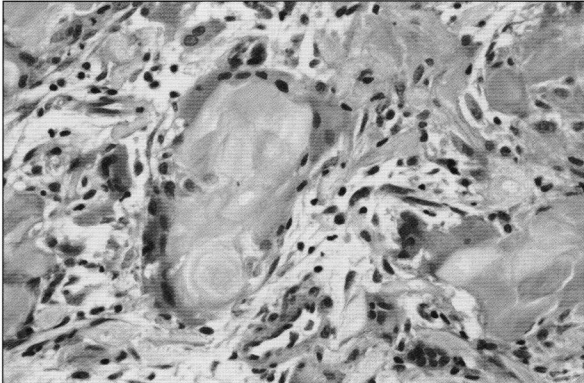

Fig 13-33f High-power view of ghost cells within a fibrous stroma containing numerous multinucleated giant cells. The keratin exuded by the ghost cells has provoked a foreign body response within the connective tissue.

pattern. In addition, a *developing odontoma* and an *ossifying fibroma* also appear well circumscribed and mixed radiolucent-radiopaque, as would a *calcifying epithelial odontogenic tumor*. When the calcifying odontogenic cyst presents as an extraosseous cyst, it will bear a resemblance to a *gingival cyst of the adult*, a *peripheral ossifying fibroma*, and a *chronic periodontal abscess*. More rarely, other extraosseous odontogenic lesions, such as the *peripheral ameloblastoma* and the *extraosseous calcifying odontogenic tumor*, may present in this fashion.

DIAGNOSTIC WORK-UP AND TREATMENT ▶

Periapical radiographs and a panoramic radiograph are the only studies required before surgical removal with an enucleation procedure.

HISTOPATHOLOGY ▶

Calcifying odontogenic cysts are usually unilocular cysts, the lining of which contains a distinct basal cell layer. This layer consists of cuboidal to columnar cells with hyperchromatic nuclei that may be polarized away from the basement membrane (Fig 13-33c). Overlying this, the epithelium proliferates to a variable extent and shows morphologic diversity (Fig 13-33d). The lining may be only a few cells thick or may proliferate to occupy most of the lumen. As with the adenomatoid odontogenic cyst, this may give the impression of a solid tumor. The cells are often in loose arrangement, resembling stellate reticulum, but may be admixed with more densely cellular areas. A characteristic finding is the presence of ghost cells (Fig 13-33e). These are eosinophilic epithelial cells that occur singly or in clusters. The cell outlines are usually distinct but may merge with their neighbors. The nuclei have degenerated, usually completely, so that only a small round void remains. These cells appear to represent an abnormal keratinization process and are subject to dystrophic calcification. This may be seen as fine basophilic granules, but when sufficiently extensive there may be broad sheets of calcification.

If ghost cells lie in contact with the connective tissue wall, a foreign body reaction is elicited due to their exudation of keratin. Numerous multinucleated giant cells can be seen (Fig 13-33f). Occasionally, dysplastic dentin may be deposited in the wall adjacent to the epithelium. An odontoma is seen with some frequency in conjunction with these cysts. An earlier designation for the calcifying odontogenic cyst was *calcifying and keratinizing odontogenic cyst*; because the keratinization is often extensive and the calcification less prominent, this may actually be a more accurate description.

The diagnosis of the calcifying odontogenic cyst, like that of the odontogenic keratocyst, depends on its pathognomonic histopathology.

PROGNOSIS ▶

Enucleated calcifying odontogenic cysts do not recur. Calcifying odontogenic cysts have a limited biologic behavior. However, some ameloblastomas have ghost cell differentiations, giving rise to the concept that calcifying odontogenic cysts may occur in association with an ameloblastoma. Ameloblastomas with ghost cells are the same as any ameloblastoma and require the appropriate treatment for an ameloblastoma. They are not collision lesions of both an ameloblastoma and a calcifying odontogenic cyst. Such ameloblastomas have also falsely suggested a more aggressive biologic behavior for the calcifying odontogenic cyst, prompting a suggestion that *odontogenic ghost cell tumor* should replace the term *calcifying odontogenic cyst*. There are no data to support the use of this term and no justification to treat a calcifying odontogenic cyst with anything more aggressive than enucleation.

Adenomatoid Odontogenic Cyst

CLINICAL PRESENTATION AND PATHOGENESIS ▶

The adenomatoid odontogenic cyst (AOC) (Fig 13-34a) is a cystic hamartoma arising from odontogenic epithelium. It will characteristically have a lumen lined by epithelium from which proliferations fill much and sometimes all of the lumen space, then mimicking a solid tumor.

This cyst will present as an expansile lesion usually in the anterior region of either jaw. It has sometimes been referred to as the "two-thirds tumor" because about two thirds occur in the maxilla, two thirds occur in young women (preteen and teenage years), two thirds are associated with an unerupted tooth, and two thirds of those teeth are canine teeth. The two-thirds statistics vary slightly, but the rough distribution is accurate. The cyst's clinical emergence may be subtle and discovered only as an incidental clinical or radiographic finding, or it may be discovered by rapid clinical expansion causing alarm and pain. Some will reach very large sizes (10 cm) and distort facial contours (Fig 13-34b).

The cyst's appearance on a panoramic radiograph will be that of a well-demarcated, unilocular radiolucency usually associated with an impacted tooth (Fig 13-34c). Almost all will have histologically identifiable dentinoid calcifications, but in only 50% of cases will they be sufficiently large or coalesced to appear on a panoramic or periapical radiograph. They will frequently displace the roots of adjacent teeth, but only rarely will they induce a regular smooth resorption of roots.

DIFFERENTIAL DIAGNOSIS ▶

Adenomatoid odontogenic cysts that appear without radiographic evidence of calcification will be most suggestive of the more common *dentigerous cyst*. In this young age group, other strictly radiolucent lesions worthy of consideration include an *odontogenic keratocyst*, an *ameloblastic fibroma,* an *odontogenic myxoma*, or a *central giant cell tumor* as well as an *ameloblastoma* as the age increases beyond 14 years.

Cysts in which calcifications can be observed resemble a *calcifying odontogenic cyst*. Other mixed radiolucent-radiopaque lesions possible in this young age group include an *ameloblastic fibro-odontoma* and an *ossifying fibroma*. As the age increases beyond 14 years, a *calcifying epithelial odontogenic tumor* (CEOT)

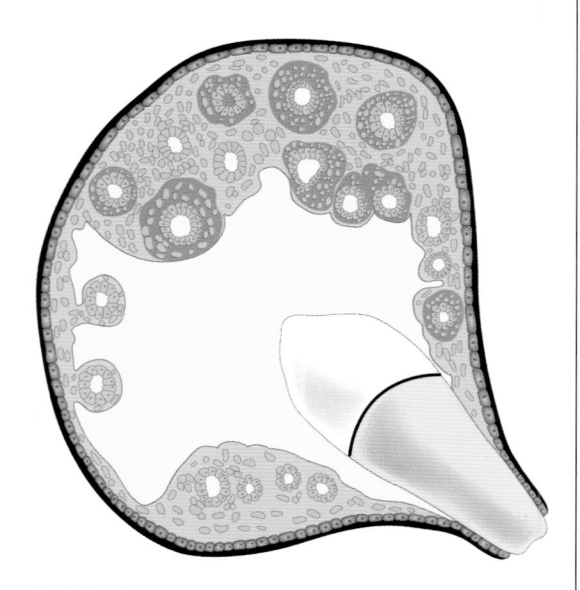

Fig 13-34a Illustration of an adenomatoid odontogenic cyst. Note the extensive intraluminal proliferation, the duct-like structures in the lining, and its emergence from Hertwig epithelial root sheath.

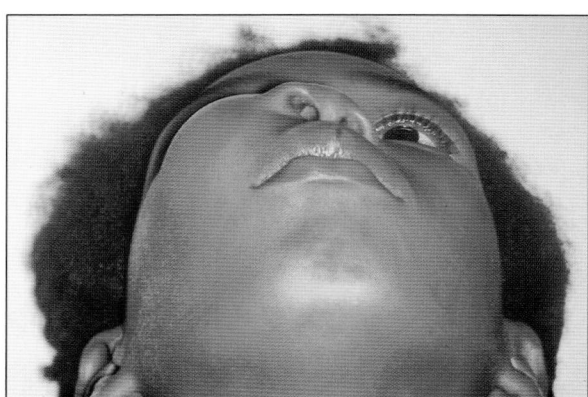

Fig 13-34b The adenomatoid odontogenic cyst may rapidly attain a very large size, causing facial distortion.

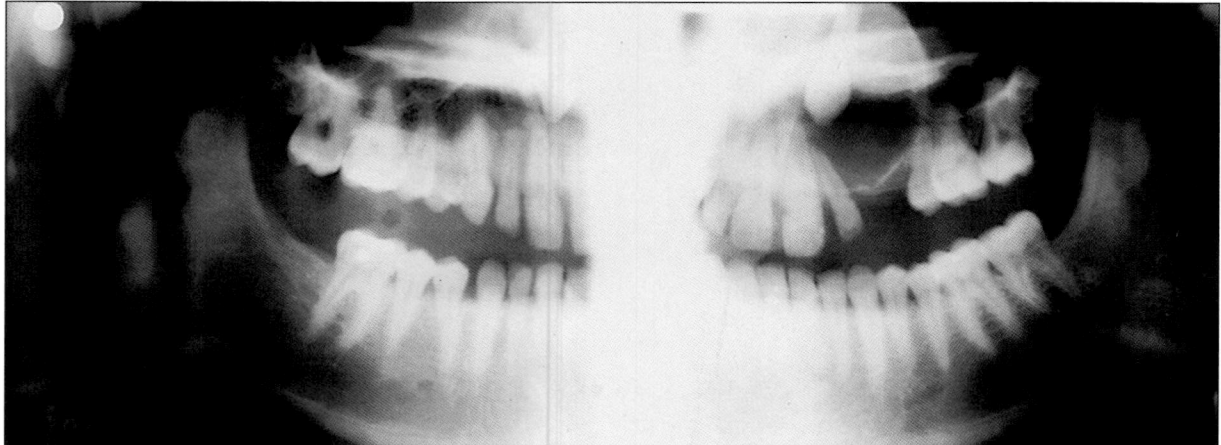

Fig 13-34c Typical radiographic picture suggestive of an adenomatoid odontogenic cyst. Specifically, it is a large, well-demarcated radiolucency in the canine-premolar area, and it has a canine tooth within it. The impacted tooth is completely within the lesion rather than the lesion arising from the cementoenamel junction area.

DIAGNOSTIC WORK-UP AND TREATMENT ▶

may also be considered even though a CEOT is uncommon at any age and even less common in individuals younger than 25 years.

An AOC is diagnosed and treated by direct exploration and enucleation from its bony crypt. If the lesion is aspirated, it will usually return a straw-colored fluid indicative of its cystic nature. The lesion readily separates from its bony crypt because it has a thick connective tissue capsule. If the specimen is cut open, the lumen will be readily apparent and the thick cyst lining will be rough textured like carpet piles (Fig 13-34d). A specimen radiograph, which can be readily obtained on an occlusal radiograph, will show the calcifications not often apparent on the patient's preoperative radiographs (Fig 13-34e).

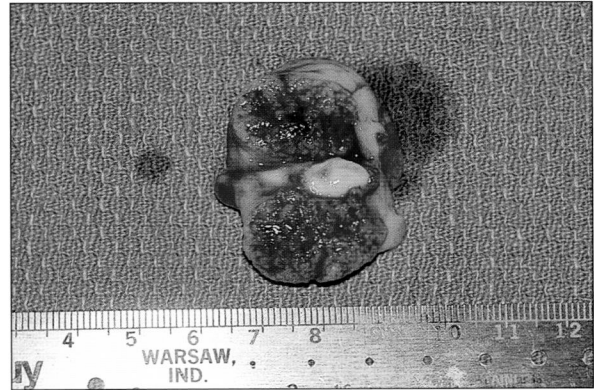

Fig 13-34d The adenomatoid odontogenic cyst arises from the root sheath epithelium and has a thick connective tissue wall and an exophytic epithelial lining growing into the lumen. At times the lining may be so prolific as to make the cyst seem like a solid tumor.

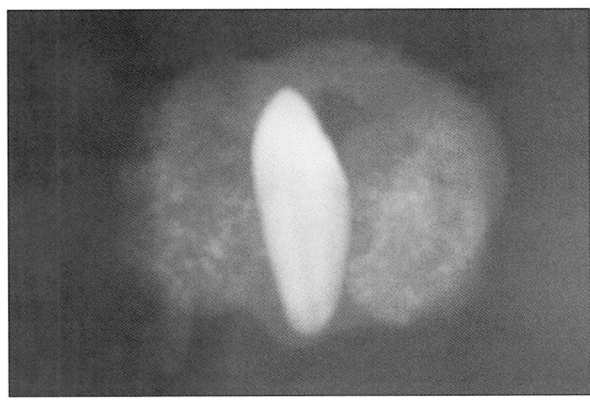

Fig 13-34e Most adenomatoid odontogenic cysts will contain small dentinoid calcifications too small to appear on a panoramic radiograph but readily visible on a specimen radiograph.

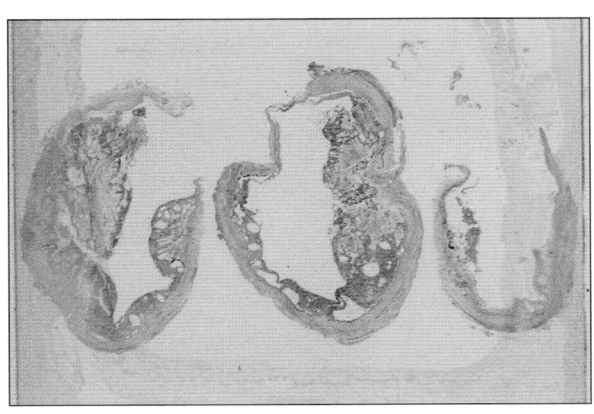

Fig 13-34f Low-power view of an adenomatoid odontogenic cyst showing its cystic configuration.

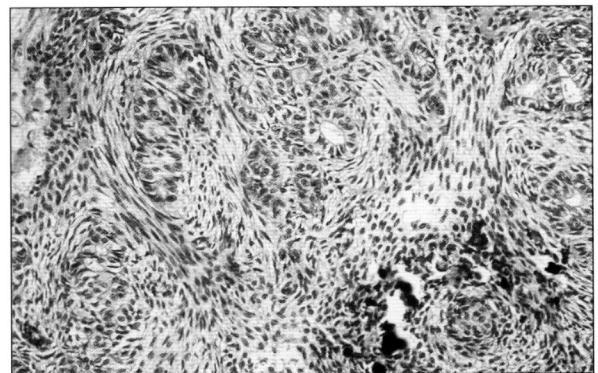

Fig 13-34g An adenomatoid odontogenic cyst showing a proliferation of spindled epithelial cells and small duct-like structures lined by cuboidal to columnar cells. Some eosinophilic globules can be seen, and dark-staining droplet calcifications are also present.

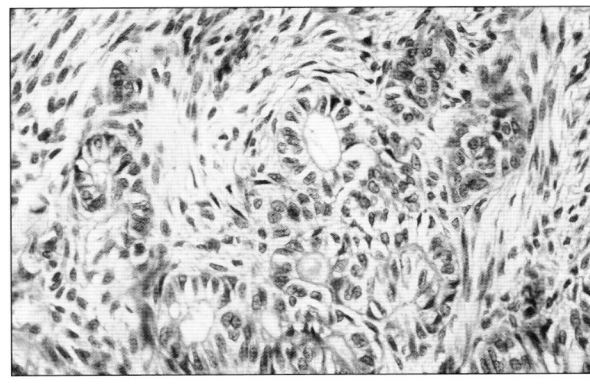

Fig 13-34h The duct-like structures containing some eosinophilic material are surrounded by columnar cells.

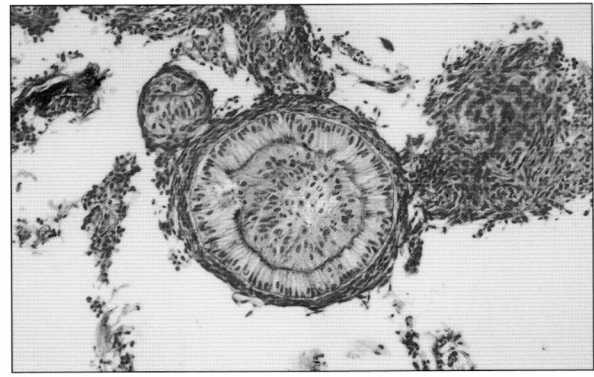

Fig 13-34i Trichrome staining of an adenomatoid odontogenic cyst in which the polarity of the columnar cells is evident. These cells do not always exhibit polarity, as is shown in Fig 13-34h. In addition, the thin blue line within the structure corresponds to the eosinophilic material seen in the hematoxylin & eosin (H&E) stain. This indicates that the material is collagen.

Because the lumen is associated with an impacted tooth, there has been some consideration given to marsupializing the lesion to gain tooth eruption. Since the AOC is a cyst rather than a tumor, this is biologically possible, but it is surgically impossible because the tooth is completely within the lumen. The AOC does not arise from the follicle of the tooth crown but instead arises from Hertwig epithelial root sheath, which would explain the finding of the tooth being completely within the lumen rather than the tooth root being within a bony crypt.

HISTOPATHOLOGY ►

These are well-demarcated cysts that typically appear with intraluminal masses (Fig 13-34f). They are very cellular with a scant fibrous stroma. The epithelial cells are bimorphic. Spindle-shaped cells lie in streams, whorled nodules, and rosettes (Fig 13-34g). Within some of these rosette-like structures, eosinophilic material may be seen. This material is periodic acid–Schiff (PAS) positive and appears to represent replicated basal lamina. In addition, there are cuboidal to columnar cells that usually line small duct-like spaces or larger cyst-like spaces, which are actually blind spheres (Figs 13-34g and 13-34h). When the nuclei are polarized, it is toward the basement membrane (away from the lumen) (Fig 13-34i). There is typically a thin layer of eosinophilic material at the periphery of the lumen. The epithelial cells may also form a plexiform pattern, particularly at the periphery of the cyst. Calcifications are present in varying quan-

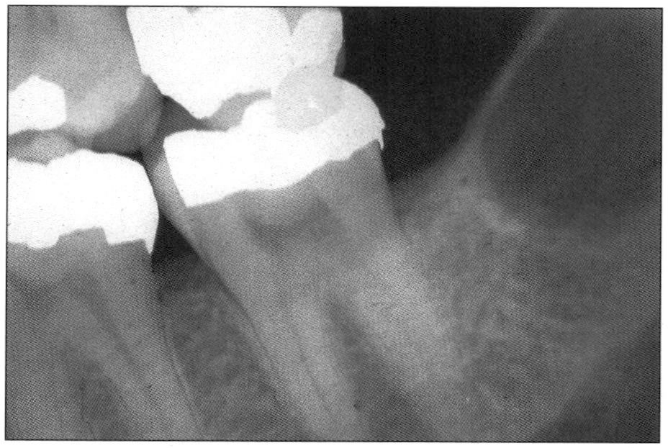

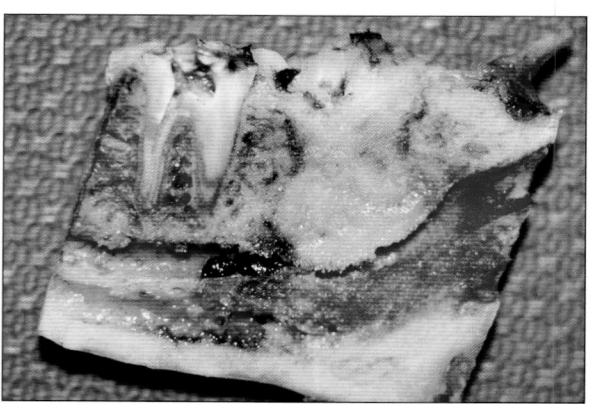

Fig 13-35a Unilocular radiolucent lesion of the mandible that was removed and diagnosed as a glandular odontogenic cyst.

Fig 13-35b Four years after removal, this supposed glandular odontogenic cyst recurred as a solid mass that was diagnosed as a low-grade mucoepidermoid carcinoma.

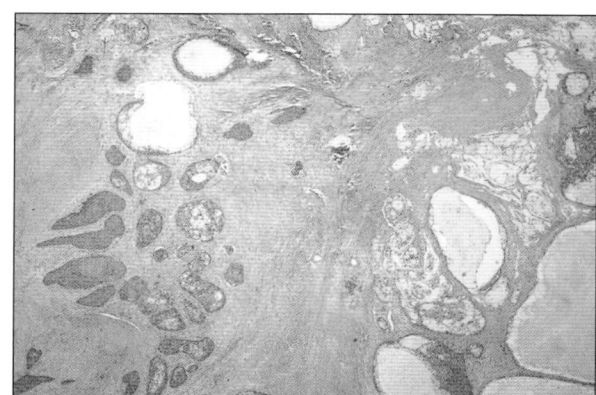

Fig 13-35c Histopathology of a low-grade mucoepidermoid carcinoma originally diagnosed as a glandular odontogenic cyst. Mucous cell–lined cystic spaces and a clear epidermoid component are evident.

tities and usually occur as small droplets (see Fig 13-34g). There may be Liesegang ring formations, and sometimes the calcifications resemble dentin or cementum, which further confirms its histogenesis from Hertwig root sheath.

PROGNOSIS ▶

Simple enucleation is curative for an AOC. Recurrences are not seen. The resultant bony cavity is best closed with the mucoperiosteal flap, and there is no need for packing or for drains. Bony regeneration is usually complete in young patients, taking about 9 to 12 months.

Rarely, peripheral AOCs are reported. Almost always occurring in the maxillary gingiva, they tend to be small proliferations in the canine region. They are excised directly and closed.

Glandular Odontogenic Cyst (Sialo-Odontogenic Cyst)

CLINICAL PRESENTATION AND PATHOGENESIS ▶

The glandular odontogenic cyst may not be a cyst or even a real entity. However, since 1990, several reports have appeared identifying jaw cysts with either numerous mucinous glandular elements in the lining or complete glandular linings. Previously, odontogenic cysts were noted to be lined with clear cells and were accepted as glandular prosoplasia from the squamous cell linings having no special clinical significance. More recently, there has been an attempt to identify these cysts as individual glandular odontogenic cysts with a notably more aggressive behavior and larger size. Some authors have suggested treatments that are even more aggressive than the enucleation and curettage recommended for most other cysts. Most studies have had limited follow-up, and in some cases the cysts themselves have recurred while in others the recurrences have been identified as low-grade mucoepidermoid carcinoma. Therefore, the status of the glandular odontogenic cyst as an unequivocal pathology remains uncertain. This author (REM) has treated three low-grade mucoepidermoid carcinomas 3 to 5 years after they were initially diagnosed as glandular odontogenic cysts (Figs 13-35a to 13-35c).

Therefore, the glandular odontogenic cyst represents one of three possibilities: (1) a true cyst of glandular origin from either entrapped salivary gland primordia or undifferentiated primitive epithelial rests that differentiate into glandular epithelium; (2) an odontogenic primordial-origin cyst in which the epithelial lining undergoes prosoplasia (metaplasia from a less specific differentiation to a more specific differentiation) into glandular epithelium. Such processes are seen in other diseases such as basaloid squamous cell carcinoma and adenosquamous cell carcinoma; or (3) a low-grade mucoepidermoid carcinoma that forms an initial single cystic space instead of the usual multicystic spaces.

HISTOPATHOLOGY ▶

Glandular odontogenic cysts are often multilocular. They are lined by epithelium of varying thickness, which usually has a flat epithelial-connective tissue interface. The epithelium is often squamous, but a dis-

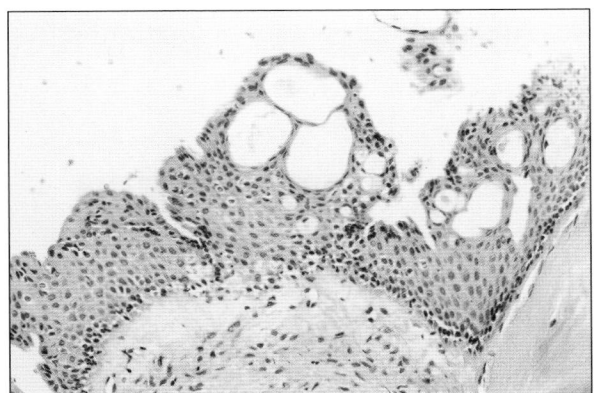

Fig 13-36a Glandular odontogenic cyst with a flat epithelial–connective tissue interface and cystic spaces within the squamous epithelial lining.

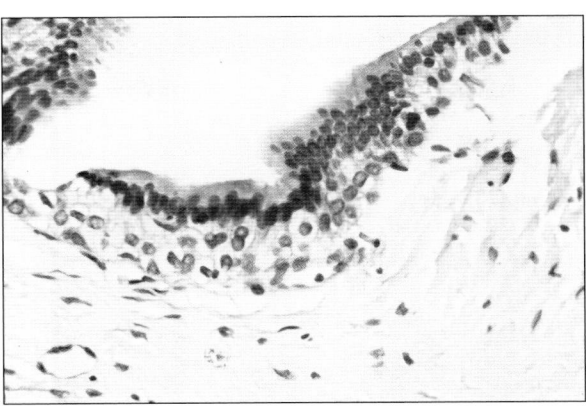

Fig 13-36b A portion of a glandular odontogenic cyst showing the luminal columnar layer of epithelial cells with eosinophilic cytoplasm.

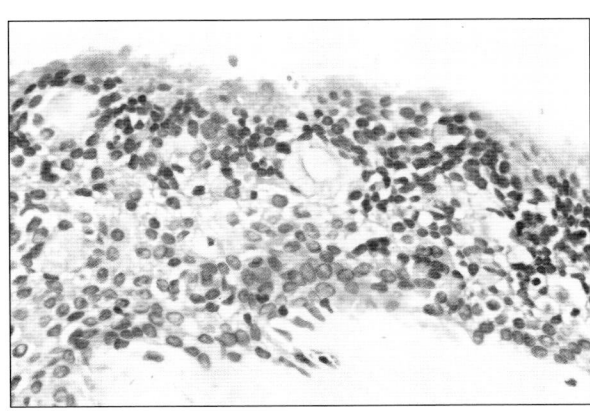

Fig 13-36c A portion of the cyst shown in Fig 13-36b showing mucous cells within the epithelial lining.

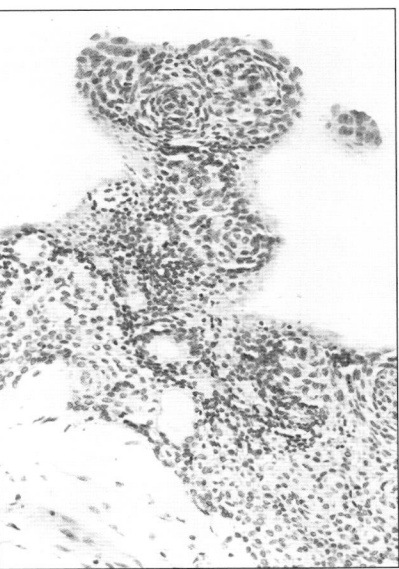

Fig 13-36d The cyst shown in Figs 13-36b and 13-36c showing the whorled cells in a nodule protruding into the lumen. This is similar to the plaques in lateral periodontal cysts. Mucous cells can also be seen in the deeper epithelial layers.

tinctive feature is that on the surface there is often a layer of cuboidal to columnar cells with eosinophilic cytoplasm. Some cells may be mucous producing and some may have cilia. Crypts that are lined by these types of cells can also be found within the deeper layers of the lining (Figs 13-36a to 13-36c). These cysts may also show features of lateral periodontal or gingival cysts in that there may be the same plaque-like thickenings and clear, glycogen-positive cells (Fig 13-36d). The mere presence of mucous cells or cilia does not confirm the diagnosis since these features are seen in other odontogenic cysts, particularly the dentigerous cyst. The wall is fibrous, usually without an inflammatory component.

TREATMENT AND PROGNOSIS ▶

Until more clear-cut data from longer follow-up studies are available, these so-called cysts are best treated as cysts with enucleation and curettage procedures. However, a thorough review of the histopathology by more than one oral and maxillofacial pathologist is recommended, as are serial sections to assess for any evidence of a mucoepidermoid carcinoma. If no more than a cyst is found, these patients are still recommended to be placed on a follow-up protocol similar to the those recommended for a malignancy—that is, an examination and panoramic radiograph every 4 months for the first 3 years and every 6 months thereafter. If a diagnosis of a low-grade mucoepidermoid carcinoma is made from the enucleated "cyst," a follow-on resection of the jaw with 1.0- to 1.5-cm margins and some overlying mucosa is recommended.

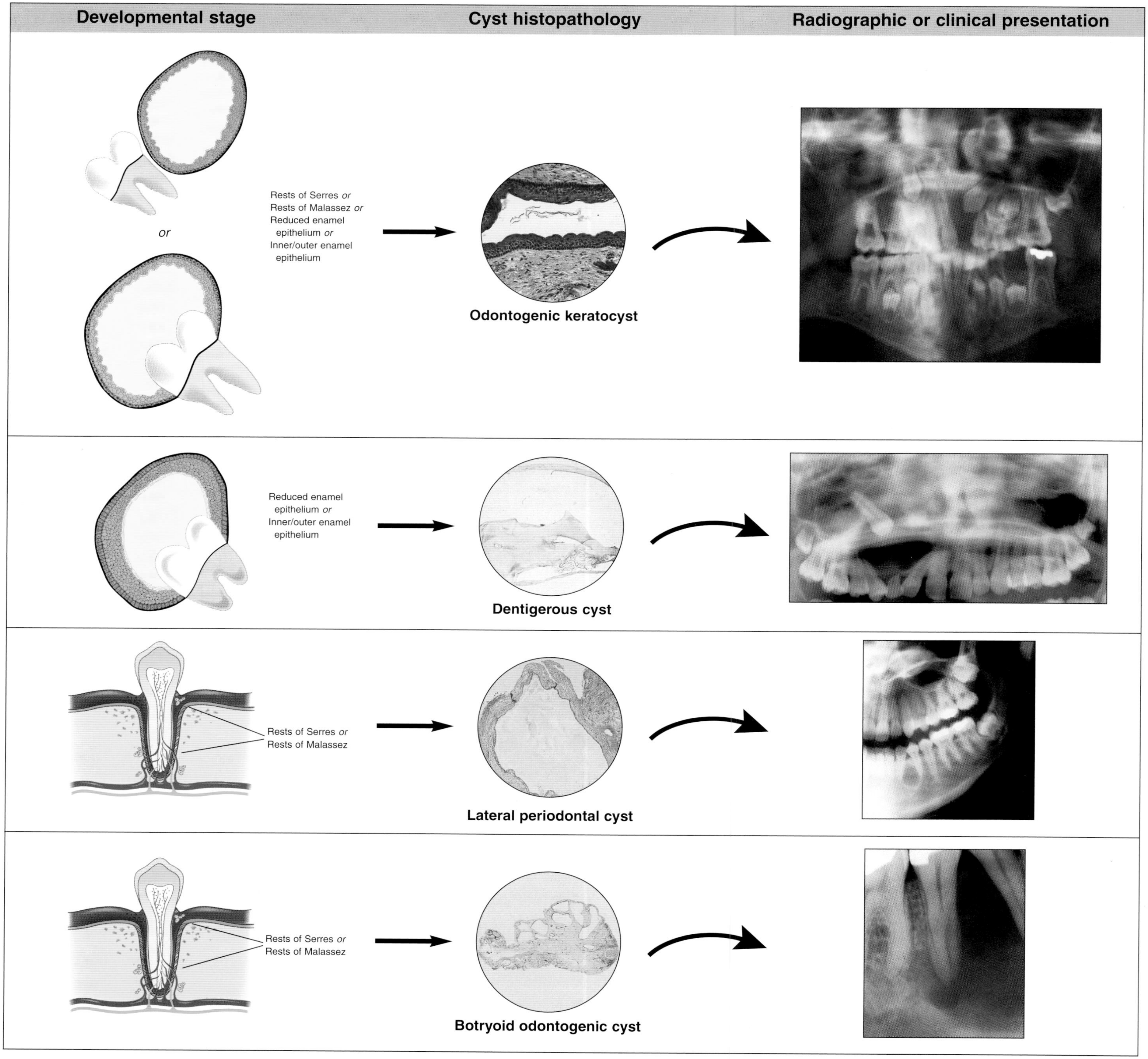

Developmental stage	Cyst histopathology	Radiographic or clinical presentation

or

Rests of Serres *or*
Rests of Malassez *or*
Reduced enamel
epithelium *or*
Inner/outer enamel
epithelium

Odontogenic keratocyst

Reduced enamel
epithelium *or*
Inner/outer enamel
epithelium

Dentigerous cyst

Rests of Serres *or*
Rests of Malassez

Lateral periodontal cyst

Rests of Serres *or*
Rests of Malassez

Botryoid odontogenic cyst

Fig 13-37a Origin, histology, and clinical/radiographic presentation of odontogenic cysts.

Developmental stage	Cyst histopathology	Radiographic or clinical presentation

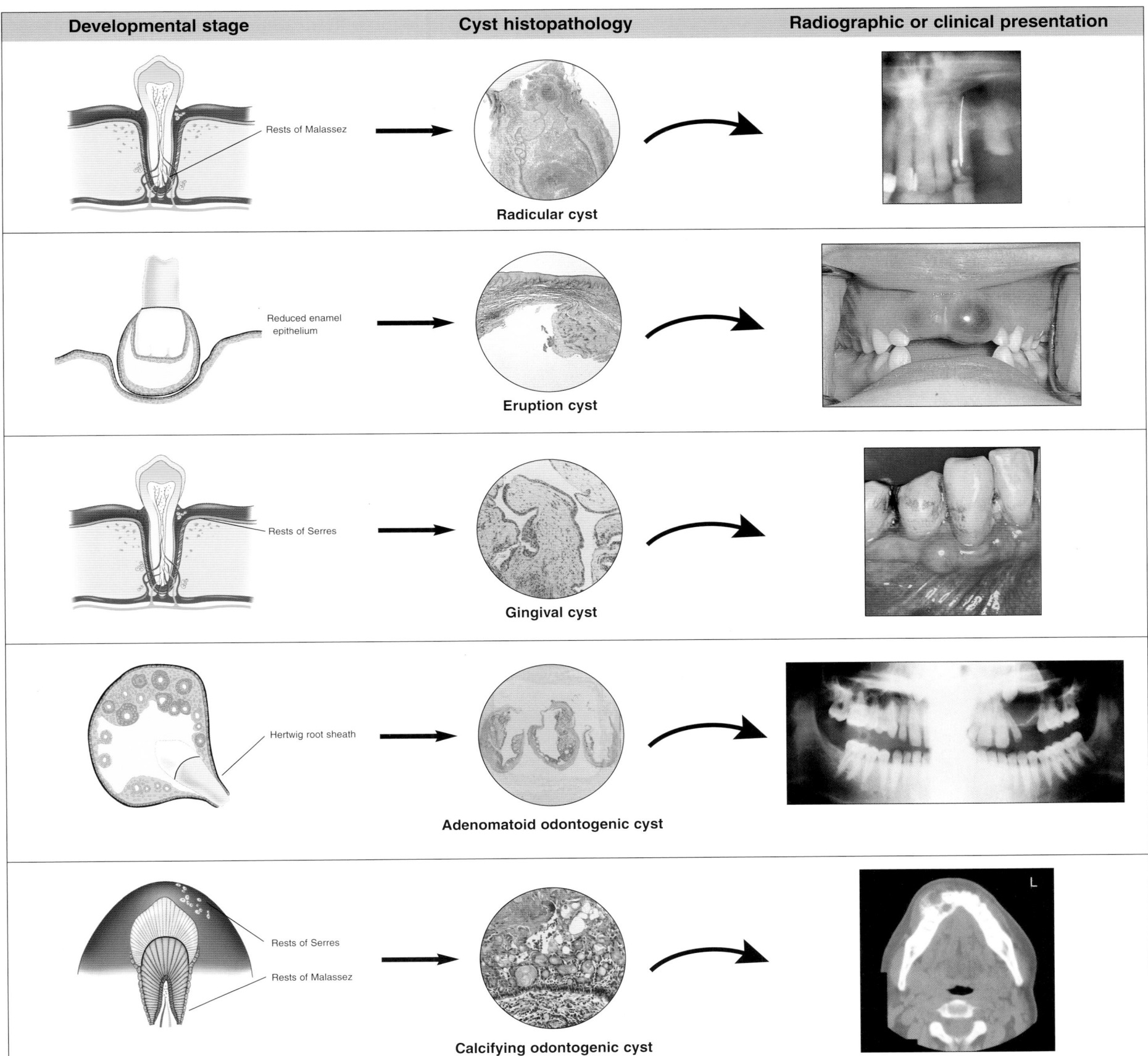

Fig 13-37a Origin, histology, and clinical/radiographic presentation of odontogenic cysts (*continued*).

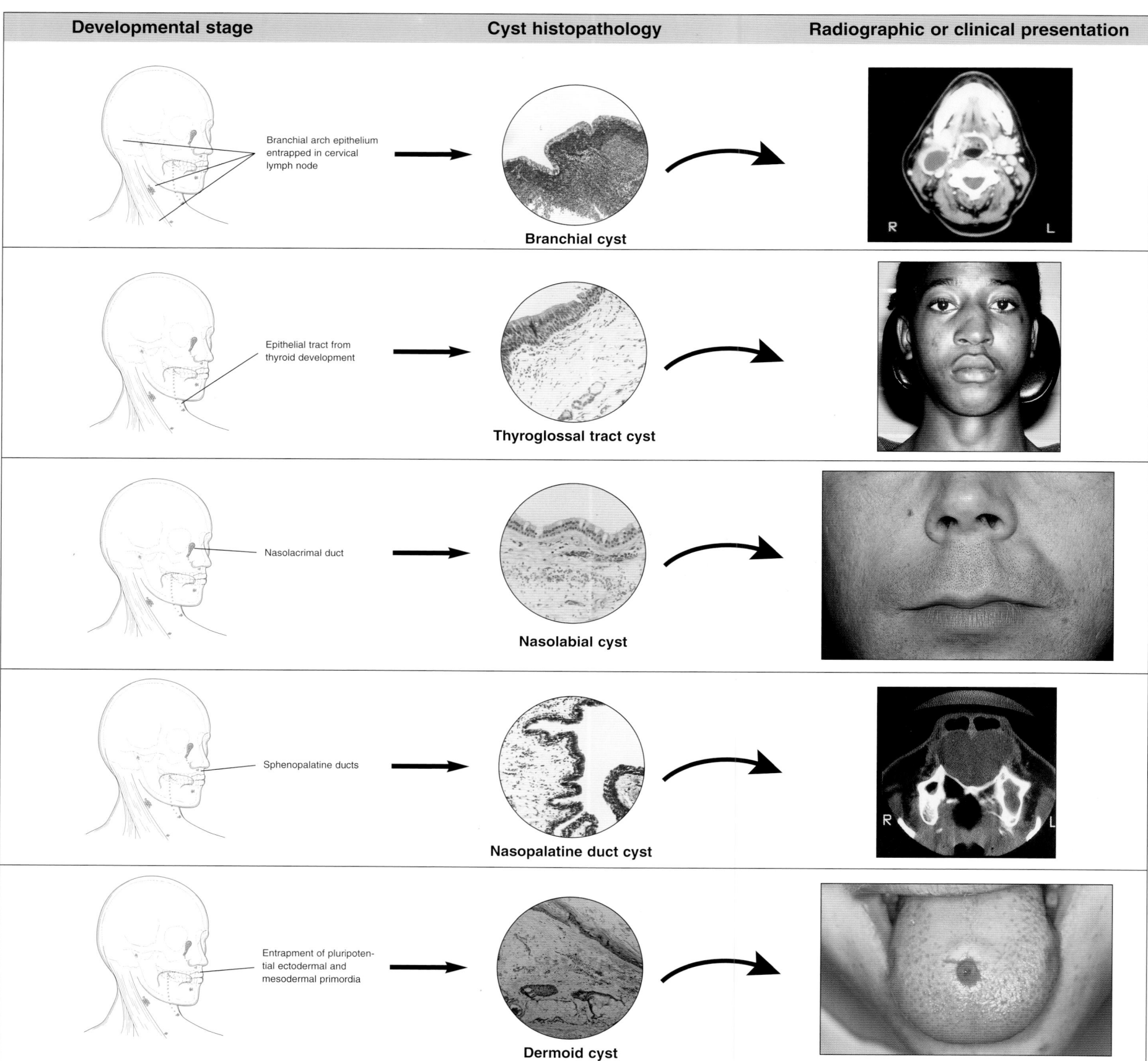

Developmental stage	Cyst histopathology	Radiographic or clinical presentation
Branchial arch epithelium entrapped in cervical lymph node	**Branchial cyst**	
Epithelial tract from thyroid development	**Thyroglossal tract cyst**	
Nasolacrimal duct	**Nasolabial cyst**	
Sphenopalatine ducts	**Nasopalatine duct cyst**	
Entrapment of pluripotential ectodermal and mesodermal primordia	**Dermoid cyst**	

Fig 13-37b Origin, histology, and clinical/radiographic presentation of nonodontogenic cysts.

Developmental stage	Cyst histopathology	Radiographic or clinical presentation

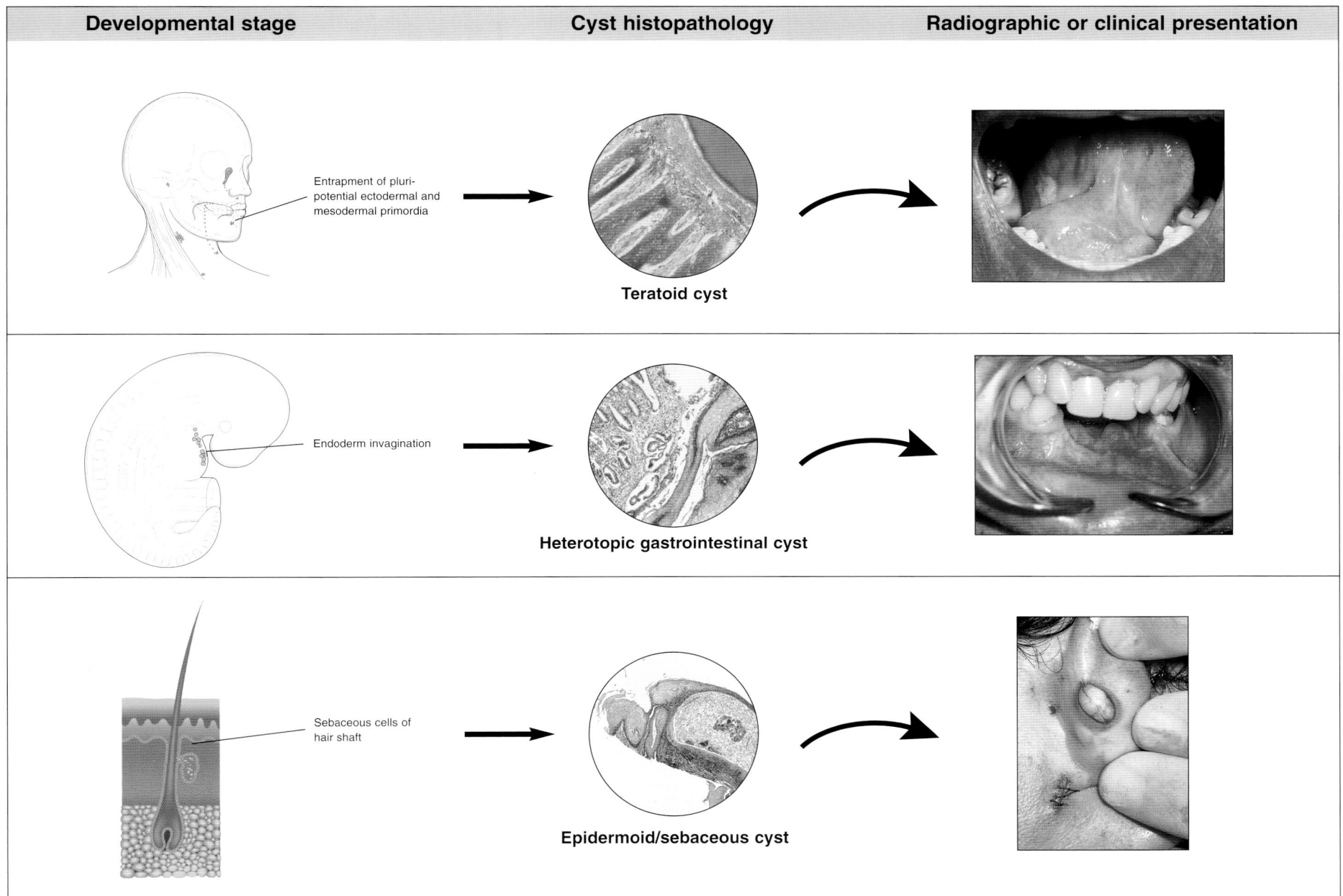

Entrapment of pluri-potential ectodermal and mesodermal primordia

Teratoid cyst

Endoderm invagination

Heterotopic gastrointestinal cyst

Sebaceous cells of hair shaft

Epidermoid/sebaceous cyst

Fig 13-37b Origin, histology, and clinical/radiographic presentation of nonodontogenic cysts (*continued*).

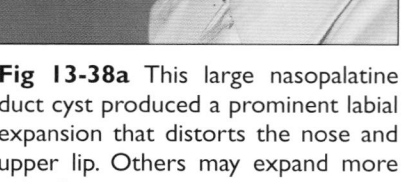

Fig 13-38a This large nasopalatine duct cyst produced a prominent labial expansion that distorts the nose and upper lip. Others may expand more palatally.

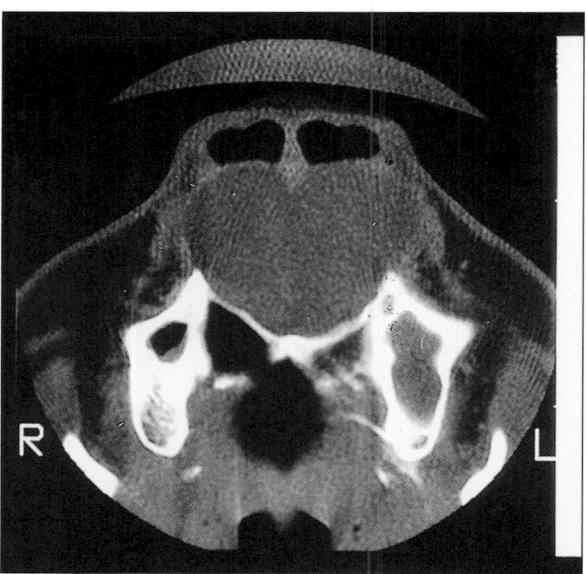

Fig 13-38b The nasopalatine duct cyst will usually be heart shaped and located in the midline. Here the nasal distortion is also visible.

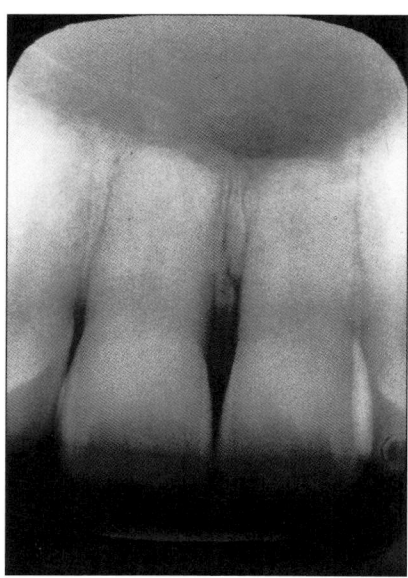

Fig 13-38c Smooth, regular root resorption of the incisor teeth. The four incisors were unresponsive to pulp testing because of pressure from the cyst. They regained responsiveness at 9 months.

Nonodontogenic Cysts

Nasopalatine Duct Cyst (Incisive Canal Cyst)

CLINICAL PRESENTATION AND PATHOGENESIS ▶

The nasopalatine duct cyst arises from epithelial remnants from the two embryonic nasopalatine ducts. Consequently, cysts may form anywhere along the ducts' course, which runs from the posterior palatal midline to the soft tissue palatine papilla (incisive papilla). Cysts in the posterior palatal midline (formerly termed *median palatal cysts*) and cysts limited to the soft tissue palatine papilla (formerly termed *cysts of the palatine papilla*) are now understood to represent nasopalatine duct cysts that are merely found in slightly different locations along this embryonic tract.

The cyst usually presents as a soft tissue swelling of the palatal midline. Smaller cysts and cysts limited to the palatine papilla show only a swelling just behind the maxillary central incisors. Larger cysts create a labial expansion as well as a midpalatal expansion, which is often compressible because the palatal bone is resorbed beneath the mucosa (Fig 13-38a). In some cases, an earlier infection that may have initiated cyst development is documented. Some cysts present with subtle drainage that the patient will report as a salty or unpleasant taste.

Men are affected more than women (2:1 ratio), and most individuals are in the 30- to 60-year age range.

The cyst originates from remnants of the paired embryonic nasopalatine ducts that become incorporated into the incisive canal along with the terminal extensions of the sphenopalatine neurovascular bundle as the maxillary palatine processes fuse from each side. The cells may spontaneously activate in adult life to produce a cyst, but more likely are stimulated by an infection similar to the formation of branchial cysts, thyroglossal tract cysts, and radicular cysts.

RADIOGRAPHIC FINDINGS ▶

Radiographically, large lesions revealing a midline, heart-shaped, unilocular radiolucency are apparent (Fig 13-38b). If sufficiently large, they create a smooth, regular resorption of the incisor roots (Fig 13-38c).

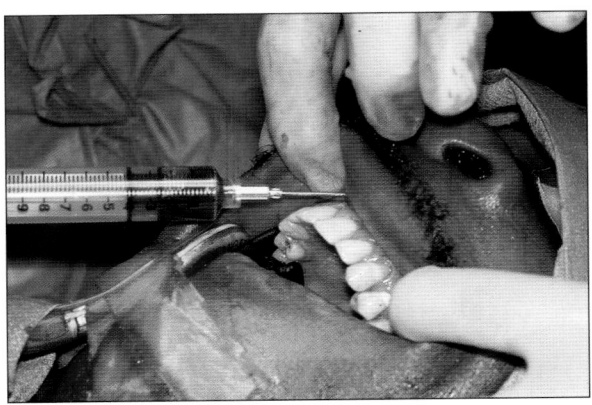

Fig 13-38d Aspiration of a nasopalatine duct cyst will usually return straw-colored fluid, confirming its cystic nature.

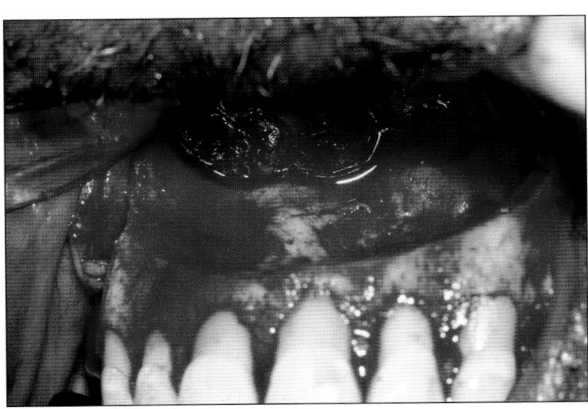

Fig 13-38e Removal of a large nasopalatine duct cyst reveals extensive bone resorption, including the palate. Shown here is the palatal submucosa from the labial view.

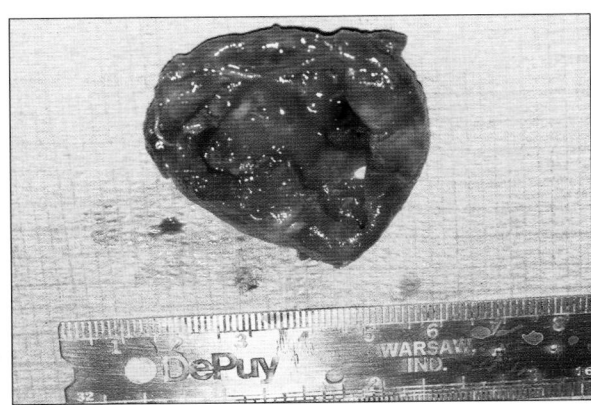

Fig 13-38f Gross specimen of a nasopalatine duct cyst, showing a thin lining with a hemorrhagic cyst wall indicative of the numerous small blood vessels within it.

Smaller lesions show either a definitive, well-demarcated unilocular radiolucency or only an expanded incisive canal. The latter presentation is diagnostically controversial because many wide yet normal incisive canals are diagnosed as incisive canal cysts (nasopalatine duct cysts). However, a wide incisive canal radiographically without a soft tissue or bony expansion or clinical symptoms is not considered a nasopalatine duct cyst and requires no exploration.

DIFFERENTIAL DIAGNOSIS ▶

A midline palatal radiolucency and expansion is believed to represent a nasopalatine duct cyst until proven otherwise. However, in this area, a simple *periapical granuloma* or *radicular cyst* from nonvital central incisor teeth may produce a similar presentation. In addition, a *primordial cyst* related to supernumerary tooth buds, such as the mesiodens, is a consideration. In patients with a small radiolucency and/or minimal swelling, the most difficult distinction may be that of a *normal incisive canal*. Although a rare entity, a *chondrosarcoma* is reasonable to consider since this is one of the preferred locations for this rare tumor of the jaws.

DIAGNOSTIC WORK-UP AND TREATMENT ▶

The incisor teeth require pulp testing, but the results should be interpreted cautiously. While it is important not to ignore a nonvital tooth that has an apical lesion, one should realize that cystic pressure, which may cause root resorption, may also cause a neuropraxia and hence nonresponsiveness to pulp testing. Endodontic therapy for a clinically sound tooth with root resorption related to a nasopalatine duct cyst encroachment is inappropriate.

Plain radiographs and aspiration of the lesion provide strong evidence of its cystic nature (Fig 13-38d). The cyst is best treated with enucleation from a labial approach. In large lesions where the palatal bone has been resorbed, the cyst wall will become adherent to the periosteum (Fig 13-38e). This area in particular requires careful and often sharp dissection to prevent a palatal tear (Fig 13-38f). In any large cyst that resorbs palatal bone, a maxillary palatal splint is advised to support the palatal mucosa. This splint should be planned for and fabricated on a premade stone cast. It may be retained by wire clasps or directly wired to the teeth. The splint can be removed in 10 to 14 days.

While marsupialization may be performed, it is unnecessary and creates a long and laborious postoperative course. It will also slow and in most cases retard bone regeneration. Similarly, packing the enucleated cavity is unnecessary and will also slow and retard bone regeneration. Less commonly, a more posteriorly located cyst will have no labial presentation. If radiographs or CT scans show a remaining thickness of labial bone above the incisor root apices, a palatal approach is best. In such cases, a palatal sulcular incision to reflect a full-thickness, posteriorly based palatal flap is recommended for best access. The cyst can then be enucleated from the bony cavity and separated from the palatal periosteum by direct vision.

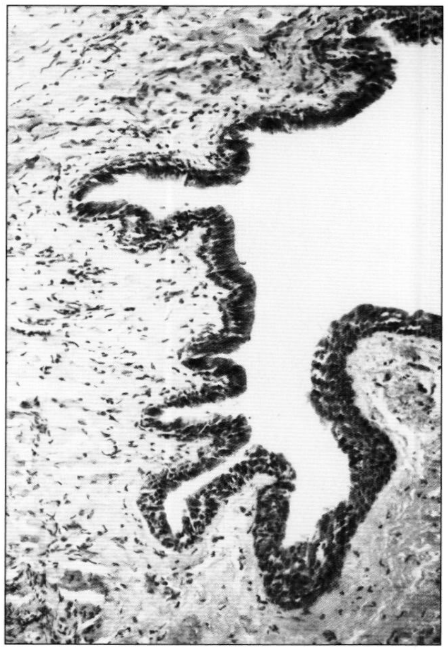

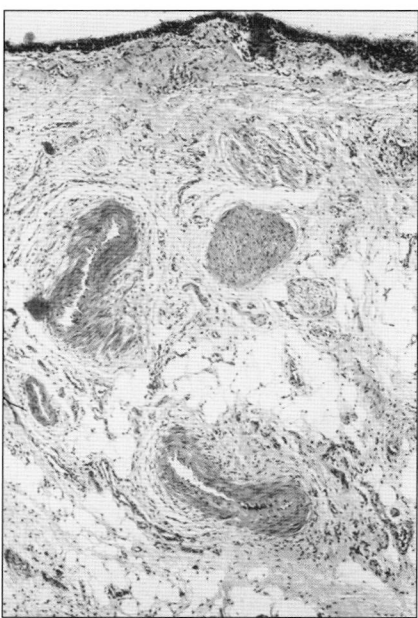

Fig 13-38g Nasopalatine duct cyst lined in part by stratified squamous epithelium and in part by respiratory epithelium.

Fig 13-38h The wall of a nasopalatine duct cyst often contains nerve and thick-walled blood vessels. A portion of the stratified squamous epithelial lining can be seen.

HISTOPATHOLOGY

The lining of the nasopalatine duct cyst may be stratified squamous epithelium, pseudostratified columnar epithelium with or without cilia, or a combination of these. Mucous cells may be prominent (Fig 13-38g). As with the thyroglossal tract cyst, these variations may be influenced by the position of the cyst within the duct. The wall consists of fibrous tissue and structures reflecting the anatomy of the area. This includes thick-walled blood vessels, nerve bundles, fat, and occasional mucous glands (Fig 13-38h). Sometimes a small amount of cartilage is seen. Inflammatory cells are variably present. Tissue removed from an asymptomatic radiolucency, representing an enlarged but otherwise normal incisive canal, will show nothing other than normal connective tissue components, including a portion of the incisive nerve.

PROGNOSIS

Enucleation of this cyst is curative without recurrence.

Nasolabial Cyst

CLINICAL PRESENTATION AND PATHOGENESIS

The nasolabial cyst is a very rare cyst limited to soft tissue that is believed to originate from embryonic epithelial elements of the nasolacrimal duct. Because no bone is involved, its former name, nasoalveolar cyst, is inappropriate.

The nasolabial cyst will present in middle-aged adults as a painless round mass within the skin adjacent to the ala of the nose around the uppermost portion of the nasolabial crease (Fig 13-39a). The mass will be doughy and sometimes compressible, suggesting a cyst. The overlying skin will be normal without areas of drainage. The cyst's location is subcutaneous and external to the facial musculature, although it may cause the oral mucosa to bulge noticeably. Nasolabial cysts have shown a 4:1 predilection for women.

The presumed origin of the nasolabial cyst has changed. In the past these cysts were thought to represent the soft tissue corollary of the globulomaxillary cyst, which was theorized to arise via entrapment of embryonic epithelium between the lateral nasal process and the maxillary processes. However, this theory has been abandoned because embryologic evidence shows that epithelium does not exist be-

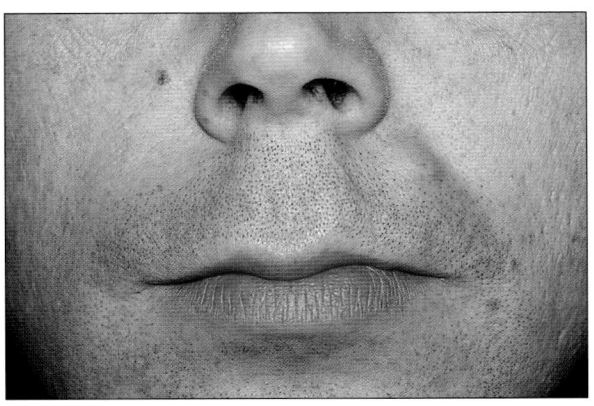

Fig 13-39a A nasolabial cyst will present as a painless soft tissue mass in the nasolabial crease.

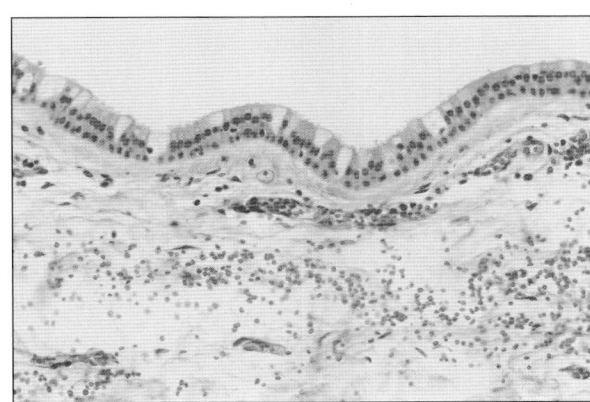

Fig 13-39b Nasolabial cyst with a pseudostratified columnar epithelium and obvious mucous cells.

tween these processes and because those cysts previously labeled as globulomaxillary cysts were actually found to be cysts and tumors of other origins. Instead, the nasolabial cyst seems to arise from epithelial rests derived from the nasal mucosal invaginations that produce the nasolacrimal duct.

DIFFERENTIAL DIAGNOSIS ▶

The most common entity to present in a similar fashion clinically is a *canine space abscess* from an odontogenic infection. In addition, a *sebaceous cyst* or an *implanted epidermal inclusion cyst* clinically and histologically resemble a nasolabial cyst. In such cases, a thorough histopathologic review of the epithelial lining is necessary to distinguish them. In the nasolabial cyst, the majority of its lining is pseudostratified columnar cells rather than stratified squamous cells as are found in the other two. Additionally, salivary gland neoplasms are located in the mucosa on the oral side of the facial musculature, but large *benign salivary gland tumors* will produce an external bulge as well, and *malignant salivary gland tumors* will infiltrate the buccinator, which can produce a nasolabial area mass.

DIAGNOSTIC WORK-UP AND TREATMENT ▶

A dental examination including pulp testing of the maxillary teeth in the affected area is needed to rule out an odontogenic infection.

Definitive resolution of the nasolabial cyst is accomplished by surgical pericapsular excision. Because the cyst is located external to the facial muscles, a transcutaneous approach is preferred. The incision is often best placed in the nasolabial crease to minimize the prominence of the scar. An ellipse of overlying surface such as is used when removing a sebaceous cyst is not required. The cyst is usually well circumscribed and possesses a connective tissue capsule that permits a straightforward pericapsular dissection.

HISTOPATHOLOGY ▶

The lining of nasolabial cysts is usually a pseudostratified, nonciliated columnar epithelium and may contain numerous mucous cells. However, stratified squamous epithelium may also be present. The wall is fibrous (Fig 13-39b).

PROGNOSIS ▶

Nasolabial cysts are eradicated by excision. Recurrence does not develop.

Thyroglossal Tract Cyst

CLINICAL PRESENTATION AND PATHOGENESIS ▶

The thyroglossal tract cyst is the most common cyst found in the neck. It will often be preceded by an upper respiratory tract infection and has a rapid ascendancy of 2 to 4 weeks. Most (60%) occur in the midline over the thyrohyoid membrane (Fig 13-40a). About 15% occur slightly off the midline and may, therefore, prevent the clinician from considering a thyroglossal tract cyst. About 2% will arise within the tongue itself deep to the foramen cecum. The remainder (23%) will occur in the midline below the level of the thyrohyoid membrane.

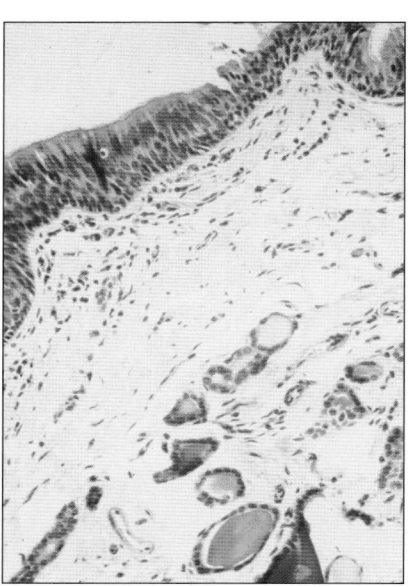

Fig 13-40a This thyroglossal tract cyst arose in 10 days following a viral flu. It moves with the hyoid upon swallowing and is located in the midline.

Fig 13-40b Thyroglossal tract cyst showing a pseudostratified columnar epithelial lining and some thyroid follicles in the wall.

Most cysts will be doughy, round masses with a smooth, rounded surface. Because they are often stimulated by an upper respiratory tract infection, many are tender to palpation, some are painful, and others may be overtly infected with a cutaneous fistula draining pus. They will classically move with the hyoid bone when the patient swallows because the tract that remains connected to the cyst also goes through the body of the hyoid bone.

About 60% of thyroglossal tract cysts occur in adolescents or in adults in their 20s. About 10% occur in children, and only 30% occur in adults older than 30 years. The incidence proportionately decreases after the age of 30 years.

Thyroglossal tract cysts arise from stimulated residual epithelial cells from the descent of embryonic oral epithelial cells that formed the thyroid gland. The source of this dormant epithelium that becomes activated in later years is the cells that invaginated from the fetal tongue area. The anterior two thirds of the tongue arises from the first branchial arch, and the posterior one third arises from the third branchial arch. The second branchial arch between the two involutes. Before it involutes, the thyroid anlage in the area destined to become the foramen cecum invaginates downward at about the fourth week of fetal life. The tract courses through the developing hyoid bone until the tenth week of fetal life and finally comes to rest at the inferior edge of the developing thyroid cartilage. Involution of the tract as well as the second branchial arch representation in the oral cavity occurs at this time. Residual epithelium and even elements of thyroid gland tissue remain after involution.

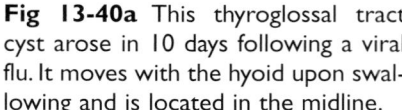

DIFFERENTIAL DIAGNOSIS ▶ The uncomplicated thyroglossal tract cyst will be strongly suggested by its rapid development, its midline or near-midline presentation, and its movement on swallowing. Other midline or paramidline solitary mass lesions include a *lipoma,* a *sebaceous cyst,* a *dermoid cyst,* or lesions related to a *lymphadenopathy* (which may be related to nonspecific infections), *cat-scratch disease,* a *lymphoma,* or *HIV-related lymphadenopathy,* among others. A branchial cyst would not be a serious consideration because although it may occur at several levels in the neck, it is always in the area of the anterior border of the sternocleidomastoid muscle or the preauricular area and not in the midline.

Those cysts with a draining fistula may still be thyroglossal tract cysts and should not be overlooked. The drainage would otherwise focus the concern on a *submental space abscess,* the drainage associated

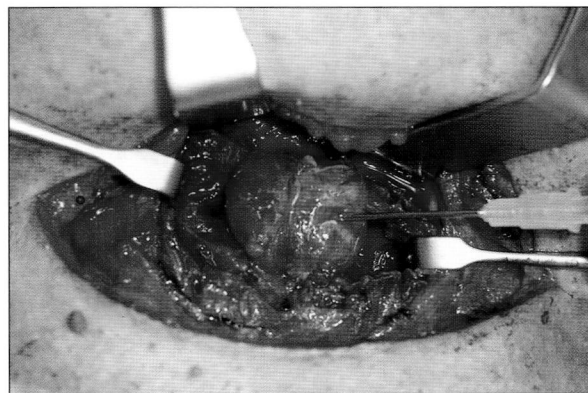

Fig 13-40c The thin wall of a thyroglossal tract cyst is implied by its blue color. The fluid contents are aspirated while the sternohyoid muscle is retracted to increase exposure.

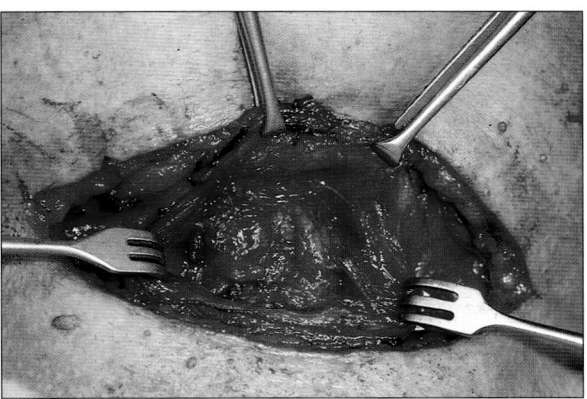

Fig 13-40d A thin-walled thyroglossal tract cyst that has deflated, whether by aspiration or by a tear in the lining, is more difficult to see and to remove.

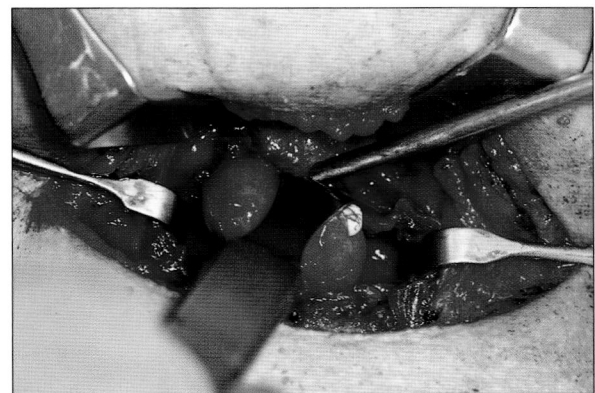

Fig 13-40e A thyroglossal tract cyst injected with Coesoft or alginate will add consistency and stabilize the cyst to facilitate removal.

with about 10% of cases of *cat-scratch disease,* a *tuberculosis-related lymphadenitis,* or even an *osteomyelitis of the mandible.*

DIAGNOSTIC WORK-UP ►

Although a CT scan or an MRI scan can confirm the cyst's fluid-filled center and its location, and a needle aspirate can suggest the diagnosis by its return of fluid, a thyroglossal tract cyst is a diagnosis suspected through clinical examination and confirmed only upon removal.

HISTOPATHOLOGY ►

Thyroglossal tract cysts are usually lined with pseudostratified columnar epithelium that may be ciliated. They are sometimes lined with stratified squamous epithelium, especially when the cyst is located more superiorly. The wall frequently contains thyroid follicles (Fig 13-40b). Malignancy rarely develops, but adenocarcinomas have been reported.

TREATMENT ►

Treatment is performed by a surgical excision called the *Sistrunk procedure.* The cyst is approached with a horizontal neck incision in the nearest available skin fold over the mass. The cyst will protrude from between the two sternohyoid muscles, which are reflected laterally to increase exposure. The cyst will have a very thin lining that can be easily ruptured during a dissection around its periphery. Therefore, it is often useful first to aspirate the fluid contents (Fig 13-40c) and then, while leaving the needle in place, to inject an equal volume of soft tissue liner material (Coesoft, GC America) or alginate (Caulk, Dentsply). This maneuver, which is appropriate only for soft tissue cysts, will prevent collapse of the cystic shape and facilitate a pericapsular dissection (Figs 13-40d and 13-40e).

As the cyst is separated from its surrounding tissues, it will remain pedicled on a stalk (the residual thyroglossal tract) to the body of the hyoid bone (Fig 13-40f). The body of the hyoid is resected and the residual tract deep to it clamped and ligated before the cyst, a portion of the tract, and the body of the hyoid are delivered. Removing the hyoid body will not destabilize the hyoid. The remaining suprahyoid and infrahyoid muscles attached to the lesser and greater horns keep this bone stable, as does the closure, in which the reflected geniohyoid muscle attachment from above is sutured to the thyrohyoid muscle below. The remaining wound is drained and closed in layers.

Because thyroglossal tract cysts are often initiated by a case of pharyngitis, a full course of antibiotics, usually oral phenoxymethyl penicillin (Pen-Vee K, Wyeth-Ayerst), 500 mg four times daily for 10 days, is recommended. Recent experiences with this classic Sistrunk procedure have indicated that maintenance of the body of the hyoid is possible without risk of recurrence. Today, it is more common to tie off the tract remnant at the surface of the hyoid bone rather than to resect the body of the hyoid bone.

PROGNOSIS ►

Excised thyroglossal tract cysts rarely recur. The specimen should be carefully inspected for thickened areas (Fig 13-40g), as rare cases of a malignancy occurring from the lining have been reported.

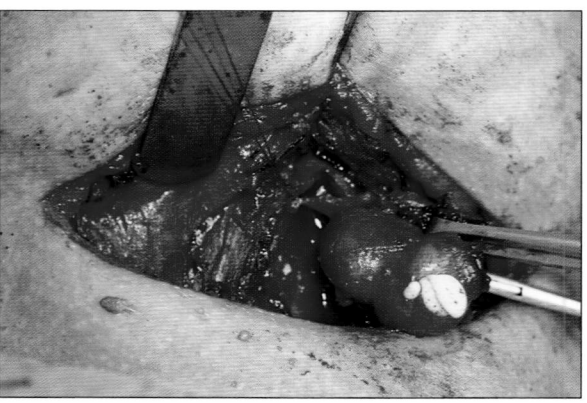

Fig 13-40f The thyroglossal tract cyst with its tract entering the hyoid bone is well exposed. The cyst lumen was injected with Coesoft.

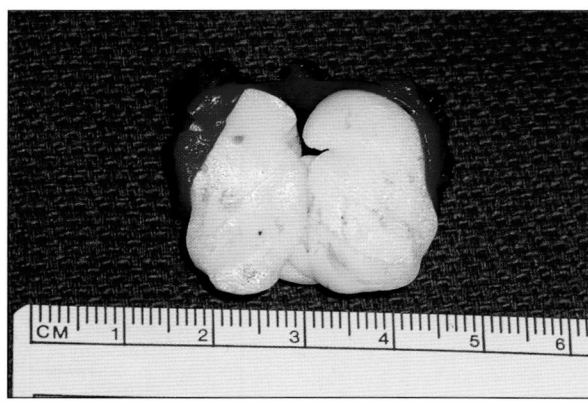

Fig 13-40g The thin walls of a thyroglossal tract cyst are well delineated against the background and support of the white Coesoft.

Branchial Cyst

CLINICAL PRESENTATION AND PATHOGENESIS

The branchial cyst will usually arise rapidly (1 to 3 weeks) as a mass in the neck just anterior and deep to the sternocleidomastoid muscle at the level of the carotid bifurcation. Less commonly, some cysts will develop higher along the sternocleidomastoid border, appearing in the preauricular-parotid area, or lower along the sternocleidomastoid border, appearing in the supraclavicular area. Most arise in preteens, teenagers, and young adults and are preceded by an upper respiratory tract infection.

Branchial cysts often attain a very large size (exceeding 8 cm) and do not move with head motion or upon swallowing (Fig 13-41a). They will feel firm and, although not fixed, they also are not readily movable. Many will be painful or at least tender to palpation since their stimulus is related to inflammation. Rare cysts will be overtly infected and may present with a draining cutaneous fistula.

Branchial cysts are believed to be related to residual or buried epithelium from the branchial clefts; hence the name sometimes used is *branchial cleft cyst*. The fact that they occur at the three levels of the branchial clefts and that at any level they have a residual tract leading to the pharynx supports this concept. Those that arise at the carotid bifurcation level are thought to be related to the second branchial cleft, which is the biggest and deepest cleft.

An alternative theory of origin is that epithelium of salivary origin becomes embryonically entrapped within cervical lymph nodes and later undergoes cystic degeneration. The histopathologic finding of lymphoid aggregates in these cysts would seem to support this theory. However, with the ubiquitousness of lymphoid elements in the neck and the usual inflammatory stimulant to this cyst, its association with lymphoid aggregates may be expected. This theory alone does not adequately explain the association with pharyngeal infection or the pharyngeal sinus tract associated with this cyst in 80% of cases. It also denies the precedent set by the thyroglossal tract cyst, which does arise from embryonic epithelium left behind from a residual tract.

Lesions similar to the branchial cyst, called *lymphoepithelial cysts*, occur in the floor of the mouth and in the parotid gland. They are identical in their histopathology and probably arise from entrapped epithelium in these locations as well. Those in the floor of the mouth tend to be less than 1 cm and readily excisable. Those in the parotid gland may be 2 to 5 cm and require superficial parotidectomies.

DIFFERENTIAL DIAGNOSIS

A large, firm mass in the neck in this location always suggests the possibility of *metastatic squamous cell carcinoma*. However, the patient's age, the cyst's rapid ascendancy, and its usual tender nature all speak against this diagnosis. In this age group, lymph node diseases are a serious consideration, especially *cat-scratch disease,* which also has a rapid ascendancy; *Hodgkin lymphoma; sarcoidosis; tuberculosis-related*

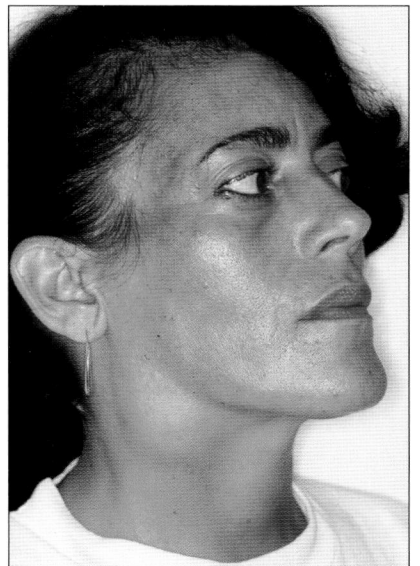

Fig 13-41a This branchial cyst grew to a size of 6 to 8 cm in 2 weeks following a pharyngitis. (Courtesy of Dr Eric Carlson.)

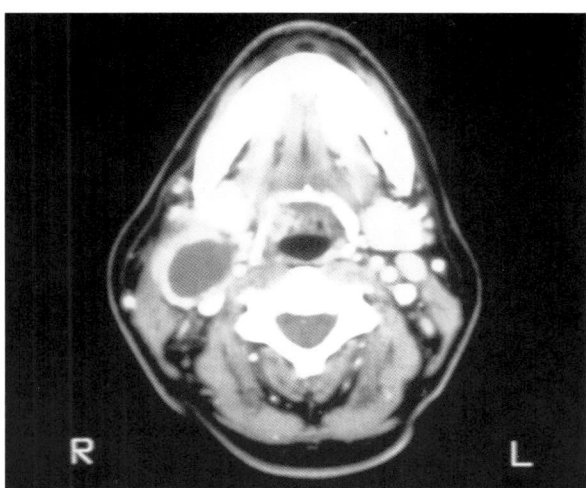

Fig 13-41b A CT scan reveals the thick, hyperdense wall and fluid-filled, hypodense lumen of a branchial cyst. Its location, deep to the sternocleidomastoid muscle and superficial to the carotid sheath, is also seen on the scan. (Courtesy of Dr Eric Carlson.)

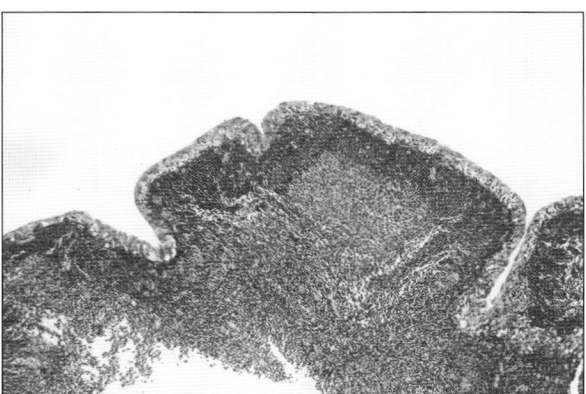

Fig 13-41c Branchial cyst (lymphoepithelial cyst) with stratified squamous epithelial lining and lymphoid tissue in the wall. A germinal center is present.

lymphadenitis (scrofula); and *HIV-related lymphadenopathy*. A thyroglossal tract cyst would not be a serious consideration because it would not occur laterally in the neck.

DIAGNOSTIC WORK-UP ▶

Masses in the neck that realistically represent the possibility of a deposit of squamous cell carcinoma should undergo a fine needle aspiration biopsy before an exploration and biopsy by removal. A branchial cyst will usually return more than 10 mL of a brown, watery fluid. A CT scan or an MRI scan is not required but will elicit a picture suggestive of a fluid-filled cyst as well as outline its size and anatomic relationships. The CT scan should also show the characteristically thick wall of a branchial cyst (Fig 13-41b).

HISTOPATHOLOGY ▶

The lining of a branchial cyst is usually a stratified squamous epithelium, although sometimes it is pseudostratified and columnar and occasionally ciliated. The lining can be ulcerated. The fibrous wall contains prominent lymphoid tissue, which often has well-developed germinal centers. In most cases, the lymphoid tissue is in close proximity to the epithelium. These histologic features are diagnostic (Fig 13-41c).

TREATMENT ▶

Branchial cysts are excised and their residual tract ligated. The cyst is approached with a horizontal neck incision in the closest natural skin crease over the prominence of the mass. Some reports describe a vertical skin incision parallel to the anterior border of the sternocleidomastoid muscle, but this approach provides no better access and produces a more pronounced scar. The cyst is found deep in the cervical fascia and is deep to the platysma muscle. Positioned anterior to and lying upon the carotid sheath, the cyst is readily separable from its surrounding tissues (Fig 13-41d). If the cyst is perforated and deflates, making its removal more difficult, the cavity may be injected with a soft tissue liner or alginate to re-inflate it. The return of contour assists the technique of blunt pericapsular dissection required for removal. However, unlike the easily torn lining of the thyroglossal tract cyst, the branchial cyst has a very thick wall that is not easily torn, and therefore this maneuver is rarely needed (Fig 13-41e). With the carotid sheath and the sternocleidomastoid muscle retracted posteriorly, a tract may be found to course from the cyst through the carotid bifurcation to the lateral pharyngeal wall. This tract is ligated as deep as possible before the cyst and a portion of its tract are delivered. The resultant wound is usually drained because of the dead space it represents. The patient is also treated with a 10-day course of antibiotics to eradicate any pharyngitis and to reduce the population of the pharyngeal flora. Aqueous penicillin G (Wyeth Ayerst), 1.2 million U intravenously every 6 hours, is usually used until discharge, followed by oral

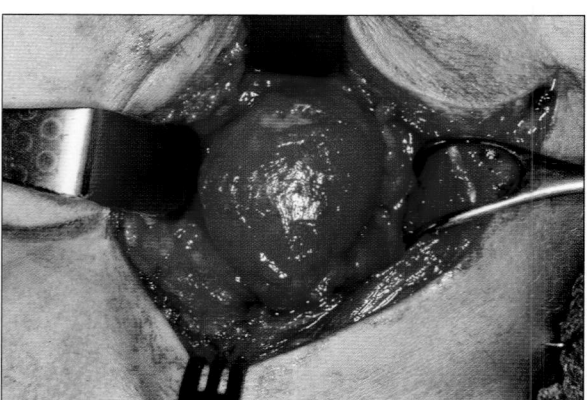

Fig 13-41d Branchial cysts are removed with a pericapsular dissection except for the pharyngeal tract, which requires ligation. (Courtesy of Dr Eric Carlson.)

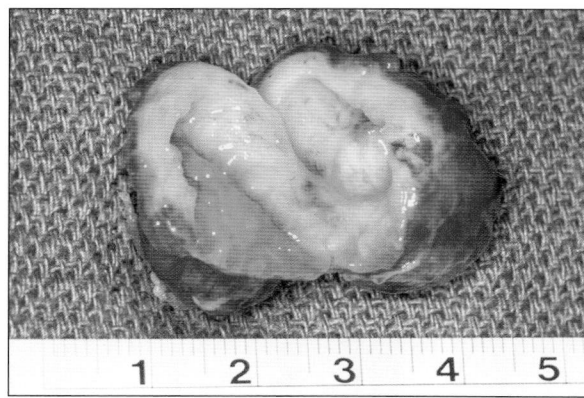

Fig 13-41e Gross specimen of a branchial cyst showing its very thick connective tissue wall and its thin epithelial lining. (Courtesy of Dr Eric Carlson.)

phenoxymethyl penicillin (Pen-Vee K, Wyeth-Ayerst), 500 mg four times daily for 5 to 7 more days. In the penicillin-allergic patient, erythromycin, 1 g intravenously every 6 hours until discharge, is suggested followed by erythromycin ethyl succinate, 400 mg three times daily for 5 to 7 more days.

PROGNOSIS ▶   Branchial cysts are permanently eradicated by surgical excision. Rarely, a recurrence may develop at another level, which probably represents a new cyst. A rare carcinoma within or associated with the cyst has been reported.

Epidermoid Cyst/Sebaceous Cyst

CLINICAL PRESENTATION AND PATHOGENESIS ▶   Epidermoid and so-called sebaceous cysts may arise in any part of the facial skin or neck, but they are most common in the midcheek and preauricular area. They arise more commonly in individuals with irregular complexions indicative of active or past acne. About 80% are painless, solitary masses, and the other 20% are painful because of secondary infection. Most are freely movable within the skin, but some are fixed because of fibrosis from repeated infections.

   Sebaceous cysts arise from hair follicle epithelium, which includes sebaceous cells, and/or have the potential to form sebum on their own. They are believed to be caused by a plugging phenomenon that results in the subsequent build-up of sebum and proliferation of the epithelium. Epidermoid cysts are thought to arise from epithelium in the upper portion of the pilosebaceous unit and, therefore, do not produce sebum (Fig 13-42a).

DIFFERENTIAL DIAGNOSIS ▶   Most cases are suspected from the history of acne and of past cysts with infections, but less apparent epidermoid cysts will present in a manner similar to a *lymph node enlargement*. In various locations, they may be confused with entities more specific to that location. In the preauricular area an epidermoid cyst may resemble a *parotid tumor*, in the midlateral neck a *branchial cyst*, in the midline of the neck a *thyroglossal tract cyst*, and in the submental triangle a *dermoid cyst*.

DIAGNOSTIC WORK-UP AND TREATMENT ▶   Epidermoid/sebaceous cysts are usually treated when the pain and swelling related to secondary infection leads the patient to seek care. While antibiotics to eradicate staphylococcal organisms and moist heat will alleviate symptoms over time, re-infection is common. It is therefore best to excise such cysts and to treat the excisional wound with staphylococcal antibiotic coverage for a 10-day period.

   The removal of an epidermoid/sebaceous cyst is usually more difficult than expected because of its fibrosis to surrounding tissues (Fig 13-42b). A small elliptical portion of overlying skin should be excised to include the drainage point or hair follicle of origin (Fig 13-42c). The cyst's adherence to surrounding tissues often requires meticulous, sharp dissection. An electrocautery to control small bleeding points is

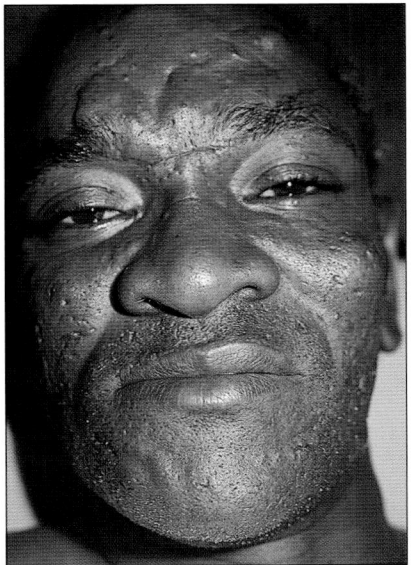

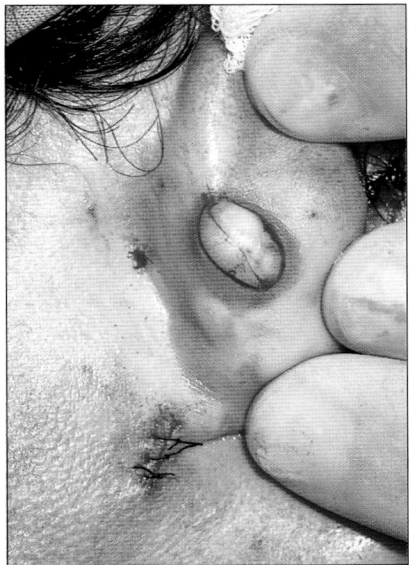

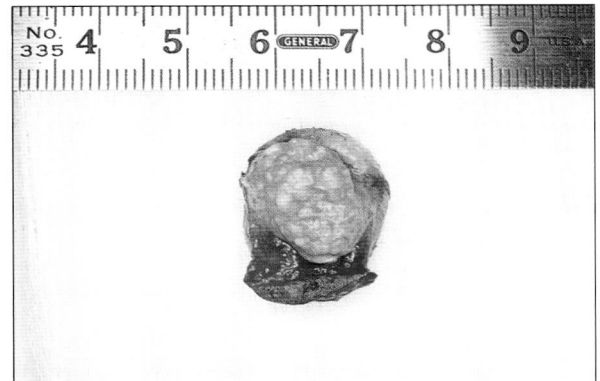

Fig 13-42a An individual with several true sebaceous cysts of the forehead as confirmed by the sebum contained in the lumen.

Figs 13-42b and 13-42c Although encapsulated, a sebaceous cyst may be difficult to remove because of its fibrosis to surrounding tissues.

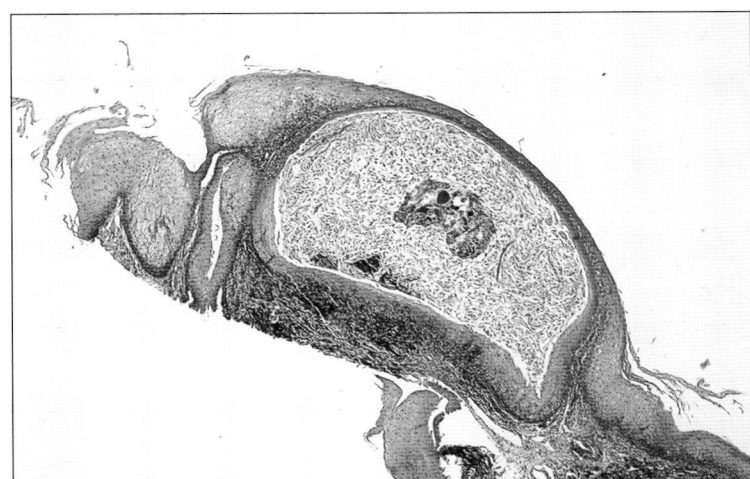

Fig 13-42d Epidermoid cyst with a thin keratinizing stratified squamous epithelial lining and keratin in the lumen.

recommended, as an avascular pericapsular plane found in many other cysts is usually not present. If the cyst ruptures during removal, its complete excision will be more difficult and less probable. If this occurs, injecting the cyst with a volume of soft tissue liner or alginate will reinflate it, facilitating its removal. The resultant wound should be thoroughly irrigated and closed in layers, and a pressure dressing applied. Antibiotic therapy should continue for 10 days and is recommended to include coverage of the anticipated staphylococcal organisms. Dicloxicillin (Dynapen, Wyeth-Ayerst), 500 mg by mouth four times daily; cephalexin (Keflex, Dista), 500 mg by mouth four times daily; and ciprofloxacin (Cipro, Bayer), 500 to 750 mg orally twice daily, are reasonable antibiotic choices for this indication.

HISTOPATHOLOGY ▶

Epidermoid/sebaceous cysts are lined by keratinizing stratified squamous epithelium. Sebaceous cells may be present in the wall and inflammatory cells and fibrosis may be apparent. Keratin and/or sebum may fill the lumen (Fig 13-42d).

PROGNOSIS ▶

True sebaceous cysts are more recurrent than simple epidermoid cysts and other cysts because of their greater difficulty to remove. In addition, new cysts often arise in the same patient because of a predisposition related to skin anatomy.

Epidermal Inclusion Cyst

Epidermal inclusion cysts are histologically defined as cysts of the skin lined only by stratified squamous epithelium. They are caused either by traumatic implantation of epithelium into the dermis or by embryonic inclusion. From either genesis, the cyst will present at any age as a smooth, freely movable, painless mass in the subcutaneous-dermal level of the skin. The skin surface will be intact, with no apparent drainage point.

A solitary, movable skin nodule is suggestive of the more common *sebaceous cyst* or an *epidermoid cyst* arising from the pilosebaceous unit. However, sebaceous cysts are associated with an irregular skin complexion, acne lesions, and other sebaceous cysts. Lymph node enlargements are another consideration that includes entities such as *nonspecific lymphadenopathy, cat-scratch disease,* and *HIV-related lymphadenopathy,* among others. Depending on anatomic location, other specific entities might include a *dermoid cyst* in the submental triangle; a *branchial cyst* in the midlateral neck; and a *thyroglossal tract cyst* in the midline of the neck.

Epidermal inclusion cysts are diagnosed and treated by simple pericapsular excision without the need to excise overlying epithelium. The only major surgical consideration is the placement of the incision: either a natural skin crease or a resting skin tension line produces a minimally noticeable scar.

Epidermal inclusion cysts are lined by keratinizing stratified squamous epithelium. The wall is fibrous, and as the name suggests, there is a resemblance to the epidermis because no skin appendages are present. Keratin typically fills the lumen (see Fig 13-42d).

Epidermal inclusion cysts only rarely recur because of their uncomplicated complete removal, unlike sebaceous cysts, which often recur from the residual lining of an incompletely removed cyst, or from new cysts arising in predisposed individuals.

Dermoid Cyst

Dermoid cysts are developmental cysts in young adults that are uncommon in the oral and maxillofacial area (accounting for only 2% of all dermoid cysts). In this region the cysts are mostly found in the submental triangle external to the mylohyoid muscle or in the floor of the mouth oral to the mylohyoid muscle. On occasion, a larger cyst will present both oral and external to the mylohyoid muscle. Some will occur in the midline of the tongue (Fig 13-43) or in the submandibular triangle.

The cyst presents as a painless compressible mass, which is movable unless prohibited by its size. Most are small, but some have exceeded 12 cm. They will frequently distend the mucosa so thoroughly that some of the yellow fluid contents may be seen. When they present in the floor of the mouth, they displace the tongue upward, which may interfere with speech. In the submental triangle, they will create a double-chin appearance.

Dermoid cysts in these locations arise from epithelial entrapment when the branchial arches of each side fuse in the midline. Because the branchial arches form both oral and extraoral structures, epithelium may become entrapped in either location, resulting in mainly midline dermoid cysts in either type of structure. Because there are other facial areas in which embryonic processes fuse, one would expect dermoid cysts to occur in these locations as well. Orbital dermoid cysts arise in the naso-optic groove and are commonly associated with hemifacial microsomia (Fig 13-44). Nasal dorsum dermoid cysts occur from inclusions between the developing nasal bones.

A dermoid cyst that occurs in the floor of the mouth will most closely resemble a *ranula.* Additional considerations include its sister lesion, the *teratoid cyst;* a *sublingual space infection* from an odontogenic source; a *sublingual salivary gland tumor;* or a soft tissue tumor such as a *granular cell tumor,* which is noted to occur in this location as well as in the tongue.

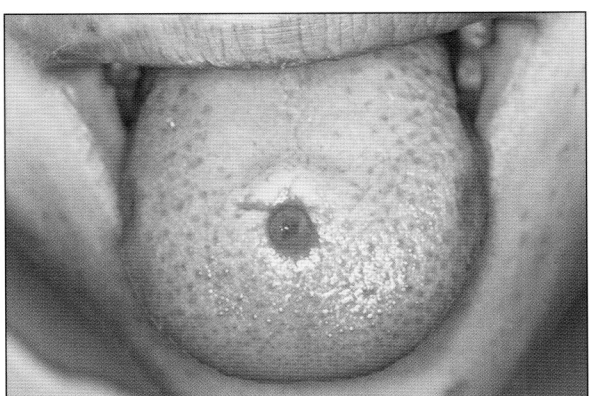

Fig 13-43 Dermoid cyst in the midline of the anterior tongue. This presentation would usually be associated with an intact mucosa. Here the ulceration is due to an earlier biopsy.

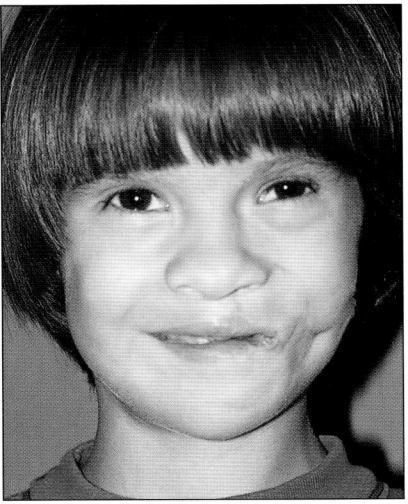

Fig 13-44 Ocular dermoid cysts are sometimes a component of hemifacial microsomia. Here a dermoid cyst in the inferior outer quadrant of the left orbit arose from epithelial remnants of the naso-optic groove.

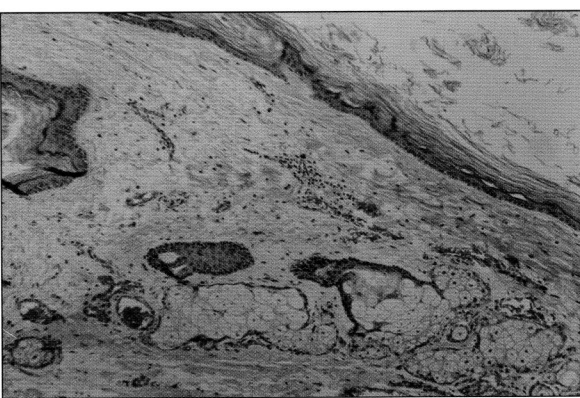

Fig 13-45 Dermoid cyst with stratified squamous epithelial lining, keratin in the lumen, and sebaceous glands and hair follicles in the wall.

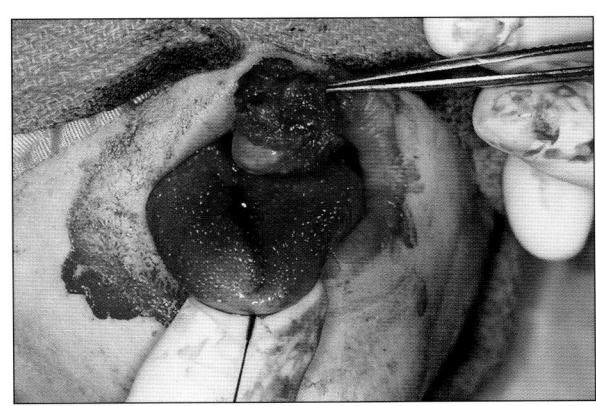

Fig 13-46 A sharp pericapsular excision of a dermoid cyst is usually required because of its fibrosis to surrounding tissues.

A dermoid cyst that occurs in the submental triangle also will most closely resemble a *ranula* (that is, a *plunging ranula*). Additional considerations in this location include a *submental space abscess,* a *thyroglossal tract cyst, cystic hygroma,* and lymph node enlargements such as those found in *cat-scratch disease, lymphoma, tuberculosis-related lymphadenitis* (scrofula), and *HIV-related lymphadenopathy.*

A dermoid cyst that occurs in the tongue may resemble a *granular cell tumor,* a *schwannoma,* a *salivary gland tumor,* or a *rhabdomyoma.*

DIAGNOSTIC WORK-UP ▶

Aspiration of the mass reveals its cystic nature by a return of straw-colored fluid or a semisolid mixture of keratin and other cell products. Large lesions may be better assessed and surgically planned by obtaining a CT scan or an MRI scan. A dermoid cyst's CT scan appearance should suggest a thick wall and a fluid center.

HISTOPATHOLOGY ▶

As suggested by its name, these cysts contain elements present within the dermis. The lining is a keratinizing, stratified squamous epithelium, with keratin present in the lumen. The wall contains skin appendages, sebaceous glands, hair follicles, and/or sweat glands. Thus sebum may also be present within the lumen (Fig 13-45).

TREATMENT AND PROGNOSIS ▶

The approach to excision is dictated by cyst location. Large lesions require a wider access, and some lesions may require both a transoral and a transcutaneous approach. With either approach, removal is difficult because of the cyst's adherence to surrounding tissues and occasionally because of its size. These cysts tend to become fibrosed to surrounding tissue, requiring sharp more than blunt dissection (Fig 13-46).

Cysts in the floor of the mouth require particular care; the submandibular ducts must be identified and retracted laterally and the lingual nerves retracted posteriorly. With large lesions, the resultant wound in the neck may represent significant dead space that will require drainage. A large oral wound may be allowed to close by granulation. Excision resolves a dermoid cyst without recurrence.

Teratoid Cyst (Teratoma)

CLINICAL PRESENTATION AND PATHOGENESIS ▶

Teratoid cysts/teratomas are developmental semicystic disturbances akin to the dermoid cyst, but by definition they include formed elements of all three germ layers. They are cystic in nature but may contain a sufficient amount of formed structures such as hair, cartilage, bone, and even teeth to make them appear solid. Clinically, they differ from dermoid cysts in one important aspect: while dermoid cysts occur in adults, teratoid cysts are congenital. When teratoid cysts develop in the oral and maxillofacial area, they are usually found in the same locations as dermoid cysts, that is, the floor-of-mouth/submental triangle area. However, they tend to be more firm, possibly even bone hard. Extremely large cysts may cause upper airway obstruction via posterior displacement of the tongue (Fig 13-47).

Radiographically, many cysts will contain calcifications that may range in appearance from fluffy opacities representing immature bone to formed teeth, most of which are of the premolar type. Such teratoid cysts also occur in the ovary, where they have given rise to dramatic radiographs and gross specimens with jaw-like formations complete with teeth and periodontal membrane spaces (Figs 13-48a and 13-48b).

Like dermoid cysts, teratoid cysts/teratomas are thought to arise from the entrapment of cells in the fusion line of the branchial arches. In teratoid cysts/teratomas, the cells are apparently multipotential stem cells, which can differentiate along nearly all cell lines.

DIFFERENTIAL DIAGNOSIS ▶

If the mass occurs in its most usual oral and maxillofacial location—that is, the floor of the mouth—other congenital conditions that must be considered are its sister lesion, the *dermoid cyst,* as well as a *cystic hygroma-lymphangioma,* and a *ranula.* Considerations such as lymph node enlargements and salivary gland tumors that would otherwise be appropriate for a firm mass in these locations are not appropriate in this clinical setting because of the mass's congenital occurrence. However, a *rhabdomyosarcoma* is an appropriate consideration since the oral and maxillofacial area is the preferred site and 2% occur congenitally.

DIAGNOSTIC WORK-UP AND TREATMENT ▶

For congenital head and neck teratoid cysts, a work-up is usually impossible because of the age of the child. In some instances, complete removal is required as an emergency procedure because airway obstruction is a significant and progressive finding. There is a 9% mortality rate associated with this lesion mainly because of airway obstruction. Therefore, the first priority is securing an airway, which in many cases requires a neonatal tracheostomy.

Definitive treatment is complete surgical excision, which in itself may further compromise the airway through edema and tongue muscle detachments. Like the dermoid cyst, the teratoid cyst is attached primarily to surrounding tissues. In some cases, it will include the mandible in its growth. Sharp dissection is therefore required, and in some cases resection of a portion of the mandible is necessary.

HISTOPATHOLOGY ▶

More complex than the epidermoid and dermoid cysts, teratoid cysts often include bone, teeth, gastrointestinal elements, and/or muscle in addition to dermal appendages. Thus all germ layers are represented. Although these cysts are found primarily within the ovary, they have always been of considerable interest to the dental community because of their propensity to form teeth. Fully developed teeth, which are usually single rooted, may be seen within "alveolar" bone, surrounded by a periodontal ligament (Fig 13-48c). Unerupted teeth may also be found within bone. The lining of the cyst, while usually stratified squamous epithelium, is variable (Fig 13-48d).

PROGNOSIS ▶

Most cases of a teratoid cyst are resolved by surgical excision. However, because the cellular elements that form these cysts are active cells, incomplete removal will result in a recurrence. In those cases that

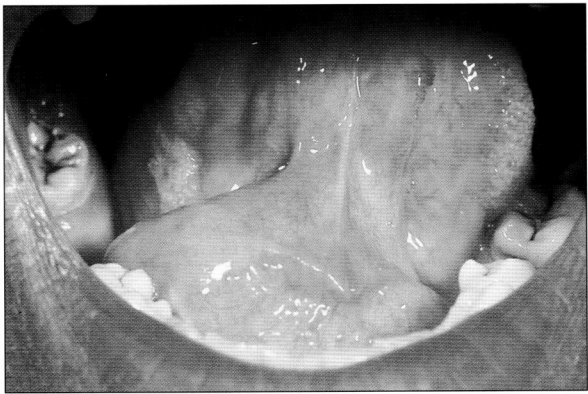

Fig 13-47 Although rare, teratoid cysts that are not congenital may form in the floor of the mouth. They are usually firm and have an intact mucosa.

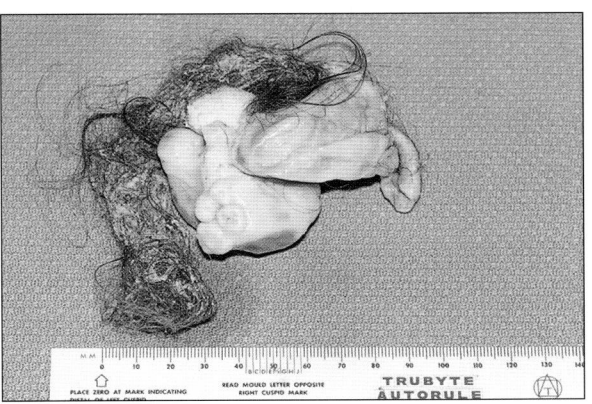

Fig 13-48a Gross specimen of a teratoma from the ovary displaying elements from all three germ layers: ectoderm—skin, hair, and enamel; endoderm—mucosa; and mesoderm—bone, dentin, pulp, and periodontal membrane of teeth.

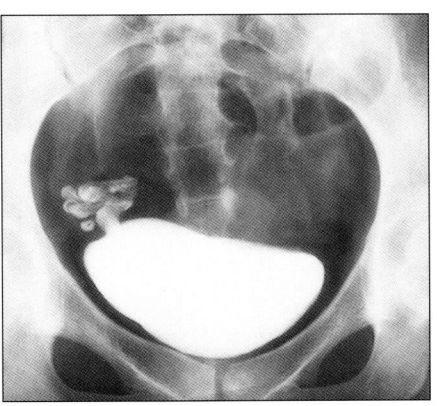

Fig 13-48b Teratoid cysts/teratomas are also seen in the ovaries. This hysterogram shows bone and teeth in the right ovary.

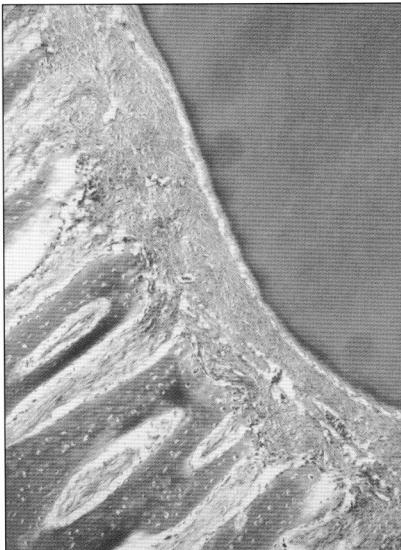

Fig 13-48c Teratoid cyst of the ovary showing a tooth root with a periodontal membrane and bone.

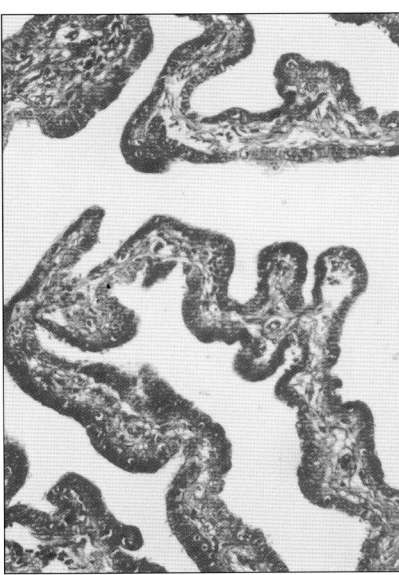

Fig 13-48d The epithelial lining of the teratoid cyst shown in Fig 13-48c.

require a mandibular resection, spontaneous osteogenesis will regenerate much if not all of the excised bone if the proximal segments are prevented from collapsing. This may be accomplished with a 2.3- or 2.4-mm reconstruction bone plate using unicortical screws placed at the inferior border to avoid impinging on developing tooth buds. Careful placement of such plates and suturing of the anterior digastrics, geniohyoid, and genioglossus muscles to the plate will reduce the risk of posterior tongue displacement and airway obstruction. This may reduce the amount of time that the tracheostomy needs to be in place. The reconstruction plate must be removed about 6 months after placement to prevent plate migration lingually and complete immersion into bone from the effects of growth. At that time, new bone formation should be evident.

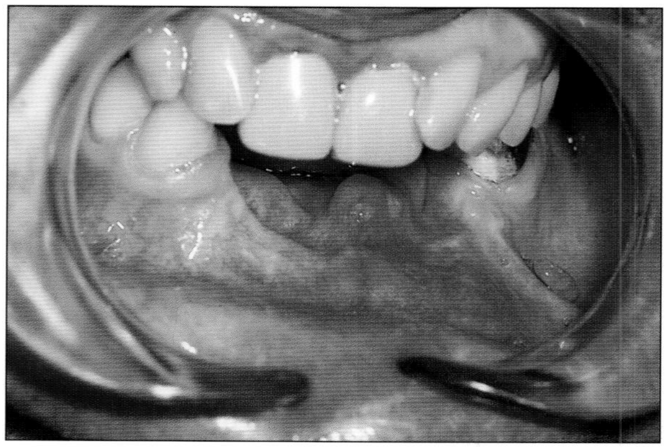

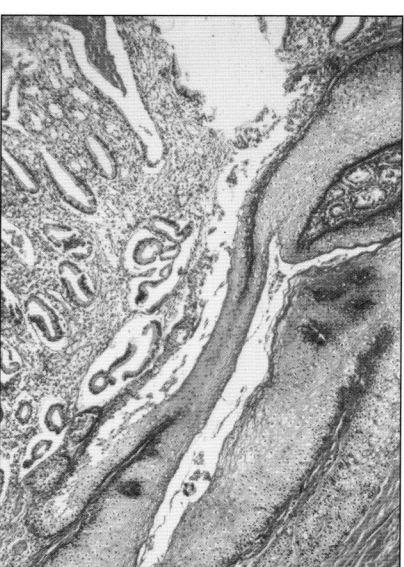

Fig 13-49a This small submucosal nodule in the midline of the floor of the mouth represented the rare finding of a heterotopic gastrointestinal cyst.

Fig 13-49b Heterotopic gastrointestinal cyst showing glandular crypts and a stratified squamous epithelial lining.

Heterotopic Gastrointestinal Cyst

CLINICAL PRESENTATION AND PATHOGENESIS ▶

Heterotopic gastrointestinal cysts are small developmental cysts that occur singly or in multiple numbers throughout the gastrointestinal tract from the mouth to the anus. Most occur in the small intestine, but 0.3% are reported to occur in the tongue and a rare few others in the floor of the mouth (Fig 13-49a). Those that have been reported in the tongue have mostly been small (less than 2.5 cm). Nearly all have been in boys ranging in age from 4 months to 12 years.

The lesion presents as a nodule or firm mass within the substance of the tongue or floor of the mouth. The mass will be asymptomatic unless it has a sinus tract, which will drain a brown, salty liquid. It may occur anywhere along the tongue from tip to base but usually is midline or near midline.

The heterotopic gastrointestinal cyst has been theorized to arise from various sources: entrapment of epithelial cells during formation of the tongue and gut, residual lacunae of fetal mucosa formed when the gastrointestinal tract forms a lumen, and primordial intestinal epithelium remaining in the submucosa. However, these theories do not explain the occurrences of the cysts from mouth to anus and the presence of gastric or intestinal cells in all of them. The currently favored theory suggests that primitive endoderm becomes misplaced by the infolding of the notochord plate as it forms the notochord proper. The infolding action is believed to drag endoderm toward the notochord and into the mesoderm, which later develops into a cyst lined by differentiated endoderm that is mostly intestinal or gastric epithelium. Because the notochord develops along the entire length of the fetus from head to coccyx, this theory explains the observation of such cysts throughout the gastrointestinal tract as well as the cell type within the lining.

DIFFERENTIAL DIAGNOSIS ▶

If the lesion occurs in the floor of the mouth or anterior tongue area in a child, the most likely differential lesions are the spectrum of other developmental cysts (*epidermoid cyst, dermoid cyst, teratoid cyst*) and salivary retention phenomenon (*mucoceles* and *mucus retention cysts*). Additionally, *hemangiomas* and *lymphangiomas* are associated with youth. If the lesion occurs more toward the base of the tongue, the clinician must also consider a *persistent lingual thyroid* and *developmental choristomas of bone or cartilage*.

Of significance is the possibility of a *rhabdomyosarcoma* developing in the tongue, as this organ contains a large population of rhabdomyoblasts and the peak age of occurrence of rhabdomyosarcoma overlaps that of heterotopic gastrointestinal cysts.

DIAGNOSTIC WORK-UP AND TREATMENT ▶

Most lesions are approached with a direct surgical exploration and excision with pericapsular margins. If the location is in the area of the foramen cecum, and therefore a persistent lingual thyroid is a realistic consideration, it is best to perform an ^{131}I radionucleotide scan to rule out the presence of thyroid tissue prior to surgery.

The capsule of the cyst is usually not well defined, and excision often includes a small cuff of surrounding muscle. The approach is via a midline incision, which offers the best potential of avoiding branches of the lingual nerve and lingual vessels. The cyst is almost always found deep within the tongue.

HISTOPATHOLOGY ▶

Heterotopic gastrointestinal cysts are lined by stratified squamous epithelium and gastric or intestinal mucosa with their specialized cells. A muscle layer may also be seen (Fig 13-49b).

PROGNOSIS ▶

Recurrences do not develop after excision. However, other cysts may be present within the gastrointestinal tract. If the individual has symptoms suggestive of obstruction or drainage into the gastrointestinal tract, a work-up consisting of a CT scan and gastrointestinal series with contrast or a fiberoptic gastroscopy may be needed.

Odontogenic Tumors: Hamartomas and Neoplasms

CHAPTER 14

▶ *"The best chemotherapy for odontogenic tumors is a jar of formalin."*
—Robert E. Marx

As a group, odontogenic tumors are cellular proliferations with a wide range of biologic potentials and behaviors. A correct understanding of each type of biologic behavior upon which to base rational treatments is required. Odontogenic tumors represent four classic biologies encompassed under the general term *tumor*, which connotes a dysmorphic increase in cellular mass.

Hamartomas Hamartomas, which are dysmorphic proliferations of cells native to the organ in which they arise, gain a certain size before ceasing their proliferation. This type of biologic behavior may be expansile and is locally resorptive of bone but does not invade adjacent tissue. It therefore can be approached for cure by enucleation and curettage procedures. Examples of hamartomas include the odontoma, the ameloblastic fibro-odontoma, and the adenomatoid odontogenic cyst (previously termed *adenomatoid odontogenic tumor*).

Choristomas Choristomas are dysmorphic proliferations of cells not native to the organ in which they arise, and like hamartomas, they gain a certain size and then cease. This biology is also curative with local excision or enucleation and curettage surgeries. Choristomas of the oral cavity may or may not be a rare finding. The relatively common finding of Fordyce granules actually represents choristomas that originate in nonfunctional sebaceous glands found in the submucosa. Yet, the rare enteric duplication cyst in the floor of the mouth and the rare osteoma in the tongue are also examples of choristomas.

Benign Neoplasms Benign neoplasms are defined as continual dysmorphic proliferations of cells native to the organ in which they arise, which also elaborate the cytokines necessary for tissue invasion but not those necessary for metastasis (Figs 14-1a to 14-1c). This type of biology generally is not curable by enucleation and curettage. Instead, curative surgery requires an en-bloc resection with tumor-free margins. Examples of this biology are the invasive ameloblastoma, the odontogenic myxoma, the calcifying epithelial odontogenic tumor, and the very rare odontoameloblastoma, which is merely a collision tumor of an ameloblastoma occurring simultaneously with an odontoma.

Malignant Neoplasms Malignant neoplasms are defined as continual dysmorphic proliferations of cells native to the organ in which they arise that may elaborate the cytokines necessary for tissue invasion and for distant metastasis. This type of biology requires consideration for en-bloc surgeries encompassing the fields of local-regional metastasis and sometimes radiotherapy or chemotherapy. Examples of odontogenic malignancies exist but are rare. The most common of this very uncommon group is the ameloblastic fibrosarcoma. Others include the ameloblastic carcinoma, the malignant ameloblastoma, and the central odontogenic carcinoma.

Consideration of these biologies together with the specific history of each odontogenic tumor, its size, its location, and its clinical presentation is the basis upon which a curative treatment approach can be planned. The authors discourage use of the terms "conservative" approaches or "radical" surgeries.

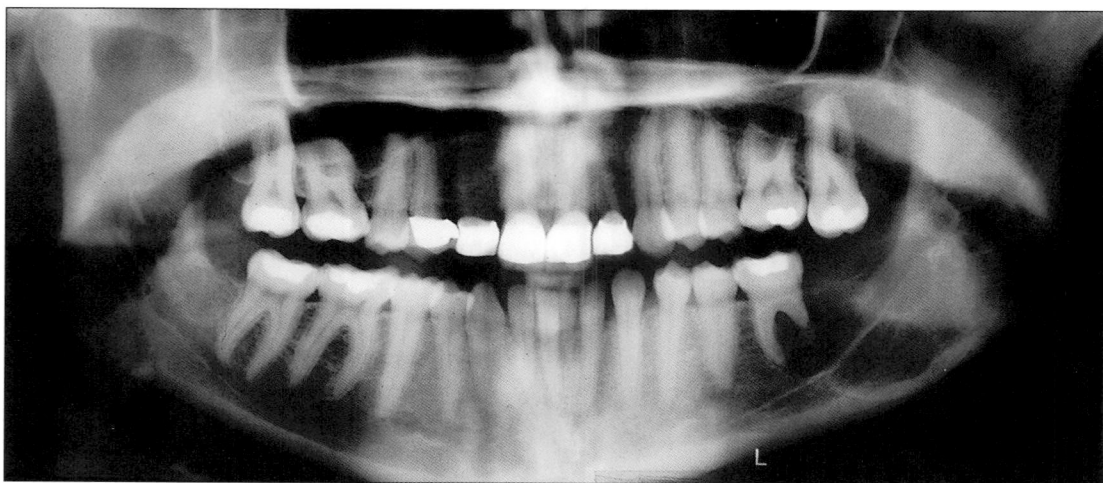

Fig 14-1a Panoramic radiograph of an ameloblastoma that was 6 cm at the time of the initial diagnosis.

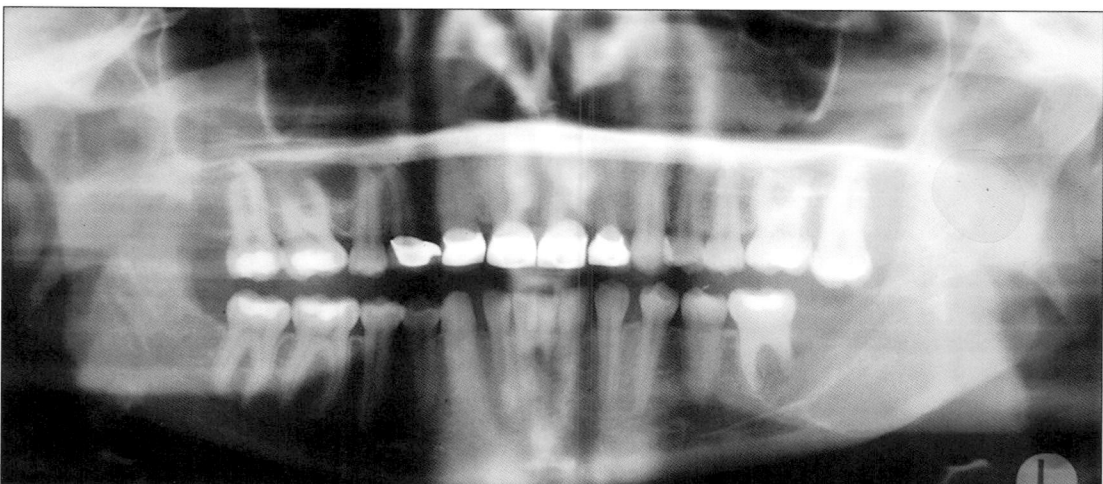

Fig 14-1b After 1 year, the ameloblastoma shown in Fig 14-1a is only slightly larger (about 0.5 cm).

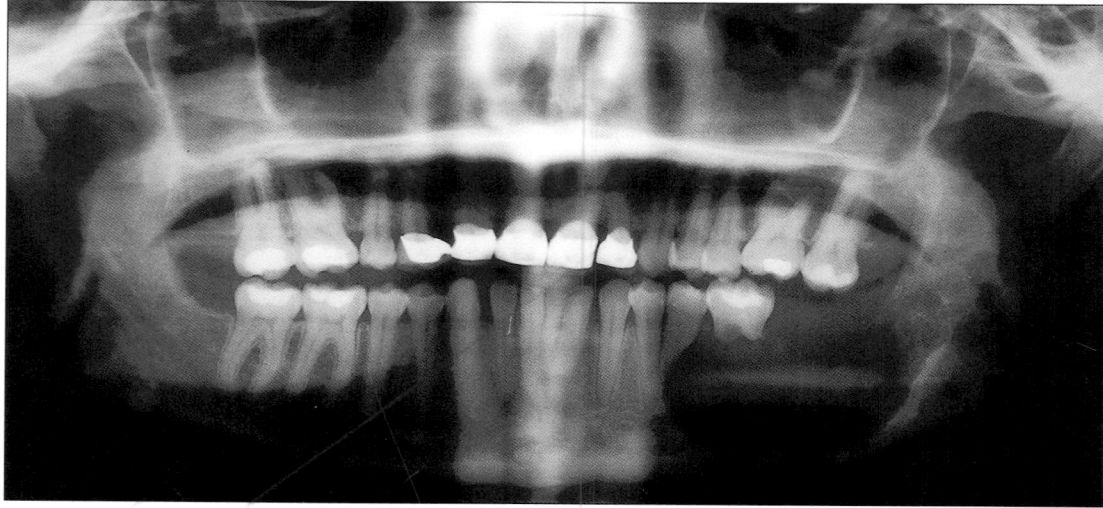

Fig 14-1c Left untreated for 6 additional years, the ameloblastoma slowly grew to further resorb bone, including most of the inferior border and nearly all of the first molar root.

These are not appropriate medical or dental terms. Too often an attempt at "conservative" treatment eventuates into a large recurrence, tissue loss, and even death that could hardly be accepted as conservative. Seemingly "radical" surgery, if curative, will in the long run be more preservative of tissues and function than lesser surgeries that require re-operation or that develop recurrences. Instead, the authors suggest the terms "curative treatment," which effects a permanent resolution of the disease greater than 80% of the time, "palliative treatment," which improves the individual patient but does not effect a cure, and "remission therapy," which places an incurable disease into a clinically undetectable state.

Odontogenesis

Odontogenic neoplasms, hamartomas, and odontogenic cysts are all lesions derived from the tooth-producing apparatus, and as such they often reflect aspects of odontogenesis. A brief summary of the events of odontogenesis will aid in an understanding of these entities.

Teeth begin development by invagination of the covering ectoderm of the stomodeum into the underlying mesenchyme of the primitive alveolus. Focal thickenings heralding the primary dentition develop in the ectoderm, and double-layered strands extend into the mesenchyme. This is the dental lamina. At the base of these extensions, an invagination begins, signifying the initial development of the enamel organ, which surrounds and causes a proliferation and condensation of the local mesenchyme to form the dental papilla. The enamel organ develops through cap and bell stages with the formation of outer enamel epithelium, stellate reticulum, stratum intermedium, and inner enamel epithelium. Around the periphery of the enamel organ and dental papilla, condensation of the mesenchyme forms the dental follicle. Thus are produced the three components of the tooth germ: the enamel organ, which is epithelial; and the dental papilla and dental follicle, which are mesenchymal.

As the odontogenic epithelium differentiates into the pre-ameloblasts of the inner enamel epithelium, they induce the mesenchyme of the dental papilla to differentiate into odontoblasts. The odontoblasts then secrete dentinal matrix, called the mantle dentin; this induces the inner enamel epithelial pre-ameloblasts to differentiate into functional ameloblasts, which then deposit enamel matrix onto the mantle dentin. The pre-ameloblasts are columnar cells with nuclei that are polarized away from the dental papilla. The ameloblasts lay down enamel, which must become anchored to the mantle dentin. Therefore, prior to enamel deposition the mantle dentin forms and develops into the dentinoenamel junction as the enamel dentin begins to be laid down.

An offshoot from the dental lamina forms the anlage for the permanent tooth. Epithelial remnants from the dental lamina form the rests of Serres, which are some of the more active rests since they are responsible for the development of many odontogenic cysts and tumors. A double layer of epithelium grows downward from the enamel organ to form Hertwig root sheath, which induces mesenchymal cells of the dental papilla to form the odontoblasts of root development. Just as the dental lamina breaks up, leaving rests in the alveolar mucosa (rests of Serres), Hertwig root sheath, which covers the root dentin, is penetrated by mesenchyme and forms epithelial rests within the periodontal membrane known as the rests of Malassez; these may also give rise to odontogenic cysts and tumors. The somatic mesenchyme adjacent to the root is induced by Hertwig root sheath to form the periodontal membrane. The odontogenic mesenchyme of the dental papilla will form into odontoblasts and produce root dentin. The residual dental papilla becomes the dental pulp. Once Hertwig root sheath disintegrates, the somatic mesenchyme comes into contact with the dentin and differentiates into cementoblasts to form the cementum.

As enamel forms, the enamel organ becomes compressed and is reduced to three layers of epithelium: outer enamel epithelium, stratum intermedium, and inner enamel epithelium. On eruption of the tooth, this reduced enamel epithelium fuses with the overlying oral epithelium and ultimately forms the gingival crevice and epithelial attachment. This process extends from the sixth week of embryonic life

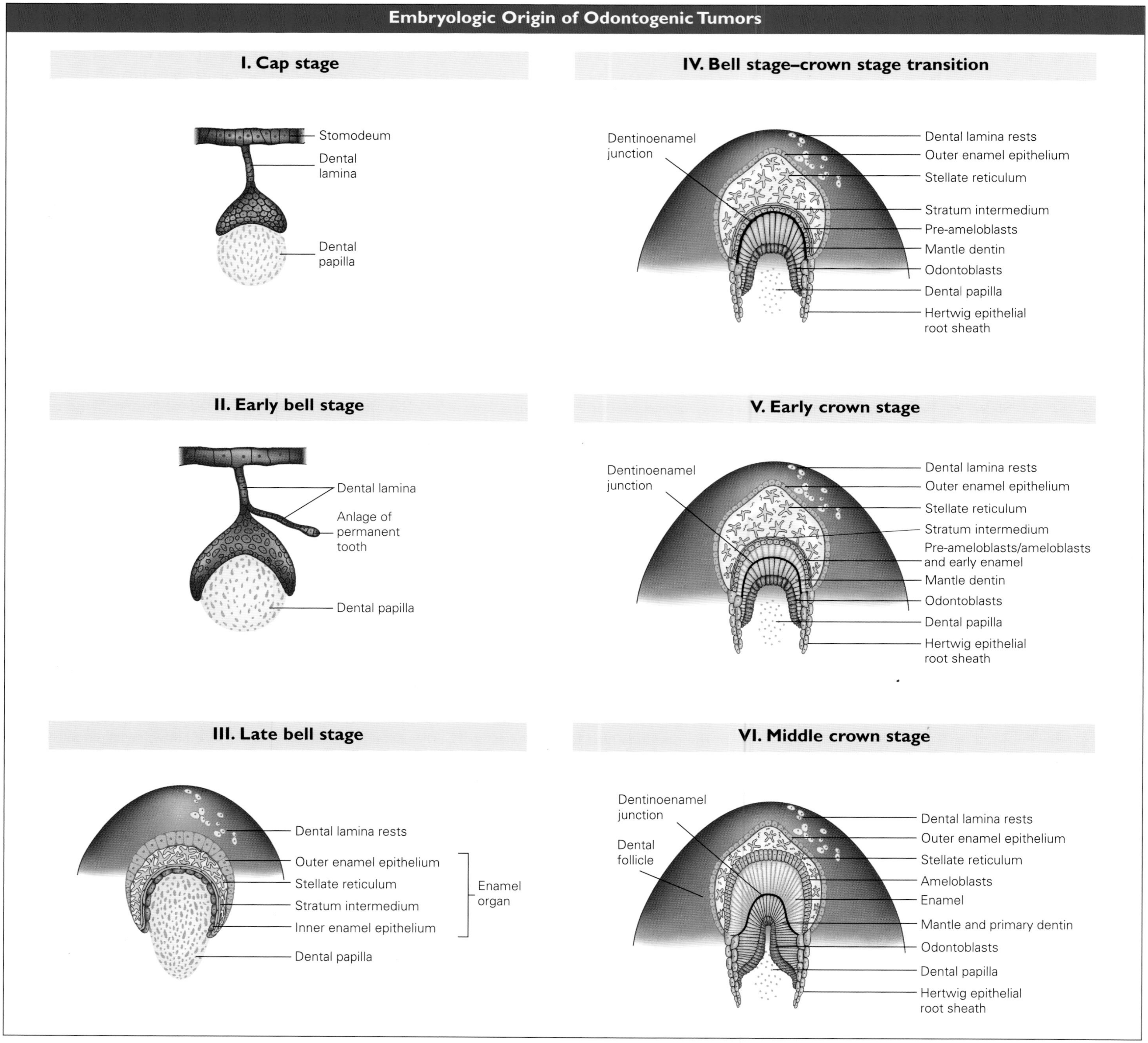

Embryologic Origin of Odontogenic Tumors

I. Cap stage

- Stomodeum
- Dental lamina
- Dental papilla

II. Early bell stage

- Dental lamina
- Anlage of permanent tooth
- Dental papilla

III. Late bell stage

- Dental lamina rests
- Outer enamel epithelium
- Stellate reticulum
- Stratum intermedium
- Inner enamel epithelium
- Dental papilla
- Enamel organ

IV. Bell stage–crown stage transition

- Dentinoenamel junction
- Dental lamina rests
- Outer enamel epithelium
- Stellate reticulum
- Stratum intermedium
- Pre-ameloblasts
- Mantle dentin
- Odontoblasts
- Dental papilla
- Hertwig epithelial root sheath

V. Early crown stage

- Dentinoenamel junction
- Dental lamina rests
- Outer enamel epithelium
- Stellate reticulum
- Stratum intermedium
- Pre-ameloblasts/ameloblasts and early enamel
- Mantle dentin
- Odontoblasts
- Dental papilla
- Hertwig epithelial root sheath

VI. Middle crown stage

- Dentinoenamel junction
- Dental follicle
- Dental lamina rests
- Outer enamel epithelium
- Stellate reticulum
- Ameloblasts
- Enamel
- Mantle and primary dentin
- Odontoblasts
- Dental papilla
- Hertwig epithelial root sheath

Fig 14-2 All odontogenic cysts, hamartomas, and neoplasms arise from cells involved with tooth formation. These are the eight recognized stages of tooth development from which different pathologies can arise.

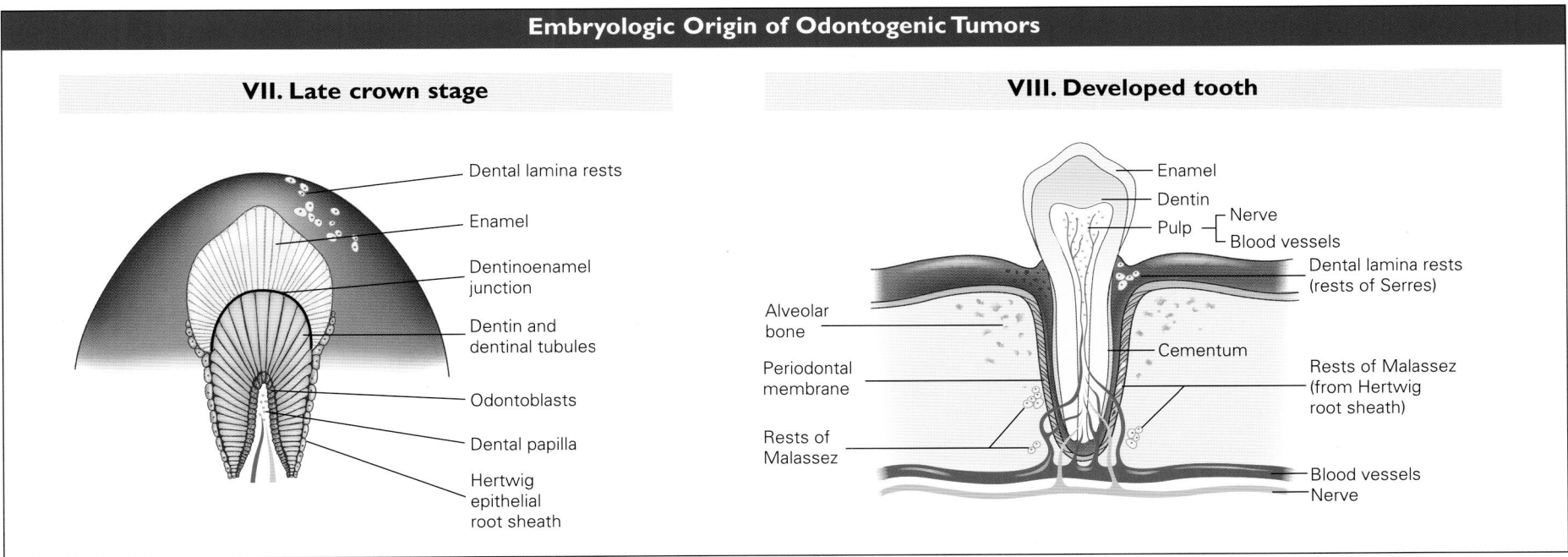

Fig 14-2 All odontogenic cysts, hamartomas, and neoplasms arise from cells involved with tooth formation. These are the eight recognized stages of tooth development from which different pathologies can arise (*continued*).

into an individual's early 20s, which explains why the potential for pathology related to odontogenesis covers a wide age range.

Classifications of odontogenic tumors have usually followed histogenesis and are divided into epithelial, mesenchymal, and mixed-origin categories. No consideration has been given to whether the lesion represents a hamartoma or a neoplasm. Because this difference has a bearing on the behavior and ultimate treatment of the tumors, this chapter will also distinguish them on this basis rather than solely on the basis of histogenesis (Fig 14-2).

Epithelial Odontogenic Tumors

The Ameloblastoma Terminology Confusion

A large body of literature has been devoted to explaining the various types of ameloblastomas that arise in association with cysts. Unfortunately, the overall effect of these publications has been to confuse rather than to clarify. Because of the imprecise use of certain terms and their overlapping meanings, the selection of inadequate treatment approaches has sometimes led to unnecessary recurrences. The term *unicystic ameloblastoma* is an important example of this problem: It has been used to describe an ameloblastoma developing within the lining, lumen, or wall of a cyst as well as an invasive ameloblastoma that has a single cystic space rather than multicystic spaces.

One of the primary sources of confusion is the frequent misapplication of the term *mural* to describe the extent to which ameloblastoma changes penetrate the connective tissue layer of a cyst. Just as a mural painting covers only the surface of a wall, a mural ameloblastoma does not penetrate the epithelial lining of a cyst. Yet in some publications the term has been used to describe an ameloblastoma limited to the cyst lining; in others, an ameloblastoma solely within the cyst lumen; and in still others, an ameloblastoma with varying degrees of invasion through the connective tissue layer of the cyst. Thus, the same term has

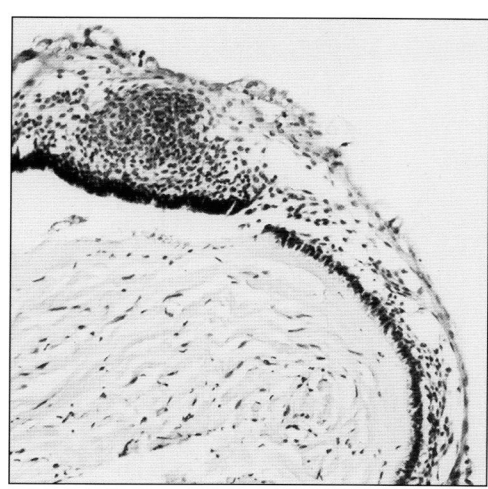

Mural ameloblastoma

Figs 14-3a and 14-3b Mural ameloblastoma developing in and limited to the epithelial lining of a cyst.

been applied to describe pathologies of limited invasive potential as well as pathologies of more aggressive invasive potential. As a result, statistics concerning recurrence rates of such so-called ameloblastomas related to the use of specific treatment approaches have been inaccurate and in some cases dangerously misleading.

To standardize the terminology of ameloblastomas associated with cysts and to recommend curative surgical approaches based on evidence of invasion, this text uses the following terms and their definitions.

I. Ameloblastoma in situ

a. *Mural ameloblastoma in situ*: Ameloblastoma developing in and limited to the epithelial lining of a cyst (Figs 14-3a and 14-3b). This pathology should be curable with cyst enucleation.

b. *Intraluminal ameloblastoma in situ*: Ameloblastoma arising from the epithelial lining of a cyst and proliferating into the lumen (Figs 14-4a and 14-4b). This pathology should be curable with cyst enucleation.

II. Microinvasive ameloblastoma

a. *Intramural microinvasive ameloblastoma*: Ameloblastoma arising from the epithelial lining and proliferating into the connective tissue layer of the cyst (Figs 14-5a and 14-5b). This represents a more aggressive pathology and requires one of the several types of resection approaches for cure.

b. *Transmural microinvasive ameloblastoma*: Ameloblastoma arising from the epithelial lining and proliferating through the complete thickness of the connective tissue layer of a cyst (Figs 14-6a and 14-6b). This represents an obviously invasive pathology and also requires one of the several types of resection approaches for cure.

III. Invasive ameloblastoma

a. *Invasive ameloblastoma arising from the lining of a cyst*: Ameloblastoma arising from the epithelial lining of a cyst and proliferating through the complete thickness of the connective tissue layer of a cyst and into the adjacent bone (Figs 14-7a and 14-7b). This represents an obviously invasive pathology and also requires one of the several types of resection approaches for cure.

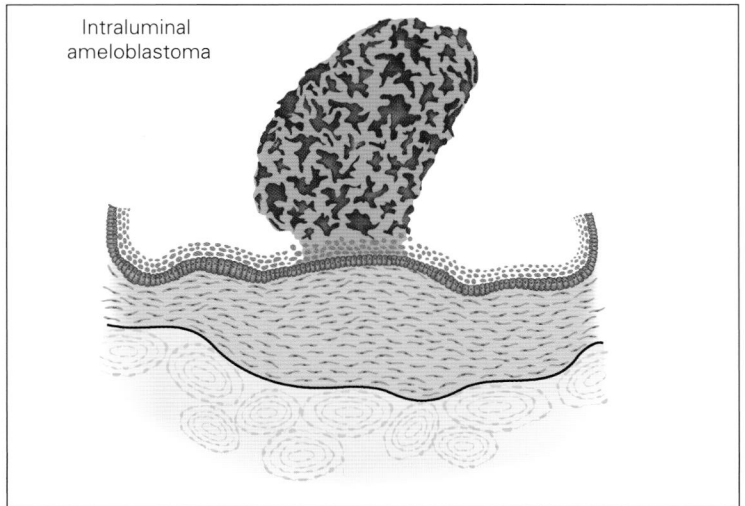
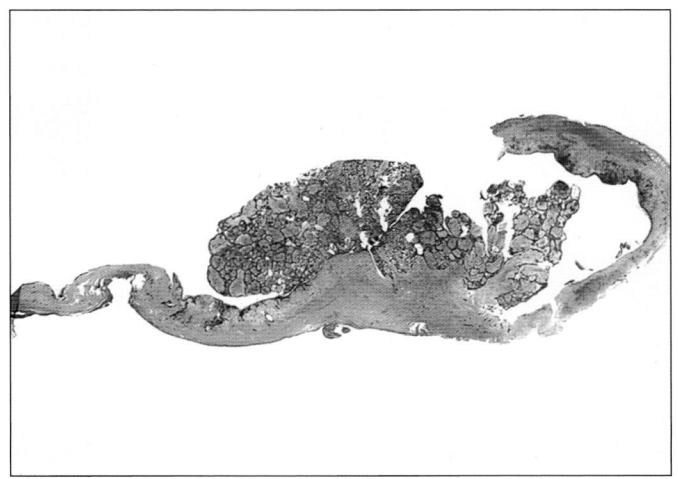

Figs 14-4a and 14-4b Intraluminal ameloblastoma in situ arising from the epithelial lining of a cyst and proliferating into the lumen.

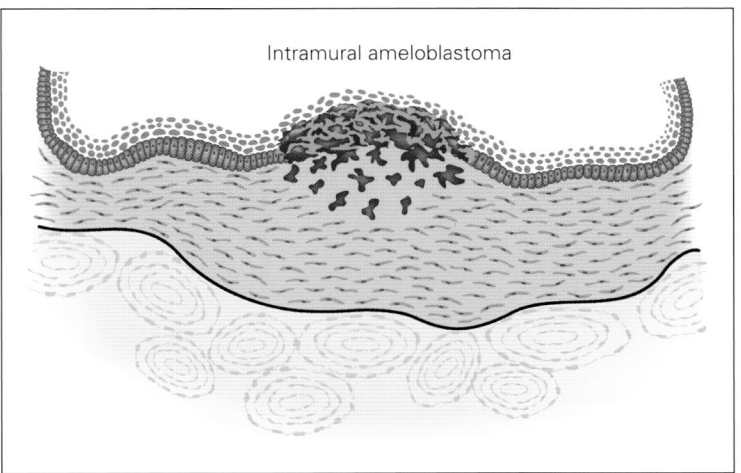
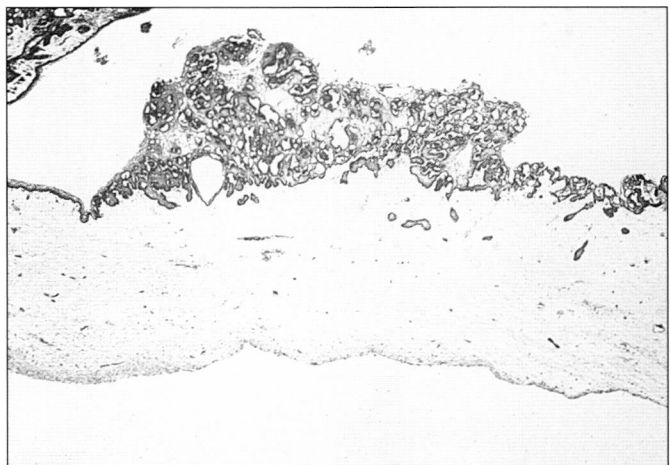

Figs 14-5a and 14-5b Intramural microinvasive ameloblastoma arising from the epithelial lining and proliferating into the connective tissue layer of the cyst.

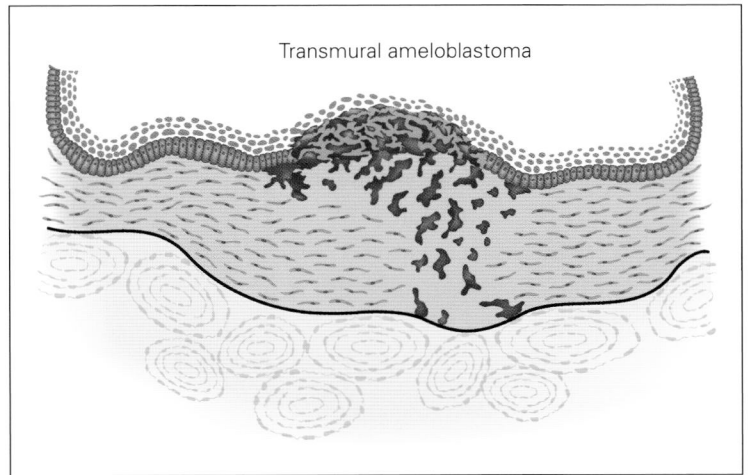
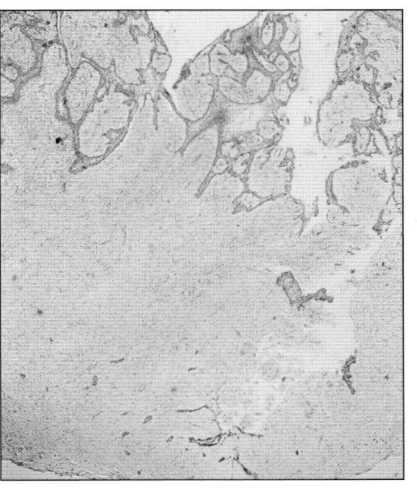

Figs 14-6a and 14-6b Transmural microinvasive ameloblastoma arising from the epithelial lining and proliferating through the complete thickness of the connective tissue layer of a cyst.

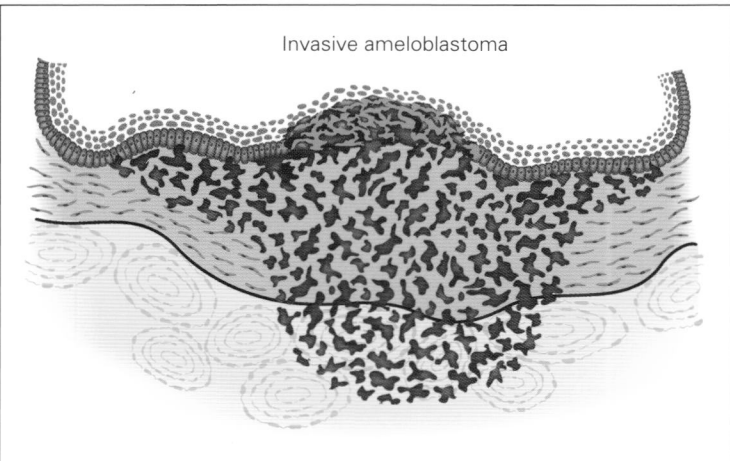
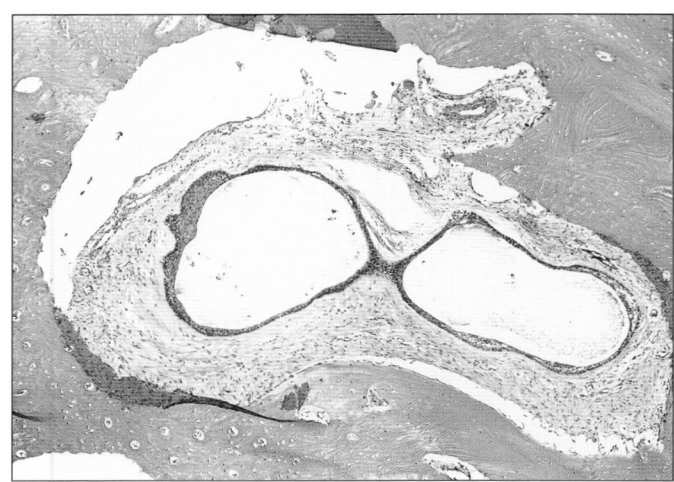

Invasive ameloblastoma

Figs 14-7a and 14-7b Invasive ameloblastoma arising from the epithelial lining of a cyst and proliferating through the complete thickness of the connective tissue layer of a cyst and into the adjacent bone.

    b. *Invasive ameloblastoma:* A solid or multicystic ameloblastoma unassociated with a cyst. This represents an obviously invasive pathology and also requires one of the several types of resection approaches for cure.

Ameloblastoma in Situ and Microinvasive Ameloblastoma

Ameloblastoma in situ is an ameloblastoma developing in the lining or into the lumen of a dentigerous cyst, because dentigerous cyst epithelium retains some primordial odontogenic cells capable of ameloblastoma expression as discussed in the preceding section. The ameloblastoma in situ may initially encompass a focal area of the cyst lining (mural ameloblastoma). It may also grow only into the cyst lumen exophytically (intraluminal ameloblastoma). A microinvasive ameloblastoma may show partial downward growth into the connective tissue (intramural ameloblastoma), or show downward growth throughout the connective tissue layer (transmural ameloblastoma). If the ameloblastoma invades the connective tissue with islands or strands of cells, it is a microinvasive ameloblastoma. If it further invades into the underlying bone, it is an overtly invasive ameloblastoma. Ameloblastoma in situ lesions and microinvasive ameloblastomas are usually discovered after cyst removal by the histopathologic review. In such cases, additional sections through the cyst should be assessed. If the ameloblastoma remains confined to the lining or to the lumen, the cyst removal will involve complete removal of the ameloblastoma in situ. If an area of true invasion is found, the ameloblastoma is beyond the in situ stage and is a microinvasive or overtly invasive tumor requiring resection for cure.

    The unfortunate term *unicystic ameloblastoma* has been used to describe these types of ameloblastoma, creating considerable confusion and leading to many recurrences. The first source of confusion is its nomenclature. The term may refer to an ameloblastoma in situ developing only in the cyst lining, either focally or throughout the lining, which is not the invasive tumor that the term *unicystic ameloblastoma* implies and is best treated with cyst removal. Yet the term may also refer to an invasive ameloblastoma that produces a single large lumen, which is best treated by resection. The second source of confusion arises from radiographic interpretation. Invasive ameloblastomas that form a unilocular radiographic appearance have been incorrectly diagnosed as unicystic ameloblastomas because of their identical radiographic appearance (Figs 14-8a and 14-8b).

    The third source of confusion arises from its treatment implications. Enucleation and curettage has led to recurrences from incisional biopsies that may have sampled an area of a dentigerous cyst show-

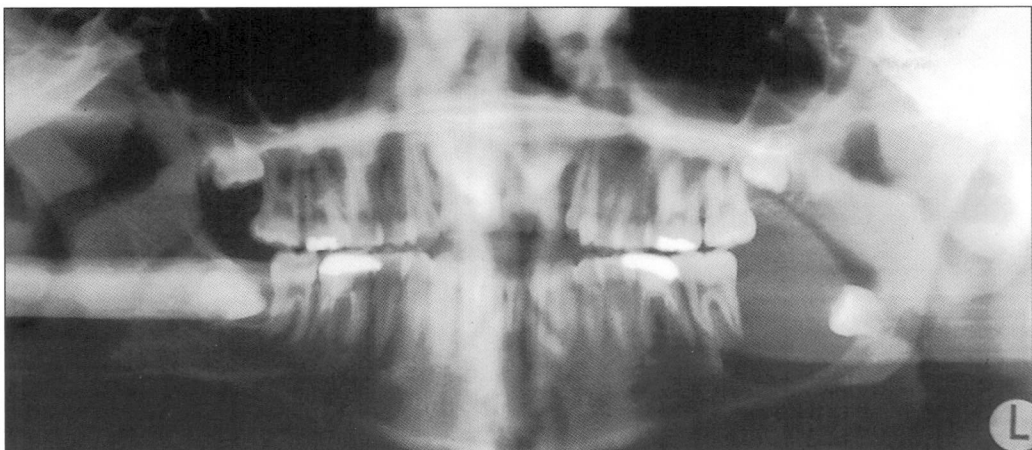

Fig 14-8a Unilocular radiolucency extending from the crown of a third molar. In this case, it represented an ameloblastoma in situ of the intraluminal type.

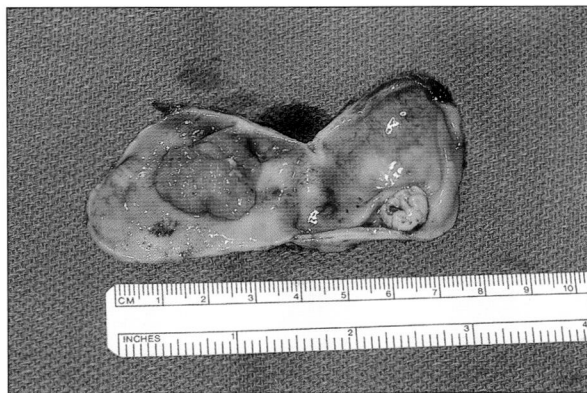

Fig 14-8b Ameloblastoma in situ of the intraluminal type showing a cyst lumen arising from the follicle's epithelium and an exophytic focus of ameloblastoma arising from the cyst lining and growing only into the lumen. Enucleation of this tumor can be expected to be curative.

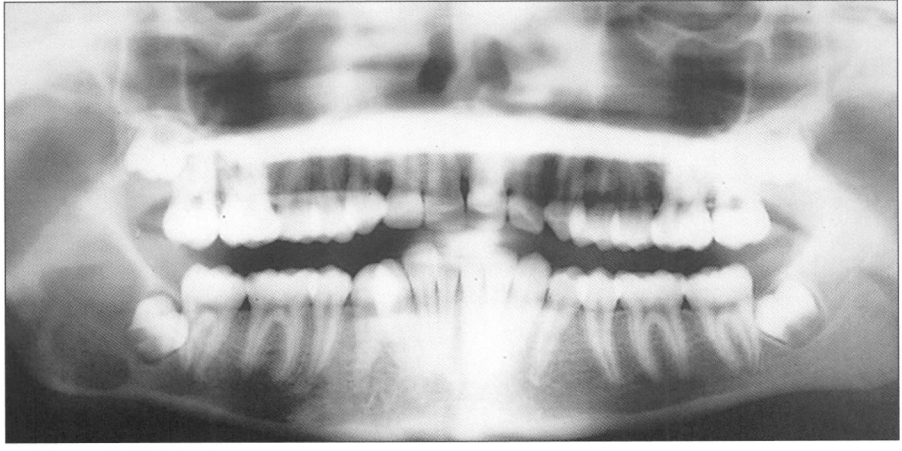

Fig 14-9a This biloculated radiolucency was explored transorally in one area and found to have a lumen. At that time, the incisional biopsy was reported as unicystic ameloblastoma. It was treated by enucleation but recurred 3 years later as a solid ameloblastoma with large internal cystic spaces (see Fig 14-9b).

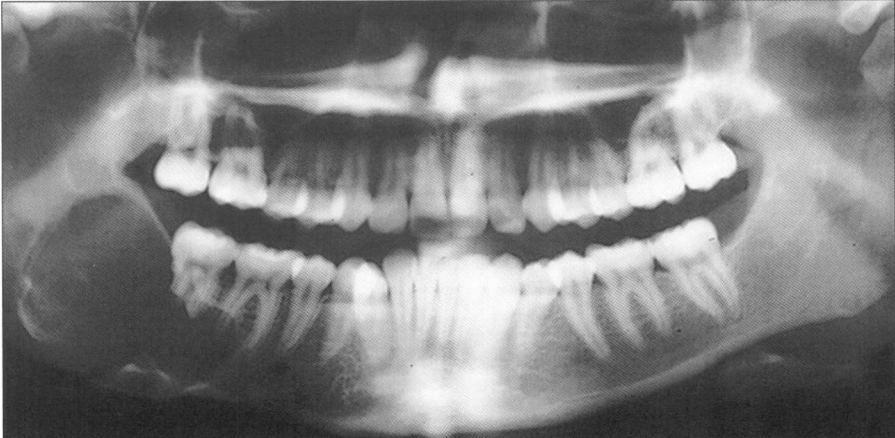

Fig 14-9b This recurrence of the invasive ameloblastoma, initially diagnosed incorrectly as a unicystic ameloblastoma, is now much larger and involves more structures than it did 3 years earlier, necessitating a much larger resection and a greater loss of bone and teeth.

ing only in situ ameloblastoma but elsewhere contained invasive ameloblastoma. Recurrences have also developed when a large unilocular invasive ameloblastoma has been biopsied, and the compressed cystic compartment of the ameloblastoma has been interpreted as a noninvasive unicystic ameloblastoma. In each situation, an invasive ameloblastoma is diagnosed as a unicystic ameloblastoma, suggesting an inappropriate treatment to the clinician (Figs 14-9a and 14-9b). The term also confuses the distinct biologies of these lesions. Invasive ameloblastomas are invasive from the outset, whereas an ameloblastoma developing in a cyst lining or lumen represents a pre-invasive stage of the invasive ameloblastoma (much like epithelial dysplasia and carcinoma in situ of the oral mucosa represent separate pre-invasive stages of squamous cell carcinoma); thus they have completely different treatment requirements.

HISTOPATHOLOGY ▶   The ameloblastoma in situ is strictly a histologic diagnosis that can be made only after careful examination of the entire specimen because there may be variation in different areas and the possibility of a more aggressive focus must be ruled out. Although there is no evidence that all solid or even multicys-

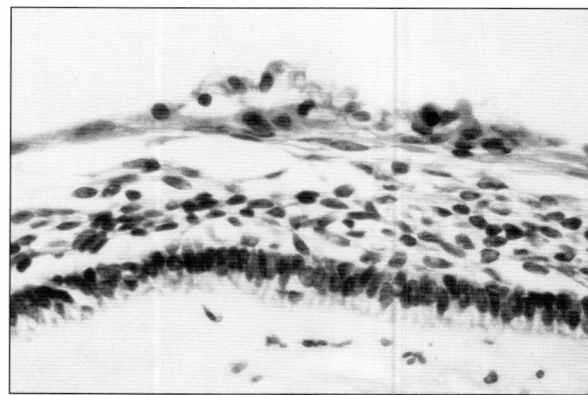

Figs 14-10a and 14-10b An ameloblastoma in situ in which there is no intraluminal or intramural proliferation and is therefore a mural type. The lining shows hyperchromatism of the basal cells, which are columnar and exhibit reverse polarity. There is also considerable separation of the epithelial cells.

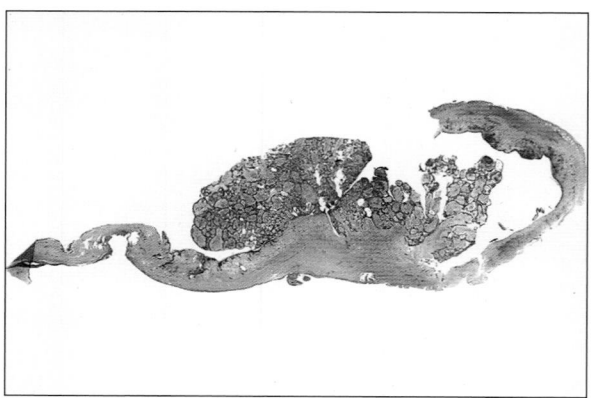

Fig 14-11 An ameloblastoma in situ with intraluminal proliferation. A portion of the cyst can be seen with a large ameloblastoma proliferating into the lumen. There is no involvement of the cyst wall.

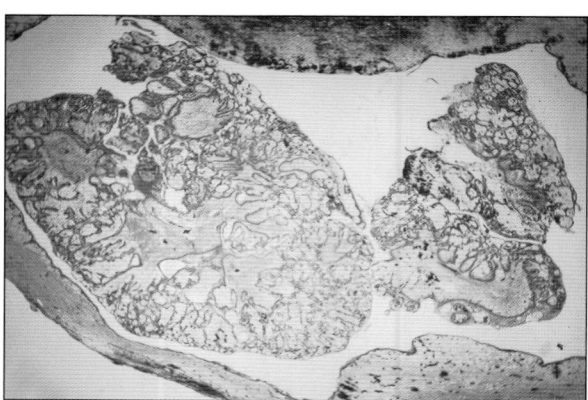

Fig 14-12 Proliferation of an entirely intraluminal ameloblastoma.

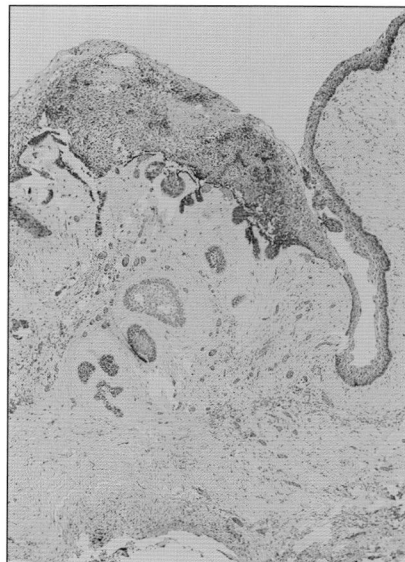

Fig 14-13 A microinvasive ameloblastoma in situ in which there is intraluminal proliferation and intramural proliferation. In this case, simple enucleation is not recommended.

tic ameloblastomas are preceded by these lesions, they do represent an ameloblastic proliferation with limited infiltrative and aggressive potential.

In the mural ameloblastoma in situ, a unilocular cyst is lined by epithelium that in whole or in part exhibits the changes described by Vickers and Gorlin for early neoplastic changes in ameloblastomatous epithelium. These features are hyperchromatism of basal cell nuclei, palisading and polarization of the basal cell nuclei, and cytoplasmic vacuolation of basal and basilar cells. Intercellular spacing of the epithelium is also present, and basal budding may occur (Figs 14-10a and 14-10b).

The intraluminal ameloblastoma in situ shows an intraluminal proliferation (Fig 14-11). This often resembles the pattern of a plexiform ameloblastoma. There is no involvement of the cyst wall (Fig 14-12). The lining of the cyst may be nonspecific and/or may show features consistent with Vickers and Gorlin's criteria. These lesions have sometimes been called *plexiform unicystic ameloblastomas.*

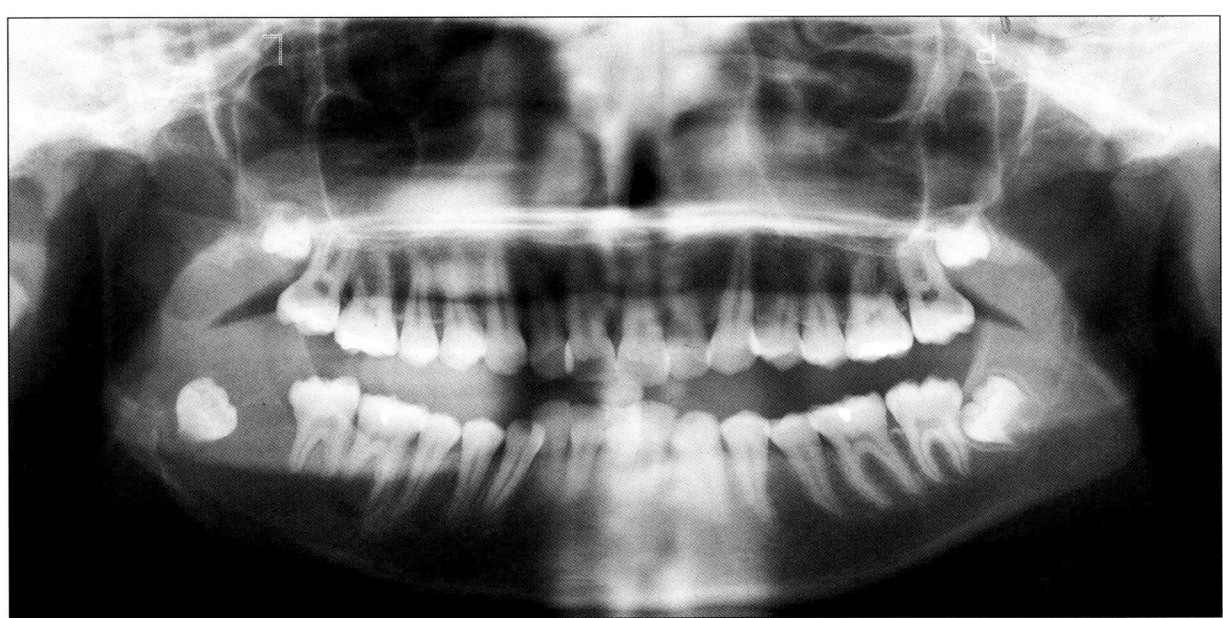

Fig 14-14 Invasive ameloblastomas often produce a multilocular expansile radiolucency with well-demarcated borders. They often displace teeth and the outline of the mandibular canal.

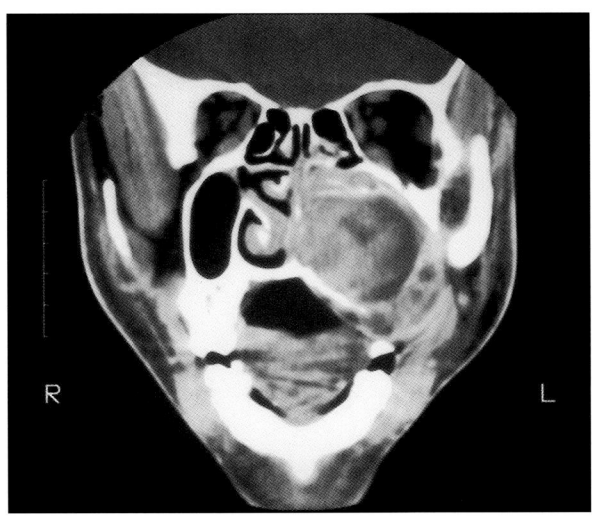

Fig 14-15 A maxillary ameloblastoma may occupy the maxillary sinus; expand into the nasal cavity, ethmoids, and orbit; and expand the palate, as shown here.

Microinvasive ameloblastomas contain islands of ameloblastic epithelium in the cyst wall (Fig 14-13). The lining of the cyst may or may not be in continuity with these islands. Features of the mural and/or intraluminal ameloblastoma may or may not be present. The significant feature is the cyst wall, which heralds a change in biologic behavior from the ameloblastomas in situ to a more invasive tumor.

Invasive Ameloblastoma

CLINICAL PRESENTATION AND PATHOGENESIS

The ameloblastoma is the prototype of a benign neoplasm: that is, it will exhibit cell replication and growth throughout its existence, but it will not metastasize. The rare cases of ameloblastomas that have metastasized are termed *malignant ameloblastomas*. Alternatively, they may represent a malignant tumor of a nonodontogenic cell line that bears a histologic resemblance to an ameloblastoma. Nevertheless, the ameloblastoma recognized as a specific odontogenic neoplasm is benign and arises from odontogenic epithelium that is involved with tooth formation. It will therefore become progressively destructive if left untreated. In many third-world countries with limited access to care and a shortage of trained oral and maxillofacial surgeons, development of extreme ameloblastomas of monstrous size is indicative of their relentless growth (see Figs 14-24a to 14-24c).

The ameloblastoma of this discussion is the invasive ameloblastoma that occurs centrally in either jaw and will usually present as an asymptomatic expansion. It has been reported in all age groups, but its peak incidence is between 20 and 35 years of age with no sex predilection. It is rare to see ameloblastomas in children younger than 12 years. The most common site is the third molar area of either jaw. The mandible is more frequently affected (75%) than the maxilla (25%).

Radiographs show an expansile radiolucency that may be either unilocular or multilocular but will have a well-demarcated border. The tumor may cause tooth displacement, displacement of the inferior alveolar canal (usually toward the inferior border) (Fig 14-14), displacement of the sinus membrane (usually toward the orbit), or root resorption (Fig 14-15). Root resorption is usually a smooth regular resorption indicative of benign disease. Despite displacement of the inferior alveolar canal, nerve sensation is not altered by the tumor because of its inability to undergo true neural invasion.

Ameloblastomas originate from the sources of residual odontogenic epithelium, including the dental lamina rests of Serres and the rests from the breakup of Hertwig epithelial root sheath (ie, the rests of Malassez). They also arise from the reduced enamel epithelium after crown formation and therefore may mimic a dentigerous cyst or arise from the epithelial lining of a dentigerous cyst. In either case, the neoplastic genetic alteration of these cells confers a biology whereby they invade and resorb bone; if they escape the confines of bone, they can invade and grow within soft tissue. This is a direct contrast to the odontogenic keratocyst, which has the ability to invade and resorb bone but cannot infiltrate into soft tissue.

DIFFERENTIAL DIAGNOSIS ▶

The two general radiographic presentations of an ameloblastoma are a unilocular radiolucency and a multilocular radiolucency. In the adult, a unilocular radiolucency is suggestive of the more common *dentigerous cyst*. It may also represent an *odontogenic keratocyst*, which is also more common than an ameloblastoma. In the anterior regions of either jaw, an *adenomatoid odontogenic cyst* may also be a consideration, particularly if the individual is younger than 20 years. Additionally, an early *calcifying odontogenic cyst*, which often will not show calcifications on a radiograph, is a consideration.

If the lesion is multilocular, the more common *odontogenic keratocyst* and *central giant cell tumor* are the most serious considerations. The *odontogenic myxoma* and the *central hemangiomas* (both cavernous and arteriovenous), although less common, may present an identical clinical and radiographic picture.

DIAGNOSTIC WORK-UP ▶

The diagnosis is made from an incisional biopsy. A CT scan is recommended as an aid in determining areas of possible tumor extension beyond the cortex as well as within the marrow space. Extracortical extension is recognized by a perforation in the cortex that is also associated with a soft tissue density.

HISTOPATHOLOGY ▶

A multiplicity of histologic subtypes of solid and multicystic ameloblastomas has burdened the literature, confusing the clinician. The variations are essentially of academic interest, allowing the pathologist an appreciation of this histologic diversity. Biologic behavior, however, is not affected by these variations.

In general, these tumors are unencapsulated, infiltrating neoplasms, although sometimes there may be areas that appear well demarcated. The most frequent pattern is follicular (Fig 14-16a). Epithelial islands are present within a variable quantity of fibrous stroma, which is generally well collagenized. The islands mimic the enamel organ. At the periphery are columnar cells, resembling preameloblasts, in which the nuclei are polarized away from the basement membrane and toward the center of the island (Fig 14-16b). Within the center of the island is a loose arrangement of the epithelial cells, resembling the stellate reticulum. Within the stellate reticulum, a variety of changes may be observed. Squamous metaplasia is not uncommon, and less frequently keratinization may be seen (Fig 14-16c). When this process is extensive, the term *acanthomatous ameloblastoma* has been applied. Cystic degeneration, possibly extensive with coalescence of cystic spaces (Fig 14-16d), is a frequent finding. This phenomenon may be carried to the extreme in large, long-standing tumors that may become virtually hollow. Marked cystic change led to the designation *cystic ameloblastoma*, a term that has also been applied to the *unicystic ameloblastoma* (vide infra). The stellate reticulum may sometimes appear more compact and show spindling, promoting the term *spindle cell ameloblastoma* (Fig 14-16e). Occasionally, the cells within the stellate reticulum are large and contain granular, eosinophilic cytoplasm (Fig 14-16f). Ultrastructurally and immunohistochemically, the granules represent lysozomes, just as they do in the granular cell tumor. This variant has been called *granular cell ameloblastoma*.

The second major pattern of ameloblastoma is plexiform. The epithelium proliferates in a network of anastomosing strands, very much as if the islands of the follicular pattern open and become confluent with their neighbors (Fig 14-17a). Consequently, the epithelial component will show peripheral columnar cells with nuclei polarized away from the basement membrane, toward the central stellate reticulum (Fig 14-17b). Some limited cystic change may occur within the stellate reticulum, but the broad spectrum of changes that may be seen within the follicular pattern are not present here. The connective tissue component is usually ill-defined and poorly collagenized (see Fig 14-17b). Occasionally, aggregates of foamy histiocytes are seen (Fig 14-17c).

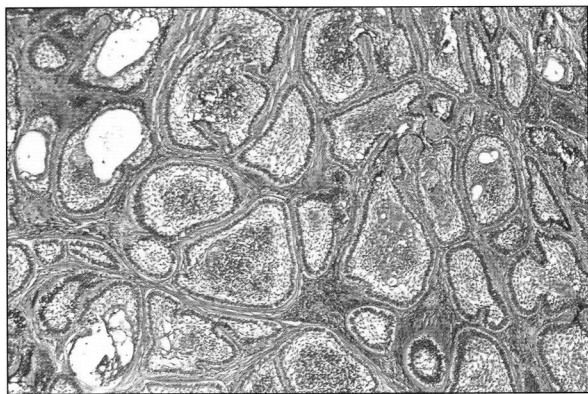

Fig 14-16a An ameloblastoma with a follicular pattern. The epithelial islands are supported by a densely collagenized tissue. The islands have peripheral columnar cells with a loose central stellate reticulum. Squamous metaplasia and cyst formation can be seen within some of these islands.

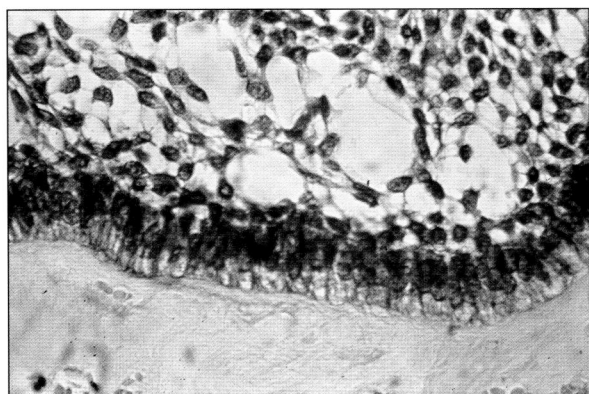

Fig 14-16b High-power view of an island within an ameloblastoma showing peripheral columnar cells exhibiting reverse polarity. The microcyst formation within the stellate reticulum is evident.

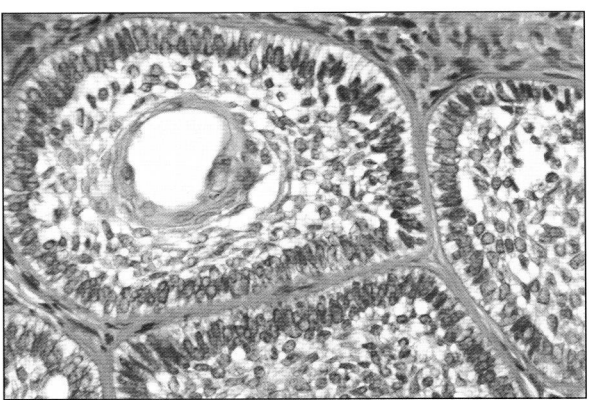

Fig 14-16c An epithelial island within a follicular ameloblastoma showing cystic change and squamous metaplasia.

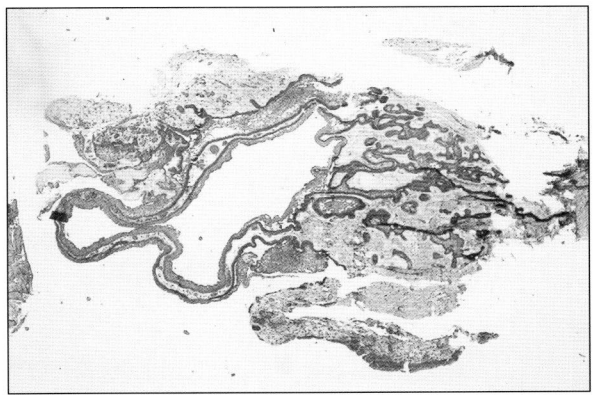

Fig 14-16d A large cystic space, achieved through coalescence, has formed within this ameloblastoma.

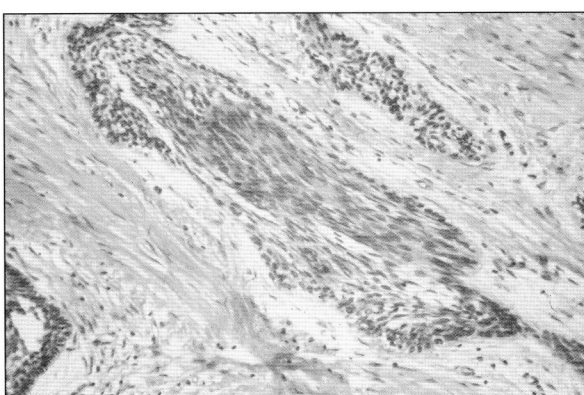

Fig 14-16e Some of the epithelial islands within this follicular ameloblastoma consist of spindle cells.

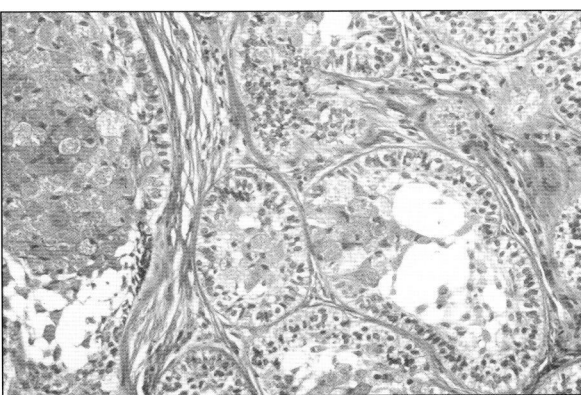

Fig 14-16f A granular cell ameloblastoma. The overall pattern is follicular, but many of the cells within the islands are large and granular.

The similarity of an ameloblastoma to basal cell carcinoma is often noted, and the designation "basal cell pattern" is sometimes given to tumors that form islands and anastomosing strands of basaloid cells in a fibrous stroma. Peripheral palisading may be seen (Figs 14-18a and 14-18b).

Again, it is important to emphasize that from the clinician's perspective there is little reason to subclassify these tumors since their biologic behavior does not vary.

TREATMENT ▶

Curative treatment of a primary invasive ameloblastoma is accomplished by bony resection using 1.0- to 1.5-cm bony margins and anatomic barrier margins of one uninvolved anatomic barrier (see pages 684 to 703). Palliative therapy may be achieved with enucleation and curettage procedures and is indicated only for individuals who prefer and request palliation over curative resection or for whom anesthetic and surgical risks are too great to undergo a curative resection. Recurrence with enucleation and curettage procedures is expected (70% to 85%) but will take about 5 years to become clinically apparent. Therefore, it may achieve effective short-term palliation (see Figs 14-1a to 14-1c).

Enucleation and curettage is not advised since recurrences develop after 5 years and frequently result in large, extensively destructive tumors. In addition, enucleation and curettage has a potential for

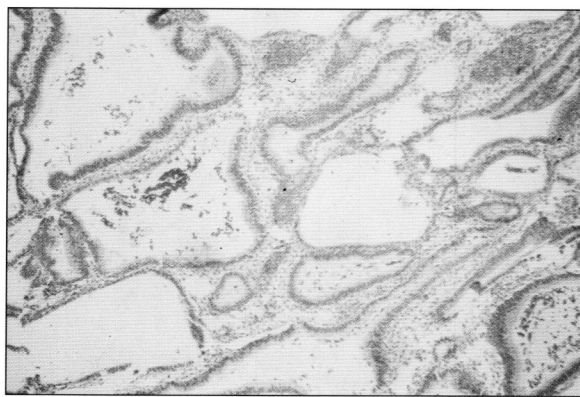

Fig 14-17a A plexiform pattern within an ameloblastoma. Here the epithelial component forms a network rather than discrete islands. Because it is very poorly collagenized, the stroma is not readily apparent.

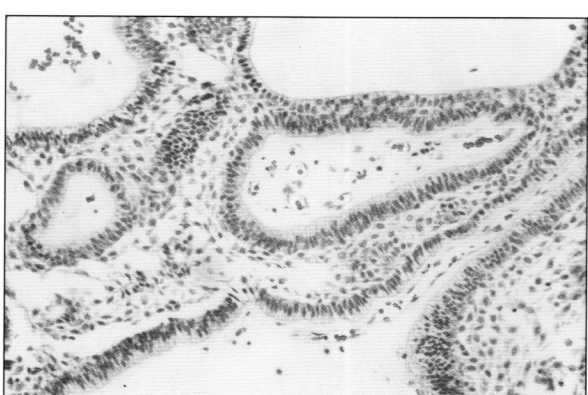

Fig 14-17b Higher-power view of Fig 14-17a showing that even though the arrangement may be different than in the follicular pattern, the peripheral columnar cells that are palisaded and polarized are still present, and the stellate reticulum pattern is seen in between. The stroma is so ill-defined that the spaces may give the impression of cystic lumina. The presence of capillaries in some of these areas indicates that they represent stroma.

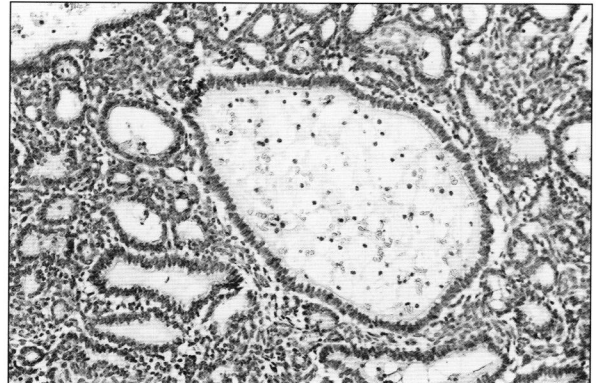

Fig 14-17c This plexiform pattern shows foamy histiocytes within the stroma.

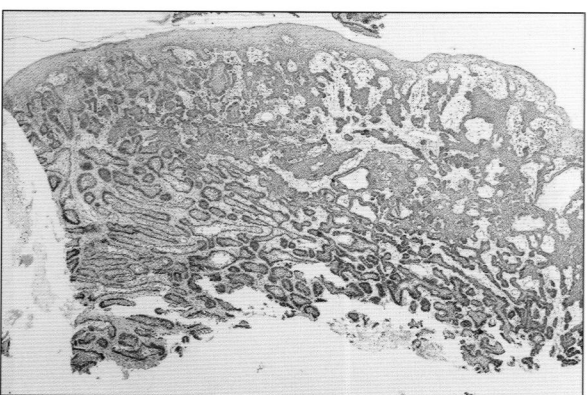

Fig 14-18a This ameloblastoma bears a striking resemblance to basal cell carcinoma. Although this particular tumor appears to arise from the surface mucosa, it is a central tumor that has broken out of bone and fused with the overlying mucosa. One must avoid assuming that such a lesion is a peripheral ameloblastoma.

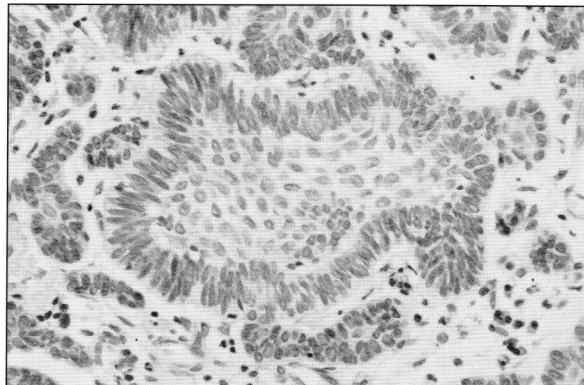

Fig 14-18b High-power view of Fig 14-18a showing the resemblance to basal cell carcinoma of skin.

PROGNOSIS ▶

tumor seeding. The particulation of an ameloblastoma by the curettage itself and the rotary action of a bur often used to remove bone is known to implant tumor cells within soft tissues, resulting in unresectable and debilitating tumor recurrences (Figs 14-19a to 14-19d).

Ameloblastomas treated by resection seldom recur (98% cure rate). Enucleation and curettage procedures are associated with a high incidence of recurrence (70% to 85%). The concern of a malignant ameloblastoma is always present if a recurrence develops. However, repeated surgeries have no real means of inducing malignant changes. Those that recur as large, unresectable tumors after enucleation and curettage procedures clinically do not metastasize and remain histologically benign. They are often life threatening by their location rather than their biology. Those that recur and metastasize represent the rare ameloblastoma that was malignant from the outset or was developing a malignant biology on its own.

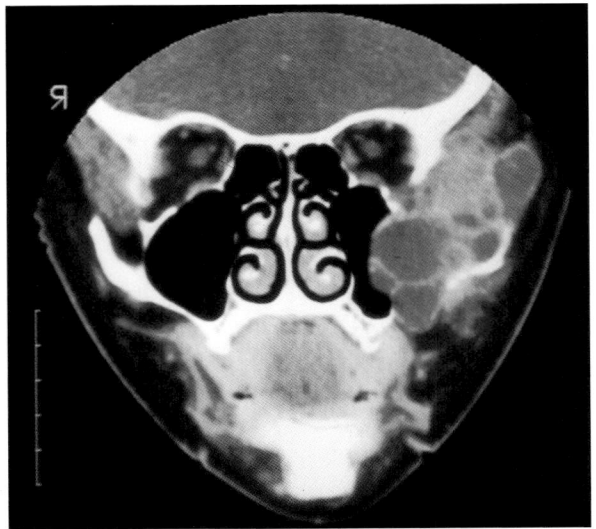

Fig 14-19a Recurrent ameloblastoma involving the entire zygoma and temporalis muscle as well as the infraorbital fissure 8 years after an incomplete removal via enucleation and curettage.

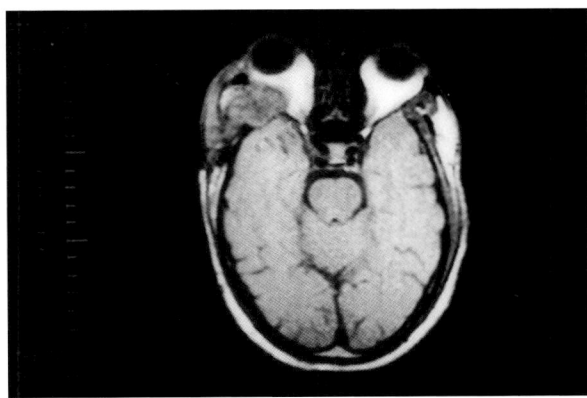

Fig 14-19b Recurrent ameloblastoma after several enucleation and curettage procedures. Tumor is in the retro-orbital space and has eroded into the temporal lobe of the brain. The radiolucent streaks in the temporal lobe represent areas of inflammation. This patient died of this complication.

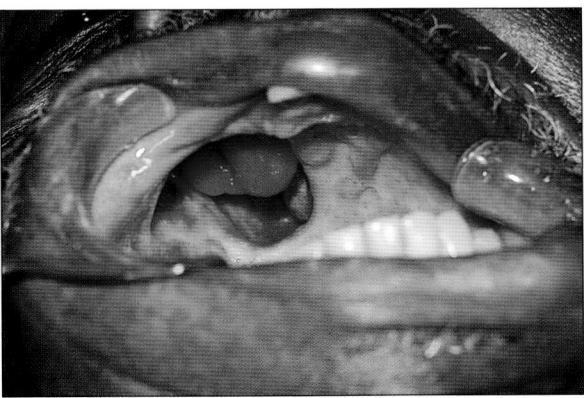

Fig 14-19c This mass represents the third recurrence of an ameloblastoma after enucleation and curettage procedures followed by a hemimaxillectomy as a salvage attempt. Tumor is extending down from the sphenoid and cavernous sinuses.

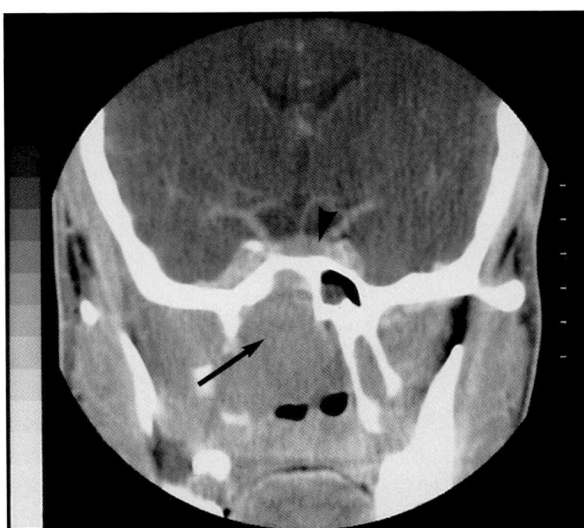

Fig 14-19d CT scan of recurrent ameloblastoma in the nasopharynx and sphenoid sinus (*arrow*), and now in the cavernous sinus (*arrowhead*) from previous enucleation and curettage attempts.

Clinical and Histologic Variations of Invasive Ameloblastomas

Peripheral Ameloblastoma

This ameloblastoma is not a true neoplasm and lacks the biologic potential of the central ameloblastoma. It is a hamartomatous proliferation of odontogenic epithelium arising from rests of Serres or perhaps from the basal cells of the oral mucosa. Usually not attaining a size larger than 3 cm, it will present as a firm single or polyploid mass arising exophytically from the gingiva (Fig 14-20). It does not invade bone, and, as a true peripheral ameloblastoma, it is not associated with a radiolucent area. Some central ameloblastomas have been misdiagnosed as peripheral types when they eroded through the alveolar bone and presented with a soft tissue mass. Peripheral ameloblastomas are managed by local soft tissue excision with 2- to 3-mm margins. Recurrence is not seen.

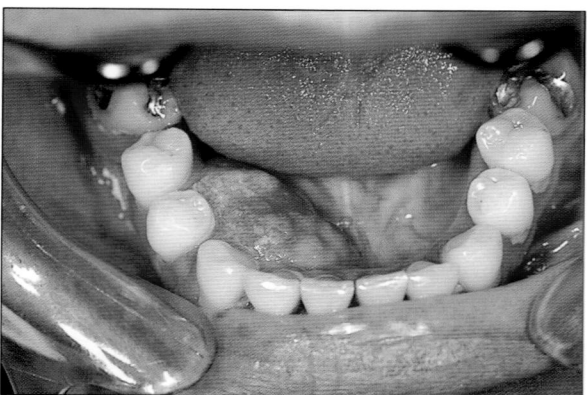

Fig 14-20 A peripheral ameloblastoma will be an unexpected diagnosis. It will present as a firm mass arising from the gingiva with no evidence of an origin in bone. (Courtesy of Dr Jorge Ravelo.)

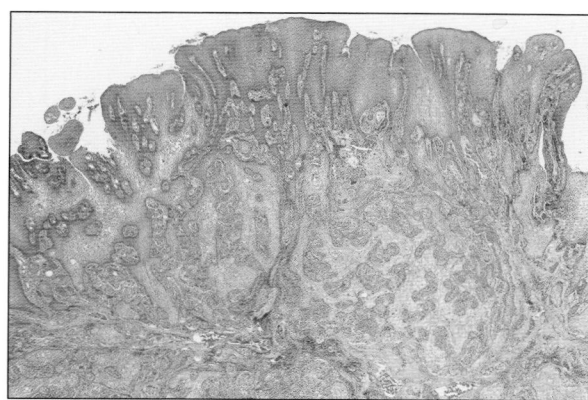

Fig 14-21 A peripheral ameloblastoma with a follicular pattern. The tumor islands can be seen below the mucosal surface. No intraosseous component was present.

HISTOPATHOLOGY ▶

The peripheral ameloblastoma cannot be distinguished histologically from the intraosseous tumors. They may develop follicular, plexiform, and basilar patterns (Fig 14-21). Squamous change is usually prominent. The ameloblastoma will frequently appear fused to the overlying mucosal epithelium. Whether this represents confluence or origin from the overlying epithelium is uncertain. Central intraosseous ameloblastomas may perforate bone and present a similar pattern (see Fig 14-18a). Because biologic behavior and treatment differ, this possibility must be excluded before the diagnosis of a peripheral ameloblastoma is made.

Desmoplastic Ameloblastoma

The desmoplastic ameloblastoma is a rare but histopathologically and radiographically unique ameloblastoma. It is otherwise identical to the more common central ameloblastoma and is treated in the same fashion. Its unique radiographic appearance is that of a mixed radiolucent-radiopaque lesion unlike the strictly radiolucent quality of other ameloblastomas (Fig 14-22). Therefore, it is usually a surprise diagnosis from a differential list composed mostly of fibro-osseous diseases and odontogenic cysts and tumors that are characteristically radiolucent-radiopaque. These include *ossifying fibromas*, *fibrous dysplasia*, *osteoblastomas*, *osteosarcomas*, *calcifying epithelial odontogenic tumors*, and *calcifying odontogenic cysts*. Histologically, they are unique by virtue of their thickened bony trabeculae and dense, scar-like fibroblastic stroma. The strands and islands of a desmoplastic ameloblastoma are sparse compared to the stroma, but invasion and continued slow growth are the same as in other ameloblastomas.

HISTOPATHOLOGY ▶

This variant seems to have at least a different radiologic appearance. Histologically, these tumors elaborate a large quantity of densely collagenized stroma within which islands and cords of odontogenic epithelium are found. This component often appears hyperchromatic and compressed (Figs 14-23a and 14-23b). Some well-developed islands, like those seen in the follicular pattern, may be observed.

Recurrent Ameloblastoma

Recurrent ameloblastomas present the clinician with some unique challenges. In tertiary institutions to which individuals are referred for care, recurrent ameloblastomas represent 60% of all ameloblastomas seen. Most of these are related to incomplete removals in which enucleation and curettage was the mode of therapy. The average time lapse between the first surgery and the detected recurrence is about 5 years, but many recurrences are not recognized until 9 or more years have passed. Fortunately, most are recurrences within bone, which allows for curative salvage by resection. In such resections, it is help-

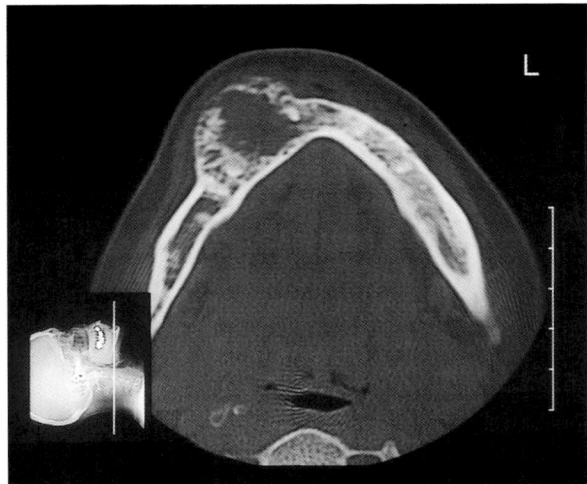

Fig 14-22 Although this CT scan is suggestive of an ossifying fibroma, a calcifying epithelial odontogenic tumor, or a calcifying odontogenic cyst, it nevertheless represented a desmoplastic ameloblastoma.

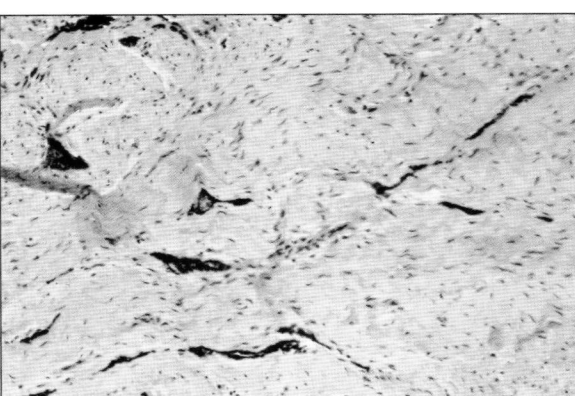

Fig 14-23a A desmoplastic ameloblastoma in which an abundant, densely collagenized stroma can be seen. In this area, the epithelial islands appear to be compressed.

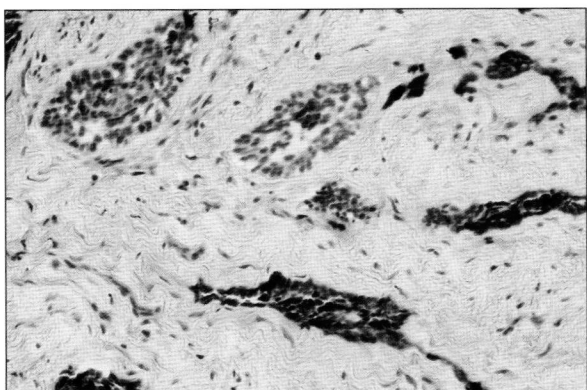

Fig 14-23b The same tumor as in Fig 14-23a. While many islands are compressed, others are not, and a more characteristic ameloblastomatous pattern can be recognized.

ful to have access to the original radiographs. The salvage resection should be based on the original radiographs rather than on those of the recurrent tumor. If only the area of recurrence is treated, a risk of further recurrences remains within the original tumor area, which cannot be addressed by a salvage surgery based solely on the location of the recurrence.

Some recurrences develop in anatomic spaces outside of bone in areas such as the infratemporal space, deep temporal space, lateral pharyngeal space, base of skull, retropharyngeal space, and retro-orbital space; these are unresectable and, therefore, unsalvageable (see Figs 14-19a to 14-19d). In these instances, the tumor mass effect will cause functional compromise and in rare cases may cause death due to airway obstruction or intracranial spread. Since regrowth of the tumor remains slow, a palliative debulking procedure is useful. Although one can rarely remove all of the tumor, removing most of it will slow the onset of functional loss and may prolong life if the individual is young. In any recurrent lesion, but particularly in one where size and location are disturbing, a careful review of the original histopathology and current biopsy material is essential. Occasionally, one will find that the original tumor was not a benign odontogenic neoplasm, as may have been reported, but an odontogenic carcinoma, a malignant ameloblastoma, or even a malignant tumor of nonodontogenic histogenesis, such as mucoepidermoid carcinoma or squamous cell carcinoma.

Extreme Ameloblastomas

Occasionally, the oral and maxillofacial surgeon may be confronted with an extreme ameloblastoma of excessive size (Figs 14-24a and 14-24b). These patients are usually from third-world rural areas and brought to medical centers for treatment. Although these ameloblastomas are benign (Fig 14-24c), they are nonetheless life threatening. Many have eventuated in death due to airway obstruction, starvation from restriction of feeding, and complications of hypoproteinemia produced partially by the restriction of feeding and partially by protein loss into the cystic spaces of the tumor, which then leaks it out through the mouth.

The basic principles for treating these extreme ameloblastomas are the same as for other ameloblastomas. Cures can be accomplished with resection and immediate reconstruction using a titanium plate to restore continuity, function, and form. However, the surgery is technically difficult and must be approached with these cautions and modifications in mind:

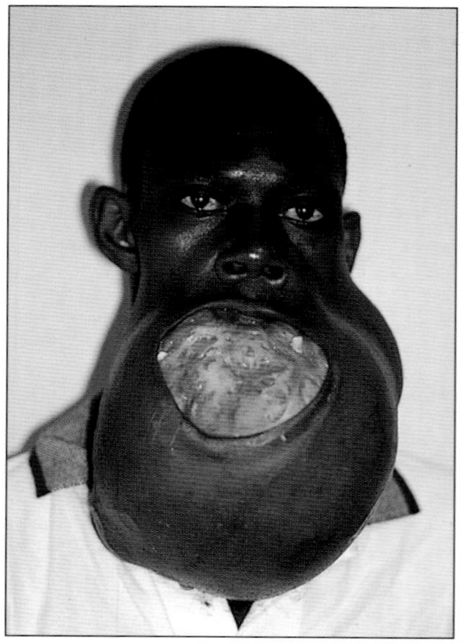

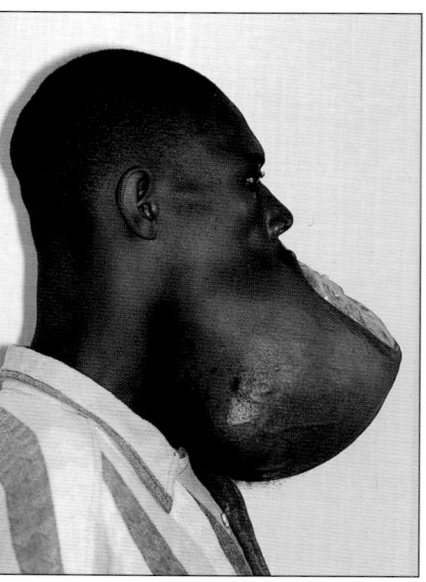

Fig 14-24a This extreme ameloblastoma of over 16 years' duration reached enormous size yet remained benign.

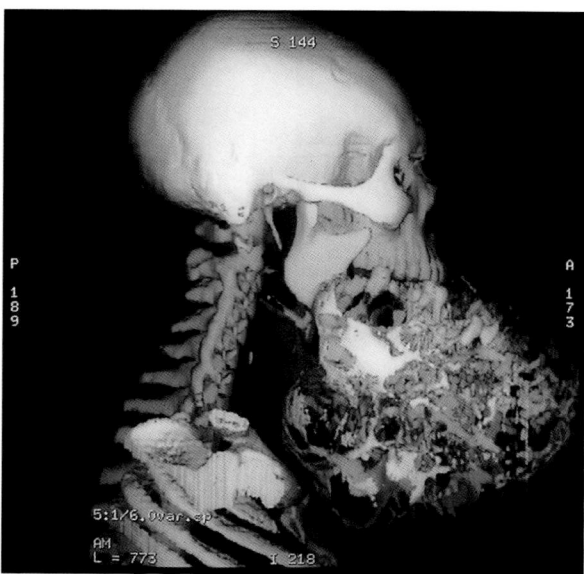

Fig 14-24b Extreme ameloblastomas will act as tissue expanders; note the increased lip length. They also have a significant nutrient demand; note the numerous dilated blood vessels.

Fig 14-24c A CT scan or plain radiographs will show the same features found in most ameloblastomas—that is, a multicystic, expansile, and well-delineated appearance.

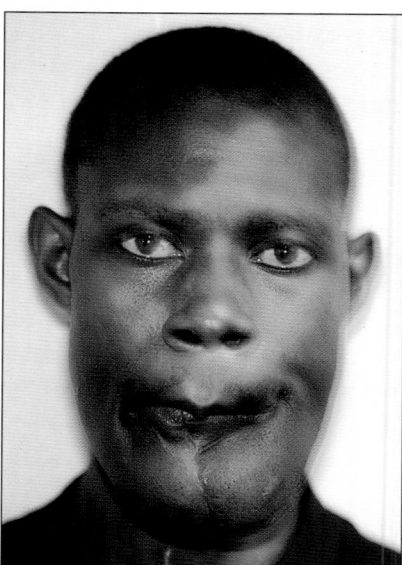

Fig 14-24d Removal of an extreme ameloblastoma is accomplished with a resection using the same bone and soft tissue margins as for any ameloblastoma, in addition to a reconstruction plate. The removal of this tumor, which weighed 8.55 lb, resulted in a dramatic improvement.

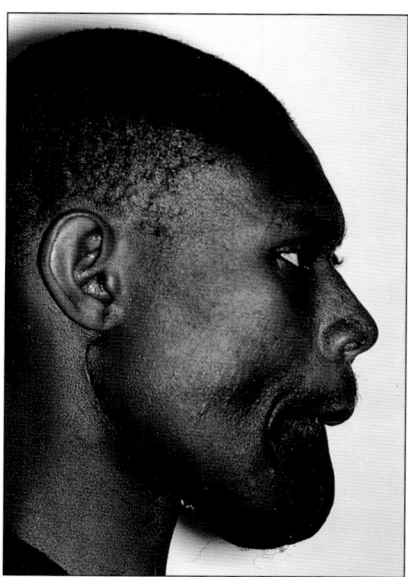

Fig 14-24e Profile of patient in Figs 14-24a to 14-24d shows the value of reconstruction plates even in the largest of jaw resections.

1. The physical size of the tumor and the degree of jaw resection will require a tracheostomy that most likely will need to be slowly decanulated over several days to perhaps several weeks postoperatively.
2. The physical size of the tumor will require an attention to neck support during surgery and the need for several assistant surgeons.
3. The patient will be hypoproteinemic because of eating restrictions and protein fluid loss from the tumor. Preoperative protein supplementation and a thorough physical examination are needed.
4. Due to its metabolic demands, a tumor of this size will have numerous feeding vessels. The surgical team must be prepared for multiple vessel ligations and cautery and have typed and cross-matched blood ready for transfusion.
5. The circumference of these tumors is great and their displacement of normal anatomy will require a longer surgical time. This together with the excess soft tissue and the placement of a reconstruction plate may require 8 to 12 hours of surgery.
6. These tumors cause significant expansion of the tissues of the skin and lip. The surgeon should develop a plan for excising some and sculpting the remainder of the excess soft tissue and lip to create a normal-appearing form (Figs 14-24d and 14-24e).

Odontoameloblastoma

CLINICAL PRESENTATION AND PATHOGENESIS ▶

The odontoameloblastoma is an extremely rare odontogenic neoplasm of which only a handful have ever been reported. It essentially represents an invasive ameloblastoma occurring simultaneously with an odontoma in what may be thought of as a "collision tumor." Neither seems to arise from the other. The unfortunate term *ameloblastic odontoma* is often used to describe this lesion as well, but its name belies the invasiveness characterized by an ameloblastoma. It instead suggests the biologic behavior of an odontoma, which is entirely misleading; therefore, it should not be used.

The odontoameloblastoma, like most ameloblastomas, presents as a painless jaw expansion. The radiograph usually shows a multilocular, mixed radiolucent-radiopaque lesion, although it can also be unilocular. The odontoma component will most likely be of a complex type because most occur in the molar ramus region, but its mineral density will be greater than that of bone. It will approach the mineral density of dentin.

This tumor is rare because of the remote likelihood of two coinciding odontogenic developmental disturbances: one an aberrant attempt at tooth formation, the other a neoplastic genetic alteration of odontogenic epithelium. There is no evidence that these two components are part of the same process.

DIFFERENTIAL DIAGNOSIS ▶

An odontoameloblastoma is so rare that it should never be a prime consideration on any differential list. Instead, odontogenic cysts and tumors such as the *calcifying epithelial odontogenic tumor*, the *calcifying odontogenic cyst*, or the *ameloblastic fibro-odontoma*, which more commonly present as mixed radiolucent-radiopaque lesions, and certain tumors of bone such as an *ossifying fibroma*, are the usual considerations.

DIAGNOSTIC WORK-UP ▶

An incisional biopsy is required and may take the form of enucleation of the soft and hard tissues from bone. After diagnosis, a CT scan is useful to assess the extent of the tumor.

HISTOPATHOLOGY ▶

The epithelial component of these tumors is identical to that of the ameloblastoma. The distinguishing feature is the presence of an ectomesenchymal component with the formation of dentin and enamel. The result is a mixture of ameloblastoma and odontoma.

TREATMENT ▶

The treatment is the same as for an ameloblastoma, which requires a resection using 1.0- to 1.5-cm bony margins and one uninvolved anatomic barrier margin (see pages 684 to 703).

PROGNOSIS ▶

The prognosis is the same as for an ameloblastoma. Resection is anticipated to be curative unless previous treatment attempts have resulted in tumor seeding. Recurrence is anticipated with enucleation and curettage, but the slow growth of this tumor, like that of an ameloblastoma, allows this approach to be palliative.

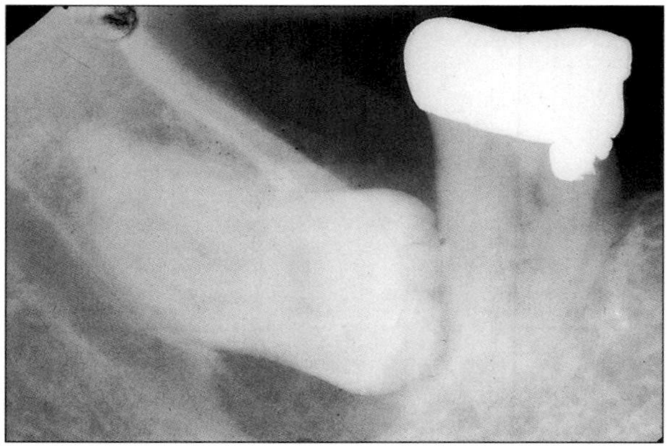

![Fig 14-25 radiograph]

Fig 14-25 This seemingly innocuous radiolucency, suggestive of a dentigerous cyst, developed in a 68-year-old man and was identified as a primary intraosseous carcinoma arising from a cyst lining.

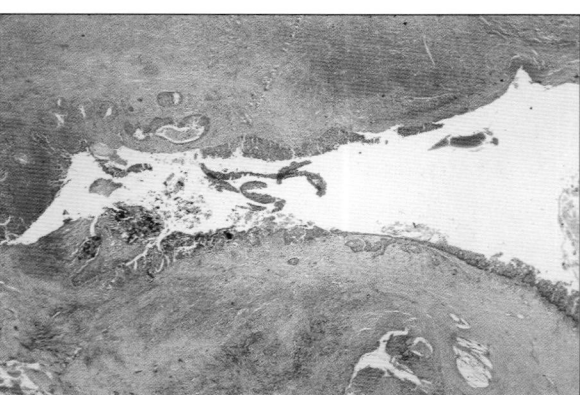

Fig 14-26a Low-power view of a residual cyst in which an area of squamous cell carcinoma can be seen.

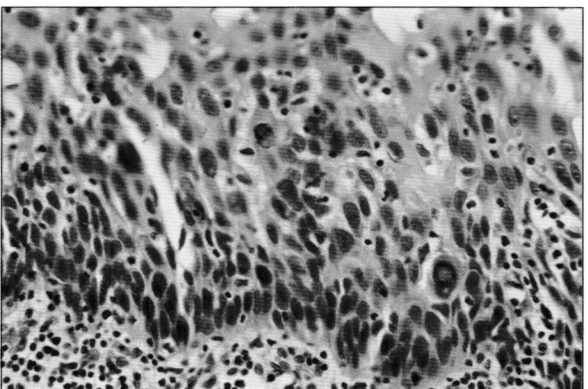

Fig 14-26b Higher-power view of a portion of the cyst shown in Fig 14-26a reveals the dysplastic change within the epithelium.

Odontogenic Carcinomas

Residual odontogenic epithelium from several sources (rests of Serres, rests of Malassez, and reduced enamel epithelium) is composed of cells that are sufficiently undifferentiated so that a series of genetic alterations can produce specific oncogenes or cause the loss of tumor suppressor genes, resulting in a malignancy. Today, we recognize four types of odontogenic carcinomas: primary intraosseous carcinoma ex-odontogenic cyst, primary intraosseous carcimona de novo, malignant ameloblastoma, and ameloblastic carcinoma.

Primary Intraosseous Carcinoma Ex Odontogenic Cyst

CLINICAL PRESENTATION AND PATHOGENESIS ▶

The primary intraosseous carcinoma ex-odontogenic cyst may present as an uncomplicated dentigerous cyst; the diagnosis can be established only when the histopathologic studies are completed. It may also present as a dentigerous cyst in which the radiolucency shows an irregular demarcation to adjacent bone. The presence of decreased sensation or paresthesia is a suspicious sign suggesting malignancy. The cyst is most often seen in individuals older than 50 years. It should be suspected when a residual impacted tooth in an older individual develops an expanded follicle appearance or seems to develop a dentigerous cyst–like radiolucency (Fig 14-25). These carcinomas can also arise in radicular and residual cysts.

HISTOPATHOLOGY ▶

This tumor is essentially an odontogenic cyst in which an invasive carcinoma arises from the cystic lining. This is a rare occurrence, and the possibility of a collision between a carcinoma and a cyst must be considered. Credence for the origin of the carcinoma is given when the cystic lining is dysplastic (Figs 14-26a and 14-26b). The carcinoma is squamous in nature and invades the surrounding tissue. It has all the regional lymph node and distant metastatic potential of mucosal squamous cell carcinoma.

Primary Intraosseous Carcinoma de Novo

CLINICAL PRESENTATION AND PATHOGENESIS ▶

The primary intraosseous carcinoma de novo presents as a more clinically aggressive and radiographically destructive radiolucent lesion in which the border with adjacent bone is irregular (Fig 14-27). It may also cause an irregular and jagged type of root resorption, in contrast to the smooth regular root resorption seen with odontogenic cysts and benign tumors. Paresthesia and anesthesia are common with this tumor.

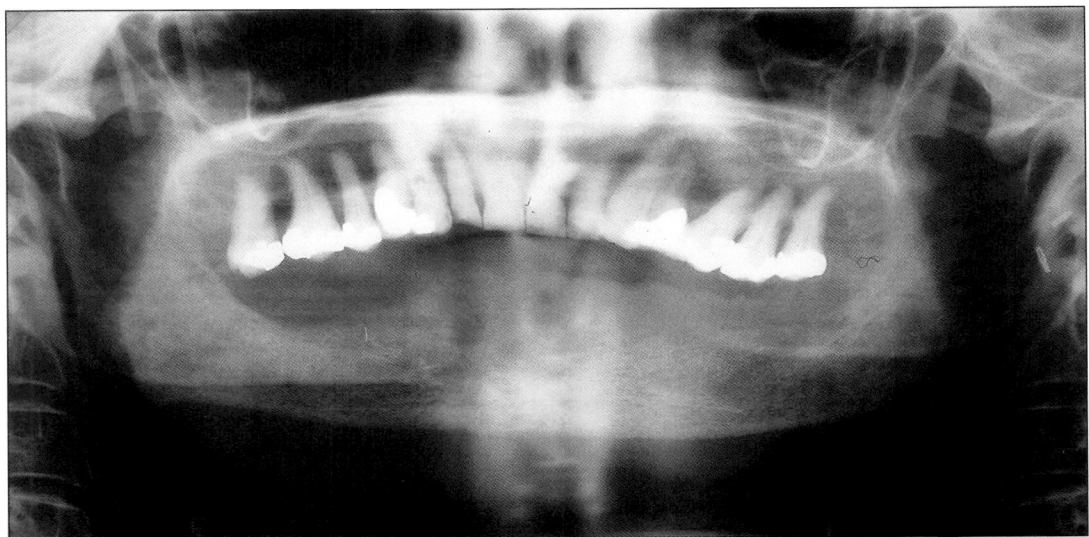

Fig 14-27 An irregular and rapidly destructive process is associated with a primary intraosseous carcinoma. This malignancy presumably arises from rests and has no communication with the overlying epithelium until it advances out of the bone.

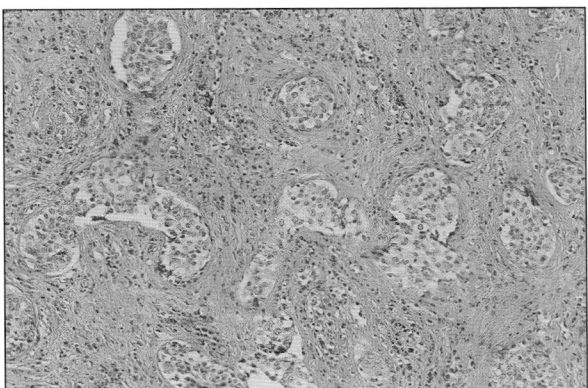

Fig 14-28a Atypical epithelial cells within bone consistent with a diagnosis of intraosseous carcinoma.

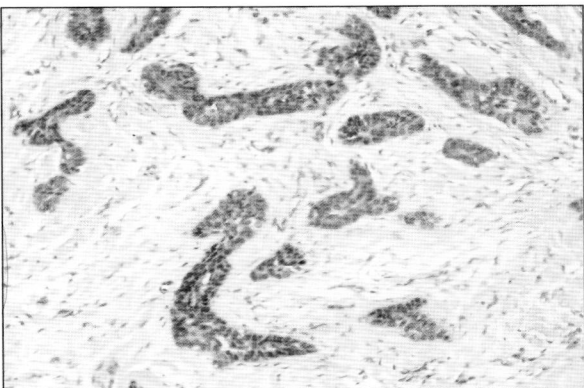

Fig 14-28b An intraosseous carcinoma with islands of malignant epithelium in a loose fibrous stroma.

HISTOPATHOLOGY ▶   This carcinoma is essentially a central epithelial malignancy of the jaws in which no clinical or histologic connection to an odontogenic cyst or overlying mucosa can be identified. It usually resembles squamous cell carcinoma and often exhibits keratinization. Because the cell of origin is odontogenic epithelium, the proliferating cells may be more basaloid, and peripheral palisading atypical cells may be present. This histology may be difficult to distinguish from ameloblastic carcinoma (Figs 14-28a and 14-28b).

Malignant Ameloblastoma

CLINICAL PRESENTATION AND PATHOGENESIS ▶ The malignant ameloblastoma will most commonly present as a multilocular radiolucent jaw expansion typical of a benign ameloblastoma (Figs 14-29a and 14-29b), but with a concomitant metastatic focus, usually in the lungs. The type of root resorption manifested by this malignancy is also suggestive of a benign process, and paresthesias may or may not be observed. The metastatic focus is often discovered on a routine chest radiograph or may be found by a site-specific complaint.

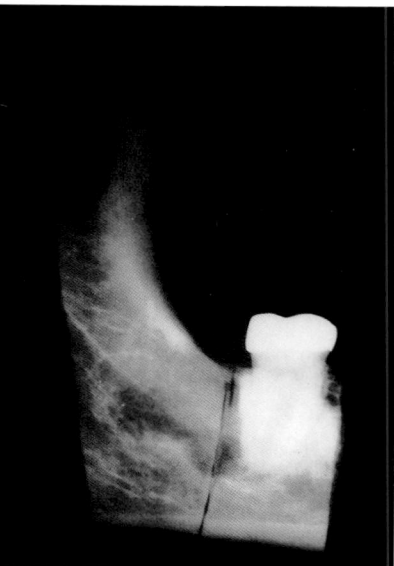

Fig 14-29a A malignant ameloblastoma will often appear to be radiographically identical to a benign ameloblastoma.

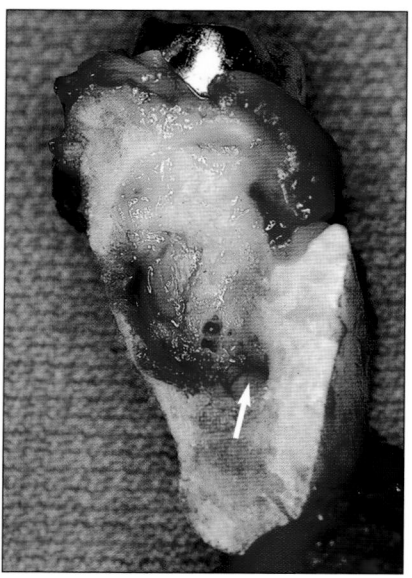

Fig 14-29b The gross specimen of the malignant ameloblastoma resection shown in Fig 14-29a reveals exophytic growth and intraneural invasion (*arrow*). This tumor also evidenced regional lymph node metastasis.

HISTOPATHOLOGY ▶

The malignant ameloblastoma represents a jaw tumor that is a benign ameloblastoma histopathologically but metastasized to a distant site or to regional lymph nodes. Although some lung metastases have been attributed to aspiration of tumor cells because of their location in the right middle and upper lung fields, some other cases have shown metastasis to lymph nodes, long bones, vertebrae, etc, where aspiration cannot be implicated as the cause. This phenomenon is indeed biologically feasible because malignant cells can undergo vessel invasion, transport, cloning, angiogenesis, and establishment of a self-sustaining colony independent of cytologic appearance and growth rate.

Ameloblastic Carcinoma

CLINICAL PRESENTATION AND
PATHOGENESIS ▶

The ameloblastic carcinoma differs from the malignant ameloblastoma in the following features. First, the pre-ameloblasts are cytologically atypical, whereas in the malignant ameloblastoma they appear cytologically benign. Second, the ameloblastic carcinoma may be locally aggressive and undergo regional lymph node metastasis, but it is not required to show metastasis to confirm the diagnosis. A malignant ameloblastoma, in contrast, must show metastasis to be a confirmed diagnosis.

Ameloblastic carcinomas are usually large tissue masses with ulcerations, significant bone resorption, and tooth mobility (Fig 14-30). Their behavior is similar to that of an aggressive squamous cell carcinoma, for which they are often mistaken until the histopathology identifies the pre-ameloblast cellular atypia.

HISTOPATHOLOGY ▶

Unlike the malignant ameloblastoma, this tumor shows cytologic features of malignancy. It has the basic pattern of an ameloblastoma but may show hypercellularity, cellular atypia, hyperchromatism, and mitoses (Fig 14-31). While metastatic deposits may resemble those of an ameloblastoma, they tend to take on the appearance of squamous cell carcinoma.

DIFFERENTIAL DIAGNOSIS
AND WORK-UP ▶

Because the lesions are usually identified after an incisional biopsy or the removal of a cyst and are a surprise finding, a differential list concerning these lesions is usually a moot point. When the diagnosis

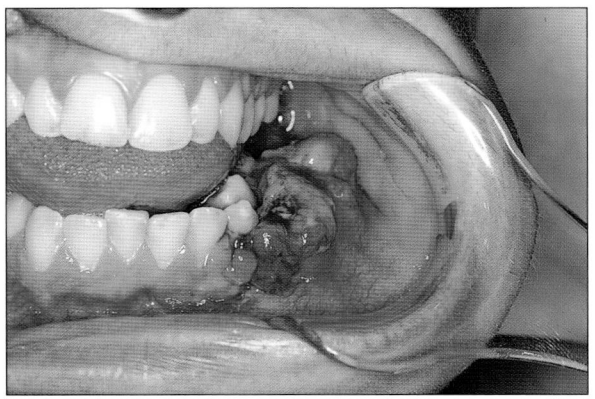

Fig 14-30 Most ameloblastic carcinomas are aggressive malignancies. This one has eroded and fungated into the buccal vestibule, causing significant mobility.

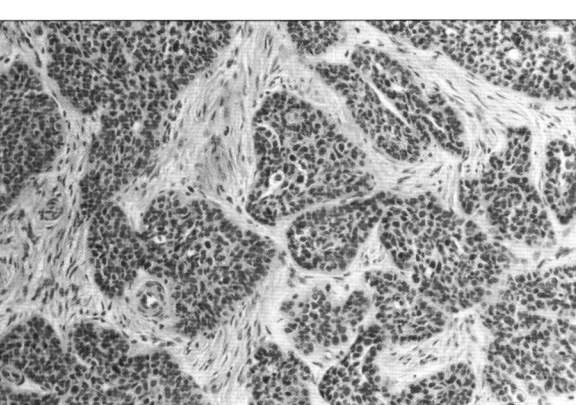

Fig 14-31 An ameloblastic carcinoma with hypercellularity and hyperchromatism.

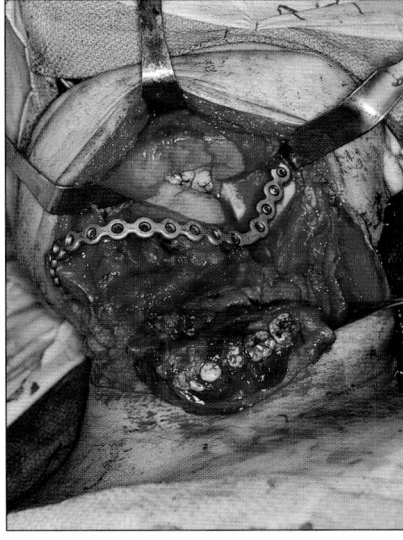

Fig 14-32a Odontogenic carcinomas have a biologic potential similar to that of mucosal squamous cell carcinomas and are thus treated in a similar manner: jaw resection, consideration for an incontinuity neck dissection (shown here), and in some cases postoperative radiotherapy.

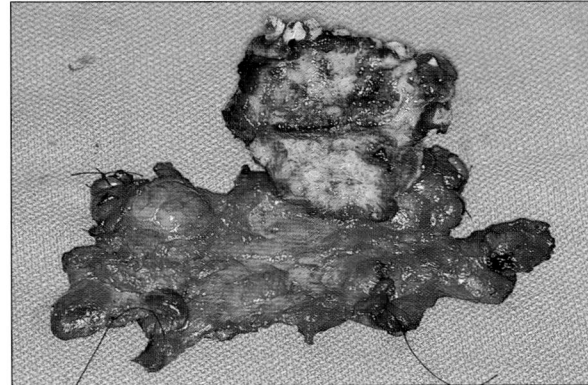

Fig 14-32b An ameloblastic carcinoma is an aggressive malignancy usually requiring resection with an incontinuity neck dissection as well as consideration for postoperative radiotherapy.

of any of these four types of odontogenic carcinomas is made, a staging work-up consisting of a neck examination, a CT scan of the area, and a chest radiograph becomes necessary. Because these are intraosseous tumors, they are T_4 lesions by location. An assessment for nodal metastasis and for evidence of distant metastasis is required.

TREATMENT AND PROGNOSIS ►

All four carcinomas tend to be aggressive and have a guarded prognosis. Treatment usually requires jaw resection with 2- to 3-cm bony margins and contiguous neck dissection, both prophylactic and therapeutic (Figs 14-32a and 14-32b). Postsurgical radiotherapy is also a consideration in many cases. The finding of distant metastatic deposits in individual cases makes them incurable, but effective palliation may be gained from chemotherapy or selective site radiotherapy. Too few cases with reliable follow-up have been reported to fully understand prognosis. However, it appears that 5-year survival rates are less than 40% and recurrence rates exceed 60% even in the face of aggressive treatment.

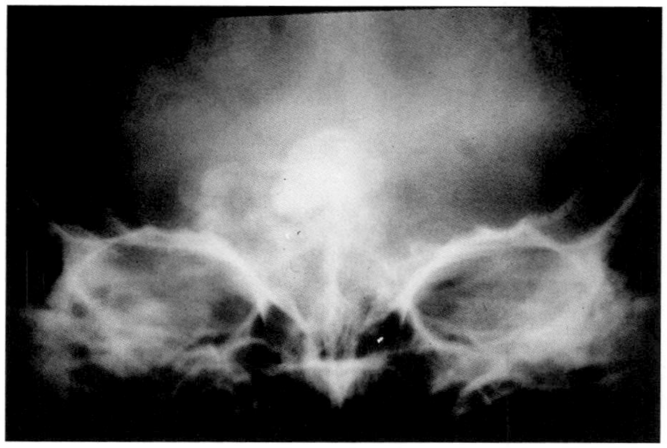

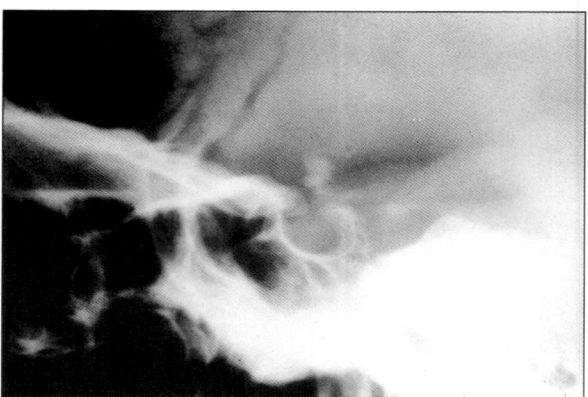

Fig 14-33a Lobular calcifications on an anteroposterior skull radiograph in the midline and paramidline areas should suggest a craniopharyngioma.

Fig 14-33b A lateral skull radiograph, CT scans, or tomograms will localize a destructive lesion usually with calcifications of the sphenoid–sella turcica area.

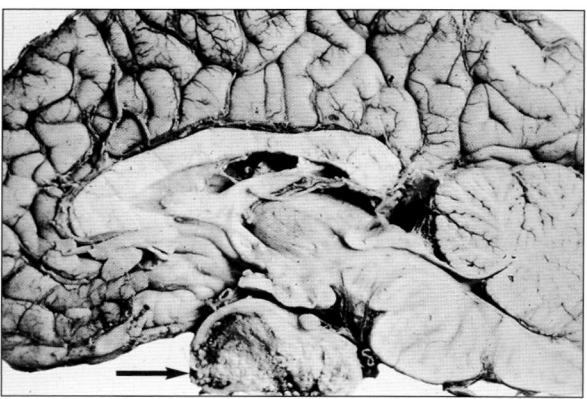

Fig 14-33c This hemisection of a brain shows a large craniopharyngioma (*arrow*) at the inferior edge of the midbrain.

Ameloblastoma-like Lesions

Craniopharyngioma

CLINICAL PRESENTATION AND PATHOGENESIS ▶

Craniopharyngiomas are benign tumors that are dangerous because of their location. They are thought to arise from primitive oral ectoderm that becomes entrapped as Rathke pouch invaginates from the fetal oral cavity to form the adenohypophysis (anterior pituitary). Therefore, these cells are rests, and like other rests they can form benign tumors years later.

Most craniopharyngiomas occur in early life, from 10 months to 20 years of age (mean, 10 years of age). The clinical presentation may include a wide range of signs and symptoms depending on whether the tumor's location is prechiasmatic (anterior to the optic chiasm), retrochiasmatic (posterior to the optic chiasm), or within or on the sella turcica portion of the sphenoid.

The most common presenting finding is headaches (68%) followed by a variety of endocrine disturbances related to the tumor's compression of the anterior pituitary (66%). Its disturbances mostly manifest as obesity, hypothyroidism (low thyroid-stimulating hormone resulting in serum thyroxine levels of less than 5 µg/dL), diabetes insipidus, and delays in the development of secondary sexual characteristics. More rarely, precocious puberty may also be seen. About 60% of patients also develop visual disturbances, the most common of which is bitemporal hemianopsia and decreased visual acuity. About one half of individuals will have concomitant hydrocephalus most often associated with retrochiasmatic tumors.

The histopathologic and behavioral similarities of the craniopharyngioma to the ameloblastoma are explained by their similarity of origin. The primitive oral ectoderm of Rathke pouch is almost identical to the primitive oral ectoderm of the dental lamina and, therefore, the other odontogenic epithelial components of the enamel organ. It is probable that in each location (cranial and jaw), entrapment of such cells is common (odontogenic rests of Malassez and Serres are already known to be common) and that only in rare cases do some cells of these rests later express oncogenes, which produce their respective tumors.

DIFFERENTIAL DIAGNOSIS ▶

DIAGNOSTIC WORK-UP AND TREATMENT ▶

The main diseases producing a similar set of symptoms are *pituitary adenoma, hydrocephalus,* and *Langerhans cell histiocytosis* (previously termed Hand-Schüller-Christian disease).

Suspicious cases require an intense multispecialty work-up. The tumor itself requires CT scans and MRI assessment. Frequently, calcifications as well as fluid-filled cystic spaces can be seen in craniopharyngiomas, which strongly suggests the diagnosis (Figs 14-33a to 14-33c). In addition, complete endocrine, ophthalmologic, and neurologic evaluations are required.

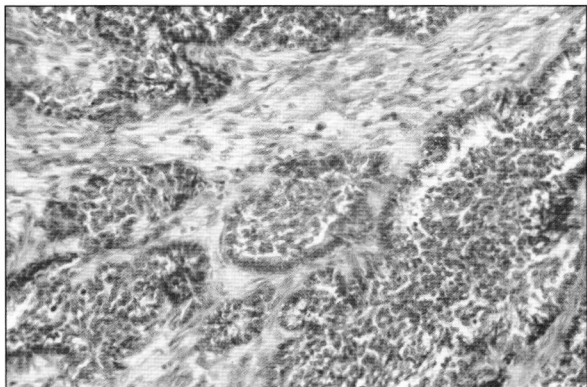

Fig 14-34 A craniopharyngioma resembles an amelo-blastoma with epithelial islands and peripheral palisaded cells.

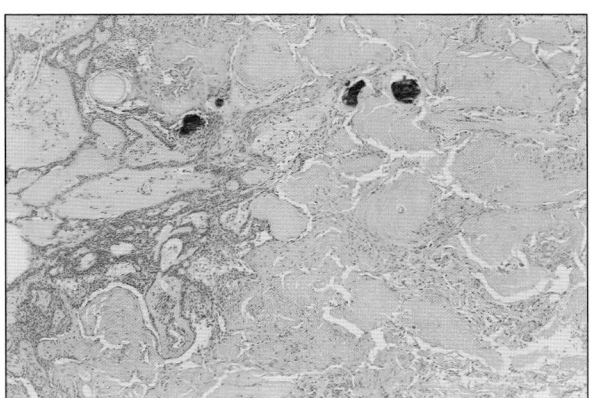

Fig 14-35a This craniopharyngioma shows a prolifera-tion of epithelium, extensive keratinization, and some calcification.

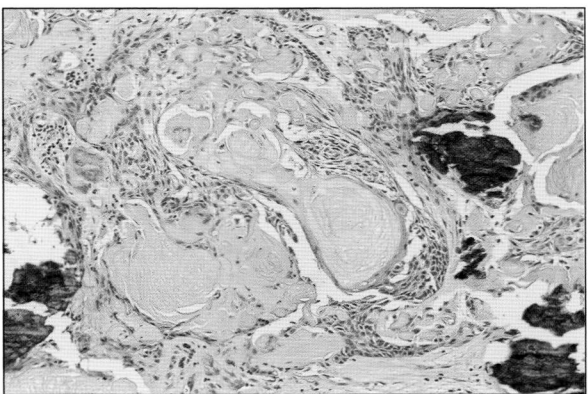

Fig 14-35b High-power view of Fig 14-35a showing keratinization, ghost cells, and calcification. This pattern of craniopharyngioma bears a striking resemblance to the calcifying odontogenic cyst.

Treatment usually consists of a neurosurgical right frontal craniotomy approach to gain access to the tumor. If the tumor is retrochiasmatic, access is more difficult and requires removal of the pterion (a 3-cm area where the frontal, temporal, parietal, and greater wing of sphenoid join) and sometimes the tu-berculum sellae (the transverse ridge on the upper surface of the body of the sphenoid).

HISTOPATHOLOGY

The histologic similarity of the craniopharyngioma to the ameloblastoma is well-known; as in amelo-blastoma, a follicular or plexiform pattern of epithelial cells is often seen (Fig 14-34). The craniophary-ngioma is often cystic. It will frequently show keratinization with ghost cells and calcified material so that it will mimic a calcifying odontogenic cyst (Figs 14-35a and 14-35b). It is an infiltrative but slow-growing tumor.

PROGNOSIS

Despite what surgeons report as "complete removal," the recurrence rate is 40%. This is due to com-promised access and the nature of the tumor, which, like ameloblastomas, undergoes local invasion and infiltration with no encapsulation. Recurrences are clinically recognized within 3 to 4 years by a return of symptoms (66%) or by routine radiographic follow-up (34%) in individuals who are asymptomatic. Recurrences are most often managed by additional surgery and occasionally with radiotherapy. About 50% recur a second time, and about 15% of patients die of the tumor or of complications of treatment.

Retrochiasmatic lesions have a higher recurrence rate because of the difficult surgical access. Tumors with significant calcifications also have a higher recurrence rate due to adherence to brain tissue.

Adamantinoma of Long Bones

The adamantinoma of long bones bears no relation to the ameloblastoma and does not arise from any oral ectoderm or enamel organ cells. It is included here as an ameloblastoma-like lesion only because of its historical reference and its unfortunate nomenclature.

CLINICAL PRESENTATION AND PATHOGENESIS

Adamantinomas of long bones are low-grade malignant tumors, 80% of which occur in the tibia and another 7% in the fibula. The tumors occur in all age ranges but have a peak incidence between 20 and 40 years of age. Their name and confusion with the ameloblastoma are related to their histopathologic appearance of epithelial basal-like cells in nests and islands, their multilocular radiolucent appearance, and their tendency to recur. This very rare tumor is associated with trauma in 60% of cases. The tumor pro-duces an expansion of the involved bone, which creates a multilocular destructive appearance as well as a sclerosis of adjacent bone (Fig 14-36). Most are asymptomatic or produce only dull pain unless they undergo a pathologic fracture, creating significant pain.

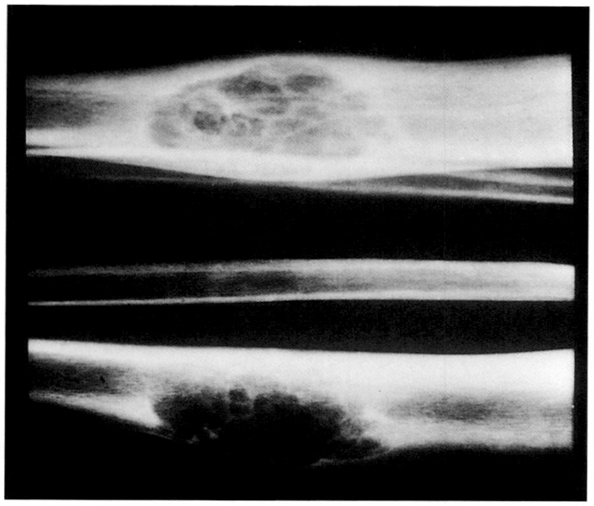

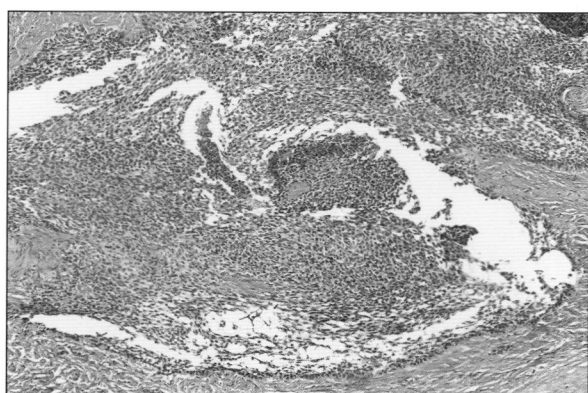

Fig 14-37a An adamantinoma of the tibia with an area bearing a slight resemblance to the ameloblastoma.

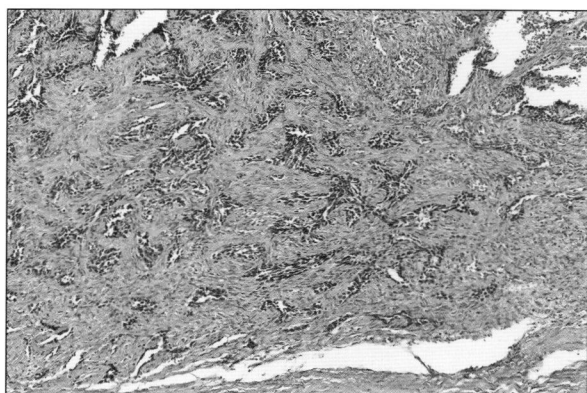

Fig 14-37b The same tumor as shown in Fig 14-37a with a more angioblastic pattern.

Fig 14-36 An adamantinoma of the tibia or other long bone is not a true ameloblastoma but rather a tumor of basal cell epithelium. As shown in this tibia, it will, however, present a radiographic picture similar to that of an ameloblastoma of the jaws.

This tumor is analogous to the ameloblastoma in that it arises from entrapped epithelium (embryonic rests), in this case skin ectoderm. This genesis explains in part its preference for the tibia and for locations in the tibia (anterior shaft) and other bones where the periosteum and cortex are closest to skin. Electron microscopic studies have confirmed the basal cell nature of their epithelial component, and immunohistochemical studies have documented the presence of basal lamina and tonofibrils, which confirm these cells as epithelial in origin. Immunohistochemical study results have also been consistently negative for factor VIII, which is characteristic of endothelium, disproving the once advanced hypothesis that these tumors were endothelial cell tumors.

DIFFERENTIAL DIAGNOSIS ▶

The adamantinoma of long bones is included only in a differential diagnosis of radiolucent expansile lesions of the tibia. Benign tumors known to produce an identical presentation include the *central giant cell tumor,* the *central hemangioma of bone,* an *ossifying fibroma,* and a *chondroma.* Other malignant tumors, such as a *chondrosarcoma* and an *osteosarcoma,* may also produce this presentation.

HISTOPATHOLOGY ▶

Occasionally, these tumors show a superficial resemblance to ameloblastomas, although there is no evidence of a common histogenesis (Fig 14-37a). Ultrastructurally and immunohistochemically, however, these tumors appear to be of epithelial origin. Even when the appearance is similar, the columnar cells are irregular and lack reverse polarity of their nuclei. These tumors may also be composed of small, dark-staining cells or may be angioblastic in appearance (Fig 14-37b).

TREATMENT ▶

Most adamantinomas of long bones are treated with en-bloc types of resections and are found to extend well beyond their radiographic margins. Recurrence rates approach 30%, and mortality is about 20%.

Calcifying Epithelial Odontogenic Tumor

CLINICAL PRESENTATION AND PATHOGENESIS ▶

The calcifying epithelial odontogenic tumor (CEOT) is an uncommon odontogenic neoplasm with a variable biologic behavior ranging from very mild to moderate invasiveness. Occurring in individuals over a wide age range but peaking in incidence in the 40s, it will present as a hard, painless expansion that, like other benign odontogenic tumors, will not cause an alteration of nerve sensation. The mandible is affected two to three times more frequently than the maxilla, and the molar region of each jaw is the preferred site.

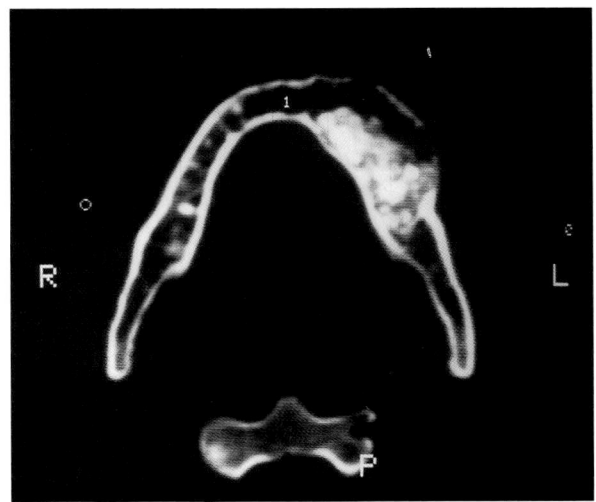

Fig 14-38 A calcifying epithelial odontogenic tumor will be expansile and will have a mixed radiolucent-radiopaque quality with a variable amount of radiopacity.

An early tumor may be completely radiolucent. As the tumor matures and becomes larger, most will become mixed radiolucent-radiopaque, although some larger tumors will remain radiolucent. Moreover, the radiographic picture will present a spectrum ranging from a unilocular radiolucency to a very multilocular one, suggestive of a "soap bubble" appearance. Most are associated with the crown of an impacted tooth, but others may appear in place of a tooth. In some, the radiopacity is so complete that it resembles a bone tumor (Fig 14-38). The demarcation of the CEOT with adjacent normal bone also is quite variable. Some will have distinct and even sclerotic borders, while others will appear to interface diffusely and imperceptibly with adjacent bone.

Odontogenic epithelium is evidently the origin of this tumor but the particular cell remains unknown. The original hypothesis of Pindborg, who first described this tumor in 1956 as arising from the stratum intermedium of the enamel organ, remains the most likely one. Its reduced invasiveness compared to the ameloblastoma may then be explained by the reduced invasive potential and reduced activity of the stratum intermedium compared to the potential of the dental lamina, reduced enamel epithelium, or epithelial rests thought to be the more likely and common origins of the ameloblastoma.

DIFFERENTIAL DIAGNOSIS ▶ The minority of CEOTs that present strictly as a radiolucency resemble the presentation of other radiolucent jaw lesions, such as a *dentigerous cyst,* an *odontogenic keratocyst,* an *ameloblastoma,* and an *odontogenic myxoma.* The more common presentation of a mixed radiolucent-radiopaque lesion will suggest a *calcifying odontogenic cyst* or, if the patient is young, an *ameloblastic fibro-odontoma* and even the rare *desmoplastic ameloblastoma.* Otherwise, the radiographic picture resembles tumors in bone such as an *ossifying fibroma,* an *osteoblastoma,* or even an *osteosarcoma* if the lesion shows diffuse margins.

DIAGNOSTIC WORK-UP ▶ Because the invasiveness of this neoplasm is variable and will influence treatment, a panoramic radiograph and a CT scan are recommended. The diagnosis is best made from a transoral midcrestal biopsy deep within the lesion.

HISTOPATHOLOGY ▶ CEOTs are unencapsulated, infiltrating tumors. The characteristic epithelial component consists of sheets and islands of polygonal cells that often have distinct intercellular bridges (Fig 14-39a). The nuclei are centrally located and often have a prominent nucleolus. The nuclei may be pleomorphic, hyperchromatic, and bizarre in appearance. Binucleated cells may be frequent (Fig 14-39b). These findings do not indicate malignancy, however, and mitoses are very uncommon. Clear cells are sometimes present; these are negative for glycogen (Fig 14-39c). Rounded, pale eosinophilic masses may be found within the sheets of tumor cells and can undergo calcification, often in the form of *Liesegang rings* (see Fig 14-39b). The surrounding tissue may also contain large clumps of this homogeneous eosinophilic material. Calcium salts are often diffusely deposited within these areas (Fig 14-39d). The eosinophilic material stains positive for amyloid with Congo red, crystal violet, and thioflavine T (Fig 14-39e).

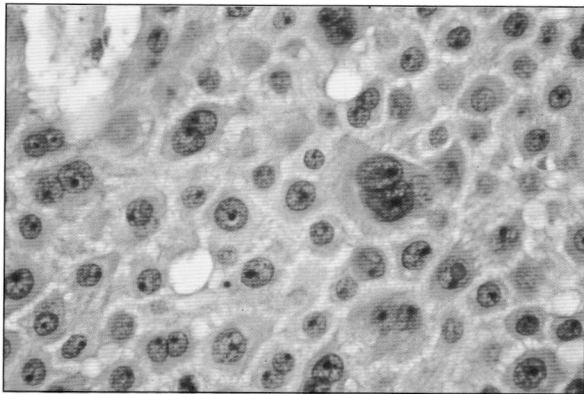

Fig 14-39a High-power view of a calcifying epithelial odontogenic tumor showing the characteristic epithelial component. The cells are eosinophilic and often polygonal, and they have intercellular bridges. Binucleated cells can also be seen.

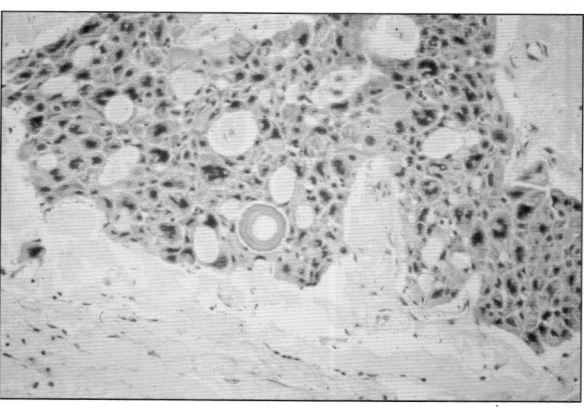

Fig 14-39b Low-power view of the calcifying epithelial odontogenic tumor shown in Fig 14-39a. In this area, the nuclei of the epithelial cells are hyperchromatic and bizarre in shape. A Liesegang ring can be seen. In addition, the abundant acellular pale pink material is amyloid.

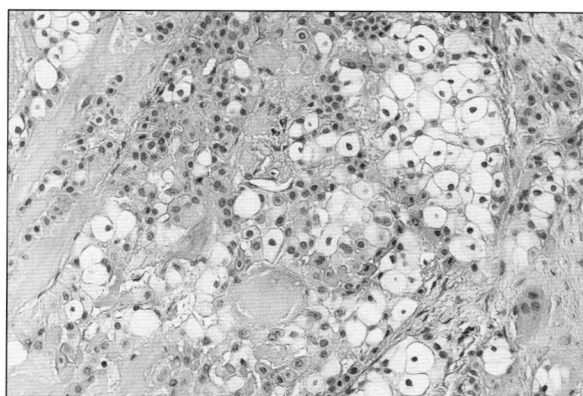

Fig 14-39c This calcifying epithelial odontogenic tumor contained numerous clear cells.

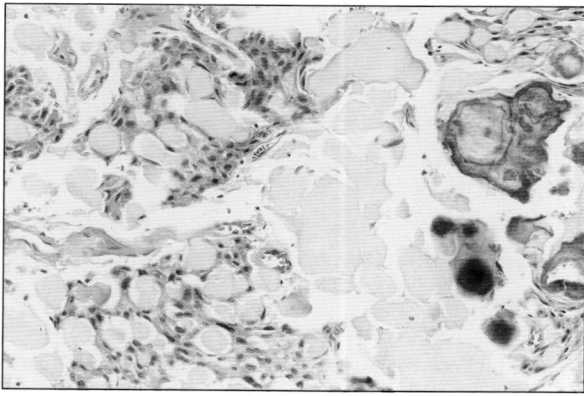

Fig 14-39d A calcifying epithelial odontogenic tumor in which dystrophic calcification of the amyloid can be seen.

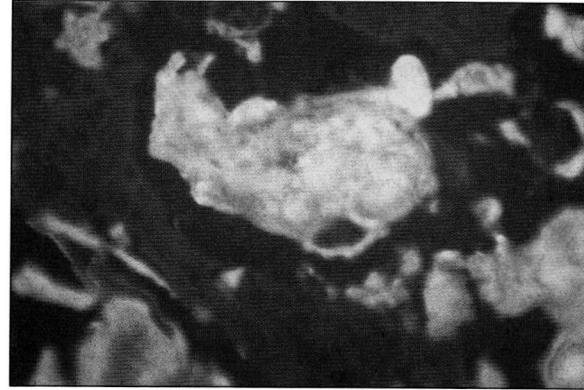

Fig 14-39e A thioflavine T fluorescent stain of a calcifying epithelial odontogenic tumor demonstrating that the acellular material is amyloid.

The diagnostic features of the CEOT are first and foremost the characteristic epithelium. The amyloid is usually abundant, the amount of calcification variable, and clear cells infrequent.

TREATMENT ▶

Although the CEOT, like the ameloblastoma or odontogenic myxoma, is a benign odontogenic neoplasm, it is less aggressive and less invasive than either. Therefore, the literature has varied regarding its treatment. Because it is an uncommon and slow-growing tumor and follow-up is often lost or only minimal, too few reports of long-term outcomes are available. Many individual reports are available with only 2- or 3-year follow-ups, but such limited follow-up times are unreliable. It seems that those treated with enucleation and curettage procedures show a recurrence rate ranging from 15% to 30% after just 2 to 4 years. Those treated with resection approaches have few if any recurrences. Therefore, the CEOT is best treated with a resection using 1.0- to 1.5-cm margins in bone and one uninvolved anatomic barrier margin.

PROGNOSIS ▶

The central CEOT is curable with resection. Follow-up must be lengthy because recurrences as late as 31 years later have been reported. While there is no malignant variant of the CEOT, a few have escaped bone or have been implanted into deep tissue spaces to present later as an unresectable recurrence.

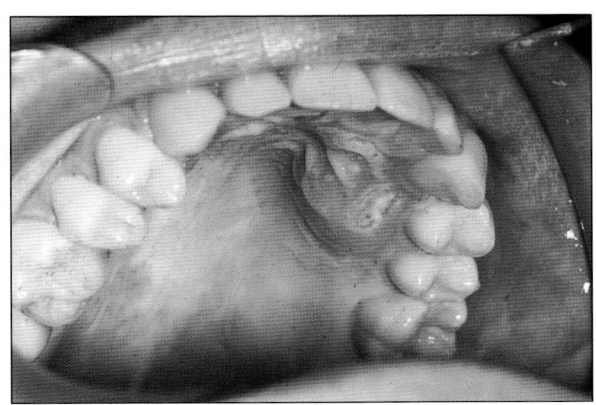

Fig 14-40 The squamous odontogenic tumor will usually present as a firm mass in the maxillary premolar region.

Peripheral Calcifying Epithelial Odontogenic Tumor

The CEOT has an even more uncommon soft tissue counterpart. These are usually small lesions (less than 2 cm) arising from the gingiva or edentulous crestal mucosa. They are also painless and tend to be firm with no evidence of surface resorption of the underlying bone. Radiographically, they will often appear to have foci of calcifications within a soft tissue density. They may, therefore, resemble a *peripheral ossifying fibroma*. If no calcifications are seen, its appearance may instead suggest a *pyogenic granuloma*, a *peripheral giant cell proliferation*, or a *gingival cyst of the adult*. As with other odontogenic neoplasms, this soft tissue counterpart to the central CEOT is a nonaggressive, noninvasive proliferation. The peripheral CEOT, like the peripheral ameloblastoma, is therefore treated by a local excision with 5-mm margins and inclusive of underlying periosteum. The resultant wound can be closed via primary closure or with a mucosal advancement.

Squamous Odontogenic Tumor

CLINICAL PRESENTATION AND PATHOGENESIS ▶

The squamous odontogenic tumor is a hamartomatous proliferation of mature epithelial cells that probably arise from the rests of Malassez. It presents as a painless expansion of the alveolar process that may displace teeth, cause tooth mobility, or resorb roots. It generally occurs in adult life around the age of 40 years, but it has a wide age range. It is a rare tumor for which statistics may not be accurate, but it has been suggested to favor the premolar-canine region of the maxilla and the molar region of the mandible (Fig 14-40). It may occur in a familial pattern in which several members of the same family have one or more lesions, or it may occur without a familial pattern as multiple separate lesions in individuals.

Radiographically, most tumors are well-demarcated, unilocular radiolucencies limited in size to 3 cm or less. In rare instances, they have grown larger. Nearly all are confined to the alveolar bone.

The location and cellularity of the squamous odontogenic tumor suggests its origin from the epithelial rests of Malassez. The fact that these stimulated rests result in a solid proliferation of squamous cells rather than a lateral periodontal cyst suggests that the lateral periodontal cyst arises from the dental lamina rests rather than the rests of Malassez. It may also be that the stimulus or the genetic alteration that causes each of these lesions is different yet may affect either the rests of Serres or the rests of Malassez.

DIFFERENTIAL DIAGNOSIS ▶

The squamous odontogenic tumor is sufficiently rare as to be an unexpected diagnosis when it is discovered. Its alveolar location in the adult suggests cysts and tumors that are more commonly seen in this area, in particular an *odontogenic keratocyst* and a *lateral periodontal cyst*. The *botryoid odontogenic cyst* variant of the lateral periodontal cyst may also be considered. In addition, early true odontogenic neoplasms such as the *ameloblastoma* and *odontogenic myxoma* are important considerations.

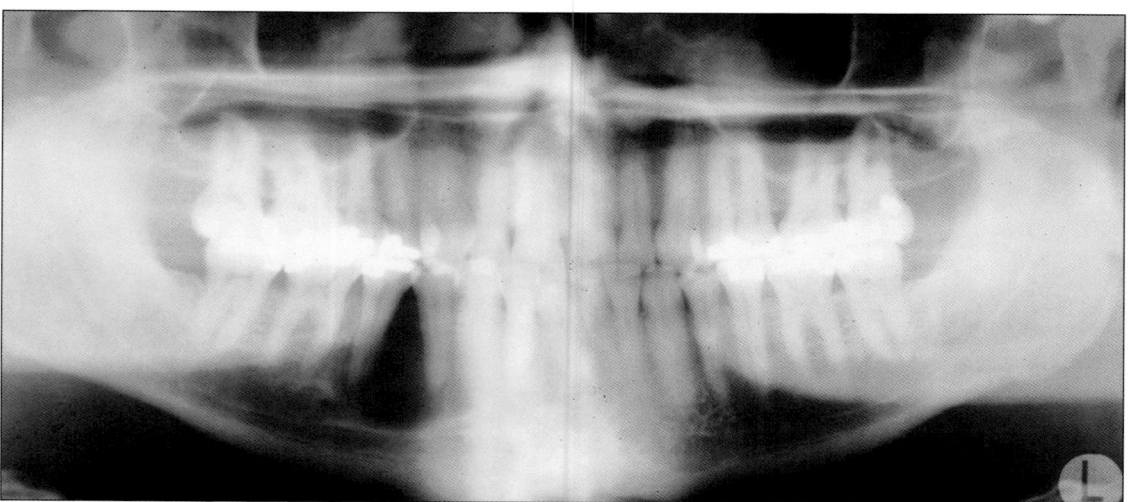

Fig 14-41 The squamous odontogenic tumor is usually unilocular but may at times be multilocular. It is curable by enucleation and curettage. However, its development in close association with tooth roots may require tooth removal or result in a periodontal defect.

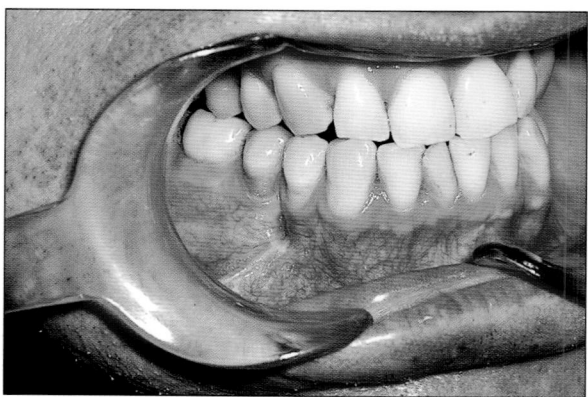

Fig 14-42 This periodontal defect and root exposure resulted from the removal of a squamous odontogenic tumor.

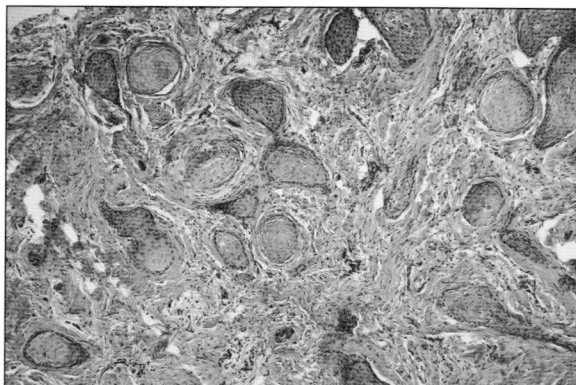

Fig 14-43 A squamous odontogenic tumor with islands of bland squamous epithelium in a fibrous stroma.

DIAGNOSTIC WORK-UP AND TREATMENT ▶

Most such presentations require direct exploration and removal by enucleation and curettage (Fig 14-41). Periapical radiographs or a panoramic radiograph is sufficient. The tumor is usually firm and encapsulated within its bony crypt. The resultant defect may create a periodontal pocket or become a residual periodontal defect (Fig 14-42). To reduce this possibility, maintenance of the crestal alveolar bone is important. If the crestal ridge of bone is lost, a membrane technique to inhibit fibrous tissue replacement may be used.

HISTOPATHOLOGY ▶

The squamous odontogenic tumor consists of islands of well-differentiated squamous epithelium that lack peripheral columnar cells. The cells are uniform and benign in appearance. There may be vacuolation and formation of microcysts. Individually keratinized cells may be present. Intraepithelial calcifications, probably dystrophic in nature, and hyalin globules that are negative histochemically for amyloid may be seen. The stroma is a mature collagenized fibrous tissue that may contain some inflammatory cells (Fig 14-43).

PROGNOSIS ▶

Recurrences are extremely rare and are related to the encumbered surgical access between and behind roots. If the entire visible portion of the lesion is removed, recurrence is not seen. However, new lesions arise in a different location in as many as 20% of patients.

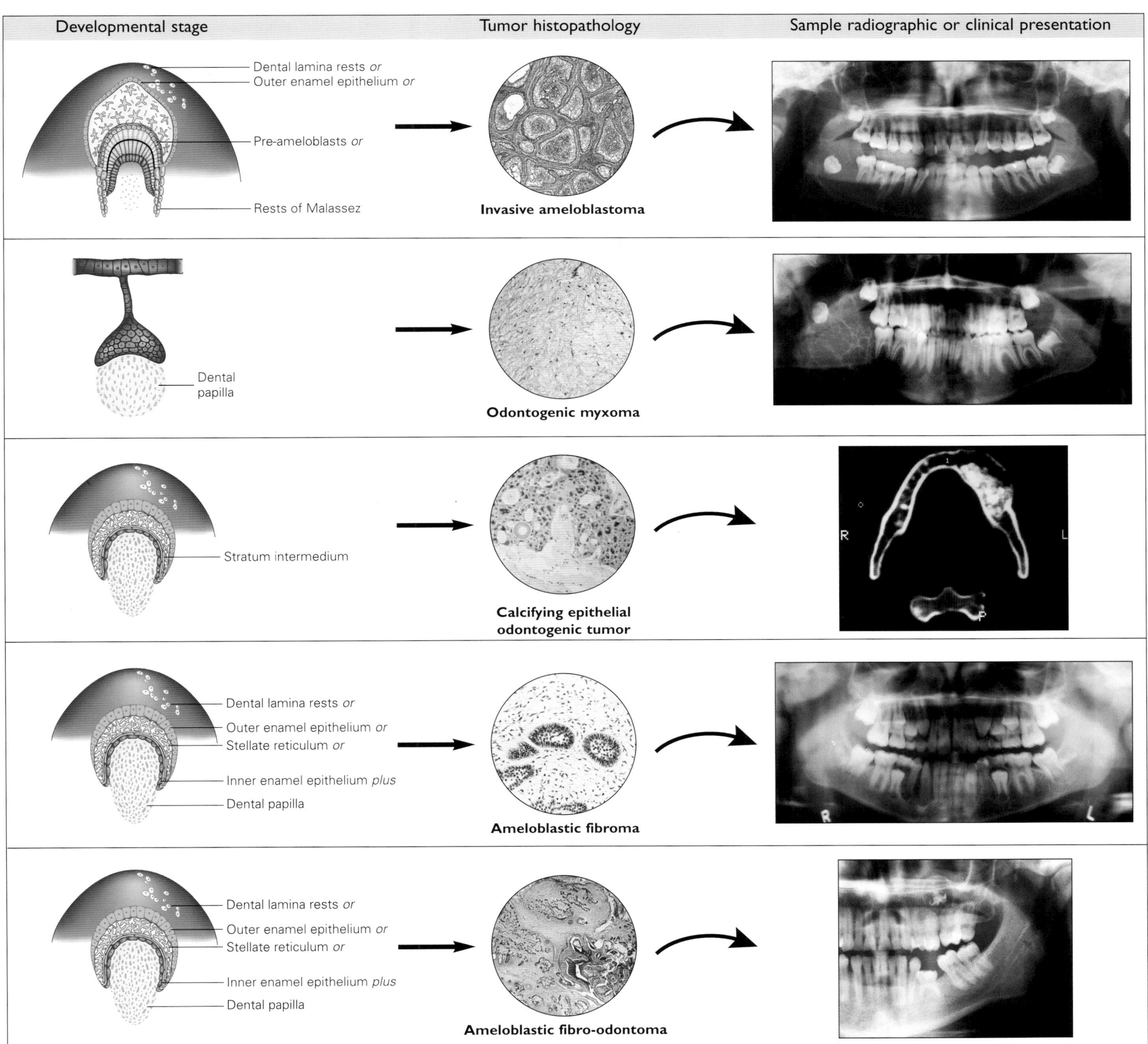

Developmental stage	Tumor histopathology	Sample radiographic or clinical presentation

Dental lamina rests *or*
Outer enamel epithelium *or*

Pre-ameloblasts *or*

Rests of Malassez

Invasive ameloblastoma

Dental papilla

Odontogenic myxoma

Stratum intermedium

Calcifying epithelial odontogenic tumor

Dental lamina rests *or*

Outer enamel epithelium *or*
Stellate reticulum *or*

Inner enamel epithelium *plus*

Dental papilla

Ameloblastic fibroma

Dental lamina rests *or*

Outer enamel epithelium *or*
Stellate reticulum *or*

Inner enamel epithelium *plus*

Dental papilla

Ameloblastic fibro-odontoma

Fig 14-44 Histogenesis of odontogenic hamartomas and neoplasms showing their suspected origins in the developmental stage of tooth development and samples of their subsequent histopathology and their associated radiographic or clinical presentation.

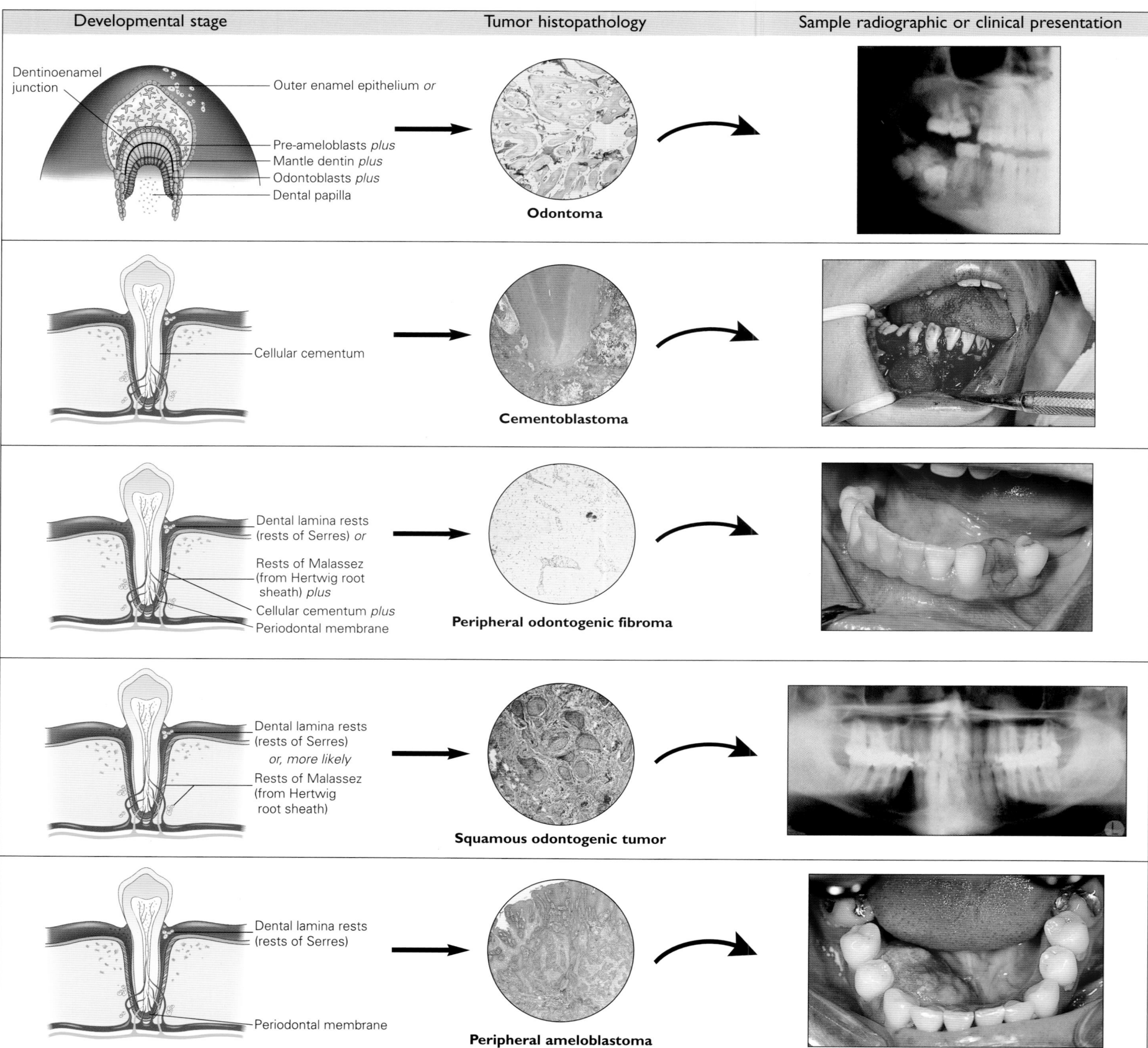

Fig 14-44 Histogenesis of odontogenic hamartomas and neoplasms showing their suspected origins in the developmental stage of tooth development and samples of their subsequent histopathology and their associated radiographic or clinical presentation (*continued*).

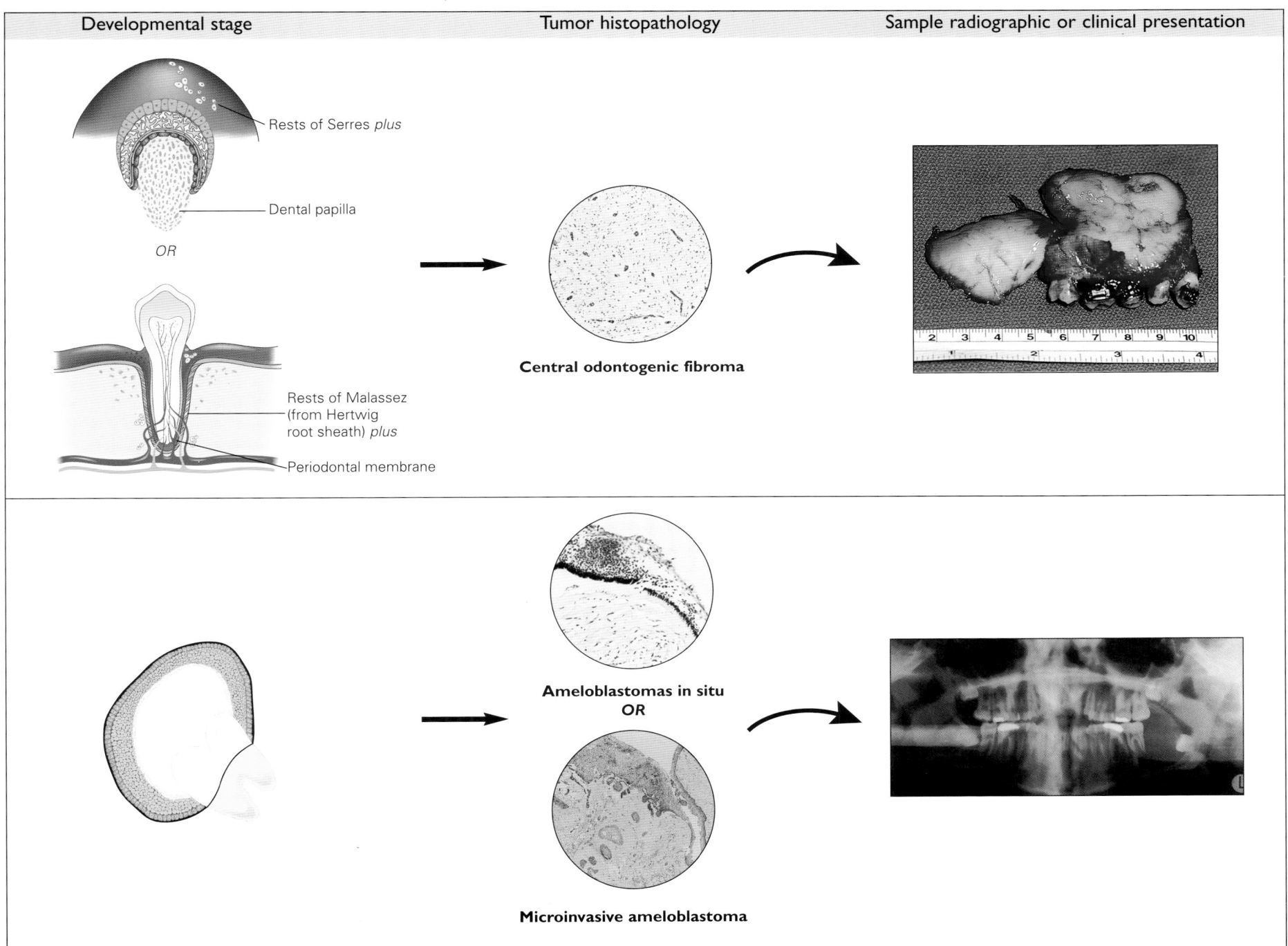

| Developmental stage | Tumor histopathology | Sample radiographic or clinical presentation |

Rests of Serres *plus*

Dental papilla

OR

Rests of Malassez (from Hertwig root sheath) *plus*

Periodontal membrane

Central odontogenic fibroma

Ameloblastomas in situ
OR

Microinvasive ameloblastoma

Fig 14-44 Histogenesis of odontogenic hamartomas and neoplasms showing their suspected origins in the developmental stage of tooth development and samples of their subsequent histopathology and their associated radiographic or clinical presentation (*continued*).

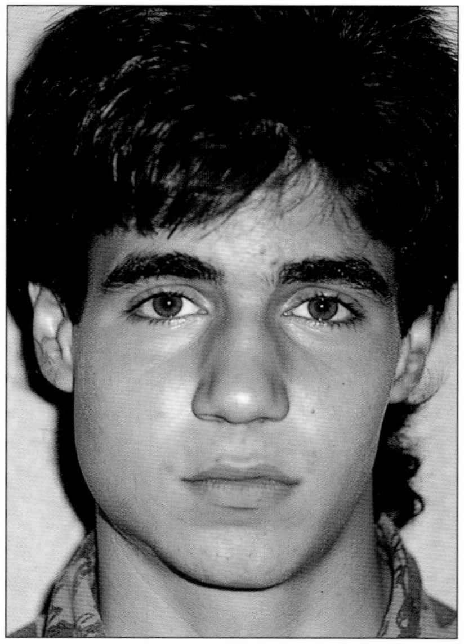

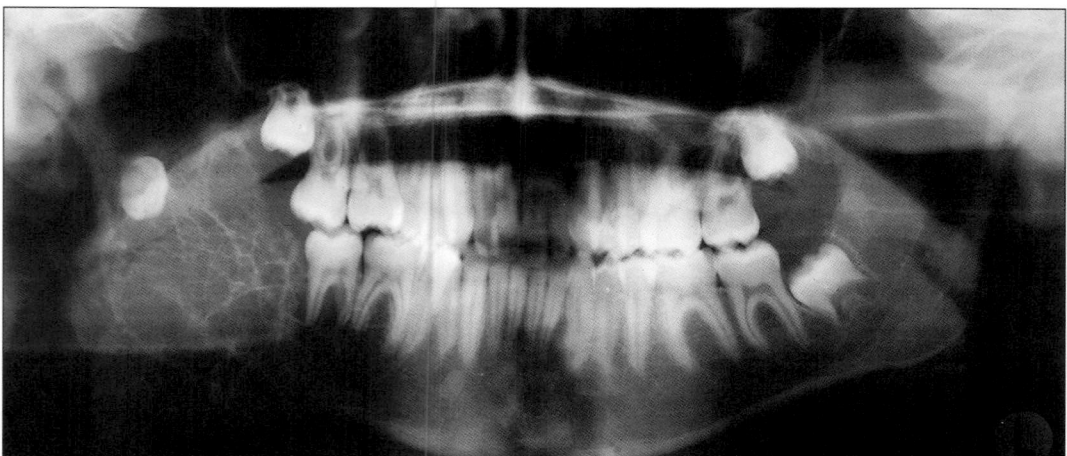

Fig 14-45a The odontogenic myxoma, like the ameloblastoma, will often present as an asymptomatic expansion in the jaws without affecting the local sensory nerve function.

Fig 14-45b Although the odontogenic myxoma may present as a unilocular radiolucency, it is more often a multilocular radiolucency with small coalesced radiolucent areas referred to as a "honeycomb" or "soap bubble" appearance.

Mesenchymal Odontogenic Tumors

Odontogenic Myxoma

CLINICAL PRESENTATION AND PATHOGENESIS ▶

The odontogenic myxoma is a benign neoplasm arising from odontogenic mesenchymal origin with growth characteristics and a clinical and radiographic presentation similar to those of the ameloblastoma. It shows infiltrative growth but does not metastasize. It presents as an asymptomatic jaw expansion without sensory nerve changes (Fig 14-45a). Radiographically, it most often presents as a multilocular radiolucency (Fig 14-45b), which has been described as "honeycombed," but it may also appear as a unilocular radiolucency. Its age distribution is very broad, ranging from 5 to 65 years, but its peak age range (15 to 30 years) is slightly younger than that for the ameloblastoma. Cases in individuals younger than 15 years are common, in contrast to the rarity of ameloblastomas in that age group.

The myxoma differs from the ameloblastoma in site preference as well. While the ameloblastoma is much more commonly seen in the third molar areas, particularly in the mandible, the odontogenic myxoma is evenly distributed throughout the jaws. Tooth displacement and root resorption may be seen, as might displacement of the inferior alveolar canal, which is indicative of its benign process.

The histogenesis of the odontogenic myxoma is thought to be the dental papilla (primitive dental pulp). While myxomas do occur in long bones, these are rare and are thought to arise from pluripotential mesenchymal stem cells. The jaws also contain a small population of nonodontogenic pluripotential mesenchymal stem cells that may give rise to a myxoma. However, the much greater incidence of myxomas in the jaws parallels the much greater amount of primitive mesenchyme associated with 20 primary and 32 permanent tooth formations, increasing the likelihood of a myxoma. Though unproven, myxomas in the jaws are thought to originate from odontogenic mesenchyme rather than from somatic mesenchyme and are thus termed *odontogenic myxomas*.

A note of caution: Many neurosarcomas and some osteosarcomas histopathologically show a myxomatous character. Several of these malignancies have been diagnosed as an odontogenic myxoma based

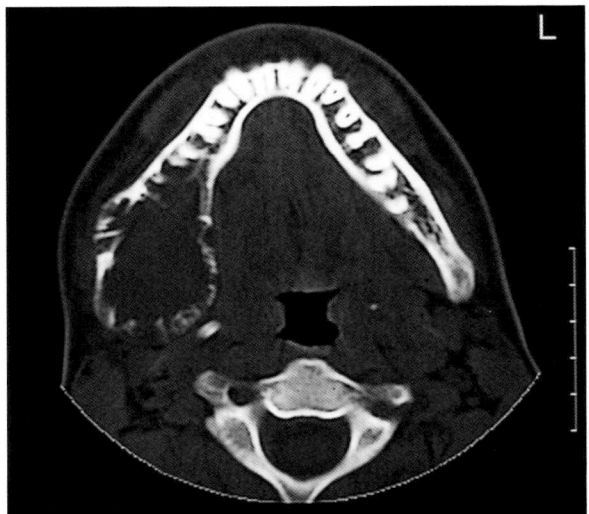

Fig 14-46 A CT scan is valuable in the presurgical work-up for an odontogenic neoplasm. Here the expansion, the medullary extension, and areas of possible cortical perforation can be assessed.

on the preoperative impression of an odontogenic myxoma recorded on the clinician's pathology request. It is critically important to review radiographs and scans carefully to ensure they are consistent with the disease diagnosed by histopathologic studies. It is also useful to copy selected radiographs and CT scans for the pathologist to review with the specimen slides.

DIFFERENTIAL DIAGNOSIS ▶

The most common presentation of the odontogenic myxoma is a multilocular radiolucent expansile lesion in a young adult or teenager. The multilocular quality strongly suggests an *ameloblastoma* or an *odontogenic keratocyst*. If the individual is younger than 15 years, the possibility of an *ameloblastic fibroma* increases. Other multilocular radiolucent lesions include a *central giant cell tumor* (increasingly likely in individuals between 5 and 15 years of age) and the *central hemangiomas* (cavernous or arteriovenous types), which also may present as "honeycombed" radiolucencies.

DIAGNOSTIC WORK-UP ▶

The diagnosis of an odontogenic myxoma can be made from a deep incisional biopsy through the sockets of removed teeth that were rendered mobile by bone resorption. In edentulous areas or where teeth are not mobile, a sulcular or midcrestal incision is used to access the medullary portion of the jaw. A CT scan is valuable in planning the surgery, particularly in locating areas where the tumor may have resorbed cortical bone and infiltrated soft tissues (Fig 14-46).

HISTOPATHOLOGY ▶

Odontogenic myxomas are unencapsulated, infiltrating, gelatinous tumors that are sparsely cellular (Fig 14-47a). The cells are spindle-shaped or stellate with long cytoplasmic processes (Fig 14-47b). Ultrastructurally and immunohistochemically, these cells seem to be myofibroblasts because they are vimentin- and actin-positive. They probably give rise to the abundant stroma, which is composed of acid mucopolysaccharides, rich in hyaluronic acid and chondroitin sulfate. This gives the tumor its gelatinous consistency and may be responsible for its infiltrative nature. Little collagen is typically present. Tumors that are somewhat more collagenous have been called *myxofibromas* or *fibromyxomas* (Fig 14-48), but their behavior does not appear to differ appreciably. Occasionally, inactive rests of odontogenic epithelium may be seen.

Odontogenic myxomas must be distinguished from other myxoid tissue that may be seen in dental follicles or developing dental pulp, which may be extruded during surgical procedures. This is particularly pertinent to the removal of incompletely developed third molar teeth where the dental papilla is still present. The clinical picture and the discrete, noninfiltrative nature of the latter should prevent misdiagnosis (Fig 14-49).

TREATMENT ▶

Curative treatment of an odontogenic myxoma is accomplished by resection with 1.0- to 1.5-cm bony margins and one uninvolved anatomic barrier margin (see pages 684 to 703). Palliation may be achieved with enucleation and curettage for those individuals who prefer and request palliation over curative resection, or for those whose anesthetic risk is too great to undergo curative surgery. Recurrence

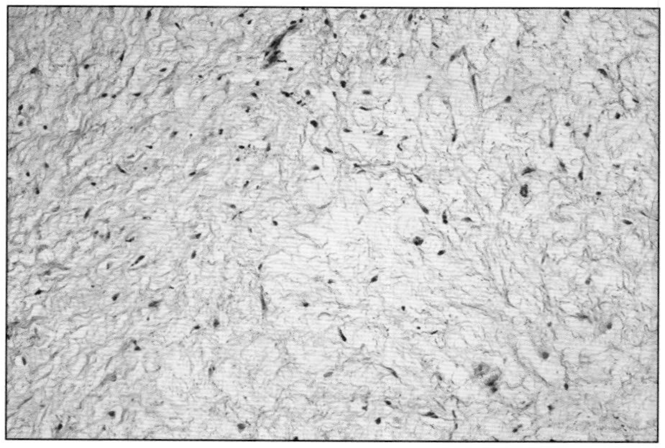

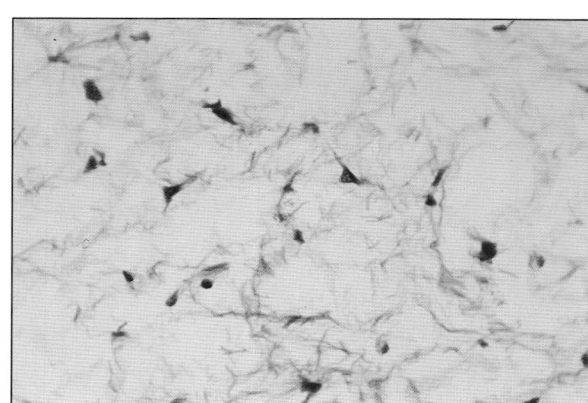

Fig 14-47a Myxomas are typically sparsely cellular with some fibrils and abundant ground substance.

Fig 14-47b High-power view of Fig 14-47a showing that myxomatous cells may be fusiform, stellate, or tripolar.

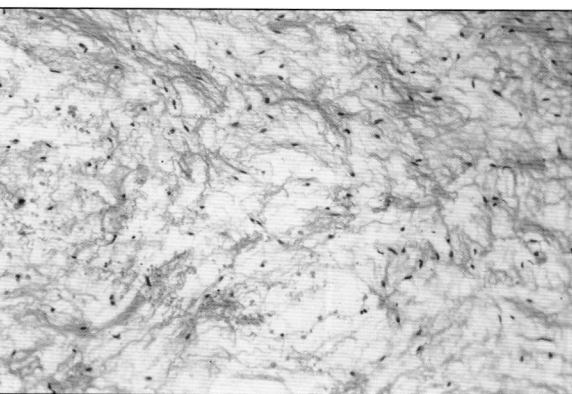

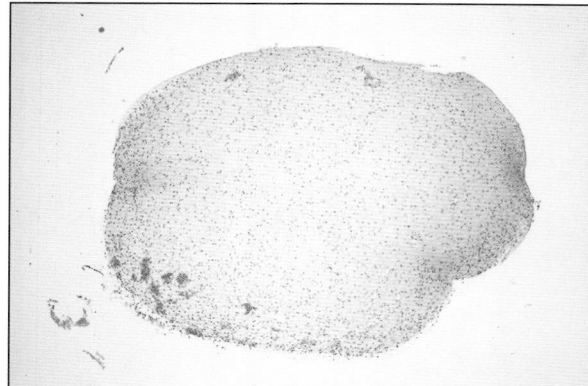

Fig 14-48 Some myxomas have a more collagenized background, as shown here. There is no evidence to support a different behavior or treatment for these myxomas.

Fig 14-49 An extruded dental papilla or developing dental pulp can be mistaken for a myxoma. This low-power view of a dental papilla, removed along with an incompletely developed tooth, shows a discrete mass of tissue that is not characteristic of a myxoma.

is expected with enucleation and curettage procedures but may not be clinically detected for 5 years or more. As with the ameloblastoma, seeding of tumor cells can occur, especially given the loose gelatinous consistency of an odontogenic myxoma, resulting in unresectable recurrences. Therefore, enucleation and curettage is not advised if cure is the goal.

PROGNOSIS ▶ Odontogenic myxomas treated with tumor resection seldom recur. Cases treated by enucleation and curettage procedures are expected to recur; almost all recurrent tumors are reported to have been first treated with enucleation and curettage. As with the ameloblastoma, recurrent odontogenic myxomas in bone are salvageable for cure with resection based on the original size and extent of the tumor. Tumors that recur from extension or seeding into unresectable anatomic spaces may require extensive cancer surgery–like procedures to attempt cure and may be indicated in young individuals. In older individuals, it may be best to accomplish palliative debulking procedures to preserve function and prolong life if the tumor is completely unresectable or the risk of surgical morbidity too great.

Cementoblastoma

CLINICAL PRESENTATION AND PATHOGENESIS ▶ The cementoblastoma is a hamartomatous proliferation of cementoblasts forming disorganized cementum around the apical one half of a tooth root. It will usually present as a hard expansion in the pre-

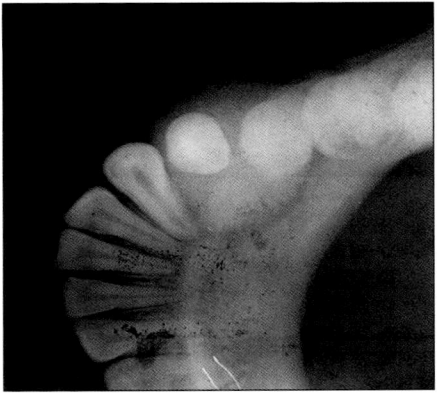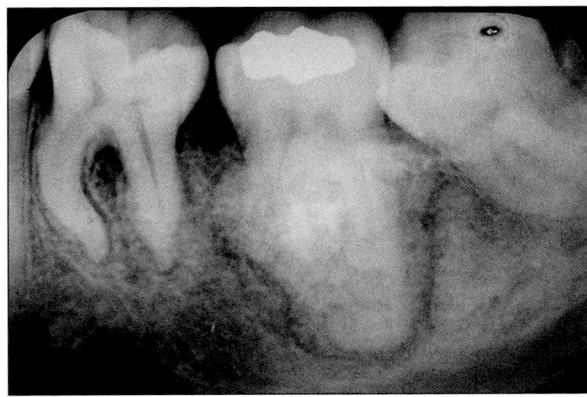

Figs 14-50a and 14-50b The cementoblastoma occurs in the premolar-molar regions and has a distinctive radiographic appearance. It will arise from the apical one half of the root as a lobulated but symmetric radiopacity with a distinctive radiolucent periphery, mimicking a periodontal membrane space.

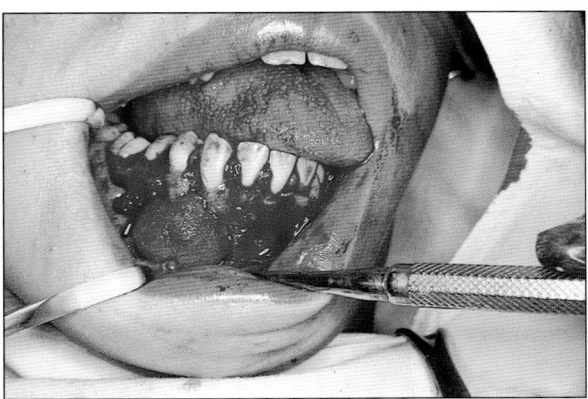

Fig 14-51 Removal of a cementoblastoma requires removal of the tooth and a pericapsular dissection. There may be some areas where the tumor has lost its capsule and is therefore fused to the surrounding bone.

molar or molar region of either jaw. There is frequently a deep, dull pain associated with the expansion. The overlying mucosa is intact, and the associated teeth are not mobile. More lesions occur in the mandible than in the maxilla. Most occur in teenagers or adults younger than 30 years.

Radiographically, the lesion characteristically shows a spherical, radiopaque mass encompassing and essentially replacing the apical half of the root. This mass is not periapical per se but arises from and obliterates the outlines of the root's apical half instead. There is a characteristic radiolucent margin around the mass, giving the impression of a periodontal membrane space (Figs 14-50a and 14-50b). The tooth is vital unless it is nonvital for other reasons.

This lesion arises from the cellular cementum. It produces a disorganized and vascular cementum that seems to recapitulate a periodontal membrane–like encapsulation.

DIFFERENTIAL DIAGNOSIS ►

The distinguishing features of a cementoblastoma are its peripheral radiolucent margin to adjacent bone and its obliteration of one half of the root. These features distinguish it from other radiopaque lesions that may become superimposed over tooth roots, such as an *osteoblastoma*, an *ossifying fibroma*, and an *odontoma*. These features also distinguish a small cementoblastoma from *hypercementosis* and *focal bone sclerosis*, so-called condensing osteitis.

DIAGNOSTIC WORK-UP ►

A cementoblastoma is diagnosed and treated by removal of the associated tooth with the lesion attached. Because of its capsule, the apparently bulbous mass is readily separated from the surrounding bone. The buccal cortex around this tumor may be absent or severely thinned. The tumor can then be removed in one unit with the tooth attached (Fig 14-51). The lesion and tooth is removed toward the buccal aspect. If the lesion has gained sufficient size as to abut adjacent teeth, its cementum may fuse to the adjacent tooth, making the removal of that tooth necessary as well.

The resultant bone cavity is closed at the mucosal level without the need for a drain or packing. A long-term resorbable membrane or a permanent membrane requiring later removal placed over the buccal cortical opening may be used to inhibit fibrous tissue ingrowth and to ensure a more complete bone regeneration.

HISTOPATHOLOGY ►

The cementoblastoma has a thin fibrous capsule that is usually continuous with the periodontal membrane (Fig 14-52a). The tumor consists of sheets of cementum-like material continuous with the tooth root (Fig 14-52b). Frequently, there is root resorption with replacement by cementum. Invasion of the root canal is common. The proliferating cementum is lined by numerous plump cells (Fig 14-52c). Cementoclasts may also be present, and reversal lines are prominent (Fig 14-52d). Some of the cemental material may be uncalcified, particularly at the periphery of the mass. The tumor cementum is often arranged in struts perpendicular to the capsule (see Fig 14-52a). The fibrous stroma is highly vascular (see Fig 14-52d).

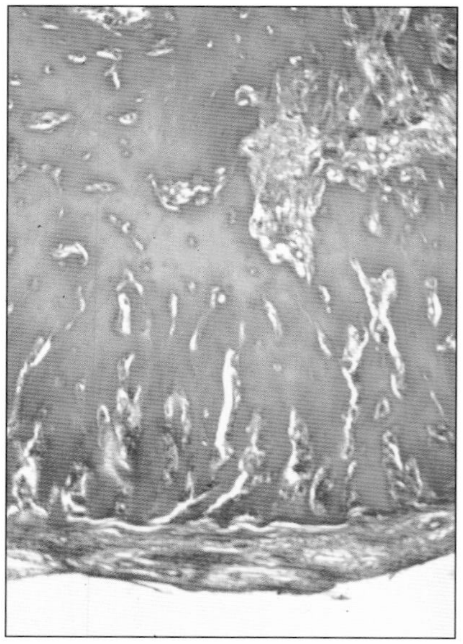

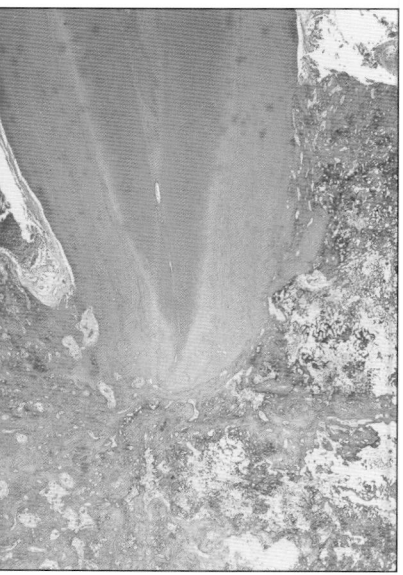

Fig 14-52a A peripheral portion of a cementoblastoma shows the fibrous capsule and the perpendicular struts formed by the tumor cementum.

Fig 14-52b Cementoblastoma showing the continuity of the tooth root with the tumor cemental material.

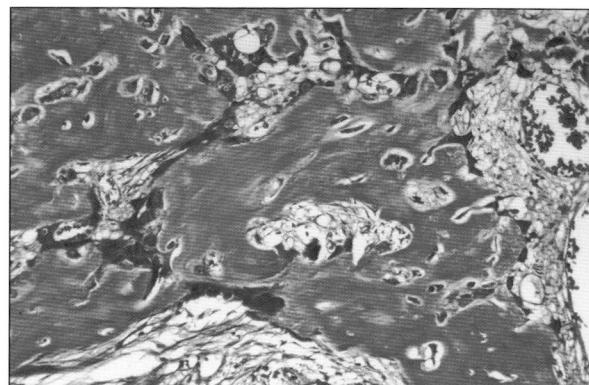

Fig 14-52c This cementoblastoma shows the plump, active cementoblasts that lay down the cementum.

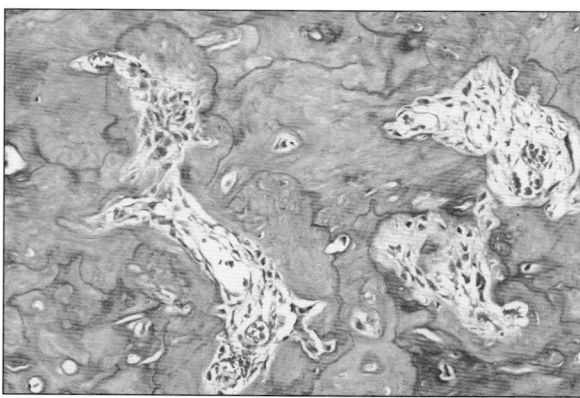

Fig 14-52d In this field, the reversal lines, vascularity of the stroma, and proliferating cementoblasts can be seen.

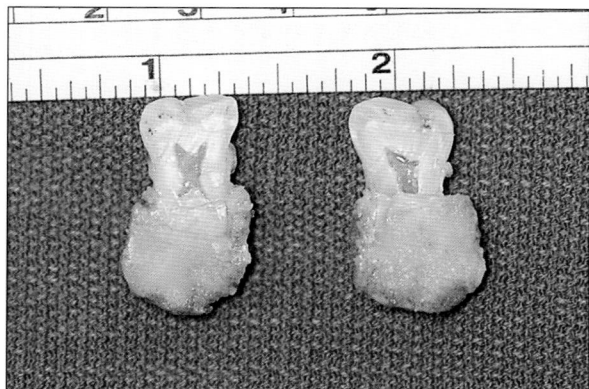

Fig 14-53 Sagittal section of a cementoblastoma showing its capsule and its involvement with at least one half of the root, including the furcation and the pulp.

PROGNOSIS ▶

Tooth removal with the lesion attached is curative without risk of recurrence. Theoretically, one could also effect a cure with a root resection, removing the lesion attached to the resected apical one half of the root. However, this is impractical as the resulting crown-root ratio would be insufficient for retention of the remainder of the tooth (Fig 14-53).

Central Odontogenic Fibroma

CLINICAL PRESENTATION AND PATHOGENESIS ▶

The central odontogenic fibroma is a very rare proliferation of mature odontogenic mesenchyme. It is sufficiently rare that locations and sex and age distributions cannot be accurately determined. Those reported have occurred over a wide age range in each jaw, with no sex predilection noted. It will present as either a unilocular or multilocular radiolucent lesion with well-demarcated borders. The radiolucency itself is not associated with the crown of an unerupted tooth but may appear so in young individuals by

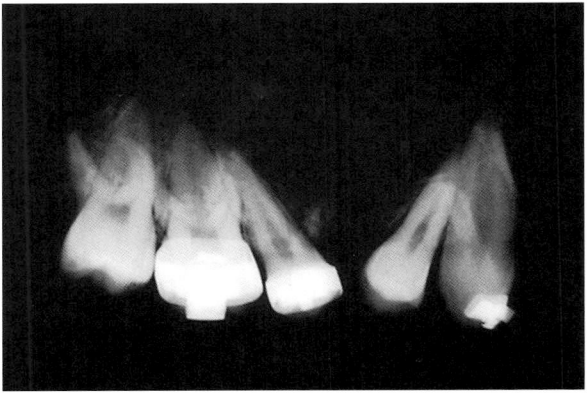

Fig 14-54a Specimen radiograph of a large odontogenic fibroma showing a soft tissue mass with no calcified product and displacement of teeth.

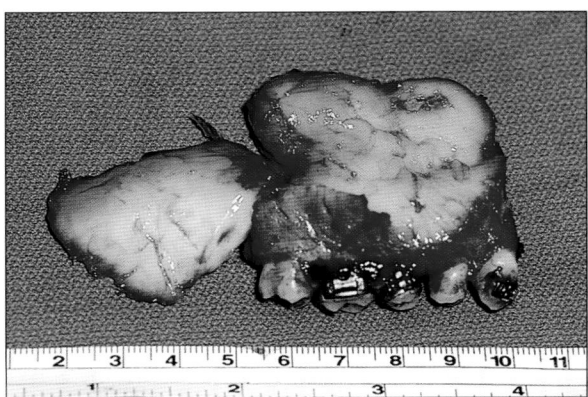

Fig 14-54b Large, solid soft tissue tumor had a well-defined capsule. Histologically, it showed a delicate, loose, fibrous tissue with sparse collagen consistent with the rare odontogenic fibroma.

its expansion into areas of developing teeth. It causes a painless expansion that may displace tooth roots or resorb portions of them (Figs 14-54a and 14-54b).

The central odontogenic fibroma is believed to be the counterpart to the peripheral odontogenic fibroma that arises from the periodontal membrane. Indeed, the central odontogenic fibroma may also arise from the partially induced somatic mesenchyme otherwise destined to become periodontal membrane. However, this origin would not be from the odontogenic apparatus per se; instead, it could be said that it arises from the somatic mesenchyme influenced by the odontogenic apparatus. The alternative theory is that it arises from the true odontogenic mesenchyme of the dental papilla, like the odontogenic myxoma, but that it differs from the myxoma by the maturity of the mesenchyme and its limited growth potential and invasive capability.

DIFFERENTIAL DIAGNOSIS ▶

The rarity of the central odontogenic fibroma excludes it from most differential lists. When it is diagnosed, it is an unexpected finding that usually requires expert second opinions for confirmation. Most presentations will suggest the more common radiolucent odontogenic cysts and tumors such as an *odontogenic keratocyst*, an *ameloblastoma*, or an *odontogenic myxoma* as well as an *ameloblastic fibroma* in children and teenagers. In younger individuals, the presentation will also suggest a *central giant cell tumor*. Lesions such as a dentigerous cyst or an adenomatoid odontogenic cyst are not strong possibilities because they are unilocular and associated with the crown of a developing tooth (in the adenomatoid odontogenic cyst about 65% of the time).

DIAGNOSTIC WORK-UP ▶

Most central odontogenic fibromas require an incisional biopsy because their presentation suggests more aggressive disease. Once the diagnosis is established, a panoramic radiograph is sufficient for treatment planning.

HISTOPATHOLOGY ▶

Two histologic patterns occur within the current rubric of odontogenic fibroma. One consists of delicate fibrous tissue, which may contain various amounts of collagen. Some rests of odontogenic epithelium may be present. The second type, which has been referred to as the WHO (World Health Organization) type, is usually well demarcated or encapsulated. It consists of cellular fibrous tissue often with myxoid areas within which are found islands and strands of inactive odontogenic epithelium. The quantity of epithelium may be striking. In addition, dysplastic dentin and cementum-like material may be present (Fig 14-55).

The granular cell odontogenic fibroma consists of sheets of large granular cells with an appearance similar to the cells of the granular cell tumor of soft tissue. In between these cells are round islands of odontogenic epithelium (Fig 14-56). Although the granular cells are S-100 protein negative, ultrastructurally they are mesenchymal. As in the odontogenic fibroma, some calcified material may be present.

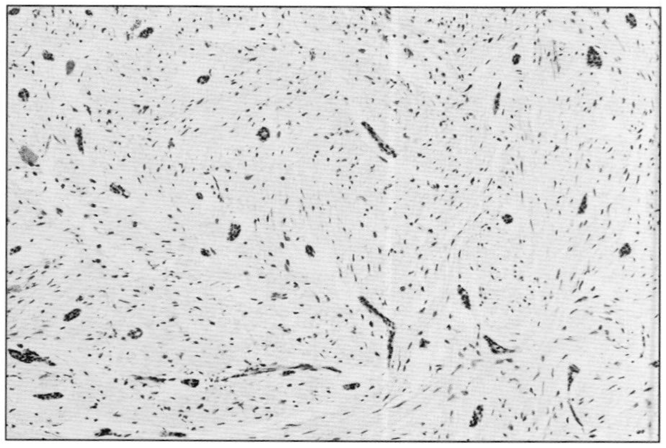

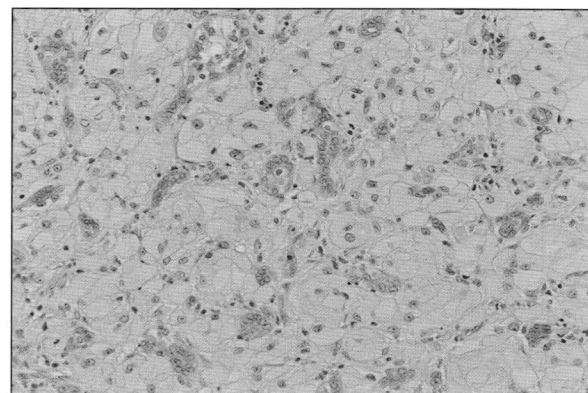

Fig 14-55 A central odontogenic fibroma with scattered odontogenic epithelial rests and a loose fibrous stroma.

Fig 14-56 A granular cell odontogenic fibroma consisting of prominent granular cells between which some epithelial islands can be seen.

TREATMENT ▶

Central odontogenic fibromas can be treated by enucleation and curettage for cure. They readily separate from their bony crypt and show no evidence of bony infiltration. The resultant bony cavity is closed at the mucosal level without the need for drains or packing.

PROGNOSIS ▶

Recurrence should not develop. If a recurrence is observed, the original pathology specimen as well as a biopsy specimen of the recurrence should be reviewed. It is possible that an odontogenic myxoma with fibrous features, often termed a *fibromyxoma*, was interpreted as a central odontogenic fibroma. It is also possible that an ossifying fibroma with few bony or cementum-like components was interpreted as the type of central odontogenic fibroma that has its usual mature fibrous connective tissue and its own calcific deposits, which are believed to be either cementum or dentin.

Peripheral Odontogenic Fibroma

CLINICAL PRESENTATION AND PATHOGENESIS ▶

The peripheral odontogenic fibroma is a firm soft tissue mass clinically indistinguishable from other fibromas such as the peripheral ossifying fibroma and the giant cell fibroma. It will present as a painless mass on the gingiva that will at times prolapse over a tooth, thus resembling an operculum. Close inspection often reveals its emergence from the gingival crevice or periodontal membrane (Fig 14-57). The overlying mucosa usually is intact and of normal color unless secondarily ulcerated because of trauma. These lesions are seen somewhat more frequently in women than in men and are most commonly found in the premolar-canine region. Radiographs will not show bony resorption or sclerosis as a reaction to the presence of this lesion.

This fibroma appears to originate from the periodontal membrane. The odontogenic epithelia usually found within it are either dental lamina rests (rests of Serres) or rests from the breakup of Hertwig epithelial root sheath (rests of Malassez). Whether this fibroma represents a reactive fibrous proliferation from some minor, often clinically unrecognized stimulant or a hamartomatous proliferation of limited growth potential remains unknown. Because it is neither destructive nor invasive and reaches a size of only 2 cm or less, it is not considered a true neoplasm but rather a hamartoma.

DIFFERENTIAL DIAGNOSIS ▶

Gingival mass lesions most likely are fibromas or reactive lesions that can be specified only by histopathology; each should be included on a differential list. The other fibromas include the *peripheral ossifying fibroma* and the *giant cell fibroma* (also called *giant cell fibrous hyperplasia*). The reactive lesions include the *pyogenic granuloma* and the *peripheral giant cell proliferation*, although each tends to be less firm and more friable and may appear reddish-blue. The peripheral giant cell proliferation also may cause a cupped-

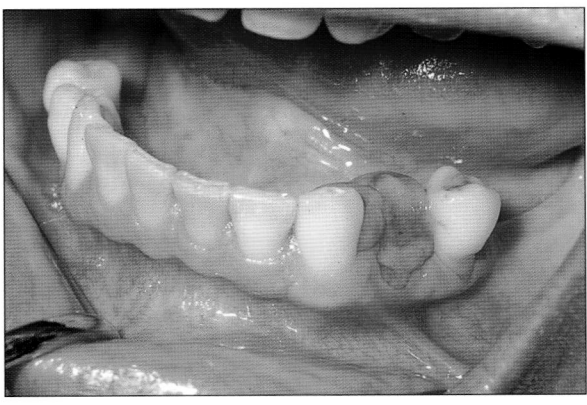

Fig 14-57 The peripheral odontogenic fibroma will be firm and of limited size and will arise from the periodontal membrane.

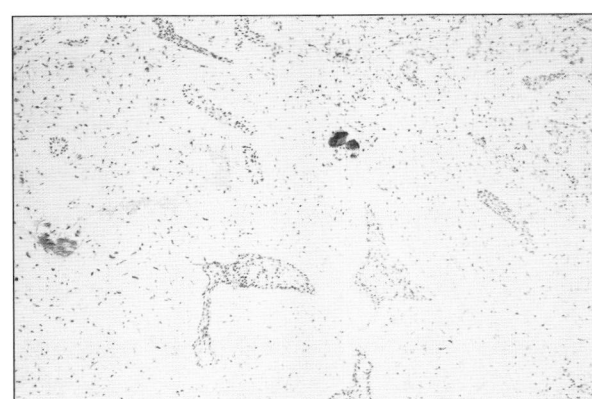

Fig 14-58 A peripheral odontogenic fibroma with epithelial islands, a loose fibrous stroma, and some calcifications.

out surface resorption of the underlying bone. It is also worthwhile to suspect either a *primary malignancy* or a *malignant metastatic focus* seeded into bone and emerging through the alveolus.

Peripheral fibromas and gingival masses require a local excision with only 1- to 2-mm mucosal margins for diagnosis and treatment. It is important to include the lesion's base and the area of periodontal membrane from which it arises, which often results in a periodontal defect that must be accepted or reconstructed. The tooth may require removal if the lesion is large. Periapical radiographs or a panoramic radiograph is useful to assess for surface bone erosion or a central radiolucency indicating that the gingival lesion may be arising from within bone.

HISTOPATHOLOGY ▶ The histology is essentially the same as in the central odontogenic fibroma. Peripheral odontogenic fibromas consist of cellular fibrous tissue that may be intermixed with more myxoid areas. Strands or rests of odontogenic epithelium are typically present and may be very prominent, suggestive of a peripheral ameloblastoma. The epithelium, however, appears to be inactive. The epithelial cells may sometimes be vacuolated, and calcifications may be seen (Fig 14-58).

PROGNOSIS ▶ The peripheral odontogenic fibroma has a low recurrence potential. While its recurrence rate is unknown, it recurs somewhat less than the 20% rate noted for the peripheral ossifying fibroma. Recurrences apparently result from local excisions that do not include the base of the fibroma in the periodontal ligament. A complete excision including this point of origin should prevent recurrence.

Mixed Epithelial and Mesenchymal Odontogenic Tumors

Ameloblastic Fibroma

CLINICAL PRESENTATION AND PATHOGENESIS ▶ The ameloblastic fibroma may behave either as a true neoplasm or as a hamartomatous proliferation of odontogenic epithelium of the enamel organ and odontogenic mesenchyme of the primitive dental pulp. It will usually grow to a certain size, sometimes large, then cease growth and not be invasive beyond its own capsule. Less commonly, it will exhibit continued slow growth. It is essentially a proliferation that occurs in children and teenagers. The mean age range is 6 to 12 years, and only a very few cases are seen after the age of 25 years. The mandibular molar area is the preferred site, but the tumor may occur in any location. There is no sex predilection.

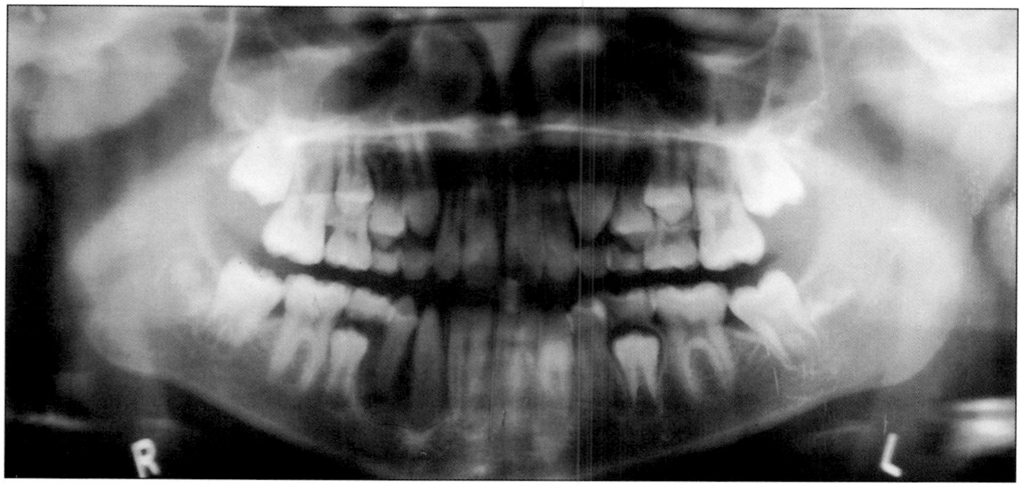

Fig 14-59 An ameloblastic fibroma in the late mixed-dentition stage. It will usually cause a well-demarcated radiolucency in a child, teenager, or young adult.

The tumor presents as an asymptomatic expansion of the jaws. Radiographically, it is completely radiolucent, but it will have a well-demarcated border with bone (Fig 14-59). It may be either unilocular or multilocular, and it may be associated with the crown of an impacted tooth and mimic a dentigerous cyst or be unassociated with the crown of an impacted tooth. Because of the age of occurrence, the mass will frequently displace developing teeth. It may also resorb roots and displace the inferior alveolar canal.

The ameloblastic fibroma has the same histogenesis as the odontoma. It arises from odontogenic epithelium of the enamel organ and odontogenic mesenchyme of the primitive dental pulp. It, too, represents an aborted attempt at tooth formation, but one that occurs prior to any enamel or dentin formation. Intermediate in this spectrum of aborted tooth formation attempts is the ameloblastic fibro-odontoma, which actually forms some dentin and enamel, but not as much nor in as organized a manner as an odontoma.

DIFFERENTIAL DIAGNOSIS ▶

A strictly radiolucent lesion in the jaws of a child in which a well-demarcated margin within bone is observed usually suggests a cyst. If it is associated with the crown of an impacted tooth, a *dentigerous cyst* is likely. If it is unassociated with the crown of an impacted tooth, an *odontogenic keratocyst* is likely. At this age, a *central giant cell tumor* is also a distinct consideration. Less commonly presenting as a radiolucency in children and young adults are an *odontogenic myxoma*, a *central hemangioma* (cavernous or arteriovenous type), a *calcifying odontogenic cyst* that has not formed sufficient calcified material so as to appear on a radiograph, and rarely, an *ameloblastoma*.

DIAGNOSTIC WORK-UP ▶

Most ameloblastic fibromas are sufficiently large and destructive to strongly suggest some of those entities that are treated with resection rather than enucleation and curettage. Therefore, an incisional biopsy for diagnostic confirmation is the best approach. A CT scan is also extremely useful in determining the extent of the mass and its association with developing teeth.

HISTOPATHOLOGY ▶

Ameloblastic fibromas are circumscribed tumors that fail to show inductive changes and calcified products. They consist of both active mesenchymal and epithelial components (Fig 14-60a). The mesenchymal portion is myxoid in appearance and not collagenized. It resembles the dental papilla. The epithelial portion is scattered in the form of islands and strands but can occur in a clustered arrangement. The islands are relatively small and resemble those of an ameloblastoma with peripheral columnar cells and a central stellate reticulum (Fig 14-60b). Some limited cystic change may be seen within the islands, but other variations that may occur in ameloblastomas, such as squamous metaplasia, are not present. The connective tissue is the feature that readily distinguishes the ameloblastic fibroma from the follicular ameloblastoma: In the former it is myxoid, whereas in the latter it is fibrous tissue with readily apparent collagen stained pink with eosin. The islands may sometimes be surrounded by hyalinized

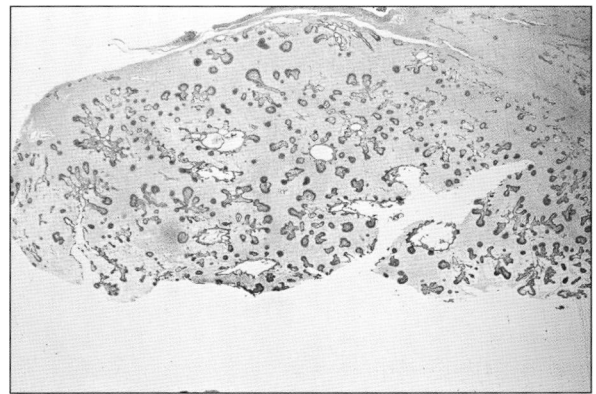

Fig 14-60a Low-power view of an ameloblastic fibroma showing numerous ameloblastic islands.

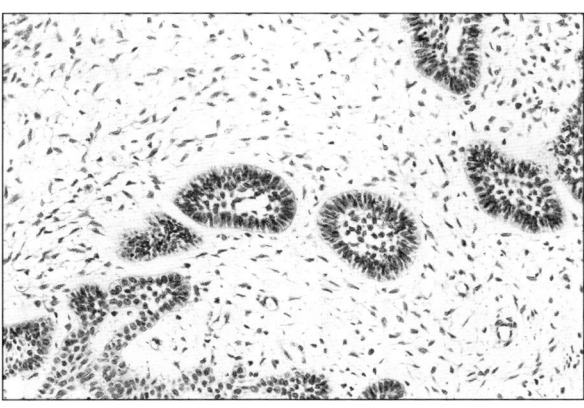

Fig 14-60b High-power view of an ameloblastic fibroma showing ameloblastic islands with peripheral palisaded columnar cells and reverse polarity. The stroma is myxoid in appearance, showing a resemblance to the dental papilla. This helps to distinguish this entity from the ameloblastoma, in which the stroma is collagenized.

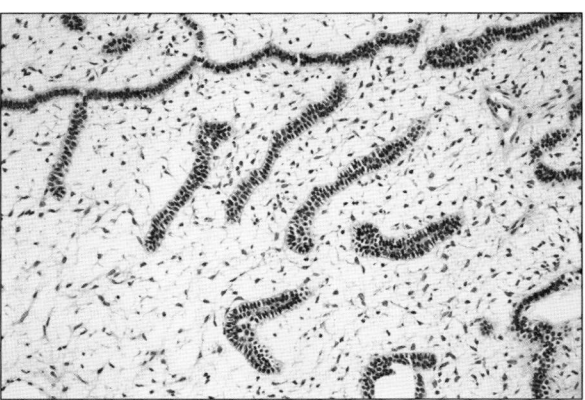

Fig 14-60c An ameloblastic fibroma in which the epithelial component resembles dental lamina. The mesenchymal portion is myxoid.

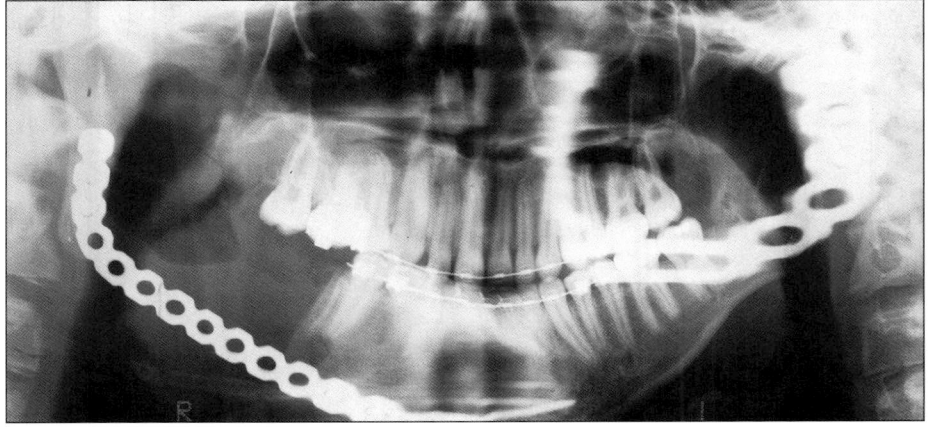

Fig 14-61a Resection of odontogenic hamartomas or neoplasms in children and teenagers may be reconstructed with a rigid titanium plate with the expectation of significant spontaneous bone regeneration.

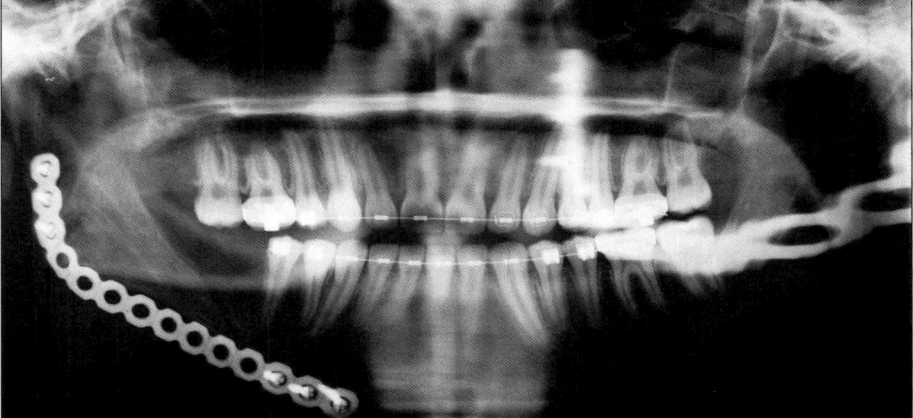

Fig 14-61b The resection shown in Fig 14-61a here shows complete bony regeneration of the continuity defect. This occurred in a 15-year-old patient over a 10-month period.

eosinophilic material that represents basal lamina. Alternatively, the epithelial component may lie in strands, usually two cells wide, that resemble dental lamina (Fig 14-60c).

TREATMENT ▶

The ameloblastic fibroma usually requires only enucleation and curettage to effect a cure. It is an encapsulated, noninvasive mass that is readily removed. The tumor will not invade the inferior neurovascular bundle or even the inferior alveolar canal. Therefore, nerve preservation is usually achieved. The resultant wound is closed at the mucosal level without the need for drainage or packing. Because of the patient's youth, regeneration of bone in the cavity will occur within 9 to 12 months. In cases of extremely large tumors, a resection is reasonable. A 2.3- or 2.4-mm reconstruction plate should be placed at the inferior border to avoid damage to developing tooth buds. Spontaneous complete bone regeneration in these young individuals often occurs, eliminating the need for bone grafting at a later date (Figs 14-61a and 14-61b). The plate should be removed after about 1 year to prevent bone from developing over the plate, at which time either no bone grafting or a smaller bone graft will be required.

PROGNOSIS ▶

Ameloblastic fibromas have a low recurrence rate. Simple enucleation and curettage is expected to be curative. The very few tumors that have recurred may have been significant portions of the original lesion left behind as an incompletely removed mass. Some may have been subtle ameloblastic fibrosar-

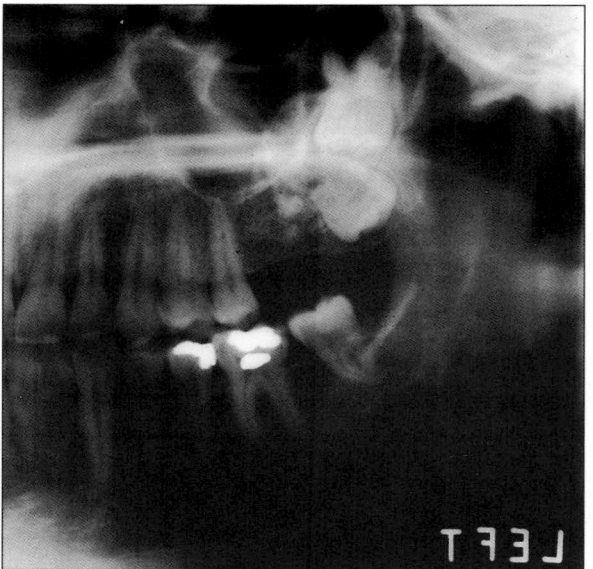

Fig 14-62 This developing odontoma is actually a mixed radiolucent-radiopaque lesion, which may also mimic the closely related ameloblastic fibro-odontoma. Here it has prevented the eruption of a molar tooth.

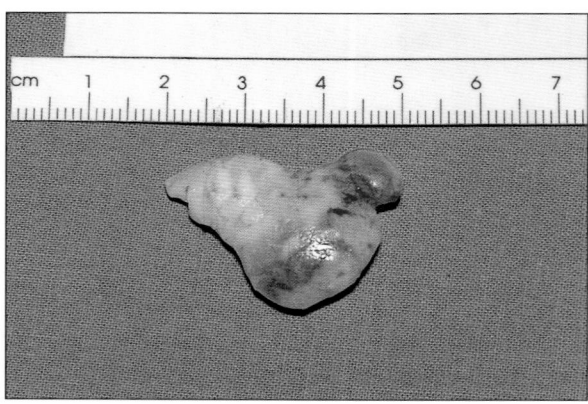

Fig 14-63a This odontoma shows the distorted attempt at tooth formation.

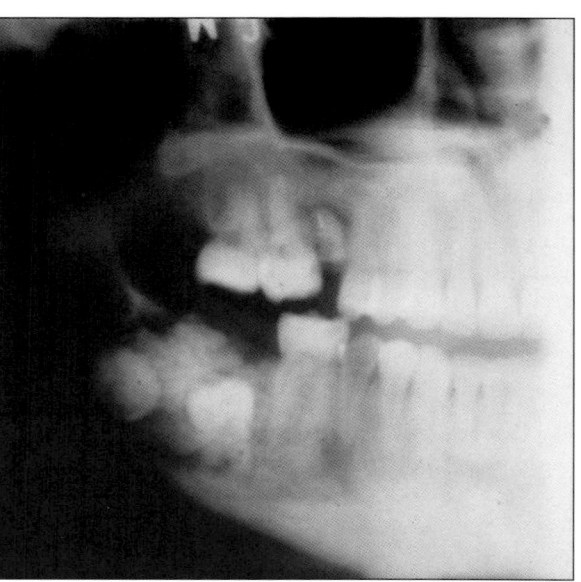

Fig 14-63b An odontoma becomes more radiopaque as it matures and can be identified by its well-demarcated borders and a radiographic density that is greater than that of bone.

comas not recognized in the original histopathology. If an ameloblastic fibroma does recur, ameloblastic fibrosarcoma, the most common odontogenic malignancy, should be considered, especially if the patient is an adult.

Odontomas

CLINICAL PRESENTATION AND PATHOGENESIS ▶

Odontomas are hamartomas of aborted tooth formation, of which there are two general types. One type, which forms multiple small tooth-like structures, is called the *compound odontoma*. The other type forms an amorphous calcified mass and is called the *complex odontoma*. Both types may get somewhat large (up to 6 cm) but will reach a maximum size and cease growth. Most are incidental radiographic findings observed on a dental examination. Others are radiographic findings discovered if clinical suspicion is aroused when a tooth fails to erupt, a primary tooth fails to exfoliate, or an expansion of bone is observed (Fig 14-62).

Whereas compound odontomas occur slightly more often anterior to the mental foramen, complex odontomas occur more often posterior to the mental foramen. However, each type may occur in any location in either jaw without a sex predilection. Most occur in children and young adults; it is doubtful whether new odontomas arise after the age of 25 years.

Radiographically, the compound odontoma will present a gravel-like appearance in which the outline of miniature teeth may be noticed. The complex odontoma will present as a dense amorphous and irregularly shaped mass. In both, a well-demarcated border with adjacent bone can usually be seen. On occasion, a radiograph will reveal an odontoma in its early stage of formation when calcification of its distorted dentin is incomplete. In such cases, it will appear mixed radiolucent-radiopaque but have a well-demarcated border with bone.

Odontomas are actually mixed odontogenic hamartomas. They arise from both odontogenic epithelium, which produces enamel, and odontogenic mesenchyme, which produces dentin via odontoblast differentiation. Because they are composed of both cell types and form products of both cell types, they

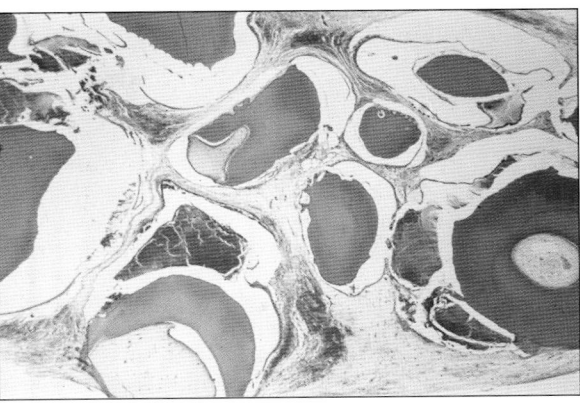

Fig 14-64 Discrete tooth-like structures are apparent, consistent with a compound odontoma.

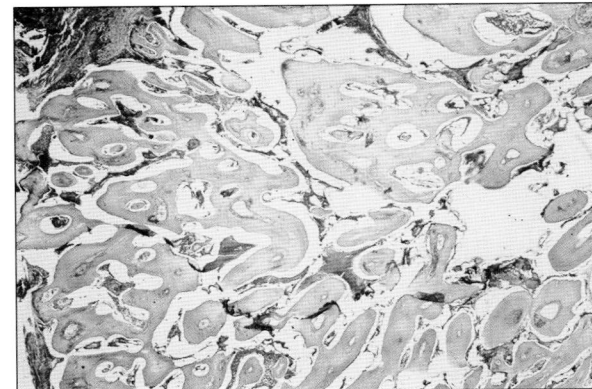

Fig 14-65 A complex odontoma with the dental hard tissues forming a solid mass rather than individual teeth.

have previously been termed "composite" odontomas. This unnecessary redundancy of nomenclature has been abandoned, since it is assumed that they are composites of two tooth-forming cell lines, as are all teeth. Odontomas represent an attempt to duplicate tooth formation but in a distorted fashion (Figs 14-63a and 14-63b).

DIFFERENTIAL DIAGNOSIS ▶ Mature compound odontomas with identifiable tooth-like structures are readily recognized. However, early in their development, the mixed radiolucent-radiopaque appearance will closely mimic that of a related lesion, the *ameloblastic fibro-odontoma*. Compound odontomas, as well as complex odontomas if superimposed over roots, also may suggest a *cementoblastoma* and, if not discovered until after the age of 30 years, *periapical cemento-osseous dysplasia* or *florid cemento-osseous dysplasia*. In addition, complex odontomas bear a radiographic resemblance to *osteoblastomas, ossifying fibromas,* and even *lingual tori* or *osteomas* that are projected over the mid-mandible and therefore appear as a central lesion.

TREATMENT ▶ The odontoma and the lesions on its usual differential list are curable with enucleation and curettage. These calcified masses are not adherent to bone and can be enucleated from the bony cavity with hand curettes. In larger compound or complex odontomas that may have multiple components, it is useful to take an intraoperative radiograph to ensure that all of the small calcified masses have been removed. The resultant bony cavity is closed at the mucosal level. Spontaneous osteogenesis in these usually young patients will result in bone regeneration in 9 to 12 months.

HISTOPATHOLOGY ▶ Odontomas are composed essentially of mature dental tissues—that is, enamel, dentin, cementum, and pulp tissue—and may be arranged in discrete tooth-like structures (compound odontoma) (Fig 14-64) or as unstructured sheets (complex odontoma) (Fig 14-65). In addition, components of the enamel organ may be present. The bulk of the tumor usually consists of dentin that is normal in appearance. Cementum may be cellular or acellular, and enamel may be mature or consist only of matrix. Occasionally, epithelial ghost cell keratinization may be seen. There is a fibrous capsule and a small amount of supporting fibrous tissue.

PROGNOSIS ▶ Enucleation and curettage of odontomas is curative. Recurrence does not develop, but portions of the lesion have occasionally been left unexcised. Such residual odontomas remain unchanged throughout the years. However, a wound infection becomes a possibility after an incomplete removal because the avascular odontoma portion acts like a foreign body.

Ameloblastic Fibro-odontoma

CLINICAL PRESENTATION AND PATHOGENESIS ▶ The ameloblastic fibro-odontoma is not a neoplasm but, like the cementoblastoma and the odontoma, a hamartoma. It represents a limited proliferation of odontogenic epithelium of the enamel organ and

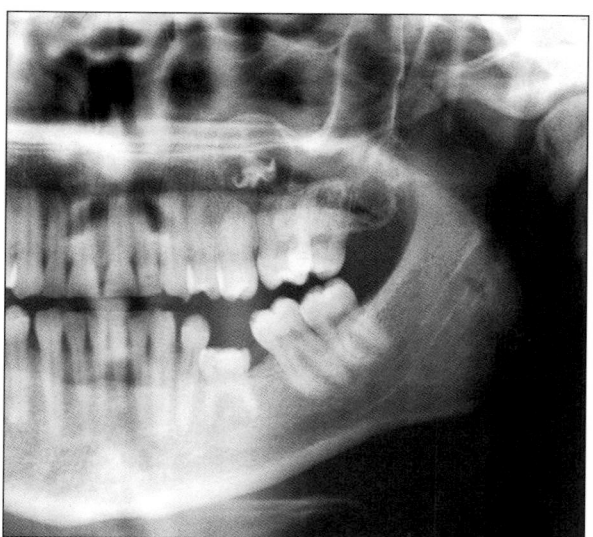

Fig 14-66 An ameloblastic fibro-odontoma will appear as a well-demarcated, mixed radiolucent-radiopaque mass.

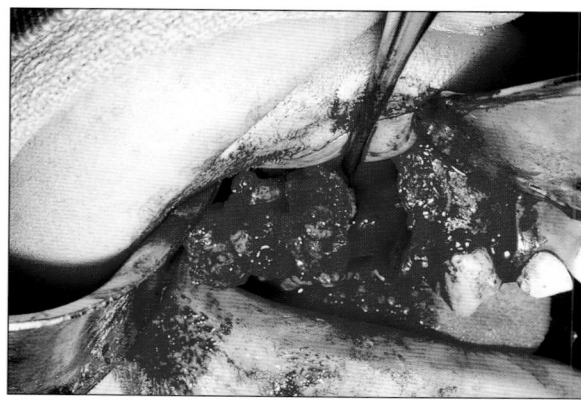

Fig 14-67a As a hamartoma, the ameloblastic fibro-odontoma will readily separate from its bony crypt. (Courtesy of Dr Eric Carlson.)

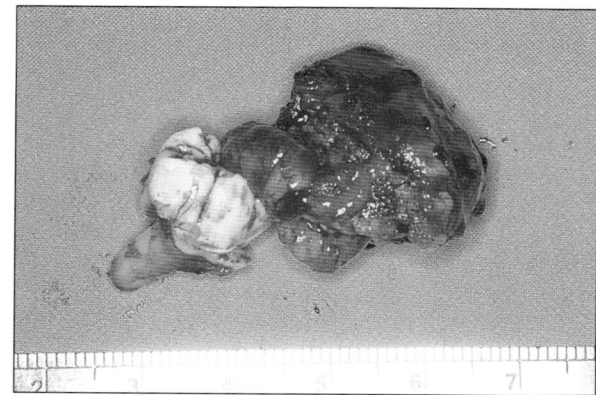

Fig 14-67b Because the ameloblastic fibro-odontoma has components of both an odontoma and an ameloblastic fibroma, it will consist of both soft and hard tissues. (Courtesy of Dr Eric Carlson.)

odontogenic mesenchyme of the primitive dental pulp. This proliferation comprises the soft tissue recapitulation of the dental follicle, which then produces some enamel but mostly dentin. It is not an invasive proliferation and will reach a maximum size, which at times may be quite large, and then cease growth.

The ameloblastic fibro-odontoma will present as an asymptomatic jaw expansion that may resorb tooth roots, displace developing teeth, and displace the inferior alveolar canal. Radiographically, it is characterized by a mixed radiolucent-radiopaque appearance in which the irregular calcifications are more dense than bone and approach the density of the adjacent teeth. It will also show a distinct demarcation from the adjacent bone (Fig 14-66). Like the ameloblastic fibroma and odontoma, it is mostly seen in children and teenagers. It is rare to see any new tumors develop after the age of 25 years; those found in older patients often can be shown to have been present earlier. The tumors are more common in the mandibular molar area but can occur anywhere in either jaw with no sex predilection.

The ameloblastic fibro-odontoma is a hamartoma representing an aberrant or aborted attempt at tooth formation. This aborted attempt at tooth formation or aberrancy occurs during the formation of enamel and dentin. This is in contrast to the ameloblastic fibroma, in which the aborted attempt occurs before hard tissues are formed; and to the odontoma, in which the aborted attempt occurs during the formation of enamel and dentin. Therefore, all three lesions behave like developmental disturbances of tooth formation. They show none of the invasive characteristics of true neoplasms but rather exist as malformations of their intended structures with limited growth potential.

DIFFERENTIAL DIAGNOSIS ▶

The presentation of a mixed radiolucent-radiopaque lesion in the jaws of a child or young adult narrows the differential list to a few odontogenic lesions and bone tumors. The most likely differential lesion is a *developing odontoma* followed by a *calcifying odontogenic cyst*. If the lesion is in the anterior portion of the jaws, an *adenomatoid odontogenic cyst* would also be considered. A calcifying epithelial odontogenic tumor is not likely since most occur in the late 30s or older, and few if any occur in childhood. The main bone tumor to consider in this age group is an *ossifying fibroma*. Fibrous dysplasia is not a likely inclusion since it would not be well demarcated from adjacent bone and would not have the distinct areas of radiolucency found in the ameloblastic fibro-odontoma.

DIAGNOSTIC WORK-UP AND TREATMENT ▶

The mixed radiolucent-radiopaque nature of an ameloblastic fibro-odontoma places it with a differential of other lesions that are treated by enucleation and curettage. Indeed, the area is usually explored and the lesion removed by enucleation and curettage (Figs 14-67a and 14-67b). A CT scan will show the

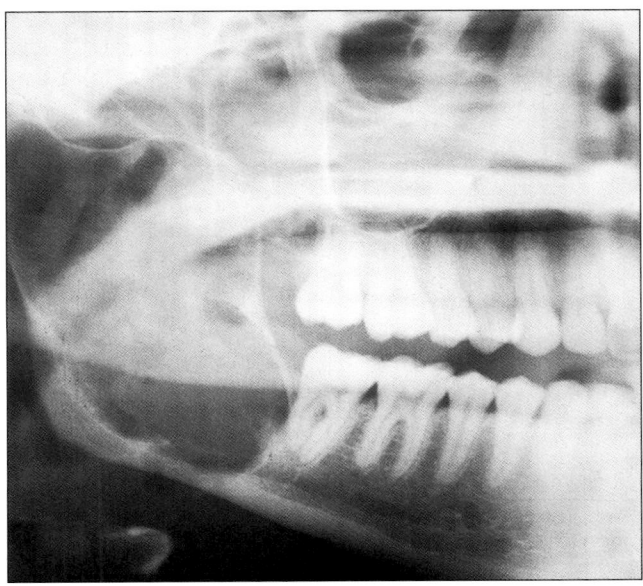

Fig 14-68a A large defect after removal of an odontogenic lesion in a 12-year-old patient. It was treated with only a mucosal closure and a soft diet recommendation for 6 weeks.

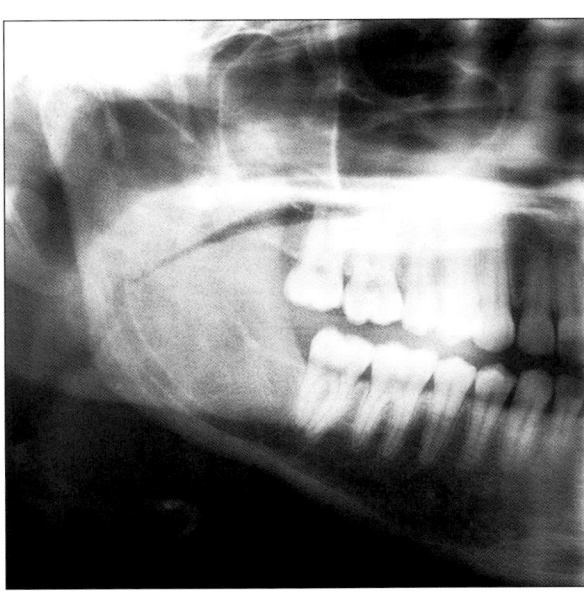

Fig 14-68b The large defect shown in Fig 14-68a here has completely regenerated bone within 9 months.

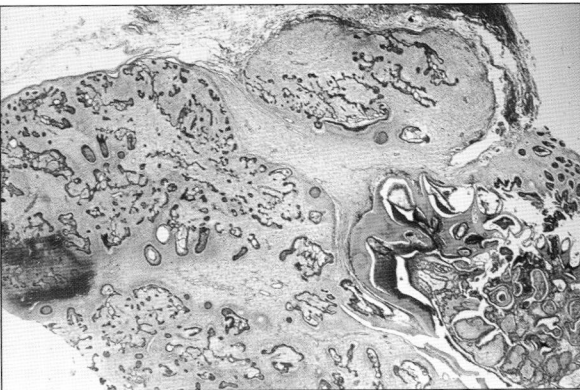

Fig 14-69a An ameloblastic fibro-odontoma. The soft tissue component is identical to that of an ameloblastic fibroma with islands of epithelium in a myxoid background. In addition, hard dental structures in the form of enamel and dentin are also present.

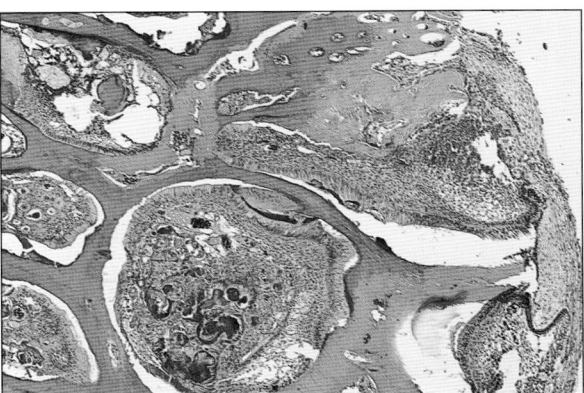

Fig 14-69b The predominantly calcified product of an ameloblastic fibro-odontoma is dentin. Here odontoblasts form dysmorphic dentin and some odontoblastic tubules.

extent of the lesion and may help in surgical planning if it has caused the displacement of developing teeth but is not necessary in every case. The lesion is neither infiltrative nor adherent to bone. It separates easily from the bone and will appear encapsulated. The resultant bony cavity is closed at the mucosal level without the need for drainage or packing. Bone will regenerate completely in the defect at this age (Figs 14-68a and 14-68b). Full bony regeneration may take 9 to 12 months.

HISTOPATHOLOGY ▶ These circumscribed tumors combine the histologic features of ameloblastic fibroma and odontoma. Thus, in addition to the presence of dental papilla–like tissue with epithelial strands and islands, as seen in the ameloblastic fibroma, there is inductive change with the formation of dentin and enamel (Figs 14-69a and 14-69b). Occasionally, tumors may show inductive changes limited to the formation of dentin. These have been called *ameloblastic fibrodentinomas*, but they merely represent a minor variation of an ameloblastic fibro-odontoma.

PROGNOSIS ▶ Simple enucleation and curettage is curative. No recurrence is expected.

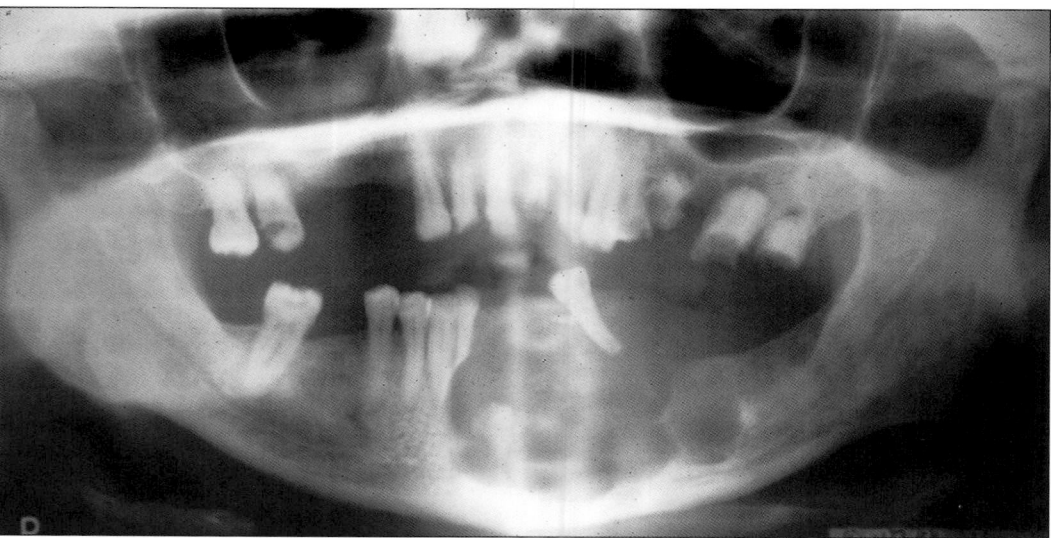

Fig 14-70 The ameloblastic fibrosarcoma is usually a low-grade malignancy with extensive local destruction and invasion. Its radiographic appearance will be similar to that of a large ameloblastoma or myxoma.

Ameloblastic Fibrosarcoma

CLINICAL PRESENTATION AND
PATHOGENESIS ▶

The ameloblastic fibrosarcoma, though rare as an individual entity, is the most common malignant odontogenic tumor. While it is capable of metastasis, it rarely undergoes distant metastasis. Instead, it is a low-grade malignancy as ascertained by its cytologic atypia and mitotic figures within the fibroma component of an otherwise benign ameloblastic fibroma. Apparently the malignant counterpart of a benign ameloblastic fibroma, its behavior becomes locally aggressive and infiltrative, resembling that of an ameloblastoma or an odontogenic myxoma (Fig 14-70).

The ameloblastic fibrosarcoma occurs approximately 20 to 30 years later than the ameloblastic fibroma, with a peak incidence at 30 to 40 years of age. Some arise from a pre-existing ameloblastic fibroma; others seem to arise de novo as an ameloblastic fibrosarcoma. It will present much like the more aggressive but benign ameloblastoma and odontogenic myxoma—that is, as a multilocular radiolucent lesion causing jaw expansion. As a malignant tumor, it is capable of neural invasion and may therefore include paresthesia in its presentation. Even though the tumor is malignant, its low-grade nature produces only slow growth with little tendency to ulcerate the overlying mucosa.

The malignant component of the ameloblastic fibrosarcoma is the fibroma arising from the primitive odontogenic mesenchyme of the dental papilla. Such a malignancy is readily understandable as a de novo malignant expression from a genetic alteration of this mesenchyme. The odontogenic epithelium (pre-ameloblasts), not sharing any further genetic alteration, remains in place without the infiltrative capacity or unlimited growth capacity of the mesenchymal component. The transformation of a pre-existing ameloblastic fibroma that is residual or recurrent is also understandable, but realistically many result from two separate situations. One is a true transformation of a benign mesenchymal component by one or two further gene changes in a single mesenchyme cell that clones to develop the malignant fibrosarcoma component. This phenomenon of spontaneous malignant transformation has its precedent in other benign neoplasms, such as the pleomorphic adenoma, the neurofibroma, and even some nonneoplastic conditions like Paget disease and fibrous dysplasia. The other is a de novo ameloblastic fibrosarcoma that was falsely interpreted as a benign ameloblastic fibroma because of the sparseness of mitotic figures and lack of cellular atypism (sort of a wolf in sheep's clothing). The recurrence of what appears clinically

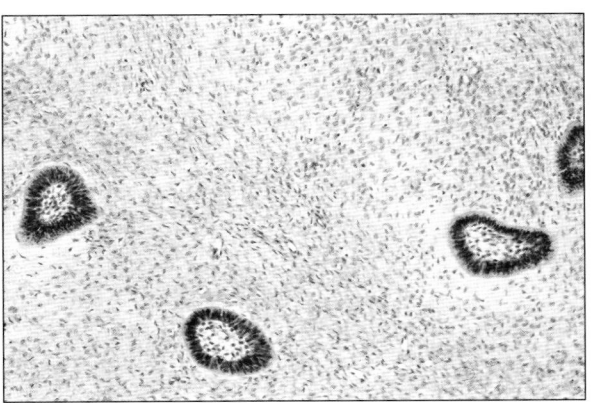

Fig 14-71a An ameloblastic fibrosarcoma. The epithelial islands are benign in appearance, but the mesenchymal component is greatly increased in cellularity and in quantity.

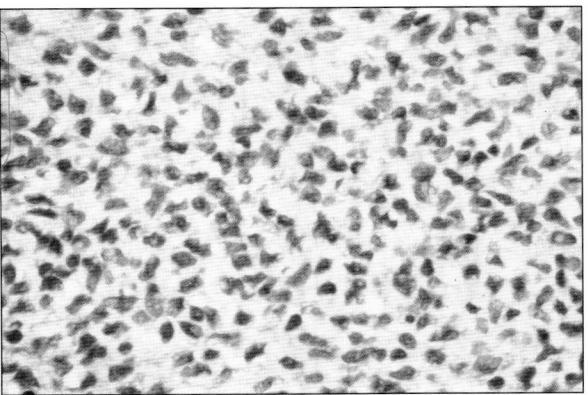

Fig 14-71b High-power view of Fig 14-71a showing the sarcomatous appearance of the mesenchymal component.

and histopathologically to be a benign ameloblastic fibroma should be looked upon as suggestive of an ameloblastic fibrosarcoma.

DIFFERENTIAL DIAGNOSIS ▶

Because the presentation is one of a multilocular, expansile jaw lesion, the prime differential considerations are the more common odontogenic cysts and tumors as well as the tumors in bone that present in this manner: the *odontogenic keratocyst*, the *ameloblastoma*, the *odontogenic myxoma*, and the *central giant cell tumor*. If paresthesia is apparent, the concern shifts to the known central malignant tumors of the jaw, such as a *primary intraosseous carcinoma,* a *central mucoepidermoid carcinoma,* an *osteosarcoma* producing very little tumor osteoid, or the rarer malignancies, such as a *malignant fibrous histiocytoma* or a *neurosarcoma.*

DIAGNOSTIC WORK-UP ▶

The diagnosis must be established by an incisional biopsy deep within the lesion from a midcrestal approach. Once the malignancy is diagnosed, a CT scan is valuable in determining the extent of the disease, and a chest radiograph is required.

HISTOPATHOLOGY ▶

The tumor resembles the ameloblastic fibroma histologically. The epithelial nests remain as a benign component, but the mesenchymal component is malignant (Fig 14-71a). This is demonstrated by hypercellularity, pleomorphism, and mitoses, as well as infiltration (Fig 14-71b). Particularly in recurrent lesions, the epithelial component can be inconspicuous since the sarcomatous element dominates.

TREATMENT ▶

Because an ameloblastic fibrosarcoma is a low-grade malignancy, its treatment is nearly identical to that of an ameloblastoma or an odontogenic myxoma. It is best treated with resection using 1.0- to 1.5-cm bony margins and one uninvolved anatomic barrier margin. Frozen sections documenting tumor-free margins in soft tissue as well as the marrow space are of great value. In the mandible, the resultant continuity defect is best managed by a rigid reconstruction plate. In the maxilla, the surgery is usually a submucosal partial maxillary resection resulting in a central defect over which the mucosa may be closed and a denture-like splint for support may be placed.

Radiotherapy is of little value in this tumor, but chemotherapy protocols similar to those used for malignant fibrous histiocytoma and fibrosarcoma may be considered as an adjunct to surgery in the rare case that shows more aggressive behavior.

PROGNOSIS ▶

The prognosis associated with ameloblastic fibrosarcoma is very good when treated with surgical resection. Too few have been reported with sufficient follow-up to produce reliable statistics, but recurrence after resection is uncommon. However, if the lesion is treated with enucleation and curettage, recurrence is frequent and predictable because of its infiltrative nature. Follow-up must be prolonged because of the slow growth rate. Tumors may not evidence recurrence until several years after treatment.

Management of Odontogenic Tumors

Definition of Terms

Odontogenic tumors, benign bone tumors, and fibro-osseous diseases are treated by a variety of procedures. Each has its own terms and modifications. A single procedure may vary from one geographic location to another and from one clinician to another. This section provides a practical definition of terms as applied to central lesions within bone.

1. *Enucleation:* Removal of all soft tissue and hard tissue produced by the lesion from its bony cavity.

2. *Curettage:* Removal of all soft tissue and hard tissue produced by the lesion from its bony cavity, including removal of some thickness of the bony wall itself (usually 1 to 3 mm).

   Curettage of the bony wall may be accomplished by a number of means: physical, thermal, or chemical. Each may be effective. Physical removal is usually via a sharp curette or a rotary bur. To prevent overlooking an area of the bony wall, methylene blue can be painted on its surface and the curettage continued until all of it is removed. Such procedures, however, should be undertaken with the knowledge that particulation of any neoplasm and especially the displacement of cells by a rotary bur may implant tumor cells into the surrounding soft tissue.

   In thermal removal (cryotherapy), a gel is placed into the bony cavity and frozen with a cryoprobe. The freezing process will crystallize water in the cells of the bony cavity wall, thereby disrupting and lysing them. Chemical removal is usually via Carnoy's solution, which contains 1 g of ferric chloride ($FeCl_3$) in 24 mL of absolute alcohol, 12 mL of chloroform, and 4 mL of glacial acetic acid. Essentially a tissue fixative, Carnoy's solution is secondarily a good topical hemostatic agent. It is soaked into a gauze sponge until it is dripping wet and placed into the bony cavity for 5 minutes. Studies have indicated that this length of exposure will not cause sensation changes in the inferior alveolar nerve distribution, even if placed in direct contact with the neurovascular bundle. There is also no known systemic toxicity despite the nature of these agents, probably because of the coagulation of protein limiting systemic uptake and the limited time it is used. This fact underscores its limited tissue penetration and, therefore, its limited usefulness.

   It is important to note that curettage is not a procedure consistent with principles of tumor removal because it is uncontrolled and not en bloc. It is best applied to cysts and hamartomatous lesions rather than to neoplasms. Additionally, cryotherapies and Carnoy's solution used in the treatment of odontogenic keratocysts and central giant cell lesions have not shown reduction in recurrence rates.

3. *Peripheral resection:* Resection of tumor en bloc within bone, which does not interrupt continuity; the margins may vary depending on the type of tumor. This usually implies preservation of the inferior border of the mandible or a subsinus or subnasal resection in the maxilla.

4. *Resection:* Resection of the tumor en bloc within bone, which interrupts jaw continuity; the margins may vary depending on the tumor. This implies a continuity resection of the mandible inclusive of the inferior border and a resection extending into the sinus and/or nasal cavities in the maxilla.

   Either type of resection may include teeth or overlying mucosa as dictated by tumor invasion. It may also include the periosteum or other anatomic barriers appropriate for the tumor extension. If the resection requires removal of the mandibular condyle, the procedure remains a resection. Some have termed this a *disarticulation resection.*

5. *Osseous sculpture:* Removal of excess surface bone to improve contour. Osseous sculpture is often a "shaving of bone," which is accomplished in quiescent fibrous dysplasia or mature cherubism in which

margins are neither important nor required. It can be accomplished with saws, osteotomes, burs, or a powered bone file.

Surgical Principles

What we loosely call odontogenic tumors involves a spectrum of biologies ranging from aberrant attempts at tooth formation (eg, odontoma) to hamartomas (eg, ameloblastic fibro-odontoma) to true neoplasms (eg, ameloblastoma). The onus is on the clinician to apply the treatment most appropriate to the biology of the lesion. Too often, the discussion concerns "conservative" vs "radical" approaches. These are unfortunate terms that have little meaning in the science of surgical therapy. So-called conservative approaches, in a well-meaning attempt to preserve teeth, bone, or native soft tissue, may lead to recurrences, with further loss of tissue and occasionally even death. Conversely, "radical" approaches inappropriate for a particular tumor but accomplished in a well-meaning attempt to prevent recurrence may lead to unnecessary removal of native tissue, compromising function and requiring extensive reconstruction.

The more appropriate terms are *curative* vs *palliative* approaches. A curative approach for a benign tumor may be empirically defined as a procedure that resolves the lesion at least 80% of the time. A palliative approach is one in which function and preservation of form are prolonged at the expense of cure. Palliation may be preferred by the patient or it may be a necessity if systemic health makes curative approaches unacceptably risky.

Based on the known biology of benign odontogenic tumors, there are only four primary tumors for which cure requires a resection; the others may be treated with enucleation and curettage for cure. These four are neoplasms with continued growth potential and invasive properties. They are the *ameloblastoma, odontogenic myxoma, calcifying epithelial odontogenic tumor,* and the rare *odontoameloblastoma,* which is actually an ameloblastoma occurring together with an odontoma. The remaining benign odontogenic "tumors" (odontomas, ameloblastic fibromas, ameloblastic fibro-odontomas, squamous odontogenic tumors, and odontogenic fibromas) are hamartomas or aborted attempts at tooth formation that, although they can reach a large size, do not have a continued growth potential or invasive properties. These masses are treated with enucleation and curettage for cure. The rare malignant variants of odontogenic tumors are treated as malignancies, which in these cases involve resection and consideration of a neck dissection for all except the ameloblastic fibrosarcoma.

Benign Odontogenic Neoplasms of the Mandible

Continuity Resection

When one of the four odontogenic neoplasms is found in the mandible, resection principles require a resection with 1.0- to 1.5-cm bony margins, one uninvolved anatomic barrier margin, and frozen sections documenting tumor-free margins (Figs 14-72a to 14-72c). Such resections may be accomplished either from a transoral or a transcutaneous approach but should plan for stabilization of the mandible, preferably with rigid plate fixation (Fig 14-72d). The rigid fixation plate should be at least 2.4 mm or preferably 2.7 mm and made of titanium. Three or four bicortical screws on each segment is ideal; however, two bicortical screws on a proximal segment consisting only of the condylar neck and condyle may suffice where the resection margins are at the condylar neck and leave sufficient bone for only two screws (Fig 14-73).

When the tumor extirpation includes the condyle, a reconstruction plate with a condylar replacement is used (Fig 14-74). Because of the absence of a proximal segment, such metal condylar replacements have long-term functional success without complications if they articulate against a native disc or against reconstructed soft tissue or cartilage. Placement of the metal condyle directly against the bone

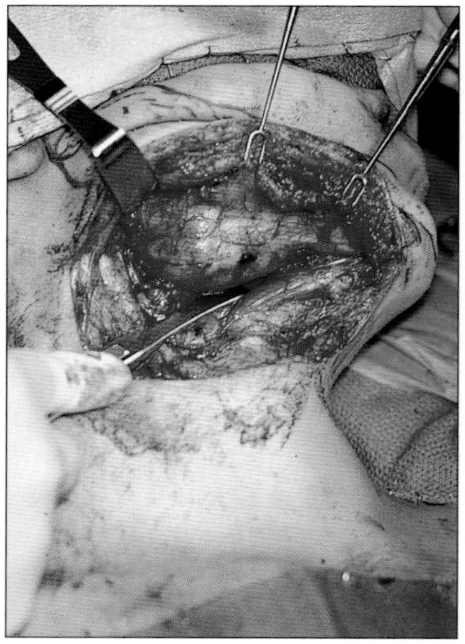

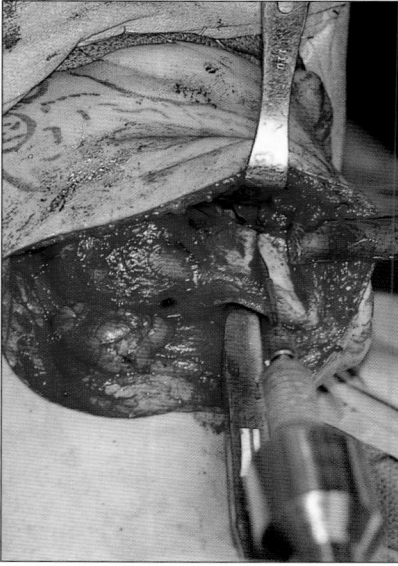

Fig 14-72a Here, an odontogenic myxoma is dissected in the supraperiosteal plane. The periosteum will serve as a tumor-free anatomic barrier necessitated by the cortical erosion and perforation of this tumor.

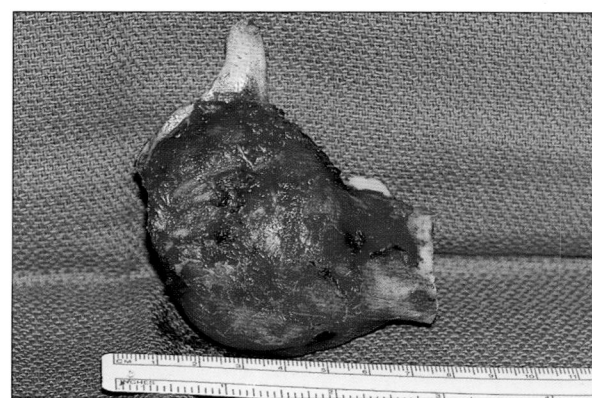

Fig 14-72b The anterior resection should be accomplished first at 1.0 to 1.5 cm from the clinical and radiographic tumor edge.

Fig 14-72c The resection specimen of a benign odontogenic neoplasm should be encased in one tumor-free anatomic barrier (here periosteum) and requires 1.0- to 1.5-cm bony margins.

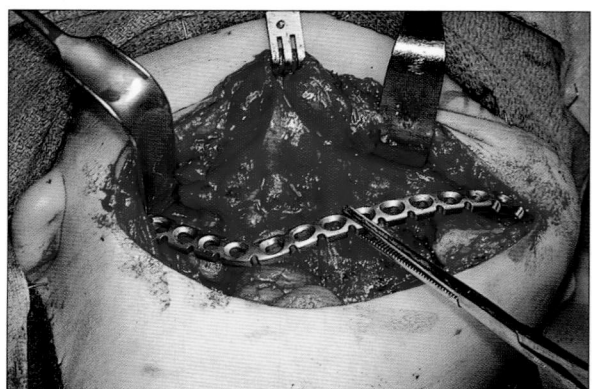

Fig 14-72d After the tumor resection is accomplished and the patient's occlusion is indexed with maxillomandibular fixation, a reconstruction plate is adapted to the contours to allow for three or four bicortical screws on each segment.

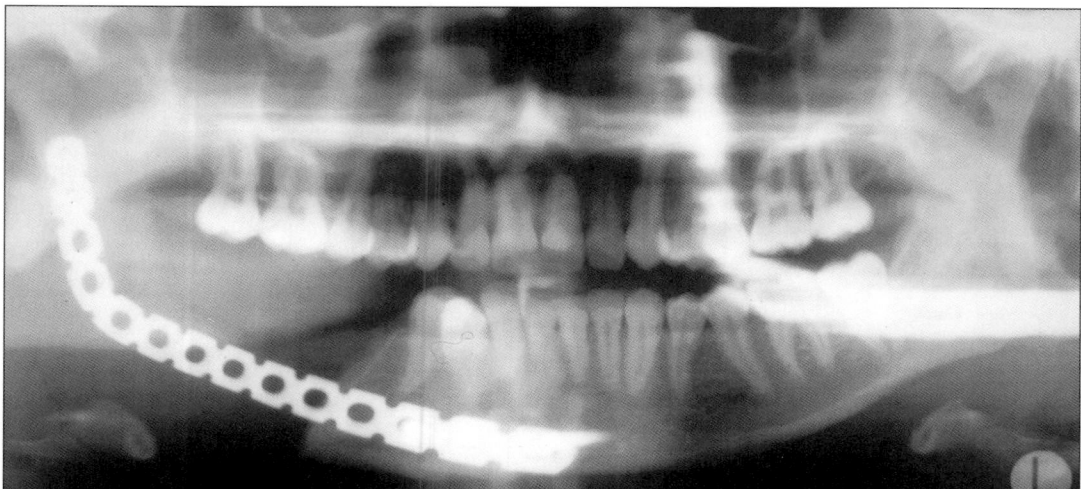

Fig 14-73 Reconstruction plate that was placed with three bicortical screws in the distal segment but only two in the proximal segment because of limited bone. Note that one-half to one socket width of distance exists between the resection edge and the nearest tooth.

of the temporal fossa invites bony erosion, pain, and displacement into the temporal fossa. Use of a so-called total TMJ metal articulation prosthesis or of a metal condyle articulating against another nonbiologic substance creates microscopic particles that induce pain, foreign body reactions, and fibrosis. Therefore, only a metal condylar replacement articulating against a biologic soft tissue in the temporal fossa is acceptable in tumor patients. In these situations, five or six bicortical screws must be placed in the distal segment in order to gain sufficient stability (Figs 14-75 and 14-76).

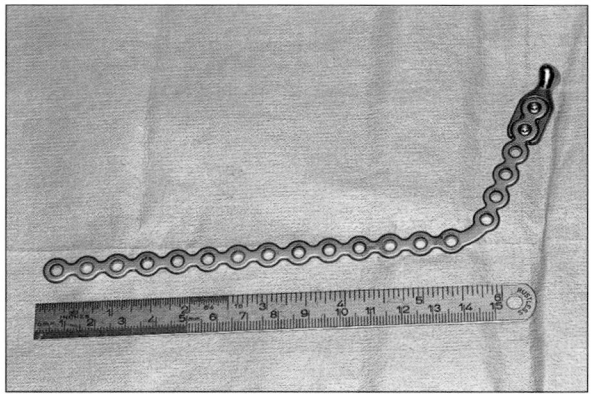

Fig 14-74 Titanium reconstruction plate with a condylar replacement. Condylar position and ramus height can be adjusted by removing one plate hole at a time.

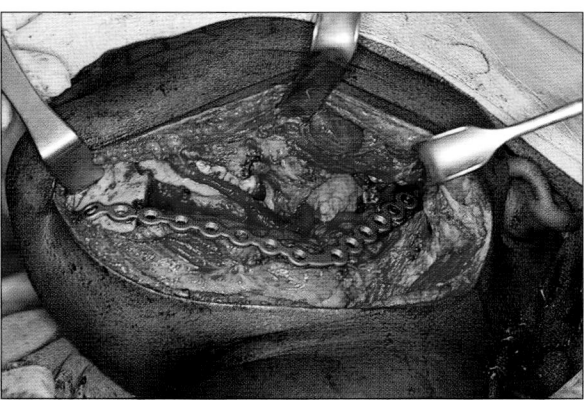

Fig 14-75 Following a tumor resection that required removal of the condyle, a reconstruction plate is placed with a titanium condylar replacement. The plate must overlap the distal segment and be fixated with five or six bicortical screws.

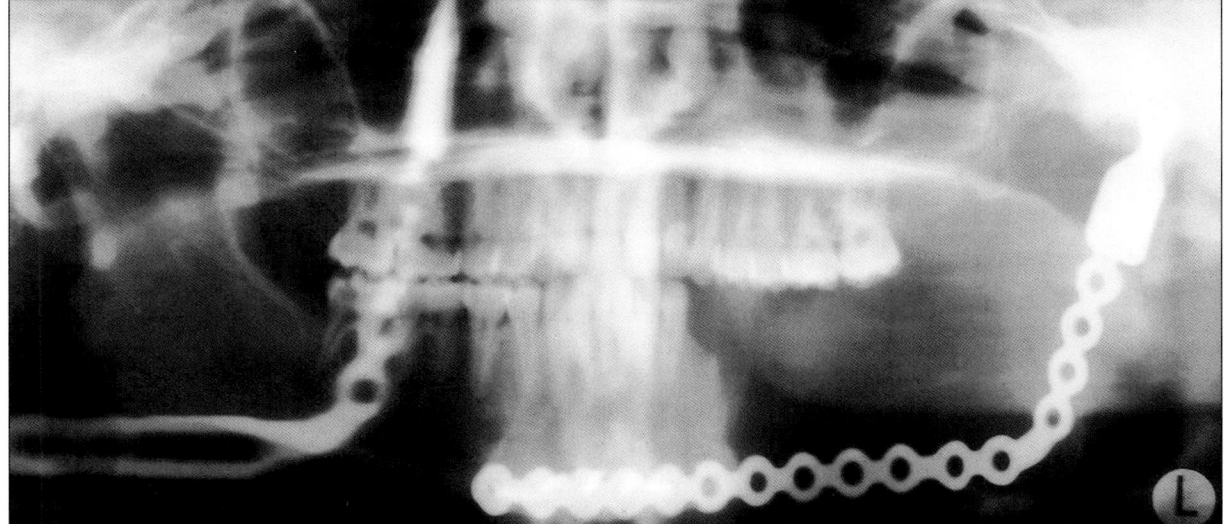

Fig 14-76 Titanium reconstruction plate with a condylar replacement is ideally positioned in the temporal fossa and fixated with five bicortical screws at the distal segment.

External skeletal pins, maxillomandibular fixation, or immediate bony reconstruction may be planned. Because of their limited longevity and the resultant deviation of the mandible after their removal, external skeletal pin fixation and maxillomandibular fixation are less ideal than an internal rigid fixation plate. Immediate reconstruction is not advised if there is a communication into the oral cavity. Even if such communications can be closed well, the contamination of the tissue bed and the microscopic leakage of additional organisms through even the best closure results in an unacceptably high infection rate. When a resection can be accomplished without a communication through the oral mucosa, immediate reconstruction is strongly advised. Internal spacers other than rigid plates are to be avoided because of their frequent exposure by tissue dehiscence and the avascular scar that forms around them.

When a mandibular neoplasm is removed via a transcutaneous approach, the dissection plane is deep to the superficial layer of the deep cervical fascia, deep to the common facial vein, and, therefore, deep to the course of the marginal mandibular branch of the facial nerve. It is superficial to the submandibu-

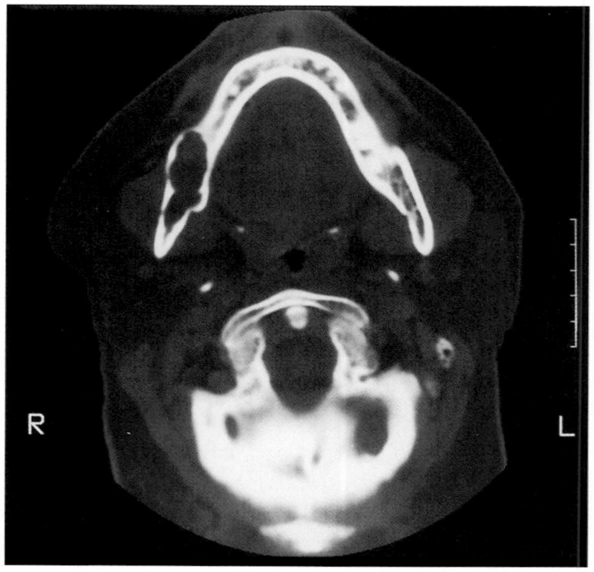

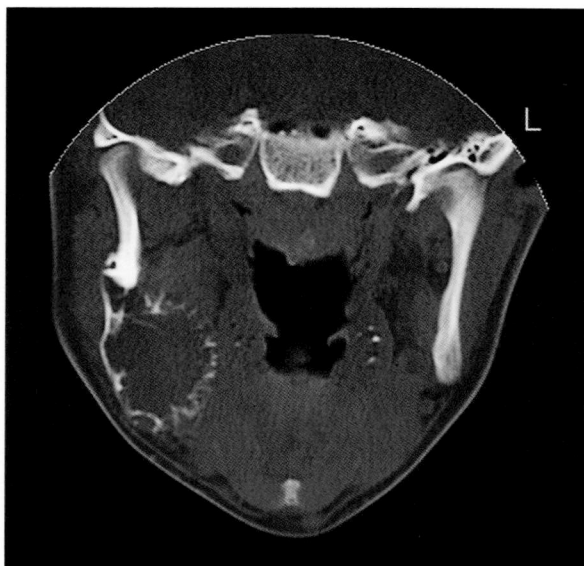

Fig 14-77a A CT scan that shows a tumor confined by an intact cortex indicates that the resections may be accomplished in the subperiosteal plane.

Fig 14-77b A CT scan that shows perforations of the cortex may be evidence of microscopic disease just beyond the cortex. This finding would indicate a resection in the supraperiosteal plane.

lar gland, the anterior and posterior digastric muscles, the sternocleidomastoid muscle, and the stylohyoid muscle. If the preoperative CT scan indicates a tumor confined within the expanded cortices with no perforations, the cortex of the mandible becomes the correct anatomic barrier and a subperiosteal dissection proceeds (Fig 14-77a). If the CT scan indicates a cortical perforation, a supraperiosteal dissection plane is performed since the periosteum then becomes the correct anatomic barrier (Fig 14-77b). In either case, identification of tumor through an anatomic barrier in a focal area requires a local excision of the next anatomic layer and frozen sections (Figs 14-78a to 14-78d).

As the dissection progresses around the lingual and buccal surfaces of the mandible, the oral cavity is entered in dentate individuals and through mucosa in cases with tumor or biopsy sites. The mucosa of these areas must be excised with the tumor. The tooth within the resection site that allows for a 1.0- to 1.5-cm margin from the radiographic extent of the tumor should be removed. The bony resection should be planned so that at least one half of a tooth socket remains between the resection edge and the adjacent tooth (Fig 14-79a). Closer resections will create periodontal pocketing, secondary infections, and bone loss around the adjacent tooth, all of which will compromise reconstructive attempts. If the dissection was in the supraperiosteal plane, an incision to bone is made in the area of bony resection, and periosteum is reflected in that area to allow for the saw cut (Fig 14-79b). If the tumor has a minimal buccal expansion, a rigid reconstruction plate may be placed on the mandible prior to resection and the resection accomplished with the plate in place. In this manner, condylar position and the occlusion are best maintained (Fig 14-79c).

If the buccal expansion caused by the tumor is significant, the resection is accomplished first and the reconstruction plate is placed secondarily with temporary maxillomandibular fixation. Before the wound is closed, it is advisable to examine the fresh resected specimen. Any areas of unexpected tumor perforation through bone can be correlated with a location in the wound and frozen sections taken. It is also advised to take curettings of the marrow space at each resection margin of host bone. The marrow is the ideal area of bone to sample as tumor extension takes the path of least resistance, which is the fibrofatty marrow. The lack of bony trabeculae in the marrow space almost always allows for frozen sections. If the trabecular bone is too dense for frozen sections, the specimen may be thinly spread on a

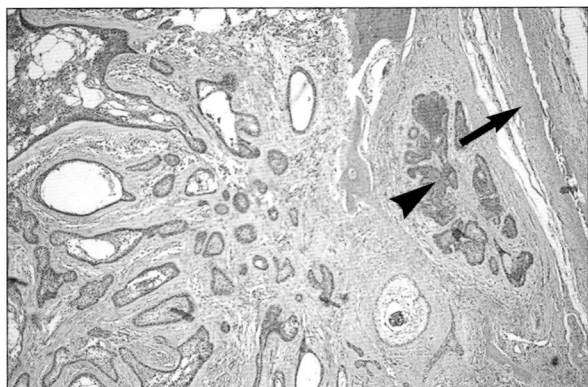

Fig 14-78a Focus of ameloblastoma beyond the cortex (*arrowhead*) and beneath the periosteum (*arrow*). A subperiosteal resection in this case would have left this ameloblastoma focus on the periosteum to develop into a recurrence.

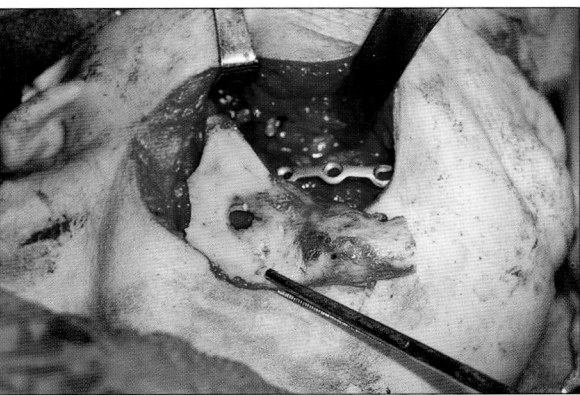

Fig 14-78b If a tumor is resected using a subperiosteal plane and the specimen shows a focal area of cortical perforation, periosteum and sometimes muscle adjacent to the perforation should be excised and examined with a frozen section.

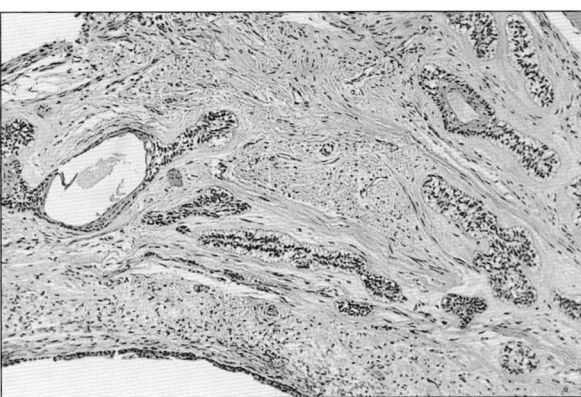

Fig 14-78c The removal of periosteum adjacent to the perforation (see Fig 14-78b) shows invading ameloblastoma (ie, a positive frozen section), indicating the need to remove further soft tissue until a clear frozen section is obtained.

Fig 14-78d Resection specimen of an odontogenic myxoma showing the proximal bony margin grossly free of tumor and the thin band of periosteum, which was microscopically found to be free of tumor.

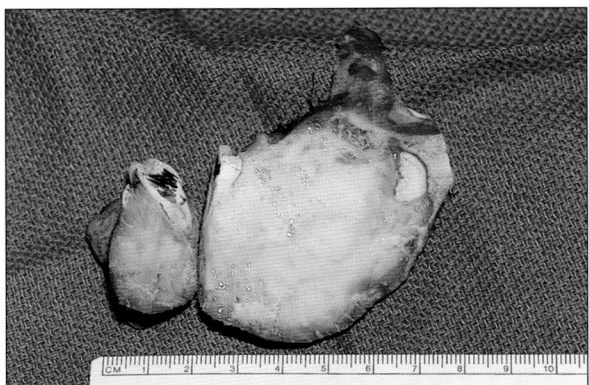

glass slide for a cytologic smear preparation. Specimen radiographs may also be helpful as they allow for a more detailed image without the shadowing of superimposed structures (Fig 14-79d). Once the neoplasm is believed to be completely removed, closure can begin. With a rigid fixation plate in place, it is advisable to close one layer beneath the plate and one immediately above the plate in addition to a mucosal and neck closure. Such internal plates can harbor microorganisms for a long time. Their envelopment by soft tissue via a precise closure minimizes the chances of infection and hence dehiscence and plate exposure.

In selected cases, the resection of an odontogenic neoplasm can be prepared for an immediate reconstruction in which oral communication can be avoided. Because odontogenic neoplasms grow slowly, this allows the clinician to remove teeth in the area planned for resection so as to permit a mature edentulous alveolar ridge to develop (Fig 14-80a). This healing takes about 3 to 4 months. The process of tooth removal does not seed tumor into the mucosa because the periodontal membrane serves as an anatomic barrier. Once the ridge mucosa is healed and mature (the thickness and color are uniform), the tumor can be resected from a transcutaneous approach and a reflection of mucosa over the edentulous bony ridge accomplished in a submucosal plane. The resultant wound defect has no oral communication and is an ideal graft bed (Figs 14-80b to 14-80e). A bone graft that achieves full alveolar height and width as well as continuity can then be placed.

This approach produces excellent reconstructive results and has not been associated with recurrences (see Figs 14-80d and 14-80e). However, it is applicable only in selected cases. The tumor must be

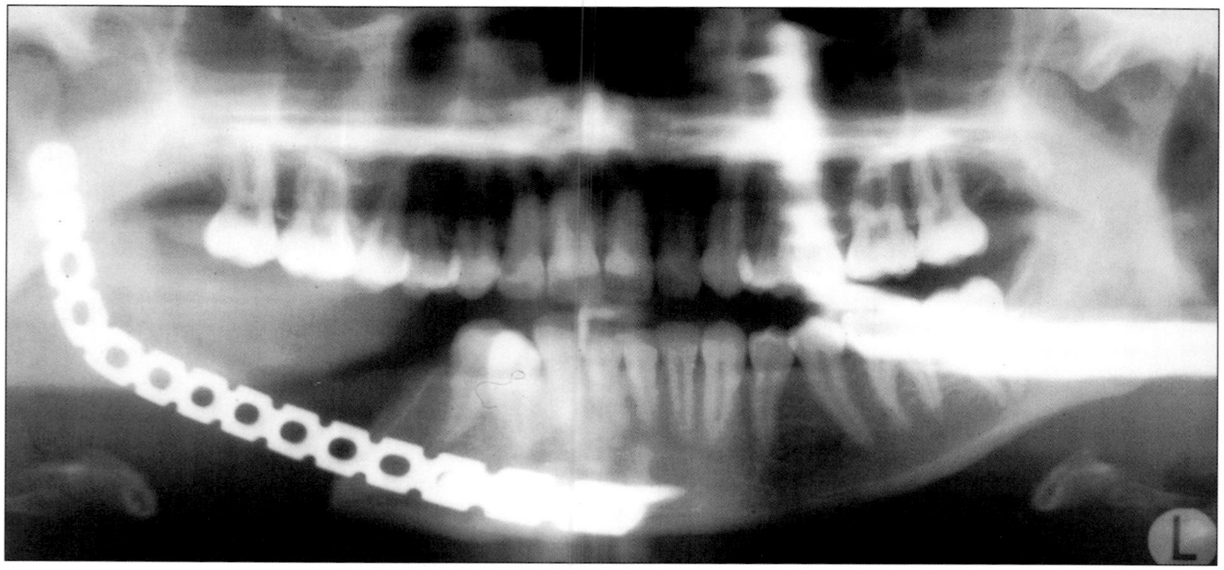

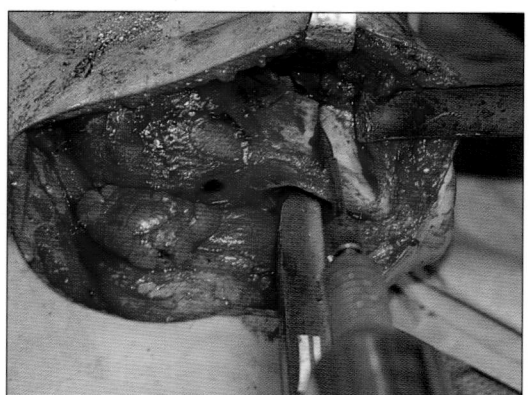

Fig 14-79a Reconstruction plate stabilizing a continuity defect after an ameloblastoma resection. Note the one-half to one complete socket width between the resection margin and the adjacent tooth.

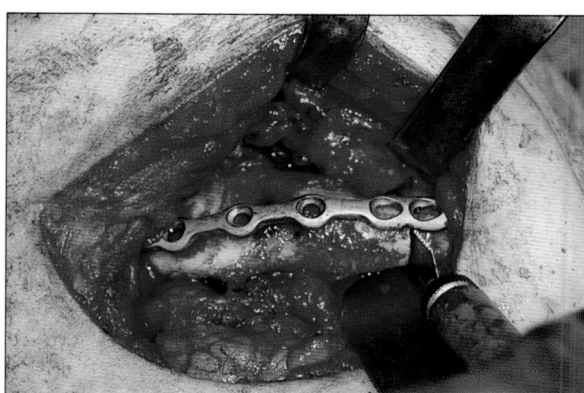

Fig 14-79b The resection is accomplished 1.0 to 1.5 cm from the clinical tumor edge where the periosteum has been reflected. The periosteum remains on the tumor as an anatomic barrier.

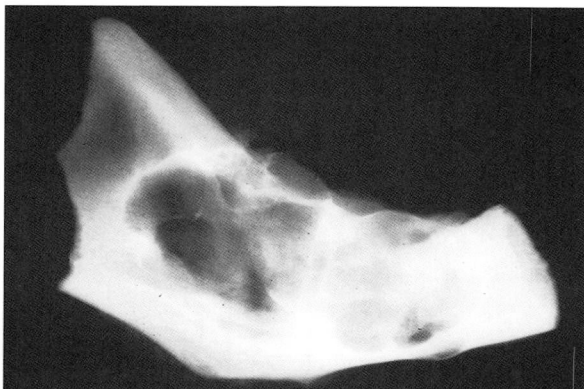

Fig 14-79c In cases where there is little or no buccal expansion, the reconstruction plate may be placed and the tumor resected from lingual to buccal without removing the plate and also without the need to index the occlusion with maxillomandibular fixation.

Fig 14-79d A specimen radiograph is highly recommended for assessing the tumor's relationship to the bony margins and its pattern of growth.

confined to the central part of the mandible without extension beyond the cortex. Moreover, it must not perforate the alveolar bone and enter the mucosa, thus requiring mucosal excision.

Mandibular resections may also be accomplished from a transoral approach. Both subperiosteal and supraperiosteal dissections may be performed in this manner (Fig 14-81). A reconstruction plate may also be placed through this access, although the working space is smaller (Fig 14-82). In such cases, bicortical screw fixation in the angle and ramus area need to be achieved via a small percutaneous incision and a tissue-protecting trocar that will allow drill and screw access.

Peripheral Resection

When one of the four odontogenic neoplasms occurs in the mandible and is sufficiently small that a 1.0- to 1.5-cm bony margin will leave at least 1 cm of the inferior border, a peripheral resection may be indicated. The peripheral resection is usually a transoral procedure. If the tumor extends into the oral mucosa, that portion of the oral mucosa is excised around its periphery and included in the resection spec-

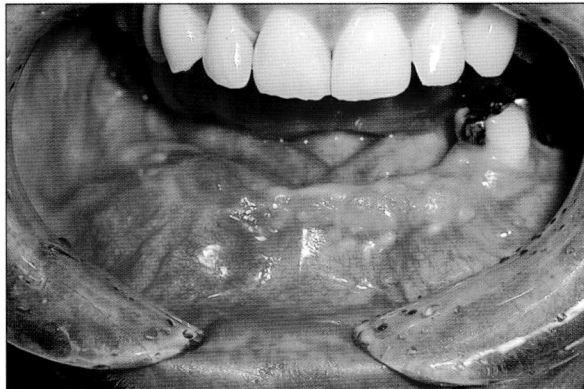

Fig 14-80a Removing the teeth in the area of the tumor and allowing an edentulous ridge mucosa to develop has shown no evidence of seeding tumor into the mucosa and may allow an immediate bone graft to be accomplished from a transcutaneous approach without an oral communication.

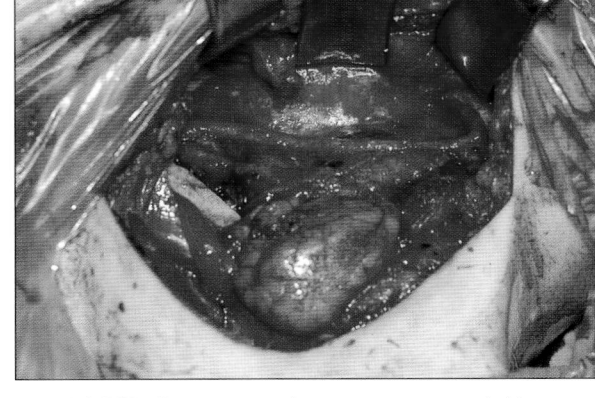

Fig 14-80b Resection of a recurrent ameloblastoma with nerve preservation and without entering the oral cavity makes an immediate bone graft possible. The teeth were removed from this area 4 months earlier.

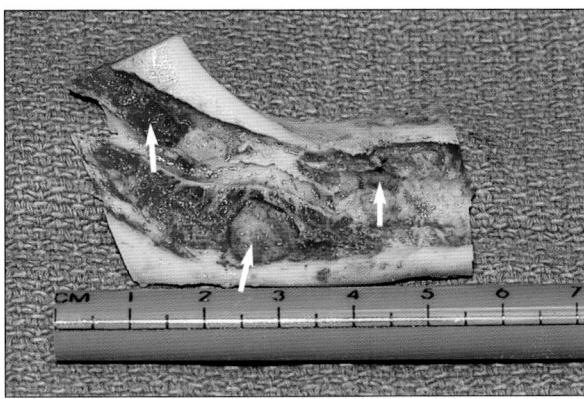

Fig 14-80c This resection specimen shows multiple foci of recurrent ameloblastoma (*arrows*).

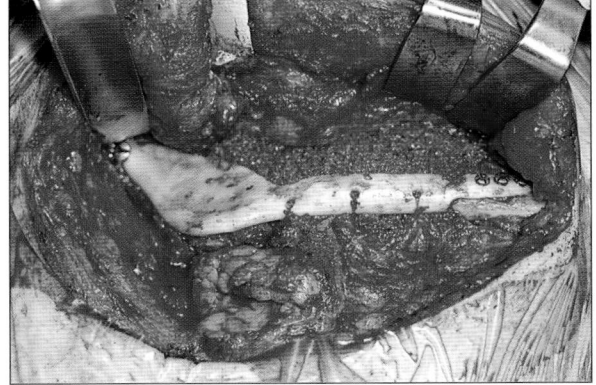

Fig 14-80d Bone graft of the resection defect shown in Fig 14-80b. Here an allogeneic hemimandible was used as a crib to contain a cancellous cellular marrow graft from the posterior ilium.

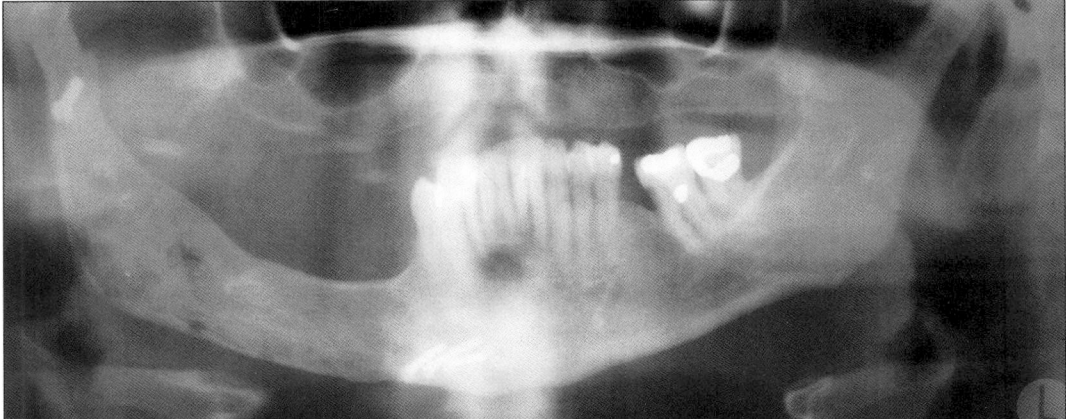

Fig 14-80e A 10-year follow-up of the graft shown in Fig 14-80d shows no evidence of recurrent tumor, excellent consolidation of the graft, and maintenance of the graft's height and contour.

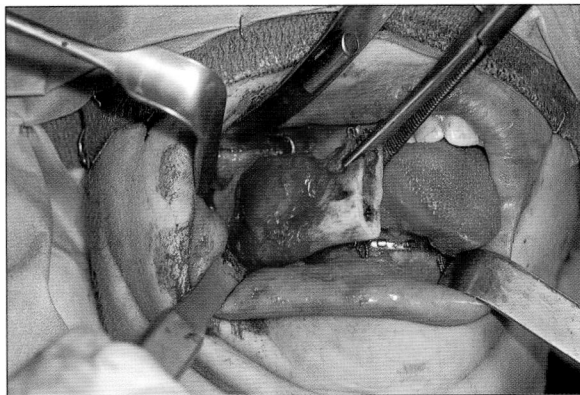

Fig 14-81 Odontogenic neoplasms may be resected from a transoral approach provided sufficient access can be obtained to accomplish an en-bloc resection with 1.0- to 1.5-cm bone margins, one anatomic barrier margin, and placement of a reconstruction plate.

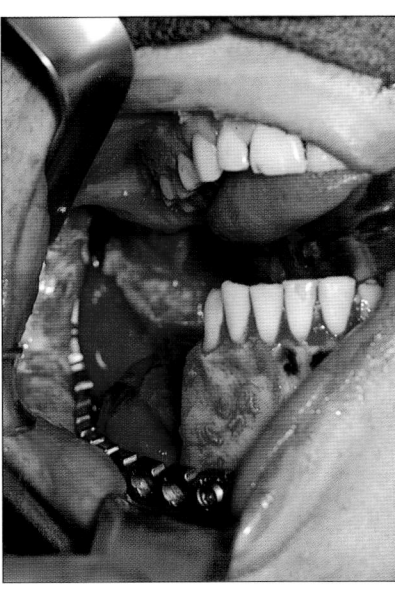

Fig 14-82 Placing a reconstruction plate for a large continuity defect requires a wide oral access. The proximal segment screws will likely be placed through a percutaneous access with a placement trocar.

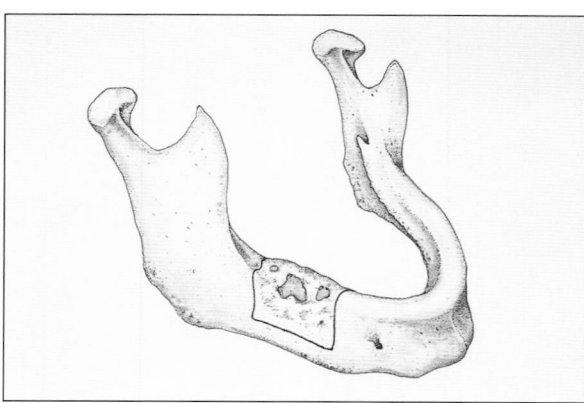

Fig 14-83a A peripheral resection in the adult should avoid this type of a right-angle box design and should leave at least 1 cm of the inferior border.

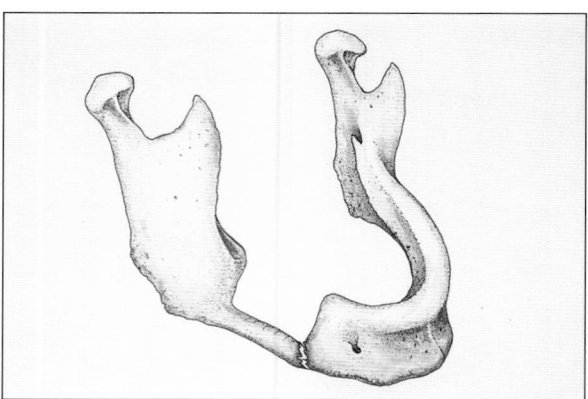

Fig 14-83b After right-angle peripheral resections, fractures of the mandible occur at the inferior border–vertical wall junctions because biting forces are transmitted and concentrated toward these corners.

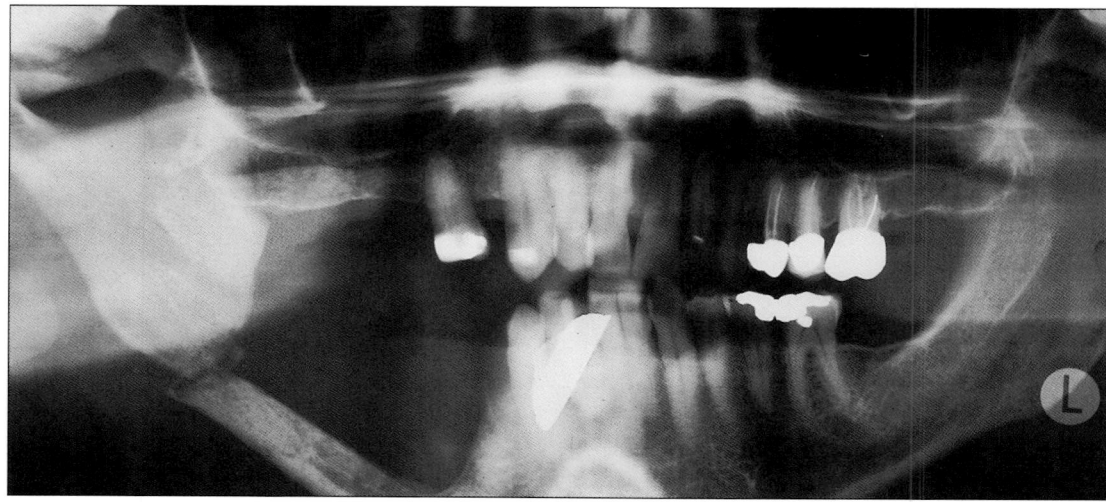

Fig 14-83c Fractured mandible at one of the predicted locations after a peripheral resection, which was at right angles and left less than 1 cm of the inferior border.

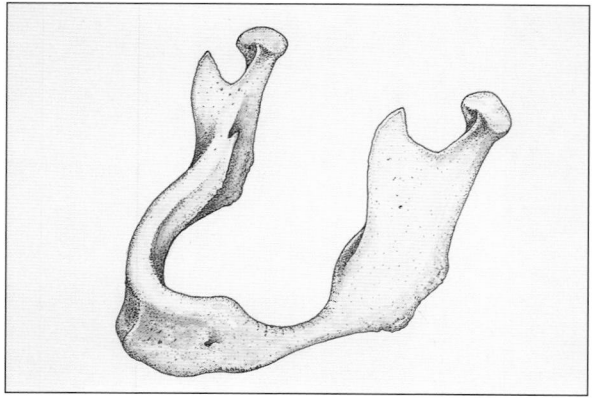

Fig 14-84a The superior design for a peripheral resection should avoid right angles, create a sloping or arch shape, and leave more than 1 cm of the inferior border.

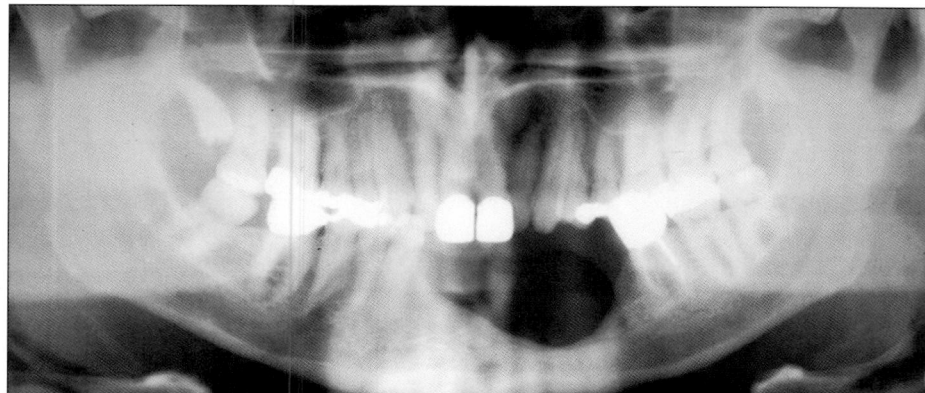

Fig 14-84b The proper design for a peripheral resection was used in this case.

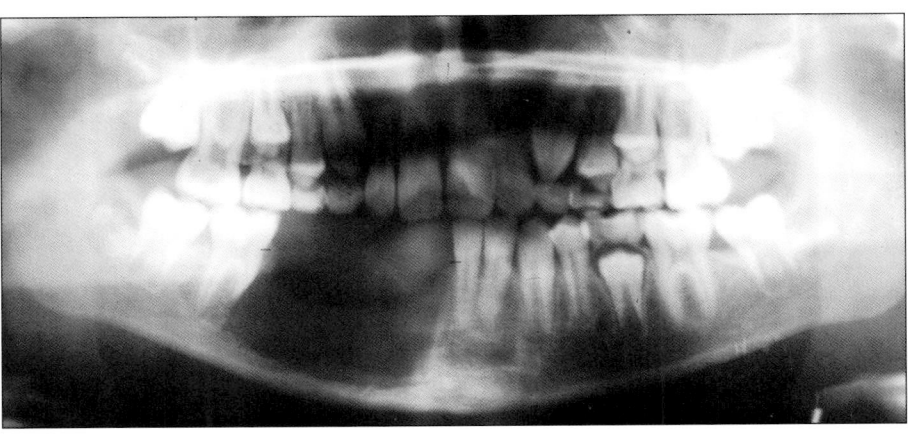

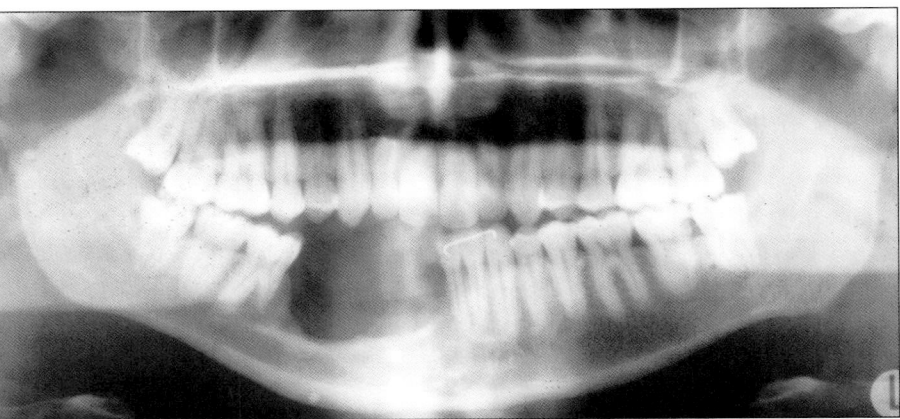

Fig 14-84c Peripheral resection for an ameloblastoma in this 10-year-old patient left minimal inferior border.

Fig 14-84d With the patient at age 18, about one half of the alveolar bone height had regenerated with grafting.

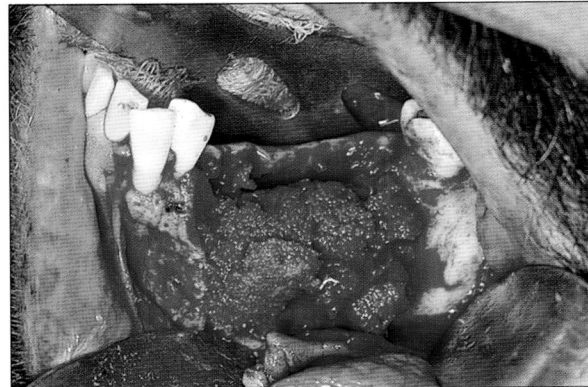

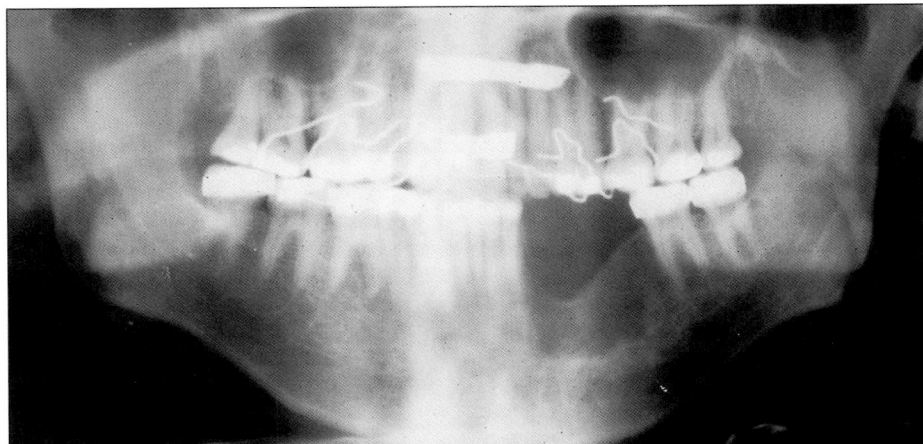

Fig 14-85a Immediate bone grafting of a peripheral resection is feasible without an increased infection rate because of minimal dead space and the stability provided by the inferior border continuity.

Fig 14-85b Consolidated transoral bone graft after a peripheral resection.

imen. The same oral incisions and planes of dissection apply in the peripheral resection as in the more commonly required continuity resection.

The actual bony resection is often conceptualized as a box with right-angle corners. This resection design is to be avoided in those older than 30 years or in those in whom the remaining inferior border is 1 cm or less. The reduced elasticity of bone in this age group, particularly at the dense inferior border, coupled with biting forces that are transmitted to the right-angle corners of the box, will frequently produce pathologic fractures (Figs 14-83a to 14-83c). To avoid this, the bony resection design should be more of a curvilinear design in the shape of the letter "U" with the top widened even further (Figs 14-84a and 14-84b).

Peripheral resections may be closed primarily. About one half of the lost bony height is regained by spontaneous osteogenesis in the adolescent (Figs 14-84c and 14-84d). In such resections, immediate bony reconstruction is possible and is associated with a greatly reduced infection potential compared to continuity resections with communication to the oral cavity. The reason is that peripheral resection wounds, by virtue of their remaining continuity, have greatly reduced dead space and less micromotion that causes seepage of microorganisms through the mucosal closure (Figs 14-85a and 14-85b).

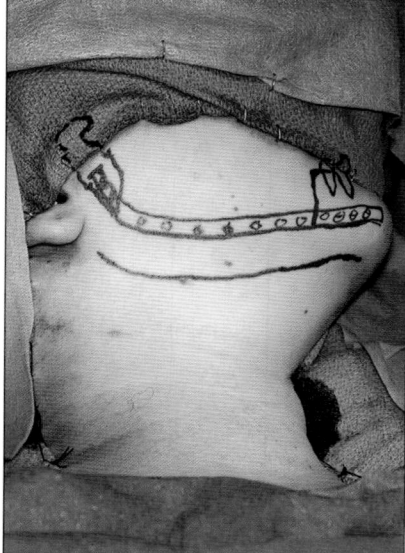

Fig 14-86a The incision for a mandibular reconstruction should be placed in a natural skin fold or parallel to the mandible, 3 cm below the inferior border and slightly curvilinear.

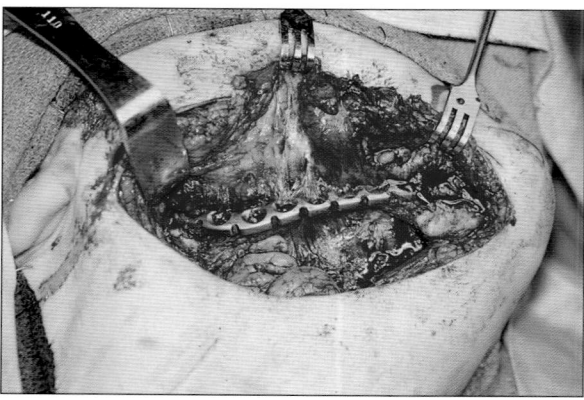

Fig 14-86b The avascular scar that forms around all reconstruction plates may look like a periosteal sheath, but it is nevertheless a scar that should be excised.

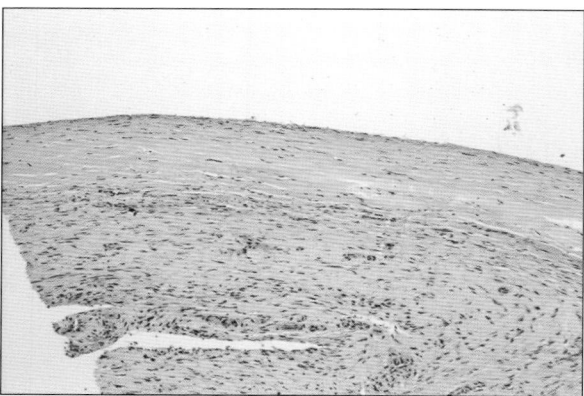

Fig 14-86c The avascular scar around reconstruction plates is consistently 440 μm. Since the diffusion distance of nutrients and oxygen from a capillary is only 180 to 200 μm, this scar will inhibit revascularization and hence bone regeneration in a graft. Therefore, it should be excised.

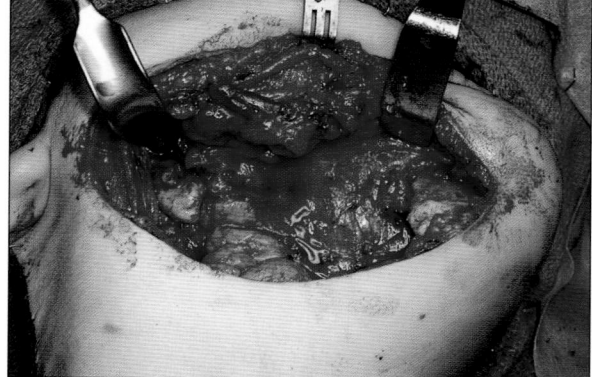

Fig 14-86d The prepared tissue bed should expose both the proximal and the distal bone segments to the height of the alveolar crest without an oral communication.

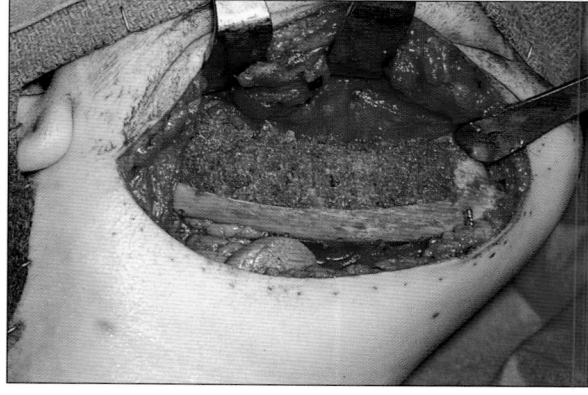

Fig 14-86e Here a freeze-dried, ethylene oxide–sterilized, allogeneic rib segment is used as containment at the inferior border for an autogenous cancellous marrow graft.

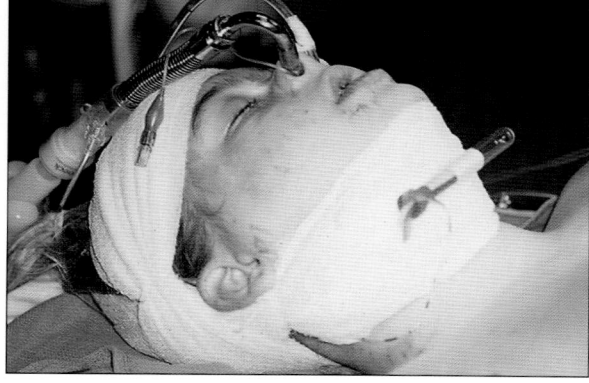

Fig 14-86f A pressure dressing and drain is recommended to stabilize and support the environment around the graft by preventing hematomas and seromas in the early course.

Reconstruction of Benign Tumor Defects of the Mandible

In most benign tumor defects, the rigid reconstruction plate provides excellent stabilization, function, and contours. It may be left in place indefinitely if there is sufficient remaining dentition and the plate itself remains stable. Therefore, bony reconstruction becomes an elective surgery that can be planned at a convenient time for the patient. The tissue itself may be re-entered when it is completely healed and mature, which takes 3 to 4 months. This permits the bone graft to be placed into a contamination-free and infection-free tissue.

In addition to an infection-free and contamination-free recipient tissue, the principles for successful bone grafting include transplantation of viable osteocompetent cells and achievement of natural contours, bone height, and stability. Therefore, autogenous cancellous marrow grafts are preferred, a transcutaneous approach is made, and maxillomandibular fixation is required.

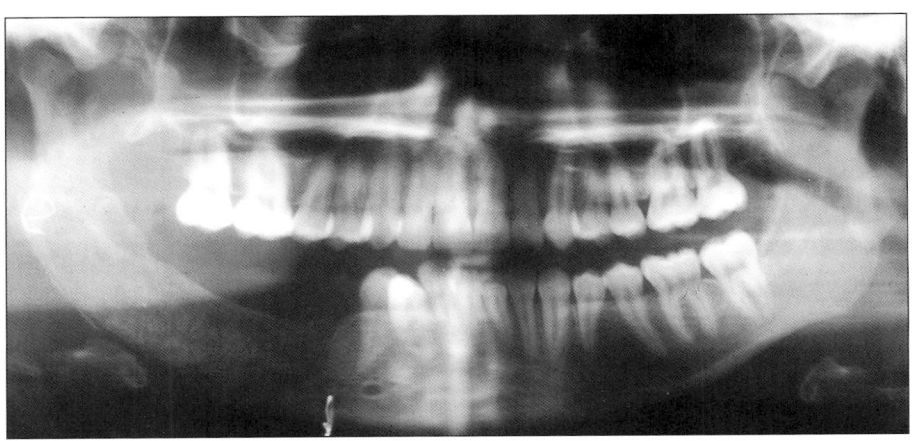

Fig 14-86g A continuity defect graft should not only reestablish continuity but also achieve a normal alveolar bone height and contour.

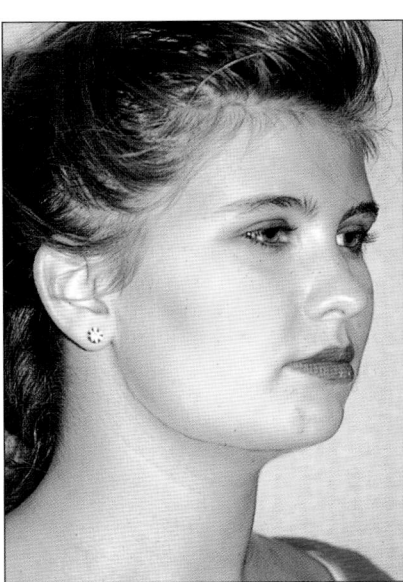

Fig 14-86h A completed mandibular reconstruction should support facial contours and appearance and at the same time provide sufficient bone for prosthetic rehabilitation.

The host bone and reconstruction plate are approached through an incision within a natural fold in the neck (Fig 14-86a). If a plate is already present, there will be an avascular scar band around the plate (Fig 14-86b). This scar band measures 440 µm (0.44 mm) in thickness (Fig 14-86c), which is more than twice the distance that oxygen and nutrients can diffuse from a capillary, and therefore should be excised. This is facilitated by removing the plate and then replacing it using the same screws in their respective holes. The periosteum on each side of the defect requires a reflection for a distance of 4 cm and should be scored to gain a maximum release for developing the graft bed (Fig 14-86d).

With the mandible in maxillomandibular fixation and a crib for graft containment in place, the cancellous marrow is compacted into the defect (Fig 14-86e). Today the rigid reconstruction plates are most often used as the crib containment because of their rigidity and the fact that they have already been in place and achieved good contours and occlusion. In this situation the neck fascia about the submandibular gland and the anterior digastric muscle are sutured to the plate holes to create the containment barrier for the graft. Because of the internal stability of the reconstruction plate in such cases, maxillomandibular fixation can be released after just 3 weeks. As an alternative, allogeneic bone cribs can be used as a resorbable graft containment. Freeze-dried allogeneic split-rib segments, ilium forms, and mandible specimens are available from tissue banks certified by the American Association of Tissue Banks (AATB). Once shaped and contoured, these serve as excellent cribs that resorb over 6 months to 3 years. The autogenous cancellous marrow graft is placed into the crib once it is in place and fixated. Such cribs should be trimmed to allow sufficient access for vascular ingrowth. Since allogeneic bone cribs are not truly rigid, maxillomandibular fixation is required for 6 weeks (Figs 14-86f to 14-86h).

Spontaneous Bone Regeneration in Youth

Individuals younger than 17 years retain sufficient native bone regenerative capability so that bone grafting may be unnecessary (Figs 14-87a to 14-87g). The younger the individual, the more probable and more complete will be the spontaneous regeneration of bone from the endosteum of each resection edge, from residual periosteum, and from circulatory stem cells attracted to the defect by the growth factors

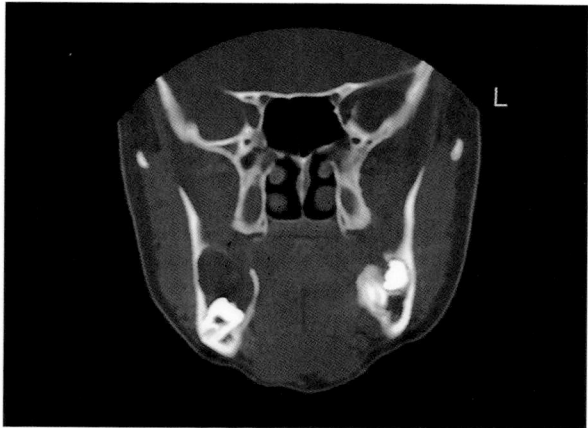

Fig 14-87a Significant bone resorption due to an ameloblastoma in a 15-year-old patient. After resection, bone grafting may not be necessary because of spontaneous host bone regeneration.

Fig 14-87b Perforation of the cortex due to ameloblastoma extension in this 15-year-old patient necessitated removal of the periosteum via a supraperiosteal resection.

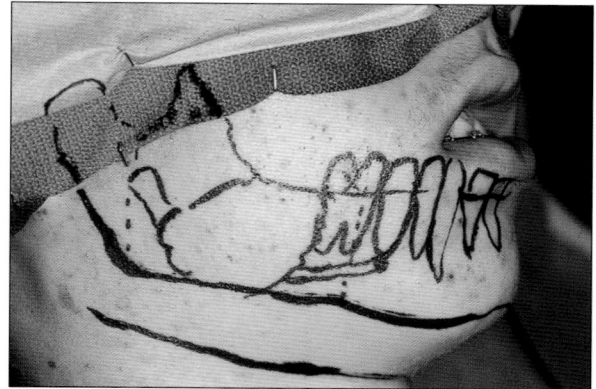

Fig 14-87c Outline of the planned resection using 1.0- to 1.5-cm bone margins and plans for nerve preservation via the pull-back approach.

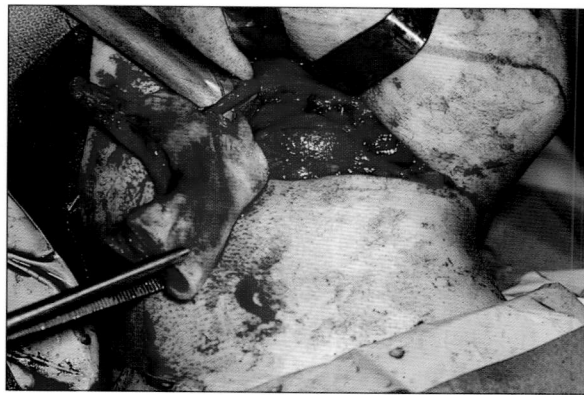

Fig 14-87d Resection of the tumor as viewed from the lingual side, where the inferior alveolar nerve is pulled back through the lingula.

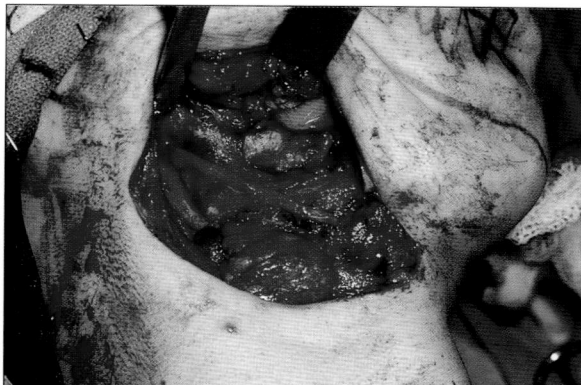

Fig 14-87e The proximal segment of inferior alveolar nerve in the defect prior to re-anastomosis to the distal nerve segment.

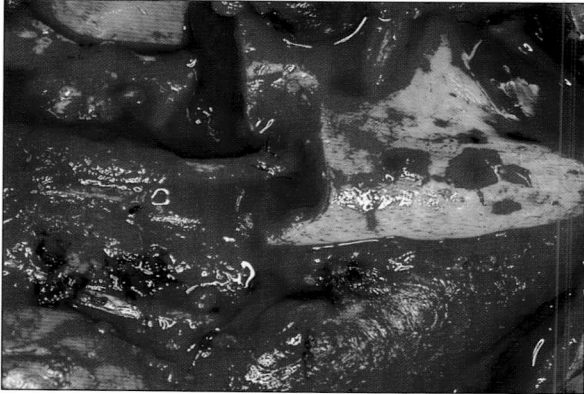

Fig 14-87f Re-anastomosis of inferior alveolar nerve with 7-0 or 8-0 nylon sutures.

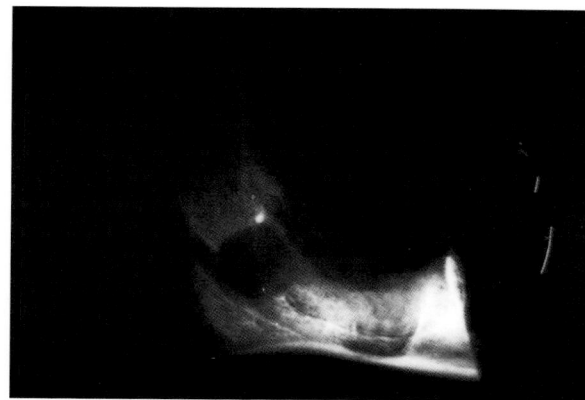

Fig 14-87g Radiograph of the resected specimen indicating radiographically clear margins.

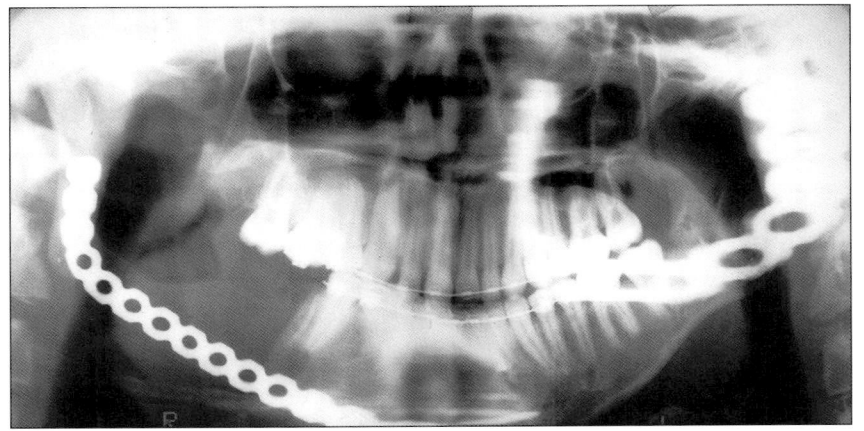

Fig 14-87h The reconstruction plate spans the defect and maintains the patient's occlusion and facial form. This radiograph, taken at 1 week, also shows the defect size.

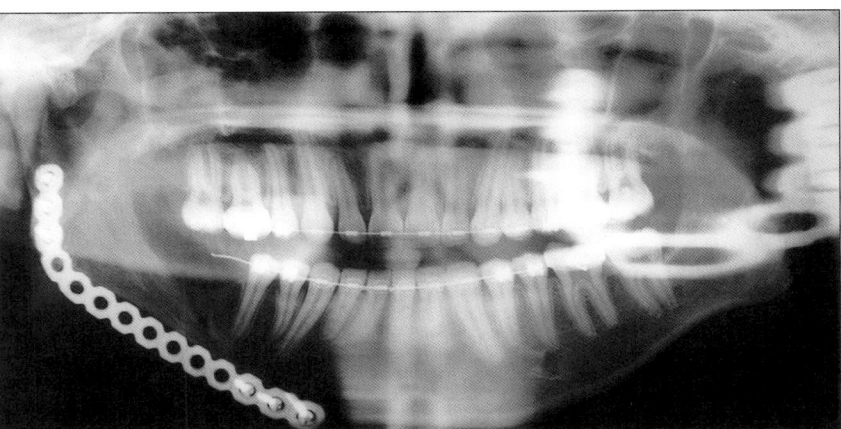

Fig 14-87i By 6 months, significant spontaneous bone regeneration is evident.

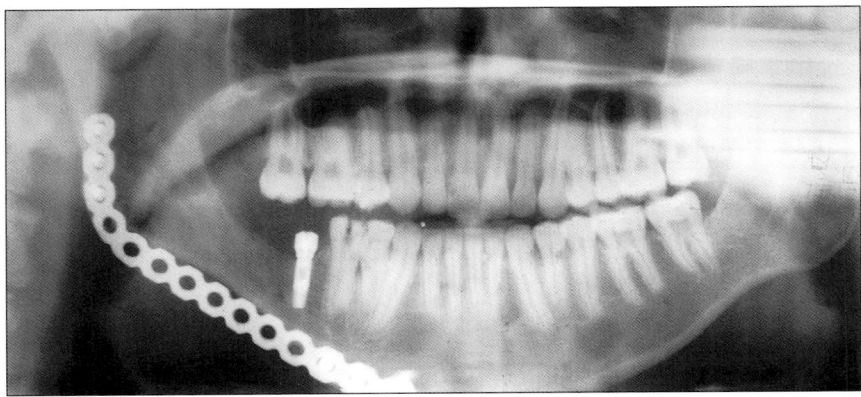

Fig 14-87j By 1 year bone has fully regenerated across the defect and has formed sufficient alveolar bone height to accommodate a dental implant.

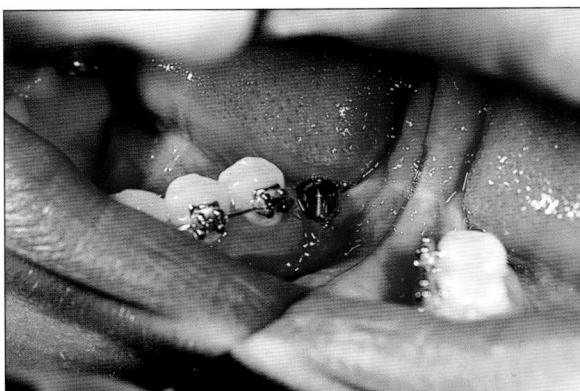

Fig 14-87k Mirror view of the dental implant shown in Fig 14-87j.

in the blood clot after resection. Therefore, in this age group the reconstruction plate is left in place for 1 year (Fig 14-87h). After 1 year the reconstruction plate is removed, and either no bone graft will be required (Fig 14-87i), a much smaller bone graft than the original defect will be required, or a complete bone graft will be required. The spontaneously regenerated native bone is fully viable and functional and may receive osseointegrated dental implants as well as grow with the patient (Figs 14-87j and 14-87k).

In cases where postresection infections have occurred, in cases of multiple surgeries, or in cases where postresection radiotherapy was used, spontaneous bone regeneration will not occur.

Preservation of the Inferior Alveolar Nerve

Decortication Approach

In peripheral resections as well as some continuity resections, the inferior alveolar nerve can be preserved. Safe tumor-surgery principles do not usually allow for preservation of the inferior alveolar nerve, and acceptance of its extirpation to maintain a curative surgery and prevent tumor seeding is the general rule. However, odontogenic neoplasms lack the enzyme processes that cause intraneural invasion; this is why these neoplasms displace the neurovascular bundle and the bony mandibular canal rather than invade them. It is also why sensory changes are not seen even in large benign tumors that completely envelop the nerve. If the neurovascular bundle is at least 1 cm from the tumor in a peripheral resection,

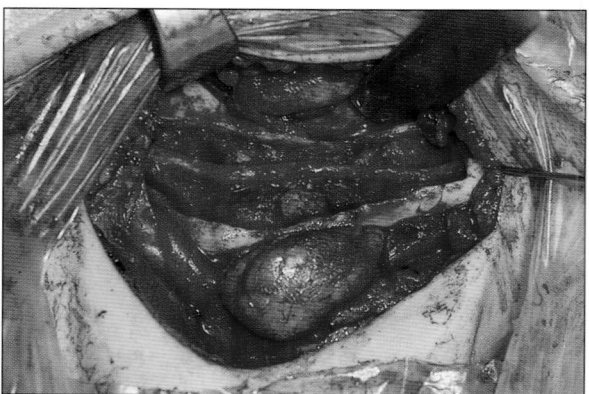

Fig 14-88a On rare occasions, the inferior alveolar nerve may be preserved by decortication and nerve displacement without dissecting through the tumor to risk tumor seeding.

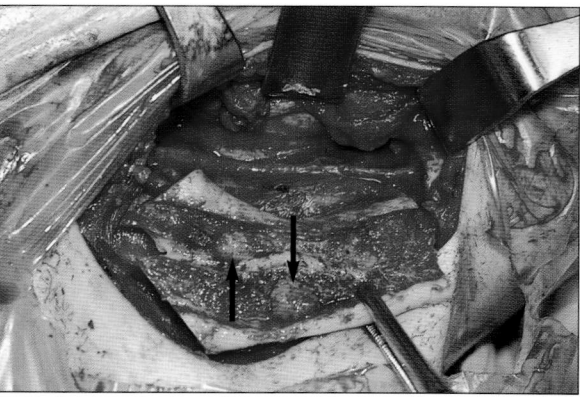

Fig 14-88b This recurrent ameloblastoma has recurred in two locations (*arrows*) and has displaced the neurovascular bundle without invading it.

it can logically be preserved. It can also be preserved if the neurovascular bundle can be isolated and displaced from the resection without dissecting through tumor (Figs 14-88a and 14-88b). This occasionally can be accomplished by a local labial decortication and nerve retraction via nerve hooks if the tumor has not encompassed the nerve, requiring dissection through the tumor. If the tumor is entered or exposed, the en-bloc principle is violated, and seeding potential followed by tumor recurrence becomes a significant concern. It is then best to include the neurovascular bundle in the resection and consider acceptance of this sensory loss or accomplish nerve grafting.

Nerve Pullout Approach

Another recently advanced resective approach has allowed a return of lip sensation superior to that of a nerve graft without the need to harvest a nerve graft. This approach also takes advantage of these tumors' inability to invade nerve epineurium. The technique requires, in applicable cases, transsecting the nerve at the mental foramen (Figs 14-89a and 14-89b). Next, a lateral decortication is accomplished posterior to the intended posterior resection margin to identify the nerve, or the nerve is identified at the lingula. In most cases, the transsected nerve can be pulled out of the specimen with ease (Fig 14-89c). If there are several teeth in the specimen, neurovascular fibers leaving the inferior alveolar neurovascular bundle to enter the root apices may not permit release of the nerve. However, the nerve can be released without the tumor contacting the tissue bed if both resections are performed so that the specimen becomes pedicled on the neurovascular bundle. A small sterile drape is placed underneath the specimen to cover the tissue bed. The specimen is then safely decorticated to transsect the fibers entering the roots so that the nerve can be pulled out of the lingula. Both the specimen and sterile drape can then be delivered from the field without spilling tumor cells onto the tissue. The native nerve is then anastomosed back to the resection stump at the mental foramen. Because the procedure involves a single epineurial anastomosis of a native nerve with an obviously matching number of fascicles and diameter, the return of sensation is superior to that of a nerve graft, and there is no donor site neurosensory loss (Figs 14-89d and 14-89e). The return of subjective and objective sensation varies with age but ranges between 80% and 95%. Odontogenic benign tumors do not adhere to the epineurium, allowing this nerve-preserving single anastomosis to be used in selected cases without risking recurrence.

Nerve Grafting

Nerve grafting is potentially possible in most resections of the mandible for benign tumors and for some malignant tumors. On one hand, patients usually tolerate a complete anesthesia of the lip and chin very

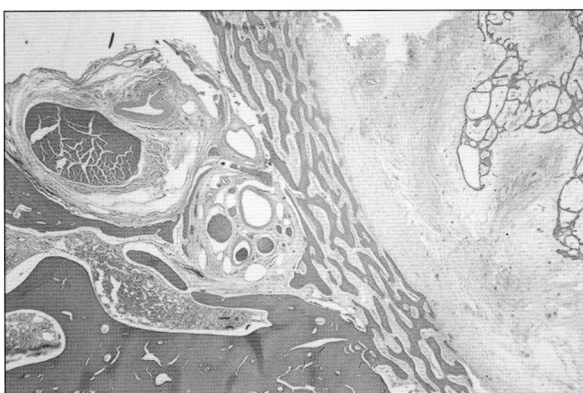

Fig 14-89a A cross-section of a resected mandible will show a displaced neurovascular bundle and the amelo-blastoma lacking direct neural invasion.

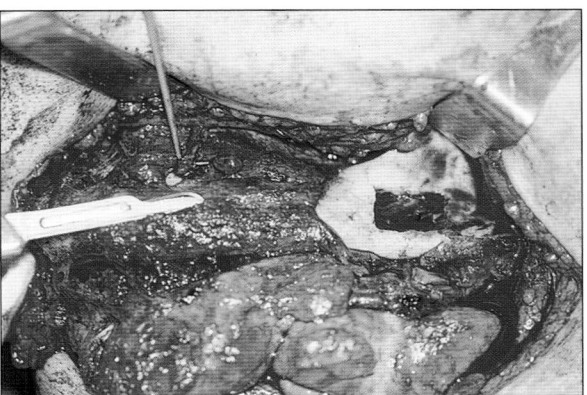

Fig 14-89b The recent development of the nerve pull-out technique at the University of Miami isolates and protects the nerve at the proximal resection margin and transsects the nerve at the distal resection margin or at the mental foramen.

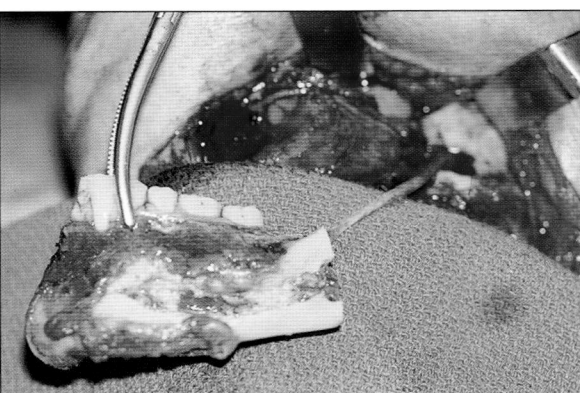

Fig 14-89c The nerve (neurovascular bundle) is "pulled out" of the specimen without tumor adherence due to lack of neural invasion.

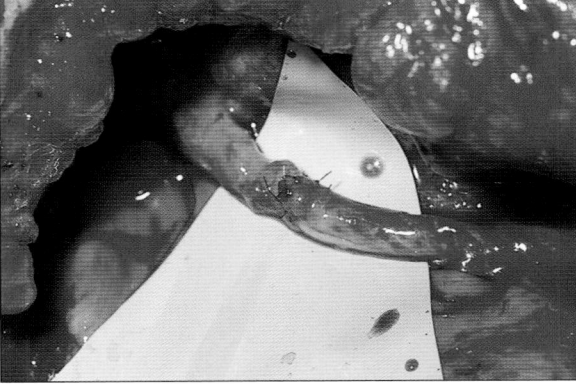

Fig 14-89d The parent nerve is then re-anastomosed under magnification using a 7-0 nylon suture on a BV-130-5 needle as an epineurial approximation.

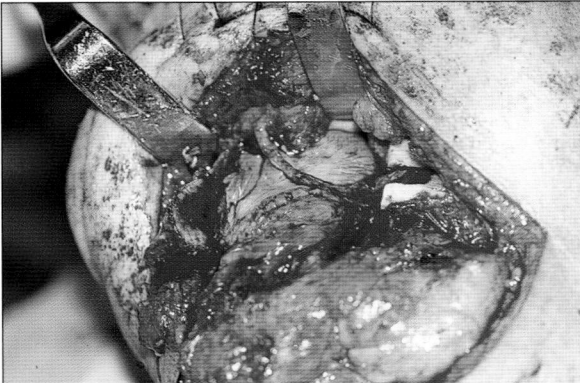

Fig 14-89e The re-anastomosed nerve is left passive in the wound while the oral and neck closures are accomplished.

well after resection, making nerve grafting an elective surgery that requires a gain-vs-loss decision by the patient. On the other hand, the ideal time to perform a nerve graft is immediately, and patients with odontogenic neoplasms are usually the best candidates because of their youth, lack of radiotherapy, and usually good systemic health. The greater auricular nerve, which can yield 6 to 8 cm of nerve length, and the sural nerve, which can yield 12 to 18 cm of nerve length, are the common donor sites.

When a nerve graft is performed, its length must be at least 1.5 times the length of the gap between the proximal and distal nerve ends (Fig 14-90a). Tension on a nerve anastomosis greatly reduces the return of sensation. The grafts themselves are usually sutured to the parent nerve with 8-0 nylon sutures with a tapered needle that has a cutting tip. A needle commonly used for these anastomoses is a BV-130-5 (Ethicon). The anastomosis is accomplished under the operating microscope or 3× or greater loops in an epineurial closure. While the greater auricular nerve is a local nerve, the sural nerve is more ideal because of its larger diameter and length. The yield is a 50% to 70% return of subjective sensation in the lip. Occasionally, the lack of 100% sensation is interpreted as a painful dysesthesia or an annoying sensation. The option of nerve grafting, with its trade-off of donor site sensory loss vs a 50% to 70% possible return of lip-chin sensation, is a matter of patient choice, but one that should be reasonably offered and discussed.

The technique to harvest the sural nerve requires a prone or lateral patient positioning. The non-dominant leg is chosen for the harvest and is prepared in a sterile manner from the foot below the ankle

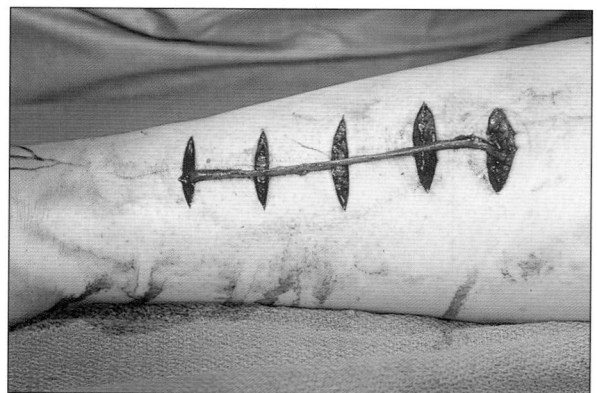

Fig 14-90a A sural nerve graft requires both a proximal and a distal epineurial approximation. The nerve graft length should be 1.5 times the defect length to assure a tension-free anastomosis.

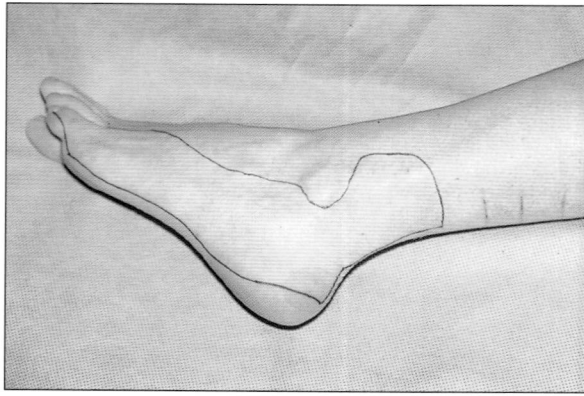

Fig 14-90b The area of anticipated sensory nerve loss is outlined and discussed with the patient prior to the harvest and use of a sural nerve graft.

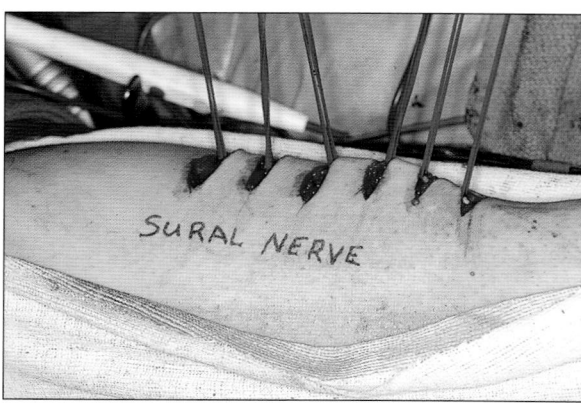

Fig 14-90c The sural nerve here is isolated and retracted with vessel loops through parallel incisions on the posterior calf.

Fig 14-90d The sural nerve has been transsected distally and separated from the subcutaneous tissues of the calf up to the most proximal incision.

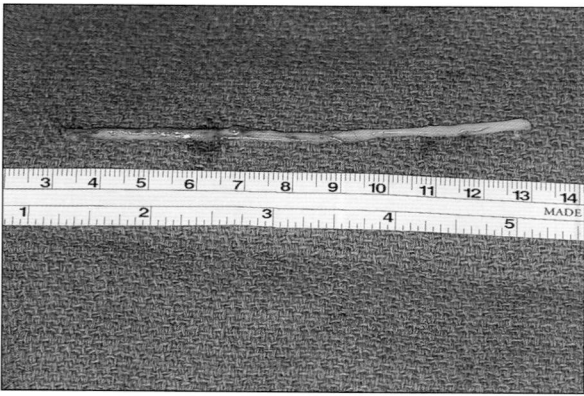

Fig 14-90e At least 11 cm of sural nerve has been harvested for the graft of a 7-cm defect.

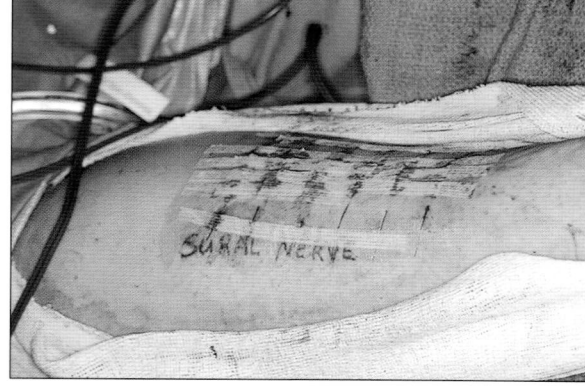

Fig 14-90f The closure and incision design will prevent a vertical scar contraction down the calf, which can be painful when walking.

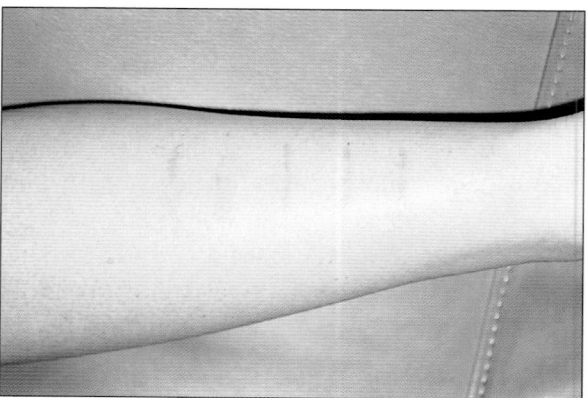

Fig 14-90g The serial horizontal incisions are also minimally visable once healed and mature.

to the popliteal fossa. The sural nerve will course down the midline of the calf. It emerges between the two heads of the gastrocnemius muscle and runs a course of about 22 cm before deviating laterally and ramifying into several branches 4 cm above the ankle. The nerve runs more superficially as it progresses down the calf and will course in the subcutaneous layer in the surgical field. Beginning in the midline 4 cm above the level of the ankle, horizontal incisions about 3 cm in length are made parallel to each other and about 3 cm apart for a distance corresponding to the required nerve graft length (Figs 14-90b and

14-90c). Vertical blunt dissection will identify a distinct round nerve just slightly larger in diameter than the inferior alveolar nerve. A small vein may course parallel to the nerve. Blunt dissection is used to free the nerve from adventitial tissues at and between the parallel incisions. The nerve is transsected at its desired distalmost point. It is then pulled proximally from the distalmost horizontal incision sequentially through each next proximal incision until the desired nerve length is freed and externalized (Fig 14-90d). The proximal end can then be transsected to deliver the graft specimen (Fig 14-90e). The transsected residual nerve stump heals without pain or the development of a neuroma. Each incision is closed in layers (Figs 14-90f and 14-90g).

Benign Odontogenic Neoplasms of the Maxilla

When one of the four odontogenic neoplasms occurs in the maxilla, the resection principles that require 1.0- to 1.5-cm bony margins, one uninvolved anatomic barrier around the bone, and frozen section documentation of tumor-free margins are the same as those used in the mandible. The procedure is often termed a *hemimaxillectomy* or a *partial maxillectomy* but differs from the maxillectomies performed for salivary gland tumors and epithelial malignancies because most of the mucosa is preserved. As with mandibular resections for benign odontogenic neoplasms, only mucosa that is directly infiltrated by tumor is removed. The procedure is thus best termed a *submucosal partial maxillary resection*.

Transoral Approach

Most maxillary odontogenic neoplasms can be approached transorally. The incision begins around the gingival sulci of the teeth in dentate individuals or the midcrest in edentulous individuals. If the tumor extends into or through the mucosa in the alveolar ridge area, it is included in the resection by directing the incision around the area. The dissection plane may be subperiosteal or supraperiosteal depending on CT scan evidence of tumor extension. Labial and palatal flaps are thus developed. The lateral bony wall of the nose, the nasal side periosteum, or in some cases the nasal mucosa can serve as the nasal anatomic barrier. The orbital floor or ethmoids are rarely involved by primary odontogenic tumors that are not recurrences caused by previous seeding into these areas; the sinus roof periosteum usually serves as an effective anatomic barrier in these situations.

The bony resection will begin through a tooth socket, which allows for a 1.0- to 1.5-cm margin from the radiographic extent of the tumor and at least one half of a tooth socket from the adjacent tooth (Fig 14-91a). It is advisable to avoid a resection through a central incisor socket or the maxillary midline suture. Prosthetic rehabilitation is greatly compromised by a resection that requires matching bone height and teeth to a single central incisor. Therefore, a general rule is either to leave or to remove both central incisors. The resection extends vertically from the chosen tooth socket to just below the infraorbital nerve or infraorbital rim and is turned laterally, preserving the infraorbital nerve; the infraorbital rim, if possible; and the body of the zygoma. The resection usually proceeds through the zygomatic-maxillary buttress to the pterygomaxillary fissure. The maxilla is separated from the pterygoid plates with curved osteotomes as in a Le Fort I osteotomy. The resection specimen with the tumor in it can then be downfractured, again as in a Le Fort I osteotomy, to complete the posterior bone separation with osteotomes to deliver the specimen (Fig 14-91b). The removed specimen should be carefully examined for areas that may indicate residual tumor in the wound. If there is an area where the tumor seems to have been cut through or entered, the corresponding area in the wound bed needs to be excised and documented as tumor-free with frozen sections.

The resultant wound is best closed primarily by reapproximating the labial and palatal flaps with a layered closure and supported by a maxillary-palatal splint. Placement of an immediate bone graft or a tissue spacer may be tempting but is not advised. This type of wound has significant dead space. With dead space and the forces of gravity, small tissue dehiscences are not uncommon. If the wound bed has no foreign body or graft material within it, a dehiscence usually granulates and heals rapidly. If there is a tissue

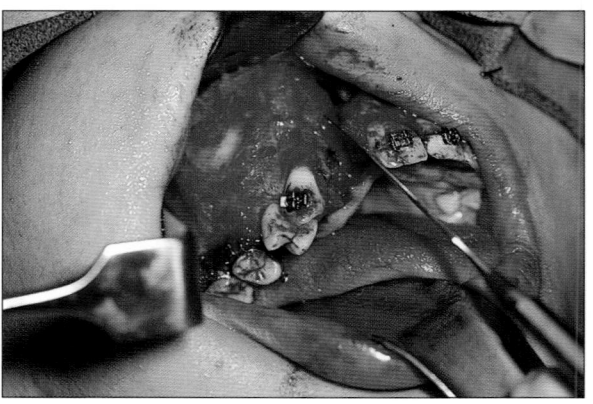

Fig 14-91a A transoral submucosal maxillary resection preserves the uninvolved mucosa overlying the tumor with buccal and palatal flaps. The resection begins through a tooth socket appropriate for 1.0- to 1.5-cm margins and leaves one half of the socket adjacent to the anterior teeth.

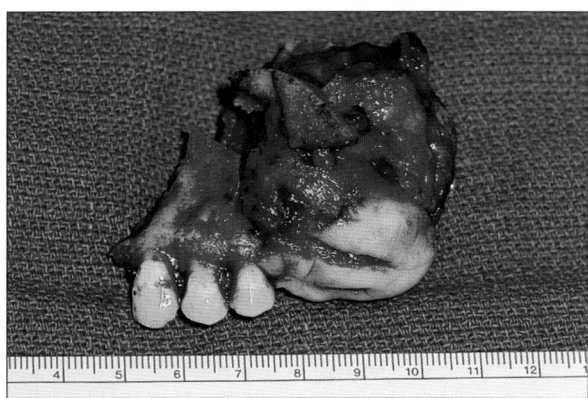

Fig 14-91b In a transoral maxillary resection, the specimen is delivered once the buccal and palatal ostectomies are made, and the pterygoid plates are either included or separated from the maxilla as in a Le Fort I osteotomy.

spacer or graft material within it, infection and persistent drainage usually continue until the wound bed is debrided. After the soft tissue heals, an early bony reconstruction can be performed, most often about 3 months after the resection, with reduced infection risks.

Transcutaneous (Weber-Ferguson) Approach

A transcutaneous or Weber-Ferguson approach to a benign odontogenic neoplasm is called for less frequently than is a transoral approach. The three primary indications for this approach are when the tumor threatens extension into the ethmoids; when it extends beyond the posterior wall of the maxillary sinus into the pterygomaxillary space; or when it extends into the orbit (Fig 14-92). In such cases, the extended access afforded by a Weber-Ferguson approach is of great value and worth the cosmetic compromise that may result. To minimize the problems of concave cheek deformity, retraction of cupid's bow, and the lip notching sometimes seen, the surgeon must adhere to certain principles of this incision. The basic Weber-Ferguson approach is an upper lip–split approach in which an infraorbital incision is carried medially to the nasal bone area and then extended around the lateral curvature of the nose and alar base to split the upper lip and join an oral incision. A precise Weber-Ferguson incision should take advantage of the highest infraorbital skin fold and be placed above the level of bony resection. If the skin incision is placed over bone that is later resected, it will tend to contract into the defect. As the incision progresses medially, the turn at the nasal bone area should be rounded. Pointed geometry in this location may result in loss of the tip of this flap. As the incision courses around the nose and alar base, it is best to keep it 1 to 2 mm away from the alar crease. Although it is tempting to keep incisions in skin creases, an incision in the alar crease will contract greatly, creating an asymmetry of the alar flare (Fig 14-93). As the incision splits the lip, it is better to course through the ridge of the philtrum rather than the midline. The para-alar incision is thus carried to the philtrum ridge, where a 90-degree turn is made to vertically course through the lip to the height of cupid's bow. At this point, another 90-degree turn is made along the vermilion-cutaneous margin to the midline, where the vermilion is split (Figs 14-94a and 14-94b). In this fashion, the healing will have a reduced retraction of the lip and cupid's bow because the incision design acts somewhat like a Z-plasty, breaking up the contraction vectors. It is also important to ensure that the transsection of the orbicularis oris muscle is precisely reapproximated during closure and if possible leaves some bony support at the alar base area (Figs 14-94c and 14-94d).

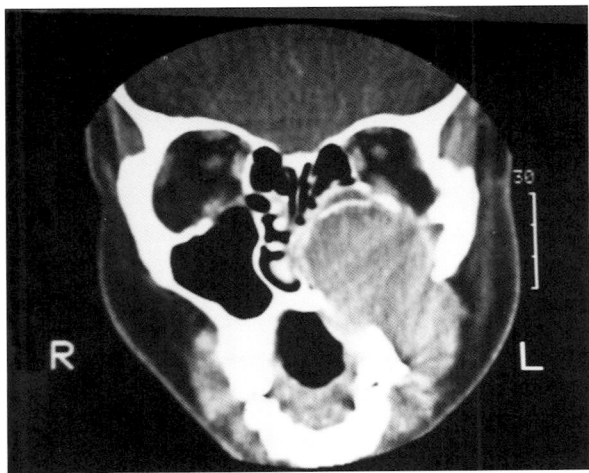

Fig 14-92 A Weber-Ferguson approach is indicated because of the tumor's extension into the ethmoids and orbit.

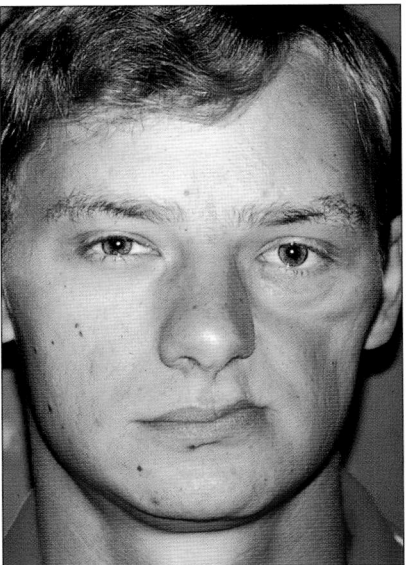

Fig 14-93 Prominent nasal-alar retraction and asymmetry resultant from a Weber-Ferguson incision incorrectly placed into the alar crease, and a lip-split through the midline rather than the philtrum ridge and vermilion-cutaneous junction.

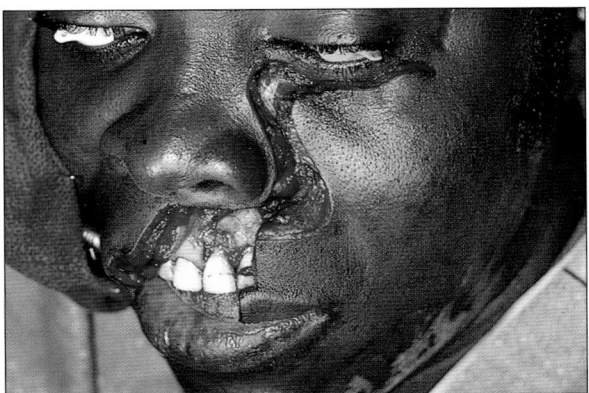

Fig 14-94a Correct design and placement of a Weber-Ferguson incision to approach a large benign maxillary neoplasm.

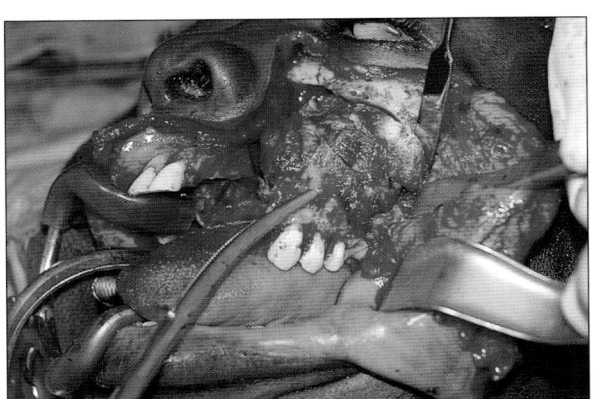

Fig 14-94b The Weber-Ferguson incision provides wide and direct visual access for the resection of a large maxillary ameloblastoma.

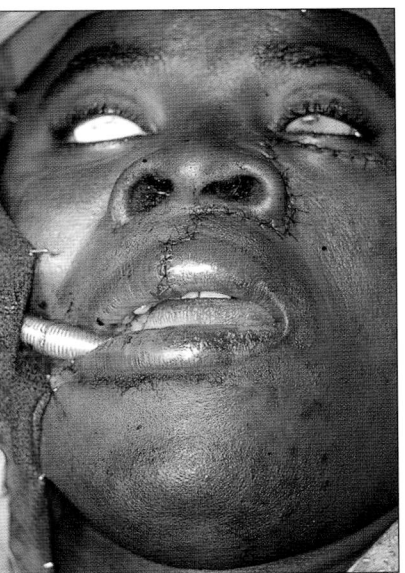

Fig 14-94c The lip closure of a Weber-Ferguson incision must accurately approximate the orbicularis oris muscle and align the vermilion-cutaneous junction.

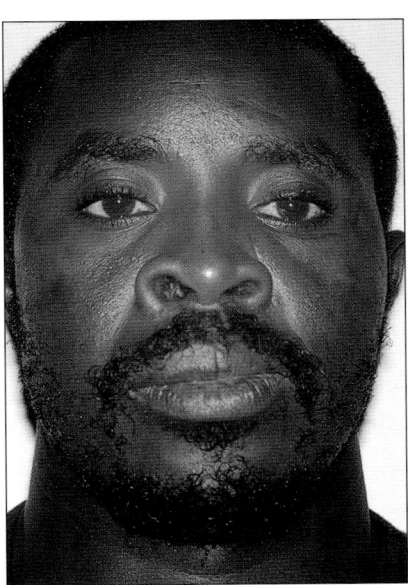

Fig 14-94d A well-designed Weber-Ferguson approach to a maxillary tumor will result in only minimal lip retraction and reduction of the alar flare.

These external incisions are connected to the mucosal incisions at the midline area. The oral mucosal incisions are the same as those used for a transoral approach; therefore aside from the Weber-Ferguson approach, the tumor extirpation remains a submucosal maxillary resection.

Pigmented Lesions of Mucosa and Skin

▶ "A good surgeon is not a cosmetic surgeon but one who prevents the need for a cosmetic surgeon."
—*Robert E. Marx*

Pathologies with abnormal coloration related to the presence of pigment occur most commonly in skin and less commonly in the oral mucosa. They will span a spectrum ranging from innocuous lesions, such as the amalgam tattoo and the oral melanotic macule, to various benign nevi to life-threatening melanomas on skin or within the oral cavity. Melanocytic lesions represent the classic spectrum of pathologies that can arise from a single cell line of precursor cells. Originating from the embryonic neural crest, these precursor cells may give rise to a number of melanocytic-related pathologies of varying biologic potential, such as those noted above. This chapter describes the full range of these pathologies, from the less aggressive to the more aggressive, and, where appropriate, relates their management to their inherent biologic potential.

Pigmented lesions are a consequence of the presence of extrinsic or intrinsic substances. Of those lesions caused by extrinsic factors, the most common affecting oral mucosa is the amalgam tattoo. Other foreign substances, such as graphite, may have a similar appearance. Another type of pigmented lesion caused by extrinsic materials is that resulting from exposure to heavy metals, either by ingestion or from the environment. Substances such as bismuth, arsenic, mercury, silver, lead, and platinum are deposited as sulfides, usually in areas of inflammation such as the gingiva as a result of the metal's reaction with hydrogen sulfide, which is produced by bacterial action on organic material. Clinically, these lesions appear as a gray or blue-black line when the black granules of the sulfide are deposited within the connective tissue (Fig 15-1). Development of these lesions is influenced by the individual's level of oral hygiene. Similar dark pigmentations occur around titanium reconstruction plates over time. These are usually observed at second surgeries when the titanium plate is removed or once again uncovered. The dark pigment represents titanium oxide particles that become embedded in the avascular encapsulation around such plates (Fig 15-2).

While intrinsic pigmentation may be due to iron such as that seen in hemosiderosis or hemosiderin deposition secondary to hemorrhage, the term *pigmented lesion* usually refers to melanin pigmentation. Melanotic lesions are significant because they may represent, clinically or histologically, a potential or developing melanoma.

Melanin pigment is formed within melanocytes, which have a small, deeply staining nucleus surrounded by clear cytoplasm. Melanocytes migrate to the epidermis, dermis, hair follicles, mucosa, leptomeninges, uveal tract, and retina, where they create varying clinical shades of brown color. Within the skin, the melanocytes are found at the epidermal-dermal junction and sometimes within the dermis. Within the mucosa, they are found at the basement membrane–lamina propria junction and, to a lesser degree, in the submucosa. The relative number of melanocytes in all individuals is the same, regardless of race or degree of pigmentation, and the ratio of melanocytes to keratinocytes is 1 to 10. Differences in skin color can be attributed to more rapid melanin synthesis, coarser melanin granules, and more active melanin dispersal. Melanin synthesis takes place within melanosomes contained in the cytoplasm of the melanocyte. Within the melanosomes, tyrosinase converts tyrosine to dopamine and ultimately to

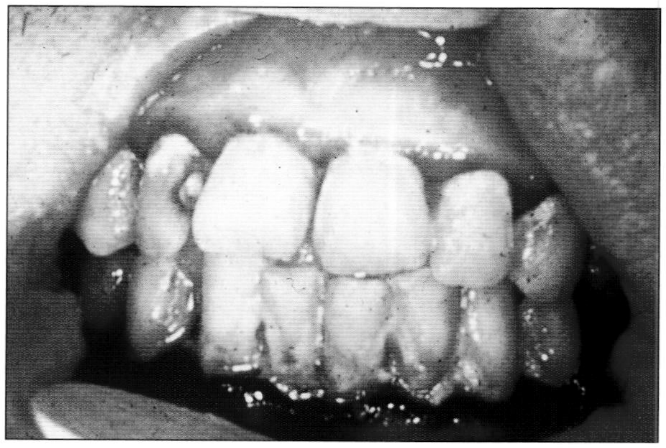

Fig 15-1 Metal sulfides of lead, silver, mercury, etc, are deposited in areas of inflammation because the hydrogen sulfide is a bacterial by-product. Here it appears as a black line on the marginal gingiva.

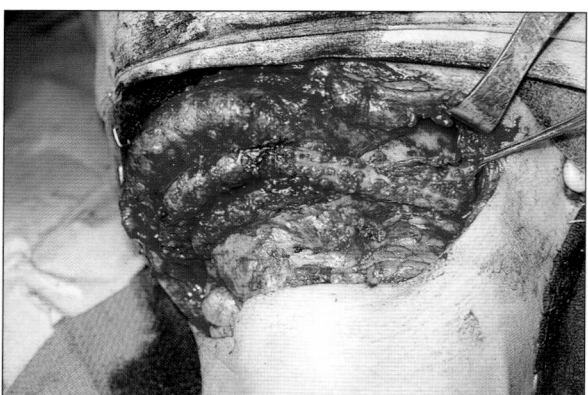

Fig 15-2 Oral and maxillofacial surgeons often observe black pigmentation in the avascular encapsulation around rigid titanium plates. This represents titanium oxide particles.

melanin. Once the melanosomes are filled with melanin, they move into the dendrites, where the tips of the dendrites are then engulfed by adjacent keratinocytes. This process is known as *apocopation*. The melanin is therefore normally transferred to the keratinocytes to produce normal skin color. Thus, in the normal production, transfer, and dispersal of melanin, melanocytes and keratinocytes function together as a unit.

There are two basic pathologic mechanisms by which melanocytic lesions develop. One mechanism relates to the excess production or the abnormal dispersal of melanin. An example of this type of lesion is the melanotic macule, which is primarily an excess of melanin production. Another type of lesion, the pigmented basal cell carcinoma, is caused by a loss of keratinocytes. These lesions are clinically pigmented because the melanin in the lost keratinocytes either remains free in the tissue or is taken up by macrophages (which are then called melanophages). Both types of lesions will feature brown-pigmented areas.

The second mechanism of melanocyte lesion development is a result of hyperplasia or neoplasia of melanocytes. In such cases, the cells involved may be epidermal melanocytes, nevus cells, or dermal melanocytes. Nevus cells are altered melanocytes that lack dendrites, retain pigment, lie in contiguity with each other, and form thèques (nests). The innate migratory nature of the melanocyte, first manifested in its journey from the neural crest, is seen in the melanocytic nevus, where migration of cells from the epidermis into the dermis is more a process of maturation than one of aggression and malignancy. The neural crest origin of melanocytes has additional significance because these precursor cells also give rise to Schwann cells and peripheral neurons. Consequently, neurogenic tumors may on occasion be pigmented. The melanocytic-neurogenic relationship is also seen in the neurotization of acquired melanocytic nevi and in the tumor's common immunohistochemical-positive reaction for S-100 protein, which is positive in nearly all nerve tumors.

The evolution of melanoma has been studied extensively, and it is generally believed that in most instances it evolves through a radial (in situ) growth phase with proliferation along the epidermal-dermal junction, in which the cells do not have a metastatic potential. It culminates in a vertical (invasive) growth phase in which a more aggressive population of cells, capable of metastasis, invades the dermis. Classifications of melanoma relate to the extent and duration of the radial growth phase. At the polar ends of the spectrum, lentigo maligna melanoma may have a prolonged radial growth phase that can extend to decades, while nodular melanomas have either an extremely short radial growth phase or none at all. Understanding these differences is extremely important, since prognosis and treatment differ significantly based on whether or not tumors are in a radial growth phase.

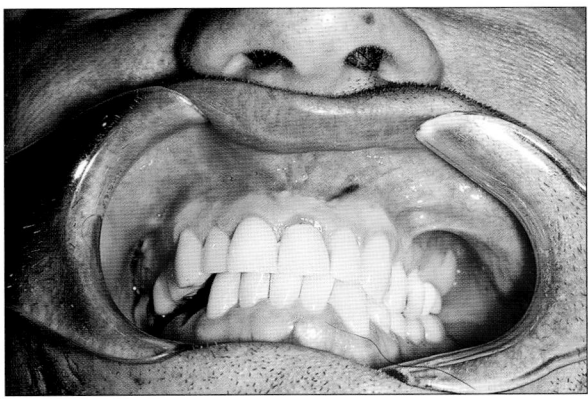

Fig 15-3a Amalgam "tattoos" associated with the high-speed handpiece removal of amalgam restorations are seen when rubber dam is not used or when amalgam particles escape during apicoectomy/retrofill surgery.

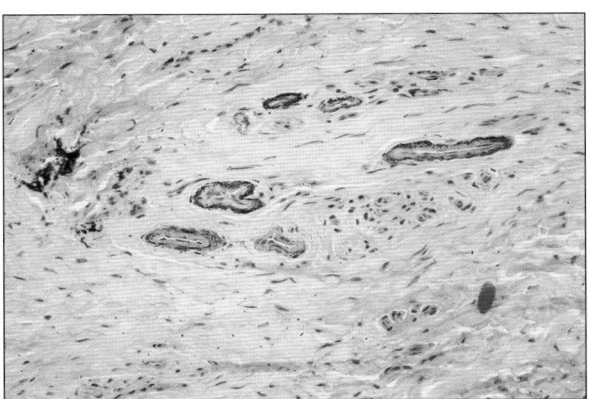

Fig 15-3b Amalgam tattoo containing amalgam particles within the connective tissue, with a concentration in the walls of blood vessels.

There is considerable disagreement concerning lesions that precede the radial growth phase. Much of this has to do with terms such as *dysplastic nevus, melanocytic dysplasia*, and *melanoma in situ*. The problem is somewhat akin to that of distinguishing oral leukoplakia and dysplasia: Some histologically aberrant lesions will proceed to carcinoma, while others will not.

Most of our understanding of melanomas has been derived from cutaneous pathology. Oral mucosal melanomas occur very infrequently, and our understanding of their biologic behavior lags far behind that of the biologic behavior of cutaneous tumors. In addition to biologic differences, the anatomy of the area presents singular problems.

Amalgam Tattoo

CLINICAL PRESENTATION AND PATHOGENESIS ▶

Nearly every dentist is familiar with the innocuous amalgam tattoo, in which fine particles of amalgam removed by high-speed dental handpieces are implanted into the mucosa below the basement membrane (Fig 15-3a). Some amalgam tattoos are actually larger coarse particles that may have become implanted or fallen into a concomitant surgical or traumatic wound during amalgam placement. Because molar amalgam restorations are often removed and replaced with cast gold restorations, most occur on the posterior alveolar ridge or gingiva. Other affected areas are the palate and buccal mucosa and more rarely the tongue and floor of the mouth.

Nearly all amalgam tattoos are asymptomatic and go unnoticed by the patient. A few rare cases have caused pain that has been traced either to peripheral nerve injury caused by the implantation of larger particles, or to local inflammation caused not by the amalgam itself but probably by surface microorganisms that became implanted with it.

Clinically, the amalgam tattoo is gray-blue and appears as part of an irregularly bordered macular lesion. The lesion is stable over time, but since most patients are unaware of its presence, only serial observations can confirm this. Occasionally, periapical radiographs confirm their metallic nature, but most amalgam tattoos are composed of particles that are too fine for plain radiographic detection.

DIFFERENTIAL DIAGNOSIS ▶

Amalgam tattoos may appear clinically similar to an early *melanoma*. Although *oral mucosal melanotic macules* are more common than *oral melanomas*, each should be considered on a differential list with melanoma primary. Other pigmented lesions worthy of consideration, though rare, are *mucosal nevi, heavy-metal pigmentations* such as lead or bismuth, and *therapeutic drug–related pigmentations* that may result from zidovudine, cyclophosphamide, or minocycline. If the lesion is located on the tongue or buccal

DIAGNOSTIC WORK-UP
AND TREATMENT ▶

HISTOPATHOLOGY ▶

PROGNOSIS ▶

CLINICAL PRESENTATION AND
PATHOGENESIS ▶

DIFFERENTIAL DIAGNOSIS ▶

DIAGNOSTIC WORK-UP
AND TREATMENT ▶

mucosa, a *mucocele* might be a consideration as might other small, diffuse, blue lesions, such as *hemangiomas* and even *low-grade mucoepidermoid carcinomas*.

As a general rule, all pigmented mucosal lesions should undergo biopsy; the amalgam tattoo may represent the only exception to that rule. Provided that the lesion is not elevated, increasing in size, or darkening, it may be clinically diagnosed and observed by the experienced clinician. Any doubtful or suspicious lesions require biopsy.

Although amalgam particles constitute a foreign body, there is usually no tissue reaction to their presence. Fine black particles can be found along collagen fibers or in vessel walls, and gold to brown pigmentation of collagen also is seen (Fig 15-3b). Sometimes coarse black granules are seen, and occasionally an inflammatory reaction occurs, particularly when the particles are large. Reactive fibrosis may be seen, and rarely there may be a granulomatous reaction.

Amalgam particles are indigestible by tissue macrophages. Like decorative tattoos, amalgam tattoos are permanent and will not fade with time. Any movement or change in color should be looked on with some suspicion, and a biopsy should be undertaken.

Melanotic Macule

The term *oral melanotic macule* is used mostly as a descriptive term to describe flat brown-to-black mucosal pigmentations associated with diseases such as Peutz-Jeghers syndrome and Addison disease. However, a number of melanotic macules occur randomly with no association with other diseases. These melanotic macules are idiopathic and may be conceptualized as the rare mucosal corollary to the much more common skin freckle (ephelis), although the melanotic macule does not darken in response to sun exposure as does the skin freckle. Usually single or small numbers of flat brown-to-black pigmented areas, the macules are small in size (usually 2 to 4 mm) and rarely become larger than 1 cm. They are most commonly seen on the lower lip vermilion or on the attached gingiva, but they can occur on any oral site (Fig 15-4a).

Idiopathic melanotic macules are variations of normal mucosal pigmentation. They represent little more than a focal area of the mucosa where the resident melanocytes have produced a greater amount of melanin. Because the melanocytes are mature and do not dedifferentiate, they are not premalignant and cannot transform into a melanoma.

The most important lesion to distinguish from a melanotic macule is an early *melanoma*. Although most oral melanomas will be black or blue and will more characteristically have varying shades of brown to black within them, early melanomas may appear as homogeneous as melanotic macules. The most common lesion that may appear similar to a melanotic macule is an *amalgam tattoo*. The *oral nevus* is also a consideration and will be clinically identical, but this lesion is very rare.

Single lesions should undergo excisional biopsy to rule out melanoma. The early identification of a small melanoma would dramatically improve the prognosis in a case with an otherwise poor prognosis. If the biopsy confirms the diagnosis of a melanotic macule, its value is piece of mind for patient and practitioner as well as the elimination of doubt.

When multiple lesions are present, it is often prudent to biopsy one or two lesions. Choose the largest, darkest, most raised (if any are raised), and most irregularly bordered ones to undergo biopsy. If the biopsy confirms more than one melanotic macule, a screening work-up for Peutz-Jeghers syndrome and Addison disease is required. For Peutz-Jeghers syndrome, an upper gastrointestinal contrast series and endoscopy from esophagus to ileum will identify the presence or confirm the absence of hamartomatous polyp formation. For Addison disease, the patient's skin color may be generally bronzed and the patient may show signs of weakness, fatigue, and orthostatic hypotension. Generally, their resting blood pressure is also low (90/70 is not uncommon), and they are usually hyponatremic ($Na^+ < 130$ mEq/L [< 130 mmol/L]), hyperkalemic ($K^+ > 5.0$ mEq/L), hypoglycemic (fasting blood glucose < 70 mg/100

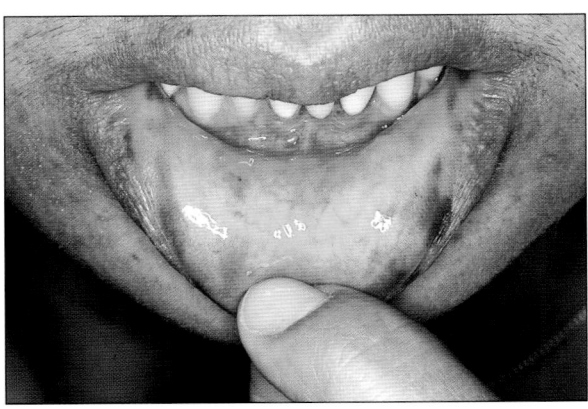

Fig 15-4a The lower lip vermilion is the most common location for a melanotic macule, which will appear as a small, flat, brown-black area.

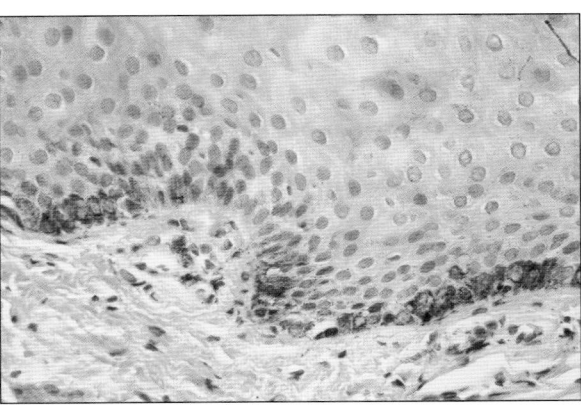

Fig 15-4b A melanotic macule showing increased melanin pigment within the basal keratinocytes. Some pigment may also be seen within melanophages of the underlying connective tissue.

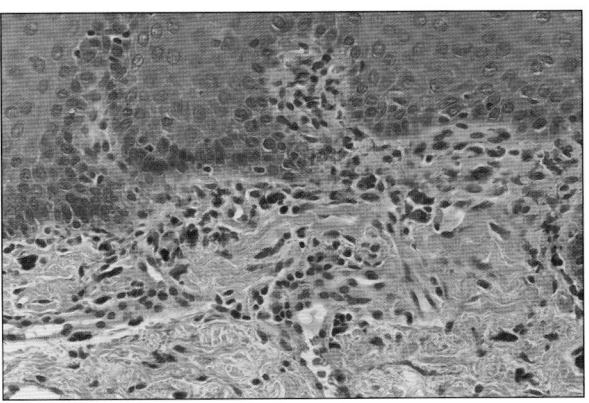

Fig 15-4c A melanotic macule showing only numerous melanophages within the corium.

dL), and often have an elevated blood urea nitrogen (BUN) (> 20 mg/100 dL) due to their adrenocortical insufficiency.

HISTOPATHOLOGY ▶

Melanotic macules are characterized by an increase in the production of melanin by a normal number of melanocytes. Consequently, there is pigmentation of the basal keratinocytes, which are increased in relation to the normal adjacent epithelium (Fig 15-4b). Melanophages may also be seen within the lamina propria and may sometimes be the only location of the melanin pigment (Fig 15-4c). The epithelial architecture is normal. The melanotic macule is distinguished from lentigo simplex, which more commonly affects the skin and only rarely the mucosa and shows a benign hyperplasia of melanocytes, pigmentation of basal keratinocytes, and elongation of rete ridges.

PROGNOSIS ▶

Excision is diagnostic but may also result in removal of idiopathic melanotic macules. Macules associated with Peutz-Jeghers syndrome or Addison disease may seem to recur from newly emerging lesions related to the parent disease.

Peutz-Jeghers Syndrome

CLINICAL PRESENTATION ▶

Peutz-Jeghers syndrome is an autosomal-dominant trait that produces the general findings of skin and/or mucosal melanotic macules with intestinal polyposis. Most individuals are young (20 to 30 years) at the time of diagnosis. About 45% have a family history of both intestinal polyps and melanotic macules, and 15% have a history of melanotic macules alone. About 35% of patients have no familial history; their cases probably represent new mutations.

Polyposis of the gastrointestinal tract, the most important feature of the syndrome, may produce symptoms. Numerous polyps may produce intussusception (prolapse of one portion of the intestine into the lumen of an adjacent portion), which is usually self-resolving but may lead to intestinal obstruction, causing pain, bowel damage, bleeding, or even death. About 80% of individuals develop some type of gastrointestinal signs or symptoms (intermittent pain, 85%; melena, 35%; and anemia from blood loss, 20%). What were once thought to be benign hamartomatous polyps limited to the small intestines are now recognized to involve all portions of the gastrointestinal tract (jejunum, 65%; ileum, 55%; large intestine, 35%; rectum, 35%; stomach, 23%; and duodenum, 15%) and to have a much higher malignant potential than previously thought. Newer studies have shown a malignancy transformation rate of 20% to 40%, and only the adenomatous polyps transformed into a malignancy. The hamartomatous polyps represent-

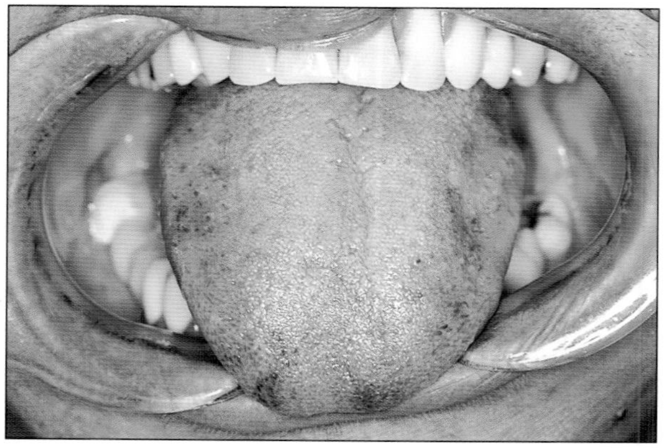

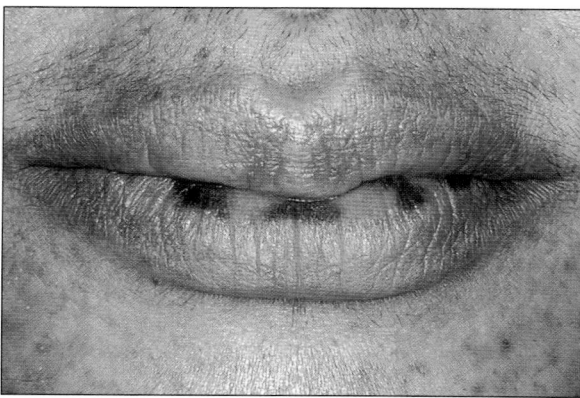

Fig 15-5a Multiple perioral skin and oral mucosal melanotic macules are common in Peutz-Jeghers syndrome.

Fig 15-5b Melanotic macules on lower lip vermilion in Peutz-Jeghers syndrome.

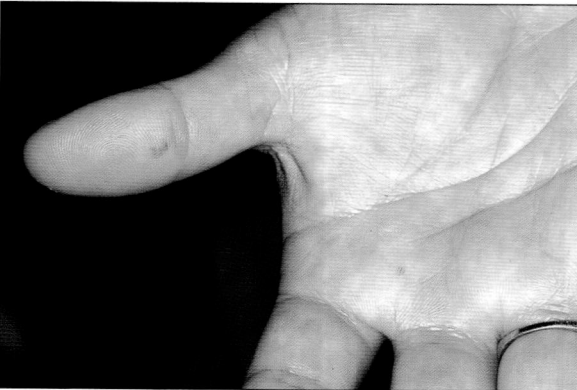

Fig 15-5c In addition to oral and perioral locations, melanotic macules are frequently seen on the hands of individuals with Peutz-Jeghers syndrome.

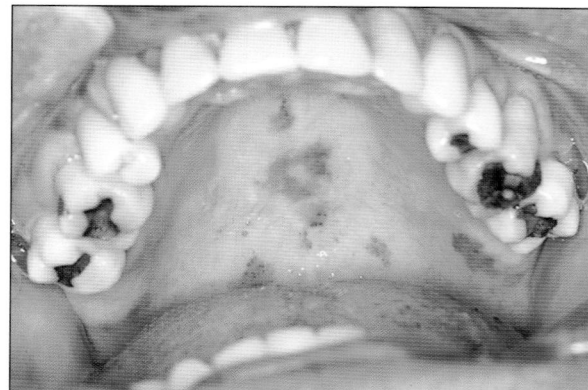

Fig 15-5d The palate is another common location to look for melanotic macules in Peutz-Jeghers syndrome.

ing focal intestinal wall overgrowths of mixed architecture do not become malignant. The adenomatous polyps that transformed into adenocarcinomas did so slowly, usually taking 15 to 30 years.

In rare cases, polyps will also form in unexpected locations such as the maxillary sinus, nose, esophagus, uterus, and gall bladder, among others. In addition, about 10% to 15% of females with this syndrome also develop ovarian tumors, some in very young children.

Melanotic macules occur in the skin in 50% of affected individuals and on the oral mucosa in more than 98% of affected individuals (Figs 15-5a and 15-5b). They will appear in each location as a brown to blue-gray flat area between 2 and 12 mm. Those on the oral mucosa tend to be slightly larger than those on the skin. On the skin, they are mostly found in the perioral regions and the hands (Fig 15-5c). The perianal and perigenital areas also may have a prominent number of macules. On the oral mucosa, most are on the lips and buccal mucosa; others appear less frequently on the palate or gingiva (Fig 15-5d).

Melanotic macules can appear at any time, but usually begin in infancy. They fade somewhat beginning at puberty, but rarely disappear completely. In some cases, the melanotic macules are the only manifestation of the syndrome.

DIFFERENTIAL DIAGNOSIS ► *Normal variation* vs syndrome with or without polyposis is the most common differential. In those individuals without intestinal polyposis, a familial history or sufficient numbers of melanotic macules in the common locations must be demonstrated for a diagnosis of Peutz-Jeghers syndrome. This may be particularly difficult in blacks or other dark-skinned individuals who have melanotic oral macules normally. *Addison disease* is the other serious differential because of its oral and cutaneous macule hyperpigmen-

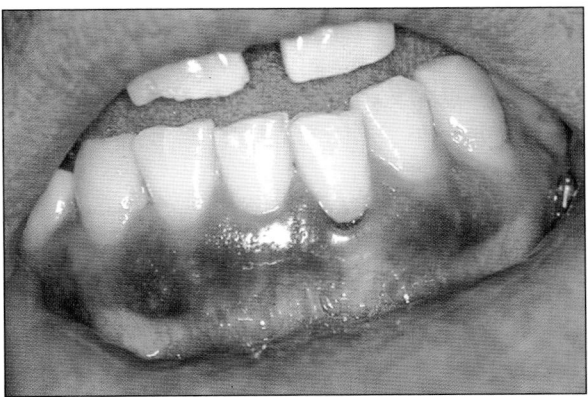

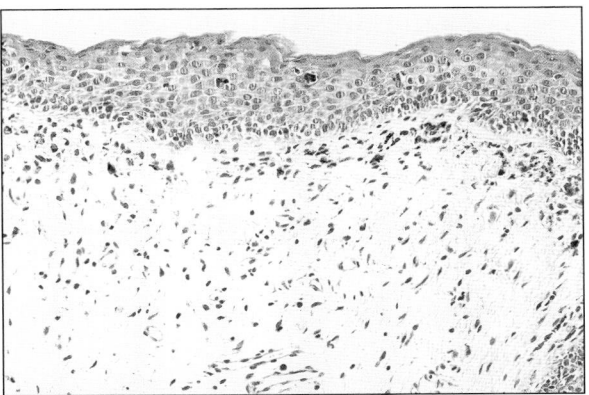

Fig 15-6a Diffuse brown pigmentation and darker pigmented areas resembling melanotic macules in a heavy smoker representing smokers' melanosis. (Reprinted from Laskaris G, *Color Atlas of Oral Diseases* 2nd ed, with permission from Thieme Medical Publishers.)

Fig 15-6b Smokers' melanosis from the floor of the mouth showing melanin within the connective tissue as well as within the upper layers of the epithelium. Note the hyperparakeratosis.

tation. Although hereditary polyposis is known to occur in Gardner syndrome, juvenile polyposis, and familial polyposis coli, none of these is associated with skin or oral melanotic macules and all have polyps limited to the colon. Albright syndrome and hereditary neurofibromatosis both manifest melanotic macular areas called *café-au-lait macules*. However, neither is associated with intestinal polyposis, and their melanotic macules are usually larger and found in areas other than the perioral, hand, perianal, and perigenital areas common to Peutz-Jeghers syndrome.

DIAGNOSTIC WORK-UP AND TREATMENT ▶

The number and locations of melanotic macules should be recorded and compared to the expected distribution. In addition, upper and lower gastrointestinal dye radiologic series are required. Because the malignant transformation incidence of adenomatous polyps is as high as 20% to 40%, flexible fiberoptic examinations and polyp biopsy also are valuable.

HISTOPATHOLOGY ▶

The lesions of Peutz-Jeghers syndrome resemble the melanotic macule with increased melanin production but no melanocytic hyperplasia. Giant melanosomes do not occur and are more likely to be seen in café-au-lait macules, nevi, and lentigines.

PROGNOSIS ▶

The overall prognosis associated with Peutz-Jeghers syndrome is considered to be good, but intense long-term follow-up is required because of a malignancy rate that is higher than previously thought and possible gastrointestinal complications.

Smokers' Melanosis

CLINICAL PRESENTATION AND PATHOGENESIS ▶

Smokers' melanosis is a focal increase in melanin pigmentation in the oral mucosa found in cigarette, pipe, and cigar smokers who smoke frequently (Fig 15-6a). The melanosis is either a diffuse patch of brownish discolored mucosa or numbers of small melanotic macules. The lesion is not dysplastic or premalignant, but its presence indicates a continual and frequent smoking habit that places the patient at an increased risk for oral carcinoma. Most lesions are seen on the labial mucosa and floor of the mouth, but the tongue, gingiva, and buccal mucosa may also be involved. The lesion is asymptomatic and flat (macular), as if the mucosa were painted a light brown beneath its surface. It is more common in premenopausal women and those on oral contraceptives, suggesting a relationship to female hormones.

Some smokers believe that the melanosis is a stain, but it is actually an increase in melanin pigment synthesis and disbursement within the cytoplasm of melanocytes. Some suggest that tobacco products stimulate this melanocytic reaction, which is enhanced by female hormones. The heat related to smoking may also play an important role since this reaction is not observed in smokeless tobacco users.

DIFFERENTIAL DIAGNOSIS ▶

Any brown, black, or blue oral pigmentation may be suggestive of *melanoma*. In addition, brown macules and patches that look like a submucosal stain may be present in *Addison disease* (adrenal cortical insufficiency), where increased corticotropin levels stimulated by low serum cortisol levels have a melanocyte-stimulating hormone–like effect on melanocytes. They may also be present in *Peutz-Jeghers syndrome*, in which there is genetic coding for oral as well as perioral and other skin-area melanotic macules.

DIAGNOSTIC WORK-UP AND TREATMENT ▶

Most cases of smokers' melanosis are identifiable by history and observation. Only lesions suggestive of melanoma by virtue of induration, thickening, ulceration, or darkening in color require biopsy. Because these lesions are not themselves dangerous, no specific treatment is required. However, smoking reduction or cessation is strongly advised, which, in turn, will often result in a lightening of the pigmentation and in some cases elimination of it.

HISTOPATHOLOGY ▶

The lesions of smokers' melanosis present a histologic appearance similar to that of the melanotic macule in that melanocytes are not increased in number, but there is an increase in melanin production with increased pigmentation of basal keratinocytes. Pigment may also be seen higher in the epithelium. Melanophages are often present in the underlying tissue. There is usually an accompanying hyperkeratosis or hyperparakeratosis (Fig 15-6b).

Melanotic Neuroectodermal Tumor of Infancy

CLINICAL PRESENTATION AND PATHOGENESIS ▶

The melanotic neuroectodermal tumor of infancy (MNTI) is a clinically distinctive benign neoplasm of neuroectodermal origin. With only rare exceptions, the tumors arise from the anterior maxilla (the rare exceptions are in the anterior mandible, skull, scapula, and epididymis). They are never congenital but will emerge sometime within the first year of life and usually at less than 6 months of age. They often first appear as a blue gingival mass that is mistaken for an eruption cyst. The mass will grow rapidly, raising the concern of a malignancy. It is not uncommon to see the mass double in size in 1 week.

The mass characteristically will be round with a bluish-black coloration and will carry one of the primary central incisor teeth outward with it (Fig 15-7a). It will not carry both central incisors since these tumors arise from one side of the midline. The central incisor is visible in most cases, seeming to erupt from the mass (Fig 15-7b). More rarely, the central incisor is within the mass just beneath the surface and will be readily apparent on an occlusal radiograph. Larger lesions are often secondarily ulcerated by trauma from the hands of the infant, but the lesion itself does not ulcerate.

The lesion is destructive. Occlusal radiographs show an irregular resorption of the anterior maxilla and displacement of developing tooth buds (Fig 15-7c). The lesion has no radiopaque components except for the developing teeth, particularly the ipsilateral central incisor, which is often displaced and located within the tumor.

The MNTI, which originates from neural crest cells, represents an overgrowth of these cells rather than their usual involution. Normally, neural crest cells originate from a mantle around the developing spinal cord and project out to the periphery along sympathetic nerves. In other parts of the body, they populate the primordia of sympathetic ganglia and the adrenal medulla to become neurosecretory cells of these respective structures. In the maxilla and most peripheral sympathetic neural pathways, they involute. Those that develop into the MNTI are the rare failures of involution, which instead proliferate into a tumor.

DIFFERENTIAL DIAGNOSIS ▶

The rapid development and, at times, frightening growth of the MNTI suggest a malignancy. In particular, the *neuroblastoma* is a distinct and serious consideration. The few cases of so-called "malignant MNTI" that have recurred or metastasized have probably represented neuroblastomas, which are the most common early childhood malignancy and the fourth most common malignancy in the head and neck area. Other infancy tumors with aggressive behavior and possible blue colorations are *rhabdomyosarcomas*, which have a predilection for the head and neck area in children, and *hemangiomas* or *lymphangiomas*, which may indeed present with a bluish color and often appear within a few months after

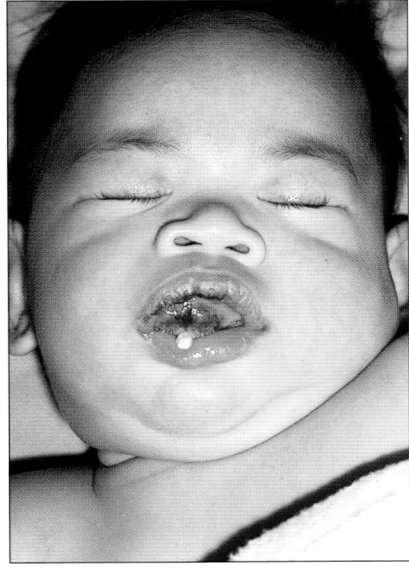

Fig 15-7a The expected presentation of a melanotic neuroectodermal tumor of infancy is in a child younger than 1 year with a pigmented anterior maxillary mass containing a central incisor tooth.

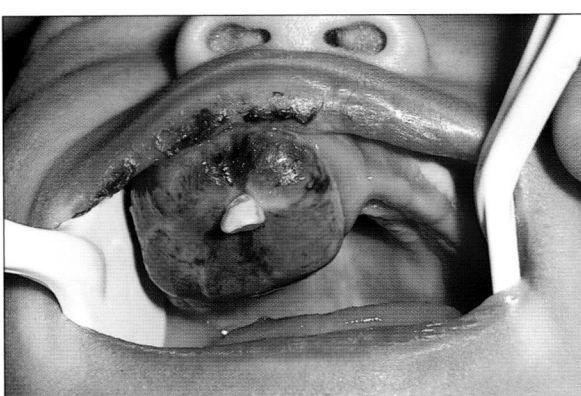

Fig 15-7b The central incisor tooth will seem to erupt from the melanotic neuroectodermal tumor of infancy mass and will create a "candle in a cupcake" appearance.

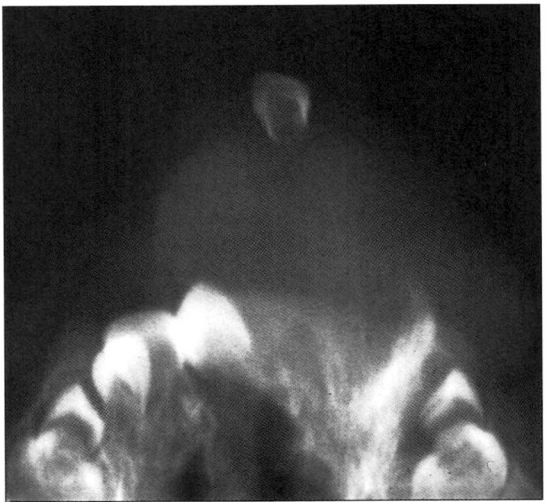

Fig 15-7c Occlusal radiographs of a melanotic neuroectodermal tumor of infancy will show irregular bony borders, a soft tissue mass, adjacent tooth displacement, and usually one central incisor carried outward with the mass.

birth with rapid development. The congenital granular cell tumor, which also frequently arises from the anterior maxilla (65%) and is seen in infants, is not a consideration because it is always congenital (present at birth) whereas the MNTI is never congenital. Questioning the parent or the birthing team about the presence of an oral mass at birth will distinguish between the two.

DIAGNOSTIC WORK-UP ▶

The most important diagnostic step is a confirmatory incisional biopsy. However, an occlusal radiograph that shows the central incisor displaced to the periphery of a mass that itself shows destruction of the anterior maxilla is pathognomonic. About 10% to 15% of MNTI will elaborate vanillylmandelic acid (VMA or 3-methoxy-4-hydroxy mandelic acid), which is a soluble metabolic breakdown product of norepinephrine. It is indicative of the neuroectodermal cell origin of this tumor. VMA levels from a 24-hour urine collection may be compared to normal values but have no real diagnostic value. This is because increased VMA levels may imply a neuroectodermal cell origin, but normal VMA levels do not rule out a neuroectodermal cell origin because not all the cells are involved in neuroepinephrine synthesis.

HISTOPATHOLOGY ▶

These infiltrating, unencapsulated tumors have irregular alveolar spaces and a dense, fibrous stroma (Fig 15-7d). The spaces contain two types of cells. The larger cuboidal cell usually lines the space and has a pale nucleus and abundant cytoplasm, which often contains melanin. These cells are S-100 negative, however. The more centrally located cells are smaller and round with a deeply staining nucleus and scant cytoplasm, resembling neuroblasts (Fig 15-7e). Mitoses are not seen. These tumors appear to be of neural crest origin, and neuroblastic and melanocytic cell lines have been identified ultrastructurally. Both cell types are positive for neuron-specific enolase and synaptophyisn and negative for S-100. The larger cells are cytokeratin positive and HMB (human melanoma block)-45 positive, features that are noted in pigmented retinal epithelium. In the rare instances in which these tumors have behaved in a malignant fashion, their histologic appearance and clinical behavior have paralleled those of the neuroblastoma.

TREATMENT ▶

The melanotic neuroectodermal tumor of infancy should be treated by a peripheral excision with 2- to 5-mm margins (Fig 15-7f). Although the destructive nature of this tumor and its growth rate are significant, total maxillectomies and maxillary resections with margins greater than 5 mm are unnecessary.

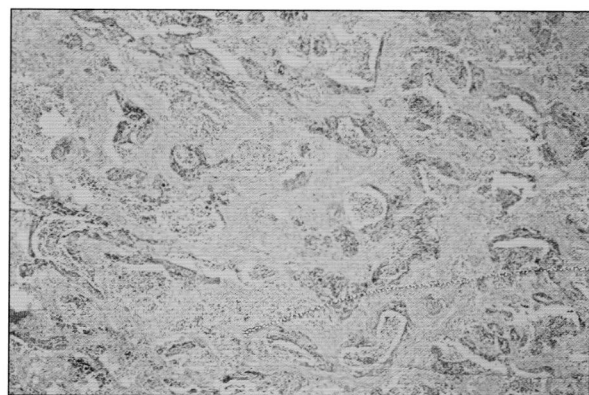

Fig 15-7d Melanotic neuroectodermal tumor of infancy with scattered tumor islands within dense fibrous stroma. Pigmentation at the periphery of many of the islands is readily seen.

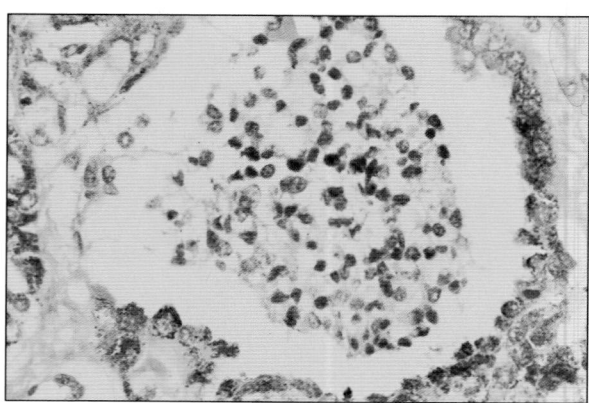

Fig 15-7e High-power view of the tumor shown in Fig 15-7d. The larger peripheral cells contain melanin pigment. Within the center of the tumor islands, some of these larger cells are seen, but small, round, dark-staining cells are also noted.

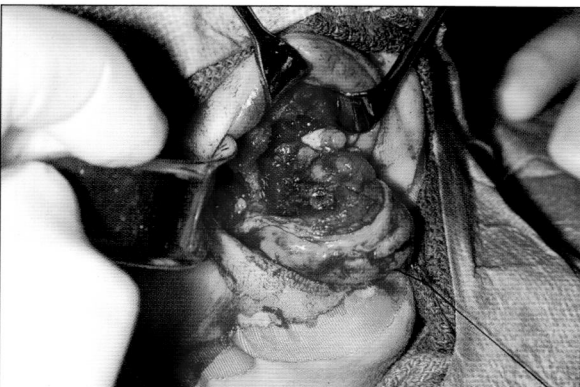

Fig 15-7f A melanotic neuroectodermal tumor of infancy is treated with a peripheral resection using 2- to 5-mm margins.

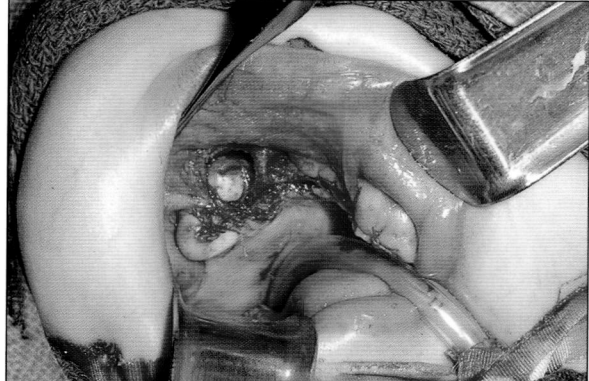

Fig 15-7g Resultant surgical defect following excision of a melanotic neuroectodermal tumor of infancy.

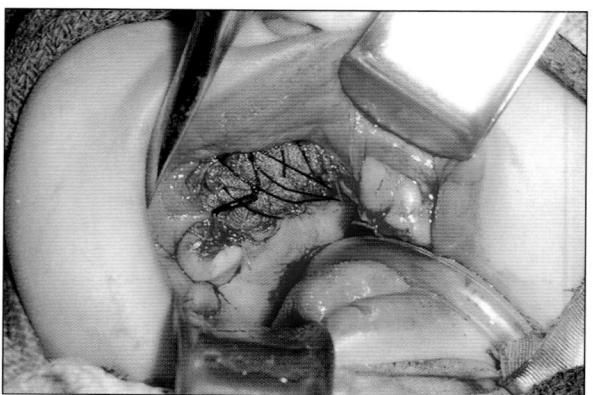

Fig 15-7h A tie-over dressing applied to the wound will maintain hemostasis and protect the wound from direct trauma.

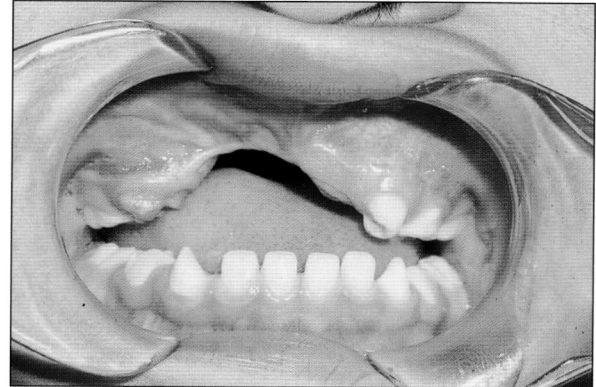

Fig 15-7i The surgical defect resultant from the removal of a melanotic neuroectodermal tumor of infancy will seem to become smaller over the years as growth makes the defect size a smaller percentage of the total maxilla. This defect is residual from surgery 5 years earlier.

Early excision is of great value. Limiting the destruction that the tumor causes in the anterior maxilla will lessen the deformity and preserve developing teeth. The excision should include the overlying mucosa. The resultant wound may be packed with a tie-over pressure dressing (Figs 15-7g and 15-7h) for 5 to 7 days to reduce oozing. The wound itself heals rapidly by granulation tissue and secondary epithelialization.

PROGNOSIS ▶

The excised MNTI in which gross tumor is not allowed to remain should not recur. Recurrent MNTI should be looked on as suggestive of an unrecognized malignancy and followed by a review of multiple sections of the excised specimen and a systemic review for neuroblastoma elsewhere.

The maxillary defect becomes relatively smaller as the child grows (Fig 15-7i). Nevertheless, primary and permanent teeth will be missing and a permanent concave defect in the canine to midline area will be present. Most children adapt to this very well, but some will require speech therapy and serial removable appliances. The resultant scarring will usually eventuate in an anteroposterior deficiency of the maxilla as well as a crossbite relationship more severe on the affected side. Therefore, as the child develops, orthodontic care and possibly orthognathic surgery may be required.

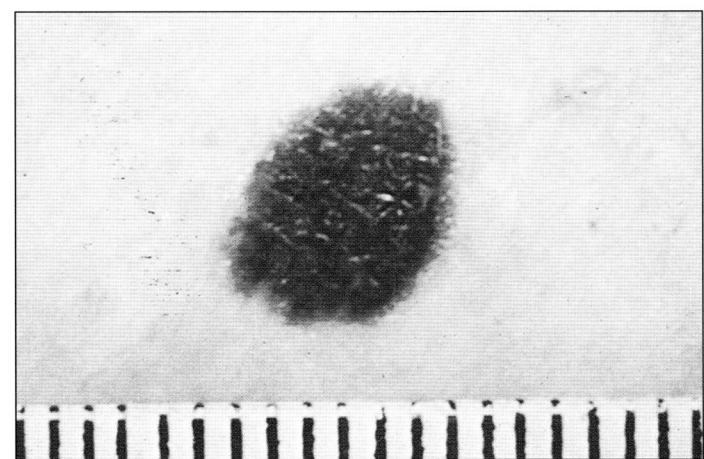

Fig 15-8 A typical junctional nevus is flat, small (here about 7 mm), homogeneous in color, and has regular borders.

Melanocytic Nevi

CLINICAL PRESENTATION AND
PATHOGENESIS ▶

Nevi, also called moles, are benign collections of nevus cells that are derived either from melanocytes or from the same neural crest precursors as melanocytes. Nevi on skin are very common; nearly every person has at least one. Nevi on the oral mucosa are very uncommon, with less than 1% of individuals possessing a true mucosal nevus. About 1% of newborns have a nevus. The number of individuals with nevi increases and the number of nevi on each individual increases to a peak at puberty. Although nevi can occur on any skin surface, greater numbers appear on sun-exposed surfaces.

The concern of both the patient and the practitioner is differentiating a nevus from a melanoma (so-called black-mole cancer). Nevi are far too numerous and melanoma far too uncommon to biopsy all nevi. Therefore, only those with suspicious deviation from the usual appearance are excised. The nevus may be either brown, black, or blue, but the color is uniform throughout. Although nevi have different outlines, the outlines are regular and basically symmetric. Additionally, unlike melanomas, nevi do not change color, shade, or texture over time. Despite these characteristics, uniformity cannot always be relied on to differentiate a nevus from a melanoma. Early melanomas may appear quite uniform with an oval shape and a uniform brown color. In such cases, repeat examinations, often using a magnifying glass or loop magnifications and noting changes in color, shape, and texture, will draw suspicion to a developing melanoma.

Nevi are classified into three types—*junctional, compound,* and *dermal*—based on the location of nevus cells in the skin. The three types reflect the evolution of the nevus to some degree. During childhood, the nevus cells are located in the area of the basement membrane both suprabasilar and infrabasilar. Clinically, these nevi appear flat. Over time, some of the nevus cells migrate into the dermis, resulting in a compound nevus. Migration of all the nevus cells into the dermis results in a dermal nevus. When this occurs, the nevus cell collection results in smooth-surfaced elevated nodules. Because this process takes several years, nearly all dermal nevi are found in adults.

Junctional Nevus

Junctional nevi are flat or only slightly elevated. Most are hairless and small, varying in size from 1 to 10 mm (Fig 15-8). They are only rarely seen as a congenital nevus. Most arise at about age 2 years and evolve into compound nevi in the teen years. Junctional nevi on the palms, soles, and genital areas remain junctional and never seem to convert to a compound nevus. Transformation into a melanoma is very rare.

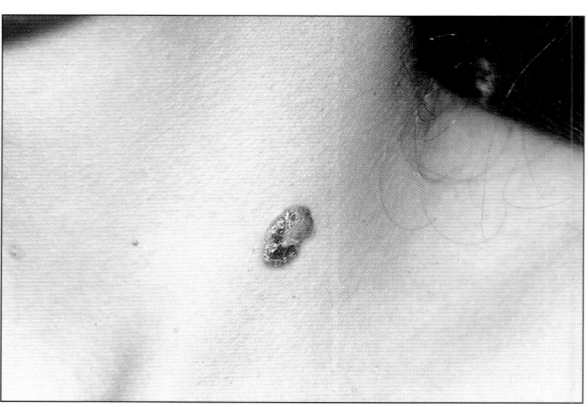

Fig 15-9 A compound nevus is also small, oval, has regular borders, and may be slightly raised.

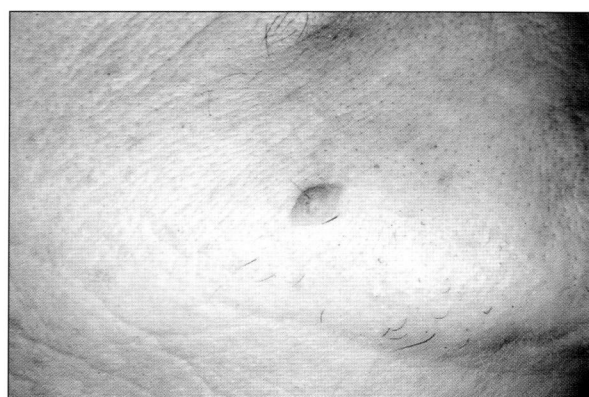

Fig 15-10 Some compound nevi will become more elevated and may develop a warty appearance with a few isolated hairs.

Compound Nevus

Compound nevi tend to be elevated with a uniformly round or oval shape. Many are natural skin color, others are somewhat darker. Hair is often present arising around a compound nevus. With increasing age, nevi become more elevated and may develop a warty appearance (Figs 15-9 and 15-10). Melanoma transformation is also rare.

Dermal Nevus

Dermal nevi may also be of natural skin color or darker. All are elevated nodules and become firm as fibrous tissue replaces degenerated nevus cells. Most are described as dome shaped, but others may be warty (Fig 15-11). Like the warty surface texture of some compound nevi, the warty surface is regular and symmetric throughout the lesion. Some dermal nevi will also develop a stalk and produce a pedunculated lesion resembling a skin tag, particularly in the groin, axilla, and neck (Fig 15-12). Transformation into a melanoma is very rare, but the dermal nevus itself may resemble a nodular melanoma. The unchanging appearance of the nevus is the best way to differentiate the two.

DIFFERENTIAL DIAGNOSIS ▶

Any nevus can resemble a *melanoma*. Junctional and compound nevi may resemble *superficial spreading melanomas*, and dermal nevi may resemble *nodular melanomas*. On sun-exposed skin, nevi may also be confused with *actinic keratosis, sebhorrheic keratosis,* and *pigmented basal cell carcinomas. Cutaneous hemangiomas* appear blue as do some deep dermal nevi. Some dermal nevi will appear blue (blue nevus) due to the phenomenon whereby only the higher-energy blue range of the light spectrum penetrates to this depth; the otherwise brown melanin will appear blue by the absorption of all other colors, leaving only the higher-energy blue spectrum to be reflected. A cutaneous hemangioma may also resemble a nevus by appearing brown because of accumulation of hemosiderin.

TREATMENT AND PROGNOSIS ▶

Any skin nevus with signs suggestive of a melanoma requires excision down to and including the subcutaneous level. All mucosal nevi require excision down to and including the submucosal level. Excision of such nevi eradicates the lesion and may lead to diagnosis of an early melanoma. Static nevi without features suggestive of a melanoma do not require excision and may be followed.

HISTOPATHOLOGY ▶

Melanocytic nevi form a spectrum that begins as a melanotic macule (lentigo simplex). Nondendritic, enlarged, and rounded melanocytes are seen in linear and contiguous arrangement along the basal layer. The melanocytes and keratinocytes are heavily pigmented. There is elongation of rete ridges secondary

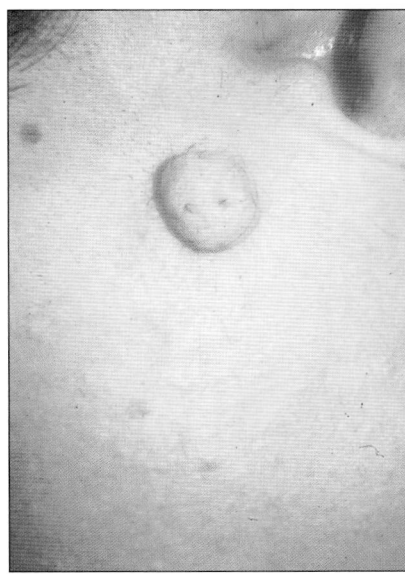

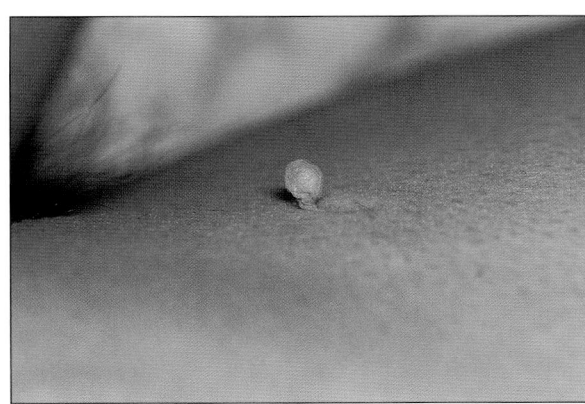

Fig 15-11 A dermal nevus is usually less dark, nodular, dome-shaped, and firm.

Fig 15-12 Some dermal nevi become pedunculated and resemble a skin tag. These are more common in the groin, axillary, and neck areas.

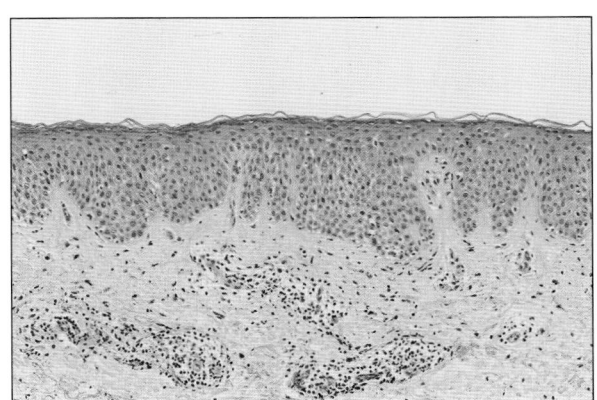

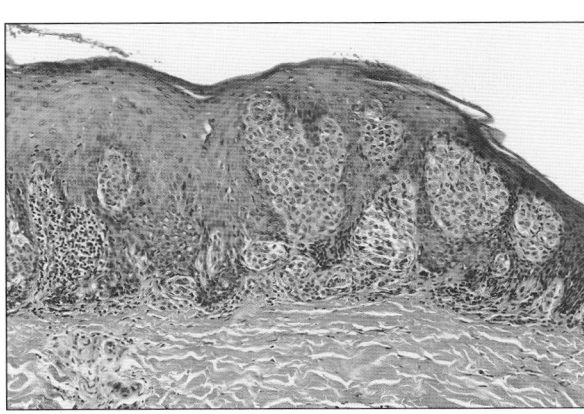

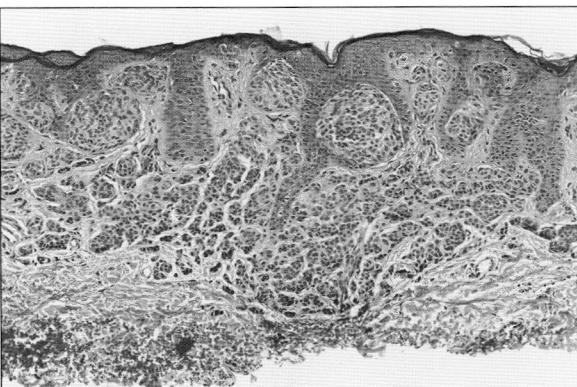

Fig 15-13 Melanotic macule (lentigo simplex) showing heavily pigmented melanocytes and keratinocytes in the basal layer with a hyperplasia of the epithelium.

Fig 15-14 Junctional nevus of the palate in which clusters of nevus cells are seen at the epithelial–connective tissue interface.

Fig 15-15 A compound nevus in which clusters of nevus cells are seen at the interface and nests of cells are seen within the connective tissue.

to proliferation of keratinocytes. Melanophages and lymphocytes are often present within the dermis (Fig 15-13).

The junctional nevus resembles lentigo simplex except that nests of melanocytes are seen at the epidermal-dermal junction, often at the tips of the elongated rete ridges. These lesions tend to be less heavily pigmented than those of lentigo simplex, and there are fewer melanophages and lymphocytes in the dermis. Contiguous rounded melanocytes are usually present in linear arrangement in the basal layer. Lesional cells are not present within the dermis (Fig 15-14).

The compound nevus maintains the pattern of the junctional nevus, but additionally there is extension of the nevus cells into the papillary dermis and sometimes into the reticular dermis as nests and anastomosing cords (Fig 15-15). A pattern of maturation may be seen within these nevus cells. The more superficial, known as type A, are large and rounded and contain melanin (epithelioid). The deeper cells,

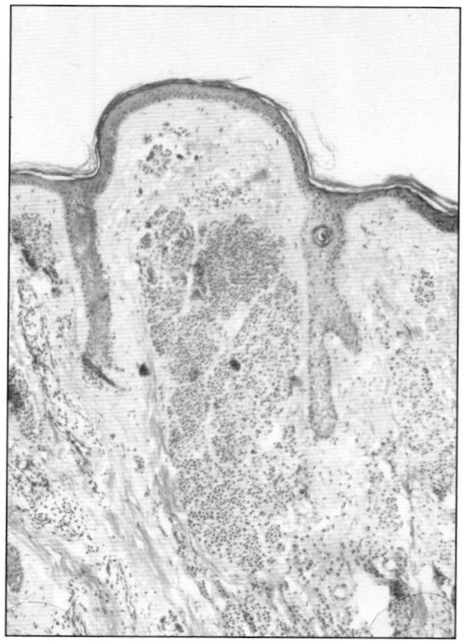

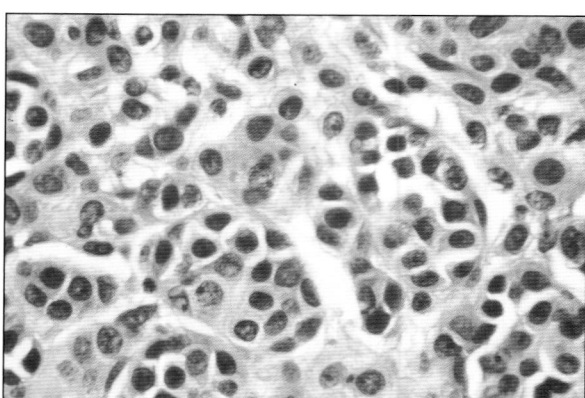

Fig 15-16a A dermal nevus showing all of the nevus cells within the dermis. There are no remaining junctional cells. At low power, the nevus cells can look much like an inflammatory infiltrate.

Fig 15-16b Higher-power view of Fig 15-16a revealing the nesting arrangement of the cells. Melanin pigment is frequently lacking, as it is here.

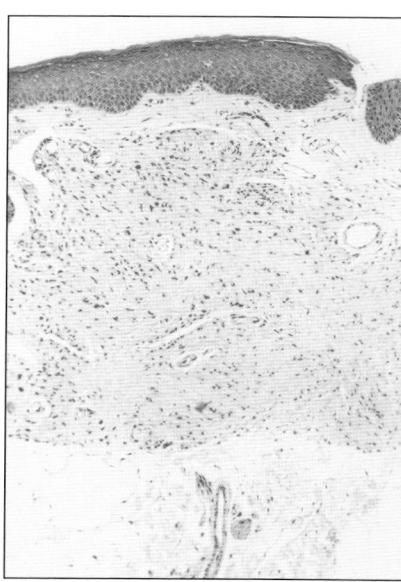

Fig 15-17 In this nevus, the nevus cells become more spindled, and the lesion takes on a neurogenic quality.

known as type B, are smaller and lack pigment (lymphoid). Older lesions may contain type C cells at their base; these are spindled and have a neurogenic appearance.

The dermal nevus (Fig 15-16a) has nevus cells only within the dermis and lacks an epidermal component. Rete ridges are not elongated. The preponderance of nevus cells is more likely to be of types B or C (Fig 15-16b). Sometimes only the spindle cells remain so that the nevus has a completely neurogenic appearance (Fig 15-17). The dermal nevus may undergo involution, in which case nevus cells are absent and are replaced by fibrous tissue and fat.

The appearance of these lesions is the same when they occur on mucous membranes.

Blue Nevus

CLINICAL PRESENTATION ▶

The blue nevus, a blue dermal nevus, is usually small (less than 5 mm) and appears as a regular, round elevated nodule. It appears blue because the melanin pigment, which is naturally brown, is located deep within the dermis (Fig 15-18a). The brown pigment and the thickness of skin absorb the longer wavelengths of light (eg, reds, oranges, yellows) and reflect the more penetrating, shorter wavelengths, such as blue (ie, the Tyndall effect).

The blue nevus will appear in childhood on the dorsum of hands, extremities, and scalp. It has a low potential for malignant transformation. However, a larger, rare variant, called the *cellular blue nevus*, has a higher melanoma transformation rate. It is frequently larger than 1 cm and most often located on the buttocks.

DIFFERENTIAL DIAGNOSIS ▶

The blue nevus will closely resemble a small *hemangioma*, a *venous varix*, or even a *lymphangioma*. Compressing the lesion (diascopy) will blanch such vascular lesions but will not change the appearance of a blue nevus.

DIAGNOSTIC WORK-UP AND TREATMENT ▶

Unless there are signs suggestive of melanoma, blue nevi may be followed without excision. However, if the clinical diagnosis is uncertain or such changes as blackening, induration, surface irregularity, outline irregularity, or ulceration occur, excision including the subcutaneous level is required.

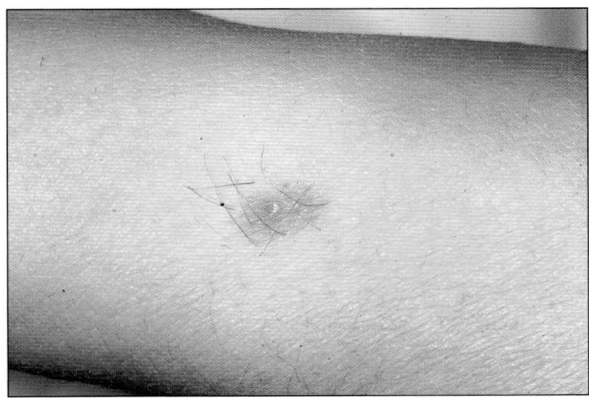

Fig 15-18a A blue nevus is usually small. It is blue because the melanin is located deep in the dermis. It will be somewhat elevated and have regular borders. The blue color may fade over time because of a dispersal of or reduction in melanin.

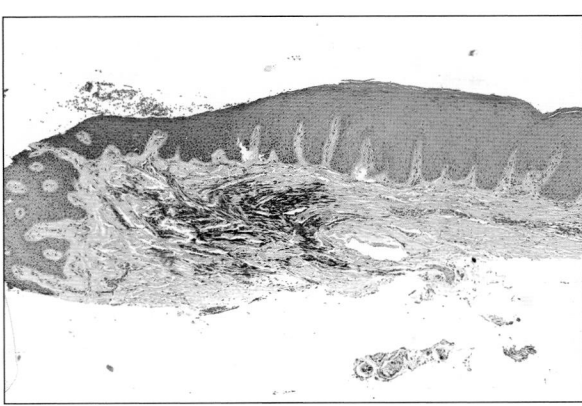

Fig 15-18b A blue nevus of the palate. Note the spindle cell proliferation and the orientation of the cells, which is generally parallel to the surface.

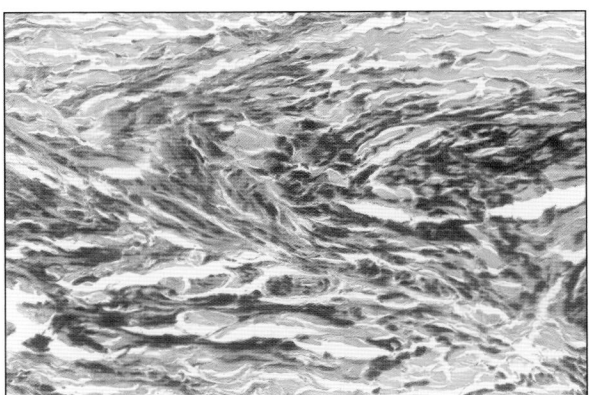

Fig 15-18c Intense pigmentation of the cells in the blue nevus.

HISTOPATHOLOGY ►

Blue nevi consist of groups of elongated dendritic or spindle cells, which sometimes have a wavy appearance and often lie parallel to the epidermis (Fig 15-18b). They contain abundant melanin granules, which often obscure the nucleus (Fig 15-18c). The cells are usually within the reticular dermis and lie between the collagen fibers, which are often thickened. A reactive fibroblastic proliferation may also be seen. The melanocytes are sometimes found within nerve or vessel walls. Melanophages may be present. The epidermis is unremarkable unless the lesion is a combined nevus, in which case there may be a concomitant junctional, compound, or dermal nevus.

The cellular blue nevus typically is biphasic with pigmented cells alternating with clear cells.

Mucosal blue nevi have the same histologic appearance as those on the skin.

Nevus of Ota

CLINICAL PRESENTATION AND PATHOGENESIS ►

The nevus of Ota is a unique nevus that represents a melanocytic disorder following the distribution of one or more divisions of the trigeminal nerve (Fig 15-19). About 48% are congenital or appear within a few weeks of birth, and 36% arise at puberty, thereby creating a bimodal incidence peak. The nevus will appear as a diffuse brownish discoloration or a cluster of small, blue-black, well-demarcated spots. The skin over the maxillary division of the trigeminal nerve seems to be involved more frequently than the other divisions, and corresponding nevi simultaneously appear on the oral mucosa, nasal mucosa, and sometimes on the conjunctiva of the ipsilateral eye.

The nevus of Ota is most common in Asians and dark-skinned individuals and has a marked predilection for women (80%).

Neither the cutaneous component nor the oral mucosa membrane component of the nevus of Ota is associated with melanoma. The nevus of Ota is thought to represent a developmental anomaly of excess melanocytes residual from neural crest cells that migrated along a trigeminal nerve distribution. In those arising during puberty, it may be a hamartomatous proliferation of these residual cells stimulated by hormonal increases.

DIFFERENTIAL DIAGNOSIS ►

Facial hyperpigmentation occurring unilaterally in children or teenagers of Asian descent is characteristic of the nevus of Ota. Other entities that may appear similar are *encephalotrigeminal angiomatosis* (Sturge-Weber anomaly), *progressive systemic sclerosis* (scleroderma), and a *melanoma*.

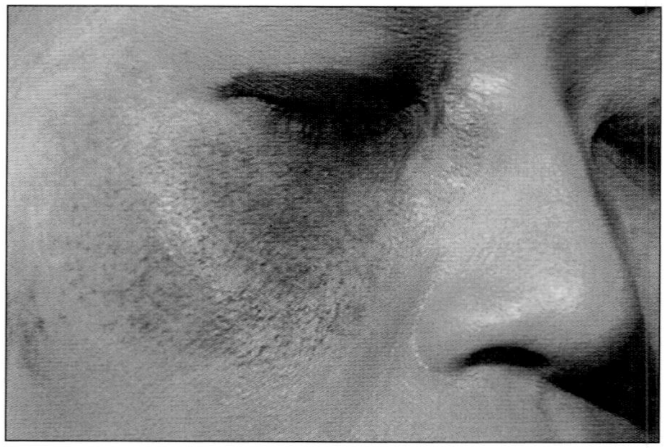

Fig 15-19 The nevus of Ota will appear as a blue or darkened patch over one or more distributions of the trigeminal nerve. It will resemble an area of ecchymosis.

DIAGNOSTIC WORK-UP AND TREATMENT

The nevus of Ota is merely a matter of cosmetic concern; rarely does it undergo transformation to melanoma, nor does the nevus usually progress throughout life. However, patients with ocular involvement have a high incidence of secondary open-angle glaucoma due to melanocytes collecting at the angle, causing obstruction of drainage. They also have a higher incidence of retinal, iridic, and cerebral melanomas. Therefore, patients with cutaneous lesions suggestive of nevus of Ota should undergo an ophthalmologic evaluation.

Various cosmetic procedures are used to remove these nevi. The argon laser is used to ablate the nevi, but this procedure often results in a lighter-colored area of equal cosmetic distraction due to permanent loss of pigment and scarring. Alternatively, the Q-switched ruby laser, which uses short pulses of high energy (8 to 10 j/cm^2 at 40 nanoseconds and 694 nanometers wavelength), has been used to damage melanocytes and melanosomes more than surrounding tissue. Partial clearing of nevi is reported in 50% of patients, complete clearing in 25%, and residual nevi in another 25%. Other approaches use microsurgical excision of each focal spot or dry ice packing combined with argon laser ablation. Many lesions are left untreated.

HISTOPATHOLOGY

A proliferation of elongated dendritic and stellate melanocytes containing melanin is seen between the collagen bundles of the reticular dermis. These lesions are less cellular than the blue nevus, but the cells may also lie parallel to the epidermis. There is no epidermal component.

Nevus of Ito

The nevus of Ito is similar to the nevus of Ota; however, it mostly occurs in the deltoid region. It may be seen on the upper chest, back, or supraclavicular area as well. Like the nevus of Ota, this nevus forms along peripheral nerve fibers. Clinically, it will present as a bluish hyperpigmentation, which on fine sensory testing may be associated with a local paresthesia. On occasion, the nevus has been associated with reduced sweating presumably because of its association with small sympathetic fibers, which innervate facial sweat glands.

The nevus of Ito is primarily an adult nevus but is rare. Because it mostly occurs in the deltoid region and other areas of low cosmetic index, it may be managed by local excision and primary closure or by laser ablation. Because it represents a benign nevus, its recurrence potential is low, and only very rare cases undergo melanoma transformation.

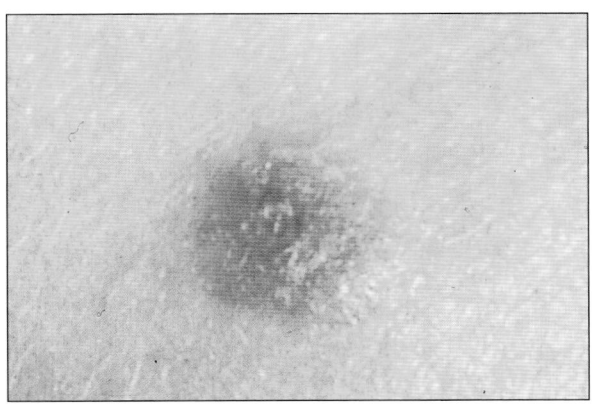

Fig 15-20a The Spitz nevus will present as a reddish-brown nodule with a rapid onset. These features, together with its vascularity and occasional bleeding, suggest a melanoma.

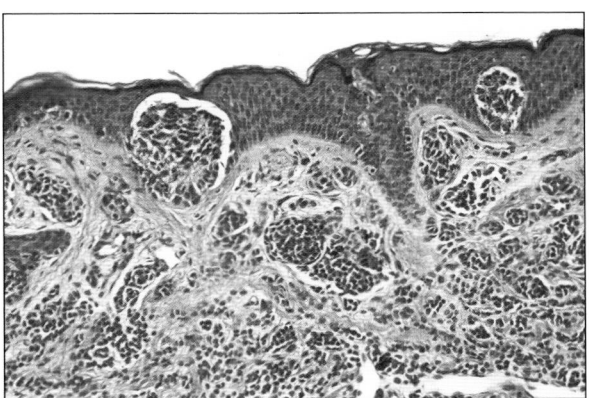

Fig 15-20b A Spitz nevus with the arrangement of a compound nevus. As is typical of this lesion, there is little melanin, inflammatory cells are present, and artifactual clefts are seen above the clusters of nevus cells.

Spitz Nevus

CLINICAL PRESENTATION ▶ The Spitz nevus has clinical and histologic features mimicking those of a melanoma. The nevi present as red or reddish-brown, smooth-surfaced nodules, usually between 0.5 and 1.5 cm. Clinically, Spitz nevi may suggest a melanoma because they emerge suddenly, unlike other nevi that develop slowly as macular lesions and evolve into nodular dermal nevi. They may also be suggestive of a melanoma because of their vascular nature, which may lead to bleeding following minor trauma (Fig 15-20a).

Most Spitz nevi occur in children as single, fast-developing nodules. However, multiple nevi can also occur, and adults may develop them as well.

DIFFERENTIAL DIAGNOSIS ▶ The rapid development of a small nodule on the skin of a child or a young adult suggests common *acne lesions, sebaceous cysts,* or *furuncles.* In addition, their reddish color and vascularity may suggest a small *hemangioma* or *lymphangioma. Melanoma* remains a serious consideration due to the lesion's color and rapid emergence.

TREATMENT AND PROGNOSIS ▶ Spitz nevi usually require excision to rule out melanoma and other diseases on the differential list. Excision is accomplished with 1- to 2-mm margins and includes the entire subcutaneous level. If the pathologist identifies the lesion as a Spitz nevus, no further excision or treatment is required. The Spitz nevus does not recur, not even in the case of incomplete excision. Therefore, in equivocal cases in which the histopathologic distinction between melanoma and a Spitz nevus is uncertain, follow-up is recommended. Any evidence of clinical recurrence is interpreted as evidence of melanoma.

HISTOPATHOLOGY ▶ Spitz nevi have the overall architecture of an intradermal or compound nevus. The overlying epithelium may show considerable hyperplasia with elongated rete ridges, and the papillary dermis may be edematous and contain dilated capillaries and lymphocytes. This vascularity contributes to the red color clinically. There are usually well-circumscribed nests of large cells, which may be plump spindle cells or large, round epithelioid cells. They are believed to represent a single cell population. The epithelioid cells have eosinophilic cytoplasm and may be multinucleated and atypical in appearance. Spindle cells are usually seen in whorls but may permeate the reticular dermis and show a single-file pattern at the base. Mitoses may be seen. Because of the pleomorphism, mitoses, and infiltrative pattern, as well as the presence of lymphocytic infiltrates, these nevi may be extremely difficult to distinguish from melanoma. Unlike melanoma, however, the Spitz nevus usually will show maturation (cells decrease in size in the deeper areas) and single-file infiltration rather than infiltration by nests and fascicles of cells. In addition, the presence of eosinophilic globules within the epidermis, which are periodic acid–Schiff (PAS) positive and

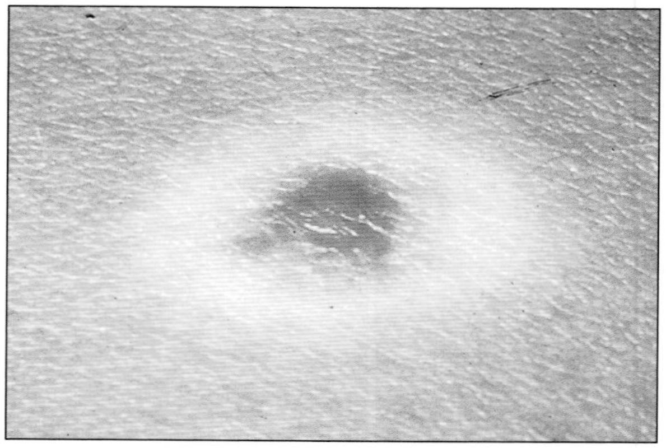

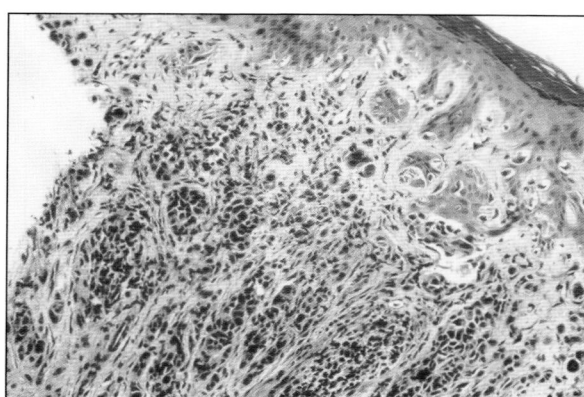

Fig 15-21a The halo nevus is very recognizable. It will usually develop during the teenage years from a pre-existing nevus with a white depigmented area at its peripheral circumference.

Fig 15-21b A halo nevus showing destruction of the nests of nevus cells by lymphocytes.

diastase resistant, are seen in a high percentage of Spitz nevi, but are very uncommon in melanoma. These are known as Kamino bodies and probably represent apoptotic cells. Melanin pigment is not usually prominent. Artifactual clefts often separate the cell nests from the keratinocytes (Fig 15-20b).

Halo Nevus

CLINICAL PRESENTATION ▶ The halo nevus is a type of compound or dermal nevus that develops a regular, symmetric white border. The white halo, which represents an area of depigmentation, is well demarcated from a normal skin edge. Halo nevi develop spontaneously from pre-existing nevi, most commonly during the teenage years (Fig 15-21a). Most occur on the trunk, some occur more rarely on the neck, but none has ever been reported on the palms or soles. Most occur singly, but on occasion several nevi may show halo characteristics around the same time.

Most halo nevi retain their halo. Some will show repigmentation of the white halo and in some others the halo will envelope and eradicate the nevus, resulting in a white circle.

DIFFERENTIAL DIAGNOSIS ▶ The main differential is a *melanoma* with halo formation. Halo areas do indeed form around some melanomas, but these halos are asymmetric and have jagged borders with the adjacent, normally pigmented skin. If the nevus is small or the halo has replaced most of the nevus, it may resemble an area of *vitiligo*. However, vitiligo lesions are also irregular, usually larger, and have several areas of depigmentation.

TREATMENT AND PROGNOSIS ▶ Removal of a halo nevus is unnecessary unless the nevus or halo shows irregularity or variations of pigmentation suggestive of melanoma. Atypical lesions require excision of the halo area as well as the nevus, including the subcutaneous level.

The halo nevus, per se, does not have a high potential for melanoma transformation. In fact, an immune system that is attacking and destroying nevus cells is associated with a reduced melanoma potential. In the past, the incidence of halo nevi transforming into melanoma has been overestimated because of the cases of melanoma that have shown halo formation. These melanomas with halos, however, arise de novo rather than from a pre-existing halo nevus.

HISTOPATHOLOGY ▶ The appearance of the halo nevus is essentially one of a compound nevus heavily infiltrated by lymphocytes, which tend to mask the nevoid pattern (Fig 15-21b). Melanophages may be present. Over time, the dermal nevus cells are destroyed. In the area of the clinical halo, there is reduced melanin production.

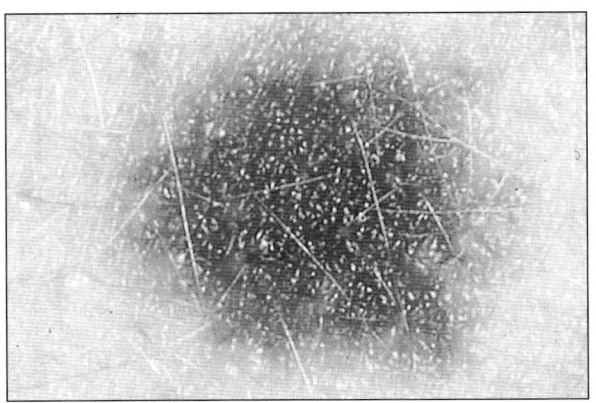

Fig 15-22 A dysplastic nevus transforming into a superficial spreading melanoma. It is clinically suspicious by its size and irregular borders and because the color at the borders gradually fades into the color of the surrounding skin.

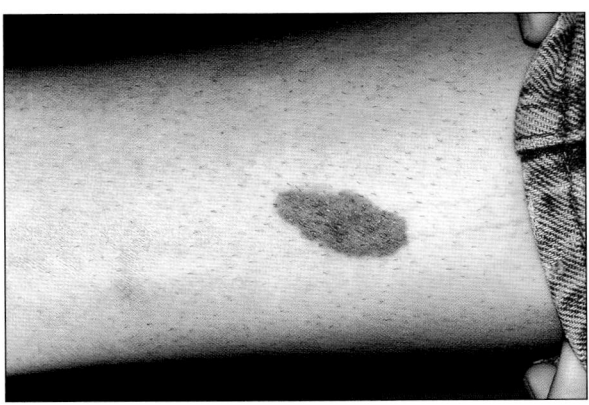

Fig 15-23 A dysplastic nevus is suggested by its larger size (greater than 1 cm), irregular borders, and variegated color.

Dysplastic Nevus (Nevus with Architectural Disorder)

CLINICAL PRESENTATION AND PATHOGENESIS ▶

The dysplastic nevus is a clinically and histologically atypical nevus representing the single most important precursor to a cutaneous melanoma. More than the congenital nevus, it is the primary pigmented lesion that transforms into a melanoma. Dysplastic nevi appear either sporadically or in an autosomal-dominant inherited condition called *dysplastic nevus syndrome* (DNS).

Clinically, the dysplastic nevus differs from the ordinary nevus. It is usually larger, and many are greater than 1 cm, whereas the common nevus rarely exceeds 0.6 cm. Its borders are irregular, with the color fading gradually into the surrounding skin, in contrast to the well-demarcated and regular borders of the ordinary nevus (Fig 15-22). It is variegated in color, usually a mixture of brown, black, and red, whereas common nevi are uniform in color (Fig 15-23). Common nevi have a site preference for sun-exposed areas, while dysplastic nevi tend to occur at unusual sites such as the scalp, buttocks, and breast.

The frequency of sporadic dysplastic nevi is unknown. However, 8% of melanomas unassociated with a familial inheritance have at least one concomitant dysplastic nevus, and serial examinations have revealed the progression of dysplastic nevi into melanoma of the superficial spreading type.

Dysplastic nevi associated with dysplastic nevus syndrome have an exceedingly high melanoma potential. Dysplastic nevi are found concomitantly on the skin of 90% of melanoma patients who have a family history of melanoma. The lifetime incidence of cutaneous melanoma among whites in the United States is about 0.6%. Those with sporadic (nonfamilial) dysplastic nevi have a tenfold greater risk and therefore an incidence of 6%. Those with a family history of DNS or melanoma who have a dysplastic nevus have an incidence of melanoma of 15%. The risk of melanoma approaches 100% for those who have a dysplastic nevus and two or more first-degree relatives with a cutaneous melanoma.

Dysplastic nevi of either the sporadic type or the familial DNS are not congenital but appear in mid-childhood as a common mole. They begin to take on the clinical features of dysplastic nevi in the early teens, and new nevi continue to appear even past the age of 40 years.

Dysplastic nevus syndrome and/or familial melanoma is estimated to affect 32,000 people in the United States, accounting for about 85.5% of all melanomas. The autosomal-dominant inheritance is localized to the distal end of the short arm of chromosome 1. This gene locus seems to be related to skin pigmentation regulation only. There is no association with or greater risks for other dysplasias or carcinomas.

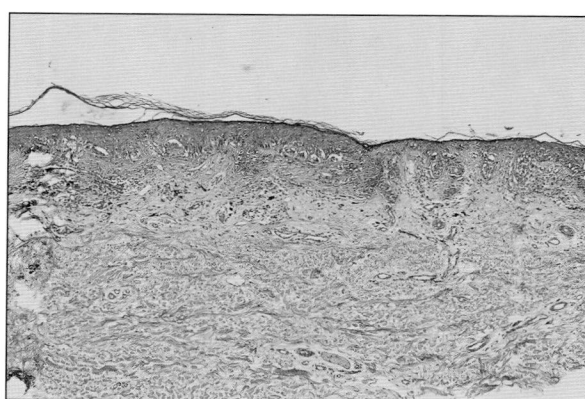

Fig 15-24a A dysplastic nevus showing a proliferation of single and nested nevus cells along the basal layer. There is a relatively regular elongation of rete ridges.

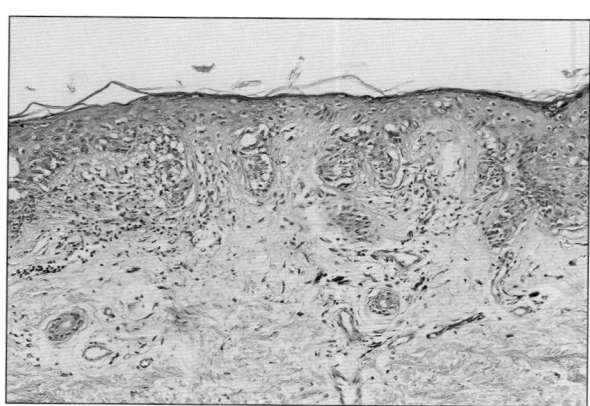

Fig 15-24b High-power view of Fig 15-24a showing nests along the sides and between the rete ridges.

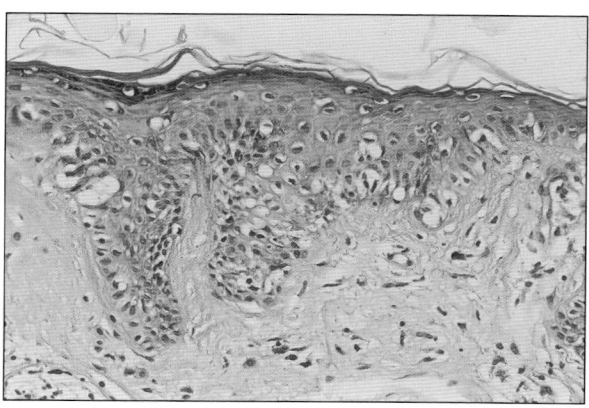

Fig 15-24c High-power view of the dysplastic nevus shown in Fig 15-24a. There is some mild atypia.

DIFFERENTIAL DIAGNOSIS ▶

Dysplastic nevi must be distinguished from common *melanocytic nevi* on one end of the spectrum and from *melanoma* on the other end. In addition, the overall presentation of multiple brown-black macular lesions may suggest syndromes associated with café-au-lait macules or other hyperpigmented lesions, including *Albright syndrome, hereditary neurofibromatosis, Peutz-Jeghers syndrome*, and *Leopard syndrome*.

DIAGNOSTIC WORK-UP AND TREATMENT ▶

Individuals who have two or more lesions clinically consistent with dysplastic nevi require a complete topographic skin examination, as do their family members. The purpose is to identify others who may have dysplastic nevi or melanomas and are therefore also at risk, as well as to assess the familial tendency. Photographs of lesions are highly recommended, as not all nevi can or should be excised. Baseline photographs enable comparisons and an assessment of change during future examinations.

The general approach is to excise two to four of the most suspicious nevi to establish a histopathologic diagnosis. The excision uses 2- to 5-mm margins to and inclusive of the subcutaneous level. If the diagnosis confirms dysplastic nevi, the general rule is to excise all new nevi that arise thereafter and all of those in the scalp because of the difficulty of monitoring scalp lesions. Prophylactic excision of all remaining nevi is neither practical nor indicated if there are more than 10. Such lesions should be followed with serial examinations and compared to baseline photographs.

HISTOPATHOLOGY ▶

Histologic features associated with dysplastic nevi include architectural, cytologic, and stromal changes.

Architecturally, there is a fairly regular elongation of the rete ridges and a lentigo simplex–like proliferation in the basal layer of single or nested nevus cells. The nests may coalesce or form bridges between adjacent rete ridges (Figs 15-24a to 15-24c). A "shouldering" pattern may be seen in which the epidermal melanocytes extend singly or in nests beyond the dermal component.

Cytologically, most cells have the appearance of a regular nevus, but scattered atypical cells are present. These are epithelioid cells, which are larger, have more abundant cytoplasm, and may contain fine, dusty pigment. These cells can show variation in size and shape of the nuclei, and nucleoli may be prominent. The degree of atypism may range from mild to severe. Mitoses are rare.

Stromal changes include a patchy perivascular lymphocytic infiltrate and eosinophilic fibroplasia, which is a condensation of collagen around the rete ridges.

PROGNOSIS ▶

Dysplastic nevi require continued surveillance. Those with a nonfamilial sporadic dysplastic nevus have a tenfold increased risk of melanoma; the greater the number of family members who have dysplastic nevi or melanomas and the greater the number of such lesions on each family member, the greater the risk.

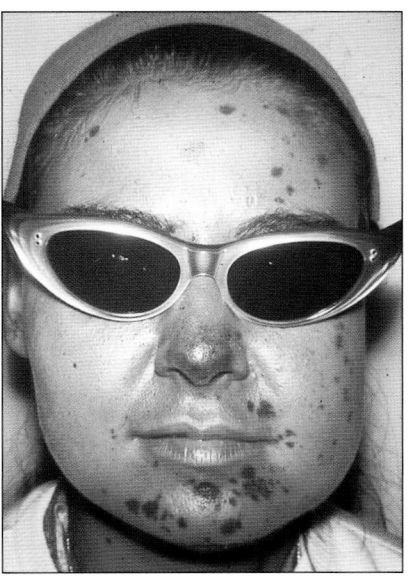

Fig 15-25 Diffuse metastatic deposits of melanoma in the skin and in internal organs, termed *melanomatosis*.

Table 15-1 Characteristic features of the nevus vs the melanoma

Nevus	Melanoma*
Symmetry	**A**symmetry
Borders regular	**B**orders irregular
Color uniform	**C**olor variegation
Diameter static	**D**iameter enlargement
Color stable	**D**arkening

*The features of the melanoma are referred to as the ABCDs.

Cutaneous Melanoma

CLINICAL PRESENTATION ▶ Melanomas, which are always malignant, represent one of the most life-threatening cancers known. Arising from melanocyte precursors, they have the ability to invade and readily metastasize, mostly via blood-borne routes but also through lymphatic channels. They are somewhat unique in their ability to metastasize to any organ, including the heart; at times they metastasize to nearly every organ in a condition called *melanomatosis* (Fig 15-25). Therefore, it is important that all clinicians be familiar with the risk factors and the appearance of early melanomas. It is also imperative that complete skin examinations be included in patient evaluations. Today, the expectation is that all practitioners are aware of the signs suggestive of melanoma and that referral or excisional biopsy of suspicious lesions be accomplished promptly. The previous practice of waiting for a change to occur in an already suspicious lesion is no longer valid, as metastasis and deeper invasion occur during this period.

RISKS ▶ Cutaneous melanomas are increasing, presumably because of the increase in recreational sun exposure and the effects of fluorocarbons on the protective atmospheric ozone layer. In 1987, the lifetime risk of cutaneous melanoma for whites in the United States was 1 in 123 (0.8%); in 2000, it approached 1 in 100 (1%).

The groups at highest risk are those with DNS or familial melanoma histories, followed by those with sporadic dysplastic nevi, followed by those with congenital nevi. Among the non–nevus-related group, the highest risk groups are those who overexpose themselves to the sun or sunburn easily (blond or red-haired individuals and/or those with blue or green eyes) or those who have had multiple, severe sunburns, particularly in childhood and the teenage years. Therefore, sunburn protection is imperative in childhood via sunblocks and limited exposures. Repeated severe sunburns spaced 1 or more years apart increase risk for melanoma more than do regular occupational exposures.

RECOGNITION ▶ When is a lesion suggestive of melanoma? The ABCDs of melanoma recognition are *a*symmetry, *b*order irregularity, *c*olor variegation, and *d*iameter enlargement. A darkening in color and an elevation of the surface are particularly suspicious; these are early melanoma signs. The more easily recognizable signs of ulceration, bleeding, or induration are late signs. Benign common nevi (moles) are uniform in color throughout and may be tan, brown, black, or blue. Their borders are regular and well demarcated from normal skin and the lesions are roughly symmetric (Table 15-1).

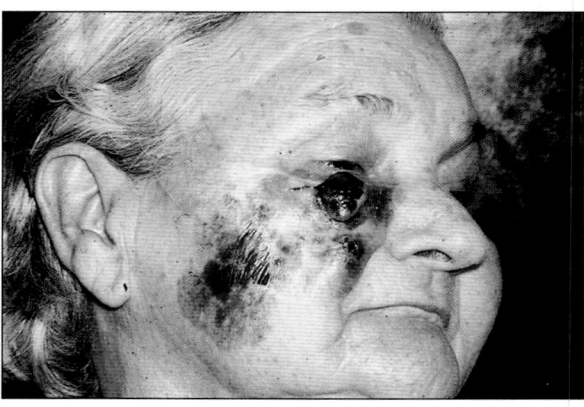

Fig 15-26 This rare photograph captures several independent lesions that together represent a clinically identifiable spectrum of a lentigo maligna to a lentigo maligna melanoma to a superficial spreading melanoma to a nodular melanoma.

PATHOGENESIS ▶

Melanocytes are normally located among the basal cells of the epidermis. They cause pigmentation by the synthesis and dispersion of melanin throughout the epidermis by their many dendritic processes, which extend between the keratinocytes (squamous cells) in the lower prickle cell layer and its basement membrane zone. They also release melanin, which is picked up by keratinocytes (squamous cells) and basal cells as well as macrophages (then called melanophages), contributing to the pigmented appearance. When melanocyte precursors become melanomas, they lose some of their constraints, which normally would keep them at the basal cell layer. Therefore, a well-differentiated melanoma or a premelanoma will retain some of its preference for the basal cell layer. It will proliferate laterally rather than downward, contained at its advancing edge by its limited growth potential and the host's immune response. Such entities that progress for years with tumor cell advancement, but with the host-induced immune response holding them in check, are well-known to occur on the face. These are termed *lentigo maligna melanoma*.

Clinical Progression and Classification

Most melanomas develop de novo, but others develop from pre-existing nevi, particularly dysplastic and congenital nevi. There are generally four clinical types of cutaneous melanomas, which correlate to characteristic histopathologic patterns at the lesion's periphery: lentigo maligna–lentigo maligna melanoma, superficial spreading melanoma, nodular melanoma, and acral lentiginous melanoma. In the superficial spreading melanoma type of cutaneous melanoma, the cells are somewhat less differentiated, and therefore they proliferate more aggressively than the host immune response can beat them back. They retain some of their affinity for the basal cell layer, but not as much as in lentigo maligna–lentigo maligna melanoma, leading to some downward invasion as well. Such melanomas may spread laterally with a limited level of downward invasion (radial growth phase) for months or even years before manifesting a pattern showing deeper levels of invasion (vertical growth phase).

The even more poorly differentiated nodular melanoma type proliferates even more aggressively. It usually has completely lost its affinity for the basal cell layer and, therefore, shows an immediate downward vertical growth phase. It will even proliferate upward to form a deep but exophytic mass.

Lentigo Maligna and Lentigo Maligna Melanoma

Lentigo maligna melanomas are most commonly found on facial skin (90%), particularly in the midcheek area in individuals 40 to 70 years of age. Representing premelanoma or melanoma in situ conditions, they have an exceedingly long radial growth phase at the basal cell level. As long as they show no downward invasion, they are termed *lentigo maligna* (also called *Hutchinson freckle*). When downward invasion begins, the condition is termed *lentigo maligna melanoma*. However, a lentigo maligna transforms into a lentigo maligna melanoma at a maximum 5% transformation rate (Fig 15-26). When transformation occurs, the prognosis depends, as it does in other melanomas, on thickness and depth of invasion. The prognosis is not inherently any better or worse when it arises from a pre-existing benign melanocytic condition.

Superficial Spreading Melanoma

The superficial spreading melanoma is most common among those 40 to 60 years of age. It is most frequently located on the mid-upper back in either sex and on the legs in women. In the oral and maxillofacial area, it is most frequently seen on the infraorbital skin, forehead, and posterior triangle of the neck. It will begin looking much like a nevus with uniform color, symmetry, and a well-demarcated regular border. After a few months, a typical superficial spreading melanoma will develop an irregular jagged border, a mixture of shades and colors, and an odd shape (Figs 15-27 and 15-28). These changes are characteristic of melanoma and of the radial growth phase in particular. The radial growth phase, which remains flat or is associated with only a slightly raised appearance, may last for just a few months or for up to 10 years before the vertical growth phase begins (Fig 15-29). The correlation best heralding nodularity and the vertical growth phase is size; when the superficial spreading melanoma attains a size of 2.5 cm, nodularity and the vertical growth phase can be expected (Fig 15-30).

Nodular Melanoma

The nodular melanoma is most common in those between 50 and 70 years of age. More frequent in men than in women by a 2:1 ratio, it will present as a dark-brown to black dome-shaped or polypoid mass (Fig 15-31). Ulceration of a melanoma is a sign of deep invasion and advanced disease (Fig 15-32). It is occasionally flesh colored and has therefore given rise to the term *amelanotic melanoma*. It is misdiagnosed more frequently than any other melanoma because it resembles small hemangiomas, dermal nevi, basal cell carcinomas, and even skin tags as a result of its nodular mass (Fig 15-33).

Acral Lentiginous Melanoma

Acral lentiginous melanomas are not found on the head and neck area, ocurring instead on the palms, soles, and distal phalanges (Fig 15-34). Occasionally they occur on mucous membranes, including those of the oral cavity. Like lentigo maligna and lentigo maligna melanomas of the face, they have a latency period of many years. Acral lentiginous melanoma is most frequently seen in Asians and blacks. When the lesions are flat, the prognosis is very good. However, when they have some elevation, an unseen aggressive downward growth has occurred, worsening the prognosis. A sudden pigmentation band appearing in the nail bed, called *Hutchinson sign*, is strongly suggestive of an acral lentiginous melanoma (Fig 15-35).

DIAGNOSTIC WORK-UP ▶

Excisional biopsy is the diagnostic procedure of choice. Where this is not possible (often around the nose or periorbit), an incisional or punch biopsy should be performed. Because diagnosis and treatment planning require a knowledge of the melanoma type, its thickness, and its level of invasion, the biopsy should allow the pathologist to assess all three features. Therefore, all biopsies should extend through the thickest part of the tumor to the underlying muscle fascia. If the lesion is flat, the biopsy should extend through the darkest area. It has been suggested that incisional or even punch biopsies dislodge malignant cells and increase the risk of metastasis, but there is no evidence to support this. Although incisional biopsies and even punch biopsies are not contraindicated from a tumor-seeding perspective, they are less ideal than an excisional biopsy because of the small size of the specimen and the difficulty in orientation.

In few other lesions is photography as important as in cutaneous melanomas. Lesions suggestive of cutaneous melanoma should be photographed before biopsy for documentation of size, color, shape, and location.

HISTOPATHOLOGY ▶

Primary melanomas originate at the epidermal-dermal junction. In radial growth phase melanoma, there is a proliferation of atypical melanocytes in the epidermis and sometimes in the superficial papil-

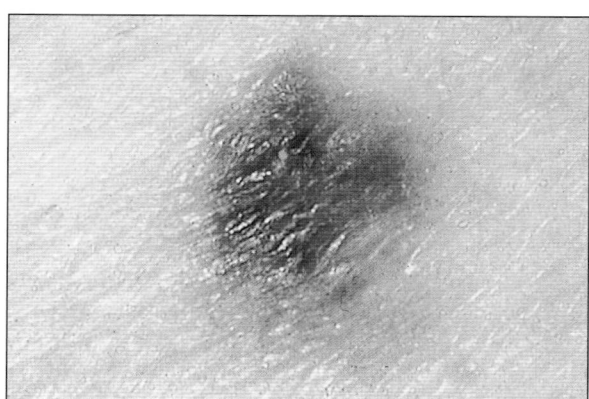

Fig 15-27 The superficial spreading melanoma is recognizable by its ABCDs: It is *asymmetric*, the *borders* are irregular, the *color* is variegated, and the *diameter* is larger than 1 cm.

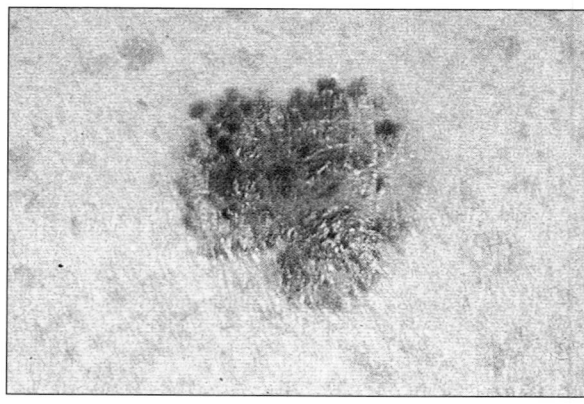

Fig 15-28 This superficial spreading melanoma also is recognized by its ABCDs. In addition, it is clinically suspicious for vertical progression by its central thickness and blue color, which is indicative of pigment deeper in the dermis.

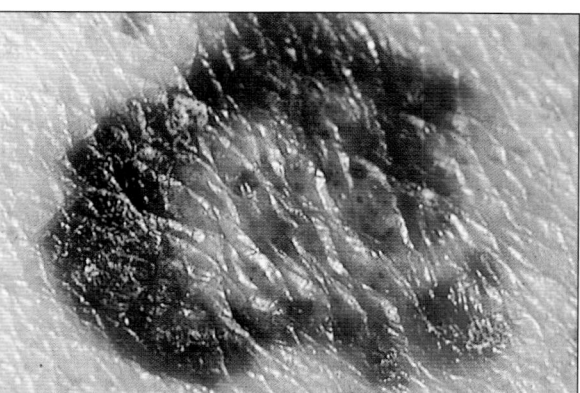

Fig 15-29 This superficial spreading melanoma in the radial growth phase is even more worrisome. The central area of regression is usually associated with progression to a vertical growth phase. (Reprinted from Elder DE, Murphy GF, *Melanocytic Tumors of the Skin*, with permission from the Armed Forces Institute of Pathology.)

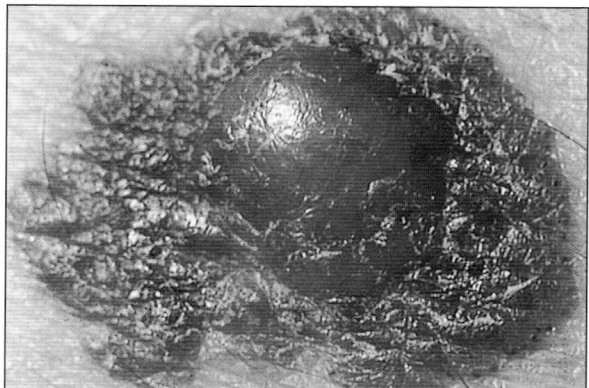

Fig 15-30 This superficial spreading melanoma has entered a vertical growth phase, apparent because of the nodule. This has formed an amelanotic melanoma. The lesion has exceeded 2.5 cm in size. (Reprinted from Elder DE, Murphy GF, *Melanocytic Tumors of the Skin*, with permission from the Armed Forces Institute of Pathology.)

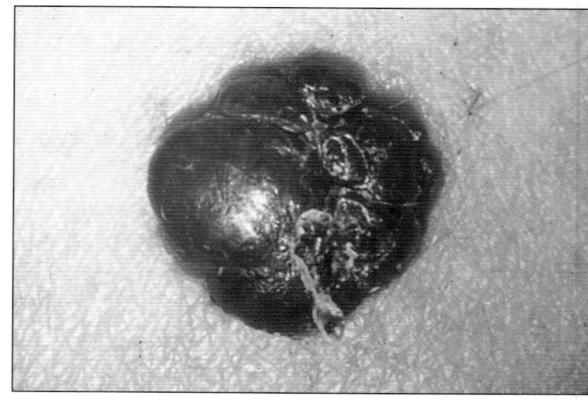

Fig 15-31 An obvious dark nodular melanoma such as this should not be dismissed because of its localized appearance. Nodular melanomas lack a radial growth phase, which gives them this well-demarcated appearance. Its exophytic growth belies deep endophytic growth and invasion.

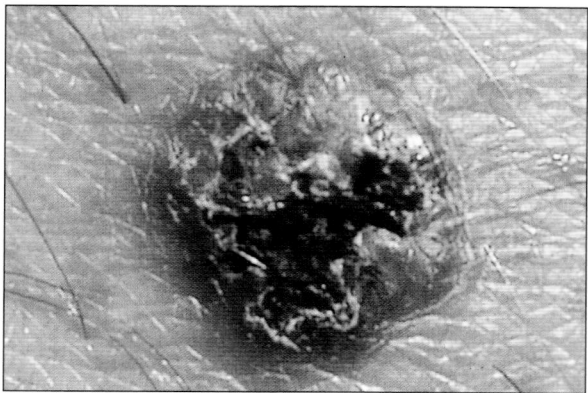

Fig 15-32 Ulceration of a nodular melanoma is a sign of deep invasion and rapid proliferation indicative of a worse prognosis.

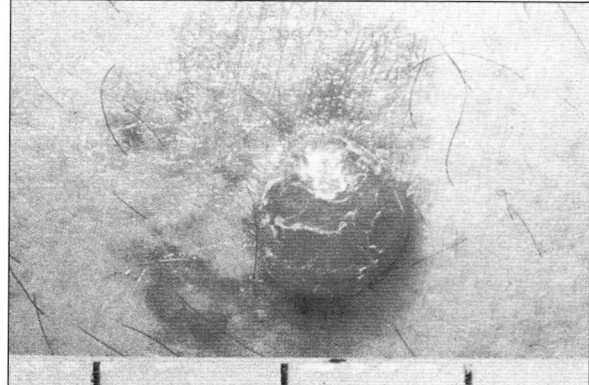

Fig 15-33 Amelanotic melanomas are just as threatening as pigmented ones. They are often misdiagnosed as hemangiomas or fibromas, and appropriate treatment is therefore delayed.

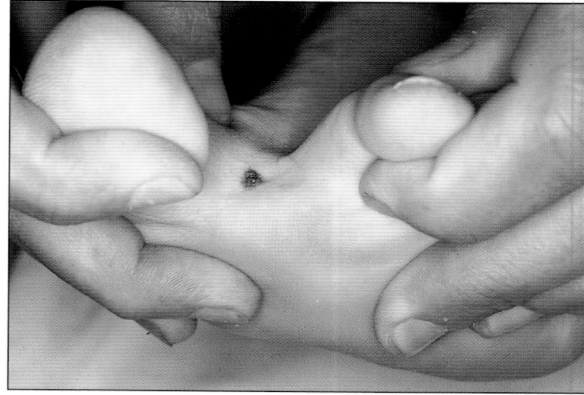

Fig 15-34 Acral lentiginous melanomas can escape detection because of their location on the palms, soles, or in webbing between fingers and toes.

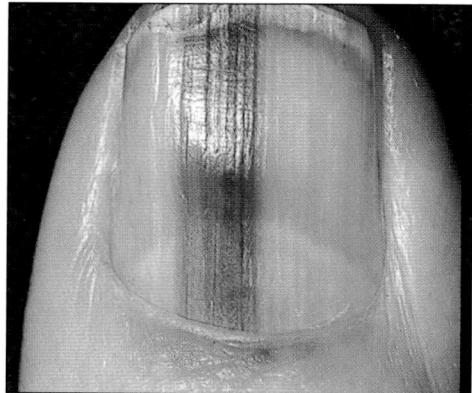

Fig 15-35 The rapid development of a pigmented lesion in a nail bed (Hutchinson sign) is strongly suspicious of acral lentiginous melanoma. (Reprinted from Cox NH and Lawrence CM, *Diagnostic Problems in Dermatology*, with permission from Mosby Publishing Co.)

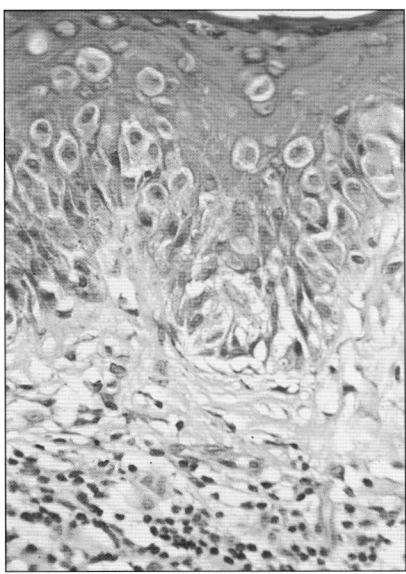

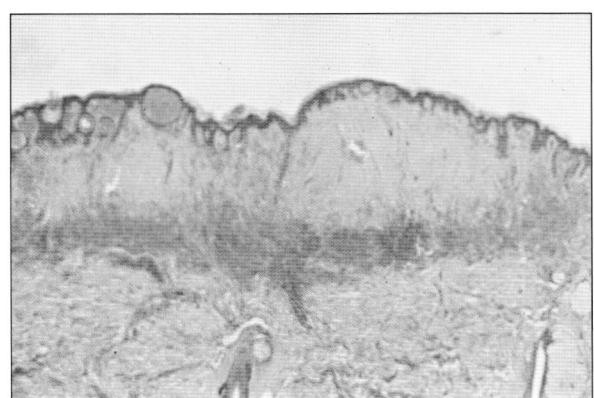

Fig 15-36 In this radial growth phase superficial spreading melanoma, pagetoid cells can be seen migrating up through the epithelium. A portion of a banded lymphocytic infiltrate within the dermis can also be seen.

Fig 15-37 Regressive changes within a melanoma, showing fibrosis, inflammation, and melanin incontinence.

lary dermis. The dermal component, however, does not proliferate as a mass to compress adjacent tissue, nor does it show mitotic activity. These lesions are asymmetric and may show thickening and elongation of the rete ridges. The clinical result is a plaque rather than a nodule. A banded lymphocytic infiltrate is present in the papillary dermis. Single enlarged, pale melanocytes, sometimes called pagetoid cells because of their resemblance to cells seen in mammary and extramammary Paget disease (Fig 15-36), may grow upward to the stratum corneum. The melanocytes also form nests of variable size, which may become confluent. The cells have abundant cytoplasm that frequently contains dusty melanin pigment. Nuclear atypism and hyperchromatism are present, and mitoses may be seen but are not numerous. Regressive changes, including lymphocytic infiltration, fibrosis, and melanin incontinence, are features of radial growth–phase melanoma (Fig 15-37). These changes are reflected clinically by notching and color variegation. The red component is a result of inflammation and the blue-gray component a result of fibrosis and melanin incontinence. Usually, however, the regressive changes are associated with vertical tumor progression.

In vertical growth phase melanoma, a tumor nodule, which is usually associated with radial growth phase changes, is formed. The nodular component is often hyperkeratotic and shows compression of the epidermis, sometimes with ulceration. Nests of tumor cells are present within the dermis; larger than the epidermal nests, they compress the surrounding tissue. Consequently, the base of the lesion may have a flattened rather than an infiltrative margin. There is no maturation of cells within the dermis, as is seen in benign melanocytic nevi. Compared to radial growth–phase melanoma, the tumor cells have less pigment but show more atypia and mitoses, although the latter are not numerous. The lymphocytic component also is diminished.

Because the prognosis associated with melanoma primarily depends on tumor thickness, measurements are indicated as part of the pathology report. Originally, Clark's levels of invasion were employed (Table 15-2); these were based on anatomic structures. Later, Breslow introduced the objective measurement of the lesion using a micrometer in the ocular of the microscope; measurement is taken from the top of the granular cell layer to the deepest extent of the tumor (Fig 15-38 and Table 15-3). In ulcerated lesions, the measurement is taken from the base of the ulcer to the deepest area of invasion.

Table 15-2 Clark's levels of invasion

Level	Degree of invasiveness
I	Tumor cells confined to epidermis and skin appendages
II	Tumor cells in papillary dermis
III	Tumor cells throughout papillary dermis and impinging on reticular dermis
IV	Tumor cells within reticular dermis
V	Tumor cells within subcutaneous fat

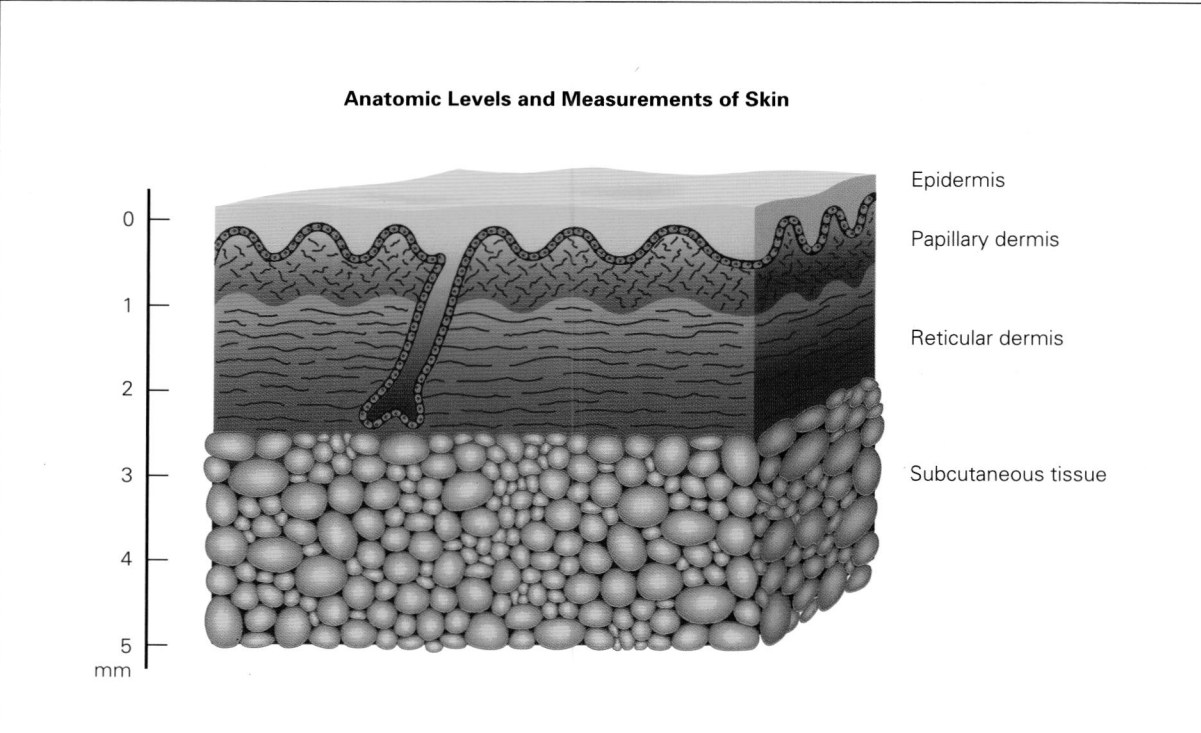

Anatomic Levels and Measurements of Skin

Fig 15-38 Approximate anatomic levels and measurements of average normal skin upon which Clark's levels and Breslow's measurements of invasion are based.

Table 15-3 Breslow's measurement of tumor thickness

Thickness (mm)	Risk of recurrence
< 0.76	Low risk
0.76 to 1.50	Low to intermediate risk
1.50 to 3.99	Intermediate to high risk
> 4.00	High risk

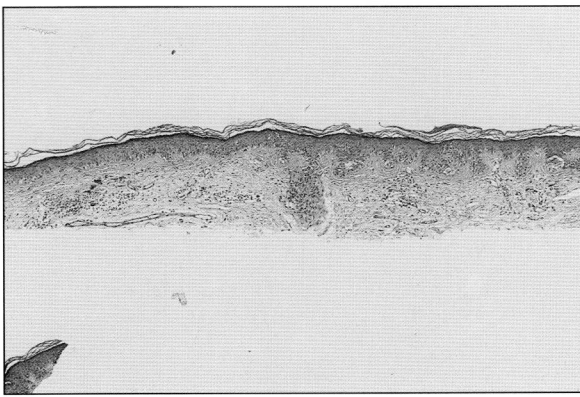

Fig 15-39a A lentigo maligna melanoma showing the extensive involvement of the basal cell layer. This finding indicates the prolonged radial growth phase of these tumors.

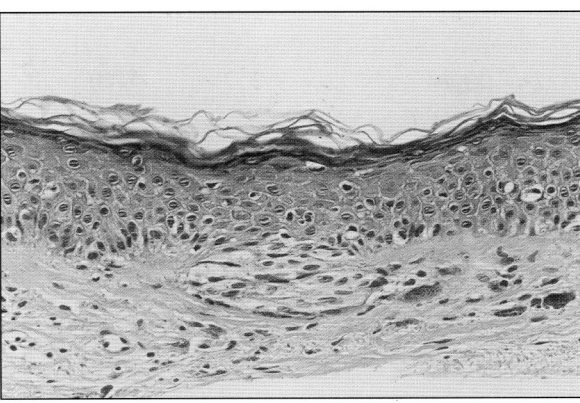

Fig 15-39b High-power view of the tumor shown in Fig 15-39a showing some spindle tumor cells.

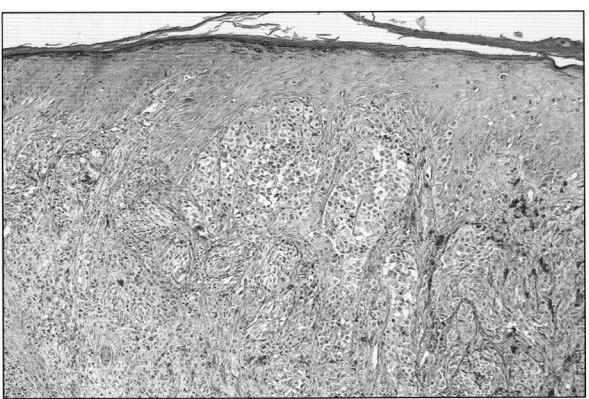

Fig 15-40a A portion of a superficial spreading melanoma showing the proliferation of nests of rounded, epithelial-like cells.

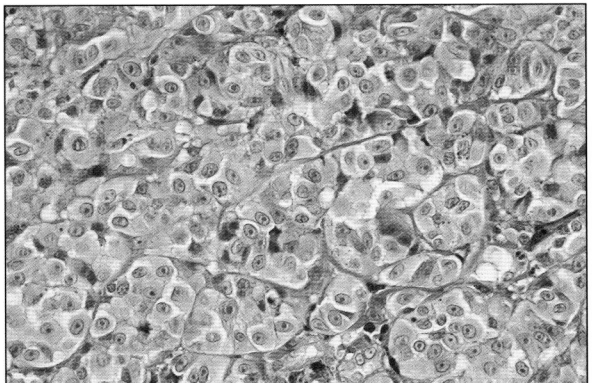

Fig 15-40b High-power view of Fig 15-40a showing the clusters of tumor cells with delicate fibrous tissue separating the nests. Melanin pigment, though present, is sparse.

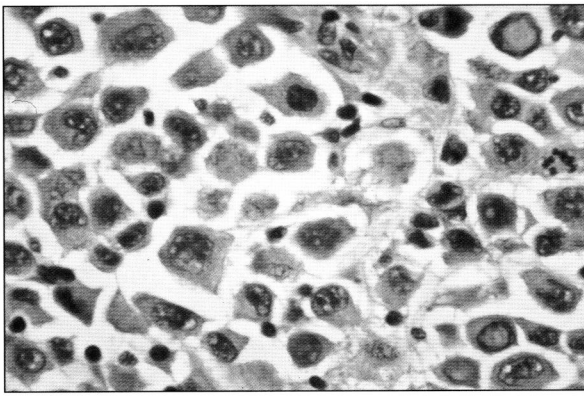

Fig 15-41a Cutaneous melanoma in which the areas closer to the epithelial surface show typical nests. In the deeper area shown here, no such pattern is found. Instead, a population of highly anaplastic cells is seen.

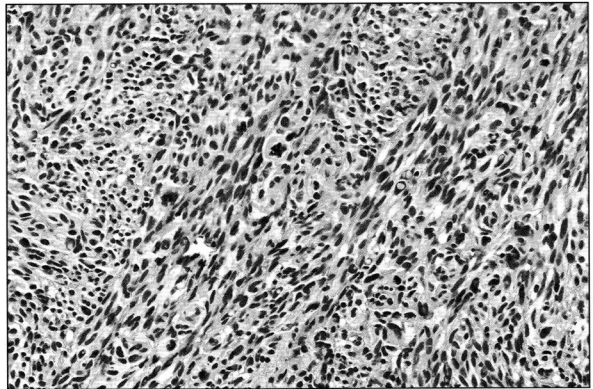

Fig 15-41b Melanoma from the maxillary mucosa showing a more sarcomatous pattern with spindle cells and mitoses.

Histologic differences in the various types of melanoma may sometimes be appreciated, but these have no direct bearing on prognosis. In general, melanomas are biphasic tumors showing spindle and epithelioid cells. Lentigo maligna melanoma and acral lentiginous melanoma tend to be predominantly spindle cell tumors (Figs 15-39a and 15-39b) and are more likely to exhibit neurotropism. Nodular and superficial spreading melanomas are usually more dominantly epithelioid. These cells tend to form an alveolar pattern with thin fibrovascular trabeculae surrounding the cell clusters (Figs 15-40a and 15-40b). They have abundant cytoplasm, often with prominent eosinophilic nucleoli. Lentigo maligna melanoma and superficial spreading melanoma will show contiguous epidermal changes, whereas in nodular melanomas the only portion of epidermis showing changes overlies the dermal component. Melanin, the quantity of which varies greatly, may be found within tumor cells or within melanophages. Even in amelanotic melanomas, the use of a Fontana-Masson stain will often reveal the presence of melanin.

The histologic appearance of melanomas is highly variable and may mimic that of a host of tumors, including anaplastic carcinomas, spindle cell sarcomas, and lymphomas (Figs 15-41a and 15-41b). Usually, the melanin pigment, biphasic cellular pattern, and prominent eosinophilic nucleoli are helpful features. It is customary to confirm the diagnosis (or to make the diagnosis) by immunohistochemistry. S-100 protein and HMB-45, which is a marker for premelanosomes, are both typically positive. Lack of keratin markers will usually distinguish melanomas from carcinomas. They are also leukocyte common antigen–negative, which distinguishes these tumors from lymphomas.

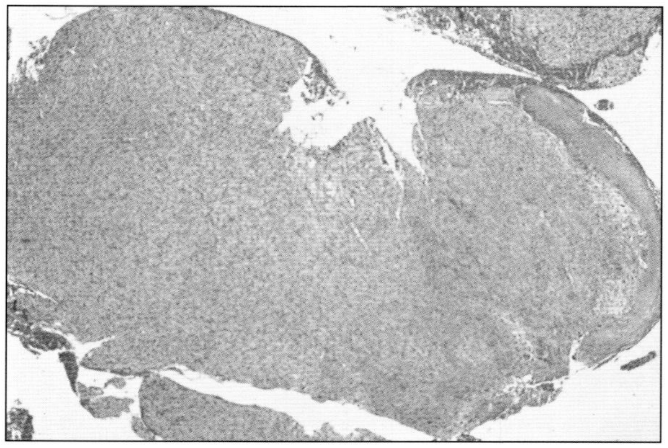

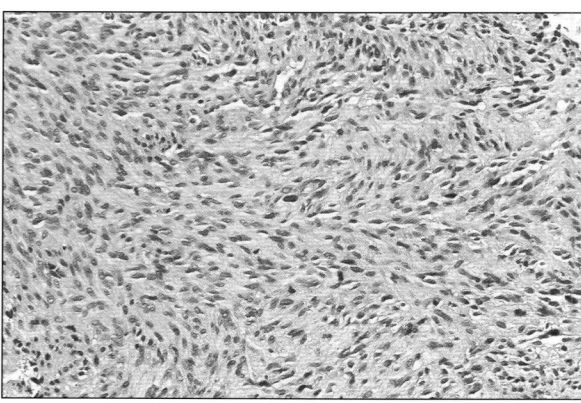

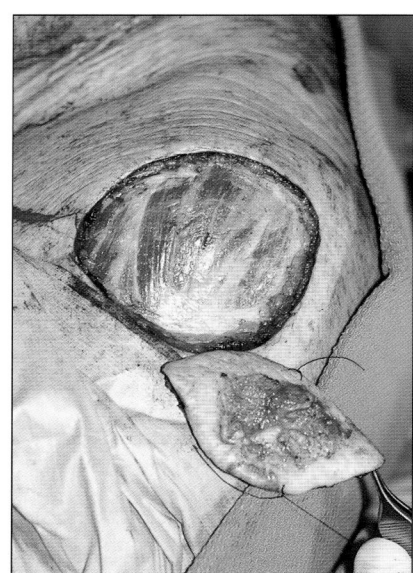

Fig 15-42a A desmoplastic melanoma of the maxillary mucosa showing a spindle cell proliferation and prominent nuclei.

Fig 15-42b High-power view of Fig 15-42a showing a spindle cell proliferation suggestive of a neurogenic tumor. Some atypia is present.

Fig 15-43 Surgical excision of a primary cutaneous melanoma requires wide margins based on the greatest depth of invasion (about 1 cm of margin per 1 mm of invasion) and to a depth inclusive of the subcutaneous layer.

Desmoplastic melanomas are predominantly spindle cell tumors that may have scant or absent pigment. Atypia is not marked, and mitoses are rare. Often the cells occur in wavy bundles and have serpentine nuclei so that they resemble peripheral nerve sheath tumors. Others are very desmoplastic and resemble fibromatoses (Figs 15-42a and 15-42b). These tumors are neurotropic and may exhibit endoneural and perineural invasion. While these neoplasms are usually S-100 positive, they are typically HMB-45 negative. Although uncommon, these tumors have arisen in oral mucosa.

CLINICAL STAGING AND WORK-UP

The work-up of a cutaneous melanoma requires only a history, a thorough physical evaluation including all skin and mucous membrane areas, clinical photographs, and a chest radiograph. More invasive studies or complex scans do not better detect metastatic melanoma.

Much of the treatment and prognosis will be based on the pathologist's assessment of the initial biopsy, particularly as it relates to Breslow's measurement of thickness or Clark's level of invasion. The pathologist also will assess the type of growth phase, the mitotic index, the degree of lymphocytic response, lymphocytic invasion into the melanoma, and histologic regression. However, each melanoma is also assigned a clinical stage that has a bearing on prognosis: stage I, local disease only; stage II, local disease with palpable lymphadenopathy; and stage III, clinical or test evidence of distant metastasis.

TREATMENT

Surgery is the focus of therapy for all types of melanoma. Neither radiotherapy nor chemotherapy has a significant impact on melanomas and is thus not usually part of the primary care.

The surgery requires two difficult treatment decisions in stage I: determination of the resection margins and whether or not to perform a regional lymph node dissection. Because thicker lesions will in general spread more laterally, the approximate peripheral margins are 1 cm if the lesion thickness is less than 2 mm, 2 cm margins if the lesion thickness is between 2 and 3 mm, and 3 cm if the lesion thickness is greater than 3 mm. The depth of excision should extend to the underlying muscle fascia (Fig 15-43). A prophylactic neck dissection is indicated only if the depth of invasion is greater than 1 mm. In the maxillofacial area, a prophylactic neck dissection is a functional neck dissection (see Chapter 7, page 301). A treatment neck dissection for palpable neck nodes would be a modified radical or full radical neck dissection (see Chapter 7, pages 298 to 301).

Table 15-4 General prognosis of melanoma in terms of location

Extremities and shoulders
Back
Skin of head and neck
Palms and soles
Subungual
Mucosa
Internal organs

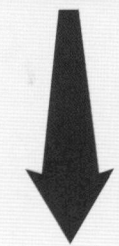

Decreasing prognosis

PROGNOSIS AND FOLLOW-UP

Melanoma prognosis encompasses an 8-year survival curve, unlike the 5-year survival curve for oral squamous cell carcinoma. The prognosis associated with cutaneous melanomas excised in the radial growth phase approaches 100% survival. However, melanomas in the early vertical growth phase up to nodular melanomas require analysis of six independent variables: tumor thickness, mitotic rate, lymphocytes infiltrating tumor, histologic regression, site of occurrence, and sex. Duration of the radial growth phase progressively decreases from nodular melanoma to superficial spreading melanoma to acral lentiginous melanoma and finally to lentigo maligna melanoma. In general, men have a worse prognosis than women. A poorer prognosis is associated with thicker tumors, a greater mitotic rate, smaller numbers of infiltrating lymphocytes, and, paradoxically, greater tumor regression. The head and neck area (cutaneous maxillofacial area) has a better prognosis than the vulvar or subungual areas of the extremities but a poorer prognosis than other areas of the extremities (Table 15-4).

Follow-up should be lifelong. Melanomas are well-known for late metastases, some more than 10 years after the primary tumor, hence the longer (8-year) survival curves on which statistics are based. The period of time between primary tumor and metastasis is inversely related to the tumor thickness; thicker tumors recur and metastasize sooner than do thinner ones. However, one should not assume that a flat or thin melanoma is cured after 5 or 6 years; it is just this type of melanoma that will emerge with a late metastatic focus.

Follow-up should consist of examinations, including a chest radiograph, at least every 6 months.

Mucosal Melanoma

CLINICAL PRESENTATION AND PATHOGENESIS

Oral melanomas and melanomas arising on other mucous membranes, such as the nose, pharynx, and conjunctiva, are termed *mucosal melanomas*. As a group, they invade and spread more quickly, metastasize more quickly and frequently, and therefore are associated with a much poorer prognosis than cutaneous melanomas. Like cutaneous melanomas, they arise from melanocyte precursors and nevus cells. Mucosal melanomas are much less common than cutaneous melanomas. They have no sex predilection and occur in somewhat older individuals, generally in those older than 50 years, than do skin melanomas.

The most common site for an oral melanoma is the palate (Fig 15-44). Other less common sites include the gingiva, lips, floor of the mouth (Fig 15-45), and buccal mucosa. Its appearance on mucous membranes follows the same ABCD recognition algorithm as skin melanomas (asymmetry, border irregularity, color variegation, and diameter enlargement).

Most clinical types of cutaneous melanoma—superficial spreading, nodular, and acral lentiginous—may also occur on mucous membranes. However, lentigo maligna and lentigo maligna melanoma do not.

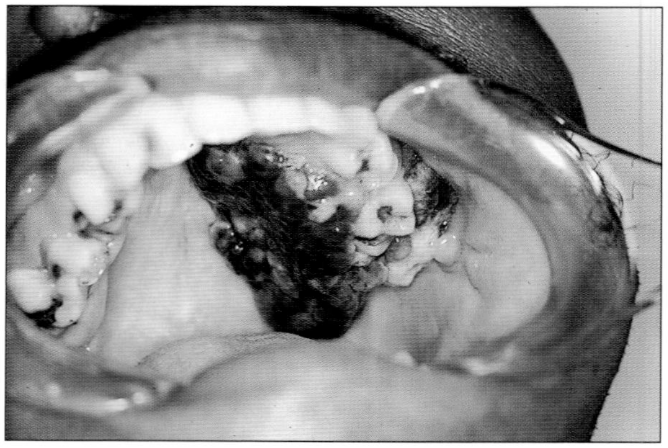

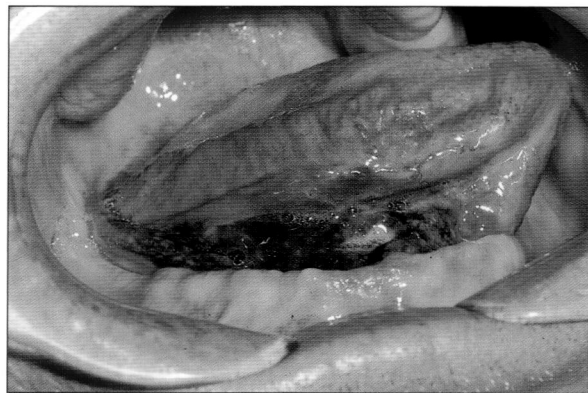

Fig 15-44 The palate is the most common location for an oral melanoma. These are, of course, unrelated to sun exposure and occur equally among all races.

Fig 15-45 Oral melanomas also may occur on other mucosal surfaces, including the floor of the mouth. Note that the ABCDs of clinical recognition, including a blue-black color, are represented here.

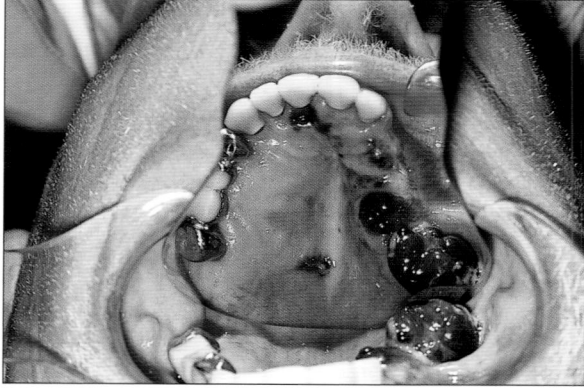

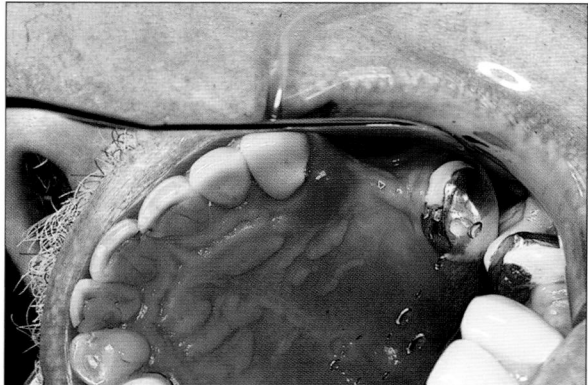

Fig 15-46 Oral mucosal melanomas frequently show multifocal clinical sites and satellite lesions, as seen here.

Fig 15-47 A desmoplastic melanoma is more localized and more subtle than other mucosal melanomas and may appear as an inflammatory process.

It is much more difficult to clinically type mucosal melanomas because of their rapid advancement and spread. Mucosal melanomas usually are not divided into subtypes because such a differentiation has little relevance to treatment or prognosis. Also, because mucous membranes are thinner than skin and do not have as many levels of anatomic distinction, most mucosal melanomas progress more quickly to the vertical growth phase. Whereas skin layers consist of epidermis, papillary dermis, reticular dermis, and subcutaneous fat, mucous membranes consist only of an epithelial layer; a lamina propria, which is also thinner than the corresponding papillary dermis of skin; and a submucosal layer. The thin lamina propria and the absence of a reticular dermis allow mucosal melanomas to spread peripherally and to gain access to the richest lymphatic and vascular networks more quickly.

Commonly accompanying mucosal melanomas are satellite lesions that are located adjacent to but separate from the main lesion (Fig 15-46). Hard palate mucosal melanomas are often associated with satellite lesions on the soft palate and/or tonsillar pillars. Such lesions represent local metastases through small lymphatic or vascular channels. Such findings are common to oral mucosal melanomas and are associated with a poor prognosis. Mucosal melanomas also may have a poorer prognosis than do cutaneous melanomas because they have a different stimulus of malignant transformation.

The oral and maxillofacial surgeon may be confronted with a pathology report diagnosing a desmoplastic melanoma in locally excised tissue from what was speculated to be a peripheral odontogenic fibroma, a peripheral giant cell proliferation, or another similar, relatively nonaggressive pathology. The desmoplastic melanoma is a very rare finding in the oral cavity and therefore will be an unexpected diagnosis. The few reported cases have usually been a small red (rather than brown or black) nodule on the maxillary edentulous ridge (Fig 15-47) or gingiva in males older than 50 years. Indeed, the nodule is nonpigmented and usually less than 1 cm in diameter. It may be associated with adjacent pigmented macules.

The importance of this diagnosis is that, while it does indeed represent a melanoma, it has a better prognosis than do other oral melanomas. It is treated with a wide soft tissue excision that does not include excision of the underlying bone if the deep margin is free of tumor. If the deep margin has tumor in it or very close to it, a local excision of the alveolus is recommended.

As discussed in Chapter 7, cancer of the same histologic type may be generated by different gene-damaging carcinogens, and different carcinogens and/or loci of gene damage result in cancers with different behavioral patterns and aggressiveness. The relationship of skin melanomas to sun-damage effects suggests a carcinogenesis of ultraviolet light; yet, the history of dysplastic nevus syndrome and its increased melanoma risk suggests a hereditary or chromosomal influence in some. The fact that oral mucosal and other mucosal melanomas arise without a sun-damage carcinogenesis already distinguishes them from skin melanomas. Therefore, their basic biologic behavior is expected to be different; unfortunately, it is one that is much more aggressive.

DIFFERENTIAL DIAGNOSIS ▶ Oral mucosal melanomas appear blue, black, or a mixture of each. Blue melanomas have less melanin and the lesion is relatively deep. Black melanomas have a higher density of melanin and a more superficial location. Blue melanomas, therefore, may resemble a *hemangioma* or a *lymphangioma*, mucus-producing salivary gland lesions such as a *low-grade mucoepidermoid carcinoma* or a *mucus retention phenomenon*, or *Kaposi sarcoma*. Black melanomas, which are more distinctive, also can resemble a *lymphangioma*. Smaller melanomas may be difficult to distinguish from the common *amalgam tattoo*, the *oral melanotic macule*, or even a *heavy-metal pigmentation*.

DIAGNOSTIC WORK-UP ▶ Because of the rapid spread and poor prognosis associated with mucosal melanomas, suspicious pigmented lesions should be removed by excisional biopsy. Large melanomas may be diagnosed by an incisional biopsy. Each biopsy should include the full thickness of mucosa and include the thickest portion of the lesion. Before biopsy, examination of the oropharynx and the neck are indicated. If a melanoma is diagnosed, a chest radiograph is required to complete a metastatic work-up.

HISTOPATHOLOGY ▶ Because oral mucosal melanomas are so infrequent, they are not yet as well understood as cutaneous melanomas. Attempts have been made to fit them into existing classifications, and reference is often made to their similarity to acral lentiginous melanoma. Often falling into this category are melanomas of the lip, which frequently have atypical dendritic melanocytes proliferating in a lentiginous pattern, with lichenoid lymphocytic infiltrates and a spindle cell proliferation with desmoplasia and neurotropism in their vertical growth phase. About one third of tumors in the oral cavity have precedent areas of pigmentation, suggesting an initial radial growth phase that can be of widely varying duration. Most other tumors appear to be nodular melanomas, since they do not seem to have a radial growth component. Clark's levels are not appropriate within the oral mucosa, and Breslow's measurements have not been used in meaningful numbers; therefore, correlation of depth of invasion and prognosis has not yet been established in the oral mucosa.

TREATMENT ▶ Early oral melanomas are treated the same as more advanced skin melanomas, with 3-cm margins. If the lesion was removed by means of excisional biopsy, the biopsy site is removed with 3-cm margins. Unfortunately, many oral melanomas are deeply infiltrative at the time of diagnosis and require bone and other deep tissue extirpation. Although each case must be treated based on clinical and CT scan evidence of its invasion, 3- to 5-cm margins are generally required with these advanced lesions. For the most common site, the palate, surgery will consist of a type of maxillectomy with 3- to 5-cm margins (Fig 15-48). Sometimes excision extending to the soft palate, tonsillar pillar, and into the pterygomaxillary space may be justified.

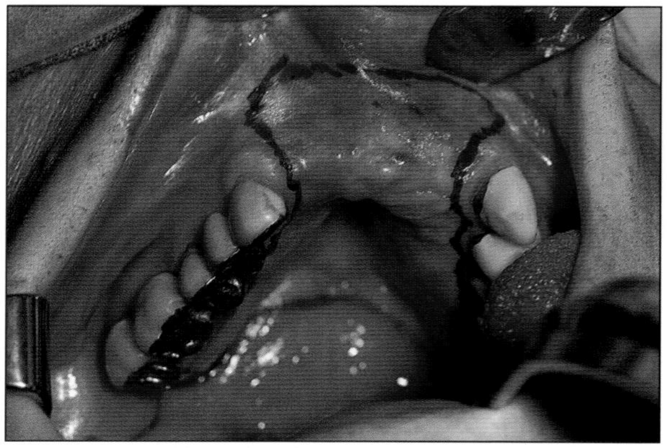

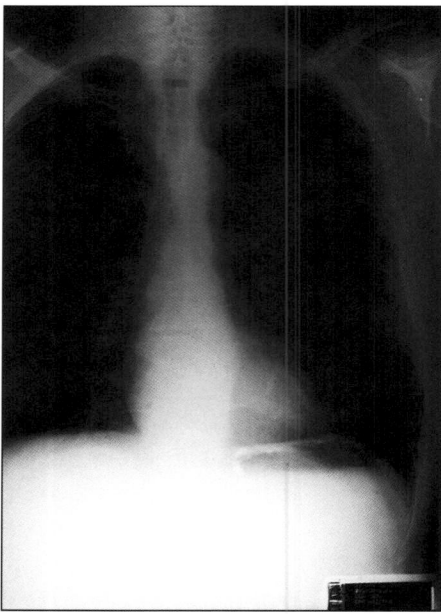

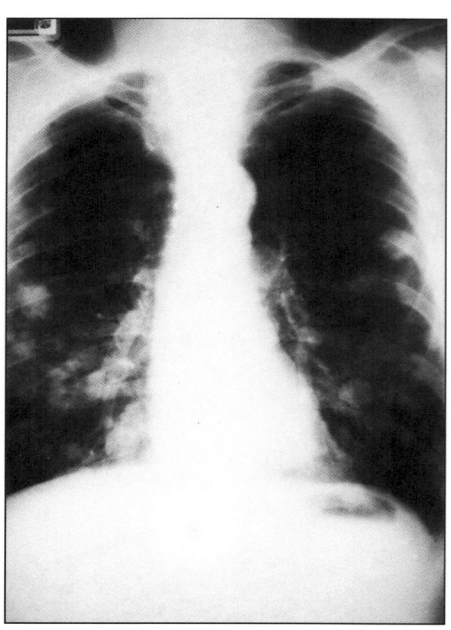

Fig 15-48 A very wide excision of oral mucosal melanomas is necessary. Margins of 3 to 5 cm are frequent. The resection may either be limited to the soft tissue mucosa or take the form of a maxillectomy.

Fig 15-49a This chest radiograph, taken at the time the palatal melanoma shown in Fig 15-46 was diagnosed, is free of metastasis.

Fig 15-49b The clear chest radiograph shown in Fig 15-49a now shows multiple metastatic deposits of melanoma in this radiograph taken 10 months later.

PROGNOSIS AND FOLLOW-UP ▶

The indications for neck dissections are as uncertain for mucosal melanomas as they are for cutaneous melanomas. However, because of rapid advancement to dense lymphatic networks, prophylactic neck dissection is a strong consideration in oral melanomas.

The 8-year survival rate for all oral melanomas is about 20%, which is less than half the 8-year survival rate for all cutaneous melanomas (about 60%). Follow-up involves a thorough oral and pharyngeal examination every 4 months and a chest radiograph every 6 months (Figs 15-49a and 15-49b). For individuals who present with significant metastasis or unresectable primary tumors, traditional chemotherapy and/or radiotherapy offer only slight palliation. However, numerous research protocols recruit such patients, offering them some hope and at times palliation. The National Cancer Institute (1-800-4-CANCER; www.cancer.gov) and the National Institutes of Health (www.nih.gov) provide lists of research protocol opportunities.

Congenital Nevi

CLINICAL PRESENTATION ▶

Congenital nevi account for only 1% of all nevi. More usual is a junctional nevus developing at age 2 years and progressing to a compound nevus through the teenage years and then to a dermal nevus in adulthood. Congenital nevi are significant because of their much higher incidence of melanoma transformation.

Congenital nevi, also called *birthmarks*, may occur in any location but most commonly are seen on the buttocks and trunk (Fig 15-50a). Some contain hair, which is usually coarse in texture. Rarely, an individual will present with an extremely large nevus, called a *giant hairy nevus*, which imparts a focal, so-called werewolf appearance. Most are flat, smooth, and uniform in color (brown to black). As the child ages, the nevus tends to become thicker and the surface verrucous or nodular. The potential for melanoma development even as early as childhood increases with the size and thickness of the congenital nevi.

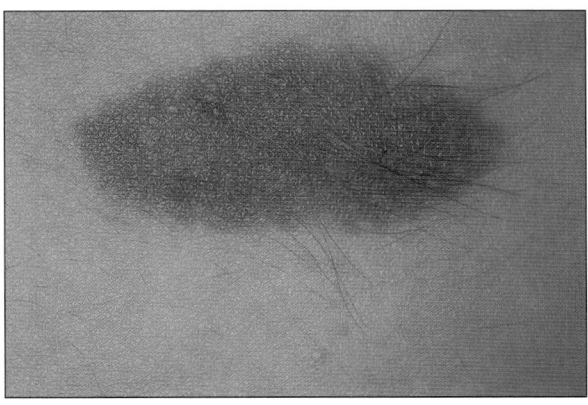

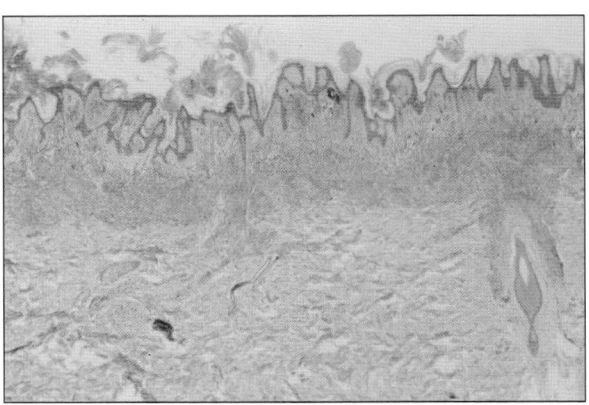

Fig 15-50a This 3.5-cm congenital nevus is located on the right buttock of a 2¹/₂-year-old boy. Present at birth, the lesion initially appeared reddish but has deepened in color and developed some dark, coarse hair.

Fig 15-50b A congenital nevus showing considerable thickness of nevus cells and concentration around a hair follicle.

DIFFERENTIAL DIAGNOSIS ▶

Most congenital nevi are recognizable clinically, but café-au-lait macules associated with *Albright syndrome* and *hereditary neurofibromatosis* may also occur congenitally. Rare syndromes such as *Leopard syndrome* (*l*entigines, *e*lectromyographic disturbances, *o*cular hypertelorism, *p*ulmonic stenosis, *a*bnormal genitalia, *r*etarded growth, and *d*eafness) and *lipatrophic diabetes with acanthosis nigricans* will manifest large areas of brown hyperpigmentation congenitally.

DIAGNOSTIC WORK-UP
AND TREATMENT ▶

Small congenital nevi require only observation. Larger, thicker lesions should be excised. Some authors have recommended excision of all congenital nevi because of the high melanoma transformation rate. This view, however, is not universally accepted; some reports show that only 8% of melanomas have features suggesting that they arose from congenital nevi. However, careful and watchful follow-up of all congenital nevi is recommended.

HISTOPATHOLOGY ▶

Congenital nevi may be indistinguishable from acquired nevi. However, they often involve the lower third of the reticular dermis and the skin appendages. Giant nevi typically involve reticular dermis, subcutaneous tissue, and fascia (Fig 15-50b). A splaying of cells is seen between the collagen bundles in the reticular dermis. Within the fat, the nevus cells often resemble fibroblasts. Abnormalities of neural crest–derived tissues, including schwannian proliferations and cartilage formation, may be seen within the giant nevi.

Fibro-Osseous Diseases and Systemic Diseases Affecting Bone

▶ "Although ego and economics drive our everyday lives, it is ideals and ideas that build our future."

—*Robert E. Marx*

Primary Hyperparathyroidism

▶

Primary hyperparathyroidism is caused by hypersecretion of parathyroid hormone (PTH), most commonly by the subset of four hyperplastic glands, less commonly by a parathyroid adenoma, or very rarely by a true carcinoma. Most cases today are identified by hypercalcemia (≥10.5 mg/dL [2.6 mmol/L], after correction for serum albumin) on routine multipanel serum testing. Less than 5% of cases are recognized by the presence of an osteolytic defect with giant cells, a condition referred to as a *brown tumor*. Some cases are suspected by the presence of renal "stones" (nephrocalcinosis). However, only 5% of people with nephrocalcinosis have primary hyperparathyroidism.

Primary hyperparathyroidism is more common in women and in those older than 50 years. Most gland hyperplasias are of unknown cause, but some are related to the multiple endocrine neoplasia syndrome of familial inheritance types I and IIa (MEN I and MEN IIa). Because most cases are due to an idiopathic hyperplasia of each gland, a neck mass is usually not palpable. In addition, most cases are asymptomatic. However, as serum calcium levels increase, symptoms may occur that are related to the hypercalcemia per se or to the disease's effects on bone and on the urinary tract.

The pathogenesis of hypercalcemia is the oversecretion of active PTH. This polypeptide hormone increases serum calcium levels by the following three mechanisms (in order of decreasing effect): (*1*) increasing osteoclastic bone resorption; (*2*) reducing renal excretion of calcium; and (*3*) increasing calcium absorption in the small intestines. The resultant abnormal laboratory test results are, therefore, hypercalcemia, a compensatory hypophosphatemia, and an alkaline phosphatase level that is usually normal but can be elevated in widespread lytic disease.

Hypercalcemia-Related Signs and Symptoms

The symptoms most commonly associated with hypercalcemia include thirst, nausea, and vomiting. In addition, constipation, weight loss, anemia, and peptic ulcer disease, as well as hypertension, may develop. If the hypercalcemia is severe (>15 mg/dL [3.75 mmol/L]) or long-lasting, depression and psychosis may result. Higher serum calcium levels also are associated with fatigability, muscle weakness, and paresthesias.

Bone-Related Signs and Symptoms

Bone pain is the main symptom and occurs primarily in the vertebrae, tibias, and joints. Long-standing disease can produce kyphosis and multiple small vertebral fractures that can lead to loss of height. Radiolucencies (brown tumors) may develop in bones, commonly in the jaws, or a diffuse

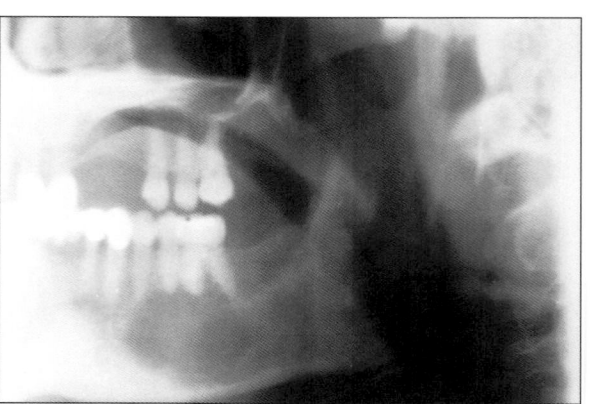

Fig 16-1a This mandibular radiolucency was asymptomatic and caused a slight expansion. It was thought to be another entity but was confirmed to be a brown tumor by biopsy and a serum calcium determination, which identified a 14.1 mg/dL value.

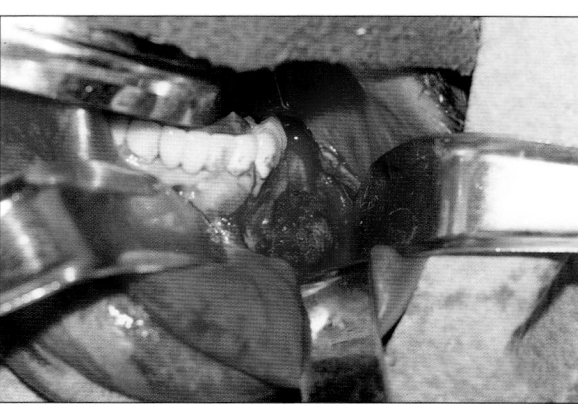

Fig 16-1b This known brown tumor of hyperparathyroidism was identical to the more common giant cell tumor. It was friable, hemorrhagic, and reddish brown.

demineralization, sometimes called *osteitis fibrosa cystica*, may result. Both entities evidence a fibrovascular stroma replacing mineralized bone, while "giant cells," which are presumably osteoclasts, are seen resorbing bone. These areas appear as a friable, red-brown mass, hence the term *brown tumors* (Figs 16-1a and 16-1b). Clinicians often seek discrete unilocular or multilocular radiolucencies representing brown tumors in the jaws; these are, however, rare. More common are subtle changes in the trabecular bone pattern resembling age-related osteoporosis. On occasion, tooth mobility occurs and sometimes loss of the lamina dura is seen, but this feature is rare and may be associated with only a few teeth.

Urinary Tract–Related Signs and Symptoms

Polyuria and a resultant increase in thirst (polydipsia) are related to hypercalcemia. Renal calculi in the calyces or ureters or calcifications within the renal parenchyma (nephrocalcinosis) are deposits of calcium oxalate or calcium phosphate. Obstructive nephropathy or nephrocalcinosis leading to renal failure may develop in long-standing disease.

DIFFERENTIAL DIAGNOSIS AND WORK-UP ▶

The most common presentation is one of hypercalcemia without radiographic evidence of bone lesions. Other entities that cause hypercalcemia and therefore must be ruled out are *multiple myeloma*, *hypercalcemia of malignancy*, *sarcoidosis*, *overingestion of calcium and/or vitamin D*, *adrenal insufficiency*, and *familial hypocalciuric hypercalcemia*.

Primary hyperparathyroidism should be confirmed by radioimmunoassays (RIAs) of the circulating parathyroid levels. Such RIAs are sufficiently specific to determine levels of normal PTH. Malignant tumor products of PTH-related polypeptides will not be registered on RIAs. If necessary, multiple myeloma can be ruled out by serum protein electrophoresis, sarcoidosis by an incisional parotid biopsy, overingestion of calcium or vitamin D by history, familial hypercalciuric hypercalcemia by history and by 24-hour urine collections showing more than 50 mg/24 hr (1.25 mmol/d) of calcium, and adrenal insufficiency by serum sodium levels and an adrenocorticotropic hormone (ACTH) challenge.

HISTOPATHOLOGY ▶

Jaw lesions of hyperparathyroidism exhibit a picture that is virtually identical to that of the central giant cell tumor. A proliferation of spindle cells with extravasated blood and haphazardly arranged, variably sized multinucleated giant cells is seen (Figs 16-1c and 16-1d). These are osteoclasts, the action of

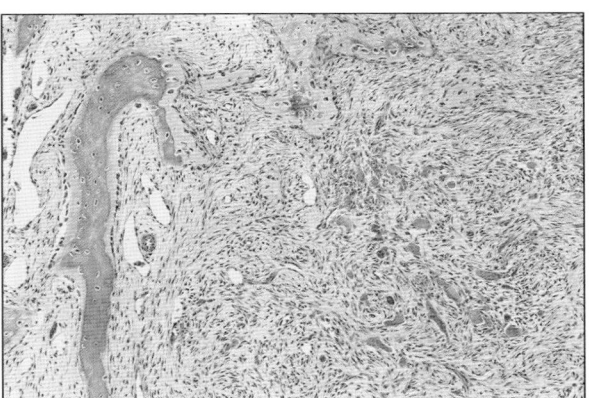

Fig 16-1c A lesion of hyperparathyroidism showing resorption of bone with deposition of osteoid and a fibrous stroma with multinucleated giant cells.

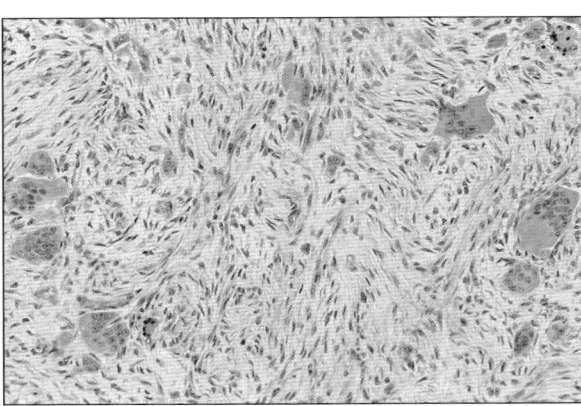

Fig 16-1d High-power view of Fig 16-1c with the fibrous stroma and scattered osteoclasts. Both the osteoclasts and hemorrhage occur haphazardly throughout the lesion.

which is influenced by PTH. Osteoid formation may also occur (see Fig 16-1c). All types of hyperparathyroidism present similar histologic findings.

TREATMENT ▶

Medical treatment for primary hyperparathyroidism is indicated only in those in whom surgery is contraindicated and in those with mild hypercalcemia (< 11 mg/dL [2.75 mmol/L], albumin corrected) who show no evidence of organ dysfunction. Treatment consists of increased fluids, exercise, avoidance of prolonged inactivity, and avoidance of thiazide diuretics, because these drugs decrease calcium excretion and raise serum calcium levels. For postmenopausal patients, estrogen hormone therapy also may be considered.

Most patients with primary hyperparathyroidism require surgery. Today, this surgery involves removal of at least three of the four glands and, in some cases, a subtotal resection of the fourth. The success of surgery is closely related to the experience level of the surgeon. If the disease has been isolated to a specific adenoma or carcinoma, excision of only that particular tumor is the rule. However, it should be noted that most pathologists report a diagnosis of "adenoma" for all parathyroid glands removed because of primary hyperparathyroidism. This does not mean that the glands were adenomatous, that is, that they were enlarged and would continue to grow if not removed. Instead, the use of the term is based on historical precedent, in which "adenoma" refers to any pathologic gland. In fact, primary hyperparathyroidism represents a more complex systemic disease of which hypersecretion of the parathyroid glands is a central component.

After surgery, most patients are expected to become hypocalcemic within 12 to 24 hours. This course should be checked with determination of serum calcium and serum albumin levels as well as eliciting a positive Chvostek sign. This assessment is required because a rapid fall in serum calcium to subnormal levels may produce a hypocalcemic tetany. A positive Chvostek sign is facial muscle twitching elicited by tapping a facial nerve component. It is also prudent to recall that early tetany may be manifested as carpopedal spasm and that hypocalcemic tetany is associated with reduced ionized calcium levels. Therefore, hyperproteinemia or respiratory alkalosis (hyperventilation) in particular may precipitate a tetanic episode by driving ionized calcium to a bound form.

Some patients require large amounts of calcium, vitamin D_3 (cholecalciferol), and increased dietary magnesium in the first 1 week to 1 month following surgery while the residual parathyroid gland responds to the hypocalcemia with its own hyperplasia. Efforts should be made to keep serum calcium levels above 8.0 mg/dL (2 mmol/L).

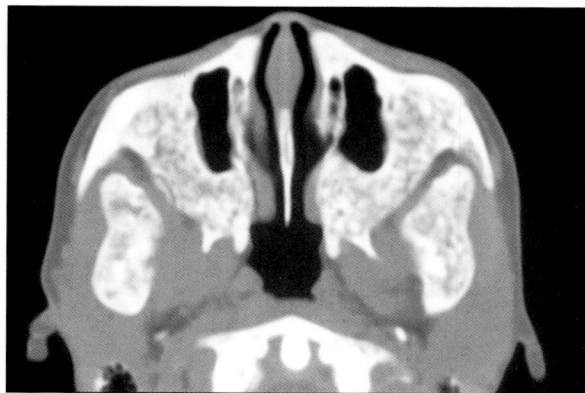

Fig 16-2a Secondary hyperparathyroidism will affect all bones with a moderate expansion and a diffuse mottled radiopacity.

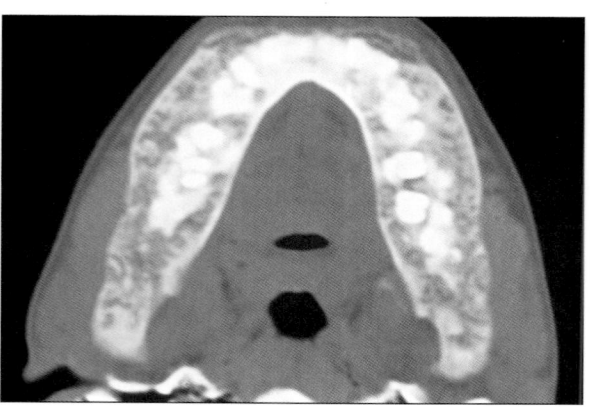

Fig 16-2b Secondary hyperparathyroidism also affects the mandible with a moderate expansion and a diffuse mottled radiopacity.

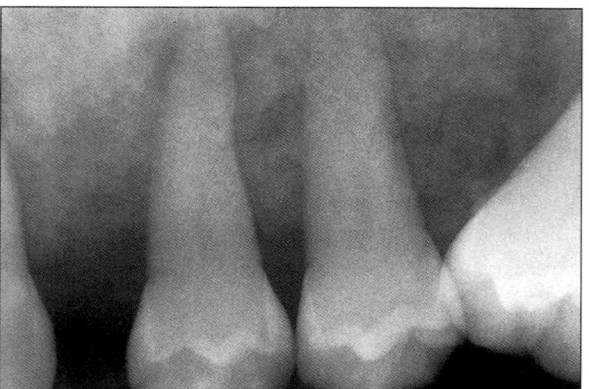

Fig 16-2c Secondary hyperparathyroidism frequently produces tooth mobility, loss of the lamina dura, and a diffuse radiopacity similar to the radiographic appearance of fibrous dysplasia.

PROGNOSIS ▶

The prognosis after surgery is very good as the remaining parathyroid gland adapts to the increased demands placed on it. Supplemental calcium, vitamin D, or magnesium is rarely needed after the first few months. The disease may recur, often many years after surgery. Most of these recurrences are hyperplasias of glands not excised at surgery. Such recurrences have been reduced by the current approach of removing three and sometimes three and one half of the four native glands.

Secondary Hyperparathyroidism

CLINICAL PRESENTATION AND
PATHOGENESIS ▶

Secondary hyperparathyroidism occurs secondary to renal failure. In fact, most patients on dialysis have some element of secondary hyperparathyroidism. In secondary hyperparathyroidism, the patient is hypocalcemic and has hyperphosphatemia, which are conditions opposite to those seen in primary hyperparathyroidism. In both, alkaline phosphatase enzyme levels are normal unless significant osteolysis occurs and circulating levels of PTH are elevated. However, in secondary hyperparathyroidism, PTH levels are elevated as a result of a normal set of parathyroid glands continuously secreting PTH in response to the hypocalcemia created by renal loss of calcium, while in primary hyperparathyroidism, hyperplastic autonomous glands fail to reduce secretion of PTH in response to hypercalcemia. Therefore, patients with secondary hyperparathyroidism lack the symptoms related to hypercalcemia but do have PTH–related signs, such as brown tumors and osteitis fibrosa cystica, which is termed *renal osteodystrophy* and referred to in older literature as von Recklinghausen's disease of bone. These symptoms are usually coupled with the signs and symptoms of their existing renal failure.

DIAGNOSTIC WORK-UP ▶

Secondary hyperparathyroidism is suspected when a patient presents with a history of dialysis and/or renal failure. It is confirmed by demonstrating hypocalcemia, hyperphosphatemia, and elevated PTH levels. Radiographs may show involvement of all bones with a patchy and mottled radiolucent/radiopaque appearance. Expansion in the areas of brown tumors also is seen. Loss of the lamina dura and tooth mobility are seen more commonly in secondary hyperparathyroidism than in primary hyperparathyroidism (Figs 16-2a to 16-2c).

TREATMENT ▶

Secondary hyperparathyroidism is managed by closely controlled dialysis or by a renal transplant. In addition, significant bone disease associated with the condition may be prevented or reduced by medical management. In particular, phosphate binders such as calcium carbonate and aluminum hydroxide antacids can reduce the hyperphosphatemia. A reduction in the excess phosphate will raise serum calcium levels, while compensatory mechanisms attempt to maintain the product of serum calcium and serum phosphate at a constant level. In addition, several forms of vitamin D may be administered until the most useful preparation for that patient is found. Even a slight increase from the low serum calcium levels found in secondary hyperparathyroidism causes the normally functioning glands to reduce secretion of PTH.

PROGNOSIS ▶

Secondary hyperparathyroidism may be totally incurable even with renal transplantation and effective dialysis. Most patients with renal failure have some element of chronic disease and undergo more active therapy to treat symptoms as they occur.

Hypercalcemia of Malignancy (A Paraneoplastic Syndrome)

CLINICAL PRESENTATION AND PATHOGENESIS ▶

The clinical presentation of hypercalcemia of malignancy usually takes one of two forms. One presentation is that of a clinically large primary or recurrent carcinoma with signs and symptoms of hypercalcemia. Often, such patients have serum calcium levels in excess of 14 mg/dL (3.5 mmol/L) and are confused, constipated, nauseated, and somewhat cachectic. The other presentation is that of a small or unseen primary carcinoma with either asymptomatic hypercalcemia or symptoms of nausea, confusion, and constipation.

Certain epithelial malignancies, most notably small cell carcinoma of the lung and to a lesser extent squamous cell carcinomas of the foregut, including some oral carcinomas, will secrete a PTH-related peptide (PTHrP). This PTHrP usually will not be identified as normal PTH by radioimmunoassays but will mimic all the physiologic functions of PTH on bone, kidneys, and the small intestines, resulting in an increase in serum calcium levels. Biochemically, both normal PTH and this PTHrP secretion have the same first 13 amino acids, and they share a similar tertiary structural configuration. However, there are differences in their amino acid sequences, and the PTHrP secretion arises from a gene on the short arm of chromosome 12, whereas the normal PTH gene is located on the short arm of chromosome 11.

DIFFERENTIAL DIAGNOSIS AND WORK-UP ▶

A case of overt carcinoma and paraneoplastic hypercalcemia is straightforward. However, in a case with no obvious tumor but unquestionable hypercalcemia, a differential diagnosis similar to that of primary hyperparathyroidism must be considered. That is, *primary hyperparathyroidism, multiple myeloma, sarcoidosis, overingestion of calcium or vitamin D, familial hypocalciuria hypercalcemia,* and *adrenal insufficiency* must be considered. Therefore, laboratory testing may need to include a radioimmunoassay for PTH; serum immunoelectrophoresis; and a 24-hour urine collection determination for calcium and serum sodium, potassium, ACTH, and cortisol levels. In addition, an incisional parotid biopsy may be needed to rule out sarcoidosis, and a thorough dietary review may be required to assess calcium and vitamin D intake. As part of the work-up, a search for a primary carcinoma may require a chest, head, and neck computed tomography (CT) scan or a magnetic resonance imaging (MRI) scan, in addition to oral, pharyngeal, and even "triple endoscopic" examination. Hypercalcemia of malignancy is confirmed when a histopathologic confirmation of a malignancy is made in the presence of PTH-negative hypercalcemia.

TREATMENT AND PROGNOSIS ▶

Paraneoplastic hypercalcemia of malignancy is primarily treated when the malignancy is treated. However, many of these malignancies are not curable, requiring the clinician to manage ongoing hypercalcemia palliatively. Although mild hypercalcemia can be managed with an increased fluid intake, paraneoplastic hypercalcemia of malignancy usually requires more aggressive management. This may include increased intravenous fluid intake and administration of furosemide, with measurements of both fluid intake and urine output. If this method is used, it is important to hydrate the patient fully before administering furosemide to avoid dehydration and exacerbation of the hypercalcemia. It is not prudent to substitute thiazide diuretics for furosemide because thiazides decrease renal excretion of calcium and will quickly exacerbate the hypercalcemia. As an alternative, a 30-mg dose of disodium pamidronate, a potent anti-osteoclastic drug, in 500 mL of normal saline may be administered intravenously over 4 hours. Such therapy will induce a decline in hypercalcemia over 2 to 4 days and last for 4 to 8 weeks before a repeat dose is needed.

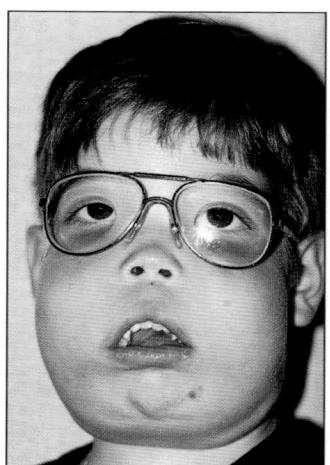

Fig 16-3a The facies of type III cherubism reflects expansion of the mandible and maxilla. Note the upward-turned eyes caused by maxillary expansion into the orbital volume and the open bite caused by nasal obstruction and subsequent mouth breathing.

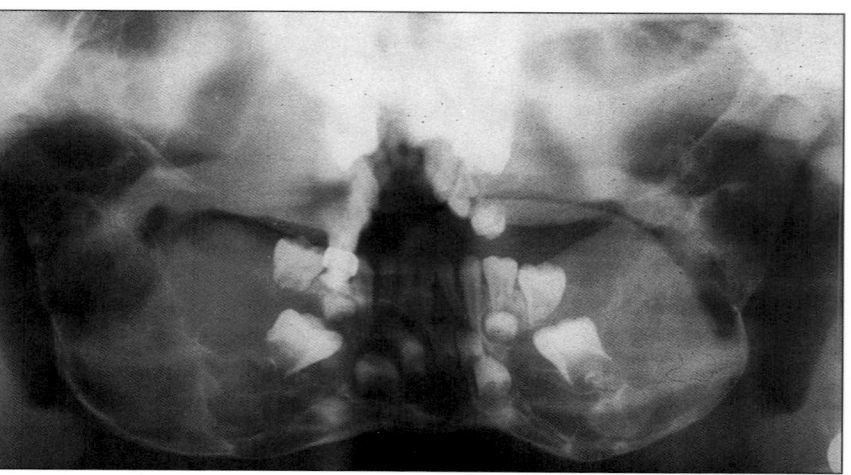

Fig 16-3b Radiographically, type III cherubism is mostly symmetric. It is a multilocular radiolucency that spares the condyle and the upper condylar neck.

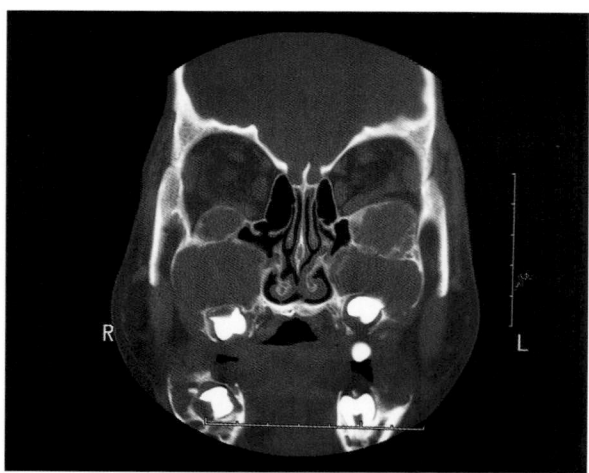

Fig 16-3c This CT scan of type III cherubism shows symmetric maxillary expansion and asymmetric expansion into the orbital volume, which had clinically displaced the left eye more upward than the right eye.

CLINICAL PRESENTATION AND
PATHOGENESIS ▶

Cherubism

Cherubism is an autosomal-dominant genetic defect that affects bone remodeling in the specific anatomically confined limits of the embryologic mandible and sometimes of the mandible and maxilla (Figs 16-3a to 16-3c). Cherubism does not occur in any other bone and will not cross a bony suture to an adjacent bone.

Cherubism first begins to manifest itself by the age of 2.5 years and is fully expressed by the age of 5 years. It affects males slightly more than females because of a 100% genetic penetrance in males and only a 50% to 70% genetic penetrance in females. Its relatively rapid progression between the ages of 2.5 and 5 years is often associated with regional lymphadenopathy and, if the maxilla is involved, nasal obstruction with resultant mouth breathing. Nasal obstruction is caused by enlargement of the middle concha. Because the genetic defect is expressed on the embryologic maxilla or mandible only, the other conchae—the inferior concha, which is an independent bone, and the superior concha, which is part of the ethmoid bone—are not involved. The rapid evolution of the disease often creates significant concern in the parents, particularly if the defect is a mutation and no direct family members or ancestors are known to possess the condition. Spontaneous mutations, called "sporadic occurrences," are more common in cherubism than in most other inherited diseases and account for up to 40% of cases.

Cherubism has three levels of expression. Type I forms only in the bilateral rami of the mandible, sparing the condyle and extending only to the third molar region (Figs 16-4a to 16-4c). This form may be so subtle that it escapes clinical detection until radiographs are taken years later. It is probable that most of the reported cases of so-called bilateral giant cell lesions of the mandible actually represent this type of cherubism, often called a forme fruste or incomplete expression of the disease. Type II forms only in the mandible and also spares the condyle, but it extends to at least the mental foramen bilaterally and may extend to involve the entire mandible (Figs 16-5a to 16-5c). Type III is the form that prompted the name "cherubism." This form involves the mandible to an advanced degree as compared to type II and also includes the maxilla (Figs 16-6a to 16-6c). The involvement of the maxilla's contribution to the orbital floor and orbital rim displaces the globes upward, causing a scleral show. This feature, combined with the expansion of the maxilla, gives a child with cherubism the chubby-faced appearance and the "upward-to-

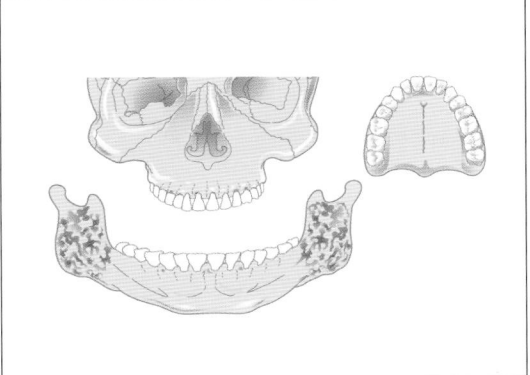

Fig 16-4a Type I cherubism involves just the bilateral rami of the mandible and may go unnoticed.

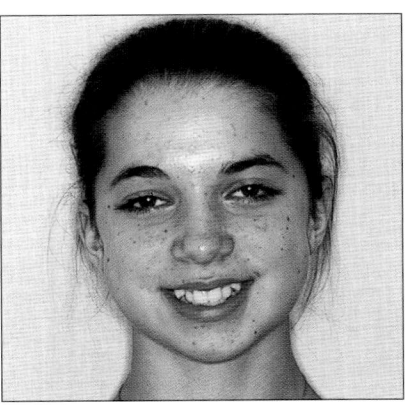

Fig 16-4b Subtle and mild expansion of the rami in a type I cherubism.

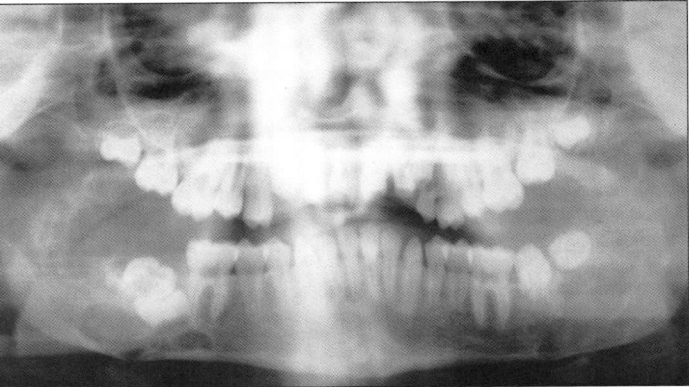

Fig 16-4c Despite the absence of obvious clinical expansion, type I cherubism will show bilateral multilocular radiolucencies in the rami and posterior body of the mandible.

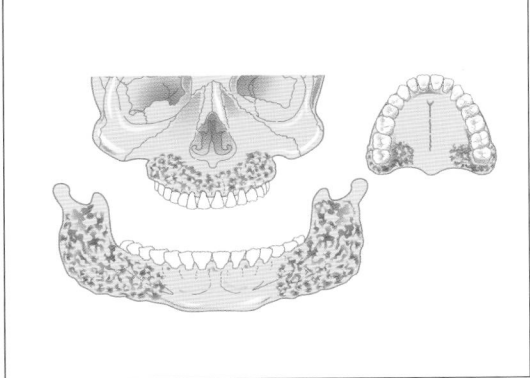

Fig 16-5a Type II cherubism involves the bilateral rami and the posterior body of the mandible as well as a small portion of the maxillary tuberosities.

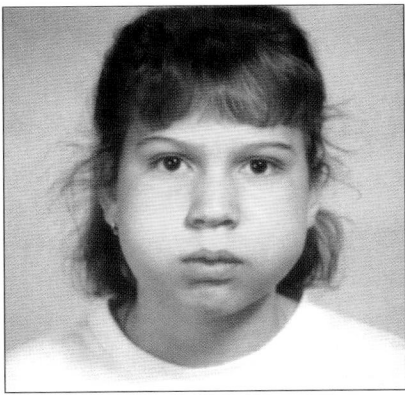

Fig 16-5b More obvious clinical expansion in an individual with type II cherubism.

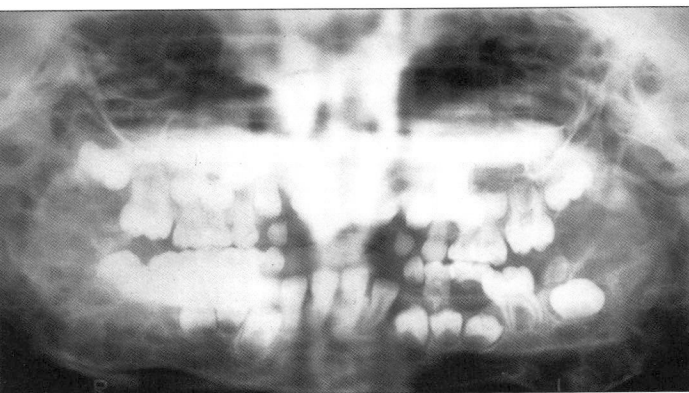

Fig 16-5c Type II cherubism will also have bilateral multilocular radiolucencies but will also show clinical expansion and may expand forward to the area of the mental foramen.

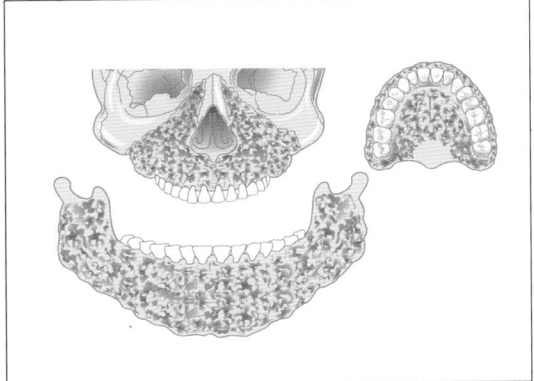

Fig 16-6a Type III cherubism involves the entire mandible symmetrically across the midline except the condyles. It also involves all the components of the maxilla and will not cross suture lines.

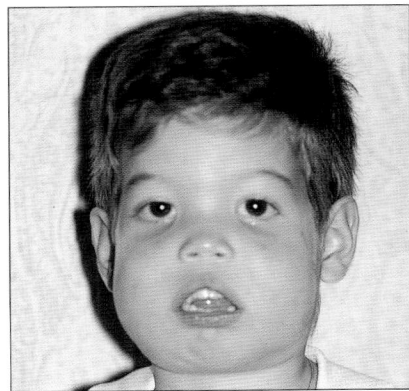

Fig 16-6b Type III cherubism will show obvious symmetrical clinical expansion of the mandible and the maxilla. The maxillary expansion will produce a scleral show and will rotate the globes upward, producing the "eyes turned toward heaven" appearance of a cherub.

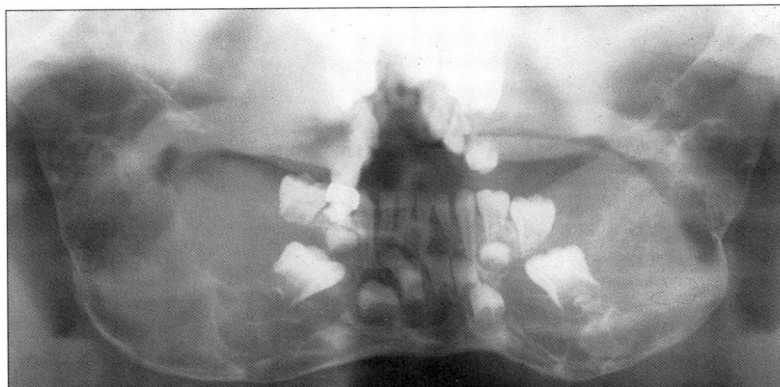

Fig 16-6c Type III cherubism will show the classic bilateral multilocular radiolucent lesions of both the mandible and the maxilla. In the mandible, the condyles will be spared. In the maxilla, the radiolucencies will not extend past the maxillary sutures.

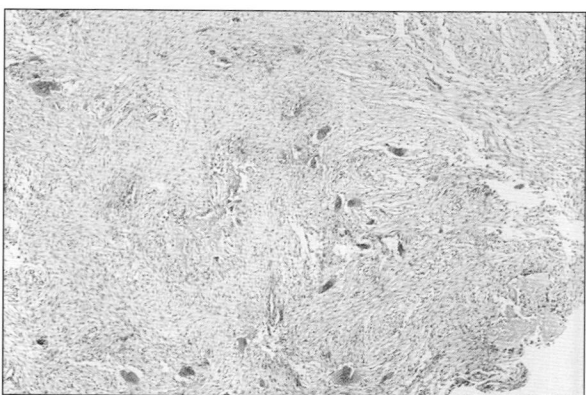

Fig 16-7a Cherubism with histologic features similar to those seen in hyperparathyroidism and central giant cell tumors. The stroma is fibrous with haphazardly arranged multinucleated giant cells and some hemorrhage.

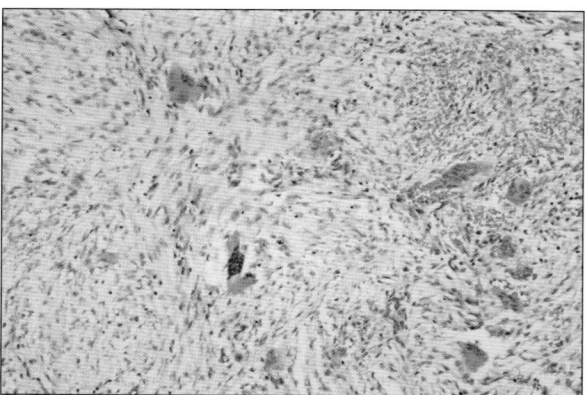

Fig 16-7b High-power view of Fig 16-7a showing multinucleated giant cells in a fibrous stroma.

heaven"–looking eyes of a cherub. The maxillary involvement includes the alveolar bone and palate but does not extend beyond the maxillary sutures. Therefore, the adjacent palatine bones, vomer, zygomas, and nasal bones are completely normal.

The child will, therefore, present with some degree of expanded facies and the possibility of nasal obstruction, lymphadenopathy, dry mouth, drooling, and rarely, pain (see Fig 16-3a). Clinically, there may be missing teeth, multiple diastemas, and misplaced teeth.

Radiographically, the involved bones show a dramatic multilocular radiolucency with thin and expanded cortices, including the inferior border. The condyle and condylar neck appear normal. Unerupted and displaced teeth are common. Radiographically and clinically, cases show symmetric involvement. Cases that do not show symmetry (ie, unilateral involvement) may not be true cherubism but similar giant cell lesions that are variable components of other diseases such as Noonan syndrome or Jaffe-Campanacci syndrome.

DIFFERENTIAL DIAGNOSIS ▶

Cherubism, like most fibro-osseous diseases, requires a clinical and radiographic diagnosis rather than a histopathologic diagnosis. It must, therefore, be distinguished from other bilateral multilocular radiolucent lesions of the jaws in young children. Other entities that may mimic this presentation are *primary hyperparathyroidism*, *Langerhans cell histiocytosis*, and *multiple odontogenic keratocysts*, perhaps as part of the *basal cell nevus syndrome*. In addition, *Noonan syndrome* and *Jaffe-Campanacci syndrome* may be considered, particularly if a fibrovascular giant cell lesion is confirmed by a biopsy.

The specific clinical and radiographic features that permit a diagnosis of cherubism are symmetric presentation, radiographic evidence of multilocular contiguous lesions, sparing of the condyle, lack of involvement of adjacent bones, middle concha enlargement (variable) in the maxilla, and emergence and expression of the disease between the ages of 2 and 5 years.

HISTOPATHOLOGY ▶

The lesions of cherubism consist of a vascular fibrous stroma, extravasated erythrocytes, and scattered multinucleated giant cells (Figs 16-7a and 16-7b). An increase in the amount of fibrous tissue and a corresponding decrease in the number of giant cells is probably associated with regressing lesions. An eosinophilic perivascular cuffing of collagen is considered characteristic of cherubism; however, this feature is frequently absent. Clinical and radiographic correlation is necessary, as the histologic features strongly resemble those seen in central giant cell tumors and the lesions of hyperparathyroidism.

TREATMENT AND PROGNOSIS ▶

As with any genetic disease, cherubism currently is not curable. However, the natural course of cherubism is one of gradual enlargement that continues until the onset of puberty. After puberty, a gradual involution begins and is often complete by age 18 to 20 years, and almost never lasting beyond age 30

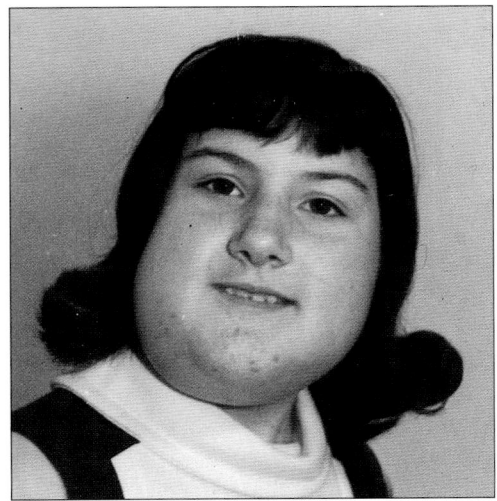

Fig 16-8a Facial expansion of cherubism at age 9 years. Here the asymmetry is the result of attempted osseous contouring of the left side. The facial expansion of cherubism is usually symmetric.

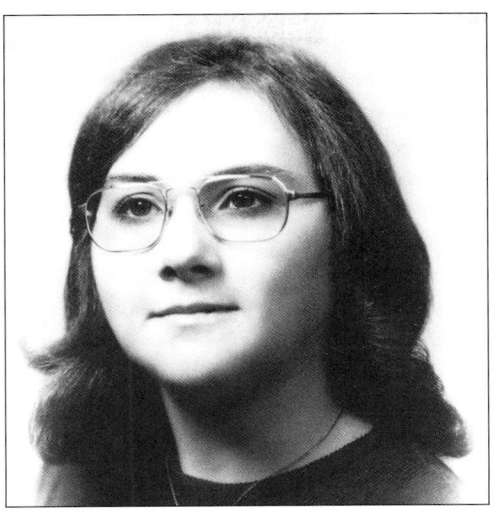

Fig 16-8b The high school graduation photograph of the individual shown in Fig 16-8a at age 17 years shows involutional clinical remodeling without further surgery.

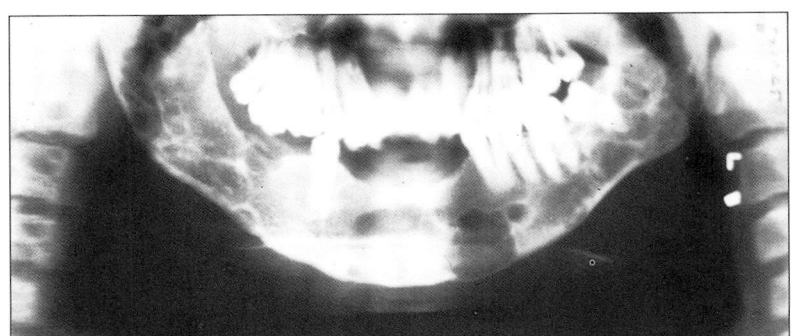

Fig 16-8c Although cherubism will clinically involute to near-normal facial contours, residual radiolucencies containing giant cell lesions are usually present, as are unerupted teeth and therefore edentulous areas.

years. The result is a nearly complete reversal of the facial expansion, which is usually very well accepted by the individual (Figs 16-8a and 16-8b). Radiographs show only partial bony regeneration as residual radiolucent areas persist. There also may be unerupted and displaced teeth (Fig 16-8c). This eruption disturbance, which occurs throughout the childhood years, may cause the patient to be partially edentulous.

The general clinical approach is to avoid surgery altogether and allow natural involution to take place or defer surgeries until after puberty. If reduction of the expanded bone (osseous contouring) is required because of pain or psychologic needs, it is done with the knowledge that the operated bone will re-expand at the same or a higher rate of expansion as before surgery. There is some concern that osseous contouring may accelerate the rate of expansion, but the limited experience with surgery on these patients does not support this concern. There is also no evidence that surgical intervention will stimulate malignant transformation. If osseous contouring is required, especially on a young patient, the surgeon must be aware of the vascular nature of the bone and proceed with the same intraoperative hemorrhage control procedures as would be used in treating a central giant cell tumor (ie, an elevated head position, hypotensive anesthesia, an accessible supply of hemostatic packs, and a preparation of autologous blood or "designated donor" blood available for transfusion).

On occasion, the nasal obstruction can become severe, leading to airway concerns or to significant mouth breathing and an open-bite deformity. In such cases, removal of the middle concha and turbinates is a reasonable and beneficial procedure.

Fibrous Dysplasia

CLINICAL PRESENTATION AND PATHOGENESIS ▶

Fibrous dysplasia is a disease of bone maturation and remodeling in which the normal medullary bone and cortices are replaced by a disorganized fibrous woven bone. The resultant fibro-osseous bone is more elastic and structurally weaker than the original bone. It is caused by the deletion of a bone maturation protein during embryogenesis. There is no evidence to suggest a hereditary influence.

Fibrous dysplasia is conceptualized into three types. Each type usually presents as an asymptomatic, slowly expanding portion of one or more bones. The condition develops in children and teenagers primarily, with few if any cases beginning after the age of 25 years. *Monostotic fibrous dysplasia,* which involves

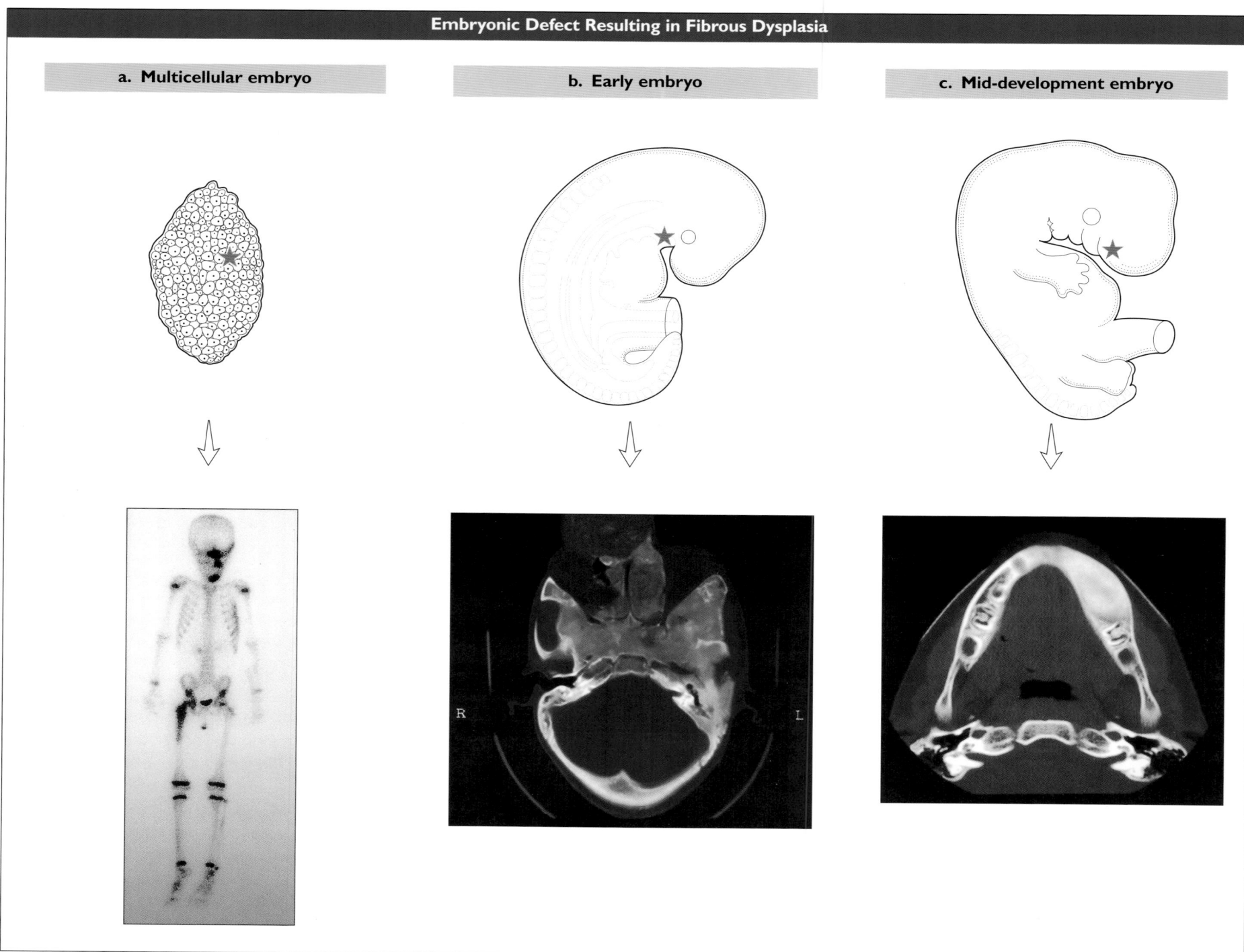

Fig 16-9 Although the clinical development of fibrous dysplasia becomes apparent between 5 and 15 years of age, it begins in the embryo with the spontaneous mutation or deletion of an intracytoplasmic transducer protein responsible for bone maturation. All daughter cells of the original aberrant cell (*star*) will produce immature bone. Therefore, the earlier this occurs in embryonic development, the more widespread will be the fibrous dysplasia (ie, polyostotic fibrous dysplasia). (*a*) For example, the loss of this intracytoplasmic transducer protein in the multicellular embryo will eventuate into polyostotic involvement similar to that seen here in the mandible, maxilla, base of skull, and right femur. (*b*) In the early embryo, the loss of this intracytoplasmic transducer protein will eventuate into craniofacial fibrous dysplasia, shown here with involvement of the maxilla, zygomas, bony conchas of the nose, sphenoid bone, and clivus. (*c*) In the mid-developed embryo, the loss of this intracytoplasmic transducer protein will eventuate into monostotic fibrous dysplasia, similar to what is seen here as a single focus in the mandible.

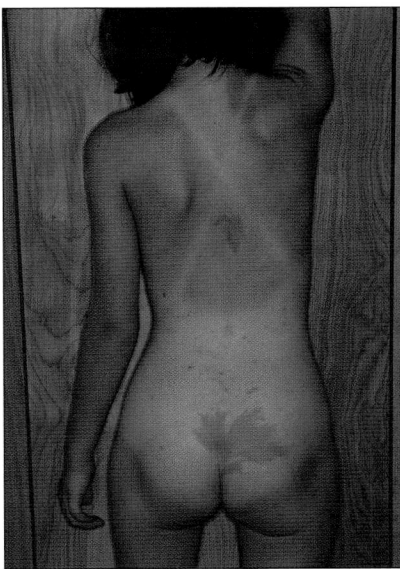

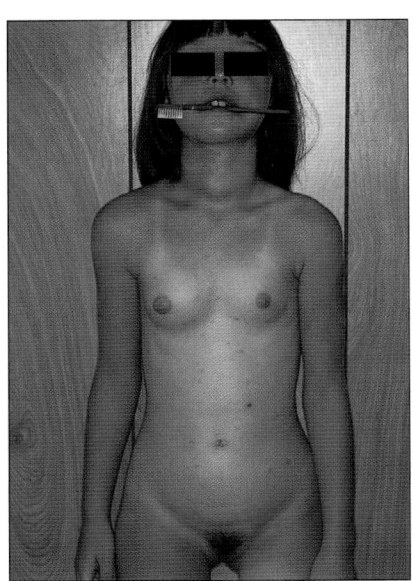

Fig 16-10a Prominent café-au-lait macules with irregular and jagged edges often likened to the "coast of Maine" contours are seen in the McCune-Albright and the Jaffe-Lichtenstein type of polyostotic fibrous dysplasia. (Courtesy of Dr Scott Wietecha.)

Fig 16-10b Precocious puberty as evidenced by mature breast development and pubic hair growth in this 6-year-old girl with the McCune-Albright type of polyostotic fibrous dysplasia. (Courtesy of Dr Scott Wietecha.)

a single focus in one bone, accounts for about 75% of fibrous dysplasia cases. In the jaws, this may be seen most frequently in the body of the mandible or in the premolar-molar regions of the maxilla.

Today it is understood that all types of fibrous dysplasia result from a defect in bone maturation that begins in the embryo. At certain times in the histodifferentiation phase of the embryo, a genetic mutation or deletion occurs in the gene that encodes for an intracytoplasmic transducer protein required for bone maturation. Consequently, all the daughter cells of this original aberrant cell will lack this signal transducer, and therefore a certain population of cells in the individual will be able to produce only fibrous dysplastic bone rather than mature bone. If the genetic defect occurs early in embryonic development, a large number of daughter cells will be affected, some of which may not yet have migrated to their eventual skeletal site. When such early term–altered cells migrate into several skeletal sites, they produce *polyostotic fibrous dysplasia*. If the genetic defect occurs in an even earlier phase of embryonic development, the original cell may produce daughter cells of divergent differentiation (Fig 16-9)—that is, some that will migrate into bone primordia, some into skin primordia, and some into endocrine gland primordia—and thus produce either the McCune-Albright syndrome or the Jaffe-Lichtenstein type of polyostotic fibrous dysplasia. The time at which these genetic alterations occur is thought to be before the sixth week of fetal life.

When the embryo is in its sixth week of development, most histodifferentiation and cell migration have already occurred. If the same genetic defect occurs around this time, the daughter cells will be localized to one region and thus may produce the craniofacial type of fibrous dysplasia, which involves several contiguous bones in a broad area. If the genetic defect occurs slightly later, the daughter cells will be even more localized and will thus produce monostotic fibrous dysplasia (see Fig 16-9).

Polyostotic fibrous dysplasia involves two or more noncontiguous bones. This form is less common than monostotic fibrous dysplasia and may involve the skull, jaws, or a facial bone together with ribs, long bones, or the pelvis. Two syndromes involving polyostotic fibrous dysplasia have been isolated. McCune-Albright syndrome encompasses polyostotic fibrous dysplasia with cutaneous melanotic pigmentations called café-au-lait macules (Fig 16-10a) and endocrine abnormalities. The most common of the endocrine abnormalities is precocious puberty (Fig 16-10b). In fact, the youngest childbirth on record occurred

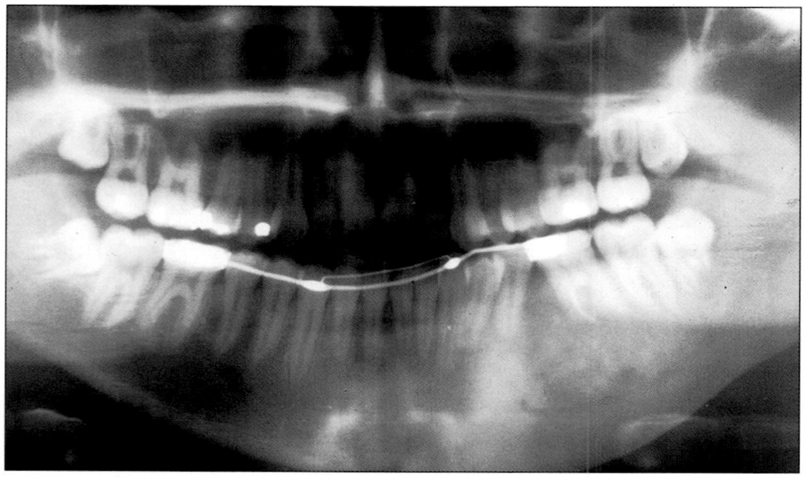

Fig 16-11a Fibrous dysplasia will produce a nondemarcated, diffuse radiopacity known as a "ground-glass" appearance. Note the diversion of the roots of the first molar and second premolar. They are divergent not because of the expansion, as would be the case with a cyst or benign tumor, but because the first molar erupted before the onset of fibrous dysplasia and the first and second premolars erupted through the expanded bone of the fibrous dysplasia 6 years later.

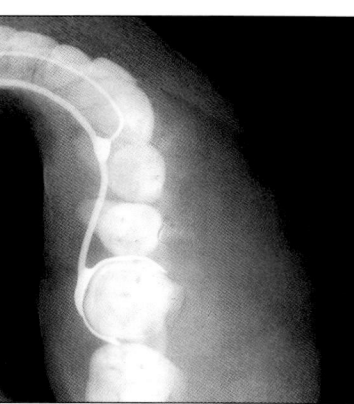

Fig 16-11b An occlusal view of fibrous dysplasia will show its diffuse "ground-glass" appearance, expansion, and fibrous dysplasia replacement of the cortical outline.

Table 16-1 Radiographic and CT scan features that differentiate fibrous dysplasia from ossifying fibroma

Feature	Fibrous dysplasia	Ossifying fibroma
Margins	Not demarcated	Well demarcated
Shape	Fusiform	Spherical or elongated
Cortices	Replaced by disease	Expanded; present or partially present
Medullary pattern	Homogeneous	Heterogeneous

when a 5-year-old Peruvian girl with McCune-Albright syndrome gave birth. Other endocrinopathies that may be part of this syndrome are hyperthyroidism, acromegaly, and hyperprolactinemia. Jaffe-Lichtenstein syndrome, less well-known than McCune-Albright syndrome, describes polyostotic fibrous dysplasia with cutaneous melanotic pigmentations in the absence of endocrine abnormalities. Craniofacial fibrous dysplasia involves two or more bones of the jaw-midface-skull complex in continuity. This type of fibrous dysplasia is seen relatively often in dental and oral and maxillofacial practices. It is frequently underestimated and thought to be a monostotic fibrous dysplasia of the maxilla, yet it often includes the zygoma, sphenoid, temporal bone, nasal concha, and clivus.

RADIOGRAPHIC PRESENTATION ▶

Nearly all cases of fibrous dysplasia will show a diffuse, hazy trabecular pattern that has been called the ground-glass appearance (Fig 16-11a). However, some reports have described this pattern as radiolucent while others have described it as mottled pagetoid. These radiographic descriptions are suspect today because these reports emerged when the diagnosis and biologic behavior of fibrous dysplasia were not well-known and CT scans were not available. Since then, more strict clinical and radiographic criteria have been developed so that fibrous dysplasia is better defined.

Today, most radiographic and CT scan pictures of fibrous dysplasia show a homogeneous, finely trabecular bone pattern replacing the medullary bone and both cortices and often the lamina dura as well (Fig 16-11b). Its shape is fusiform and its margins are indistinct, showing a gradual blend into normal bone. It shows greater buccal than lingual expansion and does not displace the inferior alveolar canal.

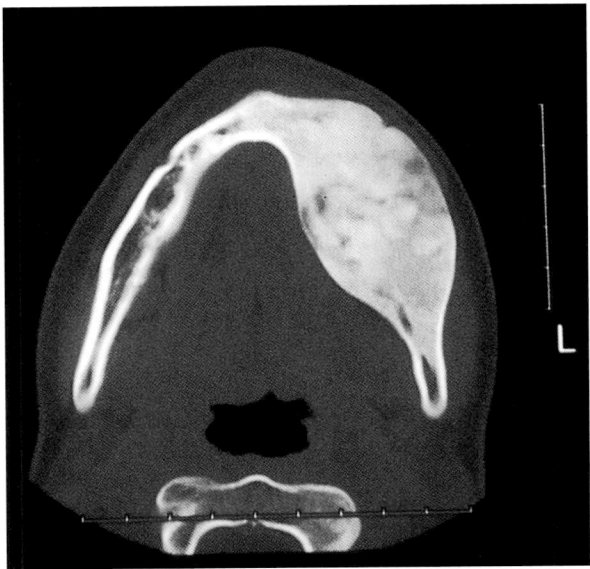 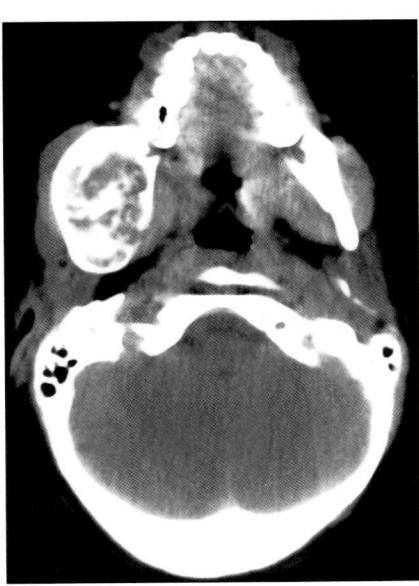

Fig 16-12a A CT scan of fibrous dysplasia shows the same features as noted in Fig 16-11a, especially the fibrous dysplasia replacement of the cortical outline as well as its generally homogeneous internal structure.

Fig 16-12b This CT scan of an ossifying fibroma can be contrasted to that of fibrous dysplasia. Its expansion is well demarcated, retains a thinned cortical outline, and has a generally heterogeneous internal structure.

DIFFERENTIAL DIAGNOSIS ▶

The single most important differential diagnosis for fibrous dysplasia is to distinguish it from an *ossifying fibroma*. Other entities that may resemble fibrous dysplasia include *chronic sclerosing osteomyelitis*, *Paget disease*, and sometimes *osteosarcoma*.

The features distinguishing fibrous dysplasia from ossifying fibroma are listed in Table 16-1. Fibrous dysplasia arises and is established by the age of 20 years. Although some ossifying fibromas also develop in youth, most begin at an older age. Radiographs and/or CT scans of axial views show an ossifying fibroma to be spherical to egg shaped, heterogeneous, and well demarcated from normal bone. Also shown are an expanded or a thinned residual uninvolved cortex and displacement of the inferior alveolar canal. The radiographs and scans support the concept advanced by Worth that an ossifying fibroma is a disease within bone while fibrous dysplasia is a disease of bone (Figs 16-12a and 16-12b).

Chronic diffuse sclerosing osteomyelitis resembles fibrous dysplasia in its diffuse and poorly demarcated radiographic appearance. It too may occur in teenagers and preteens, but it is more common in adults. However, unlike fibrous dysplasia, chronic diffuse sclerosing osteomyelitis is usually severely and constantly painful; there is frequently a history of endodontic therapy, an abscessed tooth, or some other infection; and appropriate cultures may yield *Actinomyces* species and *Eikenella corrodens*. Paget disease can be distinguished from fibrous dysplasia by its onset in individuals older than 40 years and its increased alkaline phosphatase levels. Osteosarcoma may be difficult to distinguish from fibrous dysplasia radiographically and certainly must be ruled out by histopathologic studies if the diagnosis is not clear. In general, osteosarcomas do not remodel but rather resorb a cortex and expand outward from a destroyed cortex (Figs 16-13a to 16-13c).

HISTOPATHOLOGY ▶

In fibrous dysplasia, normal bone is replaced by a generally loose, cellular fibrous tissue composed of haphazardly arranged, variably shaped trabeculae of woven bone, which typically lack osteoblastic rimming but often contain numerous osteocytes (Fig 16-14a). The osseous component thus may appear to arise directly from the fibrous stroma (Fig 16-14b). The lesion has no definable borders, and the osseous trabeculae blend into the normal surrounding bone. Aggregates of multinucleated giant cells may be present. Over time, fibrous dysplasia of the jaws may show maturation, which is characterized by formation

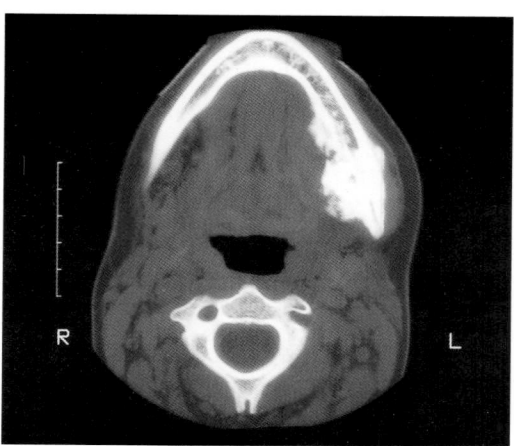

Fig 16-13a A CT scan of an osteosarcoma often shows formation of irregular endosteal and extracortical bone as well as a destroyed or obliterated cortex.

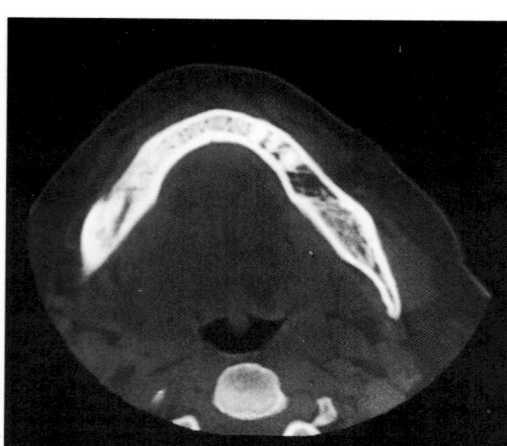

Fig 16-13b A CT scan of diffuse chronic sclerosing osteomyelitis will show endosteal sclerosis within which small areas of radiolucency may be seen.

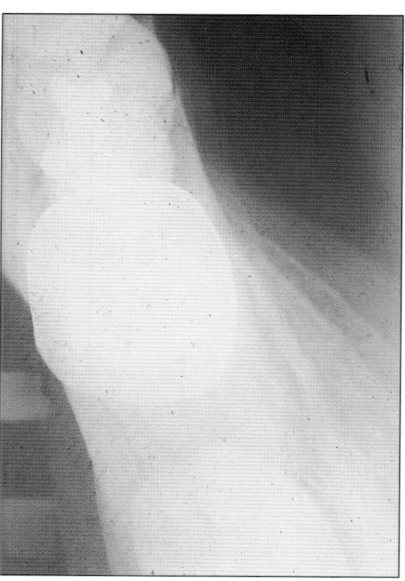

Fig 16-13c An occlusal view radiograph or CT scan of osteomyelitis with proliferative periostitis (Garré osteomyelitis) will show some expansion and extracortical bone formation outside a normal cortex. Here the extracortical bone formation is layered to produce a so-called onion-skin effect. Extracortical bone outside a normal cortex is inconsistent with osteosarcoma.

TREATMENT AND PROGNOSIS ▶

of lamellar bone and parallel arrangement of the trabeculae (Figs 16-14c and 16-14d). Histologic features alone, however, are unreliable for diagnosis; therefore, clinical and radiographic correlation is imperative.

The preferred approach to maxillofacial monostotic fibrous dysplasia and craniofacial fibrous dysplasia is no treatment. Most children adapt well to the facial expansion and do not desire osseous contouring surgery. If osseous contouring surgery is desired, it is ideal to defer it until adulthood (ages 18 to 21 years) (Figs 16-15a to 16-15c). Like cherubism, fibrous dysplasia shows less growth and its activity is reduced as adulthood approaches, although occasional late expansions and regrowth have occurred in adulthood. Regrowth is most commonly seen when surgeries are performed on patients younger than 21 years. If, because of symptoms or psychologic needs, surgery is required during this time period, it is important to remember that fibrous dysplasia undergoes episodic growth, unlike cherubism, which undergoes a slow and steady growth. Although the surgery itself does not stimulate regrowth, the earlier in life a surgery is performed, the more likely it is that a natural episode of growth will occur postsurgically. Therefore, surgery should be avoided during a period of active expansion even though that is often the time that pain or peer pressure forces its consideration. In such cases, the active phase should remit for a period of 3 months before osseous contouring is performed.

Resection is not usually indicated, even for severe craniofacial fibrous dysplasia, unless neural compression threatens vision or hearing. In such cases, local resection only around the area of the nerve compression or around the involved foramen is often necessary. Monostotic fibrous dysplasia or a focus of polyostotic fibrous dysplasia of the skull does lend itself to a local en-bloc resection. The defect is usually reconstructed with a split calvarial graft from an adjacent area. However, resection is not indicated in monostotic fibrous dysplasia of the jaws. The structural weakness of fibrous dysplasia does not functionally impair the jaws to a great extent. Therefore, jaw resection with subsequent bony reconstruction is not justified unless it is an unusual situation in which the patient's function and appearance are significantly altered and osseous contouring is not an option.

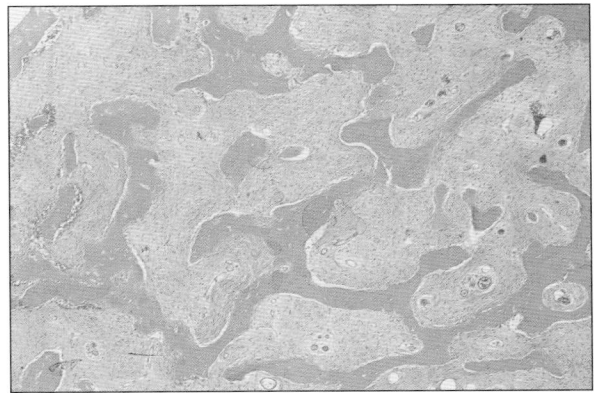

Fig 16-14a Fibrous dysplasia consisting of a fibrous stroma with haphazardly arranged trabeculae of woven bone.

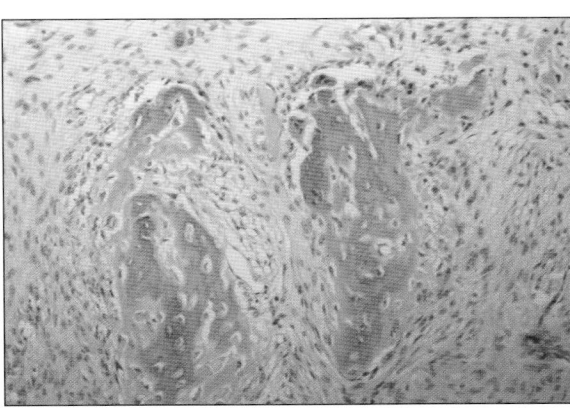

Fig 16-14b Fibrous dysplasia showing woven bone with no osteoblastic rimming and numerous osteocytes.

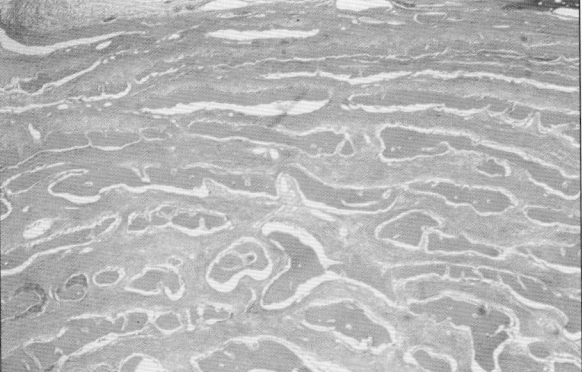

Fig 16-14c A mature lesion of fibrous dysplasia with parallel arrangement of lamellar osseous trabeculae.

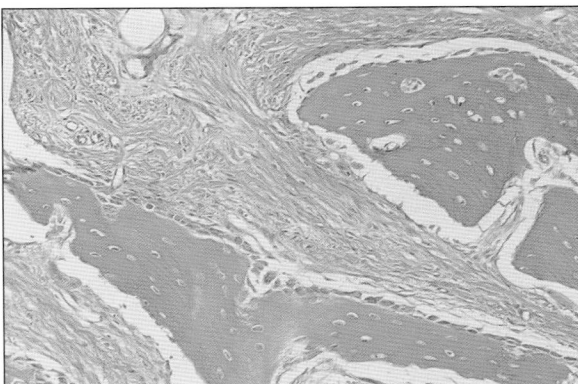

Fig 16-14d The same fibrous dysplasia lesion shown in Fig 16-14c revealing osteoblastic rimming.

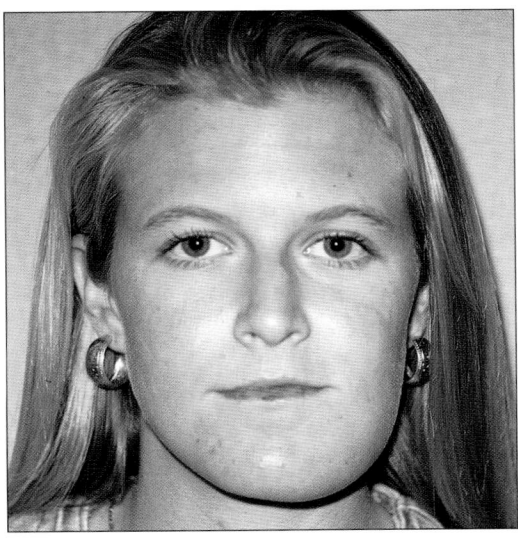

Fig 16-15a Fibrous dysplasia in a 17-year-old patient shows an expansion, which has been stable for more than 6 months.

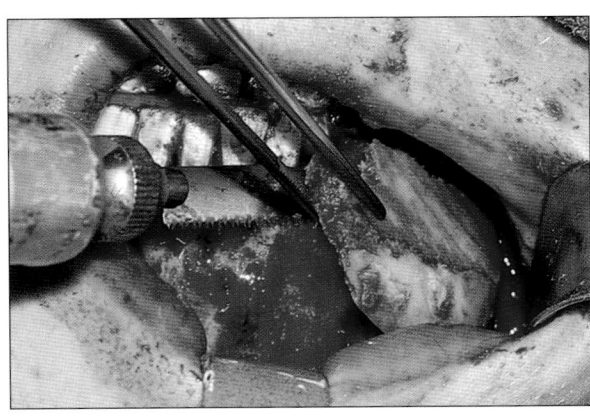

Fig 16-15b Osseous contouring of fibrous dysplasia should include the lateral and inferior border. The bone of fibrous dysplasia will have a cancellous noncortical texture. The surgeon should attempt to contour the expansion to match the opposite side.

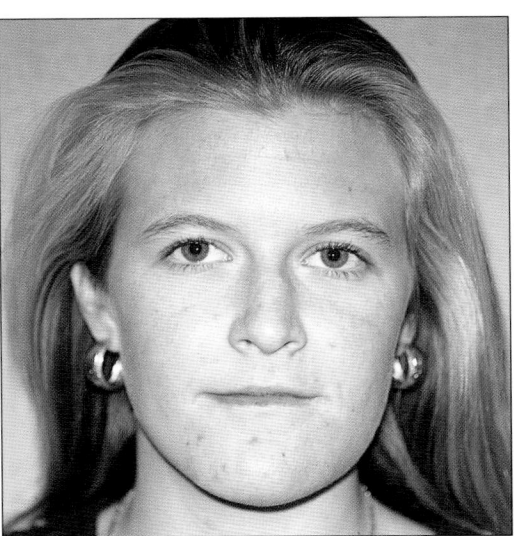

Fig 16-15c Ten years after the osseous contouring shown in Fig 16-15b, the fibrous dysplasia has remained stable and a near symmetry has been retained.

Radiotherapy is contraindicated in the treatment of fibrous dysplasias. Numerous cases of radiation sarcomas arising from radiotherapy have been documented. The time from radiation to sarcoma ranges from 10 to 35 years, with a mean at about 20 years. To date, repeated biopsies and surgeries have not been shown to be a stimulus for malignant transformation. However, about 0.8% of long-standing, usually polyostotic fibrous dysplasias spontaneously transform into sarcomas.

Cemento-Osseous Dysplasia

The term *cemento-osseous dysplasia* encompasses a spectrum of dysmorphic bone and cementum phenomena known currently as *periapical cemento-osseous dysplasia* (a localized form of dysplasia found in the anterior mandible); *florid cemento-osseous dysplasia* (a widespread form of dysplasia); and *focal cemento-osseous dysplasia* (a localized form of dysplasia found in single areas other than the anterior mandible). The use of the term *cemental* in reference to dysplasia occurring in the anterior mandible and *osseous* in reference to dysplasia occurring elsewhere is related to the inability to distinguish between cementum and bone when mineralized tissue is not covering a root surface. In fact, *cemental* and *osseous* are often used interchangeably because both cementum and bone originate from mesenchymal stem cells. The pathogenesis of cemento-osseous dysplasias involves mesenchymal stem cells that seem to have lost their ability to maintain their structural morphology and, therefore, produce what is termed *dysplastic bone*. However, these cells are not neoplastic, nor are they premalignant. Instead, these cells produce morphologically imperfect bone or cementum; therefore, the term *dysmorphic bone* is preferred.

Periapical Cemento-Osseous Dysplasia

CLINICAL PRESENTATION ▶ Periapical cemento-osseous dysplasia refers to an asymptomatic set of lesions that form around the apex of mostly mandibular, vital anterior teeth (Fig 16-16a). It is known to undergo an evolution from radiolucent to mixed radiolucent-radiopaque to completely radiopaque without a change in the root structure or tooth vitality, a process that usually takes several years. Black women of African heritage around the age of 40 years are the most commonly affected. Rarely, men, younger individuals, or members of other races also are affected. Rarely, the condition also is seen in the anterior maxilla. It is usually an incidental radiographic finding because these lesions do not induce tooth mobility or bony expansion.

DIFFERENTIAL DIAGNOSIS ▶ During the radiolucent stage, periapical cemento-osseous dysplasia may be confused with an *apical periodontal granuloma* or a *radicular cyst*. It may also resemble a *primordial odontogenic keratocyst* or the early phase of an *ossifying fibroma*. Because four and sometimes all six anterior teeth may be involved, it will also radiographically suggest a *chronic osteomyelitis*. It is, therefore, imperative that all anterior teeth undergo pulp testing and that serial radiographs are taken over time. On rare occasions, *sublingual salivary gland depressions of the lingual cortex* will produce a round radiolucency superimposed over vital apices as well.

During the mixed radiolucent-radiopaque and completely radiopaque phases, the differential diagnosis will change significantly. It will then include an *odontoma*, a sequestrum from a case of *chronic osteomyelitis*, an *ossifying fibroma*, and an *osteoblastoma*. Cementoblastomas occur only in posterior teeth and therefore are not included on this differential list.

HISTOPATHOLOGY ▶ Initially, the lesions of periapical cemento-osseous dysplasia consist of vascular fibrous tissue with no capsule. Over time, an increasing quantity of mineralized tissue develops, which may take the form of rounded, cementum-like material and/or osseous trabeculae that may show osteoblastic rimming (Figs 16-16b and 16-16c). Eventually, there is coalescence of this material with formation of a sclerotic, avascular, and acellular mass (Figs 16-16d and 16-16e). These stages are reflected in the changing radiographic picture.

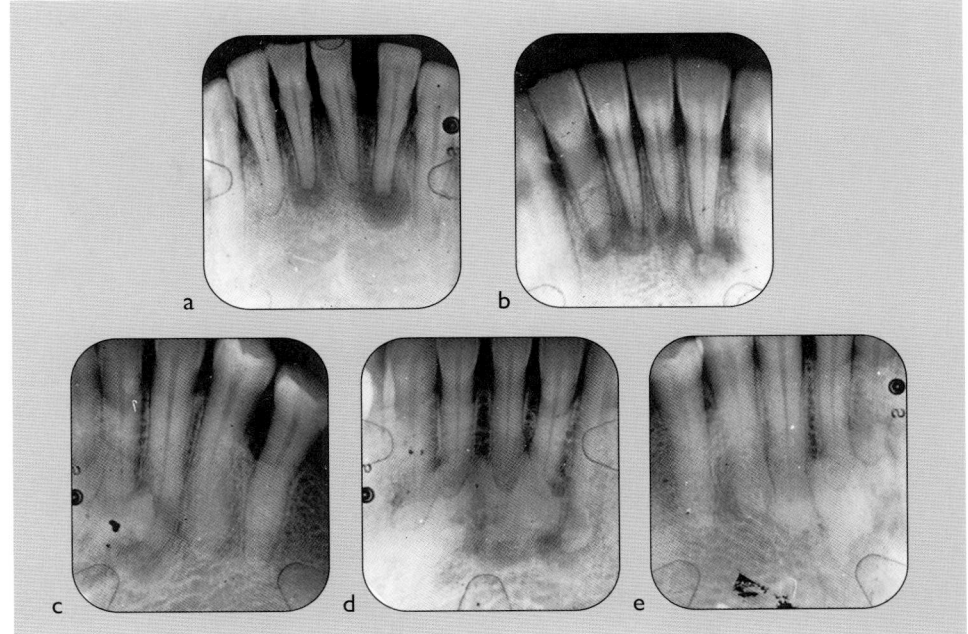

Fig 16-16a The natural radiographic course of periapical cemento-osseous dysplasia is illustrated in this series of periapical radiographs: (*a*) beginning radiolucencies; (*b and c*) beginning and more mature radiopacities creating a more dense, irregular, mixed radiolucent-radiopaque appearance; (*d and e*) mature radiopacities creating a pure, well-outlined radiopaque appearance. This sequence was recorded over a period of 18 years.

Figs 16-16b to 16-16e Photomicrographs from periapical cemento-osseous dysplasia showing the changes that occur over time. This histology is shared by all types of cemento-osseous dysplasia.

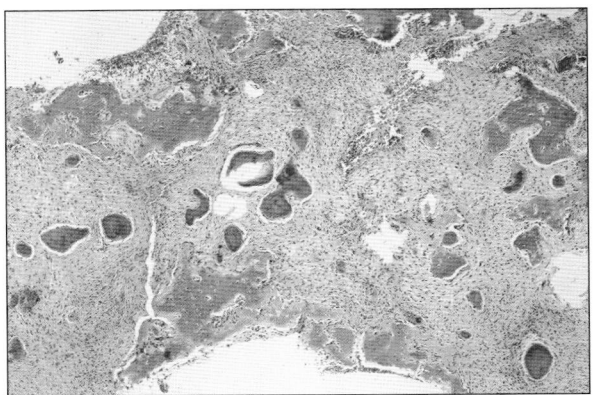
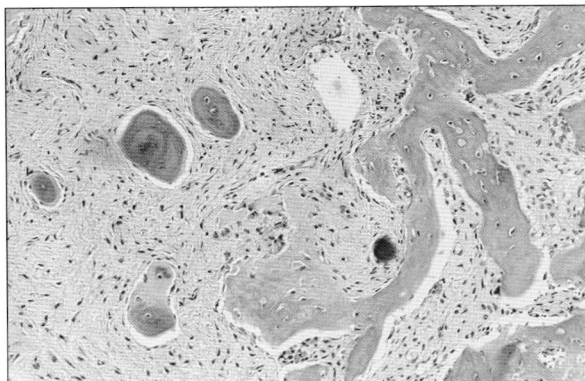

Figs 16-16b and 16-16c A fibrous stroma within which rounded and trabecular cemento-osseous tissue is randomly arranged.

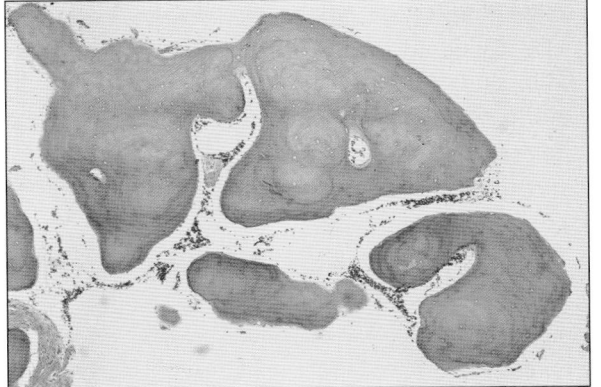
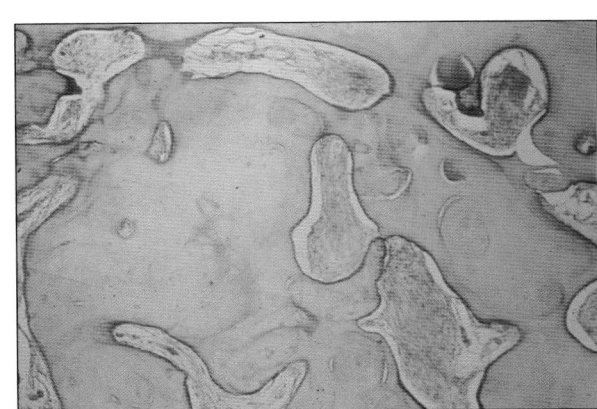

Fig 16-16d A sclerotic area with little fibrous stroma. Older lesions will exhibit this picture but, as in this case, lesions are not necessarily uniform.

Fig 16-16e Ultimately a solid sclerotic mass of tissue is formed.

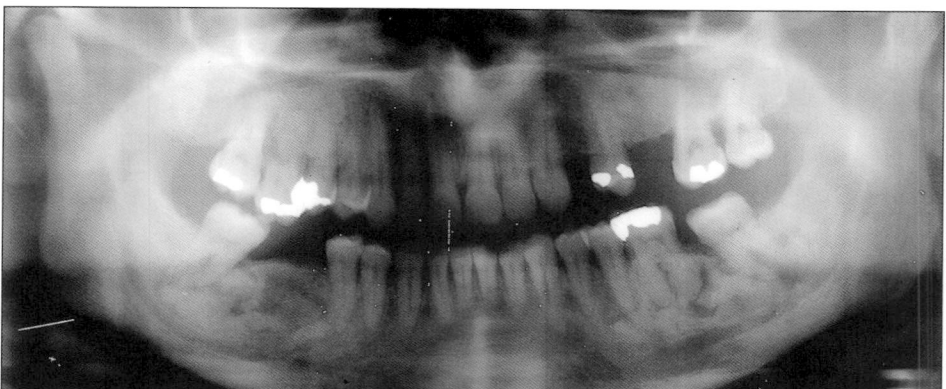

Fig 16-17 Florid cemento-osseous dysplasia will have radiopacities in several quadrants, which will obliterate tooth root outlines. However, the involvement is limited to the tooth-bearing alveolar bone and spares the rami and basilar bone.

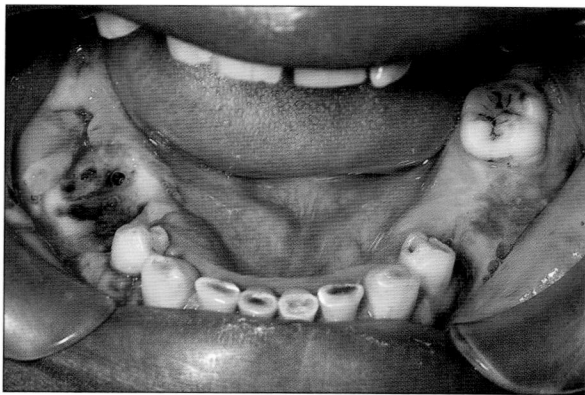

Fig 16-18 If teeth are removed from bone affected by florid cemento-osseous dysplasia, the ankylosed roots will remain in clinically hard, exposed avascular bone and will be indistinguishable from the bone itself. Bone also may become spontaneously exposed.

DIAGNOSIS AND TREATMENT ▶

Biopsy is not usually required. The clinical history, age, race, sex, and radiographic findings are sufficient to diagnose most cases.

Because this phenomenon is not progressive, symptomatic, or particularly damaging, no treatment is required. In fact, it is important to avoid well-meaning treatment attempts, such as root canal therapy or apicoectomy, merely to improve the radiographic picture. Understanding the biology of this phenomenon, its clinical-radiographic picture, and the vitality of the associated teeth will prevent unnecessary interventions that often lead to iatrogenic complications.

Florid Cemento-Osseous Dysplasia

CLINICAL PRESENTATION ▶

Florid cemento-osseous dysplasia refers to a set of radiolucent-radiopaque periapical and interradicular lesions involving the mandible bilaterally and sometimes the maxilla. It is basically an extended form of periapical cemento-osseous dysplasia (Fig 16-17). These lesions are also asymptomatic dysmorphic bone-cementum complexes. However, about 10% become exposed to the oral flora because of tooth removal, periodontal disease, or pulpal disease and become painful because of secondary infection (Fig 16-18). Some of these will also form drainage tracts intraorally or extraorally.

This presentation also has its highest incidence in women of African heritage around the age of 40 years with the same occasional occurrence in men, other age groups, and other races. Radiographs show large radiolucent, mixed, or most often dense radiopaque masses limited to the periapical alveolar bone. They do not involve the inferior border (basilar bone) except by direct focal extension and do not occur in the rami. Unlike those seen in periapical cemento-osseous dysplasia, these lesions are not always limited to the periapical alveolar bone; often, they also involve the interradicular bone up to the level of the cemento-enamel junction. Their presence is not usually associated with expansion, but rare cases may show mild expansion.

DIFFERENTIAL DIAGNOSIS ▶

Diffusely positioned, radiopaque masses in the jaws may suggest a systemic etiology, most importantly *Paget disease* or the multiple endosteomas in *Gardner syndrome*. A large *ossifying fibroma* or *chronic osteomyelitis* also may be considered. However, a true chronic diffuse sclerosing osteomyelitis should not be confused with florid cemento-osseous dysplasia, because chronic diffuse sclerosing osteomyelitis is very painful, involves the inferior border or ramus, and is seen more commonly in caucasians and Asians.

HISTOPATHOLOGY ▶

The histologic features of florid cemento-osseous dysplasia cannot be readily distinguished from those of the other cemento-osseous dysplasias. They consist of unencapsulated fibroblastic tissue with irregu-

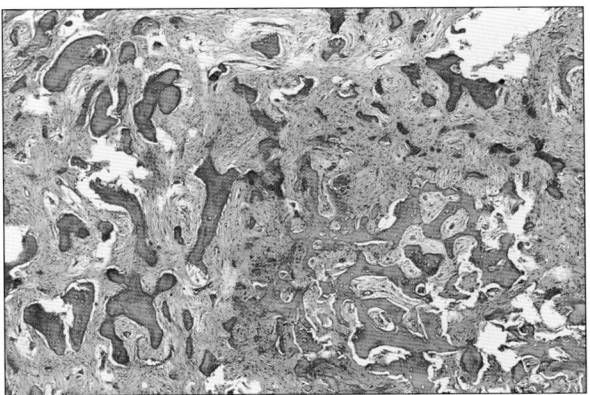 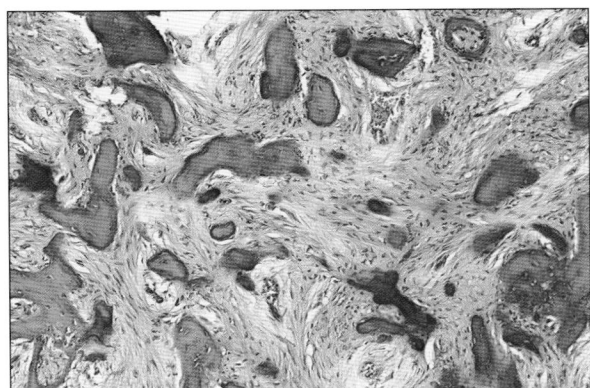

Figs 16-19a and 16-19b Florid cemento-osseous dysplasia showing a fibrous stroma with trabecular and rounded cemento-osseous tissue.

lar osseous trabeculae and acellular cementum-like material (Figs 16-19a and 16-19b). Over time, sclerotic, acellular, avascular masses develop. Idiopathic bone cavities, which consist of empty spaces lined by small amounts of fibrous tissue, may form. Once these lesions become symptomatic, inflammatory infiltrates and fibrosis also will be present.

DIAGNOSIS AND TREATMENT ▶

Florid cemento-osseous dysplasia requires a clinical-radiographic diagnosis. If it cannot be distinguished from Paget disease radiographically, an alkaline phosphatase determination is needed. If Gardner syndrome is a strong consideration, a skull series and other radiographs to search for osteomas elsewhere, as well as a colonoscopy, are recommended.

The clinician should not treat asymptomatic florid cemento-osseous dysplasia that is covered with mucosa. In fact, all attempts to salvage teeth should be exhausted before a tooth associated with opaque lesions of this type around its roots is removed. In such tooth removals, the roots are ankylosed to the bone-cementum complex, which has poor cellularity and vascularity. The result is often fractured roots that cannot be removed or even distinguished from the dysmorphic bone-cementum complex and a wound that remains exposed and does not heal. This scenario often leads to a secondarily infected wound and the onset of pain and drainage (see Fig 16-16).

Cases of symptomatic, secondarily infected florid cemento-osseous dysplasia may be alleviated with local wound care and antibiotic therapy. Persistent cases often respond better with the addition of hyperbaric oxygen to the treatment regimen, which enhances the microbicidal ability of the host defenses and antibiotics in such poorly vascular tissue. However, although these treatments often improve the symptoms, the exposed bone-cementum complex usually does not heal completely, and symptomatic exacerbations often recur. In such cases, resolution may be attained by surgery, which takes the form of an alveolar resection of the symptomatic area only (Fig 16-20a). Asymptomatic areas should not be excised because the alveolar resection leaves a significant defect to the level of the inferior border, which may require bony reconstruction at a later date.

PROGNOSIS ▶

Most individuals can live with the radiographically apparent lesions without difficulties. Those with an exposed bone-cementum complex are often helped by nonsurgical therapy. Those few who require surgery have gained disease resolution. In areas of focal resections, normal bone that does not develop the dysmorphic features of florid cemento-osseous dysplasia will regenerate, a finding that supports the concept that this entity arises as a dyscementogenesis (Figs 16-20b and 16-20c). In those patients who have undergone bone grafting after a resection, the bone graft remains normal as well.

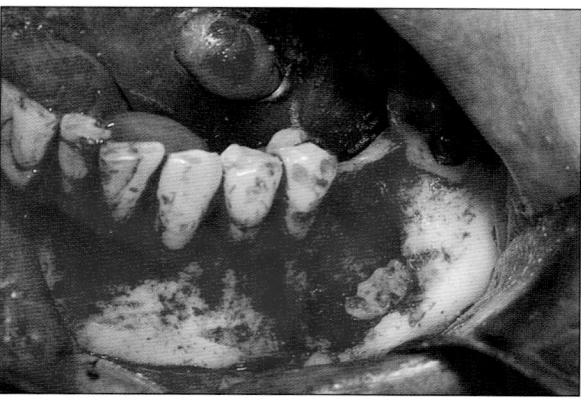

Fig 16-20a Surgery for florid cemento-osseous dysplasia will identify avascular discolored bone with some granulation tissue. The diseased bone is usually separated from normal bone by granulation tissue. When it is not, it is more difficult to remove.

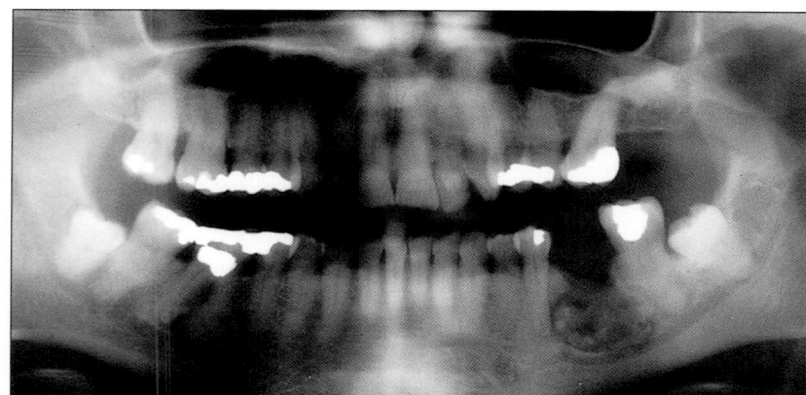

Fig 16-20b Focal cemento-osseous dysplasia will present as a single area or as two close-together areas representing a less severe form of florid cemento-osseous dysplasia but making it less distinguishable from other radiopaque lesions.

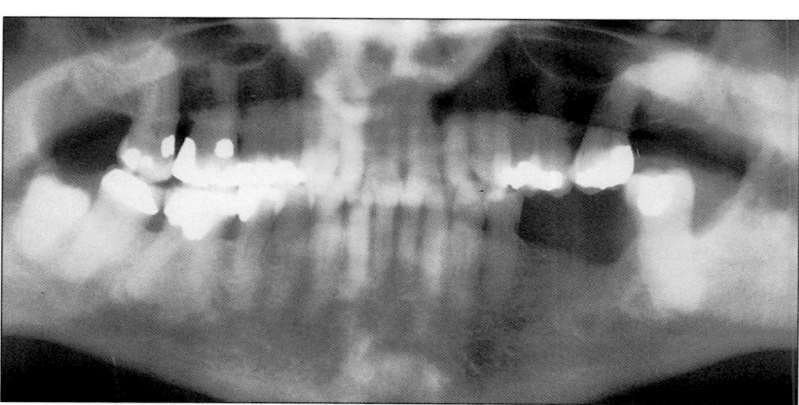

Fig 16-20c After curettage of the cemento-osseous dysplasia, the regenerated bone will be radiographically and histologically normal.

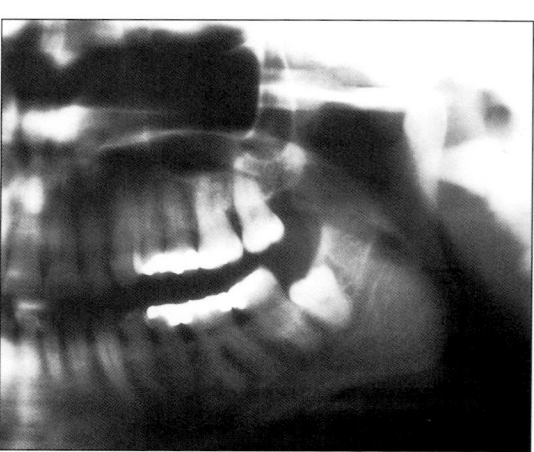

Fig 16-21 An increase in the periapical bone density related to pulpal inflammation may be termed a *condensing osteitis*, *bone scar*, or *osseous keloid*.

Focal Cemento-Osseous Dysplasia

CLINICAL PRESENTATION ▶

Focal cemento-osseous dysplasia is an incomplete form (forme fruste) of florid cemento-osseous dysplasia that is much less common. This type of dysplasia occurs when the same dysmorphic cementum-bone complex develops in a single focus in the alveolar bone of one or both jaws (see Fig 16-20b).

DIFFERENTIAL DIAGNOSIS ▶

A single radiopaque mass in the alveolar process suggests a completely different differential diagnosis than that of florid cemento-osseous dysplasia. In this case, the clinician should consider an *odontoma*, a *cementoblastoma*, an *osteoblastoma*, an *ossifying fibroma*, or even an *osteosarcoma*. In addition, there are several nonspecific entities such as a so-called *condensing osteitis*, a *residual tooth root*, or a *bone scar* from a previous injury that can produce a single asymptomatic radiopacity.

DIAGNOSIS AND TREATMENT ▶

Focal cemento-osseous dysplasia is a radiographic diagnosis that, once made, should not require treatment unless a nonhealing bone exposure or significant symptoms develop. In such cases, removal of the affected bone and teeth in the area will resolve the disease. However, because focal cemento-osseous dysplasia represents a less severe version of the genetic alteration seen in florid cemento-osseous dysplasia, a good radiographic survey of all quadrants in each jaw is necessary, as is follow-up to assess for new lesions.

Nonspecific Radiopacities of the Jaws

CLINICAL PRESENTATION AND
PATHOGENESIS ▶

Panoramic radiographs, and sometimes periapical radiographs, will identify focal radiopacities, which are relatively common. They are almost always asymptomatic, incidental radiographic findings unassociated with any bony expansion. They are usually small (less than 1 cm in diameter), single entities. They are most often a uniformly increased radiodensity with irregular borders. Alternatively, some have a small lucent center and others are lobulated.

Although they are clinically and pathologically insignificant, much has been made of these entities. Some have attributed a low-grade infectious etiology ("condensing osteitis" or "focal sclerosing osteomyelitis") and others an increase in trabecular bone density related to previous injury or infection ("bone scar" or "osseous keloid") (Fig 16-21). Indeed, some radiopacities seem to be associated with root apices affected by pulpitis or traumatic occlusion. However, others are unassociated with tooth roots or are associated with normal, caries-free teeth and may, therefore, merely represent imperfect bone.

DIFFERENTIAL DIAGNOSIS ▶

Nonspecific radiopacities may be confused with *periapical cemento-osseous dysplasia*, a *complex odontoma*, *hypercementosis*, a *cementoblastoma*, an *osteoma*, or a *superimposed exostosis*. It is, therefore, important to know that periapical cemento-osseous dysplasia involves several teeth, hypercementosis has a periodontal ligament space around its periphery, and a cementoblastoma obliterates the entire apical half of the root and has an encapsulation that produces a radiolucent band around its periphery, simulating a periodontal ligament space. A complex odontoma should be larger and more radiodense because it is mostly dentin. An exostosis can be recognized by clinical examination, and an osteoma should be palpable. Ruling out these entities and identifying the radiographic characteristics of these nonspecific radiopacities will allow the diagnosis to be made.

HISTOPATHOLOGY ▶

These radiopacities show no significant pathologic change and usually consist of unremarkable osseous trabeculae.

TREATMENT AND PROGNOSIS ▶

No treatment is required. These entities remain innocuous throughout life.

Paget Disease

CLINICAL PRESENTATION AND
PATHOGENESIS ▶

Paget disease is a condition of excessive bone resorption followed by disorganized repair. Its etiology is unknown, but several theories have been advanced, of which a slow virus theory has received the greatest support. It is not, however, a metabolic abnormality of bone as previously thought. The pathogenesis begins with overactive osteoclasis of bone. The bone responds by osteoblastic differentiation in which these osteoblasts lay down haphazard bone in many different directions. An increase in vascularity to cope with the demands of so much new bone formation develops. As the disease continues, the abundant osteoid becomes increasingly mineralized, resulting after many years in a dense, sclerotic, end-stage bone that has reduced cellularity and vascularity.

Most symptoms occur during the early and intermediate phases of Paget disease, when bone activity and vascularity are at their peak. Patients classically complain of deep bone pain as an early symptom. The pagetoid bone is structurally weak, leading to bowed tibias, kyphosis, or frequent fractures of long bones, depending on the bones involved.

Paget disease usually occurs in individuals older than 50 years (3% of the population older than 50 years is said to have at least one isolated lesion of Paget disease), although rare cases of juvenile Paget disease exist. Men are affected more frequently than women by a 3:2 margin. The bones most commonly affected are the spine, femurs, skull, pelvis, sternum, and jaws. The maxilla is affected twice as frequently as the mandible. Together, cases affecting the maxilla and/or mandible account for about 17% of all cases.

The patient with jaw involvement will present with expansion and deep bone pain. The affected area will often feel warm with visibly enlarged veins or a bluish hue because of the increased vascularity. The

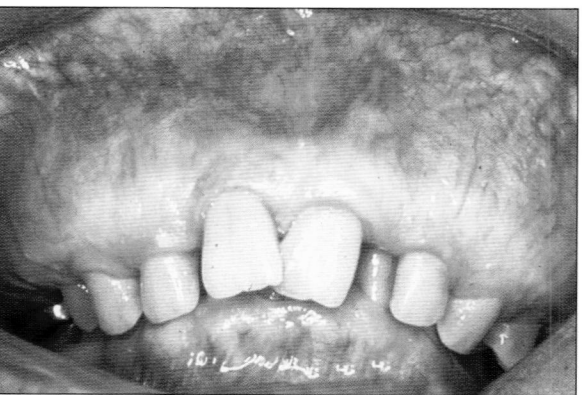

Fig 16-22 Paget disease produces a slow expansion of the involved bone; in the jaws, it creates diastemas between teeth and malocclusions. Note the increased vascularity of the area.

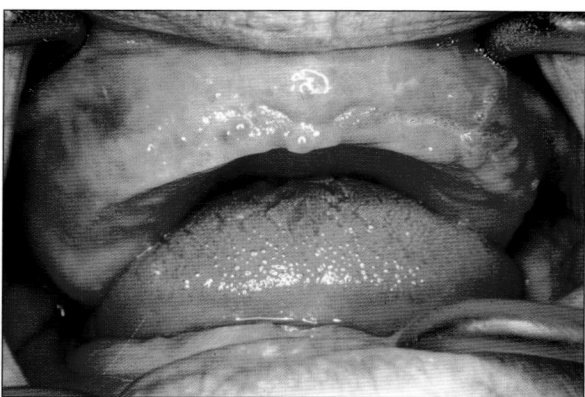

Fig 16-23 Paget disease will expand the jaws so that dentures will no longer fit in edentulous individuals. The tissue will be warm because of the excessive vascularity of pagetic bone.

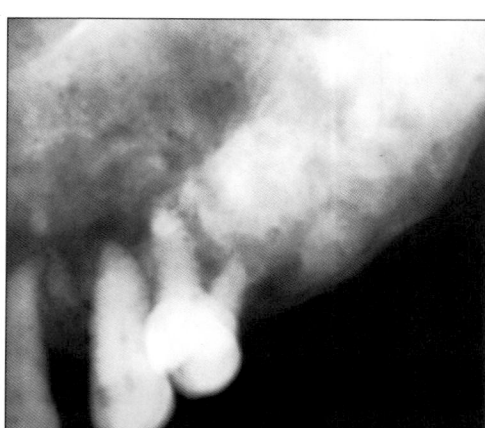

Fig 16-24a A mixture of irregular radiopacities, bone expansion, and radiolucencies give pagetic bone a so-called cotton wool appearance.

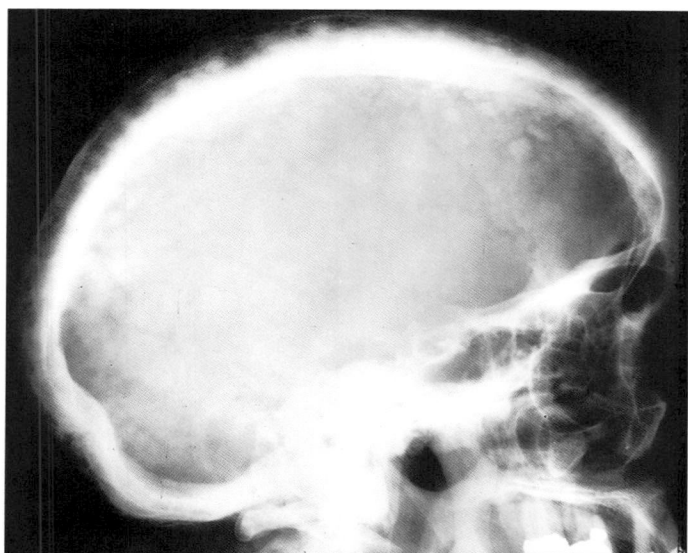

Fig 16-24b A skull radiograph of pagetic calvarium will often show the same cotton wool appearance. There is thickening of the inner and outer tables and widening of the diploe.

teeth will have diastemas and lingual inclinations because of dental compensations in response to the slow expansion (Fig 16-22). A denture wearer may present with the classic complaint of a denture that has become too small and may even have had several appliances made to keep pace with the expansion (Fig 16-23). Analogously, some of Paget's original reports described skull enlargement that necessitated ever-increasing hat sizes. Patients with jaw involvement may also complain of constant lip and associated soft tissue pain reminiscent of a neuralgia. With skull involvement, headache is the most common complaint, but neuralgiform facial pain and other neurologic complaints such as vertigo, facial paralysis, visual disturbances, and hearing loss are also reported. Such neurologic complaints are believed to be caused by pagetic bone expansion and subsequent compression around the foramina at the base of the skull or within the skull. Although pagetically weakened long bones may fracture pathologically, the jaws usually do not because of the reduced compressive forces placed on them. When such fractures heal, they heal with pagetic bone.

RADIOGRAPHIC APPEARANCE ▶ Pagetic bone appears as a mottled mixture of radiopacities and radiolucencies (Fig 16-24a). The ratio of these elements depends on the duration of the disease. The radiographic pattern has been termed the "cotton wool" appearance because it is characterized by a fluffed, radiodense, cloud-like aggregation (Fig 16-24b). In the jaws, this bone may cause root resorption as well as tooth displacement. Teeth may exhibit hypercementosis or the loss of the lamina dura.

DIFFERENTIAL DIAGNOSIS ▶ A radiopaque, painful expansion of the jaws in an adult may be suggestive of osteomyelitis, particularly *chronic diffuse sclerosing osteomyelitis*. *Osteosarcoma* is another consideration. *Fibrous dysplasia* may resemble Paget disease radiographically but would have been present from early life. An *ossifying fibroma*, particularly one that is large and mature with densely formed bone, may also resemble Paget disease radiographically and is more consistent with the age of onset. Long-standing *secondary hyperparathyroidism* will also produce expansile bone with a mottled radiopaque-radiolucent pattern and may be painful as well. Radiopacities of *florid cemento-osseous dysplasias* also mimic the "cotton wool" appearance of Paget disease and may be painful from secondary infection.

DIAGNOSTIC WORK-UP ▶ The hallmark of diagnosis for a suspected case of Paget disease is a markedly elevated serum alkaline phosphatase level. Serum calcium and phosphate values are normal unless the patient has been recently immobilized, in which case hypercalcemia will develop. Biopsy is usually not necessary unless the alkaline phosphatase levels are near normal and radiographs are equivocal. If a biopsy is performed, the most diagnostic area is the lesion's center at the point of greatest expansion. A brisk, oozing type of bleeding will occur during biopsy because of the rich vascularity. Hemorrhage can be controlled by pressure and local hemostatic agents.

HISTOPATHOLOGY ▶ Active Paget disease is characterized by repeated destruction and repair of bone with no functional organization. First is osteoclastic resorption within the haversian canals and a fibrovascular proliferation within the marrow. Subsequently, osteoblasts lay down new bone. This process continues in random fashion (Fig 16-25a). The osteoclasts are unusually large and contain numerous nuclei, sometimes more than 100 (Fig 16-25b). The repeated destruction and repair creates a pattern of irregular cemental lines that mimics a mosaic (Fig 16-25c). This finding is characteristic but not pathognomonic. The stroma is fibrous and contains a rich supply of dilated capillaries (see Fig 16-25c). This marked vascularity is of surgical significance because there may be profuse bleeding during operative procedures. Healing of this type of pagetic bone is usually uncomplicated, but the healed bone nonetheless remains pagetic bone. Paget disease may "burn out" in certain areas, in which case there may be considerable sclerosis of bone, fibrosis, and diminished vascularity (Fig 16-25d). Such areas may exhibit slow healing and complications.

TREATMENT AND PROGNOSIS ▶ Mild cases require no treatment. Paget disease is currently incurable, but the pain and deformity can be controlled with treatment. Current therapy, which is aimed at inhibiting osteoclastic bone resorption and, therefore, breaking the cycle of bone resorption–distorted repair, focuses on the anti-osteoclastic actions of calcitonin or the bisphosphonates. Synthetic salmon calcitonin (Calcimar, Aventis) is given in doses ranging from 50 to 100 IU subcutaneously daily or three times weekly over a period of months or even years. Alternatively, nasal salmon calcitonin (Miocalcin, Sandoz) may be used at 200 IU/spray once daily. A 200-mg oral dose of disodium etidronate may be given twice daily; the dosage should be modified to 5 mg/kg daily for underweight individuals. However, it is important to note that this drug is usually given for 3- to 6-month periods and then interrupted before another course is given because prolonged use of etidronate will adversely affect bone mineralization in the rest of the skeleton. Pamidronate (Aredia, Novartis) is another drug effective in Paget disease, but it must be given intravenously in 500 mL of normal saline at a dosage of 30 mg over 4 hours. Response to this therapy lasts for 3 to 6 months, then the dosage must be repeated.

Therapy with any of these three drugs results in a reduction in pain and bony expansion. Serum alkaline phosphatase levels as well as urinary hydroxyproline levels fall in response to this therapy, enabling patients to live near-normal and often active lifestyles. However, some patients with long-standing disease develop renal failure or nephrocalcinosis caused by hypercalcemia. Others undergo spontaneous malignant transformation into osteosarcoma. The incidence of this is heavily debated and mostly overstated.

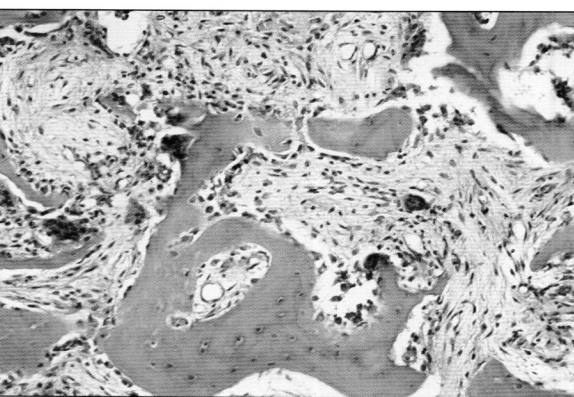

Fig 16-25a Marked osteoclastic as well as osteoblastic activity is evident in Paget disease.

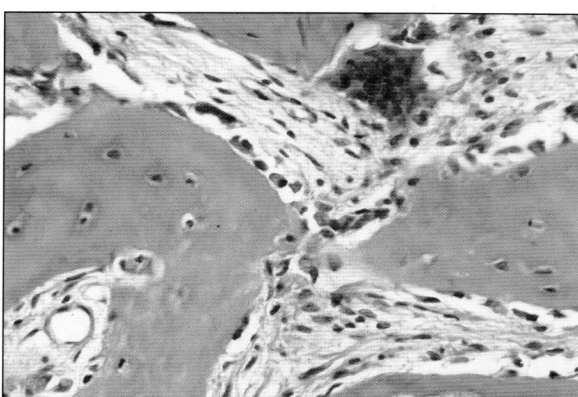

Fig 16-25b An abnormally large osteoclast is present, as are many active osteoblasts.

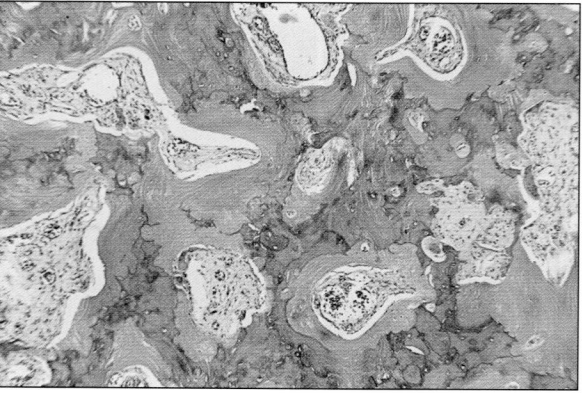

Fig 16-25c Low-power view from a case of Paget disease showing the mosaic pattern of the bone formed by the reversal lines. The vascularity of the stroma also is evident.

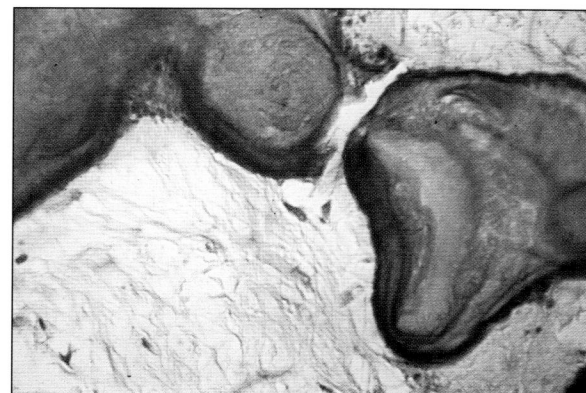

Fig 16-25d In this "burned out" area in a case of Paget disease, the bone is sclerotic and the stroma no longer vascular.

However, it is in the range of 2% to 5% of cases. Radiation in Paget disease is contraindicated because it has been proven to incite malignant transformation.

FOLLOW-UP ▶

Follow-up for patients with Paget disease is usually on a semi-annual or annual basis if the condition is stable. Radiographs and serum alkaline phosphatase levels are evaluated. Signs that may herald a sarcomatous transformation are rapid clinical expansion, surface ulceration, necrosis, development of new radiolucent areas, and an increase over previous alkaline phosphatase levels.

Osteopetrosis

CLINICAL PRESENTATION AND PATHOGENESIS ▶

Osteopetrosis is caused by an inherited defect in osteoclasts. Defective osteoclasts fail to resorb bone in the normal (0.7% per day) resorption-remodeling cycle of the skeleton. Therefore, all bones progressively become more dense, less cellular, and less vascular. Because the resorption-remodeling cycle of bone eliminates microstress lines and microfractures and maintains foramen and the marrow cavity spaces, these areas become compromised and compressed in osteopetrosis. Therefore, fractures, anemia, thrombocytopenia, and nerve dysfunction ranging from hearing loss to visual disturbance to facial palsy are possible, depending on the genetic type and level of expression of this condition.

Three inheritance patterns of osteopetrosis have been found: severe autosomal-recessive osteopetrosis, which is also known as Albers-Schönberg disease; mild autosomal-recessive osteopetrosis; and

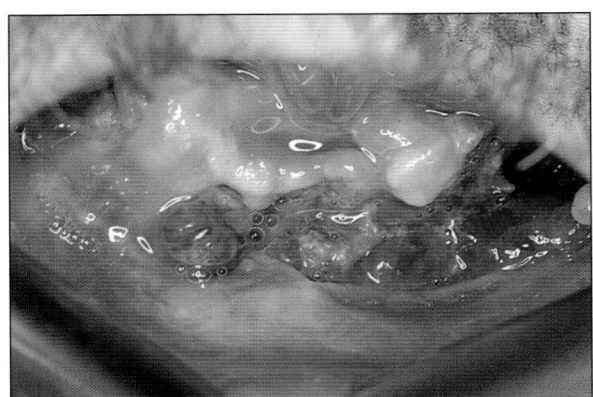

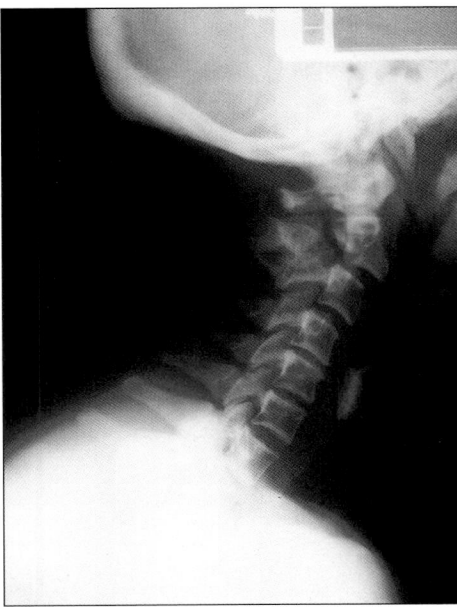

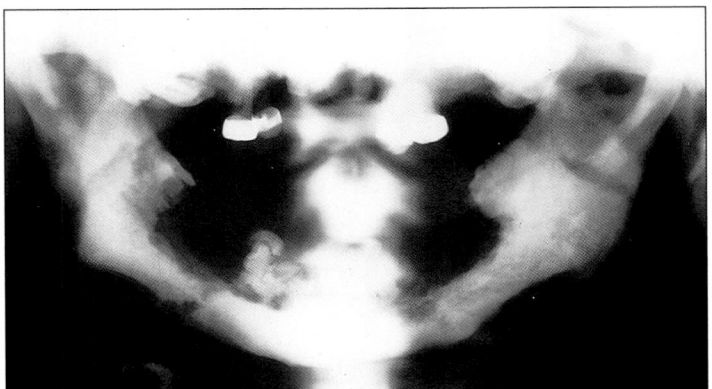

Fig 16-26a Due to the presence of teeth or the removal of teeth, osteopetrosis patients frequently have exposed bone of the alveolar ridges with granulation tissue, a finding that is not usually seen in other bones.

Fig 16-26b Early or less severe cases of osteopetrosis may be identified on a cervical- (C-) spine radiograph, which will show an increased density of the vertebral cortices, the so-called sandwich appearance. Also note the C-1 over C-2 subluxation.

Fig 16-26c Panoramic radiograph of osteopetrosis showing defects from previous surgery, a pathologic fracture, a retained tooth, and a bone sequestrum, all of which are typical of the disease.

benign autosomal-dominant osteopetrosis. Each of these inheritance patterns may produce a similar presentation clinically and will have overlapping signs because of the heterogenicity of the gene defect. Distinguishing the conditions requires genetic testing and long-term clinical observation.

Individuals with osteopetrosis often have exposed bone with granulation tissue and a low-grade osteomyelitis in the head and neck region (Fig 16-26a). Early cases may be suspected if a general increased radiographic density is seen on panoramic radiographs or skull radiographs and if unerupted teeth are present. If the radiograph shows the cervical spine, the vertebrae may appear to have the "sandwich" look, an early sign that is caused by an increased density in the superior and inferior cortices in contrast to the less dense cancellous marrow area between them (Fig 16-26b).

Long-standing cases are the rule. In most instances, these individuals have undergone well-intentioned but ineffectual bony debridements and tooth removals. Some will present with most of their alveolar bone missing from past debridements and with a pathologic fracture (Fig 16-26c). Exposed dense and discolored bone is common and almost always follows tooth extraction. Erupted teeth may be ankylosed. Cutaneous fistulae also are frequently seen. Some cases progress to a facial cellulitis.

Defective vision and nystagmus are common. However, any of the cranial nerves may be compressed at several foramina and, therefore, can present with a varied group of paresthesias and pareses.

Anemia and thrombocytopenia may be seen but are uncommon because significant bone formation within the marrow cavity of long bones and a reduced compensatory extramedullary hematopoiesis would be required for their development. Because osteopetrosis begins in the cortex of long bones and progresses inward, significant marrow cavity obliteration is a later finding.

RADIOGRAPHIC APPEARANCE ▶

Skull and jaw radiographs can be astonishing (Fig 16-27). The skull in particular will show an extreme density. The mandible should be assessed for fractures, unerupted teeth, and areas of past debridement. The maxillary sinuses may be smaller than usual and the frontal sinus obliterated altogether. Radiographs of the cervical spine in early stages will show the "sandwich" appearance. In later stages, a gen-

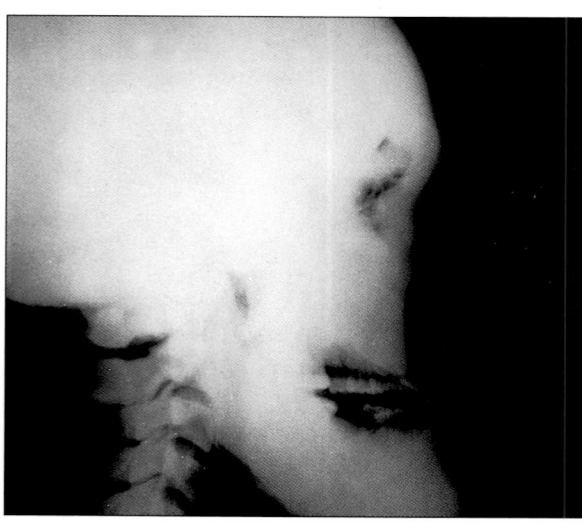

Fig 16-27 Since osteopetrosis involves all skeletal tissues, radiographs showing extreme bone densities can be astonishing.

eralized opacification is apparent. However, the most clinically important assessment of the cervical spine is for subluxations and a fracture of the odontoid process. Either may produce a serious spinal cord compression or laceration (see Fig 16-26b).

DIFFERENTIAL DIAGNOSIS ▶

A fully expressed case of osteopetrosis is radiographically pathognomonic by its involvement of all bones. However, if the presentation is one of only clinically exposed dense bone and no radiographs have been taken, the clinician should be concerned about *florid cemento-osseous dysplasia*, *osteoradionecrosis* if there is a history of radiotherapy, a later stage of *Paget disease*, and *osteomyelitis*. If only a panoramic radiograph of the jaws has been taken, osteopetrosis may resemble an advanced case of Paget disease, *secondary hyperparathyroidism*, *fibrous dysplasia*, or a *chronic diffuse sclerosing osteomyelitis*. Early cases may also produce a radiographic picture resembling the bony changes seen in severe anemias, such as *severe sickle cell anemia* and *beta thalassemia*.

DIAGNOSTIC WORK-UP ▶

Osteopetrosis is most commonly confirmed by history because the patient is usually well aware of his or her condition. Skull radiographs are useful to confirm a suspected case. Cervical spine radiographs are needed to assess for the serious complication potential of odontoid fracture or subluxations. A panoramic radiograph also is needed to rule out fractures and to identify unerupted and/or ankylosed teeth. In addition, a complete blood count is recommended either to document anemia/pancytopenia or to establish a reference point for future comparisons.

HISTOPATHOLOGY ▶

Because the underlying defect concerns osteoclastic function and bone remodeling, the pattern of endochondral bone formation is disrupted. The trabeculae have cores of heavily calcified cartilage surrounded by irregular woven bone. While the trabeculae may show little thickening in mild disease, in the severe form they may become confluent, ultimately obliterating the marrow and merging with the thickened cortex. The numbers of osteoclasts and osteoblasts vary from few to many. Ultrastructurally, the osteoclasts lack ruffled borders, which normally release lysosomal enzymes at the bone-osteoclast interface. Therefore, these defective osteoclasts fail to resorb bone in the normal resorption-remodeling cycle.

In autopsy findings reported by Younai et al, mandibles showed endosteal bone formation in three patterns: a tortuous arrangement of lamellar bone trabeculae, an amorphous globular pattern, and an osteophytic pattern. Numerous osteoclasts were noted, but there was no scalloping of bone, as would be seen when there is normal osteoclastic resorption.

Teeth in osteopetrosis may show enamel hypoplasia, defects in mineralization of dentin, and abnormal pulp chambers. Unerupted teeth show areas of ankylosis between cementum and bone with absence of periodontal membrane. The periodontal membrane has also been noted to contain fibrous tissue that runs parallel to the root surface, suggesting an abnormality. Areas of osteomyelitis involving the mandible show fibrosis with chronic inflammatory cells.

Osteopetrosis is frustrating for the clinician and the individual. Unlike in other diseases involving exposed nonviable bone, debridement is not the focus of therapy in osteopetrosis. In fact, the strategy is to avoid bony surgery and to limit the degree of surgery as much as possible. The involvement of the entire skeleton does not allow the surgeon to debride to "healthy bone," and bone grafts are not available from any site. Therefore, almost all surgeries in which bone is debrided and a soft tissue closure is obtained result in re-exposure of a greater amount of bone and further risk of fracture.

In a similar sense, tooth removal should be avoided if possible. Therefore, frequent dental visits with prophylaxis and prompt restorative and endodontic care are recommended. A removed tooth often initiates the development of persistently exposed bone and low-grade infection.

The clinician is relegated to mostly nonsurgical management even when fractures occur. The exposed bone is cultured and then best treated with the limited intervention of smoothing rough or sharp bony edges, chlorhexidine gluconate oral rinses, and frequent irrigations to reduce numbers of the microorganisms. During periods of secondary infection, culture-directed antibiotics are recommended. Hyperbaric oxygen, which produces angiogenesis in osteoradionecrosis, has been suggested for the treatment of osteopetrosis. However, its use is of limited value because osteopetrosis, unlike osteoradionecrosis, does not produce the necessary oxygen gradient loss in soft tissues. It therefore should be reserved for use as an adjunct to antibiotics and wound irrigations in episodes of secondary infection.

Should a patient with osteopetrosis require surgery under general anesthesia, the intubation should be either a fiberoptic-assisted or an awake nasal intubation. Use of a laryngoscope, which extends the neck, risks paralysis from spinal cord compression because of the high risk of cervical spine subluxation and fracture.

Effects of Calcium, Phosphate, and Alkaline Phosphatase in Fibro-Osseous Diseases

The laboratory values of serum calcium, phosphate, and the enzyme alkaline phosphatase are important to the understanding and management of many fibro-osseous diseases (Table 16-2).

Calcium

Calcium is controlled by three organs and three hormones. The organs are the gut (small intestines), the kidneys, and bone. The hormones are vitamin D, calcitonin, and parathyroid hormone (PTH). Their influences are summarized in Table 16-3. Essentially, dietary calcium is absorbed in the gut and is increased by vitamin D. Vitamin D has no influence on the kidney or bone directly. PTH also increases the gut absorption of calcium. Calcium, which is normally excreted in the urine at almost 250 mg/24 hr (6.2 mmol/day), is reduced by PTH. The most marked effect of PTH, however, is on osteoclast activation that induces bone resorption. Therefore, all of the actions of PTH result in an increased serum calcium level. PTH is the safeguard hormone of serum calcium levels; it will increase absorption from the gut, reduce its renal loss, and literally steal it away from bone. Calcitonin, which has no effect on the gut or kidneys, acts as a balance against PTH overactivity and, therefore, hypercalcemia. Calcitonin inhibits osteoclasts from resorbing bone, which is the most marked effect of PTH, and thereby lowers serum calcium levels.

As noted at the beginning of the chapter, primary hyperparathyroidism, which produces excessive PTH, creates significant hypercalcemia. Secondary hyperparathyroidism, which is related to renal failure and causes excessive urinary calcium loss, produces hypocalcemia. The hypocalcemia in turn signals the normal parathyroid glands to produce elevated levels of PTH, which is ineffective in elevating serum cal-

Table 16-2 Relative laboratory values for fibro-osseous diseases and systemic diseases affecting bone

Disease	Calcium	Phosphate	Alkaline phosphatase
Hyperparathyroidism			
Primary	High	Low	Normal
Secondary	Low	High	Normal
Paraneoplastic	High	Low	Normal
Paget disease	Normal	Normal	Very high
Cherubism	Normal	Normal	Normal*
Fibrous dysplasia	Normal	Normal	Normal*
Ossifying fibroma	Normal	Normal	Normal

*Normal for patient age, but elevated because of growth.

Table 16-3 Normal physiologic serum calcium balance

	Vitamin D	Parathyroid hormone	Calcitonin
Gut absorption	Increases	Increases	No effect
Kidney excretion	No effect	Decreases	No effect
Bone resorption	No effect	Greatly increases	Decreases

cium levels because of the constant renal loss. In both situations, PTH levels are elevated. In primary hyperparathyroidism, elevation is caused by an autonomous overproduction of PTH. In secondary hyperparathyroidism, it is caused by constantly stimulated parathyroid glands.

Phosphate

Phosphate, like calcium, is absorbed in the gut and is controlled by vitamin D. It is also excreted in the kidneys, but unlike calcium its excretion is enhanced by PTH, which prevents phosphate reabsorption. Therefore, serum phosphate concentrations are the inverse of serum calcium concentrations in each type of hyperparathyroidism. In primary hyperparathyroidism, the excess PTH produces a hypophosphatemia by increasing renal loss. In secondary hyperparathyroidism, urinary phosphate loss is reduced by the lack of glomerular filtration of phosphate and the ineffective response to PTH, resulting in hyperphosphatemia.

Alkaline Phosphatase

Bone-related alkaline phosphatase is an enzyme secreted by osteoblasts that hydrolyzes organic phosphates for bone mineralization. Elevations are a rough index of new bone formation. In all of the hyperparathyroidisms, alkaline phosphatase levels are normal because in most cases the serum hyper- and hypocalcemias and the hyper- and hypophosphatemias are unrelated to new bone formation. In Paget disease, serum calcium and phosphate levels are normal because a dynamic equilibrium exists (the same amount of each ion enters bone as it is released). However, as the new bone formation tries to keep pace with bone resorption, alkaline phosphate levels are markedly increased. In ossifying fibroma, fibrous dysplasia, and cherubism, the bone aberrations are not systemic and therefore do not affect serum calcium or phosphate levels. Moreover, the bone formation in each is independent and not directly related to serum alkaline phosphatase. However, cherubism and fibrous dysplasia mostly occur during active growth years in which there is a physiologic (normal) elevation of alkaline phosphatase.

Severe Anemias Affecting Bone

Some severe anemias will affect the jaws and facial skeleton in a clinically recognizable manner. The most common of these is beta thalassemia (thalassemia intermedia) and homozygous sickle cell anemia. Each will affect the facial bones in a different manner depending on the severity of the anemia.

Beta Thalassemia Intermedia

CLINICAL PRESENTATION AND PATHOGENESIS ▶

The reader should recall that normal adult hemoglobin is primarily hemoglobin A. It comprises about 98% of circulating hemoglobin, leaving hemoglobin A_2 and hemoglobin F to make up the rest. Normal hemoglobin A is the tetramer of two alpha chains and two beta chains and is designated as $\alpha_2\beta_2$. There are two basic types of thalassemias: alpha thalassemia and beta thalassemia. Alpha thalassemia is due to a gene deletion, which reduces synthesis of the alpha globin chains. Since all adult hemoglobins contain alpha globin chains, deficiencies in alpha globin chain synthesis do not change the ratios of hemoglobin A, A_2, or F. Therefore, alpha thalassemia is mild, is clinically normal, and has either a normal hemogram or only a mild microcytic hypochromic anemia.

Beta thalassemias are caused not by gene deletions but by point mutations on the beta globin chain. Therefore, the molecular defects leading to beta thalassemia can be numerous and are more severe. The reduced beta globin chain synthesis results in a relative increase in hemoglobin A_2 and F compared to normal hemoglobin A, as abnormal beta chains (gamma, delta, etc) substitute for the missing beta chains. This hereditary molecular change leads to damaged red blood cell membranes, which undergo intramedullary hemolysis as well as circulating hemolysis. The bone marrow attempts to compensate for this with extensive hyperplasia and bony expansion. Therefore, the patient will present as a young individual (age 2 to 20 years) with short stature, cardiomegaly, hepatosplenomegaly, and prominent bony expansion. The face and skull may be the most obvious areas of bony expansion, mimicking tumors, cherubism, or fibrous dysplasia (Fig 16-28a).

RADIOGRAPHIC FINDINGS ▶

Facial bone radiographs or CT scans may be remarkably expanded, usually in a symmetric pattern. The cortices will be thinned with little if any visible trabecular bone in the marrow space (Fig 16-28b). Skull radiographs will show a thickened cortex with vertical extracortical bone formation, often referred to as the "hair on end" effect (Fig 16-28c). All bones will be involved to some degree.

A CT scan of the abdomen will show a symmetrically enlarged spleen and liver indicative of extramedullary hematopoiesis (Fig 16-28d). A chest radiograph will show prominent cardiomegaly (Fig 16-28e).

LABORATORY FINDINGS ▶

In addition to a short stature relative to age, hemoglobinuria will produce a brown-colored urine (Fig 16-28f) and the severe anemia a tachycardia and tachypnea. The hemoglobin will usually range from 6.0 g/dL to 10.0 g/dL, the hematocrit 18% to 30%. The Wintrobe indices will be a picture of a severe microcytic hypochromic anemia. The MCV will range from 55 to 75 μ^3, and the MCH 20 to 25 pg.

DIFFERENTIAL DIAGNOSIS ▶

Most cases of thalassemia intermedia will have been diagnosed and the patient will have undergone therapy and therefore may appear normal. However, occasionally a case will have escaped medical detection and present with an expanded maxilla and mandible (see Fig 16-28a). The clinical appearance will indeed be similar to *cherubism* and the history of onset at about age 3 years will also be consistent with cherubism. Otherwise, the expansions in young individuals also mimic *fibrous dysplasia* or a benign tumor such as an *ossifying fibroma*. More rarely, other severe anemias, such as *homozygous sickle cell anemia, thalassemia major*, or *hereditary spherocytosis*, can produce a similar picture.

TREATMENT AND PROGNOSIS ▶

Alpha thalassemia individuals are clinically normal and will require no specific treatment, nor will very mild cases of beta thalassemia in which the hemogram is in the normal range. However, most beta thalassemias require a regular transfusion schedule and folate supplementation. The goal of transfusion therapy (usually 1 to 3 units per month) is to maintain the hemoglobin above 10.0 g/dL. If this is achieved, the marrow expansion will be lessened, and near normal growth and development will proceed. Since

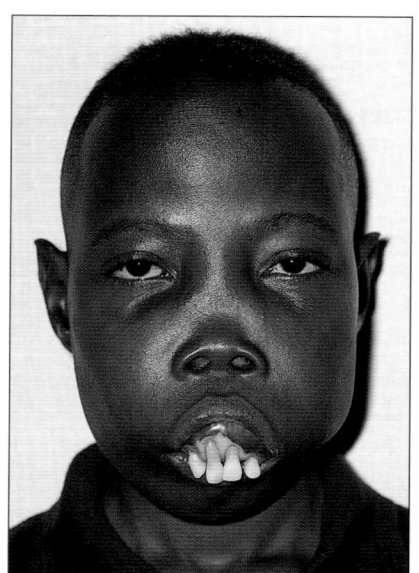

Fig 16-28a Severe maxillary expansion due to marrow hyperplasia in a 17-year-old with beta thalassemia.

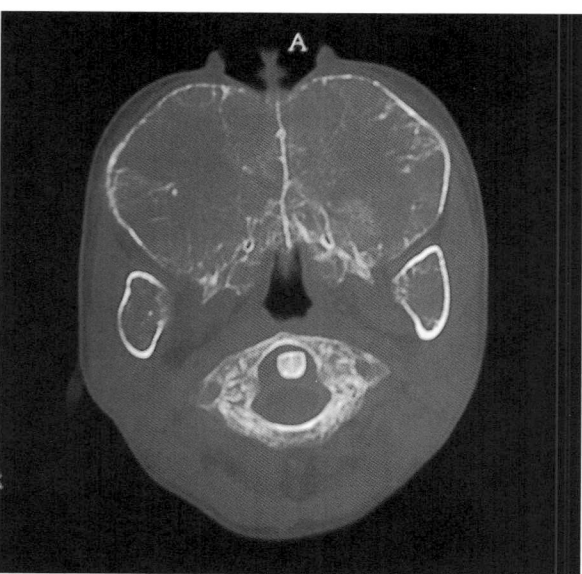

Fig 16-28b The symmetrically expanded maxilla will have a very thinned cortex and will also show elongated and thinned remnants of trabecular bone. Also note the expanded rami of the mandible and mottled arch of the atlas and odontoid process.

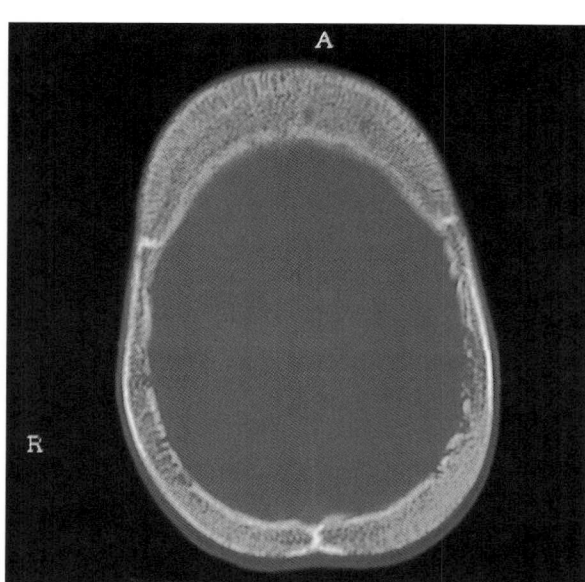

Fig 16-28c This skull CT scan shows expansion of the cranium with thin trabecular bone aligned perpendicular to the cortex to create the "hair on end" effect.

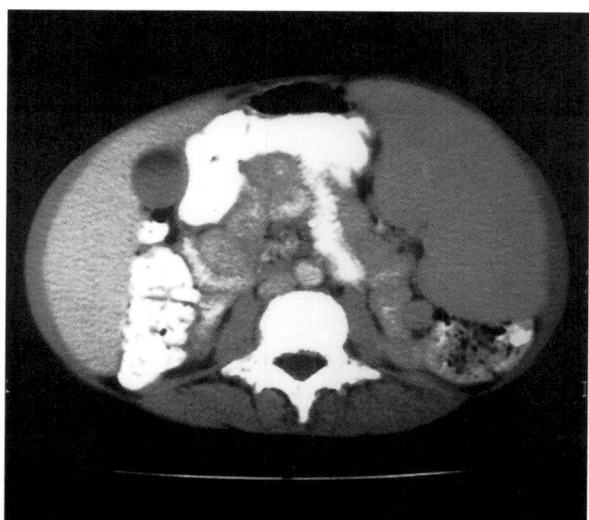

Fig 16-28d Prominent hepatosplenomegaly is seen in most beta thalassemia patients. In homozygous sickle cell anemia, hepatomegaly is common, but splenomegaly may only be observed early in its course, followed by atrophy of the spleen due to repetitive infarctions.

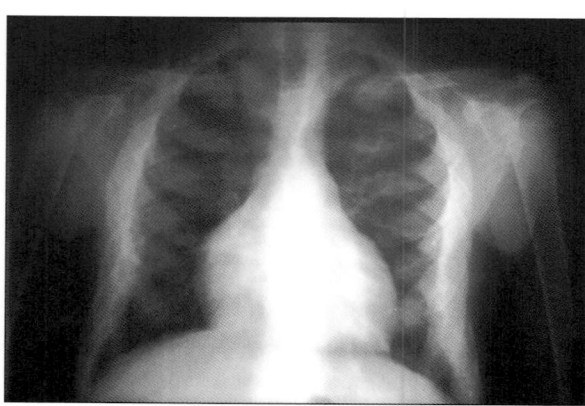

Fig 16-28e Chest radiograph in a severe anemia will usually show cardiomegaly. Note that the ribs are expanded and are mottled in appearance from marrow hyperplasia.

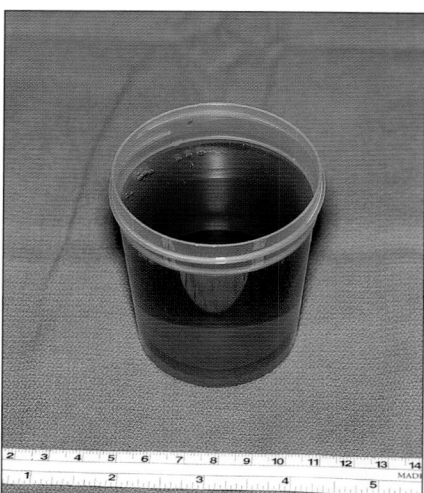

Fig 16-28f Brown urine is often observed at about 2 to 3 years of age when hemoglobin F levels fall to their lowest level and are replaced by abnormal hemoglobin A, which causes fragile cell membranes. The brown urine is due to hemoglobinuria from hemolysis.

hypersplenism also is frequently present, a splenectomy may be required to reduce the hemolysis and therefore the number of transfusions.

Iron accumulation (hemosiderosis) is an inevitable complication of beta thalassemia. It is caused by the constant hemolysis and may be contributed to by the necessary transfusions. This must be concomitantly treated with deferoxamine (Desferal, Novartis), which chelates iron and will postpone and reduce the hemosiderosis.

If iron overload and organ failure can be avoided, long-term survival can be expected and realized in about 80% of cases.

Homozygous Sickle Cell Anemia

Sickle cell anemia is an autosomal-recessive trait in which a single point mutation occurs involving one DNA base. This results in the substitution of the amino acid of valine for the normal glutamine in the sixth position on the beta chain. The abnormal beta chain is designated β^S and the hemoglobin tetramer $\alpha_2\beta_2^S$ most commonly referred to as hemoglobin S. This abnormal hemoglobin leads to a chronic hemolytic anemia that causes a variety of severe clinical manifestations.

When in the deoxy form, hemoglobin S forms polymers that damage the red blood cell membrane and cause the sickling of the cell. Physiologic factors that lead to the formation of deoxyhemoglobin, such as hypoxemia acidosis and dehydrations, are the common triggers of sickling.

The hemoglobin S gene is carried by 81% of Americans of African heritage, and 1 birth out of every 400 in African-American blacks will produce a child with sickle cell anemia. The clinical disease begins during the middle of the first year of life, when the normal beta hemoglobin F levels fall and beta globin synthesis increases.

CLINICAL PRESENTATION AND PATHOGENESIS ▶

As homozygous sickle cell anemia develops, it produces the picture of a chronically ill, poorly developed, and jaundiced child. There will be cardiomegaly and hepatomegaly; clinical splenomegaly will not be seen until well into the teenage years or not at all because of splenic infarctions. There is usually a systolic murmur. Nonhealing ulcers and retinopathy are almost always part of the picture. The skull and facial bones will not be as expanded as is seen in untreated beta thalassemia, although marrow hyperplasia is present and a "hair on end" effect is often seen on skull radiographs (see Fig 16-28c). More directly related to bone pathology are bone pain and ischemic bone necrosis due to clusters of sickle cells producing microvascular thrombi. The ischemic bone necrosis often leads to osteomyelitis, which mostly occurs in the extremities and is due to staphylococci but may also rarely occur in the jaws, where a polymicrobic infection of streptococci and anaerobes are the primary microbiology.

RADIOGRAPHIC FINDINGS ▶

Skull radiographs will show a thickened cortex with vertical extracortical bone formations as is seen in thalassemia. All bone will show a similar picture. However, those with ischemic necrosis and/or osteomyelitis may show osteolytic areas and sequestrae.

LABORATORY FINDINGS ▶

The hemoglobin will range from 6.0 mg/dL to 10.0 mg/dL and the hematocrit from 20% to 30%. A peripheral blood smear will show 5% to 50% sickled red blood cells. The reticulocyte count will be extremely elevated at 10% to 25% (normal is 1%), indicative of the marrow hyperplasia as an attempt to replace the rapidly lost red blood cells. In addition, many red blood cells will be nucleated, also indicative of marrow hyperfunction (Fig 16-29). The white blood cell count will also be high (leukocytosis) and will usually be 12,000/μL to 15,000/μL. Indirect bilirubin will also be elevated.

All of these laboratory abnormalities are indicative of the severity of a sickle cell anemia but do not actually confirm the diagnosis. A screening test for sickle cell anemia, which involves the deoxygenation of a blood sample, may be performed. If positive, it will produce a precipitate in certain media. However, the confirmatory test is hemoglobin electrophoresis, which will usually identify 85% to 98% of the hemoglobin to be hemoglobin S.

TREATMENT AND PROGNOSIS ▶

There is no specific treatment for the actual sickle cell anemia disease. However, supportive care in the form of folate supplementation and transfusions for hemolytic crises are used. Pneumococcal vacci-

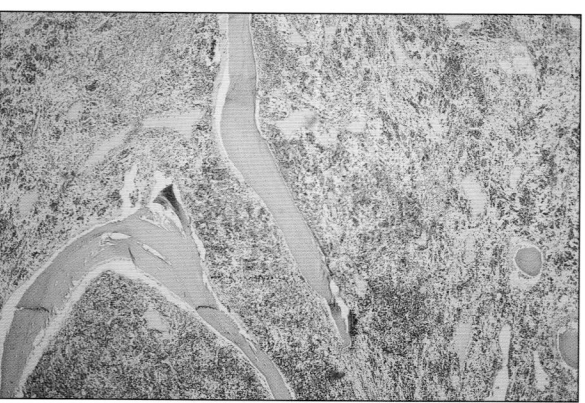

Fig 16-29 A bone biopsy of a severe anemia that affects bone will show a dramatic hyperplasia of the erythroid series. Note the elongated and thinned trabecular bone elements, which are seen on radiographs and CT scans and, if at the outer cortex of the skull, will produce the "hair on end" effect.

nation is recommended, as is avoidance of hypoxia, dehydration, and acidosis. If frequent infarction-related painful crises occur, hydroxyurea, 500 to 750 mg daily, will reduce the painful episodes. As a cytotoxic agent, hydroxyurea stimulates the synthesis of the more primitive hemoglobin F, which is one type of a normal hemoglobin.

Sickle cell anemia is a chronic disease that leads to eventual organ failure and death. With intensive supportive care, life expectancies can be extended into the 40s where they were once only into the teens.

Sickle Cell Trait

Of direct concern to the oral and maxillofacial specialist is the normal-appearing and often robust African American who may have sickle cell trait. These individuals have usually been tested or can be easily tested today. These individuals are heterozygous for hemoglobin S and will have approximately 40% of their hemoglobin as hemoglobin S. They are designated as the genotype AS. Under vigorous exertion, at high altitudes, or under hypoxic conditions, as may occur during IV sedation or general anesthesia procedures, acute painful episodes termed a *sickle crisis* may occur. Untreated, this may lead to a cardiovascular collapse or renal tubular acidosis that can lead to death or disability. Treatment of this emergency requires 100% oxygen best administered with positive pressure ventilation, intravenous fluids, and reversal of acidosis with sodium bicarbonate.

Benign Neoplasms of Bone

▶ "Ignoring or delaying a diagnosis does not change it."
—Robert E. Marx

Osteoma

CLINICAL PRESENTATION AND PATHOGENESIS ▶ Osteomas are referred to as benign neoplasms, but they are actually hamartomas that occur almost exclusively in membranous bone. Single osteomas are rare in the jaws and uncommon in the facial bones. In the oral and maxillofacial region, the skull is where most single osteomas occur, the frontal sinus being the site of predilection.

An osteoma will present as a slow-growing, painless, discrete bony mass that is palpable unless it develops within the medullary space. It will often be observed only in incidental radiographic findings as a well-defined round or oblong radiopacity. Men seem to be affected more frequently than women, and children are almost never affected unless they have Gardner syndrome, which is an autosomal-dominant trait that features osteomas, fibromatosis of the skin and fascia, and polyposis of the large intestines with a high degree of malignant transformation. In fact, the finding of a true osteoma (not an exostosis or a palatal torus) of the jaws in a child should prompt an evaluation for Gardner syndrome (Fig 17-1). On rare occasions an osteoma will be found in the tongue musculature; this represents a benign choristoma arising from mesenchymal stem cells in the tongue.

DIFFERENTIAL DIAGNOSIS ▶ Osteomas should be distinguished from *tori* and *exostosis*, which are developmental overgrowths rather than neoplasms or discrete hamartomas. Both are clinically recognizable by their broad base, which emerges from the superficial cortex of the mandible or palate. Most are lobulated or multiple. Osteomas tend to have a narrow base and appear as single lesions. *Osteoblastomas* and *radiopaque ossifying fibromas* also may mimic an osteoma. However, osteoblastomas are associated with deep, dull pain and will exhibit more rapid growth, and an ossifying fibroma will be less radiopaque than an osteoma when it is small, or, when it becomes sufficiently radiopaque, too large to be an osteoma. A *complex odontoma* could also appear radiographically similar to an osteoma.

HISTOPATHOLOGY ▶ An osteoma may consist of dense lamellar bone with little marrow, or it may show trabeculae of lamellar bone with a more prominent fibrofatty marrow and peripheral cortex. Osteoblastic activity is variably present (Fig 17-2).

DIAGNOSIS AND TREATMENT ▶ Osteomas are diagnosed and treated by local excision. Margins of more than 1 mm are unnecessary. However, the finding of a true osteoma in the jaws should prompt a search for osteomas elsewhere (ie, skull, sinuses, facial bones) and an examination for dermoid cysts, sebaceous cysts, desmoid tumors, and aggressive fibromatoses, since these may also signal Gardner syndrome (Fig 17-3). If gastrointestinal symptoms are part of the patient's history, if a second osteoma is found, or if stools are heme-positive, a colonoscopy also should be performed.

FOLLOW-UP ▶ Because osteomas do not recur, the goal of follow-up is to look for new osteomas or other signs indicative of Gardner syndrome.

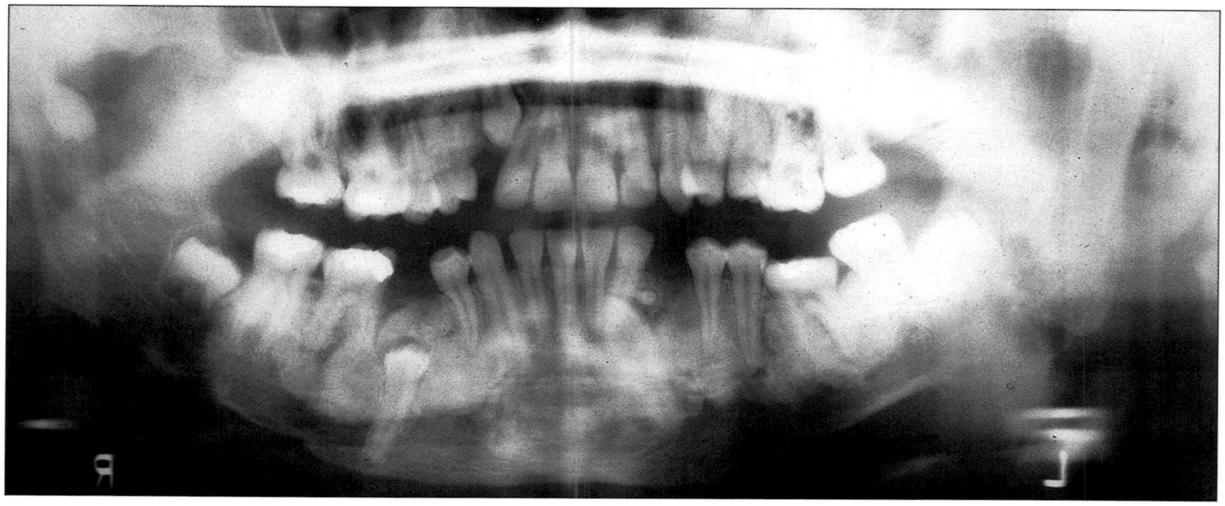

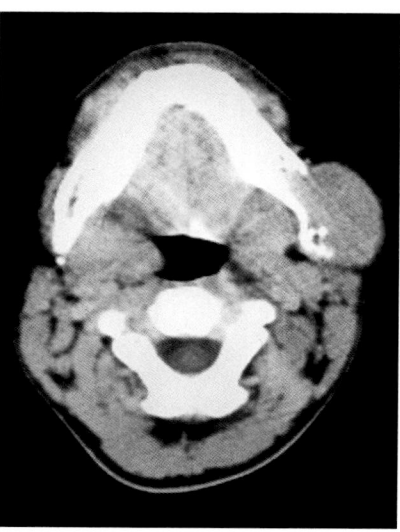

Fig 17-1 Multiple osteomas of the mandible and maxilla in Gardner syndrome. The osteoma pedicled off the right condyle should be viewed as particularly suspicious for Gardner syndrome.

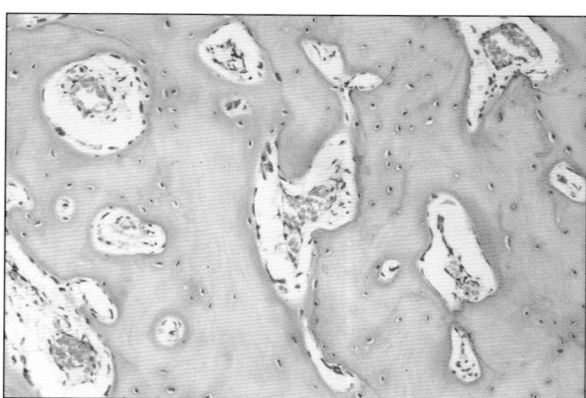

Fig 17-2 Osteoma from a patient with Gardner syndrome showing normal lamellar bone with some osteoblastic activity.

Fig 17-3 Aggressive fibromatosis arising from the periosteum of the ramus and infiltrating both the mandible and the masseter as part of Gardner syndrome.

Osteochondroma

CLINICAL PRESENTATION AND PATHOGENESIS ►

Osteochondromas are benign hamartomatous processes that result in cartilage-capped bony protrusions from the cortical surface of a bone. They arise only from endochondral bones and are, therefore, most commonly found in long bones. In the oral and maxillofacial area, they are found only in the mandibular condyle or the coronoid process. Patients are usually young (average age, 22 years), and males are affected twice as often as females.

An osteochondroma of the condyle or coronoid may be associated with dull pain, but in most cases limited jaw opening will alert the patient to its presence. Some will be palpable as a nontender, hard mass, but most are too deeply located to be appreciated clinically. If the tumor is located in the condyle, the

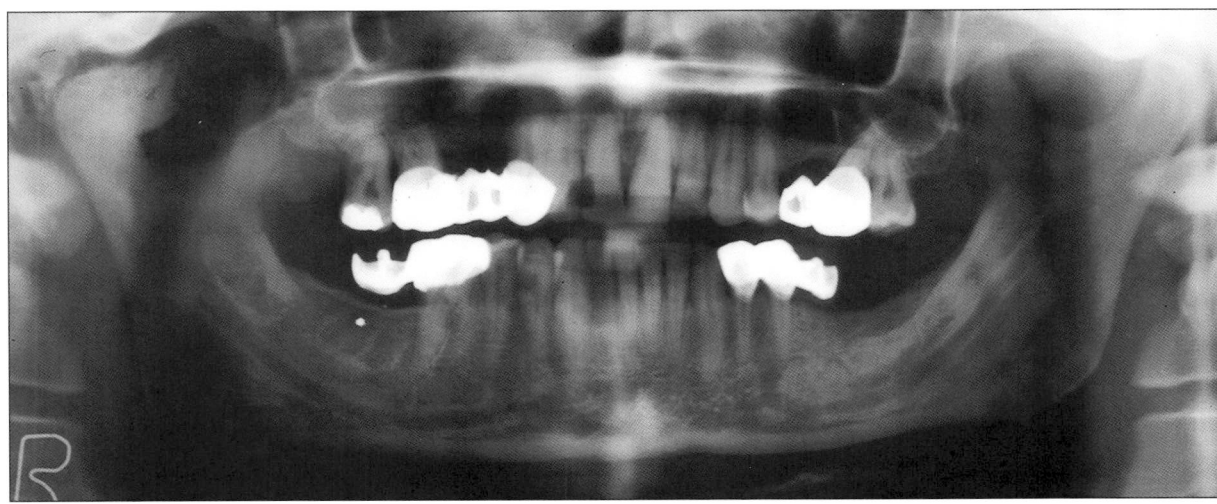

Fig 17-4a A round, radiopaque enlargement of the condyle with an anterior radiopaque projection along the lateral pterygoid tendon. This radiographic picture is pathognomonic for an osteochondroma.

tumor's slow growth may create an asymmetry, causing deviation of the dental occlusion and chin midpoint to the side opposite the tumor.

These tumors arise from epiphiseal cartilage remnants that become activated and have even been experimentally reproduced through implantation of such cells into bone cortices. Their focus of occurrence in the condyle and coronoid confirms the presence of cartilage in the development of these two portions of the mandible. This tumor's absence elsewhere in the skull, facial bones, and other portions of the mandible is consistent with the intramembranous development of these bones.

RADIOGRAPHIC FINDINGS ▶ Osteochondromas in the condyle or coronoid process have a pathognomonic radiographic appearance. In the condyle they are seen consistently as a radiopaque condylar enlargement with a tapered anteriomedial extension into the lateral pterygoid tendon (Fig 17-4a). On a panoramic radiograph, the mass will resemble a shredded flag. In the coronoid process it will project into the temporalis tendon. Most tumors arising in the coronoid process also are located on the medial edge, where the temporalis tendon attaches more densely. In some cases, small, round satellite radiopacities also are seen in the joint spaces.

DIFFERENTIAL DIAGNOSIS ▶ Fortunately, the radiographic picture of an osteochondroma allows for a provisional radiographic diagnosis. Other benign entities that may form a radiopaque mass in the condyle are an *osteoblastoma*, an *ossifying fibroma*, a *chondroma*, and *synovial chondromatosis*. Malignant entities such as *chondrosarcomas* and *osteosarcomas* may also form a similar radiographic picture. However, malignant tumors will extend beyond the condyle itself, will generally be larger, and may be associated with paresthesias or paresis. They also should project outward in all directions rather than following the course of a tendon. Synovial chondromatosis may form joint space radiopacities and induce a slight condylar enlargement that is more radiopaque than normal because of reactive bone. However, the condition is very painful, the condyle is usually not significantly enlarged, and there is no radiopaque tendon extension. Similarly, other benign tumors that may produce a roundish radiopacity in the condyle should also lack the tendon extension associated with osteochondroma.

As part of the work-up, tomograms or a computed tomography (CT) scan may be necessary to define the features of the mass and rule out larger tumors with extensions into other anatomic areas.

HISTOPATHOLOGY ▶ Osteochondromas are bony masses with a cap of hyaline and fibrous cartilage surrounded by the fibrous tissue of the perichondrium. At the deep aspect of the cartilage where it interfaces with bone, endochondral ossification is seen (Fig 17-4b).

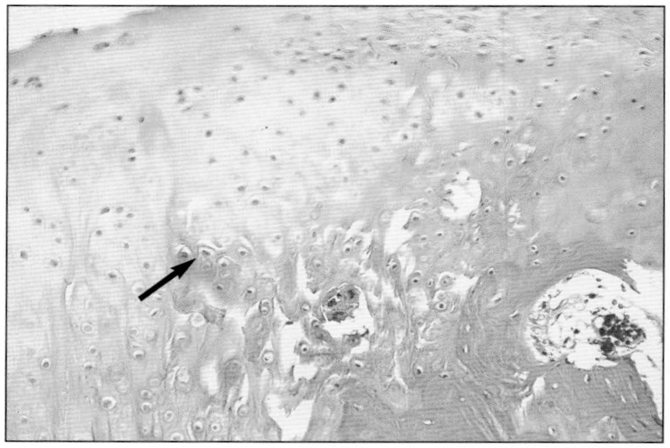

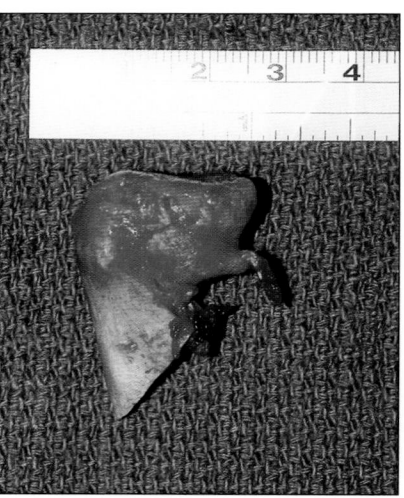

Fig 17-4b Aberrant endochondral ossification (*arrow*), hyaline cartilage, and fibrocartilage formation comprise an osteochondroma.

Fig 17-4c Gross specimen of an osteochondroma showing the mass encompassing the lateral pterygoid tendon. A resection of an osteochondroma at the condylar neck is considered curative.

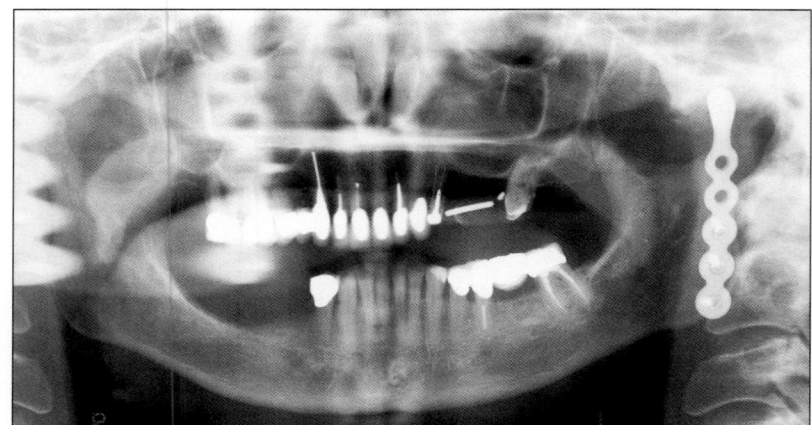

Fig 17-4d Excised osteochondroma of the condyle immediately reconstructed using a titanium plate with condylar replacement.

TREATMENT ▶ Osteochondromas require local excision (Fig 17-4c). As hamartomas, these tumors will proliferate to a certain size and then cease their growth without prominent infiltrative growth or attainment of a large size; however, their location in the joint area and/or their interference with tendons causes significant dysfunction and often causes jaw deviation. In the condyle, excision takes the form of a condylectomy at the condylar neck and a transsection of the lateral pterygoid tendon. It is often approached with a combined preauricular incision and posterior submandibular incision to enable full access to both the condylar neck and lateral pterygoid tendon. The defect lends itself well to an immediate costochondral graft reconstruction or alloplastic condylar replacement. In an autogenous chostocondral graft reconstruction, the addition of bone graft material to the condylar neck area to prevent a structural weak point in this area and suturing of the remnant of the lateral pterygoid tendon to the graft to restore some of the jaw's excursive movements are recommended. If an alloplastic reconstruction is used, a titanium plate with a condylar replacement is recommended. In such cases, at least three screws to the ramus are recommended, as is placement of the titanium condyle in the temporal fossa so as to articulate with the native disc (Fig 17-4d).

In the coronoid process, surgery takes the form of a straightforward coronoidectomy inclusive of a portion of the temporalis tendon. Reconstruction of the coronoid process is unnecessary.

PROGNOSIS AND FOLLOW-UP ▶ Excision of an osteochondroma is usually curative. Follow-up by clinical and panoramic radiographic means may be performed every 6 months for the first 2 years, then annually thereafter.

Chondroma

CLINICAL PRESENTATION AND PATHOGENESIS ▶ Chondromas of the oral and maxillofacial region are extremely rare. They are benign tumors composed of mature cartilage that may arise from cartilage rests within bone (often called *enchondromas* in reference to long bones) or from mesenchymal cells in the periosteum that undergo neoplastic cartilage cell differentiation (often called *juxtacortical chondromas* in reference to long bones). Indeed, most occur in other bones than the membranous bones of the jaws, face, and skull. The most common site is the bones

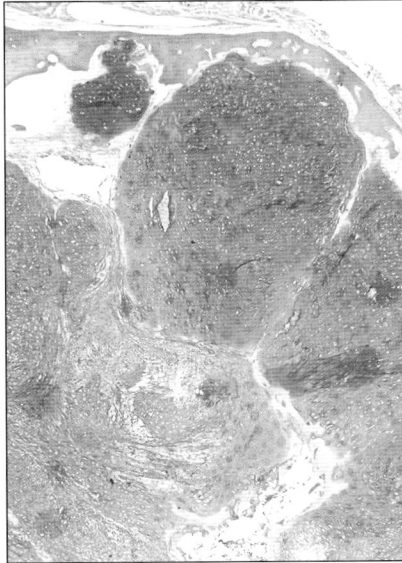

Fig 17-5 A phalangeal chondroma showing the typical lobular arrangement.

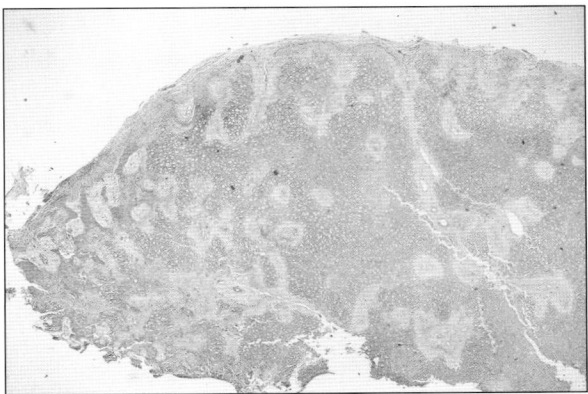

Fig 17-6 Chondroid metaplasia forming a mass on the mandibular alveolar ridge of a patient with an ill-fitting denture. Some peripheral osseous trabeculae are present at the top left.

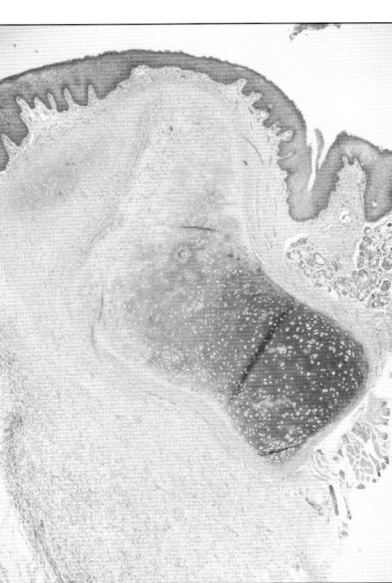

Fig 17-7 A well-defined mass of cartilage within the tongue represents a chondroid choristoma.

of the hands. Most patients are adults older than 20 years. When diagnosed in the maxillofacial area, chondromas are usually located in the anterior maxilla or nasal septum area, presumably derived from cartilage rests related to nasal cartilage development; in the mandibular condyle, presumably related to articular fibrocartilage elements; or in the body area of the mandible, possibly related to rests arising from Meckel cartilage.

Chondromas are distributed equally between men and women. They present as a well-demarcated radiolucent expansion of the bone and are usually painless. Most are unilocular but can be multilocular through lobular growth. They may also display within them foci of radiopacities caused by calcified cartilage.

DIFFERENTIAL DIAGNOSIS ▶

Because it is so rare, a chondroma will not realistically appear on a differential list. In the anterior maxilla or mandibular body region, *odontogenic cysts* and *tumors* would be more likely. In the condylar region, a *synovial chondromatosis*, an *osteochondroma*, or a *chondrosarcoma* would be more likely.

DIAGNOSTIC WORK-UP ▶

In most locations, the lesion is approached with an incisional biopsy or an exploration with an enucleation biopsy. To plan and guide the exploration, as well as to determine the extent of the lesion, a CT scan is useful.

HISTOPATHOLOGY ▶

Chondromas have a lobular arrangement of hyaline cartilage, which contains small, regular chondrocytes (Fig 17-5). Chondromas in the jaws are unusual, and the distinction between a low-grade chondrosarcoma and a chondroma can be very subtle. In fact, the diagnosis of a chondroma of the jaw is usually viewed with suspicion, as most chondroid neoplasms in this location behave aggressively because they actually represent a malignancy. Other benign chondroid proliferations that may be seen in the oral cavity include chondroid metaplasia (Fig 17-6), which can occur on the alveolar ridge secondary to chronic irritation from an ill-fitting denture, and a chondroid choristoma of the tongue (Fig 17-7). Neither of these has an aggressive potential.

TREATMENT AND PROGNOSIS ▶

The rule when confronted with a histopathologic diagnosis of a benign chondroma is to question it. The extreme rarity of this lesion above the clavicles and the benign histologic appearance of low-grade chondrosarcoma warrants second opinions and consultations. In fact, some authors, including those of this book, believe that lesions diagnosed as chondromas should be excised as low-grade chondrosarcomas with 1-cm peripheral margins. This approach is not overly aggressive considering the recurrence potential of a chondrosarcoma in this area and the rarity of chondromas. In addition, cartilage tumors, both benign and malignant, have a marked propensity to seed and grow independently in soft tissue. It is, therefore, also prudent to excise any previous soft tissue biopsy site during the excision.

FOLLOW-UP ▶

Both benign chondromas and low-grade chondrosarcomas are slow growing and may not recur clinically for several years. Follow-up clinical and radiographic examinations are recommended every 6 months for an indefinite period of time. Suspicious areas must be explored and biopsied.

Gardner Syndrome

CLINICAL PRESENTATION AND PATHOGENESIS ▶

Gardner syndrome is an autosomal-dominant trait that arises from a mutant gene on the long arm of chromosome 5. In its full expression, this gene will produce the full tetrad of findings associated with classic Gardner syndrome, while incomplete expression will produce familial colorectal polyposis (FCP). Therefore, this gene is often referred to as the GS-FCP (Gardner syndrome–familial colorectal polyposis) gene, which can produce a spectrum of findings. The tetrad of possible findings includes osteomas, particularly of facial bones and skull; intestinal polyposis with a marked malignant transformation potential; sebaceous cysts of skin; and fibromas and fibromatoses of soft tissues.

Osteomas in Gardner Syndrome

Osteomas of the facial bones and/or skull, while uncommon in general, are common in those with Gardner syndrome. They frequently will be large, multilobulated masses at the angle of the mandible. Many will be confluent with adjacent osteomas. Teardrop-shaped osteomas will seem to hang from the inferior border of the mandible or from the condyle, and medullary osteomas will resemble enostoses. About 50% of cases will exhibit three or more osteomas of the jaws in addition to those elsewhere; the frontal bone is a common location. Osteomas in endochondral bones are rare even in this syndrome. When they do occur in the tibia or femur, they appear more like a cortical thickening than a true osteoma. Of notable importance is that the appearance of osteomas will precede the other manifestations of this syndrome, including intestinal polyposis. Of lesser importance but still noteworthy is that odontomas, supernumerary teeth, and impacted teeth also are found with this syndrome at an incidence rate of 17% (see Fig 17-1).

Intestinal Polyposis in Gardner Syndrome

Polyps develop somewhat later than osteomas. Most do not develop until the patient reaches the early 20s. Their malignant transformation is assured and time dependent. At puberty, there is a 5% malignant transformation rate, which increases to 50% by age 30, and to 100% with patients older than 50 years. In addition, Gardner syndrome has an association with carcinomas of the small intestines at the ampulla of Vater as well as various other carcinomas, such as medulloblastoma, thyroid carcinomas, and hepatoblastomas.

Epidermal/Sebaceous Cysts in Gardner Syndrome

Sebaceous cysts develop in about 60% of cases. The average number of cysts is 4, but some individuals develop 20 or more. The cysts are most frequently seen on the face, scalp, arms, and legs. They also appear before puberty and the development of intestinal polyposis.

Soft Tissue Fibromas and Fibromatosis in Gardner Syndrome

These soft tissue tumors, often called *abdominal* or *extra-abdominal desmoids*, are infiltrating fibrous masses seen in 15% to 30% of Gardner syndrome cases. Such fibrous tumors are seen in only about 5% of FCP cases because of lesser penetration in the GS-FCP gene. Some of these tumors arise de novo, some following surgery (particularly abdominal surgery), and some after removal of existing desmoid tumors. Tumors in the maxillofacial area have been known to infiltrate the masticatory muscles and suprahyoid muscles (see Fig 17-3).

DIFFERENTIAL DIAGNOSIS ▶

Fully expressed Gardner syndrome will be evident from clinical and radiographic data. Other entities that may produce multiple radiodense masses or odontomas with impacted and supernumerary teeth as seen on a panoramic radiograph are *cleidocranial dysplasia, florid cemento-osseous dysplasia,* and *periapical cemento-osseous dysplasia.* Other disorders known to produce intestinal polyposis are *juvenile polyposis of the colon, Turcot syndrome, Cowden syndrome,* and *Peutz-Jeghers syndrome,* among several others. (Although most polyps in Peutz-Jeghers syndrome are located in the small intestines, some will occur in the large intestines or colon as well.) However, only Gardner syndrome has most or all of the tetrad of osteomas, fibrous tumors, sebaceous cysts, and intestinal polyposis.

DIAGNOSTIC WORK-UP ▶

To establish a diagnosis, panoramic and skull radiographs are suggested. At least one of the osteomas should undergo biopsy to confirm its identity, and a thorough examination for sebaceous cysts and masses that may represent fibrous tumors should be performed. A lower gastrointestinal barium study is suggested. Any suspicious findings or an established case of Gardner syndrome warrants colonoscopy.

HISTOPATHOLOGY ▶

Osteoma

Osteomas cannot be distinguished histologically from non–syndrome-related osteomas. The enostoses consist of compact islands of mature lamellar bone.

Polyposis and Adenocarcinoma

The polyps of Gardner syndrome are essentially adenomatous polyps occurring predominantly in the colon. However, the small bowel, particularly the duodenum, may also be involved by this process. Gastric polyps (fundic gland polyps) are also seen with frequency, but these are hamartomatous in nature. The adenomas are tubular, villous, or a combination of the two (Fig 17-8). While adenomas, particularly villous adenomas, may undergo malignant change in the general population, in Gardner syndrome patients this is inevitable and occurs early. Without colectomy, adenocarcinoma will develop. These tumors may secrete variable quantities of mucin, but prognosis is more dependent on extension of the tumor through the intestinal wall than on the specific histologic features.

Epidermal/Sebaceous Cyst

As they are in nonsyndrome cases, epidermal cysts are lined by a thin, keratin-producing, stratified squamous epithelium.

Fibroma and Fibromatosis

Patients with Gardner syndrome may have fibrous proliferations, either as discrete fibrous masses in the form of fibromas of the skin or as fibromatoses. The latter consist of a spindle cell proliferation arranged in fascicles. Pleomorphism and atypical mitoses are not present, but infiltration of adjacent tissues is seen. These tumors are locally aggressive but do not have metastatic potential.

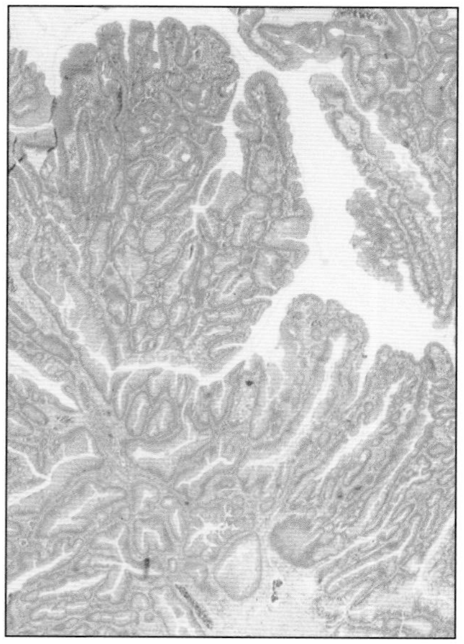

Fig 17-8 Benign tubular-villous adenoma of the colon.

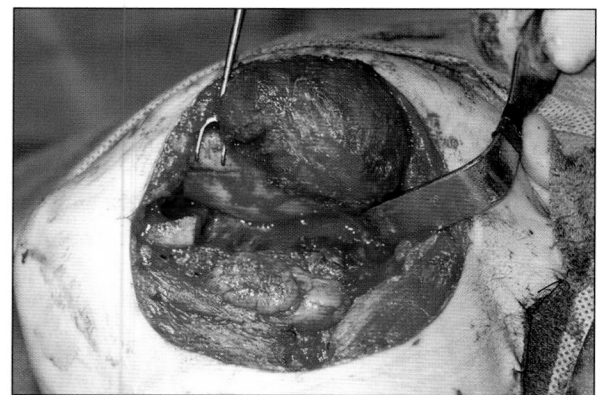

Fig 17-9 Resection of an aggressive fibromatosis requires 1-cm margins in bone and soft tissue with frozen section control.

TREATMENT ▶ The diagnosis of Gardner syndrome usually requires a prophylactic colectomy. In some cases, serial barium studies or colonoscopies are performed to delay the need for colectomy, but such studies run the risk of overlooking a malignant transformation. Although the osteomas do not require removal, they often are removed because of their appearance and interference with motion. Because Gardner syndrome is genetically driven, new osteomas can develop after several months or years. Sebaceous cysts are removed as the patient elects. The fibrous tumors and fibromatoses are usually excised, but their local infiltration requires frozen section assessment of margins and an en-bloc excision with approximately 1-cm margins (Fig 17-9).

PROGNOSIS AND FOLLOW-UP ▶ Generally, for patients with Gardner syndrome who benefit from early diagnosis and colectomy, the prognosis is very good. They go on to lead near-normal and productive lives. However, close follow-up every 4 to 6 months is required for both the patients and their relatives since the inheritance is autosomal and dominant.

Osteoblastoma

CLINICAL PRESENTATION AND PATHOGENESIS ▶ Osteoblastomas are benign neoplasms of bone. They are rare tumors throughout the skeleton, accounting for only 1% of all bone tumors. Of these, only 15% occur in the facial bones and skull, 36% occur in the vertebrae, and 30% occur in long bones of the extremities.

In the jaws and facial bones, the presentation usually consists of a local bony expansion associated with a mild, deep, dull pain. The pain is usually constant but will fluctuate in intensity. The clinical expansion is tender to palpation. Men are affected more often than women by a 2:1 ratio, and most patients are in their teens or early 20s. Very few of these tumors occur in patients older than 30 years, and those that occur in children and preteens seem to be more aggressive and recurrent.

The radiographic appearance is usually one of a well-defined, mixed radiolucent-radiopaque mass within and expanding the involved bone (Fig 17-10a). The rim may be radiolucent or sclerotic, depending on its state of activity and maturity. Rapidly expanding active lesions usually have a radiolucent bor-

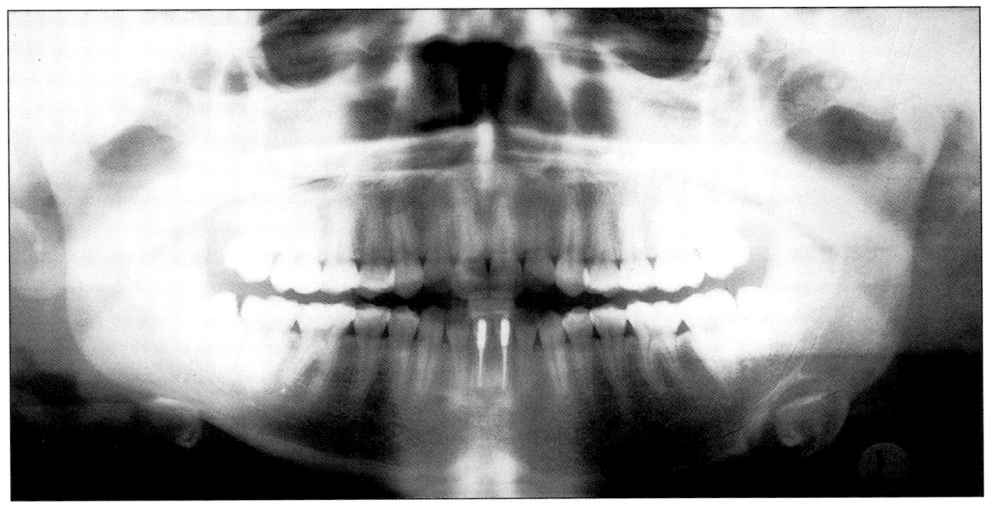

Fig 17-10a A well-demarcated, mixed radiolucent and radiopaque osteoblastoma at the angle of the mandible. It produced the deep dull pain sensation that is characteristic of an osteoblastoma.

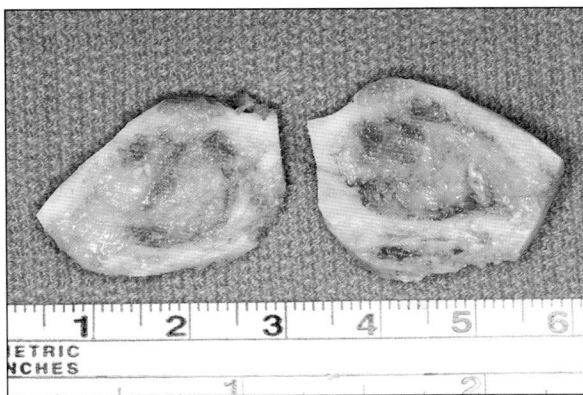

Fig 17-10b Gross specimen of an osteoblastoma showing a sclerotic periphery and a more cellular center.

der, while quiescent or slowly expanding lesions exhibit a more sclerotic border. In rare instances, this tumor is not well demarcated and induces reactivity in the surrounding bone, creating a "sun-ray" appearance suggestive of an osteosarcoma.

The pathogenesis of this tumor is purportedly a benign neoplastic proliferation of osteoblasts. Like any true neoplasm, the genetic alteration that conferred benign neoplastic development but did not confer malignant behavior spans a certain spectrum. This spectrum and variability of genetic alteration has generated the terms *osteoid osteoma* and *juvenile active ossifying fibroma* to describe what now seem to be variants of an osteoblastoma. Some literature identifies nearly identical tumors as osteoid osteomas if they are less than 2 cm in size, have a sclerotic rather than a lucent border (indicative of a capsule), and produce pain that is responsive to the anti-inflammatory action of salicylates (Fig 17-10b). Such lesions, the present authors believe, are variants of an osteoblastoma. Their sclerotic border seems to be only an initial secondary response of the adjacent bone and is caused by its slower rate of expansion. Their response to salicylates seems to be related to their central nidus of activity, which creates reactive bone and inflammation in the initial stages of this tumor. As the tumor enlarges, it resorbs the sclerotic border into a lucent rim. The dull pain continues because of continued active bone formation, but the inflammatory component is lessened, thereby lessening its response to salicylates. In the spectrum of development, this so-called osteoid osteoma type of osteoblastoma represents the most painful and yet the least aggressive and most benign behavior. Very likely, its genetic alterations from normal osteoblasts are not great.

Osteoblastomas that occur in children are more cellular, attain larger sizes, and produce less bone compared with those that occur in adults. This may be a reflection of the greater degree of osteoblastic activity in children. Some of these osteoblastomas are called *juvenile active ossifying fibroma* because of their increased cellularity and reduced osteoid production, resulting in so-called brush-stroke bone. Yet this very rare entity actually seems to represent an osteoblastoma variant on the more cellular and biologically aggressive end of the spectrum. Therefore, in this text we consider what others have referred to as osteoid osteomas and juvenile active ossifying fibromas as variants of a single pathology, that is, osteoblastoma. It is possible that they represent a spectrum of advancing neoplasms whereby osteoid osteoma represents a hamartomatous limited proliferation, osteoblastoma represents a slow-growing benign neoplasm, and juvenile active ossifying fibroma represents a biology akin to an osteosarcoma.

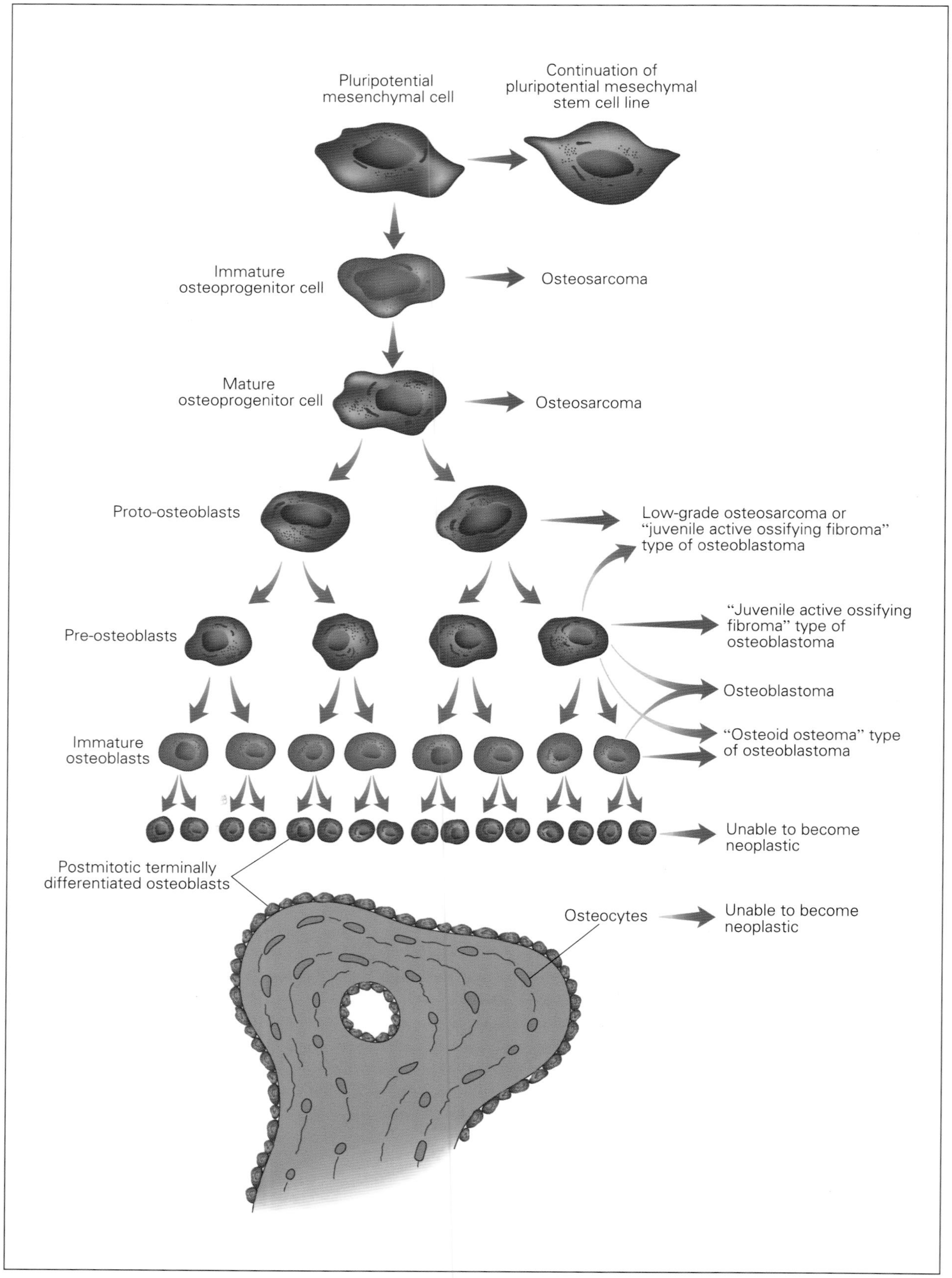

Fig 17-11 Both benign and malignant tumors of bone result from mesenchymal stem cells or their partially differentiated progeny. It is likely that the benign osteoblastoma arises from the premitotic pre-osteoblast or immature osteoblast.

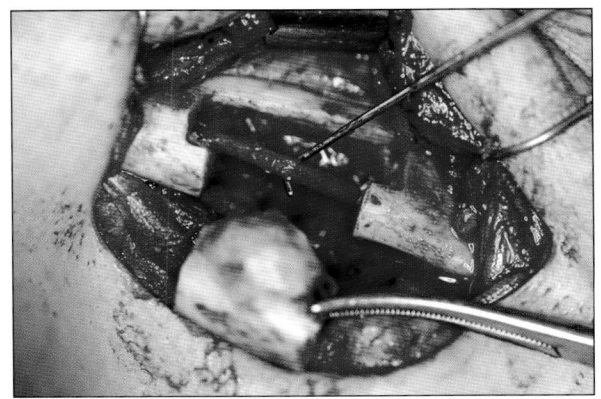

Fig 17-12 This osteoblastoma was resected with a 5-mm margin in bone. The inferior alveolar nerve was preserved.

The typical osteoblastoma represents a benign tumor of slow growth and benign behavior from a genetic alteration during osteoblastic differentiation from mesenchymal stem cells. The osteoid osteoma type represents an even more benign tumor expression, resembling an inflammatory reactive process, and arises from a genetic alteration later in the osteoblastic lineage and therefore in a more differentiated cell. Conversely, the juvenile active ossifying fibroma represents the most aggressive type of osteoblastoma. It probably possesses a more significant genetic alteration during the osteoblastic lineage sequence, or the alteration occurs earlier in the osteoblastic lineage and thus in a less differentiated cell (Fig 17-11). Therefore, what we histologically recognize as a juvenile active ossifying fibroma represents a tumor of high cellularity, rapid growth, and aggressive benign or low-grade malignant behavior. Indeed, many juvenile active ossifying fibromas exhibit multiple recurrences and disfigurement and may even result in death.

DIFFERENTIAL DIAGNOSIS ▶

A focal mixed radiolucent-radiopaque lesion in the jaws, often spherical in shape, is most suggestive of an *ossifying fibroma*. The clinical symptom of pain should, however, guide the clinician to consider osteoblastoma. A *cementoblastoma* may also resemble an osteoblastoma because of its round radiopacity and its dull pain. However, its involvement with the apical half of a single tooth should allow discernment between this entity and an osteoblastoma.

Florid cemento-osseous dysplasia may resemble an osteoblastoma if only one part of it is visible, but the multiquadrant presentation of florid cemento-osseous dysplasia should distinguish the two. Probably the most important and difficult entity in the differential diagnosis is *osteosarcoma*. Like osteoblastomas, osteosarcomas may produce dull pain, cause expansion, and seem deceptively well demarcated, at least on plain radiographs. Since the histogenesis of both lesions is the mesenchymal stem cell or its progeny into the osteoblastic lineage, this is not unexpected. However, if the presentation includes neural dysfunction, either paresthesia or paresis, then the entity must be considered an osteosarcoma unless the neural dysfunction can be attributed to a previous biopsy or trauma. A CT scan and an incisional biopsy are often required to distinguish one from the other.

DIAGNOSIS AND TREATMENT ▶

Most osteoblastomas are well demarcated and lend themselves to a peripheral resection encompassing 5-mm margins (Fig 17-12). This procedure should be curative for most osteoblastomas. If, based on the decalcified specimen, the diagnosis is an osteosarcoma, this treatment amounts to an incisional biopsy for the osteosarcoma with further extirpative surgery and chemotherapy to follow.

For osteoblastomas, the recurrence rate for a local excision in all anatomic sites is about 20%. Much of these recurrences are caused by obscured access resulting from location (the vertebrae) and the vascular nature of these tumors, which may lead to incomplete removal. Therefore, the surgical approach should enable sufficient access and the intraoperative hemorrhage controlled by hypotensive anesthetic techniques and positioning. Larger osteoblastomas and those located in less accessible areas, such as the ramus, posterior maxilla, or pterygoid plates, are best treated by a wide-access peripheral resection (Fig 17-13). If the rare juvenile active ossifying fibroma is diagnosed and confirmed by a second pathologist,

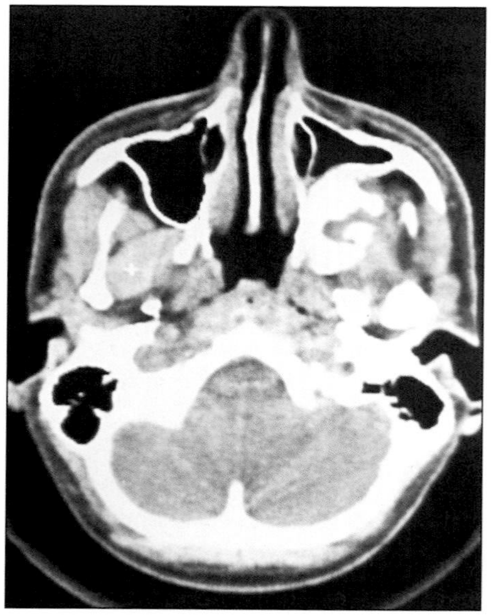

Fig 17-13 An osteoblastoma arising from the lateral pterygoid plate. Its excision required a posterior submucosal maxillary resection including the pterygoid plates.

it should be treated more aggressively than the usual osteoblastoma. This variant requires a surgical resection using 1.5-cm margins with frozen section control. Chemotherapy is not indicated. However, with recurrence, an assessment of all tissue specimens is needed to rule out an osteosarcoma, which a juvenile active ossifying fibroma can strongly resemble. Recurrent juvenile active ossifying fibromas or the identification of an osteosarcoma requires retreatment with initial chemotherapy followed by surgical resection and additional chemotherapy. (See Chapter 18 for specific treatment protocols associated with osteosarcomas.)

HISTOPATHOLOGY ▶

Osteoblastomas are well-circumscribed, nonencapsulated tumors that show consistent bone production (Fig 17-14a). Irregular osseous trabeculae are formed with broad osteoid seams rimmed by plump osteoblasts, which tend to aggregate (Fig 17-14b). The bone shows varying degrees of calcification, and reversal lines are often prominent. Osteoclasts are usually present (Fig 17-14c). The stroma is loosely fibrous with numerous dilated capillaries (see Fig 17-14b).

These neoplasms bear a histologic resemblance to those of Paget disease because of their cellular activity, reversal lines, and vascular stroma. They are similar to cementoblastomas, and there are some who believe that they represent the same entity. However, cementoblastomas have a thin, fibrous capsule and a perpendicular arrangement of the cemental struts at the periphery of the tumor, features that are absent in osteoblastomas. The most significant problem in the histologic differential diagnosis is distinguishing it from osteosarcoma. In most cases, the osteoblastoma's definition, lack of invasiveness, thick osteoid seams, and absence of cellular atypia distinguish it.

The "osteoid osteoma" is histologically identical to the osteoblastoma; in both, there is considerable deposition of osteoid by numerous active osteoblasts in a vascular stroma. The major distinction is that the lesion is small and appears as a well-demarcated nidus within the bone (Fig 17-15).

The juvenile active ossifying fibroma (also known as the juvenile aggressive ossifying fibroma and simply as the juvenile ossifying fibroma) has been a controversial lesion for many years and has no universally accepted histologic criteria. It has generally been described as having closely packed spindle and polyhedral cells that may have a whorled pattern. Within the stroma, a cellular osteoid develops (Fig 17-16a); this may have a trabecular pattern and has sometimes been described as having a "paint-brush stroke" appearance. Aggregates of multinucleated giant cells (osteoclasts) are frequently present (Fig 17-16b). Alternatively, the pattern is one in which the osteoid forms numerous uniform, rounded masses with a psammoma body–like appearance. Myxoid areas may be seen in the stroma as well as cyst-like spaces, some of which are large and blood-filled. Whatever the pattern, these tumors are unencapsulated and infiltrate bone.

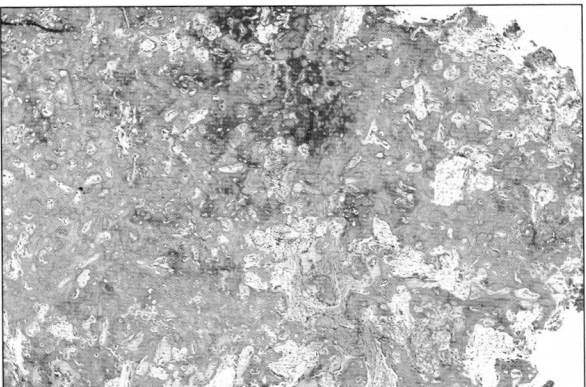

Fig 17-14a Low-power view of an osteoblastoma showing abundant bone production.

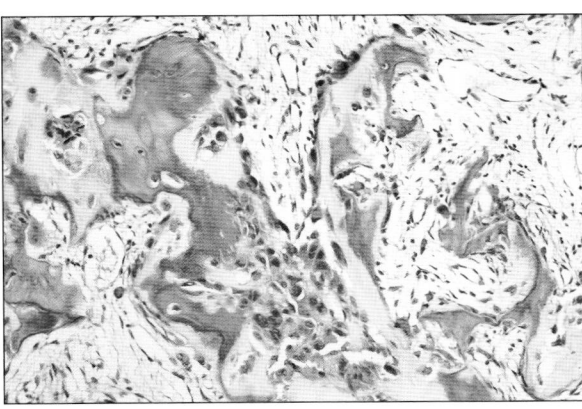

Fig 17-14b The osteoblastoma shown in Fig 17-14a here shows plump, heaped-up osteoblasts lining osteoid seams. The fibrous stroma contains numerous capillaries.

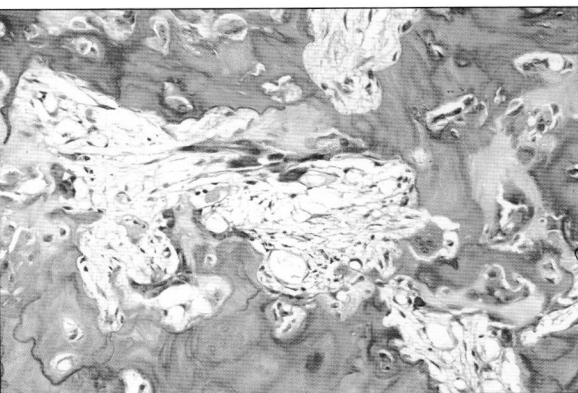

Fig 17-14c The osteoblastoma shown in Figs 17-14a and 17-14b here shows reversal lines, osteoblastic and osteoclastic activity, and a vascular fibrous stroma.

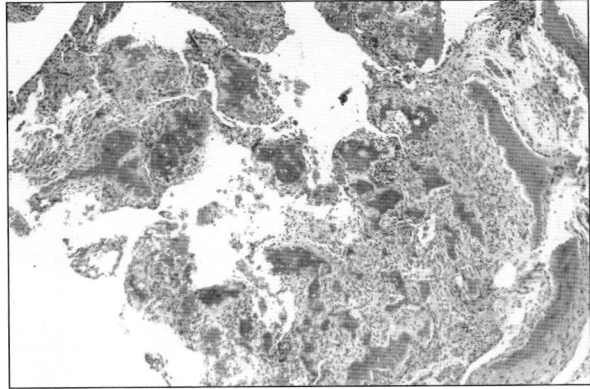

Fig 17-15 An "osteoid osteoma" with the normal bony wall on the right and the nidus of tumor in the center composed of numerous osteoblasts laying down osteoid.

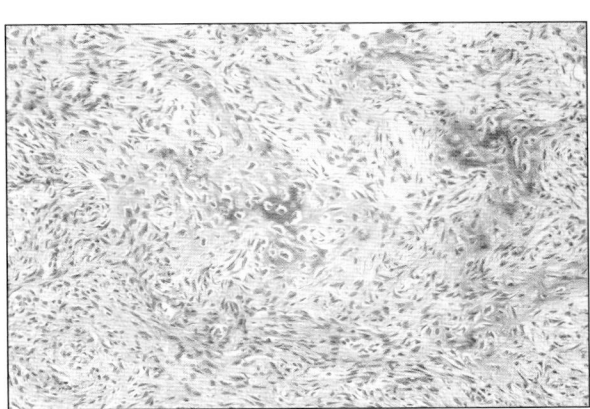

Fig 17-16a Cellular osteoid, some of which has calcified, is seen within a cellular spindle-cell stroma in this juvenile active ossifying fibroma.

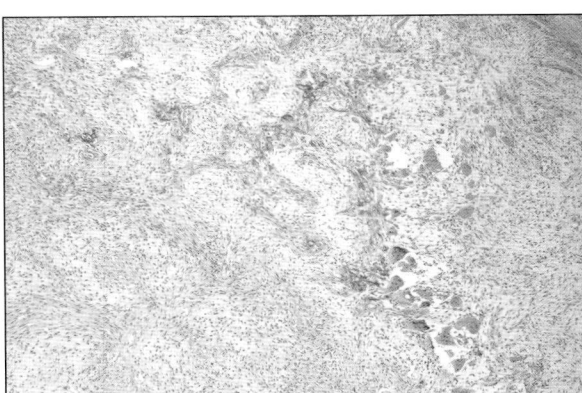

Fig 17-16b Within a cellular spindle-cell stroma, strands of osteoid may be seen. An aggregate of multinucleated giant cells is present.

FOLLOW-UP ▶ Osteoblastomas are benign tumors that may slowly recur over a period of 1 to 10 years. During the first 2 years, follow-up with clinical examinations and radiographs every 6 months is recommended. Annual follow-up is recommended after the first 2 years. The frequency of follow-up visits is not so much to follow the osteoblastoma, but to ensure that the tumor was not an osteosarcoma simulating an osteoblastoma.

Osteoblastomas have been reported to transform into osteosarcomas after radiotherapy. Therefore, radiotherapy is not indicated in the primary treatment of osteoblastomas. In addition, a few osteoblastomas have been reported to spontaneously transform into osteosarcomas. However, these few cases may have been osteosarcomas that initially simulated, and were incorrectly diagnosed as, osteoblastomas.

Central Giant Cell Tumor

CLINICAL PRESENTATION AND PATHOGENESIS ▶ Central giant cell tumors of the jaws are benign but aggressively destructive osteolytic lesions. This tumor, and biologic behavior in the jaws, is identical to that in the long bones, and the terminology related to both of them has become extremely confused (see Chapter 20). Today, these tumors seem to represent benign tumors of osteoclastic origin. They are not unique to the jaws and are not odontogenic.

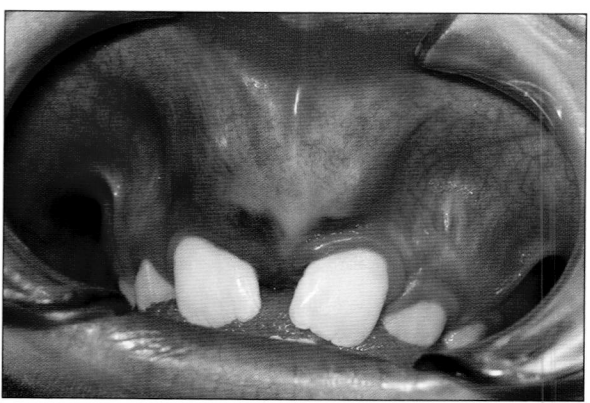

Fig 17-17 The blue color of this central giant cell tumor reveals its vascular nature. The displacement of the maxillary central incisors reveals its expansile nature. It most commonly occurs in children and young adults and will frequently cross the midline.

The giant cells have osteoclast receptors and thus represent osteoclast precursors or are themselves osteoclasts. The tumor is not a true granuloma and is not at all reparative; the use of such outdated terminology should be abandoned because it is misleading. Even the generic term "giant cell lesion" is incorrect and misleading. In addition, there is no difference in histopathologic features or biologic behavior between a central giant cell "lesion" and an aneurysmal bone cyst (which is not a true cyst either). A so-called aneurysmal bone cyst represents a central giant cell tumor that has larger vascular spaces and may attain a larger size. For the purposes of this text, central giant cell tumors will include what has also been described in the literature as an aneurysmal bone cyst. This tumor is histopathologically and behaviorally identical to the benign giant cell tumor of long bones, the most common neoplasm found in long bones; it is not to be confused with what some authors have described as malignant giant cell tumors, which may represent an osteosarcoma with prominent osteoclasts or a true malignant variant of osteoclasts.

In the jaws, a central giant cell tumor presents as a painless clinical expansion that may have a short (2-week to 2-month) ascendancy. The expanded lesion may appear blue because of its cortical and mucosal thinning and internal vascularity (Fig 17-17). Occasionally, the rapid expansion will stretch periosteum, producing pain. The peak range of occurrence is between 5 and 15 years of age, although some cases develop in the 20s and 30s as well. Women are affected twice as frequently as men. The mandible is involved three times as frequently as the maxilla. Although this lesion is one that is known to cross the midline and to occur in the anterior jaw regions, the posterior regions are affected as well.

RADIOGRAPHIC FINDINGS ▶

The central giant cell tumor will classically present as a multilocular radiolucent lesion that severely thins the cortices, including the inferior border (Fig 17-18a). It is also known to scallop the inferior border, displace teeth, and resorb interradicular bone. It may also resorb tooth roots to some degree.

DIFFERENTIAL DIAGNOSIS ▶

A multilocular, expansile, radiolucent lesion in a child or teenager is suggestive of several lesions, most notably an *odontogenic keratocyst*, an *odontogenic myxoma*, an *ameloblastic fibroma,* or *Langerhans cell histiocytosis.* If the patient is older than 14 or 15 years, an *ameloblastoma* becomes a statistically more likely consideration as well. In addition, because of the bleeding potential and generally young age of presentation, as well as a multilocular "soap bubble" radiolucency, a *central arteriovenous hemangioma* must be considered.

DIAGNOSTIC WORK-UP ▶

A clinical presentation such as that of a central giant cell tumor is approached first with the goal of ruling out a high-pressure vascular lesion. Central giant cell tumors are not high-pressure vascular lesions and will either fail to return blood or will return only a small amount. In most cases, an incisional biopsy is then performed, although it is not unreasonable to thoroughly curet the entire lesion if it is small, the access is good, and it seems consistent with the red-brown friable tissue of a central giant cell tumor (Fig 17-18b). If the lesion is determined to be any type of a giant cell tumor, it is prudent to obtain a serum calcium determination to rule out both primary and secondary hyperparathyroidism. A

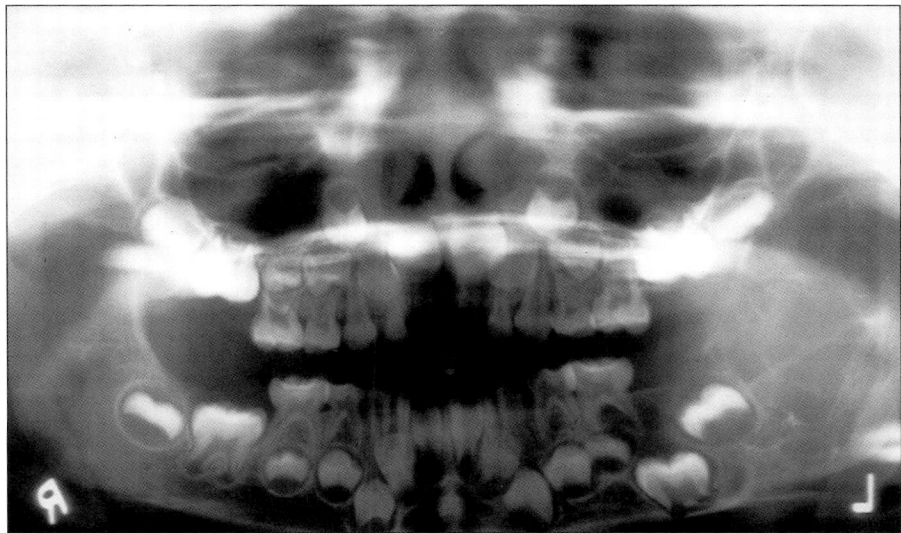

Fig 17-18a This central giant cell tumor presented in typical fashion as an expansile multilocular radiolucency displacing teeth.

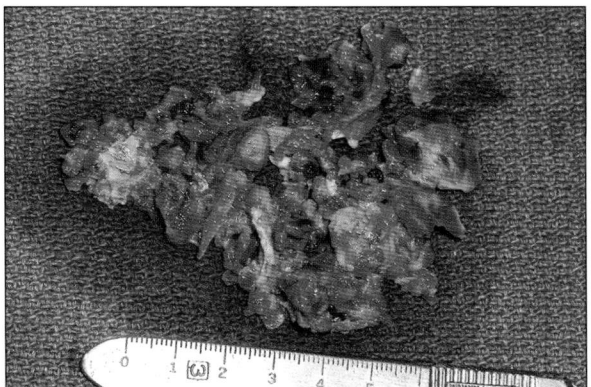

Fig 17-18b Gross specimen showing the red friable nature of a central giant cell tumor. Its texture clinically resembles granulation tissue, which gave rise to its former, inaccurate description as a central giant cell granuloma.

parathyroid hormone assay is not required because primary hyperparathyroidism of sufficient severity to produce a so-called brown tumor will evidence hypercalcemia, and secondary hyperparathyroidism of sufficient severity to produce a brown tumor will evidence hypocalcemia. An alkaline phosphatase determination also is not required because this age group frequently has growth-related elevations of this enzyme, and even in adults this study adds no further diagnostic information.

HISTOPATHOLOGY ▶

Grossly, these tumors are red to brown in color. The mass consists of a spindle cell stroma that may be quite cellular. There is a variable amount of collagen, and mitoses are sometimes seen. Extravasated erythrocytes are present, and hemosiderin may be noted. The hemosiderin may be contained within macrophages. Multinucleated giant cells are conspicuous and tend to be irregularly distributed throughout the mass, often concentrating in areas of hemorrhage. There may be considerable variation in the size of the giant cells and the number of nuclei present (Fig 17-18c). Osteoid may be deposited, particularly at the periphery of the lesion. Giant cell tumors are unencapsulated but usually delimited and frequently develop locules (Fig 17-18d). They often abut tooth roots and may resorb them (Fig 17-18e).

The giant cells have been shown to excavate bone, respond to calcitonin, and bind osteoclast-specific monoclonal antibody, indicating that they are indeed osteoclasts.

Central giant cell tumors cannot be distinguished histologically from lesions of hyperparathyroidism, and therefore this latter possibility must be ruled out. Cherubism also has the same histologic features. Occasionally, fibrous dysplasia contains a sufficient number of giant cells so that it may also enter the histologic differential.

The so-called aneurysmal bone cyst is a condition that frequently develops secondarily within another lesion of bone. Most frequently, it is associated with central giant cell tumors. Large, blood-filled spaces develop that lack an endothelial lining (Figs 17-19a to 17-19d). Solid areas of the lesion consist of central giant cell tumor with cellular fibrous tissue, extravasated blood, and multinucleated giant cells (Fig 17-19d). However, if these dilated, blood-filled spaces have developed within another lesion, the solid areas will consist of that entity. An example of this is shown in Fig 17-19e, where the primary lesion was an ossifying fibroma.

TREATMENT ▶

The most common treatment is a thorough curettage of the lesion and its bony cavity (Fig 17-20). Multiple recurrent lesions or lesions with significant destructive bone resorption to the point of near

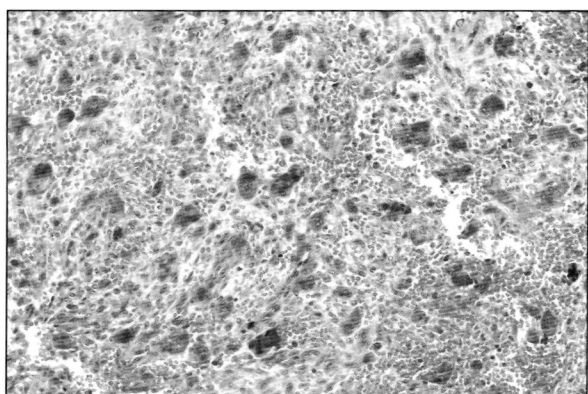

Fig 17-18c A central giant cell tumor showing a cellular stroma containing extravasated blood and diffusely scattered, multinucleated giant cells of varying size.

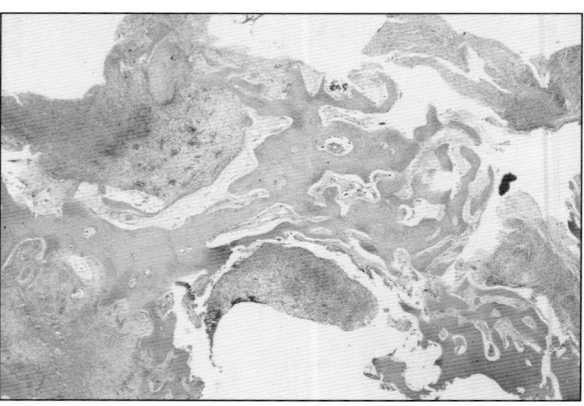

Fig 17-18d Low-power view showing the locules of a central giant cell tumor within the bone.

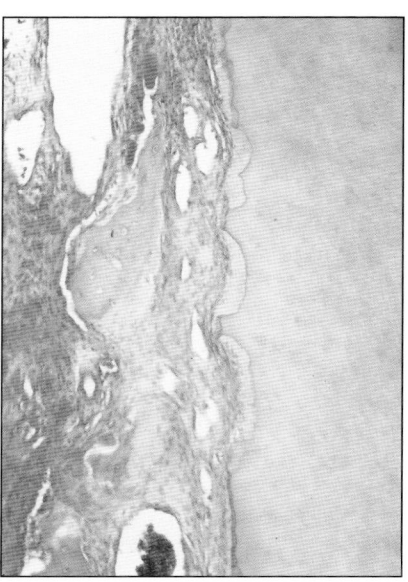

Fig 17-18e Resorption of the tooth root by a central giant cell tumor.

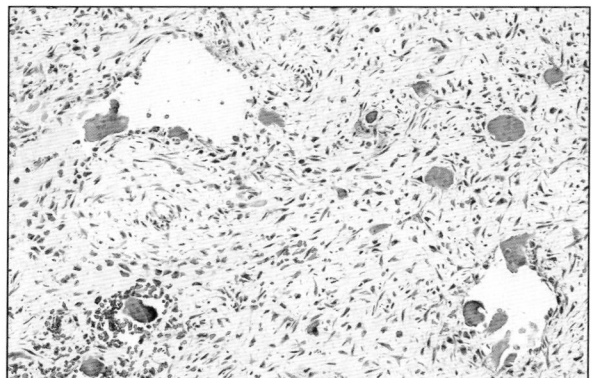

Fig 17-19a A field taken from a central giant cell tumor within which spaces lined by giant cells have developed.

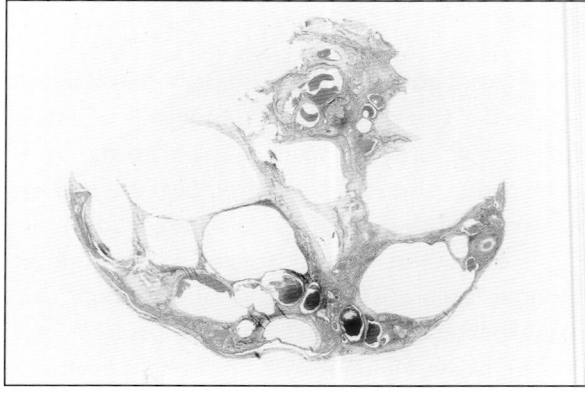

Fig 17-19b Low-power view of a central giant cell tumor with macroscopic vascular spaces. Because of this finding, this tumor was formerly termed an "aneurysmal bone cyst."

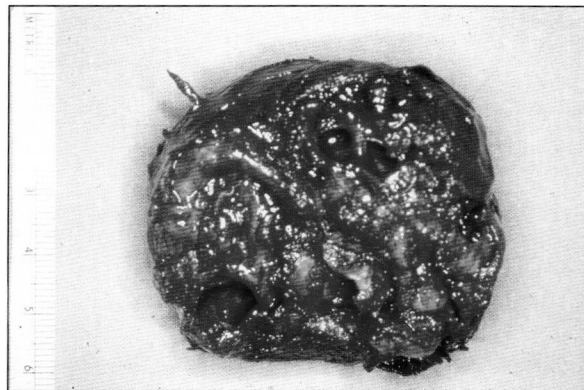

Fig 17-19c The bisected gross specimen of Fig 17-19b showing large spaces within the tumor.

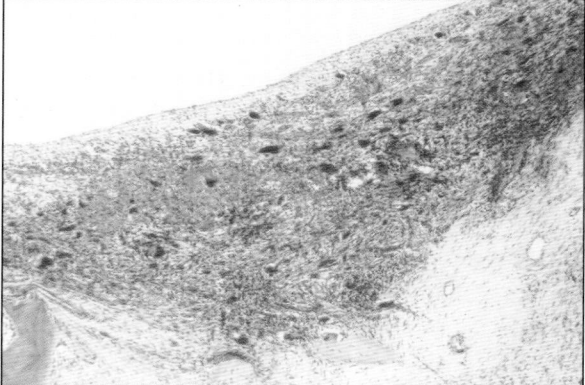

Fig 17-19d This central giant cell tumor has a large space on the upper left that is lined not by endothelium but by fibrous tissue. All spaces in these tumors are lined by fibrous tissue.

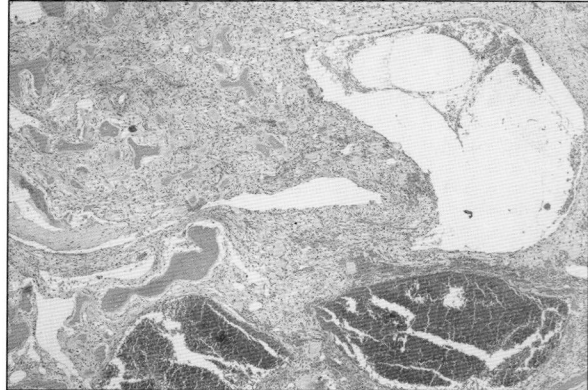

Fig 17-19e Dilated, blood-filled spaces, lined by fibrous tissue, are seen together with solid areas of an ossifying fibroma.

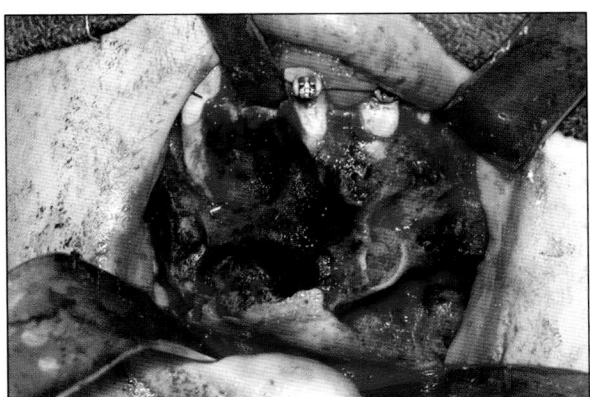

Fig 17-20 Curettage of a central giant cell tumor requires wide access and preparedness to control an oozing type of bleeding.

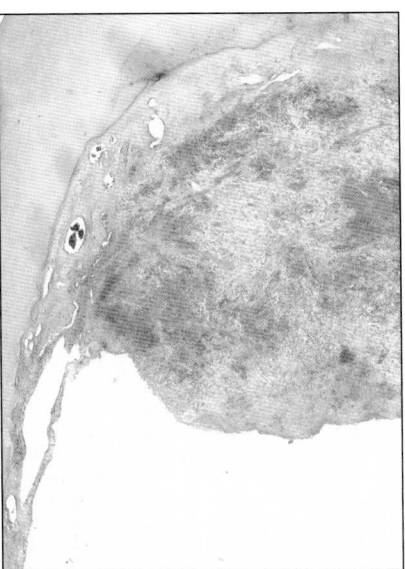

Fig 17-21 Giant cell tumor in the furcation of a molar tooth, confluent with the periodontal membrane. This is a weak point in the total removal of a giant cell tumor and a cause of recurrence.

pathologic fracture may require resection. The lesion itself is confined to and requires bone for its existence. It cannot exist outside of bone, even after possible implantation from a curettage procedure.

The central giant cell lesion does have a recurrence potential with curettage that reaches as high as 50% by some reports. Recurrences are seen more frequently with larger lesions and those that involve significant numbers of teeth. These recurrences are related to incomplete removal of a friable, bleeding lesion, which is more difficult to remove from between teeth and furcations, or to a greater possibility of incomplete excision in a larger-sized lesion (Fig 17-21). The weak points in curettage are thus the areas between teeth, the areas around unerupted teeth, and the neurovascular bundle area; additionally, the vascular nature of this lesion, which produces an oozing type of blood loss, obscures the clinician's view. To reduce the impact of these factors, the following approach to the curettage has been developed: intraoperative reduction of local blood pressure by the anesthetic technique; placement of the patient in a head-up position; local vasoconstrictor usage; and, in the case of large lesions, preparation for possible transfusion. The lesion is approached initially by a wide soft tissue reflection to obtain a direct view of the entire lesion. It is first grossly curetted to debulk its mass. This will reduce the bleeding since the residual lesion in the bone bleeds more than do normal vessels because of the absence of a muscularis around the vessels within the tumor, which normally would vasoconstrict. The remainder of the tumor is then meticulously curetted, giving special attention to the weak points associated with recurrence described earlier.

Because of the known recurrence potential and the unencapsulated vascular nature of this lesion, two other treatment concepts have been advanced. One is the use of Carnoy's solution as a cellular fixative to sterilize remaining tumor cells. However, statistics do not support a reduction in recurrences when Carnoy's solution is used. Another is to perform endodontic therapy of erupted teeth within the lesion. This also does not reduce recurrences because it is the presence of the roots, rather than their vitality, that limits curettage in this area. Endodontic therapy in otherwise healthy teeth is not recommended because the long-term function of these teeth is reduced by the extensive crown destruction created by the access preparation and the dehydration of the tooth after pulpal extirpation. Moreover, endodontic

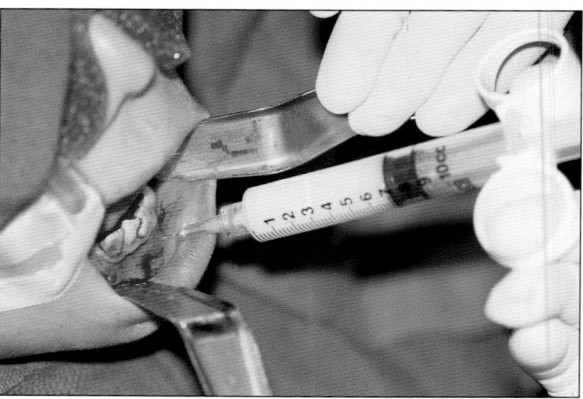

Fig 17-22a A 1% triamcinolone solution is injected into a central giant cell tumor at a volume of 1 mL per cm length of jaw involvement. Intralesional steroid injections may induce involution of some central giant cell tumors.

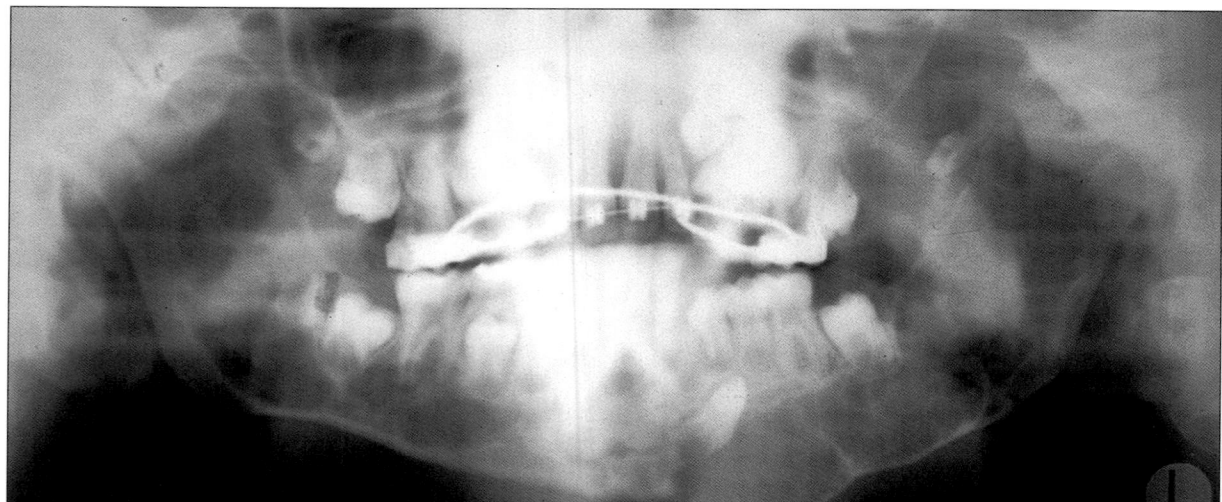

Fig 17-22b A very large central giant cell tumor that failed to respond to two series of the intralesional steroid protocol. The tumor mass was subsequently treated with curettage, which then resolved it.

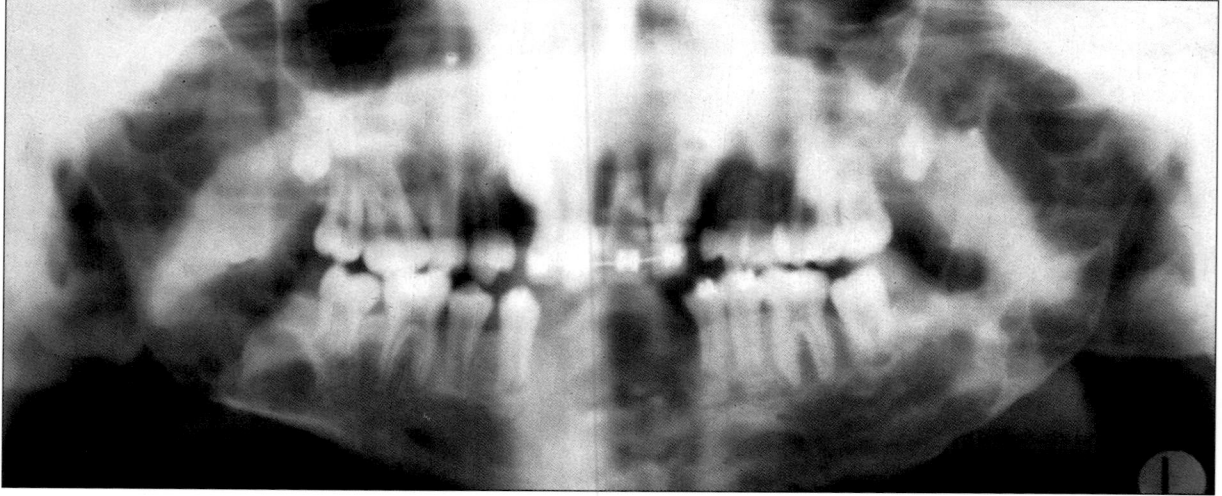

Fig 17-22c The radiolucency shown in Fig 17-22b filled in with regenerated bone and the expansion remodeled after surgical curettage.

therapy has not been shown to reduce tumor recurrence, and curettage on or around root surfaces does not truly devitalize teeth but only deinnervates them (see Fig 13-27). Even so, reinnervation is common.

More recently, intralesional corticosteroid use has shown some value, inducing complete involution in many cases and partial involution in others. The suggested treatment is triamcinolone, 10 mg/mL, of which 1 mL is injected for each 1 cm of jaw involvement throughout the lesion, once a week for 6 weeks (Fig 17-22a). Each injection sequence is performed with local anesthesia (bupivacaine) added to the injection solution. As yet, sufficient numbers and controlled studies are not available to assess the true resolution rate of this approach. In the authors' experience, 65% of central giant cell tumors have completely resolved with this therapy. The remaining 35% either recurred more aggressively or failed to respond at all, requiring either curettage or resection. Today, most cases of central giant cell tumor are initially treated with the series of intralesional corticosteroid injections. The potential value of resolving these tumors without invasive surgery is compelling. Because the treatment sequence is associated with minimal morbidity and does not preclude further therapy should it be unsuccessful, it is a reasonable first choice. If the tumor fails to respond or accelerated growth results, a population of altered osteoclasts that do not have cell membrane receptors for corticosteroids is implied. Such tumors are then treated with either curettage or a resection with 0.5- to 1.0-cm margins if they are sufficiently large (Figs 17-22b and 17-22c).

PROGNOSIS ▶

Lesions approached with wide-access, thorough curettage rarely recur. Recurrent lesions may be recuretted before resection is considered. If a recurrence develops, it is usually within the first 12 to 18 months, much sooner than recurrent odontogenic tumors. Patient age does not affect recurrence; however, the size of the lesion does seem to be related to recurrence, which is often the result of limited access caused by the tumor's infiltration between and around teeth. The biologic behavior of the giant cells varies greatly but is unrelated to patient age and the size of the lesion.

Ossifying Fibroma

CLINICAL PRESENTATION AND PATHOGENESIS ▶

Ossifying fibromas are slow-growing, benign neoplasms most commonly found in the jaws. Because of their less common but identical presence in other craniofacial bones and long bones that have no cementum (eg, the tibia is a commonly involved long bone), the term used in this text is *ossifying fibromas* rather than *cemento-ossifying fibromas*. The fact that this tumor is most common in the jaws is related to the vast amount of mesenchymal cellular induction into bone (lamina dura) and cementum (a bone layer covering tooth roots) required in odontogenesis; the probability of induction error or genetic alteration leading to a neoplasm is, therefore, greater. In the past, preoccupation with the myriad pseudonyms for this lesion (eg, osteofibroma, fibro-osteoma, cementifying fibroma, benign fibro-osseous lesion of periodontal ligament origin) created a hopelessly confusing and unnecessary terminology. Because bone and cementum cannot be distinguished by any known method, the origin of the calcified material of this tumor is a moot point, particularly when one considers that the origin of bone and cementum—that is, the mesenchymal stem cells—is the same.

Early ossifying fibromas are small and may be radiolucent. As they enlarge and mature, they will become mixed radiolucent-radiopaque, then completely radiopaque. These tumors characteristically expand slowly and asymptomatically (Fig 17-23a). Their expansion is symmetric from the epicenter of the tumor, creating a spherical or egg-shaped mass on plain radiographs and CT scans (Fig 17-23b). This tumor is seen most commonly in women in their 20s and 30s, but those younger and older, as well as men, are also affected. In the jaws, the lesions are found mostly in the tooth-bearing areas, which is consistent with the higher rate of bone and cementum induction in these areas. Ossifying fibromas also occur in the rami but at a lower incidence.

Of all the benign tumors of the head and neck area, the ossifying fibroma is one of a few allowed by patients to reach the largest and most disfiguring size (ameloblastomas, odontogenic myxomas, neuro-

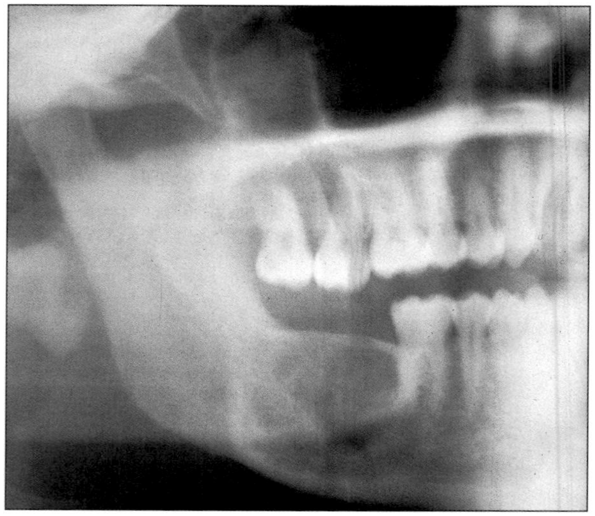

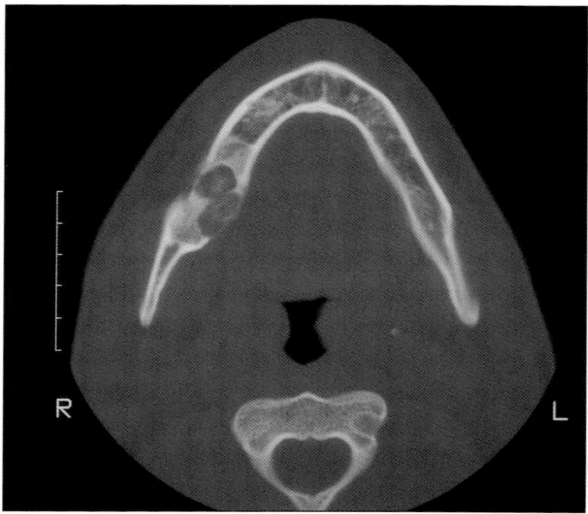

Fig 17-23a Typical radiographic picture of an ossifying fibroma as a spherical, well-demarcated, mixed radiolucent-radiopaque mass.

Fig 17-23b The spherical to ovoid, well-demarcated, mixed radiolucent-radiopaque mass typical of an ossifying fibroma may be seen on CT scans as well as plain radiographs.

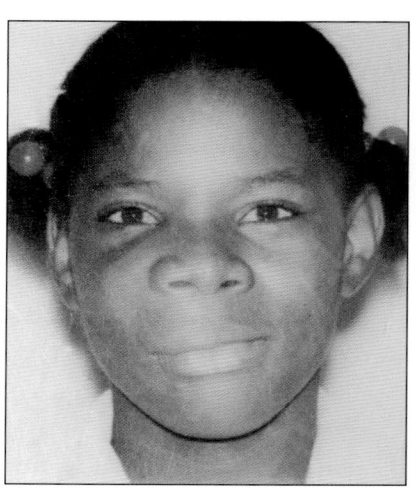

Fig 17-24a An ossifying fibroma that began at age 9 years has slowly enlarged to about 4 cm in diameter at age 13 years.

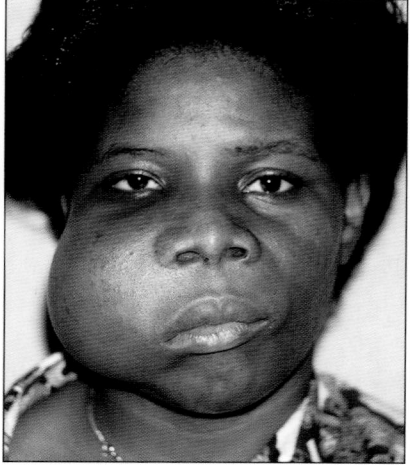

Fig 17-24b The same ossifying fibroma is 12 cm in diameter at age 19 years and has produced obvious facial distortion. Despite its large size, the ossifying fibroma has retained its spherical shape.

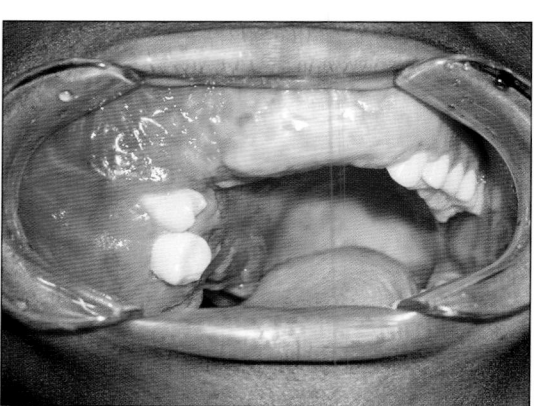

Fig 17-25 The oral examination of the patient shown in Figs 17-24a and 17-24b identified the distortion of the maxillary alveolus and the teeth. Because of the tumor, this patient could not occlude her teeth. Note the expanded but intact oral mucosa, except where her biting of the tumor has produced an ulcer.

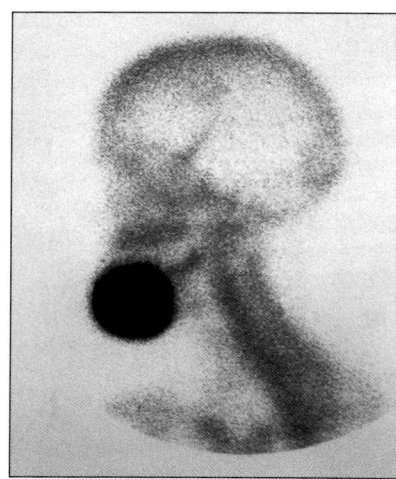

Fig 17-26 Ossifying fibromas will show an intense uptake of ^{99}Tc MDP on a bone scan; however, this type of uptake is also seen in many other bone pathologies, including fibrous dysplasia, hemangioma, osteoblastoma, and even osteosarcoma. The spherical nature of this uptake and its clear-cut margins are what make it most suggestive of an ossifying fibroma.

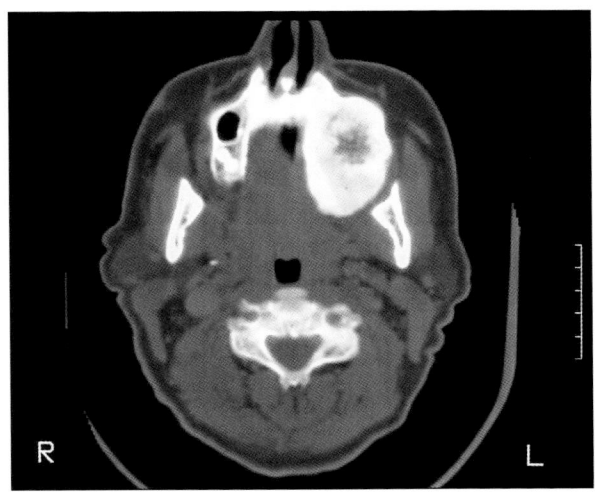

Fig 17-27 A CT scan of an ossifying fibroma showing well-delineated margins, an oval or spherical expansion, and a heterogeneous density, all of which are typical features.

fibromas, and pleomorphic adenomas are the others), probably because of its persistently steady but slow rate of growth and its painless character (Figs 17-24a, 17-24b, 17-25, and 17-26). Many will expand to the point of ulceration from occlusion by opposing teeth, but will not otherwise ulcerate. Because the tumor initially expands in bone, it remains encapsulated and therefore well demarcated radiographically. However, when it reaches a certain large size (in the range of 2 to 3 cm in diameter), it loses its encapsulation and infiltrates beyond its margins for a few millimeters. It will also induce a reactivity with the adjacent bone, making it difficult to determine the tumor edge both radiographically and visually at the time of surgery. Most of these large, mature, and very mineralized ossifying fibromas in the past have been termed *gigantiform cementomas*.

The reader should not consider a peripheral ossifying fibroma as the soft tissue counterpart of this type of ossifying fibroma. Although the term *peripheral ossifying fibroma* implies a neoplasm, it actually represents a reactive hyperplasia of periodontal membrane fibers that also may induce some bone formation (see Chapter 2).

DIFFERENTIAL DIAGNOSIS ▶

The expansile, mixed radiolucent-radiopaque quality of the ossifying fibroma often makes it resemble *fibrous dysplasia*. In addition, other benign tumors of bone, such as the *osteoblastoma*, and some odontogenic cysts and tumors that produce calcified materials, such as the *calcifying epithelial odontogenic tumor* and the *calcifying odontogenic cyst*, may radiographically resemble an ossifying fibroma. If the ossifying fibroma occurs around tooth roots, it may also resemble a *cementoblastoma* or *florid cemento-osseous dysplasia*. The latter two may be distinguished from an ossifying fibroma by their radiographic appearance. A cementoblastoma will emerge from and obscure the apical half of the involved tooth roots. Florid cemento-osseous dysplasia will exhibit not one but several sclerotic densities in the alveolar bone of one or both jaws.

DIAGNOSTIC WORK-UP ▶

Because benign tumors of bone such as ossifying fibromas cannot be accurately distinguished from several fibro-osseous lesions via histopathology, accurate clinical, historical, and radiographic data are important. A CT scan is a valuable diagnostic tool (Fig 17-27). Ossifying fibromas are spherical to egg shaped, expand cortices equally, and are heterogeneous because of an inconsistent distribution of their osseous and fibrous components. Their calcified material will be of the density of bone, not that of dentin or enamel, and there will be no air spaces or fluid spaces within them, as are found in cysts. Therefore, an ossifying fibroma can usually be diagnosed radiographically. In particular, ossifying fibromas must be distinguished from fibrous dysplasia. Because an ossifying fibroma is a benign tumor in bone, whereas fibrous dysplasia is a maturation defect of bone, they will present with distinctly different radiographic and CT scan images. As noted, ossifying fibromas will be spherical, will have expanded and thinned cortical outlines, will displace adjacent structures, and will be well-delineated from surrounding tissues (Figs 17-28 and 17-29). Fibrous dysplasia, on the other hand, will be fusiform, will expand bone but will remodel the

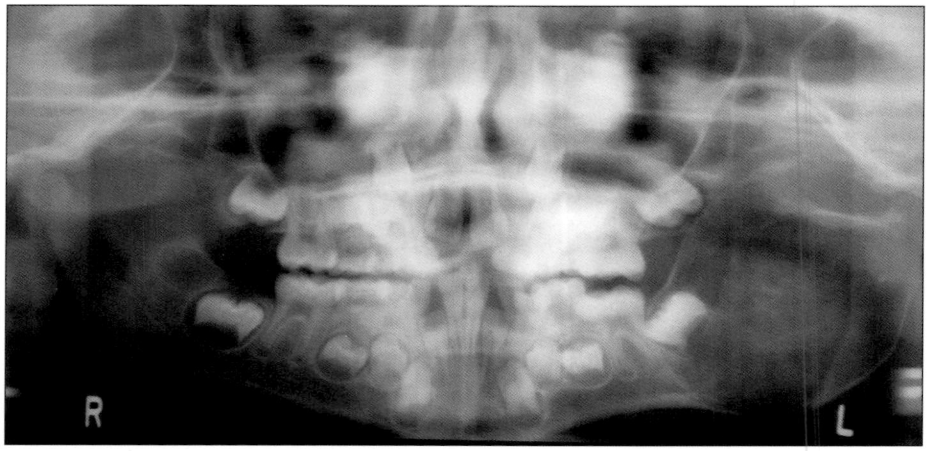

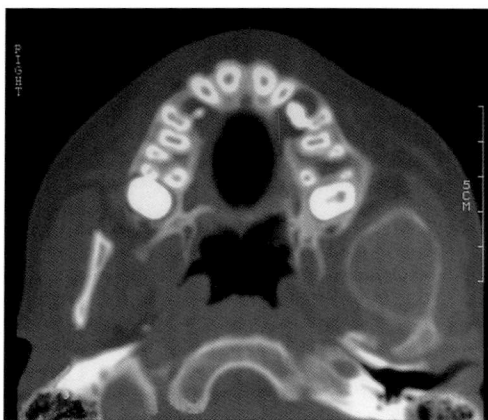

Fig 17-28 Although the age of this patient is consistent with fibrous dysplasia, the spherical shape, the obviously expanded cortex, and the well-demarcated margins rule out fibrous dysplasia and strongly suggest an ossifying fibroma.

Fig 17-29 An ossifying fibroma has a cortex that is thinned and expanded, but apparent. Note once again the spherical shape.

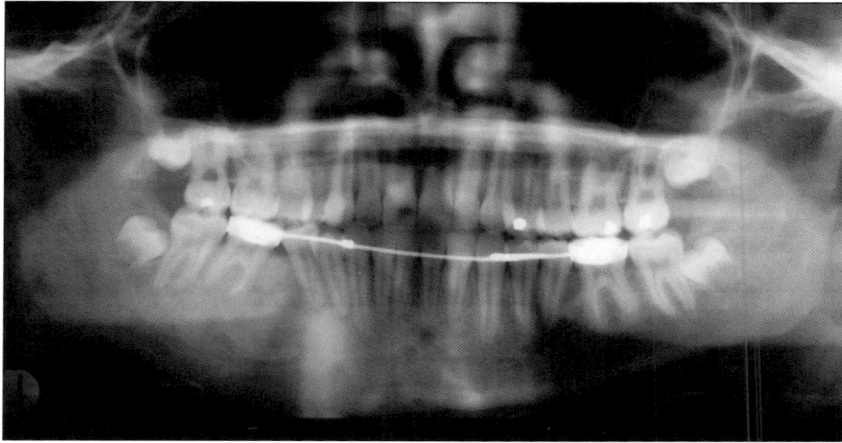

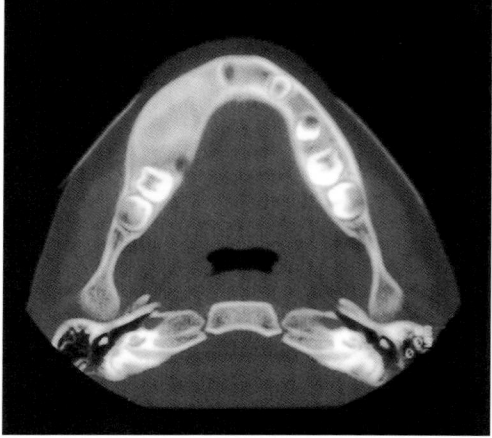

Fig 17-30 This panoramic radiograph is consistent with fibrous dysplasia by virtue of its diffuse radiopacity, absence of the inferior border cortical outline, and a nondisplaced mandibular canal. Do not be fooled by the apparent displacement of the molar and second premolar; the second premolar erupted 5 years after the first molar and therefore erupted into expanded bone.

Fig 17-31 Fibrous dysplasia is diffuse, fusiform, is not well demarcated from normal bone, and remodels the cortex so that a cortical outline is not seen.

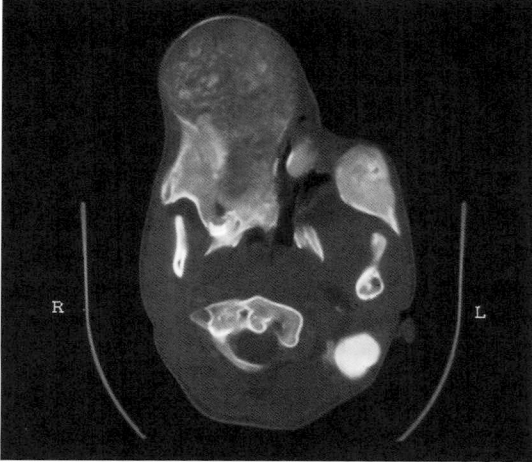

Fig 17-32a This ossifying fibroma developed within an existing craniofacial fibrous dysplasia. A distinction and contrast between their respective CT scan appearances is readily apparent. This is a rare finding of two diseases occurring simultaneously. However, ossifying fibroma is known to occasionally occur associated with other diseases, such as giant cell tumors and idiopathic bone cavities.

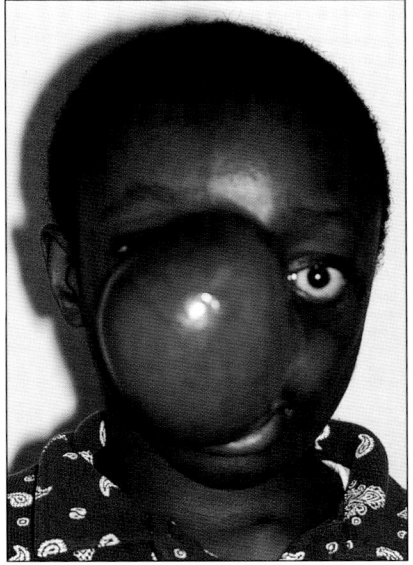

Fig 17-32b This large ossifying fibroma developed slowly from a pre-existing craniofacial fibrous dysplasia.

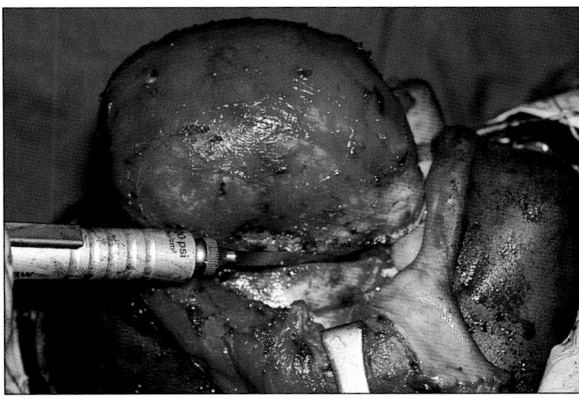

Fig 17-32c This large ossifying fibroma was resected from the fibrous dysplasia using a margin in the fibrous dysplastic bone of 5 mm.

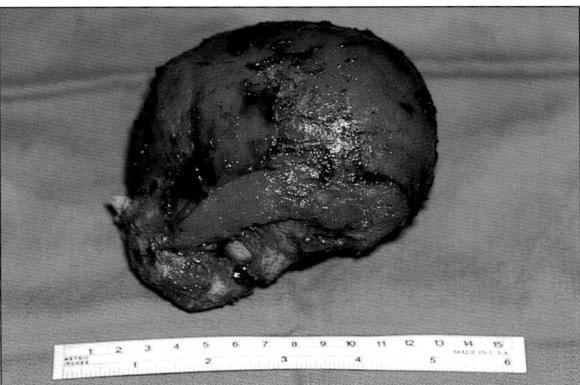

Fig 17-32d Gross specimen of the ossifying fibroma shows an encapsulation separating it from the surrounding soft tissue but a fusion to host bone.

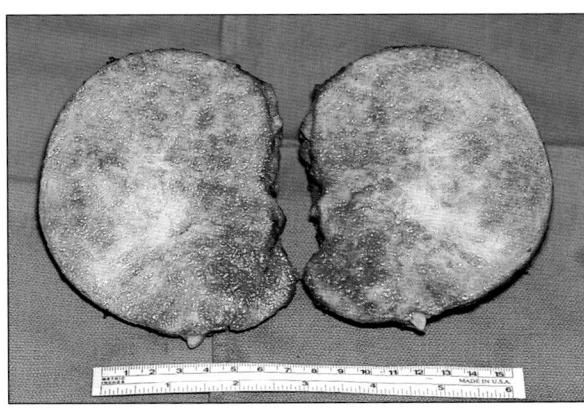

Fig 17-32e The cut gross specimen reveals the spherical nature of ossifying fibromas, the encapsulation adjacent to soft tissue, and the fusion to host bone.

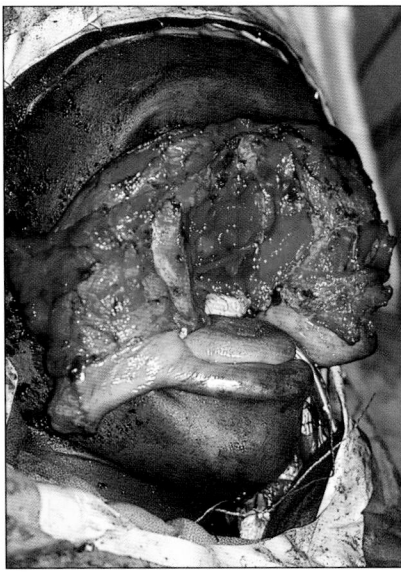

Fig 17-32f The resultant midface defect.

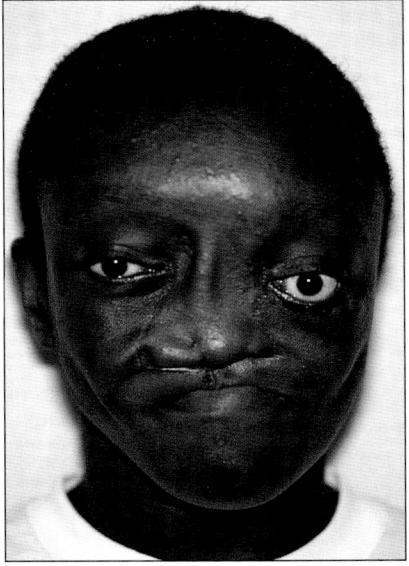

Fig 17-32g Although vastly improved, the residual eye and nasal architectural displacement requires further reconstructive surgery and is a reminder of the value of early diagnosis and treatment.

cortex to make it indistinct, will not be well demarcated, and will form around adjacent structures rather than displacing them (Figs 17-30 and 17-31). This distinction can best be seen when the ossifying fibroma develops within an existing fibrous dysplasia (Fig 17-32a). This is an uncommon occurrence that the oral and maxillofacial specialist should be careful to recognize. In such cases, a spherical mass will develop slowly and protrude from a diffuse fibrous dysplasia involvement (Fig 17-32b). These ossifying fibromas should be excised with the same 5-mm margins. However, the margins will be in fibrous dysplastic bone (Figs 17-32c to 17-32g). If osteosarcoma or Paget disease is a possibility, an incisional biopsy and/or an alkaline phosphatase determination is necessary.

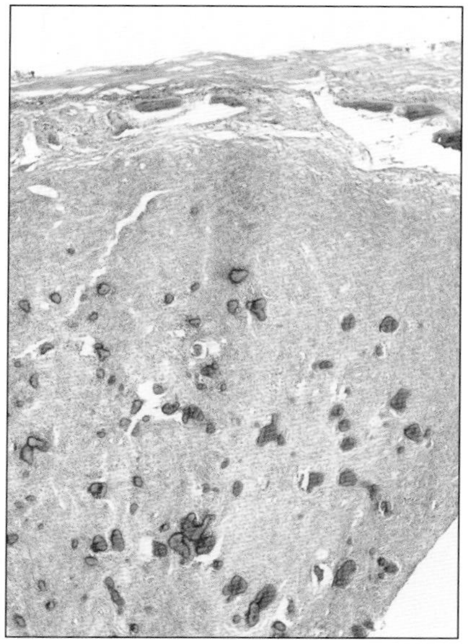

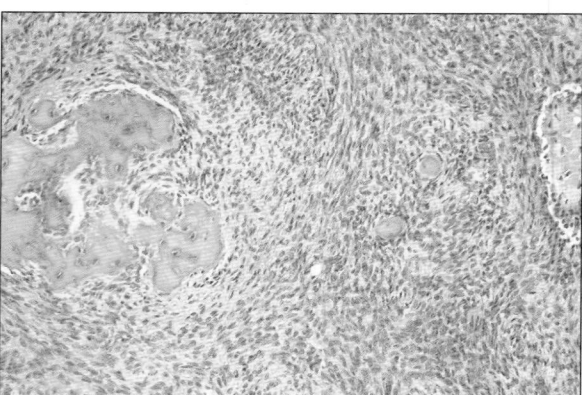

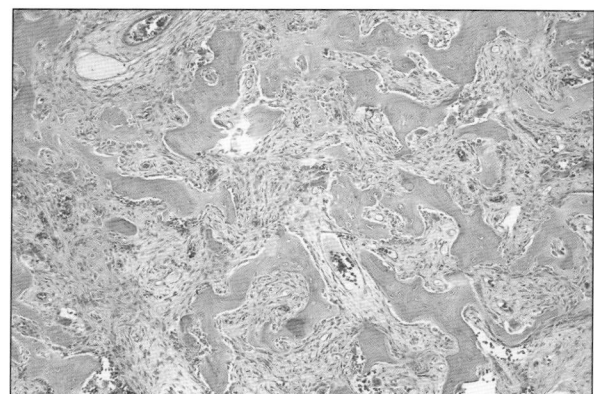

Fig 17-33a An ossifying fibroma showing some normal cortical bone on the surface and the demarcated mass below, which consists of cellular fibrous tissue with scattered rounded areas of calcified tissue.

Fig 17-33b An ossifying fibroma with a very cellular stroma containing some small, rounded calcified masses.

Fig 17-33c An ossifying fibroma showing a large number of osseous trabeculae. Some osteoblastic and osteoclastic activity may be seen.

HISTOPATHOLOGY ▶

Ossifying fibromas usually lack a capsule within bone but have minimal local bone infiltration (Fig 17-33a). This finding distinguishes ossifying fibromas from fibrous dysplasia (Fig 17-33b). The tumor itself consists of a proliferative fibrous tissue that is sometimes well vascularized. The cellularity is variable but can be considerable (see Fig 17-33b). Trabeculae of woven or lamellar bone are usually present, and osteoblastic and osteoclastic activity is variable (Fig 17-33c). Rounded, cementicle-like masses may be present, either alone or together with the trabeculae (see Figs 17-33a and 17-33b). Because of the variation in the configuration of these calcific deposits, such tumors have been referred to as both ossifying and cementifying fibromas. However, because these "cementicle-like" deposits actually represent dysmorphic osteoid, the distinction appears invalid. Thus, these tumors should be referred to as ossifying fibromas.

TREATMENT AND PROGNOSIS ▶

Early tumors that are small, well demarcated, and clinically encapsulated are treated by enucleation and curettage. However, because many patients allow this tumor to reach enormous size, resection is usually required. The decision of whether to enucleate or resect is often difficult; however, resection is generally recommended under the following conditions: involvement of (or within 1 cm of) the inferior border, extension into the maxillary sinus or nasal cavities, and/or loss of encapsulation radiographically or clinically. Often, the outcome of an enucleation procedure is the same as that of a resection. Because this tumor does not infiltrate more than 1 or 2 mm beyond its borders, when it does lose its encapsulation, resection margins need be no larger than 5 mm.

If enucleation and curettage is used, the bony cavity is best left to regenerate normal bone; there is no need to pack the cavity. Packing such cavities with iodoform gauze or other materials only delays healing and will retard and reduce normal bone regeneration. Packing the bony cavity with various hydroxyapatite preparations or bone-inductive agents has not proven to induce more or faster bone regeneration than the organized fibrin blood clot and growth factors arising from platelets within the clot. If a resection is used, stabilization with a reconstruction plate or immediate bony reconstruction may be accomplished. However, immediate bony reconstruction may be complicated by a higher incidence of infection caused by oral contamination and the dead space created by the expansion of the tumor.

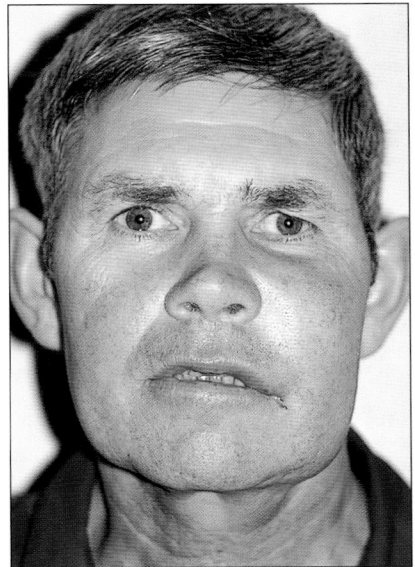

Fig 17-34a Facial expansion as the result of an ossifying fibroma that underwent slow growth over a 9-year period.

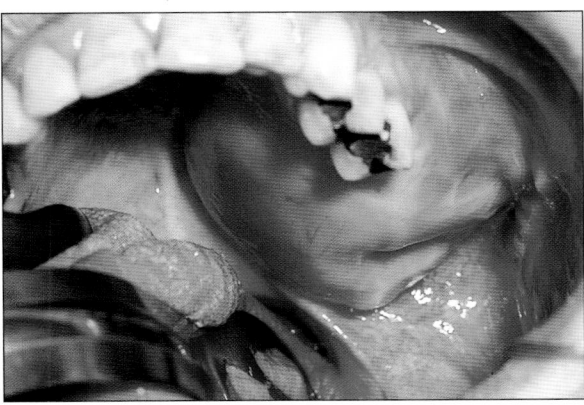

Fig 17-34b The expanded maxilla with an intact mucosa and a depression from occlusion with a mandibular molar.

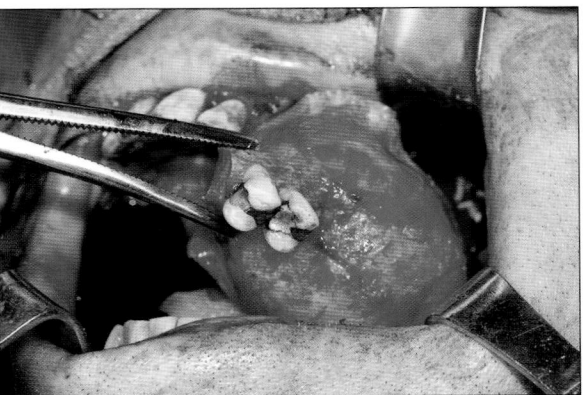

Fig 17-34c While the margin of a mature ossifying fibroma in bone may be radiographically well delineated, histopathologically there is no capsule. Here the tumor bone is fused to the adjacent normal bone. Therefore, an enucleation and curettage procedure is not as curative as a peripheral resection.

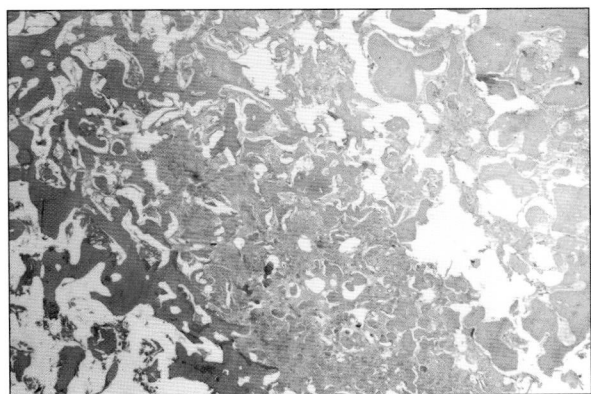

Fig 17-34d Ossifying fibroma margin to native bone. Note the absence of a capsule and the tumor's fusion to the native bone.

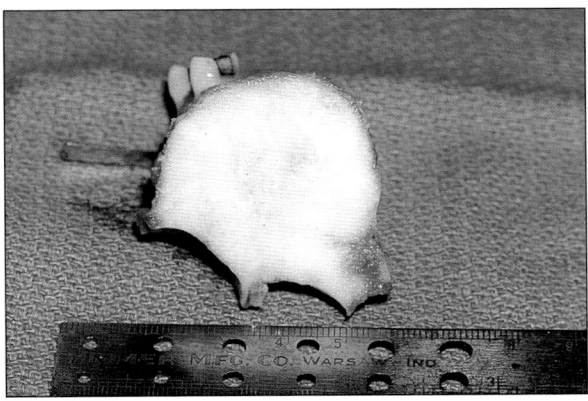

Fig 17-34e Once again, the gross specimen shows an encapsulation on the soft tissue edge and a fusion to the host bone of the maxillary sinus floor.

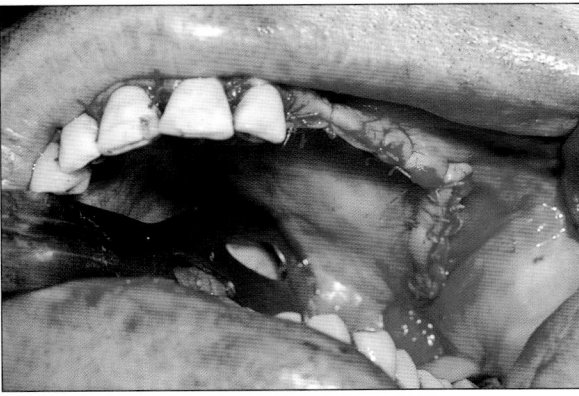

Fig 17-34f The expanded mucosa may be retained to close over the defect. However, immediate bone grafting or tissue spacers are not recommended because of the large amount of dead space and the propensity for infection.

FOLLOW-UP ▶ Resections in the maxilla do not require excision of the overlying mucosa unless it is ulcerated from occlusal injury (Figs 17-34a to 17-34e). Resections in the maxilla may be immediately reconstructed with bone if the tumor is small but are best deferred for second-stage surgery because of the thinning of the overlying mucosa, which often promotes dehiscence over the graft (Figs 17-34f to 17-34k).

By either method of therapy, the recurrence rate is extremely low. Nevertheless, the clinician should follow these patients with yearly examinations and panoramic radiographs for more than 10 years; because of the tumor's slow growth rate, there is an extended period of time during which a recurrence may develop.

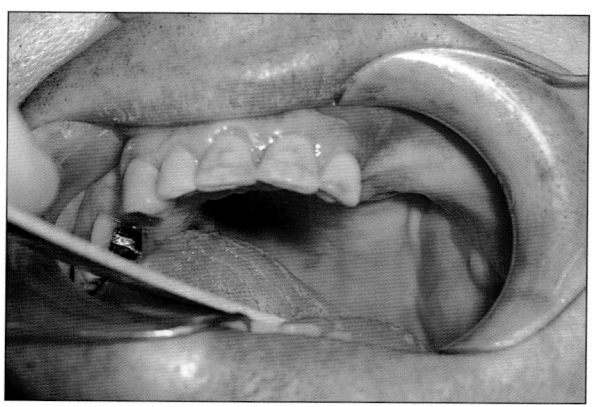

Fig 17-34g Once the tissue heals, a bone graft can be placed into an infection-free and contamination-free tissue space.

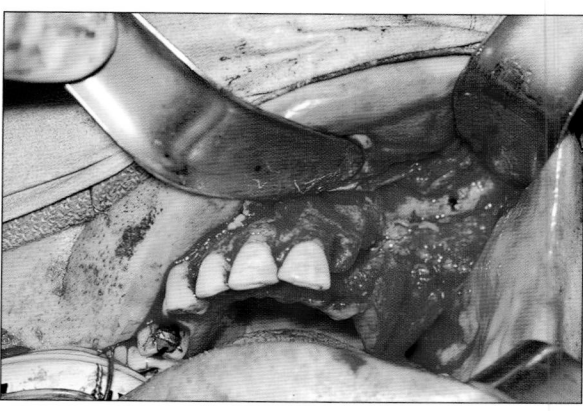

Fig 17-34h Maxillary tumor defects can be expected to partially fill in with fibrous tissue and will frequently redevelop a sinus membrane and, as seen here, a bony floor of the sinus, on which a bone graft can be placed.

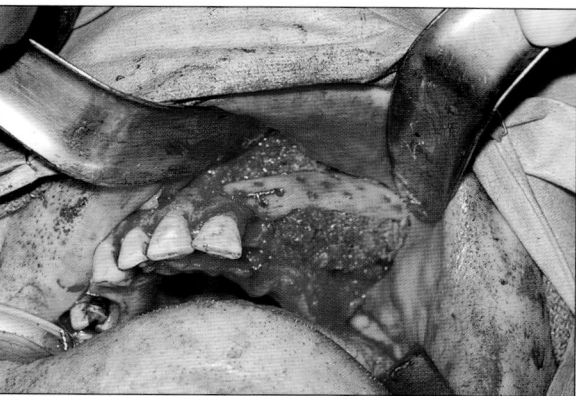

Fig 17-34i Here the maxillary defect is grafted with autogenous cancellous marrow contained by an allogeneic split-rib segment.

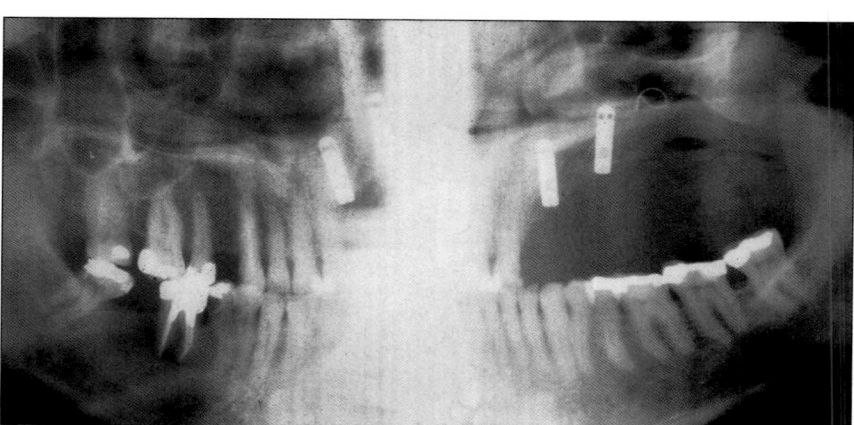

Fig 17-34j After 4 months of bone graft maturity, dental implants can be placed.

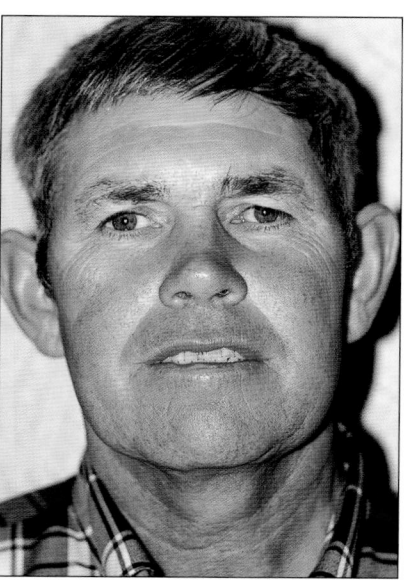

Fig 17-34k After resection of the ossifying fibroma, a secondary bone graft, and a fixed prosthesis, the facial contours and lip position have returned to normal.

Synovial Chondromatosis

CLINICAL PRESENTATION AND PATHOGENESIS

▶ Synovial chondromatosis is a hamartomatous metaplasia that occurs in synovial membranes and tendon sheaths. It is a rare condition that most commonly occurs in middle-aged individuals older than 50 years. Men are affected twice as frequently as women. The knee joint synovium accounts for 70% of cases, and most of the remaining ones occur in the elbow, hip, and shoulder joints. Very rarely it occurs in the temporomandibular joint (TMJ). When it does, it follows the same predilection for men older than 50 years.

When it occurs in the TMJ, it will present as it does in its more common areas of occurrence with pain, swelling, and limited motion (ie, jaw opening). This is due to an initial synovial proliferation, which forms multiple villous folds. Cells deep to the synovial surface are then induced to undergo cartilage

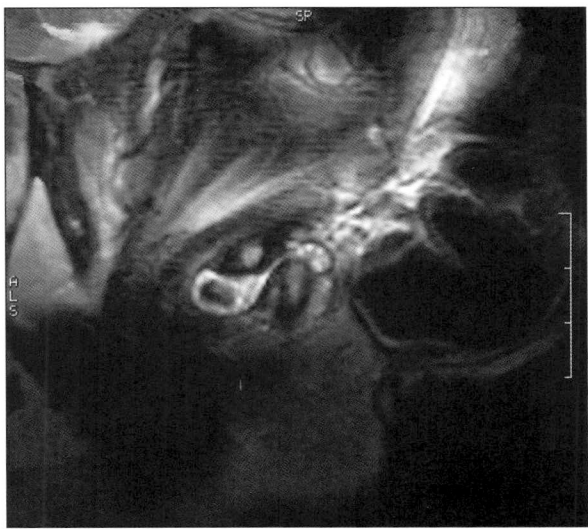

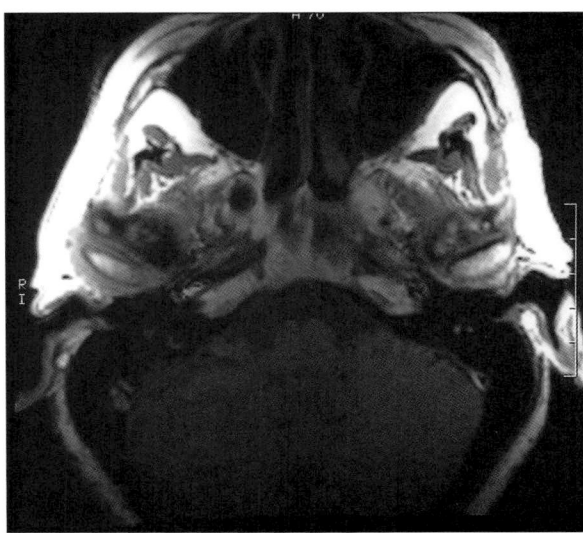

Fig 17-35a Sagittal view MRI of TMJ synovial chondromatosis. T2-weighted image shows high signal in cartilaginous bodies with central signal voids representing mineralization or ossification within areas of the cartilage. (Courtesy of Dr Andrew Slavin.)

Fig 17-35b Axial view MRI of TMJ synovial chondromatosis showing both joints with a high signal representing cartilage or hyperplastic synovium and signal voids representing mineralized areas. (Courtesy of Dr Andrew Slavin.)

metaplasia and subsequently form round, benign cartilage nodules composed of mature chondrocytes. Some of these cartilage nodules erode through the synovial surface and become loose intra-articular floating bodies. As the disease becomes long-standing, the synovial fluid nutrients and oxygen produce an actual partial or complete ossification of these cartilage nodules. These may be seen on some plain radiographs but are more apparent on tomograms, MRI scans, or CT scans. The ossifications occur from the outer surface of the cartilage inward so that many of them will appear as a target with a shell of ossification around a central radiolucency.

Initially, synovial chondromatosis does not affect the bones of the joint. However, over several years the presence of loose joint nodules and inflammation produces a superimposed osteoarthritis.

DIFFERENTIAL DIAGNOSIS ▶

The presentation of pain, swelling, and a limited jaw movement is common to many TMJ afflictions such as an *anterior displaced disc/closed lock*, a *traumatic arthritis*, or a rare *septic arthritis*. The findings of radiopacities in the joint itself or associated with the lateral pterygoid tendon sheath is also seen with an *osteochondroma* of the TMJ or the "rice bodies" seen in *rheumatoid arthritis*.

In addition, *osteophytes* formed in the progression of osteoarthritis may also appear like a synovial chondromatosis. The clinician must also remain alert to the fact that an *osteosarcoma* or a *synovial chondrosarcoma* with reactive bone formation may also mimic synovial chondromatosis.

DIAGNOSTIC WORK-UP ▶

Suspected cases of synovial chondromatosis are best studied with an MRI and/or CT scan. The MRI scan is particularly useful in early cases before ossifications of the cartilaginous nodules occur. T1-weighted images will show a signal void in the area of the lesion, and T2-weighted images will show an enhancement in each lesion and may show each individual cartilaginous nodule (Fig 17-35a). The areas of calcified cartilage or ossifications will appear as signal voids on a T2-weighted image (Fig 17-35b). The CT scan is useful in cases of longer standing because it will show the ossifications and any bony erosions from a superimposed osteoarthritis.

Despite the radiographic and scan implications of a synovial chondromatosis, its rarity and the concern over a malignancy warrant an exploration and biopsy. In years past and into the present, an open joint biopsy and removal of the synovium is indicated both to diagnose and to treat synovial chondromatosis. Today, however, a similar retrieval of diagnostic tissue and a synovectomy can be accomplished through the arthroscopy. For those well trained in TMJ arthroscopy, this is the approach of choice.

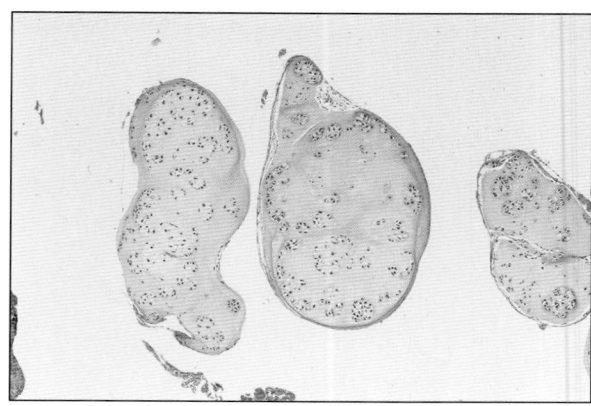

Fig 17-36 Nodules of cartilage removed from a joint space in synovial chondromatosis.

HISTOPATHOLOGY ▶

Nodules of cartilage are seen within the synovium and then lying free within the joint space. As the lesion ages, the masses are less often present within the synovium and are predominantly in the joint space. The cartilaginous nodules may ossify. Atypia of the cartilage is not considered to be significant (Fig 17-36).

TREATMENT AND PROGNOSIS ▶

A synovectomy, which is the recommended definitive treatment for synovial chondromatosis, also is accomplished during the diagnostic exploration and biopsy. If accomplished by arthroscopy, the Holmium laser has been found to be particularly useful. Once a malignancy has been ruled out, no further surgery is usually required. Synovectomy with removal of all intra-articular floating bodies usually results in a reduction of pain and swelling as well as an improved opening. Most patients will require postoperative physical therapy with jaw-opening exercises, such as chewing of soft gum and a Therabite (Therabite) device. Some patients will require postoperative nonsteroidal anti-inflammatory drugs (NSAIDs) for weeks to months.

In cases where a malignancy has already been ruled out and persistent or residual synovial chondromatosis exists, nonsurgical management with NSAIDs and the same jaw-opening physical therapy may be used. Since some synovial chondromatoses are self-limiting and essentially "burn out" after several years, this may be a reasonable approach in cases of mild symptomatology or high surgical/anesthetic risk.

Malignant Neoplasms of Bone

► "Those who say it cannot be done should get out of the way of those who are actually doing it."

—*Anders Westermark*

Osteosarcoma

CLINICAL PRESENTATION AND PATHOGENESIS ►

Osteosarcomas represent malignant neoplasms arising from mesenchymal stem cells and/or their early progeny (Fig 18-1a). Their partial differentiation leading to the production of tumor bone from a malignant cellular stroma is what defines them as osteosarcomas rather than any other malignant mesenchymal tumor that can arise from a mesenchymal stem cell (Fig 18-1b). Recent genetic findings have indicated that osteosarcoma development is related to loss of the P53 tumor suppressor gene, loss of the retinoblastoma tumor suppressor gene, and development of independence from regulation by platelet-derived growth factor (PDGF). No doubt other tumor suppressor gene losses and oncogene expressions may be involved. However, these three are known to be part of the stem cell or its early progeny's escape from its normal differentiation pathway and loss of controlled proliferation, leading to a sarcoma.

Osteosarcomas occur in the jaws at an average age of 37 years, whereas osteosarcomas occur in long bones at an average age of 25 years. However, numerous jaw osteosarcomas occur in the teen years and early 20s as well. In fact, the experience at the University of Miami Division of Oral and Maxillofacial Surgery has been that 4% occur in individuals younger than 10 years and 40% in those between the ages of 10 and 25 years. Nevertheless, it is this later-in-life average occurrence that is often used to explain the better statistical prognosis of osteosarcomas in the jaws.

Osteosarcomas may present with an expansion of bone, an incidental radiographic finding of a radiopacity, a widened periodontal ligament space (Garrington sign), a mobile tooth, a "numb lip" or other paresthesia, and/or pain. Because some of these signs and symptoms can be produced by a number of different developmental, infectious, benign neoplastic diseases, or malignancies, an osteosarcoma often goes undiagnosed for a significant period of time. No doubt its presentation, similar to that of osteomyelitis with proliferative periostitis, suppurative osteomyelitis, ossifying fibroma, osteoblastoma, and even fibrous dysplasia, has too often caused an osteosarcoma to be delayed in its diagnosis or approached with less concern than its biology would warrant.

Osteosarcomas occur evenly among males and females. Mandibular osteosarcomas are more frequent than those in the maxilla (60% vs 40%). All but a rare few arise from within the bone. *Parosteal* (also called *juxtacortical*) osteosarcomas arise from periosteum and occur outside the bone cortex. However, this type accounts for only 4% of those that occur in long bones and less than 1% of those that occur in the jaws.

RADIOGRAPHIC FINDINGS ►

Osteosarcomas may indeed produce the often-described "sun-ray" appearance (Fig 18-2). However, because of calcified cartilage or distension of reactive periosteum, other malignancies will also produce the sun-ray appearance (Figs 18-3 to 18-5). Even some benign tumors or infections causing reactive periosteal distension can produce this appearance. A widening of the periodontal ligament space, also called Garrington sign, is seen in several mesenchymal malignancies as an early finding but is most commonly seen in osteosarcoma (Fig 18-6).

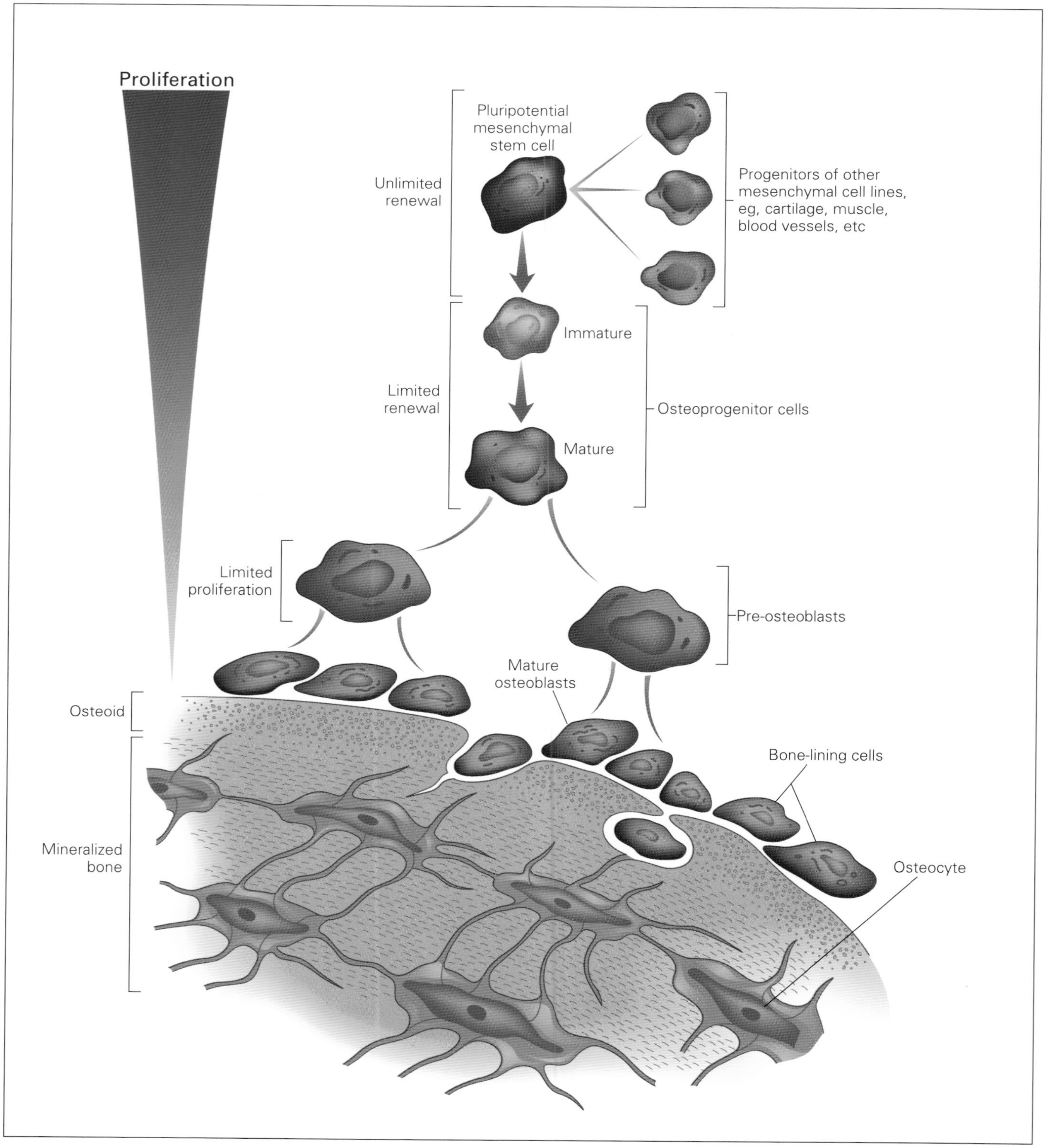

Fig 18-1a The pluripotential mesenchymal stem cell can give rise to all connective tissue lineages. The bone lineage can become neoplastic at any stage. The earlier the stage, the more malignant and high grade the tumors will be. The later the stage, the more low grade and even benign the tumors may be.

800

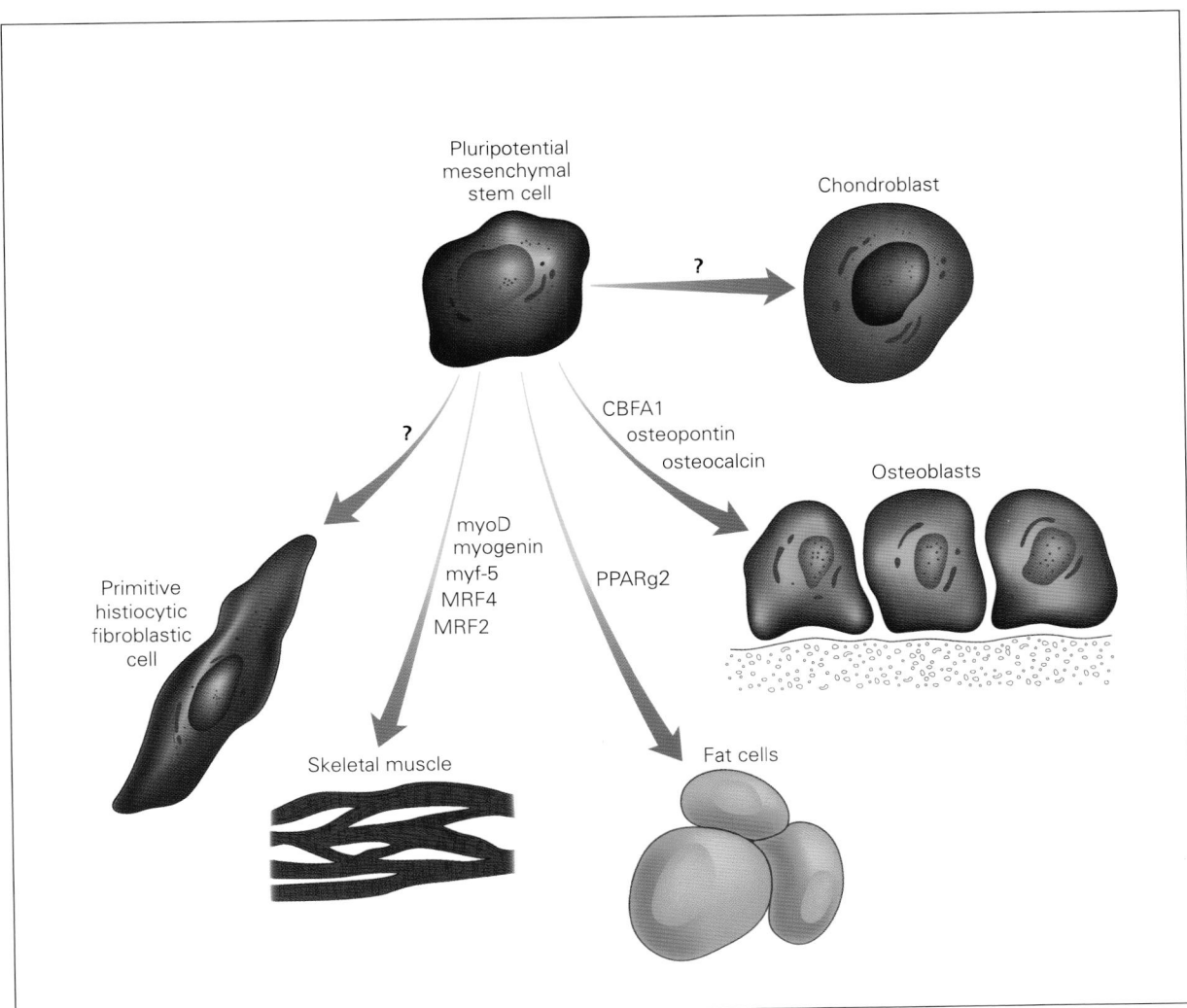

Fig 18-1b Pluripotential stem cells mature by sequential steps related to genetic expressions of differentiation proteins.

Most radiographs and computed tomographic (CT) scans show a mottled radiopaque or mixed radiolucent-radiopaque appearance in the medullary space (see Fig 18-5). Extracortical bone formation is common and may or may not produce the sun-ray appearance. However, cortical bone destruction is characteristic and should be evident (see Fig 18-5).

Maxillary osteosarcomas produce a sun-ray appearance and extracortical bone formation less frequently. Because they also grow into the air space of the maxillary sinus as a bulbous radiopaque mass, they may suggest a benign tumor of bone or a fibro-osseous disease rather than an infiltrating malignant bone tumor.

DIFFERENTIAL DIAGNOSIS ▶

The radiographic and clinical picture of an osteosarcoma can be similar to that of infections such as *osteomyelitis with proliferative periostitis, chronic sclerosing osteomyelitis,* and *suppurative osteomyelitis;* to benign bone tumors or benign tumors within bone such as *osteoblastomas, ossifying fibromas,* and *cavernous hemangiomas within bone;* to odontogenic tumors such as *calcifying epithelial odontogenic tumors* and *ameloblastic fibro-odontomas;* and to fibro-osseous diseases or systemic diseases of bone such as *fibrous dysplasia* and *Paget disease.*

An important clinical differential feature is neurosensory loss. Other than a rare osteomyelitis or neural loss from a previous biopsy or surgery, only malignancies can produce objective paresthesias. In

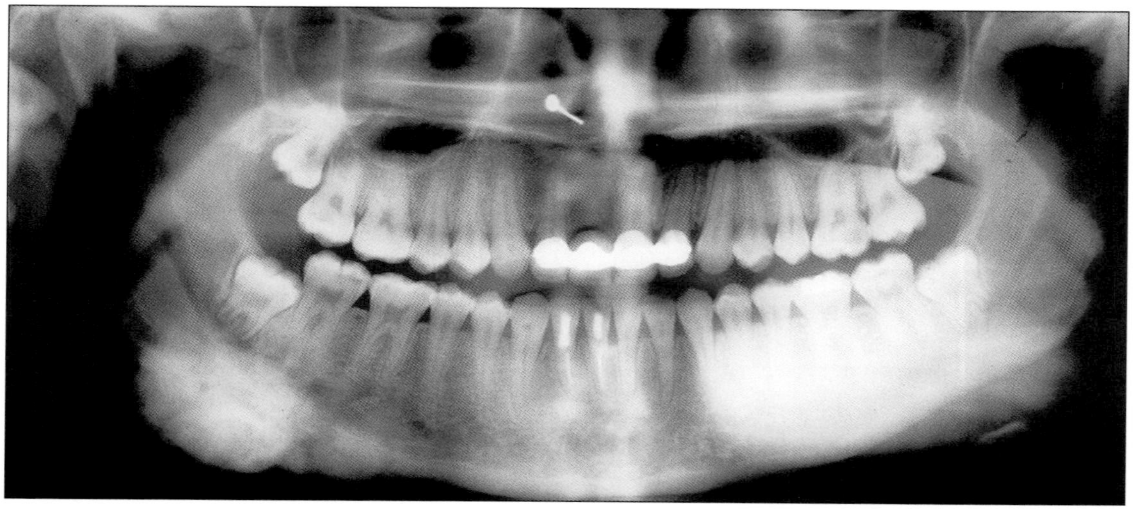

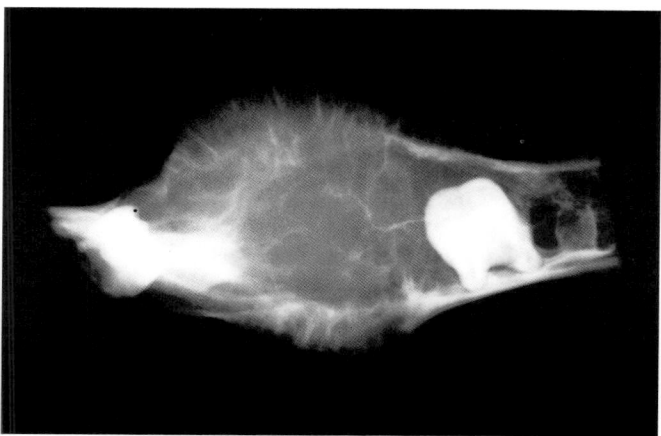

Fig 18-2 Osteosarcoma with sufficient bone to cause a radiopacity and a so-called sun-ray appearance.

Fig 18-3 Specimen radiograph of an odontogenic myxoma showing a classic sun-ray apearance. The sun-ray appearance and extracortical bone are not pathognomonic of osteosarcoma or necessarily of malignant tumors.

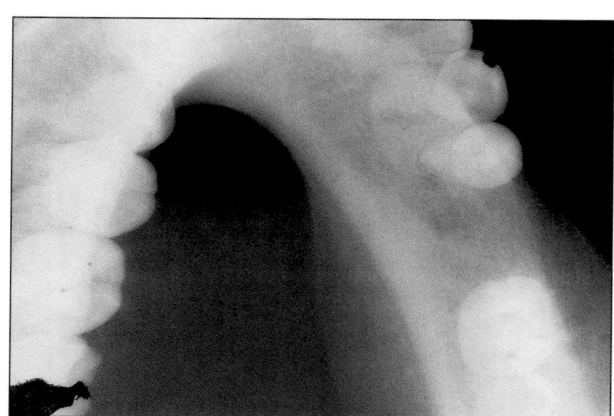

Fig 18-4 This osteomyelitis with proliferative periostitis produced extracortical bone outside a generally intact cortex. Note the homogeneous appearance and smooth outline of the extracortical bone.

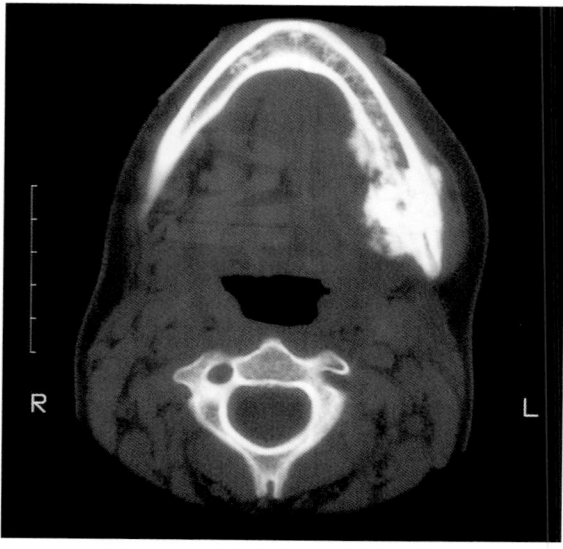

Fig 18-5 Irregular and right-angled extracortical bone formation from a disrupted cortex is strongly suggestive of osteosarcoma.

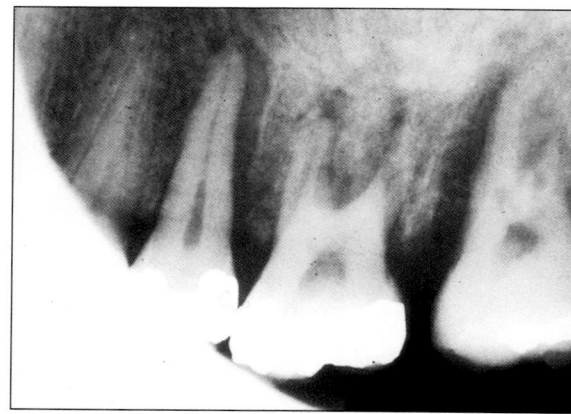

Fig 18-6 Widening of the periodontal ligament space is an early and prominent sign of several mesenchymal malignancies, including osteosarcoma.

addition, radiographs or CT scans at right angles to the cortex should show extracortical bone and a destroyed cortex. Fibrous dysplasia and ossifying fibroma will not have extracortical bone. The extracortical bone seen in osteomyelitis with proliferative periostitis will be associated with an intact cortex. Even when other osteomyelitides produce extracortical bone, it is parallel to the cortex rather than at right angles as is seen in osteosarcoma (see Figs 18-4 and 18-5).

DIAGNOSTIC WORK-UP ▶ A presentation suggestive of osteosarcoma requires a biopsy as soon as possible. A tissue biopsy is the only means of making a definitive diagnosis. The biopsy should be taken from the lesion's center to avoid missing the diagnostic portion of the tumor or including benign reactive periosteal bone in the specimen, which could lead to a misdiagnosis (Fig 18-7).

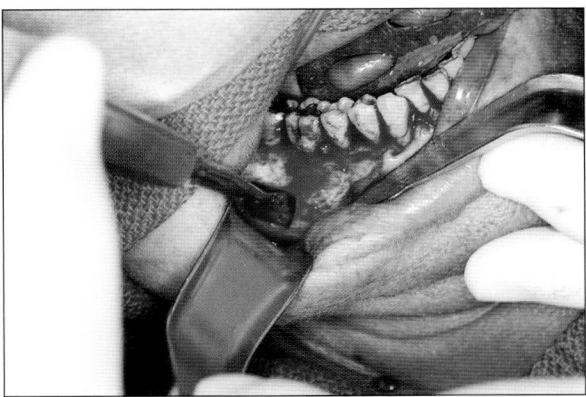

Fig 18-7 Incisional biopsies for a suspected bone malignancy need to sample the marrow space. Too superficial a biopsy will usually result in reactive bone, which may be interpreted as a fibrous dysplasia; a healing bone defect; or osteomyelitis, among others.

The remainder of the work-up requires at least a chest radiograph and perhaps a chest CT scan. Because early and small lung metastatic deposits are a concern, either will establish absence of disease or early metastasis. In addition, a CT scan of the primary site and adjacent structures is suggested for surgical planning.

HISTOPATHOLOGY ▶

The histologic appearance of osteosarcomas is highly variable. What all osteosarcomas have in common is the direct formation of osteoid from a sarcomatous stroma (Fig 18-8a). The quantity of osteoid and bone that is formed varies considerably, ranging from a sclerotic osseous tumor to one in which multiple sections may be necessary to identify some semblance of osteoid. The stromal cells may be osteoblastic, chondroblastic, and/or fibroblastic (Figs 18-8b to 18-8d). However, distinguishing osteoblastic, chondroblastic, and fibroblastic osteosarcomas based on the most prominent pattern does not seem to have any prognostic significance. In general, osteoblastic tumors are most common, but in the jaws the chondroblastic pattern prevails. A myxoid stroma is also frequently seen (Fig 18-8e), and an atypical myxoid proliferation should alert one to the possibility of osteosarcoma. The majority of tumors are not homogeneous, reflecting the pluripotentiality of the proliferating mesenchymal cell.

Some osteosarcomas are very heavily ossified, and in these cases there may be entrapment of tumor cells within the sclerotic osteoid, such that the cells appear to represent osteocytes. This process is known as *normalization* because the osteocytic cells are small and no longer retain their malignant morphologic features.

Mitoses may be present, but they are not usually numerous. Multinucleated giant cells may also be present, sometimes in large numbers, although they are unusual in the jaws. Stromal cells may be predominantly rounded, spindled, angulated, or pleomorphic with marked atypia (Figs 18-8f and 18-8g).

Other histologic variants include a telangiectatic type in which there are numerous widely dilated vascular channels and prominent multinucleated giant cells. This type is uncommon in the jaws. The small cell osteosarcoma may resemble Ewing sarcoma histologically, but unlike Ewing sarcoma, it forms osteoid. Particularly in tumors with prominent chondroblastic or fibroblastic features, or those in which identification of osteoid is difficult, the recognition of bone-specific alkaline phosphatase in fresh tissue may be helpful diagnostically.

It is important to emphasize that biopsy specimens from the superficial or peripheral aspects of the tumor—that is, from the advancing edge—are least likely to be representative of the tumor and frequently fail to demonstrate osteoid formation (Fig 18-8h).

Periosteal osteosarcomas are essentially chondroblastic osteosarcomas that expand into the soft tissue from an intact cortex.

Parosteal Osteosarcoma

Parosteal osteosarcomas develop on the surface of the bone and are well differentiated with a bland appearance. There is a hypocellular, spindle cell stroma with little atypia and irregular trabeculae of woven

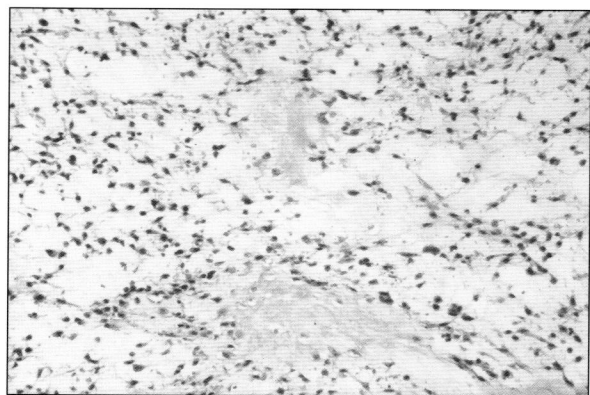

Fig 18-8a Scant, pale pink osteoid arising from a pleomorphic sarcomatous stroma.

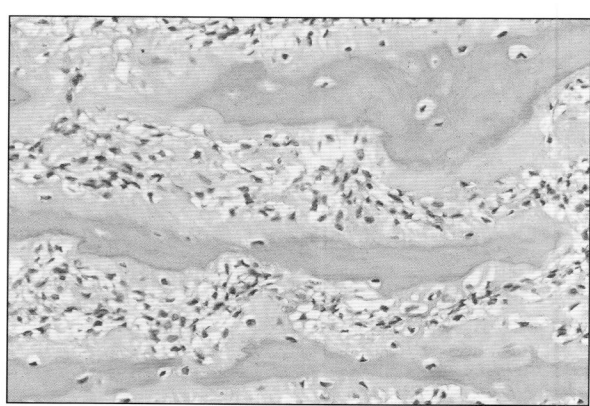

Fig 18-8b Formation of osteoid in an osteosarcoma.

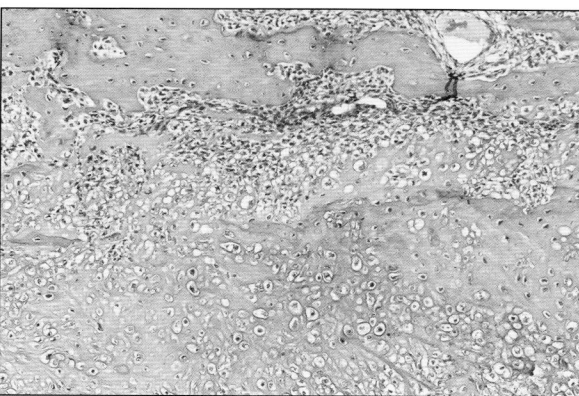

Fig 18-8c Chondroid areas in an osteosarcoma.

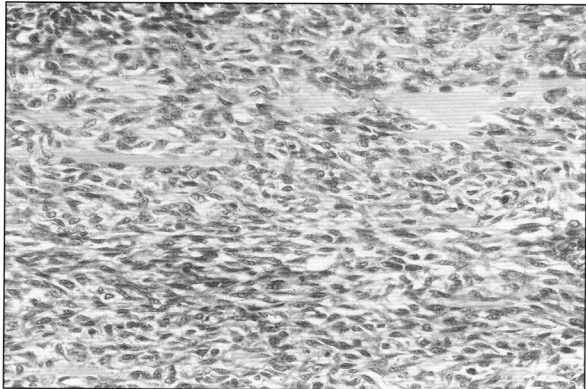

Fig 18-8d Fibroblastic areas in an osteosarcoma.

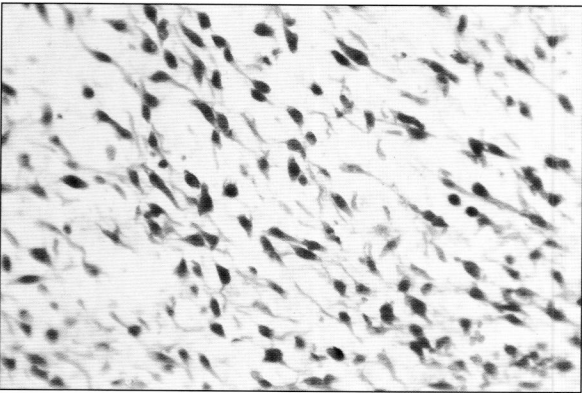

Fig 18-8e Myxoid area with plump hyperchromatic nuclei in an osteosarcoma.

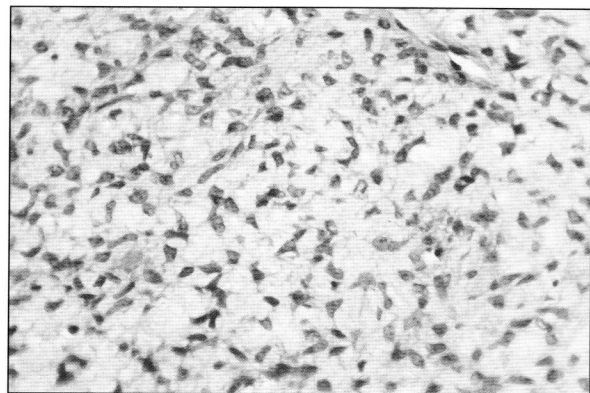

Fig 18-8f Angulated cells in an osteosarcoma with a suggestion of osteoid in one area. Other areas of the tumor revealed scant but more obvious osteoid.

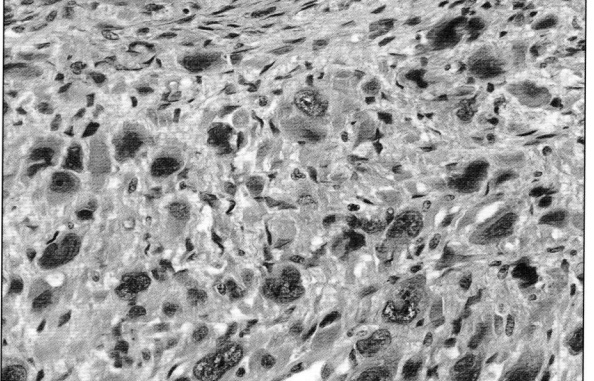

Fig 18-8g Large atypical cells in an osteosarcoma.

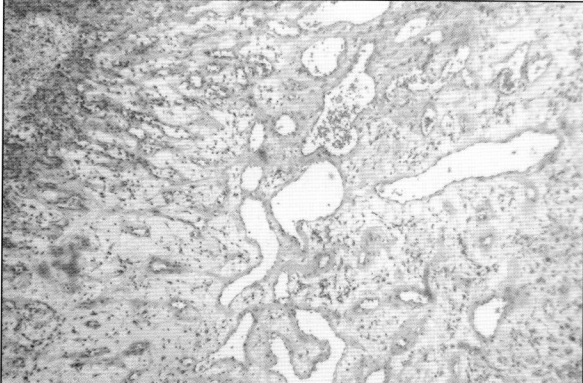

Fig 18-8h This superficial portion of an osteosarcoma shows numerous dilated capillaries with some scattered inflammatory cells. The clinical diagnosis was a pyogenic granuloma. Only the deeper tissue showed the true nature of the lesion.

bone. These tumors may be mistaken for a benign condition. Some tumors may be more histologically aggressive with more atypical stromal cells, and recurrent tumors can have increasingly atypical cytologic features.

TREATMENT AND BIOLOGIC BEHAVIOR ▶

After squamous cell carcinoma, osteosarcoma is the most common oral malignancy encountered by the dental professional. Unlike squamous cell carcinoma, osteosarcoma treatment does not involve radiotherapy except in late palliative situations, nor does it require cancer neck dissections. Instead, osteosarcomas of the jaws are ideally treated with initial chemotherapy of about five inductions, followed by surgery, which is followed by two or three additional induction doses of chemotherapy.

Treatment involves selected chemotherapy protocols to sterilize micrometastatic deposits that may already be in the lung, to test the tumor's responsiveness to the chemotherapeutic agents by assessing tumor shrinkage, and to decrease tumor bulk. Surgery involves resection of the entire tumor with wide margins. Bony margins should be at least 3 cm from the clinical-radiographic edge or to the joint or the nearest suture if in the midface (Fig 18-9a). A neck dissection is not required because, as is typical of most sarcomas, osteosarcomas do not metastasize via lymphatics except in rare instances. Instead, osteosarcomas readily metastasize via tumor emboli in the bloodstream and are most commonly filtered out in the lungs. The soft tissue margins around an osteosarcoma resection should be 2 cm or more and assessed with frozen sections. Therapeutic failure most often relates to local recurrence in the surgical area. The postoperative chemotherapy is intended to sterilize any tumor foci not excised during the surgical resection. The same chemotherapy agents used in the preoperative phase will be used in the postoperative phase if the tumor was responsive to them.

The chemotherapy protocols used for osteosarcoma will vary with each oncologist. However, doxorubicin (Adriamycin, Pharmacia and Upjohn) is usually used within every protocol, and vincristine, cyclophosphamide (Cytoxan, Mead Johnson), and prednisone are commonly used as well.

In most cases, the initial five chemotherapy inductions are physiologically and psychologically stressful. Marrow suppression will produce an anemia, thrombocytopenia, and leukopenia. A 1-month period between such chemotherapy and surgery will allow marrow recovery as well as a psychologic recovery. Vitamin C, 250 mg three times daily, and iron in the form of ferrous sulfate, 225 mg three times daily, will reduce the anemia. Surgery can be performed if the hemoglobin nears 10 g/dL, the white blood cell (WBC) count is 3,000/μL, and the platelet count has increased to 100×10^3/μL. Family support, a frank discussion of the surgery and its goals, and, at times, counseling will particularly help young individuals to cope with this diagnosis and its treatments.

If the osteosarcoma is in the mandible, the resected area is best reconstructed with a rigid titanium plate (Fig 18-9b). Bone grafting with cancellous marrow or using a free vascular bone flap is not recommended because of the necessity for postoperative chemotherapy and the general inadequacy of free microvascular fibula ilium grafts to functionally reconstruct the mandible. Because osteosarcoma resections require excision of 2 to 3 cm of surrounding soft tissue that often includes overlying skin or approaches the skin surface, myocutaneous soft tissue flaps or other soft tissue flaps may be needed (Fig 18-9c). Once the plate and flap are healed (about 6 weeks), the postoperative chemotherapy can begin (Fig 18-9d). Reconstruction of the bony defect leading to dental rehabilitation can begin after the individual recovers from the postoperative chemotherapy phase.

If the osteosarcoma is in the maxilla, the resection will take the form of a hemimaxillectomy or a variation of it (Fig 18-10a). Because an oral-nasal-antral communication is certain, the surgeon should have an obturator prosthesis ready for placement at the time of surgery. This obturator prosthesis will reduce hypernasal speech and nasal regurgitation of fluids and foods in the early postoperative phase (Fig 18-10b). It will later be replaced by a definitive denture-obturator prosthesis. The defect takes about 6 to 9 months to sufficiently mature and become dimensionally stable.

PROGNOSIS ▶

Osteosarcomas of the jaws are associated with a better prognosis than are osteosarcomas of long bones. There is about a 50% 5-year survival rate with jaw osteosarcomas compared to a 30% 5-year sur-

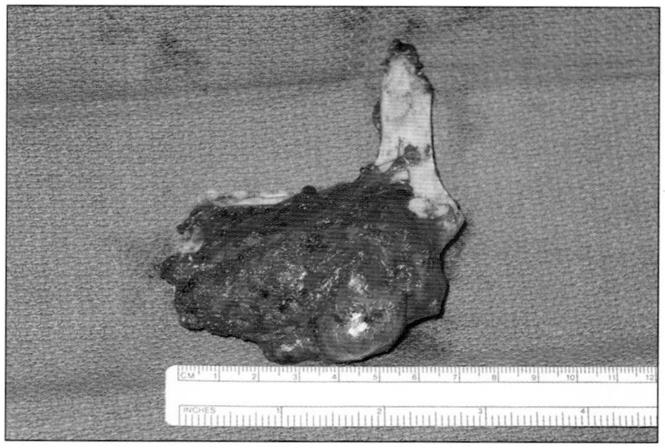

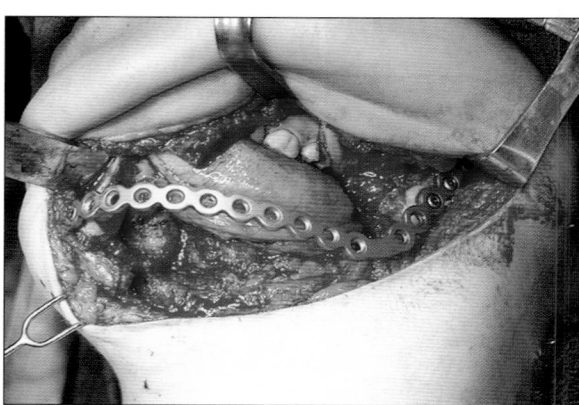

Fig 18-9a The resection principles for jaw osteosarcomas include 3-cm bony margins and 2-cm peripheral soft tissue margins. Here bone, muscle, teeth, and the contents of the submandibular triangle are part of the resection specimen.

Fig 18-9b Because a large continuity defect is anticipated, the surgeon must be prepared to rigidly stabilize the mandible. Rigid titanium reconstruction plates and predictable myocutaneous flaps are preferred.

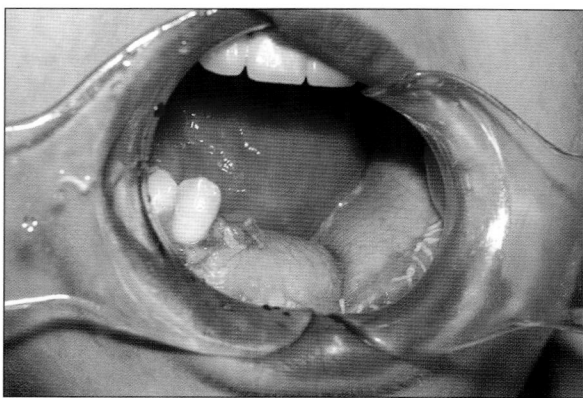

Fig 18-9c This trapezius myocutaneous flap completely reconstructed the large soft tissue defect of the osteosarcoma resection shown in Fig 18-9b.

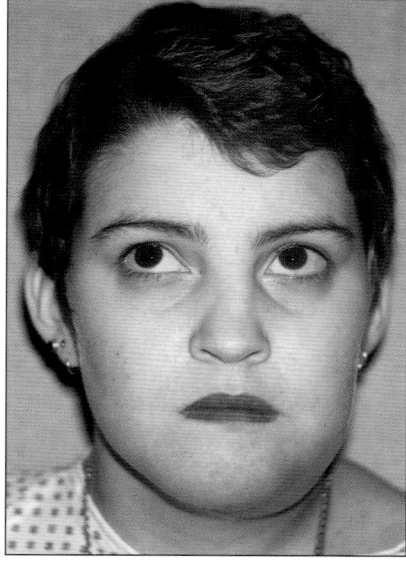

Fig 18-9d One-week postoperative appearance showing minimal deformity after a rigid reconstruction plate and trapezius flap.

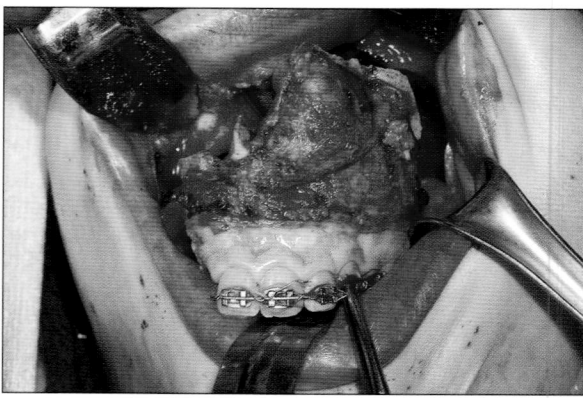

Fig 18-10a Osteosarcomas of the maxilla are treated with Le Fort I (shown here) and sometimes Le Fort II types of resection. Note the superior margin in the infraorbital rim area.

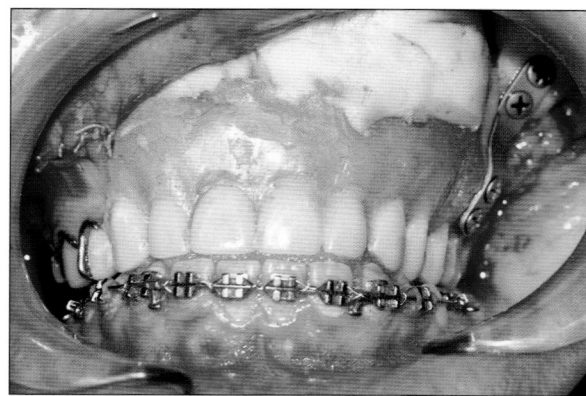

Fig 18-10b Immediate surgical obturator splints are of great value in maxillary resections. Here excellent tooth and contour matches were achieved. When defects cross the midline, a drop plate from the zygoma affords excellent short-term denture splint stability and may be used for up to 6 months.

vival rate with long bone osteosarcomas. However, 50% survival is still suboptimal. Therapeutic failure results from local recurrences followed by lung metastasis, followed by brain metastasis, and then metastasis to other bones. All of the distant metastases occur via tumor emboli in veins that either flow "downstream" to the right side of the heart, where they are pumped into and become lodged in the capillaries of the lungs, or via retrograde flow to the brain or other bones (Fig 18-11; see also Fig 7-7.)

Prognosis worsens with a delay in diagnosis and treatment, with increased tumor size, and with symptoms of pain and paresthesia. Histologically, no grading system correlates well to prognosis. However, the presence of tumor emboli in the venules within the specimen is an ominous sign. The presence of myxomatous cells, tumor giant cells, and necrosis are also associated with a poorer prognosis. The abundant

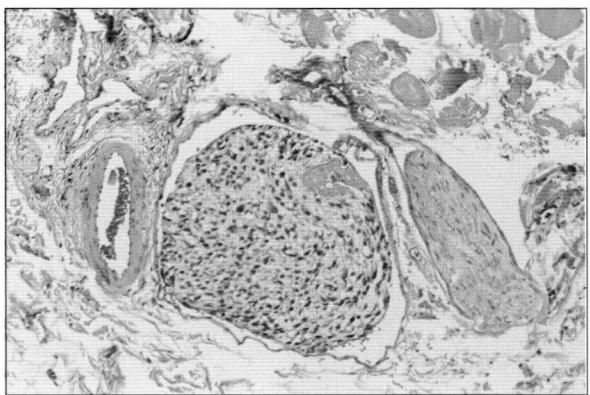

Fig 18-11 Pleomorphic malignant mesenchymal cells and a small focus of malignant osteoid in an osteosarcoma within a vein located between an artery and a nerve. Such tumor emboli are the source of distant metastases.

production of tumor bone should not be looked upon as a favorable sign or as a sign that it is "well differentiated." Osteosarcomas that produce abundant calcified bone are often associated with the poorest prognosis. The presence of numerous cartilaginous cells, however, has been found to be a somewhat favorable sign.

FOLLOW-UP

Since the concern is recurrence at the primary tumor site and/or metastasis to the lungs, a clinical oral and head and neck examination and a chest radiograph are recommended every 4 months for the first 2 years and then every 6 months for the next 3 years. Thereafter, such examinations should be carried out on an annual basis. Any suspicious changes seen on a plain chest radiograph should be further evaluated with a CT scan of the chest.

Ewing Sarcoma

CLINICAL PRESENTATION AND PATHOGENESIS

Ewing sarcoma is a genetically and histologically distinctive small round cell sarcoma of bone. It is a notoriously aggressive and destructive malignancy of bone arising from marrow mesenchymal stem cells. It is rare in the jaws but accounts for about 8% of malignancies in long bones. It was first described by James Ewing in 1920 as a "diffuse endothelioma of bone." Since then it has been documented as a distinct malignancy of primitive mesenchymal stem cells that have undergone a unique reciprocal translocation of chromosomes 11 and 22. The resultant highly malignant tumor causes extensive destruction of bone and tumor necrosis and has a strong propensity for metastasis (Fig 18-12).

In both the jaws and long bones, it is mostly seen in patients younger than 20 years (80%). The peak age of occurrence is in the teenage years (50%). It practically never occurs in black individuals. Young men are affected slightly more often than are young women (1.4:1).

In the mandible's posterior body, the angle and ramus regions are most commonly affected. It is rare in the mandible in general and even more rare in the maxilla. Its presentation will frequently involve bony expansion, mobile teeth, and fever presumably due to necrosis within the tumor and its destruction of native bone. It will, therefore, present a picture similar to that of an osteomyelitis. Its growth rate is usually rapid.

RADIOGRAPHIC FINDINGS

Panoramic radiographs and a CT scan will show an ill-defined, irregular resorption of bone with focal areas of residual bone resembling sequestra. Pathologic fractures are common, attesting to the degree of bone destruction. Ewing sarcoma has often been reported to produce a multilayered periosteal reaction that has been described as an "onion skin" appearance, similar to that commonly observed in an osteomyelitis with proliferative periostitis. However, such a radiographic appearance is almost never seen when Ewing sarcoma arises in the jaws, although it is seen occasionally when Ewing sarcoma arises within the diaphysis of long bones. Ewing sarcoma in the jaws will produce a destructive radiolucency with resorbed tooth roots and displaced teeth. On rare occasions, a Ewing sarcoma may produce a periosteal

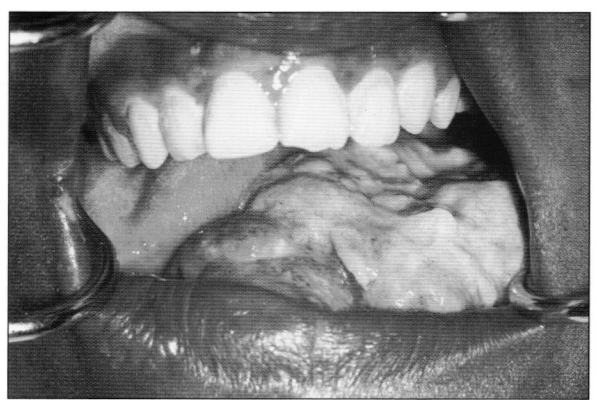

Fig 18-12 Ewing sarcoma is a highly malignant tumor with significant bone and soft tissue destruction.

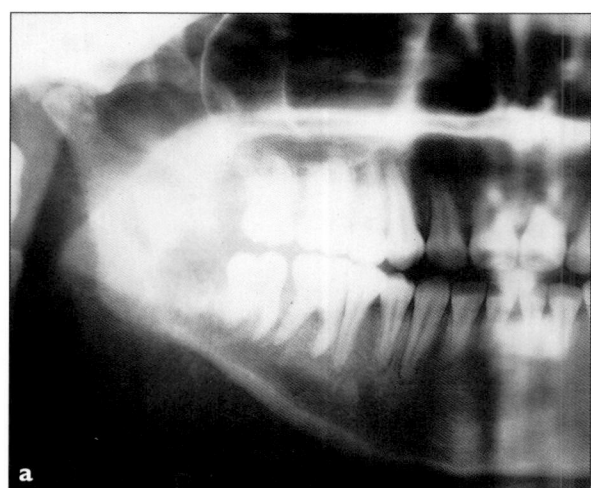

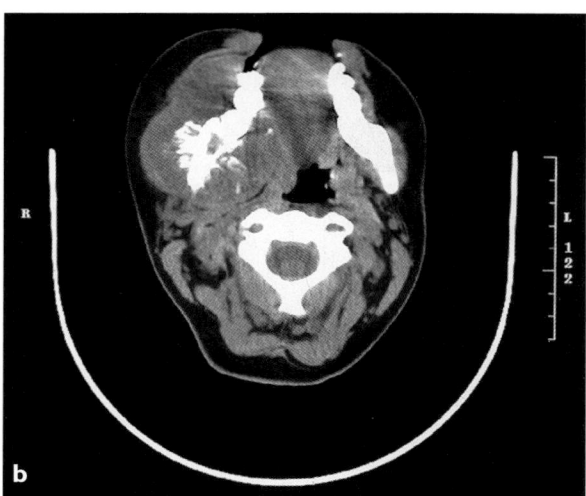

Figs 18-13a and 18-13b Ewing sarcoma of the mandible showing the typical destruction and expansion beyond the cortex along with perpendicular extracortical bone formation (referred to as "sun rays").

DIFFERENTIAL DIAGNOSIS ▶

new bone formation perpendicular to the cortex and thereby create the "sun-ray" appearance more frequently seen in osteosarcomas (Figs 18-13a and 18-13b).

The presence of pain, fever, and at times leukocytosis will suggest a *suppurative osteomyelitis*. This will be reinforced if the radiographs show a destructive bone pattern with bone foci resembling a sequestrum. If it is an early Ewing sarcoma with minimal osteolysis and with a layered periosteal "onion skin" radiographic appearance, it may resemble *osteomyelitis with proliferative periostitis*.

The usual more destructive and expansile tumors will point to an aggressive malignancy from the outset. Other aggressive malignancies that occur in this young age group include *rhabdomyosarcoma*, *osteosarcoma*, *fibrosarcoma*, and *neuroblastoma*. In the uncommon situation of an older individual developing Ewing sarcoma, one would also need to consider a *non-Hodgkin lymphoma* and a *carcinoma metastatic to the mandible*. In early presentations and in younger individuals, a seeding of leukemia cells, particularly *acute lymphocytic leukemia* and *acute myelogenous leukemia*, is a possibility.

HISTOPATHOLOGY ▶

Ewing sarcomas are composed of densely packed, rather uniform cells with little intercellular stroma (Fig 18-14a). The nuclei are rounded to oval with defined nuclear borders and a finely granular chromatin pattern (Fig 18-14b). The cytoplasm is indistinct and may be vacuolated. The cells are two to three times the size of a lymphocyte. Mitoses are infrequent. The tumors tend to grow rapidly and may undergo considerable necrosis, sometimes resulting in a perivascular pattern of viable tumor cells (Fig 18-14c). The friable consistency produced by this tumor necrosis may result in a biopsy specimen with an inadequate number and pattern of viable cells from which to make a diagnosis.

While usually arranged in broad sheets, the cells may have a filigree pattern in which infiltrating strands of tumor cells are separated by thin fibrovascular septae. There is some evidence that the filigree pattern may indicate a worse prognosis.

The histologic differential diagnosis includes other small round cell tumors, including neuroblastoma, lymphoma, small cell osteosarcoma, and embryonal rhabdomyosarcoma. Histochemical studies are of limited help. Ewing sarcoma will usually have intracytoplasmic glycogen granules demonstrated by periodic acid–Schiff (PAS) and diastase staining. However, on occasion, neuroblastoma and embryonal rhabdomyosarcomas may also yield positive staining. In recent years, Ewing sarcoma has been recognized as part of the spectrum of primitive neuroectodermal tumors (PNETs). The monoclonal antibody HBA-71 is helpful diagnostically, since it reacts with the Ewing-specific antigen MIC2 and has a high sensitivity (approximately 98%). Cytogenetic testing reveals a translocation in 95% of cases that is also shared by PNET, t(11;22)(q24;q12), that is, translocation of chromosomes 11 and 22 at their respective q24 and q12 loci. A fresh tissue specimen is necessary for this type of cytogenetic testing.

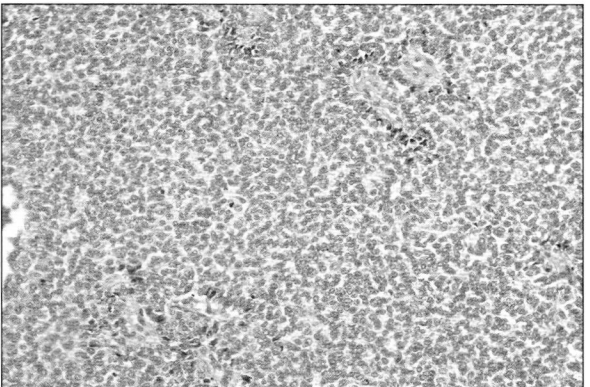

Fig 18-14a Ewing sarcoma with a monotonous infiltrate of uniform cells. There is little stroma.

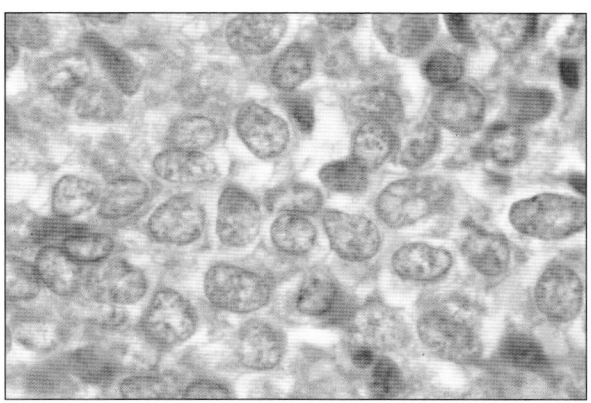

Fig 18-14b A Ewing sarcoma at 1,000× magnification shows the uniform bland nuclei of this tumor.

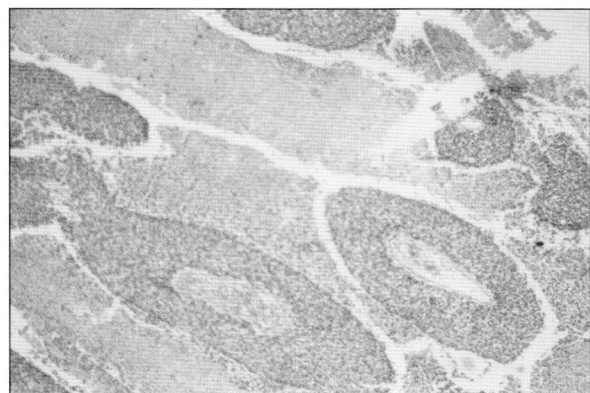

Fig 18-14c Ewing sarcoma showing viable tumor cells surrounding the blood vessels. Beyond this, the tissue is necrotic.

DIAGNOSTIC WORK-UP ►

As with all potential malignancies, a biopsy should not be delayed and it should sample tumor tissue central and deep within the bone. As with biopsies for suspected osteosarcoma, a biopsy that samples superficial aspects of the tumor may show only benign reactive bone created by periosteal distension.

A CT scan is useful to determine the local extent of the tumor in bone and soft tissue. A chest radiograph or CT scan is required to assess for metastasis to the lung, which is the most common metastatic site.

Obtaining laboratory values such as a complete blood count (CBC), WBC count, and platelet count is recommended, but the values are not diagnostic. Because the tumor necrosis produces a leukocytosis and the tumor bulk itself may produce an anemia, a baseline set of blood studies is useful. The leukocytosis usually resolves in response to treatment.

It is well for the clinician to recall that tumor necrosis will interfere with efforts to obtain a representative biopsy specimen. Therefore, the tissue to be sampled should have the firmest consistency possible. In addition, if Ewing sarcoma is part of the differential diagnosis, a portion of the specimen should be withheld from formalin fixation and submitted fresh for cytogenetic testing.

TREATMENT AND BIOLOGIC BEHAVIOR ►

Today Ewing sarcoma is treated with multimodal therapy in a manner similar to that for rhabdomyosarcoma. This approach uses all three traditional modes of cancer therapy. Although there are variations in the order of each modality, doses of radiotherapy, and choice of drugs, a commonly used protocol begins with resection of all clinically detectable disease at the primary site, followed by multidrug chemotherapy (usually vincristine, doxorubicin [Adriamycin, Pharmacia and Upjohn], and cyclophosphamide [Cytoxan, Mead Johnson]) and 5,000 cGy to 6,000 cGy of radiotherapy. The resection of this jaw tumor creates a continuity defect using bony margins of 3 cm and often includes a margin of surrounding tissue between 1 and 2 cm. If sufficient soft tissue remains, plate reconstruction is recommended. However, definitive bony reconstruction should be deferred until completion of radiotherapy and chemotherapy. In cases where there is insufficient bone to place a plate or the soft tissue loss would risk plate exposure, it may be better to let the jaw collapse into the defect rather than risk a wound-healing complication that would delay the chemotherapy/radiotherapy for more than 6 weeks.

PROGNOSIS ►

Before the advent of multimodal therapy, 5-year survival rates were approximately 15%. With multimodal therapy, patients who initially present without metastasis have a 70% 5-year survival rate. Even those with identifiable distant metastasis at presentation have a 30% 5-year survival rate. This is significant because 15% to 30% of Ewing sarcoma cases initially present with distant metastasis.

In contrast to the general rule of malignancy prognosis related to age of onset, younger patients with Ewing sarcoma have a better treatment response and 5-year survival rate than do older individuals. Generally, negative prognostic indications include larger tumor size, pain, leukocytosis, fever, and a high mitotic index. In those cases with lung metastasis, wedge resection of the metastatic deposit extends life and reduces symptoms.

Because Ewing sarcomas will usually recur within the first 2 years, initial follow-up is conducted every 3 months. The follow-up will consist of an oral and head and neck examination as well as local plain radiographs and a chest radiograph. After the first 2 years the frequency of follow-up examinations can be reduced to every 4 to 6 months.

Chondrosarcoma

Chondrosarcomas arise from mesenchymal stem cells and undergo a partial differentiation to form chondroblastic differentiation and even definable cartilage (see Fig 18-1b). A true chondrosarcoma cannot demonstrate bone formation from a malignant mesenchymal stroma. Such entities are actually osteosarcomas, which is especially important since many osteosarcomas of the jaws and facial bones have significant chondroblastic portions within them. However, if tumor bone arises from cartilage rather than from the malignant stroma, it remains a true chondrosarcoma.

Chondrosarcomas of the jaws and facial skeleton are much rarer than in other bones presumably because of the scarcity of cartilage in development and in the joint areas. Chondrosarcomas are second to osteosarcomas in their frequency as primary sarcomas of bone. Their overall incidence represents about 25% of all primary sarcomas of bone. However, of these, the face and jaw area represents only 2%.

Most chondrosarcomas of the facial skeleton and jaws occur in individuals older than 30 years with a slightly increasing frequency with advancing age. There is no race or sex predilection.

The presentation is that of a slow-growing mass. Pain may or may not be a presenting symptom. The mass will emanate from bone as an irregular lytic lesion that will palpate as a firm-to-hard lobulated soft tissue mass. Teeth involved with the lesion will be displaced and mobile. The mass is only rarely ulcerated. Most chondrosarcomas will be seen either in the anterior part of the maxilla or in the posterior body region of the mandible (Figs 18-15a and 18-15b). These areas of occurrence have been postulated to arise from remnants of embryonic cartilage precursors from nasal septal development in the anterior part of the maxilla and from Meckel cartilage precursors in the posterior aspect of the mandible.

Approximately 90% of chondrosarcomas will be slow-growing, low-grade, nonmetastasizing tumors. The remaining 10% demonstrate aggressive growth, significant local tissue invasion, and metastasis.

Because of their slow growth and their tendency to undergo neural invasion only later in their course, chondrosarcomas are often mistaken for "benign chondromas" or "cartilaginous rests." Several have presented with previous biopsies identifying "cartilage" where the patient was informed that it merely represented "ectopic cartilage." This false impression of a cartilage hamartoma or a benign cartilage-forming tumor is often supported by histopathologic features that will appear to be benign because of mature cartilage with little stroma and mostly single nuclei in each lacunae.

Chondrosarcomas will appear as irregular intramedullary radiolucencies causing cortical expansion and destruction. Punctate radiopacities may be present because of dystrophic calcifications or focal ossifications of cartilage. In the tooth-bearing areas, a widening of the periodontal ligament space (Garrington sign) may be seen as an early sign of chondrosarcoma, just as it is an early sign of osteosarcoma. Reactive extracortical bone may occasionally be seen as well.

Because of their slow growth and especially their intact overlying mucosa, most cases will initially resemble a *benign odontogenic tumor* or a *benign tumor of bone*. If the lesion is entirely radiolucent, the clinician may consider an *ameloblastoma* or *odontogenic myxoma*. If some punctate radiopacities are identifiable, the lesion will resemble a *calcifying epithelial odontogenic tumor*, an *ossifying fibroma*, an *immature osteoblastoma*, or a *cavernous hemangioma of bone*. The more obviously aggressive presentations with irregular radiolucencies and perhaps neurosensory loss would be consistent with an *intraosseous carcinoma*, an *osteosarcoma*, and a *malignant fibrous histiocytoma*. A benign chondroma or cartilage rests are not

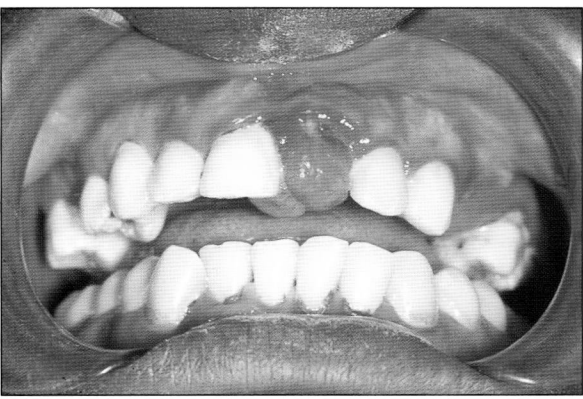

Fig 18-15a Oral chondrosarcomas are rare tumors. However, the anterior maxilla is where most develop.

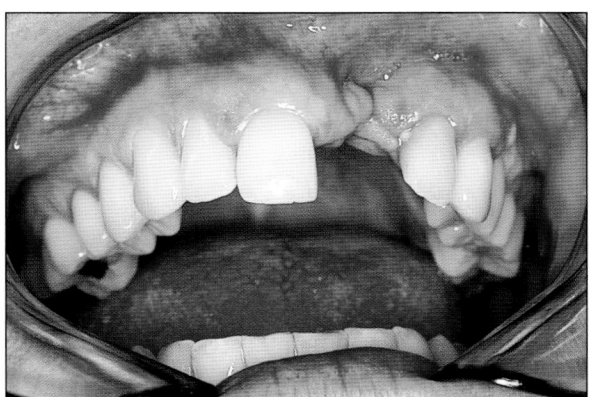

Fig 18-15b Although most oral chondrosarcomas are low grade, a simple local soft tissue excision is not curative. After an initial diagnostic biopsy, this area requires a local resection of bone.

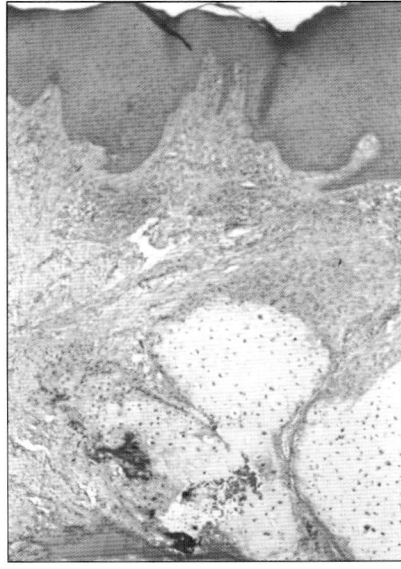

Fig 18-16a Chondrosarcoma with a lobular pattern. Large and variably sized chondrocytes also are seen.

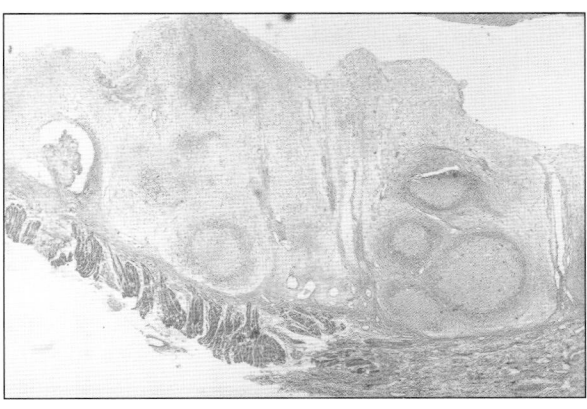

Fig 18-16b A low-grade chondrosarcoma with nodules of cartilage surrounded by less-differentiated chondroblasts.

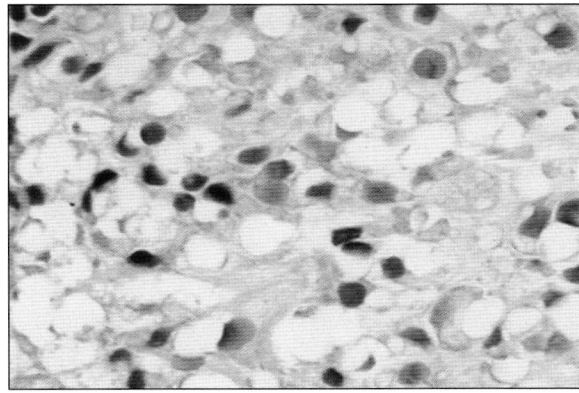

Fig 18-16c High-power view of Fig 18-16b in which hyperchromatism of the chondroblasts is apparent.

considered part of a differential diagnosis with this presentation because each is very rare and perhaps nonexistent. Accepting either of these as the final diagnosis may result in the overlooking of a true malignancy.

DIAGNOSTIC WORK-UP ▶

A deep incisional biopsy within the center of the mass is required as soon as possible. A tissue specimen is the only means of establishing a definitive diagnosis. The remainder of the work-up should include plain radiographs and a CT scan to determine tumor extent for surgical planning. Because cartilage itself and cartilaginous tumors are well demonstrated by magnetic resonance imaging (MRI), this modality may provide a better delineation of tumor extent than a CT scan. Although metastasis of chondrosarcomas is less frequent than with an osteosarcoma or other sarcomas, a chest radiograph is required to rule out this most likely place for a metastatic focus.

HISTOPATHOLOGY ▶

Chondrosarcomas are characterized by the formation of malignant cartilage without deposition of osteoid from a sarcomatous stroma. The cartilage cells have large, plump nuclei and are often binucleated or multinucleated. There is an increase in the number of cells, and lacunae often contain two or more cells. Pleomorphism and hyperchromatism also are present (Figs 18-16a to 18-16c). Histologic grading is

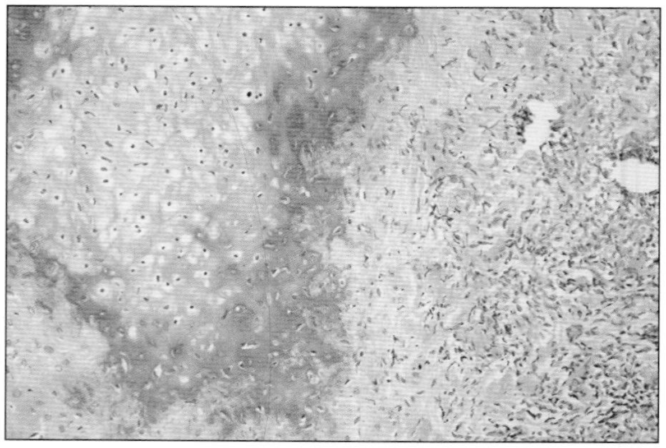

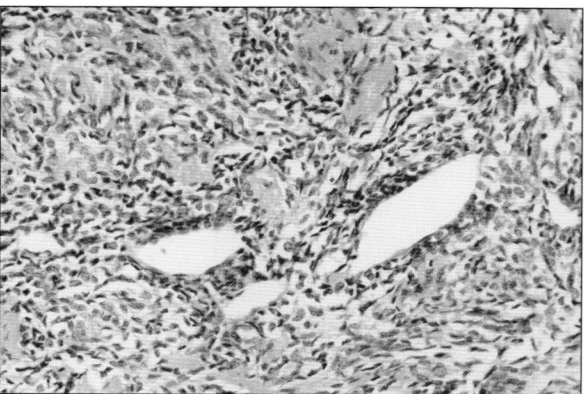

Fig 18-17a Mesenchymal chondrosarcoma showing an area of mature cartilage.

Fig 18-17b An area adjacent to that shown in Fig 18-17a showing spindle cells and poorly differentiated cells surrounding vascular channels.

important with regard to prognosis in chondrosarcoma. Grade I tumors tend to have a lobular pattern and two or more cells within a lacuna. There is endochondral ossification, and myxoid and cystic areas may develop. Grade II tumors show an increase in cellularity with retention of lobules and ossification, while grade III tumors are markedly cellular with a proliferation of spindle cells. The lobular pattern is lost. In the jaws, grade I tumors predominate.

Mesenchymal Chondrosarcoma

Mesenchymal chondrosarcomas contain islands of cartilage that may be well differentiated and circumscribed. The islands are surrounded by undifferentiated cells with round to oval hyperchromatic nuclei and a variable number of mitoses. In other tumors, the foci of cartilage may be scant. There may be a vascular stroma with branching vessels surrounded by malignant mesenchymal cells. This pattern simulates hemangiopericytoma (Figs 18-17a and 18-17b).

Mesenchymal chondrosarcomas are high-grade tumors that may metastasize to lymph nodes. Although they comprise only about 10% of chondrosarcomas, the jaws are a favored site.

TREATMENT AND PROGNOSIS ▶

The common low-grade chondrosarcomas (grades I and II) of the jaws and facial skeleton are best treated with a local resection using 1.5-cm margins for bone and soft tissue (Figs 18-18a to 18-18e). Neither chemotherapy nor radiotherapy is indicated as primary treatment. The uncommon high-grade chondrosarcomas (grade III) are treated with an initial aggressive resection of 3 cm in bone and 2 cm in soft tissue followed by chemotherapy. Because high-grade chondrosarcomas metastasize to regional lymph nodes more than do other sarcomas, an ipsilateral neck dissection also is recommended. In some cases, a high-grade chondrosarcoma can be treated with a protocol similar to that for an osteosarcoma: initial chemotherapy followed by aggressive resection surgery, which is followed by postoperative chemotherapy. However, the response of chondrosarcomas to chemotherapy is much poorer than that of most osteosarcomas.

Resultant defects in the anterior maxilla are usually obturated or reconstructed with a prosthesis (Figs 18-18f to 18-18i). Delayed reconstruction if needed with either soft tissue, usually from a temporalis flap, or bone grafting may be accomplished to provide better support for a prosthesis or to place osseointegrated implants. Defects in the mandible usually are initially reconstructed with a rigid titanium plate and soft tissue flaps if required. A delayed bone graft can be accomplished after initial healing is complete and the diagnosis is confirmed. This usually permits a definitive bone graft to be accomplished at about 3 to 4 months after extirpative surgery.

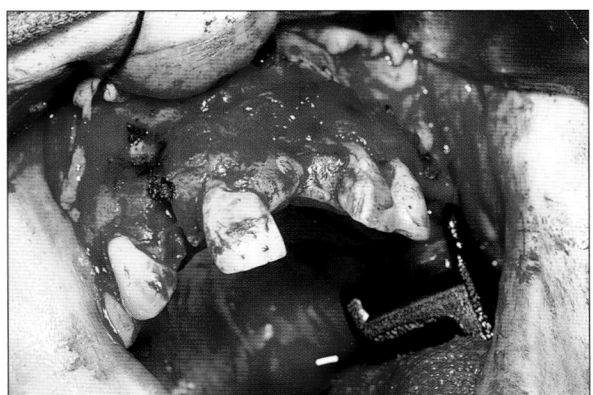

Fig 18-18a Low-grade chondrosarcoma treated with an anterior subnasal maxillary resection from the tooth socket of the right lateral incisor to the tooth socket of the left second premolar.

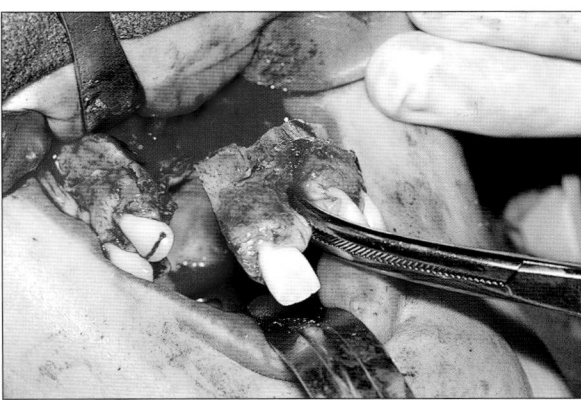

Fig 18-18b The resected bone and overlying mucosa are removed. The bone and soft tissue margins of the defect should be examined with frozen sections.

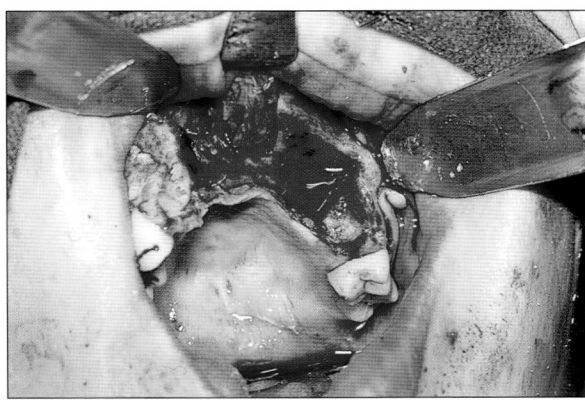

Fig 18-18c The resection defect removed the bony nasal floor and a portion of the sinus floor.

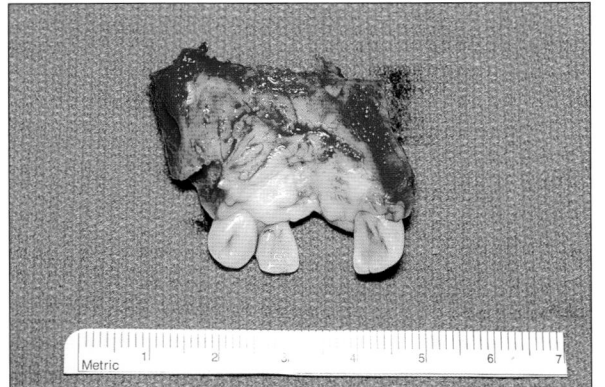

Fig 18-18d The surgeon should take the time to inspect the margins of the gross specimen.

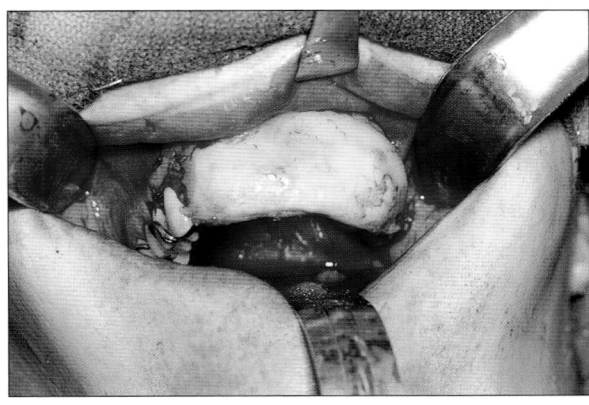

Fig 18-18e A surgical splint lined with a soft liner is fixed to the defect with a palatal screw.

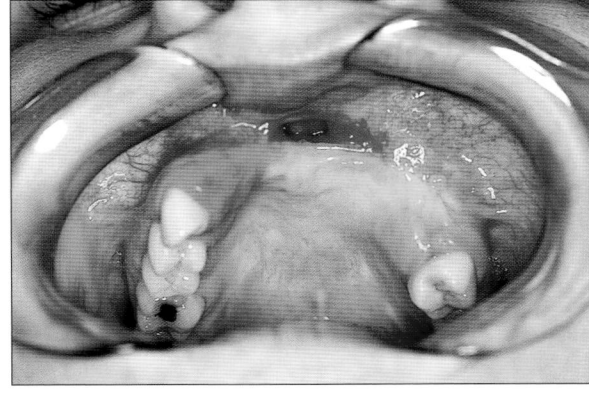

Fig 18-18f The defect will mature and become dimensionally stable at 6 months. Here the defect has mucosalized without any residual oronasal or oral-antral communication.

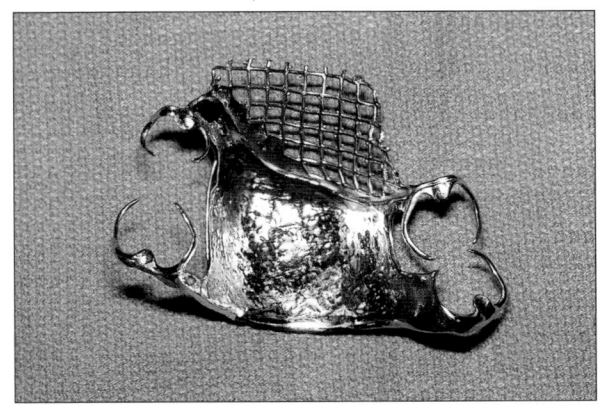

Fig 18-18g A straightforward means of reconstructing a tumor-related anterior maxillary defect of teeth, bone, and soft tissue is to use a cast framework removable partial denture. The cast palatal framework shown here will provide good stability and obviate the need for complex reconstructive surgeries.

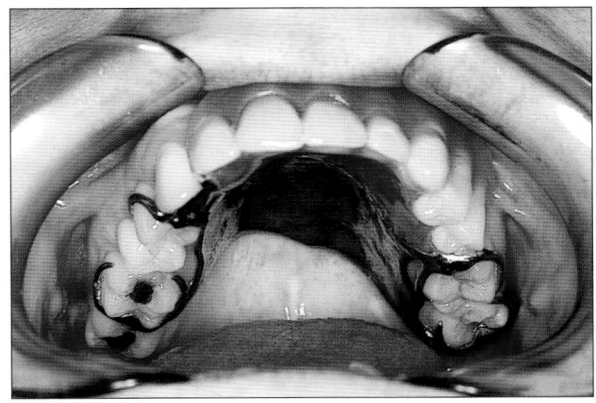

Fig 18-18h After 6 months, a definitive cast framework partial denture is used to stabilize the defect and replace the lost dentition. Without a prosthesis, the remaining teeth would tend to incline palatally and drift slightly to produce open contacts.

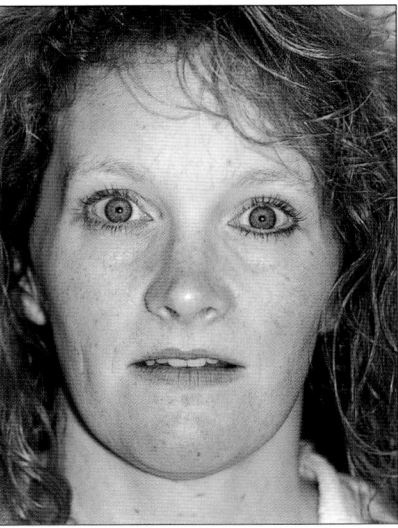

Fig 18-18i Use of an immediate surgical splint that is later replaced with a definitive partial denture prosthesis maintains the patient's lip position and facial appearance and also supports speech.

The prognosis for the more common low-grade chondrosarcoma is excellent. The 5-year survival rates are 90% for grade I and 81% for grade II. However, the less common, high-grade (grade III) chondrosarcomas are associated with a 29% 5-year survival rate.

When low-grade chondrosarcomas recur, they recur late. Most first recur between 5 and 10 years after initial treatment. At that time, a second surgery (salvage surgery) can result in a cure. However, it is best to resect with even wider margins than those used in the initial surgery. Recommended margins are 3 cm in bone and 2 cm in soft tissue. Even then, an occasional low-grade chondrosarcoma may become uncontrollable, eventuating in death despite repeated surgeries and chemotherapy. In some instances, recurrence may be associated with a more advanced histologic grade than the initial tumor. This seeming "dedifferentiation" is instead thought to represent a resistant tumor clone arising from an additional mutation within the original tumor. High-grade (grade III) chondrosarcomas more often fail cure by distant metastasis (66%), most often to the lungs. However, lymph node metastasis also can develop if the initial therapy did not include a neck dissection.

FOLLOW-UP ▶ Low-grade chondrosarcomas (grades I and II) may occur any time over several decades. Therefore, follow-up is lifelong and can be limited to an oral and head and neck examination and local radiographic studies. Semi-annual chest radiographs also are recommended.

High-grade chondrosarcomas (grade III) usually recur within the first 2 years. Therefore, follow-up consisting of an oral and head and neck examination, local radiographs, and a chest radiograph are recommended every 4 months for the first 2 years. For the next 3 years, these examinations are conducted every 6 months, and then annually thereafter.

Radiation Sarcoma

CLINICAL PRESENTATION AND PATHOGENESIS ▶ Radiation sarcomas will usually arise in an individual who mistakenly received radiotherapy for a fibro-osseous disease or a benign bone tumor. It will sometimes also arise in previously normal bone that was in the path of radiotherapy for an oral carcinoma. Though well intentioned, radiotherapy for fibro-osseous diseases such as fibrous dysplasia and cherubism, as well as Paget disease, is contraindicated. Radiotherapy also is contraindicated in the treatment of benign bone tumors. Not only is the response of these conditions to radiotherapy nontherapeutic, the risk of malignant transformation is very high. Radiation therapy is a treatment for established malignancies because it induces indirect DNA, RNA, and enzyme alterations leading to cell death. It is, therefore, mutagenic. Benign bone tumors and fibro-osseous disease are thought to be more vulnerable to malignant transformation because they already possess inherent DNA alterations and are more actively replicating, thereby permitting greater DNA exposure to the DNA-damaging effects of radiotherapy.

The histologic types of radiation-induced sarcomas are not limited to osteosarcomas, as some believe. Included are chondrosarcomas and malignant fibrous histiocytomas as well. Each of these malignancies will appear radiographically and histopathologically identical to their conventionally seen de novo types. However, radiation-induced sarcomas are known to behave somewhat more aggressively and to be less responsive to treatment.

It should also be noted that radiation can also transform a low-grade mesenchymal malignancy into a high-grade one with a higher metastatic potential. In addition, radiation therapy may also produce a delayed emergence of radiation carcinomas. Such cases have been seen in irradiated oral mucosa and are particularly noted in the thyroid gland.

The individual usually presents with a destructive soft tissue or bony mass arising from a pre-existing fibro-osseous disease focus or bone tumor (Fig 18-19). Early cases are not easily detected and may only be noted as a lytic change or an increase in the radiodensity of the area. Some cases may be suspected by the unexpected development of pain, a rapid clinical expansion, or neurosensory loss. The history of radiotherapy will almost always be a dose exceeding 4,000 cGy. Dosages less than 4,000 cGy are

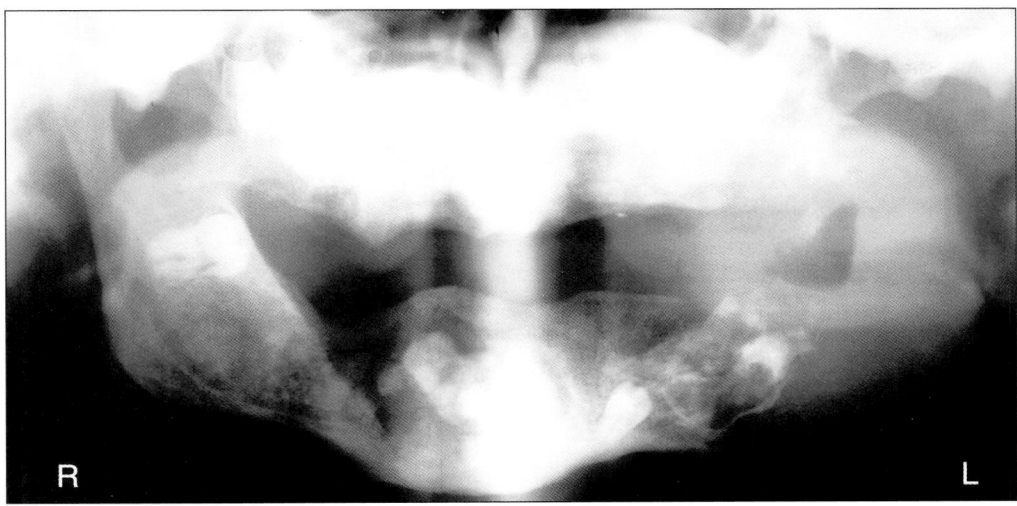

Fig 18-19 Panoramic radiograph showing the significant destruction of the left hemimandible by a radiation sarcoma. This 59-year-old underwent radiotherapy for cherubism at age 10.

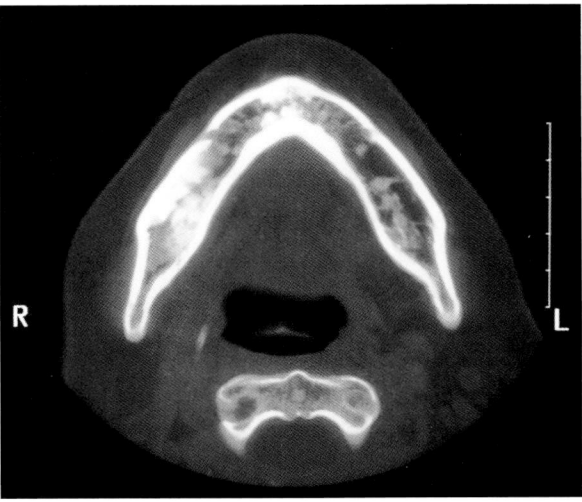

Fig 18-20 Early radiation sarcoma in the medullary space of the right body and angle regions of the mandible. This resulted from radiotherapy for an oral mucosal squamous cell carcinoma of the lateral border of the tongue.

uncommonly used for most other conditions and have not produced many reported cases. Therefore, patients who may have received lower-dose radiation therapy for acne, Kaposi sarcoma, Langerhans cell disease, etc, are presumably not at as high a risk for later development of a sarcoma as are those who received a higher dose. In either case, the history of radiotherapy is usually 5 to 10 years in the past. However, the time of past radiotherapy may be as long as 35 or even 50 years.

RADIOGRAPHIC FINDINGS

Radiation-induced osteosarcomas will have the same radiographic appearance as their de novo counterparts (see Fig 18-19). That is, they may be completely radiolucent or mixed radiolucent–radiopaque. A "sun-ray" appearance of reactive bone or tumor bone may be noted as well. Early radiation-induced osteosarcomas may appear as a more subtle endosseous diffuse radiopacity (Fig 18-20). Radiation-induced chondrosarcomas will appear as a mostly irregular lytic lesion but may also have small punctate calcifications within it. Other radiation-induced sarcomas will be expansile and lytic. Many will lead to a pathologic fracture.

DIFFERENTIAL DIAGNOSIS

The differential diagnosis of a painful, expansile mass in a previously radiated area is limited. A radiation-induced *sarcoma* would be considered first, as would possibly a radiation-induced *carcinoma with bony invasion*. However, both *osteoradionecrosis*, which is often partially radiolucent and radiopaque and may have an associated soft tissue infection causing swelling, and a true *osteomyelitis* may present with similar findings. Even a *sclerosing osteomyelitis* within a radiated mandible is possible and will present with pain and endosteal sclerosis mimicking an early radiation-induced osteosarcoma.

HISTOPATHOLOGY

The majority of radiation-induced sarcomas are osteosarcomas. The Mayo Clinic (Rochester, MN) also reported a large percentage of fibrosarcomas, whereas Memorial Sloan-Kettering (New York, NY) found a large percentage of malignant fibrous histiocytomas. It is not clear if this is related to the more recent recognition of many fibrosarcomas as malignant fibrous histiocytomas.

In general, tumors are rather poorly differentiated. The proportion of fibrosarcomas and malignant fibrous histiocytomas that are radiation induced is higher than that for osteosarcomas. All histologic types of these tumors are encountered. Other types of sarcomas, including chondrosarcomas and Ewing sarcoma, may arise, but are rare.

TREATMENT AND PROGNOSIS

Although radiation-induced sarcomas histologically appear nearly identical to their de novo counterparts, they represent a malignancy with a more aggressive clinical behavior and a greater resistance to treatment, particularly chemotherapy. Therefore, the treatment begins with a wide surgical resection using at least 3-cm margins in bone and at least 2-cm margins in soft tissue. Frozen section assessment of the margins is necessary to identify areas of particularly aggressive extension. Resultant bony defects are usually reconstructed with a rigid plate in the mandible and with an obturator-prosthesis in the maxilla. Soft tissue reconstruction with pedicled myocutaneous flaps or with free vascular transfers are often necessary. Postoperative chemotherapy is recommended, with the choice of chemotherapy agents corresponding to the histopathologic features of the tumor.

The prognosis associated with radiation-induced sarcomas is poor. Sarcomas in general have a poor prognosis, with 5-year survival statistics ranging from 30% to 50% with aggressive treatment. The survival associated with radiation-induced sarcomas is less than one half that of their de novo counterparts. Accurate survival statistics related to radiation-induced sarcomas are not available because of their low incidence. However, 5-year survival rates are estimated to be only 10% to 25%.

Fibrosarcoma

CLINICAL PRESENTATION ►

Since the 1990s, when true fibrosarcomas were first distinguished from malignant fibrous histiocytomas, they have been found to be very rare. Fibrosarcomas are distinct from malignant fibrous histiocytomas by virtue of a uniform spindle cell fibroblastic cell population arranged in parallel bands or a herringbone pattern. The malignant fibrous histiocytoma has round mononuclear cells with significant pleomorphism mixed with the fibroblastic cells and a whorled arrangement called a *storiform pattern* (Fig 18-21).

The fibrosarcoma also differs from the malignant fibrous histiocytoma by virtue of its various grades. Not all are high-grade malignancies like malignant fibrous histiocytoma. In fact, some are very low grade in behavior and in histopathology. Some of these may have an onset of more than a year's duration, indicative of slow but infiltrative growth. They occur in an even age distribution between 10 and 70 years with no sex predilection.

In the jaws, a fibrosarcoma will present as a fleshy to firm mass destructive of bone and often growing out of bone (Fig 18-22a). Bone resorption in an ill-defined, irregular pattern is common. Pain is usually not the chief complaint; instead, it is usually jaw expansion and tooth mobility (Fig 18-22b). Paresthesia and overt anesthesia are often seen if the tumor is near a nerve trunk.

RADIOGRAPHIC APPEARANCE ►

Radiographs and CT scans will show an ill-defined and irregular bone resorption (see Fig 18-22b). Early or low-grade tumors may show a widening of the periodontal membrane space (Garrington sign) or a "floating tooth" appearance due to extensive resorption of alveolar bone. There should be no extracortical bone formation. On a CT scan, the soft tissue mass will appear to gradually blend into the surrounding tissues, indicative of its infiltrative growth.

DIFFERENTIAL DIAGNOSIS ►

The destructive radiographic pattern and the fleshy to firm mass will be suggestive of both *malignant fibrous histiocytoma* and an *osteosarcoma*, which has little if any tumor bone formation. In young individuals, the presentation may resemble that of a *Ewing sarcoma* or a *rhabdomyosarcoma*. In older adults, the presentation is consistent with *carcinomas metastatic to bone* such as from the lung, prostate, breast, or kidney. If the mass is more fleshy than firm, it may clinically resemble a *non-Hodgkin lymphoma*.

Although some believe that the *desmoplastic fibroma* and *aggressive fibromatosis* represent a very low-grade fibrosarcoma (grade $1/2$), these may be part of the differential diagnosis as separate entities with an improved prognosis.

DIAGNOSTIC WORK-UP ►

The mass should undergo biopsy without delay. As with all other mass lesions in the jaws, the biopsy should be taken from the lesion's center to avoid the possibility of confusion created by overlying scar tissue or inflammation caused by exposure to the oral environment.

A CT scan is recommended to assess the degree of bony involvement and the tumor extension into surrounding soft tissues. A chest radiograph is required to rule out metastasis to the lung, which is the most common organ to which fibrosarcoma metastasizes.

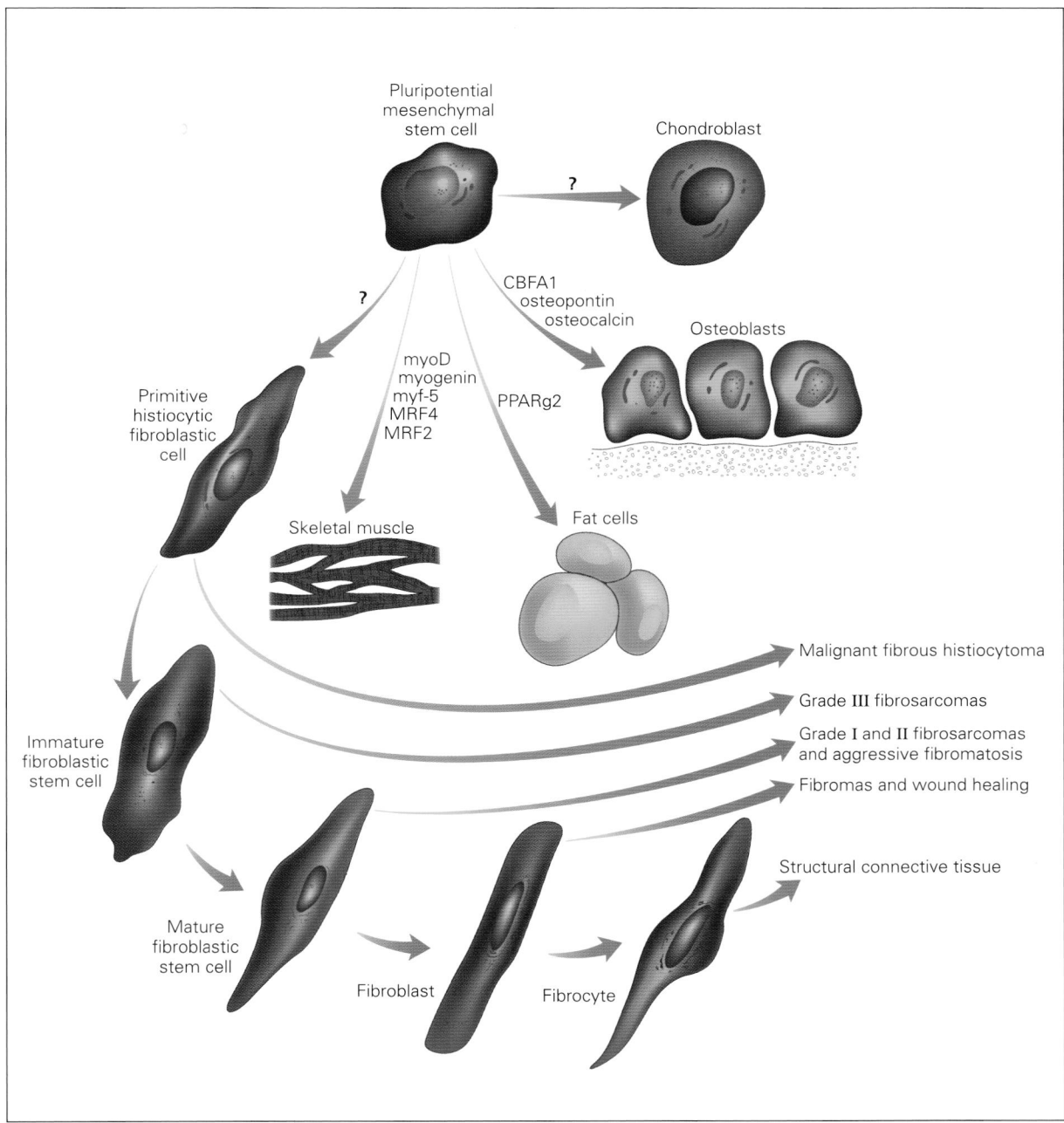

Fig 18-21 All sarcomas arise from the pluripotential mesenchymal stem cell or one of its early progeny. Each of the multiple stages in this cell maturation sequence can give rise to a neoplasia. The earlier (less differentiated) stages are thought to give rise to the higher-grade and more aggressive malignancies, such as the malignant fibrous histiocytoma and the grade III fibrosarcoma. Cells in the later (more differentiated) stages of the maturation sequence are thought to be the parent cells of the lower-grade and even benign tumors.

HISTOPATHOLOGY ▶

Fibrosarcomas are spindle cell, fibroblastic tumors that produce varying amounts of collagen but no osteoid or cartilage. Those occurring in bone are histologically identical to those occurring in soft tissue. Well-differentiated tumors demonstrate a herringbone pattern with rare mitoses (Figs 18-23a and 18-23b). More poorly differentiated tumors will show more mitoses, which are often abnormal, and less collagen production with a loss of the herringbone pattern. The less collagen that is produced, the more densely packed are the nuclei. Tumors that are less differentiated are more likely to resemble malignant fibrohistiocytomas. Immunohistochemically, alpha-1-antitrypsin, alpha-1-antichymotrypsin, and lysozyme are

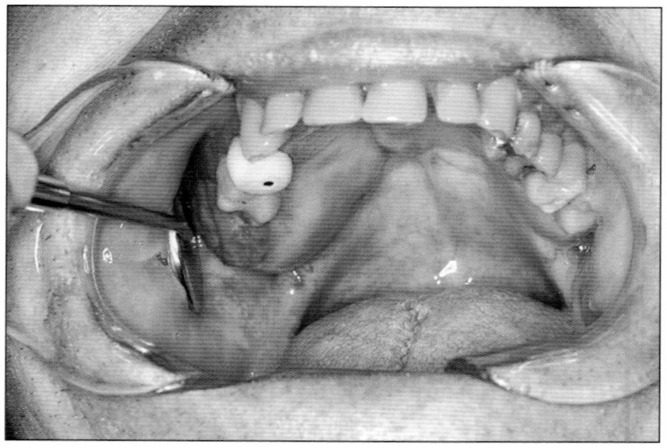

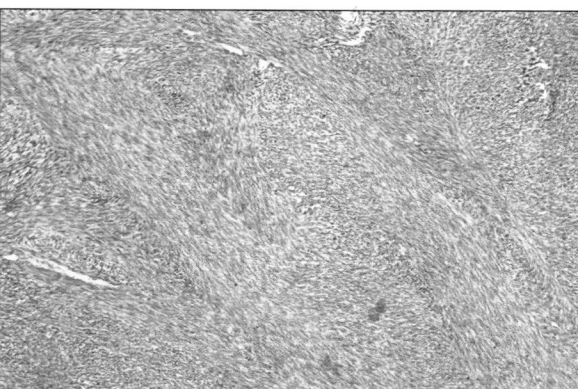

Fig 18-22a Fibrosarcomas that arise in the jaws will usually produce a fleshy or firm destructive mass arising from bone. They may ulcerate and often create significant tooth mobility.

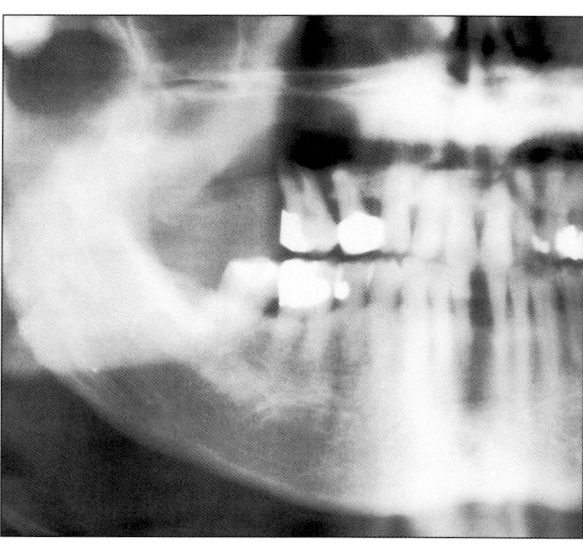

Fig 18-22b This grade III fibrosarcoma resorbed most of the posterior maxilla. Two teeth have the appearance of floating within the area of bony destruction and, of course, had 4-plus mobility.

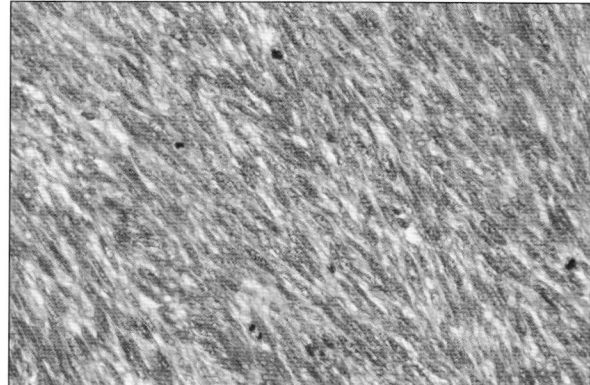

Fig 18-23a The herringbone pattern of this well-differentiated fibrosarcoma is apparent.

Fig 18-23b High-power view of Fig 18-23a showing densely packed nuclei with little collagen formation and some scattered mitoses.

TREATMENT AND BIOLOGIC BEHAVIOR ▶

negative for fibrosarcomas but positive for malignant fibrous histiocytomas. Fibrosarcomas must also be distinguished from desmoplastic fibromas and fibroblastic osteosarcomas. The latter show alkaline phosphatase activity, while fibrosarcomas do not. Reactive bone formation should not be misconstrued as tumor bone deposition.

The general consensus is that true fibrosarcomas are of only low-grade to intermediate-grade nature at most (grades I and II). Most high-grade fibrosarcomas actually represent malignant fibrous histiocytomas. Therefore, the clinician should be sure that he or she and the pathologist understand each other's definitions of the diagnosis and of the tumor grading.

If the tumor is indeed a true fibrosarcoma, chemotherapy may not be required. Rather than combined therapy, resective surgery becomes the sole treatment modality.

Fibrosarcomas in the mandible require a continuity resection with 1.5- to 2.0-cm margins in both bone and soft tissue. The bony defect can undergo immediate stabilization with a rigid plate followed by delayed bony reconstruction after the mucosa has healed. If the tumor was sufficiently large to create a significant soft tissue defect, a myocutaneous flap or free vascular flap may be used for reconstruction.

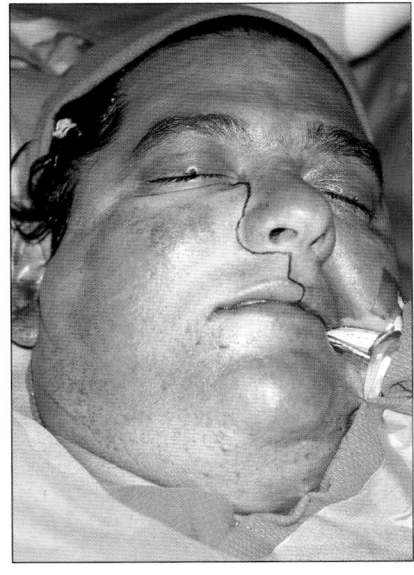

Fig 18-24a Here a Weber-Ferguson type of incision is planned to reduce scarring and prevent an upward lip retraction. This is a posterior-based cheek flap through the right philtrum ridge that is stepped to the midline along the vermilion border.

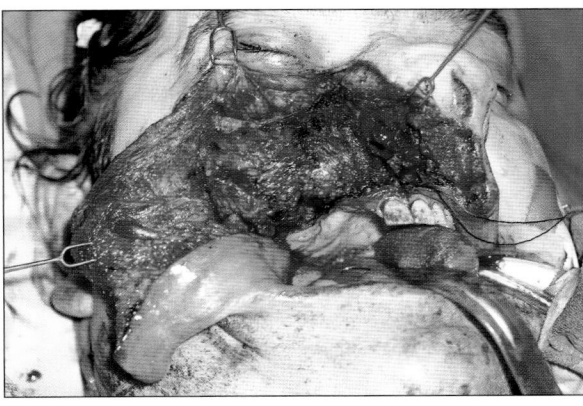

Fig 18-24b A grade III fibrosarcoma or malignant fibrous histiocytoma significantly infiltrates surrounding tissue, requiring wide access and frozen section assessments of all margins.

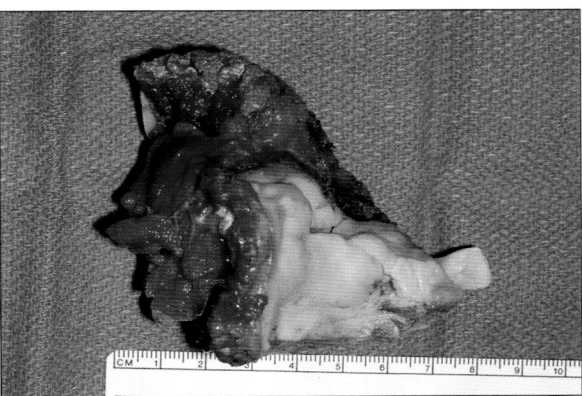

Fig 18-24c The resection specimen of grade III fibrosarcoma and malignant fibrous histiocytoma will usually include bone, adjacent soft tissue, and mucosa.

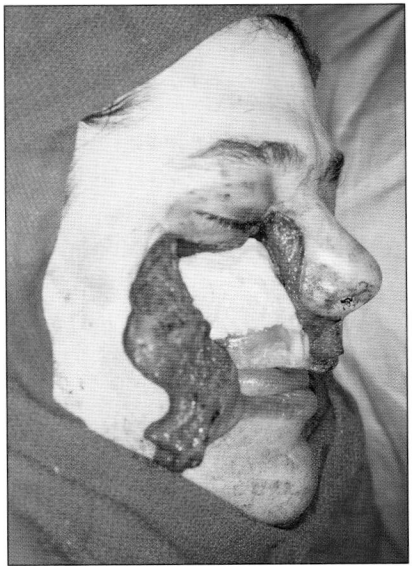

Fig 18-24d A large hemimaxillectomy defect will require an oral splint or modified denture for both obturation and cheek support.

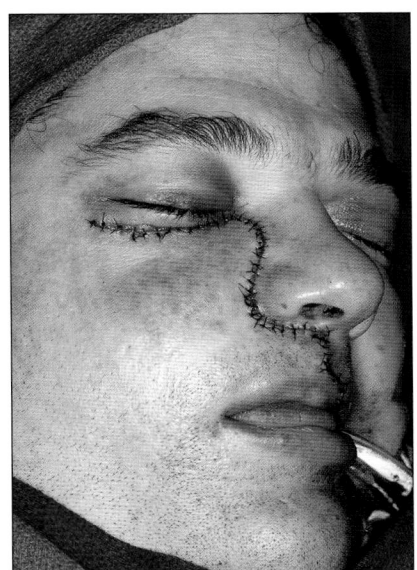

Fig 18-24e The Weber-Ferguson cheek flap is sutured over the oral splint to support the flap and provide cheek contour.

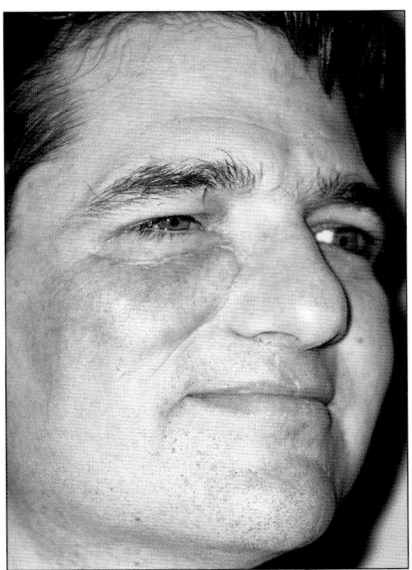

Fig 18-24f Bone and soft tissue reconstruction, along with a well-placed incision and an obturator prosthesis, allow maintenance of good function and facial contours. Note that lip retraction was prevented by the step design in the lip split.

In the maxilla, a type of partial maxillectomy is required (Figs 18-24a to 18-24c). A Weber-Ferguson type of incision is preferred when the tumor threatens the orbit or ethmoids or invades through the posterior maxilla. Otherwise a transoral approach may be used. The resultant oral-nasal-antral defect is best obturated at the time of surgery with a premade obturator splint (Figs 18-24d to 18-24f). This surgical obturator splint can be fixated at the time of surgery with either a palatal screw or with zygomatic buttress wires and then kept in place for about 2 weeks. At that time, the wires and/or screws are removed and the obturator splint converted into or replaced by a relined interim prosthesis. This interim prosthesis may have teeth, but the occlusion should be light and protected. After the first 6 months of tissue maturation and contraction, the interim prosthesis can be replaced with a final prosthesis.

A neck dissection is not required unless an obvious palpable node suggestive of tumor is present. Chemotherapy or radiation also is not required unless the tumor is high grade (ie, grade III).

PROGNOSIS ▶

The usual true fibrosarcomas, which represent a low-grade malignancy, have an 80% 10-year survival rate. Recurrences at the surgical site do occur. However, because of the tumor's low-grade, slow growth, and minimal metastatic potential, salvage surgery often effects a cure. Metastasis to the lungs does occur but much less frequently than with other sarcomas such as osteosarcoma, Ewing sarcoma, or malignant fibrous histiocytoma. Most high-grade fibrosarcomas are today diagnosed as malignant fibrous histiocytomas and have only a 30% to 40% 5-year survival rate.

FOLLOW-UP ▶

Low- to intermediate-grade fibrosarcomas (grades I and II) may occur any time over several decades. Therefore, follow-up is lifelong and can be limited to an oral and head and neck examination and local radiographic studies. Semi-annual chest radiographs also are recommended.

High-grade fibrosarcomas (grade III) usually recur within the first 2 years. Therefore, follow-up consisting of an oral and head and neck examination, local radiographs, and a chest radiograph are recommended every 4 months for the first 2 years. For the next 3 years, these examinations are conducted every 6 months, and then annually thereafter.

Malignant Fibrous Histiocytoma

CLINICAL PRESENTATION ▶

Malignant fibrous histiocytomas are aggressive infiltrating malignancies with a poor prognosis. Until the early 1990s, most were incorrectly diagnosed as high-grade fibrosarcomas. Today malignant fibrous histiocytomas are distinguished from fibrosarcomas histologically by their storiform pattern of primitive fibroblasts mixed with pleomorphic mononuclear cells resembling histiocytes or even rhabdomyoblasts. There will also be significant numbers of atypical mitoses. In contrast, the true fibrosarcoma will show only primitive fibroblasts in a parallel or herringbone pattern. Nevertheless, the histogenesis of each tumor is the mesenchymal stem cell line and/or its early progeny down the pathway to a mature fibroblast (often also called *myofibroblast*) lineage. The malignant fibrous histiocytoma actually has two cell components: one is the primitive fibroblast and the other an even more primitive mesenchymal stem cell that takes on the features of a mononuclear histiocyte.

Clinically, the malignant fibrous histiocytoma should be viewed as a high-grade sarcoma (Fig 18-25a). It will present as a destructive radiolucency in bone with expansion, and it may develop quickly. Many reports describe a duration of onset of 3 months or less. Some cases will exhibit pain, but many will not. In the jaws, mobile teeth and bony expansion are the most frequent initial complaints. Paresthesia of nerve distributions within the tumor area is not a prominent feature of this malignancy, although it has occurred.

Malignant fibrous histiocytoma is rare. It makes up only 2% of all malignant tumors in bone and has a lower incidence in the jaws than in long bones. Although it has occurred in nearly all ages, its peak incidence is in the 60-year age group.

RADIOGRAPHIC FINDINGS ▶

The typical appearance will be an ill-defined, irregular resorption of bone without new bone formation or extracortical bone formation. This completely radiolucent, destructive radiographic appearance is not distinctive of a malignant fibrous histiocytoma but is generally consistent with a high-grade malignancy. Alveolar bone resorption will create the appearance of "floating teeth," and an irregular root resorption of teeth may be seen as well.

A CT or MRI scan will demonstrate a soft tissue mass that is erosive into bone in an irregular pattern. Each should also show a gradual blending of the tumor mass into surrounding muscle and other soft tissues, indicative of its infiltrative growth (Fig 18-25b).

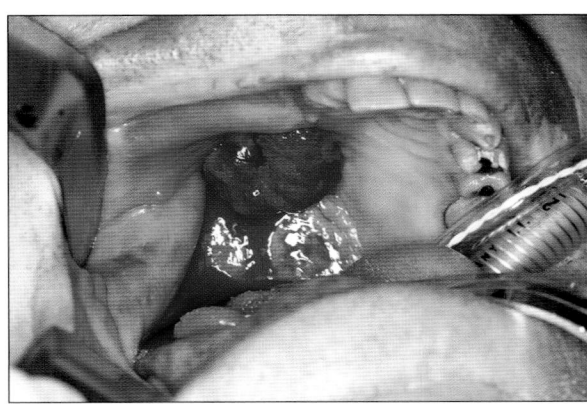

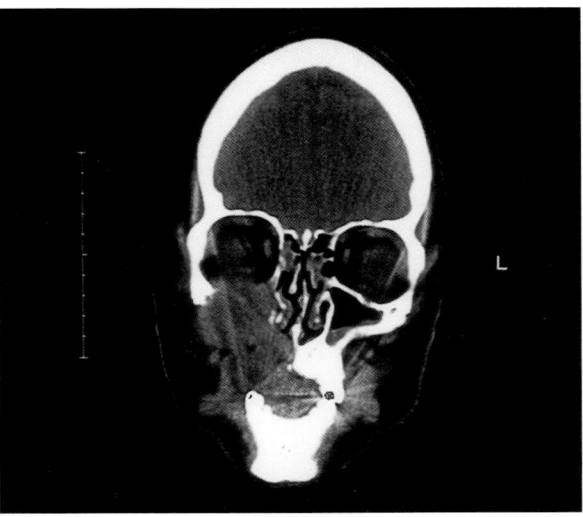

Fig 18-25a Malignant fibrous histiocytomas are high-grade sarcomas that may clinically arise from the jaws as a fleshy or, less frequently, a firm soft tissue mass.

Fig 18-25b The malignant fibrous histiocytoma shown clinically in Fig 18-25a was only a small portion of a much larger destructive tumor effacing the right hemi-maxilla and invading the nasal cavity, orbit, and zygoma.

DIFFERENTIAL DIAGNOSIS ▶

An aggressive and rapidly growing irregular radiolucency in the jaws suggests a subset of malignant tumors. Certainly other sarcomas, such as a true *fibrosarcoma*, an *osteosarcoma* with no radiographically apparent tumor bone or reactive bone formation, a *chondrosarcoma,* and some *non-Hodgkin lymphomas*, are to be considered. A *Ewing sarcoma* would not be a realistic consideration unless the patient were 25 years or younger. Metastatic malignancies to the jaws would present an identical picture. Therefore, consideration of *lung cancers*, *prostate cancers* in men, *breast cancers* in women, and *renal cancers* is also reasonable. In addition, some aggressive unencapsulated benign or low-grade malignancies of mesenchymal stem cells, such as the rare *desmoplastic fibroma* and *fibromatoses*, should also be considered. It is also well to remember that *squamous cell carcinoma* remains the most common oral cancer. A small primary squamous cell carcinoma can invade bone and produce a significant degree of destruction, mimicking a malignancy of bone without necessarily producing a noticeable surface presence.

DIAGNOSTIC WORK-UP ▶

A biopsy to confirm the suspicion of malignancy should not be delayed. The biopsy specimen should be taken from the tumor's center and sufficient tissue taken in anticipation of multiple sections for consultants and perhaps for special stains. A CT or MRI scan of the head and neck area is recommended to assess the degree of invasion, size of the tumor, and its relationship to known anatomic structures. Because this malignancy, like most sarcomas, has a marked propensity for lung metastasis, a chest radiograph is needed.

HISTOPATHOLOGY ▶

Malignant fibrous histiocytomas of bone are histologically identical to those in soft tissue. While several patterns have been described, they are all characterized by the proliferation of fibroblasts, histiocyte-like cells, and anaplastic giant cells. The most common pattern is storiform-pleomorphic, in which fibroblastic spindle cells have a whorled or cartwheel arrangement (Fig 18-26a) in the presence of multinucleated giant cells. Other types include a predominantly histiocytic proliferation with a xanthomatous component and numerous multinucleated giant cells (Fig 18-26b). Myxoid, inflammatory, and angiomatoid types have also been described.

The most notable tumor in the histologic differential diagnosis is fibrosarcoma, which, however, lacks the storiform pattern and xanthomatous cells. Alpha-1-antitrypsin, alpha-1-antichymotrypsin, and lysozyme are all positive in malignant fibrous histiocytoma and negative in fibrosarcoma.

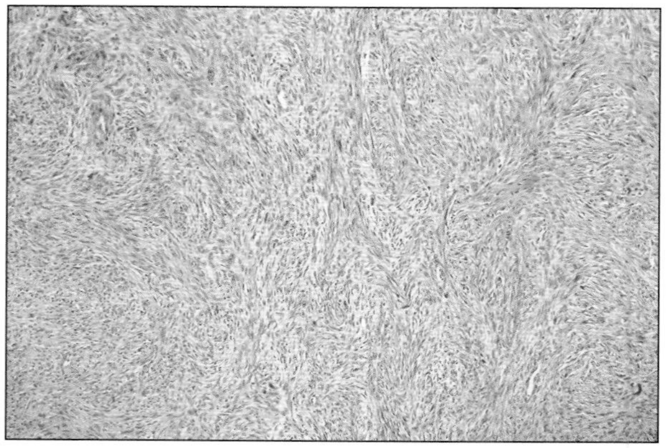

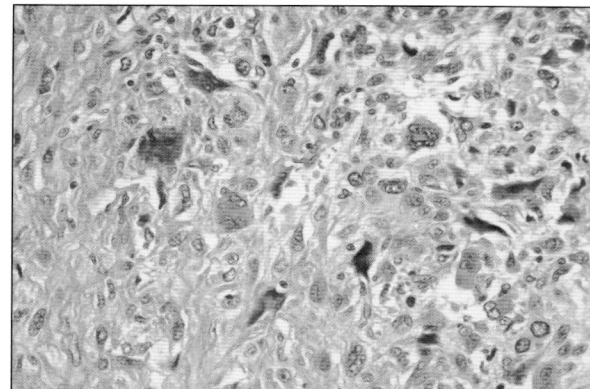

Fig 18-26a Malignant fibrous histiocytoma showing the storiform pattern formed by spindle cells. Some giant cells are present.

Fig 18-26b Malignant fibrous histiocytoma with a more pronounced histiocytic appearance and atypical multinucleated giant cells.

Prognosis relates to the grade of the tumor, which in turn reflects the degree of differentiation, infiltration, mitotic activity, and necrosis.

TREATMENT ▶

Treatment of malignant fibrous histiocytomas is a combination of initial (neo-adjuvant) chemotherapy and resection. The surgery is much like that for osteosarcomas of the jaws. That is, a resection should attempt 3-cm margins in bone and 2-cm margins in soft tissue. Bony resection in the mandible often requires extirpation of the condyle to obtain a tumor-free margin, but excision of the temporal fossa would not be likely unless there was direct tumor extension. The mandibular defect can be reconstructed with a titanium plate, and because a reasonable amount of soft tissue excision is often required, a myocutaneous or free vascular flap may be needed as well. In the maxilla, resection often extends to include the pterygoid plates, a portion of the zygoma, and, if the orbital floor is infiltrated, an orbital exenteration.

Chemotherapy agents will be selected by the medical oncologist, but doxorubicin (Adriamycin, Pharmacia and Upjohn), vincristine, cis-platinum, cyclophosphamide (Cytoxan, Mead Johnson), and prednisone are the agents most commonly used. Postoperative chemotherapy is recommended if the individual can tolerate it. Because of the rarity of the condition and hence the lack of data, the value of postoperative chemotherapy is less certain than it is for osteosarcoma. Radiotherapy may be added as a treatment modality as a postoperative option, particularly if margins were not free of tumor, but its value remains unproven.

PROGNOSIS ▶

Prognosis is poor. The 5-year survival rates associated with aggressive combined treatments are between 35% and 40%. Treatment with only one modality is associated with a 20% 5-year survival rate. Therapeutic failures most commonly result from uncontrolled local recurrences (70%). These recurrences may develop within just 3 to 6 months. Metastasis to the lungs is the second most common cause of failure.

FOLLOW-UP ▶

Because malignant fibrous histiocytomas are all high-grade, aggressive sarcomas, the early follow-up periods are frequent. An oral and head and neck examination, local radiographs, and a chest radiograph are recommended every 4 months for the first 2 years and then every 6 months for the following 3 years. After 5 years, follow-up examination should be accomplished annually.

Carcinoma Metastatic to Bone and Soft Tissue

The bones of the mandible in particular and to a lesser extent the maxilla are frequent sites for metastatic deposits from carcinomas elsewhere in the body. Statistics vary somewhat among reports, but the most common originating site is the female breast (35%) followed by the lungs (28%) and kidneys (15%).

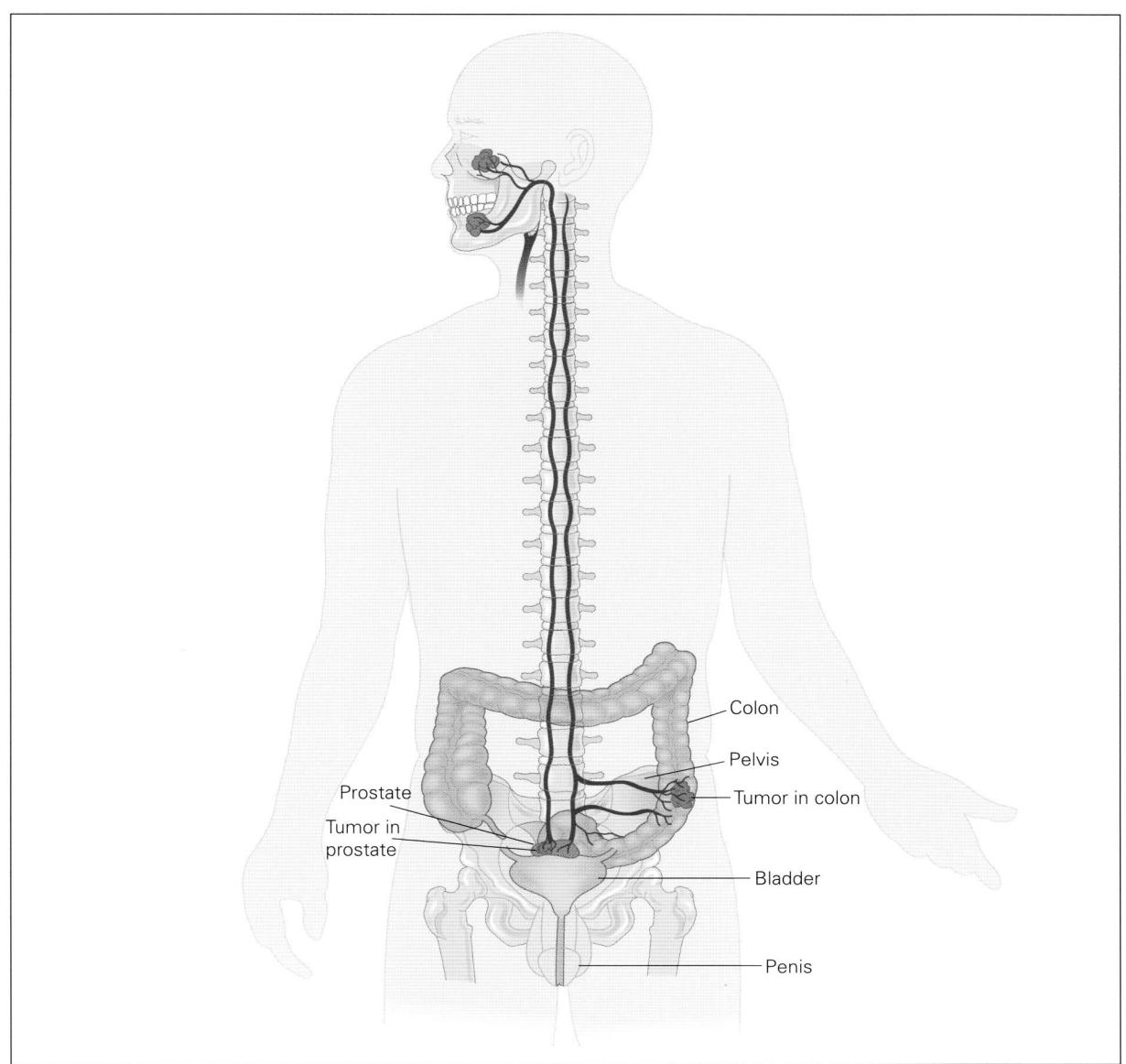

Fig 18-27 Carcinomas arising from the colon, prostate, or bladder can develop metastatic deposits in the jaws or other head and neck sites via tumor emboli that flow through the valveless paravertebral veins of Batson and thereby avoid the filtering mechanisms of the liver and lungs.

After these, several other areas deposit metastatic foci in the jaws at nearly the same relative incidence: prostate (6%), thyroid (6%), and stomach and lower gastrointestinal tract (6%).

The main mechanism for this metastatic spread is a backflow through the venous system. In 1919, Oscar Batson proved a pathway from the male genital-prostate area to the brain. He injected methylene blue into a cadaver's dorsal vein of the penis and saw it fill the paravertebral plexus to emerge in the cerebral cortex. This *paravertebral plexus of Batson* is now recognized as the main pathway for carcinomas at a distant site to settle in the jaws or any tissue above the lungs (Fig 18-27). By any other route, a carcinoma embolus would either drain from the lower abdomen into the portal vein to eventually deposit in the liver, or enter the inferior vena cava (if below the diaphragm) or the superior vena cava (if above the diaphragm) to eventually be deposited in the lungs after passing through the right side of the heart and pulmonary artery. Primarily the lungs but also the liver represent the main filters of blood flow, which is why the lungs and liver account for more than 80% of all metastatic deposits.

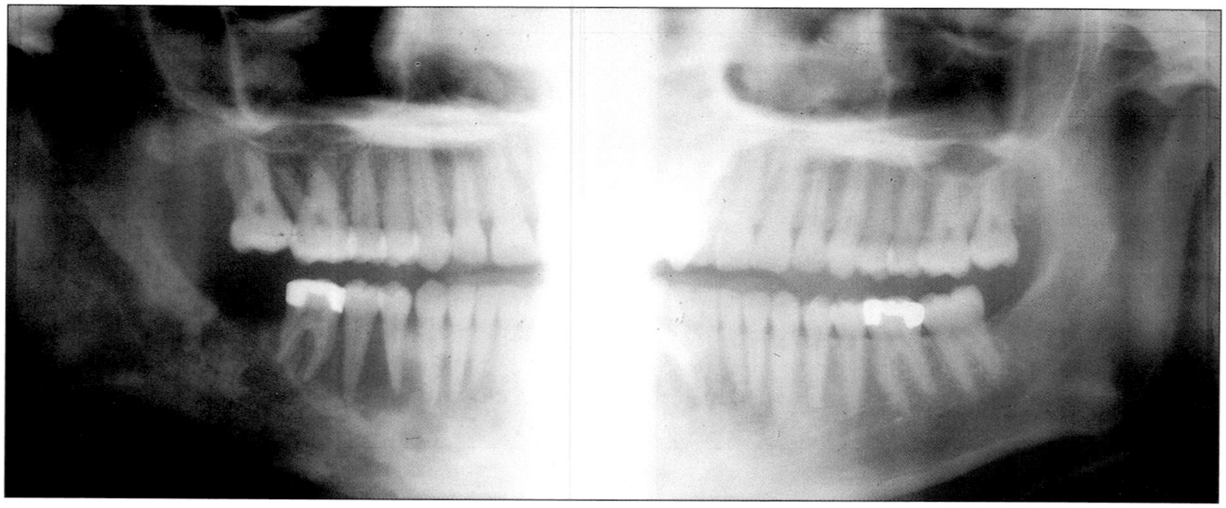

Fig 18-28 Significant alveolar bone loss from a metastatic deposit from a lung cancer. The teeth exhibited 3-plus mobility. Metastatic malignancies to the jaws are often first recognized because of tooth mobility or what appears to be local periodontal disease inconsistent with the periodontal health of the remaining dentition.

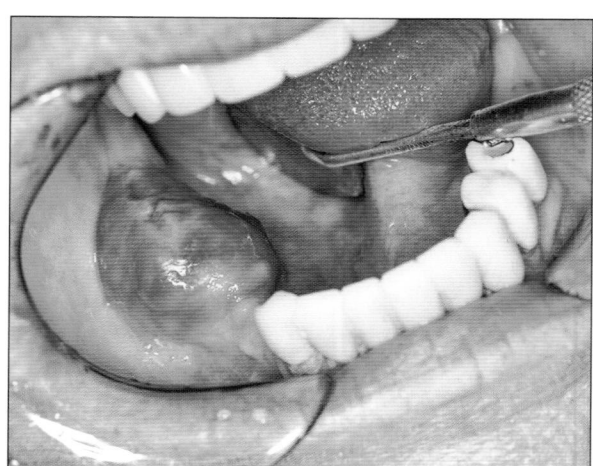

Fig 18-29 Metastatic deposit from a breast cancer that produced a soft tissue mass proliferating from the mandible.

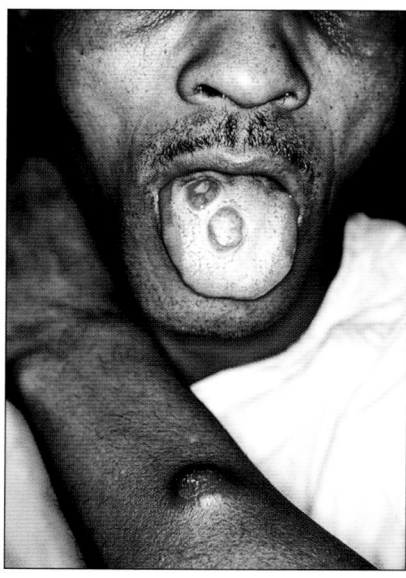

Fig 18-30 Although much rarer than metastatic deposits to bone, metastatic deposits to oral soft tissues and skin can arise, usually from the esophagus, as in this case, or from the thyroid through local venous channels.

CLINICAL PRESENTATION

The site of origin affects the clinical presentation only slightly. Metastatic deposits in the jaws will usually present as painless masses emerging from bone, most often with an intact mucosa. Only rarely are they ulcerated, and then they are the lesions of greatest duration and size. If the metastatic deposit is in a dentate area, the teeth will be mobile. In fact, extensive focal bone loss around one or several teeth inconsistent with the general periodontal status is suggestive of a metastatic tumor (Fig 18-28). A common clinical scenario has been recognized in which an individual undergoes removal of one or two "periodontally hopeless" teeth only to have a mass emerge from the socket and later be identified as either a metastatic carcinoma deposit or even a primary malignancy (Fig 18-29).

Loss of lower lip sensation or other neurosensory disturbances may be present. Pain is uncommon. When there is pain, it is most often related to mobile teeth, which may be in traumatic occlusion, or a secondary infection has occurred.

Soft tissue metastatic deposits are much less common than those in bone; in fact, there are about 20 metastatic deposits in the bony jaws for every 1 in the adjacent oral soft tissues separate from bone. Most often the tongue or lip is the site of metastatic carcinoma deposits in soft tissue, and many of these arise from the esophagus or thyroid, which ascend through the local jugular venous systems (Fig 18-30).

RADIOGRAPHIC FINDINGS ▶

The radiographic findings vary depending on the site of the primary malignancy. Most will present as an irregular radiolucency in the body region of the mandible. Other sites are less frequent. The radiographic picture may show a "floating tooth" appearance due to severe alveolar bone resorption (see Fig 18-28). Metastatic deposits, particularly from the breast and to a lesser extent from the prostate, may show a mixed radiopaque-radiolucent appearance because of reactive bone formation or bone induction. Most CT scans will show a soft tissue mass expanding bone, causing cortical destruction.

DIFFERENTIAL DIAGNOSIS ▶

The clinical radiographic presentation will be consistent with a primary malignancy. Therefore, consideration for the more common primary malignancies, such as *squamous cell carcinoma, osteosarcoma, central mucoepidermoid carcinoma*, and *malignant fibrous histiocytoma,* are warranted. The same presentation in a child or young adult would be rare. However, *Langerhans cell histiocytosis*, a *neuroblastoma*, or a *rhabdomyosarcoma* would have to be considered. If the mass is small and unassociated with symptoms or other signs, benign exophytic lesions that emerge around teeth and alveolar bone are considerations. These include the *pyogenic granuloma*, the *peripheral giant cell proliferation*, and the *peripheral ossifying fibroma*. In addition, some metastatic carcinomas are sufficiently slow growing that they may mimic *odontogenic tumors.*

DIAGNOSTIC WORK-UP ▶

A search for the primary tumor should be deferred until an incisional biopsy is accomplished. While the incisional biopsy may not provide the exact diagnosis, it should enable distinction of a metastatic deposit from a primary malignancy and a carcinoma from a sarcoma. If a metastatic carcinoma deposit is confirmed, a search for the primary focus, if not already known by history, can begin. Following the known statistics of likelihood, a woman would require a thorough breast examination and a mammogram. If negative, or for a man, the next requirement would be a chest radiograph. If the biopsy specimen revealed a small round cell carcinoma, a small cell carcinoma in the lung should also be considered, particularly if there is a significant smoking history. Because small cell lung cancers often have a small primary focus in the lung and a larger metastatic deposit elsewhere, a CT scan of the lung would be useful. Men should undergo the simple prostate-specific antigen serum test and/or be considered for a flexible fiberoptic colonoscopy. If suspicion is directed toward a renal carcinoma, an abdominal CT scan or the standard intravenous pyelogram can be performed. Similarly the suspicion of a gastric carcinoma or a thyroid carcinoma may be explored by a CT or MRI scan. Additionally, ruling out gastric carcinoma may require a gastroscopy, and ruling out thyroid carcinoma may require a [131]iodine nuclear medicine scan.

HISTOPATHOLOGY ▶

Because metastatic carcinoma does not represent a single disease, the histologic appearance is variable. In some instances, the carcinoma may be sufficiently well differentiated and visually distinctive that there is a strong indication of the primary site. Some renal cell carcinomas and thyroid tumors fall into this category (Fig 18-31). More often, however, the type and differentiation of the tumor are such that the primary site is not immediately apparent. In such cases, a complete history and thorough physical examination are extremely valuable.

Carcinomas metastasizing to bone are most frequently adenocarcinomas. They will be infiltrative, unencapsulated, and often produce an abundant desmoplastic stroma. Scattered strands, islands, and individual neoplastic cells are seen (Figs 18-32 and 18-33). Immunohistochemistry may be helpful in determining the nature of the tumor. Thyroglobulin and prostate-specific antigen may be demonstrated to identify tumors of the thyroid and prostate, respectively. In poorly differentiated tumors, cytokeratin can identify its epithelial origin. If the patient has a previously diagnosed malignancy, the histologic characteristics of the two lesions should be compared. This may assist in rendering an accurate diagnosis and in assessing any change in the differentiation of the original neoplasm.

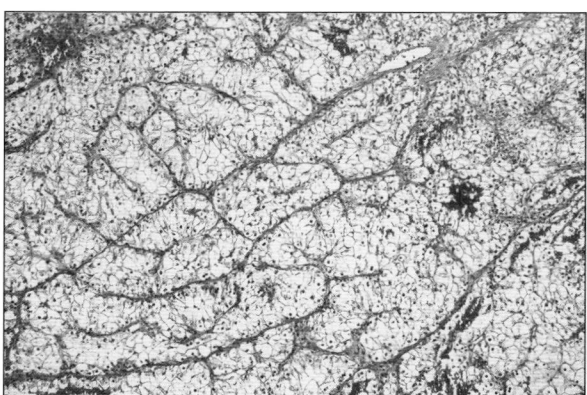

Fig 18-31 A metastatic renal cell carcinoma. The clear cells with fibrovascular trabeculae help to distinguish this tumor, but the tumor must be distinguished from other clear cell tumors such as mucoepidermoid carcinoma.

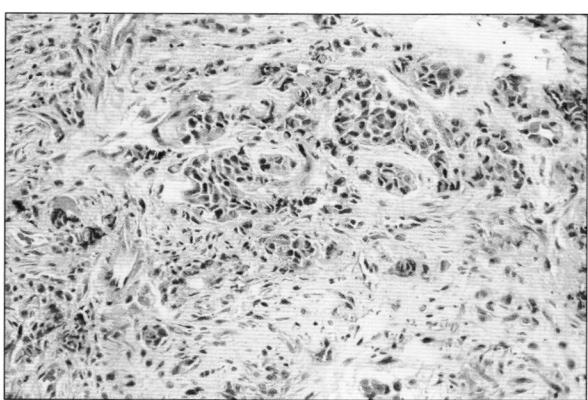

Fig 18-32 A poorly differentiated adenocarcinoma that metastasized to the posterior aspect of the mandible. The patient had a prostate carcinoma with widespread bone metastases. The cells lie randomly within the stroma.

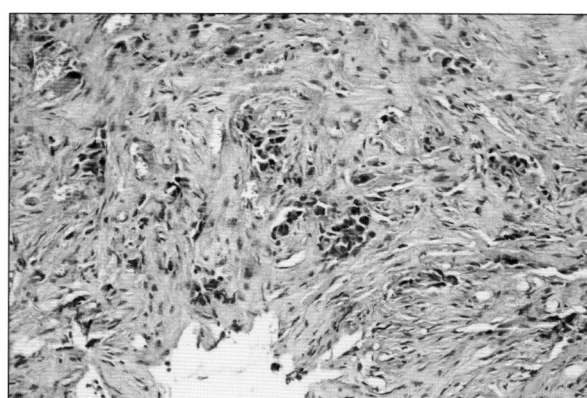

Fig 18-33 Metastatic carcinoma from a breast carcinoma. Note the abundant and densely collagenized stroma.

TREATMENT AND PROGNOSIS

It is well to remember that the identification of a metastatic deposit usually represents a terminal disease and thus a poor overall prognosis. Depending on the primary site and its responsiveness to treatment, a palliative treatment strategy for the metastatic jaw or oral deposit can be developed. The goal in palliative treatment is to reduce or eliminate pain and preserve or restore function. Sometimes this can be obtained through chemotherapy designed to reduce the size of the primary tumor as well as the metastatic deposit. Sometimes it will require a direct local excision of the metastatic deposit, particularly if the tumor has created a pathologic fracture. In these cases, the metastatic deposit is resected with approximately 1-cm margins. A radical resection as would be accomplished for a primary carcinoma will not necessarily provide better local control and may only result in a further loss of function. Defects in the mandible may be bridged with reconstruction plates. Defects in the maxilla may be obturated with a prosthesis. On occasion, radiation therapy to the metastatic deposit is the better choice. This approach may be used if the patient's overall health and risks contraindicate surgery or anesthesia or if the tumor location makes surgery unduly debilitating. It is also preferred if the tumor type is very radiosensitive, such as small cell carcinomas and myeloma deposits.

Chordoma

CLINICAL PRESENTATION AND
PATHOGENESIS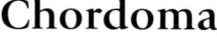

The chordoma is a low- to medium-grade malignant tumor arising from residual cell rests of the embryonic notochord. Although it is rarely seen by the oral and maxillofacial specialist, it is regarded as a relatively common malignant tumor of bone. It accounts for 3% to 4% of all primary malignant bone tumors. Over 90% occur in either the saccrococcygeal bone or the sphenoccipital/base-of-skull bone. Therefore, the oral and maxillofacial specialist may observe one either as an extension from the base of the skull or arising from the cervical vertebrae region. Even then the presentation will be of either a primary or a recurrent painful mass located deep in the neck or within the infratemporal or retropharyngeal spaces.

In human embryonal development, the notochord acts as a template for the development of the neural tube destined to become the spinal cord and becomes surrounded by the sclerotomes destined to become the vertebrae. This occurs during the first month of embryonic development. During the second month, the notochord begins its involution into residual rests located within the nucleus pulposis of the intervertebral discs, which it forms directly, and within the vertebrae, for which it acts as a scaffold

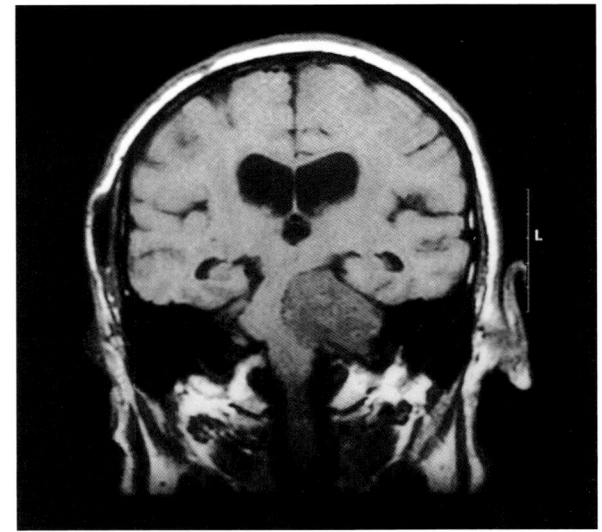

Fig 18-34a Since chordomas arise from rests of the embryonic notochord, they will occur along the vertebrae and within the cranium in the area of the third ventrical. In the head and neck area they will present as deeply located, well-demarcated masses.

to the sclerotomes. At the cephalic and caudal ends of the notochord, greater numbers of rests come to be positioned outside the vertebral bodies, and this accounts for the high incidence of chordomas in the saccrococcygeal and base-of-skull regions.

Those chordomas that develop in the head and neck area usually present as a painful, deeply located mass (Fig 18-34a). The patient is usually an adult older than 40 years. The peak incidence is about 65 years of age, but certainly a small number of chordomas have been reported in children and teenagers as well. Pertinent to the oral and maxillofacial specialist, chordomas that occur in these young individuals typically arise from the second cervical vertebrae and present as a deep neck mass or as a mass in the pharynx or tonsillar fossa. The older patient, who more frequently develops chordomas within the skull or at the skull base, may present with visual disturbances due to optic nerve compression.

DIFFERENTIAL DIAGNOSIS ▶

Because of its rarity, the presentation of a deeply located painful neck or pharyngeal mass is not likely to suggest a chordoma to the oral and maxillofacial specialist. Instead, the more common diseases such as a *fascial space infection*, a *tonsillar abscess*, or a *metastatic lymph node deposit* of a carcinoma would be the more likely considerations. If the individual is within the age range when most chordomas develop, the mass will resemble a *non-Hodgkin lymphoma*, and at any age one might consider *tuberculosis lymphadenitis* (scrofula) or *cat-scratch disease*. If a radiograph or a CT scan shows calcification in the chordoma, a *benign pleomorphic adenoma* or a *carcinoma ex-pleomorphic adenoma* from the deep lobe of the parotid would be added to the differential list.

DIAGNOSTIC WORK-UP ▶

An MRI scan is the single best tool to diagnose a chordoma. It will best identify the characteristic lobulated nature of a chordoma and its surface bony erosions. Usually, a T2-weighted image of two adjacent vertebrae shows a high signal enhancement. A CT scan and plain radiographs are also useful in delineating the mass, its size, and its association with adjacent structures. Either may show intralesional calcifications, which are very characteristic of chordomas.

HISTOPATHOLOGY ▶

These tumors are lobular with fibrous septae (Fig 18-34b). Though they often appear well contained, they are infiltrative, gelatinous tumors that have a mucoid stroma. The cells may be arranged in cords or sheets (Fig 18-34c), or the pattern may be haphazard. The tumor cells may have eosinophilic cytoplasm, but frequently the cytoplasm becomes vacuolated to form physaliphorous cells (Fig 18-34d). Atypia is rare and mitoses absent.

Myxoid chondrosarcomas may closely resemble chordomas, but chordomas bear epithelial markers and are positive for keratin and epithelial membrane antigen.

Some chordomas contain cartilaginous foci and are thus termed *chondroid chordomas*. These tumors have a more favorable prognosis.

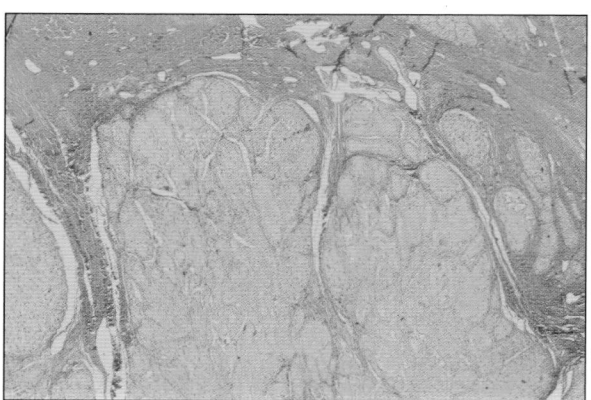

Fig 18-34b A chordoma shows the lobular pattern in which the tumor is divided by fibrous trabeculae.

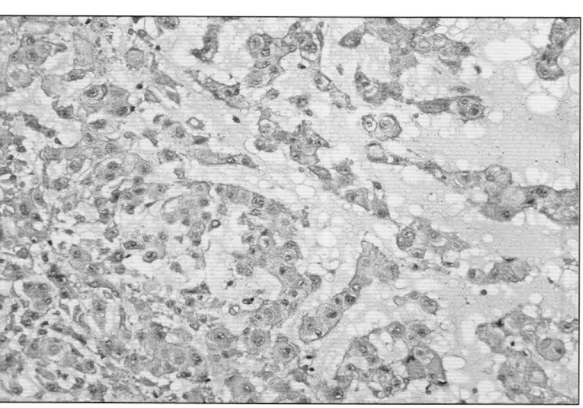

Fig 18-34c In this area, the chordoma shows rows and sheets of regular cells with eosinophilic cytoplasm. The stroma is mucoid.

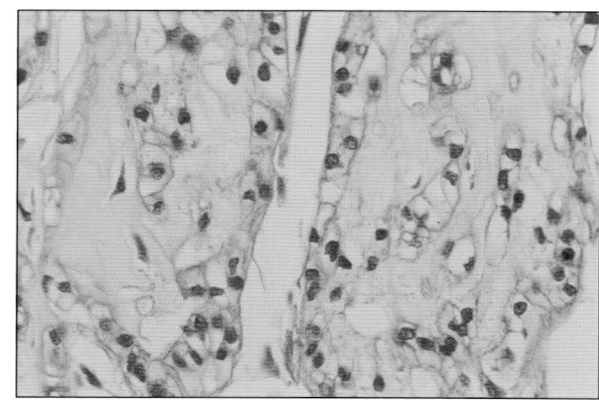

Fig 18-34d In this chordoma, the tumor cells are vacuolated (physaliphorous cells).

TREATMENT

As it is in every other location, treatment of a chordoma in the neck is extremely difficult because of its deep location and unencapsulated lobular character. Surgery, including an attempt to resect the tumor completely, is the frontline therapy. However, microscopically positive margins—even grossly positive margins—are the rule, turning the surgery into an aggressive debulking procedure. In either case, postoperative radiotherapy at doses of 5,000 cGy to 6,400 cGy is recommended.

The surgical access for tumors presenting in the neck will vary depending on their location. However, the widest possible access is recommended. The incision design will resemble that of a total parotidectomy approach with a neck dissection extension.

PROGNOSIS

Chordomas are associated with a high late-mortality rate. Tumor control is usually seen for 1 to 3 years, although some can be fulminant and recur to eventuate even more quickly in an early death. The 5-year survival rate is about 65%, but 10-year survival is rare. Local recurrence with and without regional lymph node spread is the main reason for treatment failure. Distant metastasis to other bones or as subcutaneous nodules occurs in about 10% of cases.

Neoplasms of the Immune System: Lymphomas, Leukemias, and Langerhans Cell Histiocytoses

▶ "At first I was confused on this subject. Now I am still confused but at a much higher level."

—Enrico Fermi

The oral and maxillofacial specialist does not treat lymphomas or leukemias directly; nevertheless, he or she becomes involved in the first two of the four classic phases of lymphoma and leukemia management: (1) *recognition*, (2) *diagnosis*, (3) *staging*, and (4) *treatment*. Moreover, the oral and maxillofacial specialist is often called upon to perform surgeries on individuals whose physiology has been altered by these diseases and its treatment modalities, including chemotherapy, radiation therapy, immunotherapy, and anti-angiogenic therapy. Finally, the oral and maxillofacial specialist is often called upon to treat complications of these diseases or their treatments, including but not limited to candidiasis, mucositis, xerostomia, drug-induced avascular bone necrosis, and osteoradionecrosis. This chapter focuses on the conceptualization of lymphomas, leukemias, and Langerhans cell histiocytoses as malignancies of the immune system; on recognizing their presentations; on obtaining an unequivocal diagnosis through appropriate biopsies; and on managing complications of the disease and/or its treatments. Some of the risk factors and complications of the more common treatments that the oral and maxillofacial specialist may undertake are also explored.

Cancer Cell Development, Proliferation, and Behavior: An Analogy to Quintuplets

Imagine a set of normal and genetically identical quintuplet male newborns. Each thrives and grows until the age of 2, when the growth and maturation of one is suddenly arrested. In this state he is cloned into millions, each of whom looks alike; stands about two feet, four inches tall; periodically pouts and cries; soils his clothes; and throws an occasional temper tantrum. Meanwhile, their numbers would increase to crowd out and replace all other individuals.

Imagine instead that the same event occurs at the age of 8, at which point one is arrested in his growth and maturation and also cloned into millions. These millions express the behavior of an 8-year-old: They tend to dress carelessly; show an aversion to the opposite sex; idolize sports figures; get very dirty at times; and stand about four feet, six inches tall with slight muscle development and a layer of subcutaneous fat. These also continue to multiply to overwhelm all others.

Apply this process of arrested growth and maturation at age 20, when one proliferates into millions. Each is fully grown and developed, stands six feet in height, but is not really fully matured: They tend to resist authority, exhibit nonconforming behavior, drink entirely too much beer, and have a strong attraction for the opposite sex. These millions also continue to increase in number without end.

Now imagine that this process occurs at age 35. These millions exhibit a more conforming behavior, work regular hours, have partnered with a member of the opposite sex, respect the rules of society more unquestioningly, and stand about six feet tall but are somewhat fuller in body mass. These millions also continually increase their numbers and dominate but do not replace other groups.

Let us say that one of the quintuplets, at age 55, has learned about arrested development and actually tries to induce the same process in order to "stay young." However, despite his best efforts and the use of many drugs, he cannot avoid continued maturation and cannot clone himself. At age 55 he is destined to be an individual who will continue to age; who will experience further emphasis of his present traits of increasing weight, gray hair, reduced muscle mass, regular work habits, and the caring of grandchildren; and who will then die.

This describes an imaginary human analogy to cancer development, except that cells will have even more numerous stages of development than people. At any stage, a cancer-provoking set of genetic alterations may reach its threshold to proliferate uncontrollably in that particular stage. Therefore, from a single stem cell, a larger number of histologic types of a particular cell line even than that illustrated by this analogy are possible.

Each type, like each age of a person in the analogy, will look different, will express different chemical markers and different behavior, will grow at a different rate, and will respond to external stimuli (ie, surgery-radiation-chemotherapy) differently. This sequence is best illustrated by the REAL (Revised European American Lymphoma) classification of lymphomas, though the concept is the same for all other malignancies (squamous cell carcinoma, osteosarcoma, etc). The broad and often confusing array of lymphomas and leukemias as well as sarcomas represent the many points along the differentiation pathway at which the immunohematopoetic cells or mesenchymal stem cells can go wrong and branch off into a different malignancy. This analogy also underscores the concept that genetic alterations further along in the differentiation pathway will produce tumors more histologically similar to normal cells and that a mature cell cannot dedifferentiate "back in time" to a malignant clone even if bombarded by carcinogens.

To complicate the analogy slightly more, imagine that the proliferating individuals at each arrested age begin to disagree among themselves, and some actually undergo slight physical changes. Thus, within the population of "look-alikes" a few begin to look different, and those that look different develop nasty personalities, take to carrying guns and knives, and/or proliferate even more rapidly. After a short time the majority of the population not only looks different than it did originally, but those with the nasty personalities and who carry the most weapons proliferate at the fastest rate and soon outnumber all others.

This part of the analogy highlights the fact that all cancers are continuously mutating populations of cells that obey the rules of natural selection. Those cells that are initially arrested in their maturation and then go on to proliferate will undergo further mutations. The cells with the best mutations to avoid the host immune system, to recruit blood vessels to themselves, to neutralize the growth and repair of adjacent normal cells, to resist treatments, and to replicate themselves even faster will take over the population. This explains why recurrent tumors and those that originally responded to treatment but later regrew will often progress most rapidly, demonstrate resistance to further treatments, and overwhelm the individual.

Overview and Classification of Lymphomas, Leukemias, and Langerhans Cell Histiocytoses

Lymphomas are primary malignancies of lymph nodes and the peripheral lymphatics. Leukemias are primary malignancies of bone marrow. Langerhans cell histiocytoses are usually low-grade malignancies of dendritic antigen–processing cells diffusely located in many organs. Although lymphomas and leukemias are separate organ system malignancies, they may overlap in their presentation and transition one to another. That is, lymphomas, by virtue of their origin within lymphatics, usually present with lymph node enlargements without any alteration in the count of the peripheral white blood cells. In fact, the most com-

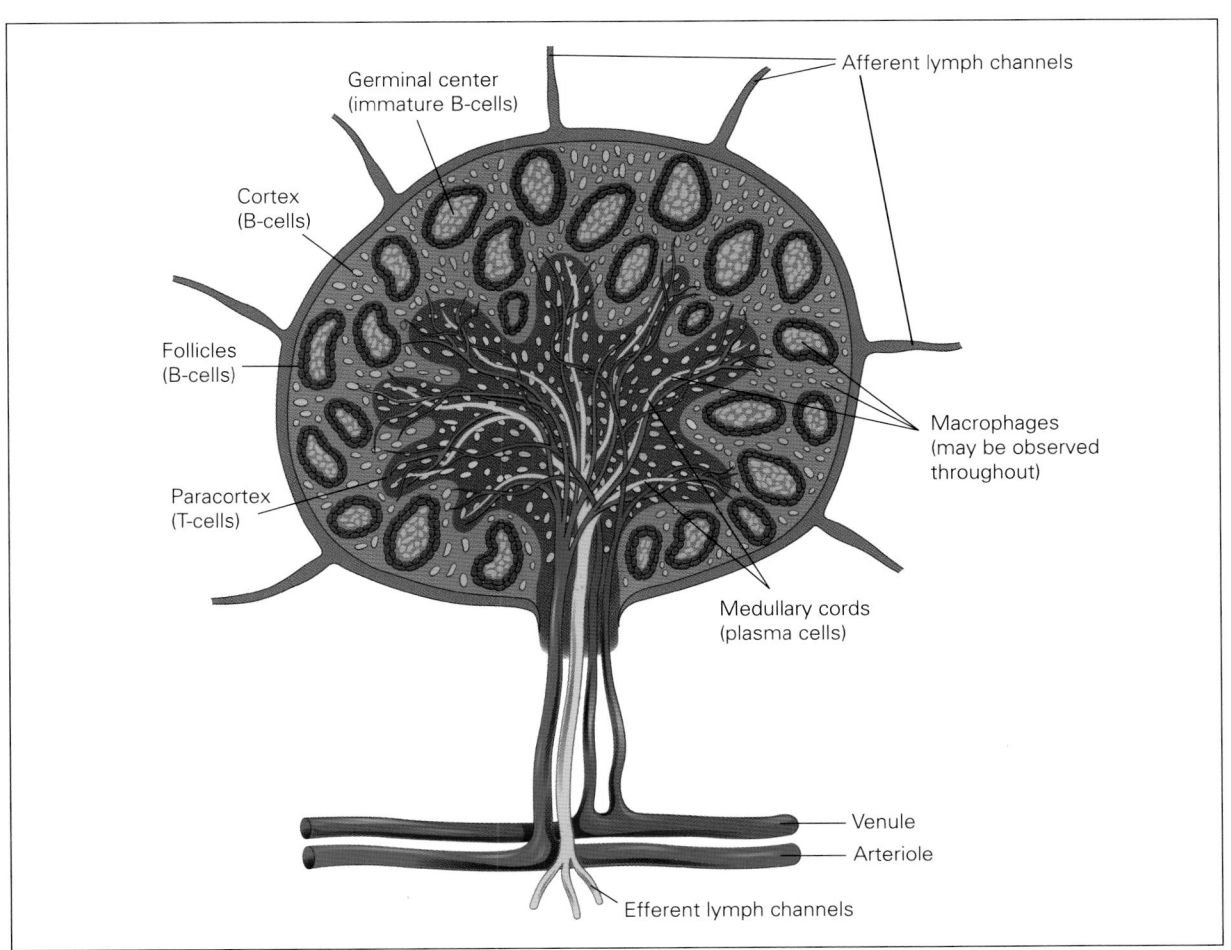

Fig 19-1 A normal lymph node is enclosed by a capsule and has germinal centers, medullary cords, and afferent and efferent blood vessels and lymphatics. The location of B cells, T cells, plasma cells, and macrophages is noted.

mon hematologic abnormality seen in lymphomas is a normochromic, normocytic anemia. However, usually later in their course or indicative of failing therapy, about 15% of lymphomas will spill malignant lymphocytes into the peripheral blood, producing a leukemic picture often termed the *Richter syndrome*. Conversely, leukemias usually present with significantly elevated peripheral white blood cell counts but do not have lymph node enlargement. However, they may seed malignant lymphocytes into lymph nodes, where their populations expand to produce lymph node enlargements. This also is more commonly seen later in the course of the leukemia and in cases where treatment responses are minimal. This type of overlap and disease transition is most commonly observed in chronic lymphocytic leukemia (CLL) and small cell lymphocytic lymphoma (SLL), a slowly progressive low-grade lymphoma of adults older than 40 years, where both often occur simultaneously.

Lymphomas are classified into two main types: Hodgkin lymphoma and non-Hodgkin lymphoma. Hodgkin lymphomas are further subclassified on the basis of lymph node histology into five subtypes (listed here in order of generally decreasing prognosis): nodular lymphocyte-predominant Hodgkin lymphoma (NLPHL) and the classic Hodgkin lymphomas, nodular sclerosing Hodgkin lymphoma (NSHL); lymphocyte-rich Hodgkin lymphoma (LRHL); mixed cellularity Hodgkin lymphoma (MCHL); and lymphocyte-depleted Hodgkin lymphoma (LDHL).

Table 19-1 Neoplasms of the immune system

Disease	Type	Subtype
I. Lymphomas		
	Hodgkin lymphomas (HL)	
		Lymphocyte predominant
		*Nodular sclerosing (cNSHL)
		*Mixed cellularity (cMCHL)
		*Lymphocyte-depleted (cLDHL)
		*Lymphocyte-rich (cLRHL)
	Non-Hodgkin lymphomas (NHL)	
		B-cell lymphomas
		T-cell lymphomas
II. Leukemias		
		B-cell leukemias
		T-cell leukemias
III. Langerhans cell histiocytoses (LCH)		
		Unifocal
		Multifocal

*Designated as "classic" Hodgkin lymphomas.

Non-Hodgkin lymphomas are further subclassified into B-cell and T-cell lymphomas. The B-cell designation refers to a cell of origin arising in the human corollary to the bursa of Fabricus in birds, where B cells were first discovered. In humans these cells are found to originate in the bone marrow, in Peyer patches in the intestinal walls, and in the germinal centers of lymph nodes. The T-cell designation refers to cells that originated from the thymus gland. B cells may evolve into plasma cells via antigen stimulation and are therefore antibody competent. T cells do not produce antibodies and cannot transform into plasma cells. They instead elaborate a host of chemical agents called *lymphokines* that neutralize, digest, or alter the function of invading microorganisms or tumor cells.

In developing an understanding of lymphomas, the clinician should also understand that both B cells and T cells exist in lymph nodes (Fig 19-1), tonsillar tissue, and peripheral lymphatics throughout the body. All of these cells begin as pluripotential precursor cells and progress through a multistage maturation process, where they appear in different sizes and shapes and express different cell membrane characteristics (markers) that identify them. Therefore, the clinician should not be surprised or intimidated by the complex nature of lymphomas and leukemias that give rise to strange names and detailed histologic descriptions (Table 19-1).

Langerhans cell histiocytoses are low-grade malignancies of Langerhans cells, which are a component of the human immune system. Normal Langerhans cells are widely distributed throughout the body as dendritic antigen-processing and antigen-presenting cells. Consequently, neoplasms arising from these cells may occur in any organ and frequently occur within bone, including the jaws and skull. Therefore, they may also be unifocal or multifocal, similar to lymphomas. Although they are destructive, they are usually only slowly progressive and are responsive to treatment.

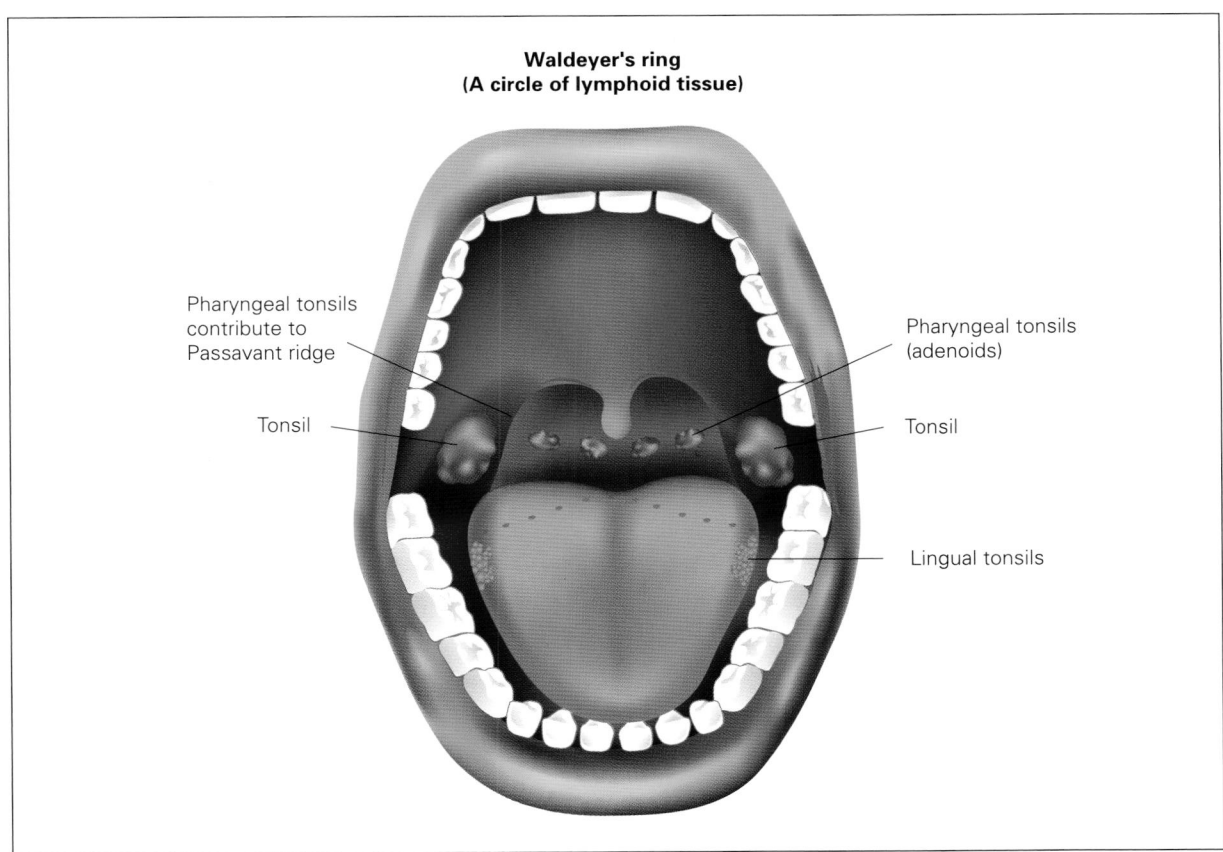

Fig 19-2 Waldeyer's ring consists of a ring of diffuse lymphoid aggregates of which the lingual tonsils, the pharyngeal tonsils, and the adenoids represent more major collections along the ring.

Characteristic Differences Between Hodgkin and Non-Hodgkin Lymphomas

All lymphomas are considered to be malignant. However, Hodgkin lymphoma (HL) and non-Hodgkin lymphoma (NHL) have significant clinical differences. NHL increases in incidence with advancing age, but HL has a bimodal peak, with the 15-to-34-years and the over-50-years populations at greatest risk. NHL is more likely to have a diffuse presentation and to spread randomly, whereas HL tends to present in a more localized fashion, involving a single or a contiguous lymph node chain. Consequently, HL is more likely to be diagnosed at an earlier stage. NHL arises in extranodal sites in more than 20% of cases, and the head and neck area particularly will present NHL as an extranodal disease more frequently than any other site.

Of these extranodal presentations, the mucosa of the hard and/or soft palate is the most common site, followed by the pharyngeal and lingual tonsils and the pharyngeal walls. These areas comprise what is often referred to as *Waldeyer's ring* (Fig 19-2). Lymphomas in these locations are almost always B-cell lymphomas and are part of what are referred to as *mucosa-associated lymphoid tissue* (MALT) lymphomas. MALT lymphomas also include most of those that arise in the stomach, lung, and parotid or lacrimal glands. In oral mucosa they present as nonulcerated, diffuse, fleshy enlargements that may be confused with swellings from dental or sinus inflammation and often cause individuals to seek a dentist because of mobile teeth or because their maxillary denture no longer fits.

HL, on the other hand, is essentially a nodal disease and only rarely involves extranodal sites. In particular, HL frequently presents in the cervical lymphatic chain. In some cases it will present as very bulky

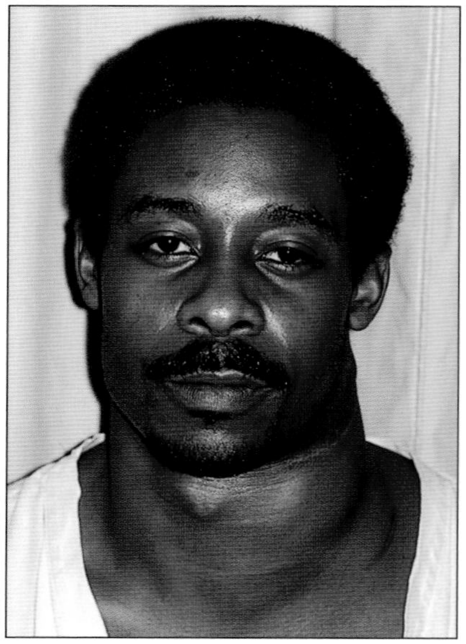

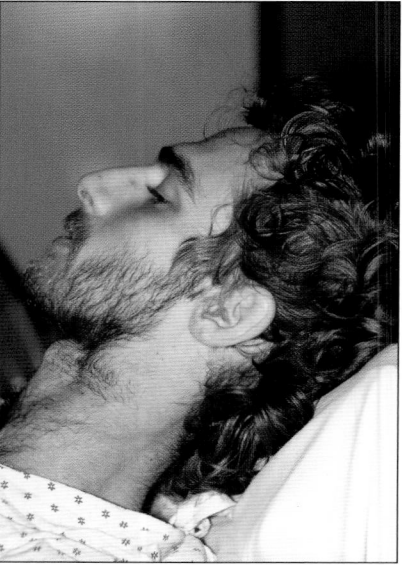

Fig 19-3 Cervical lymph nodes are a site of predilection for Hodgkin lymphoma. One common presentation is that of bulky lymph node enlargements producing a bull-neck appearance.

Fig 19-4 Another common presentation of Hodgkin lymphoma is that of enlarged but discrete lymph nodes in an individual with obvious weight loss.

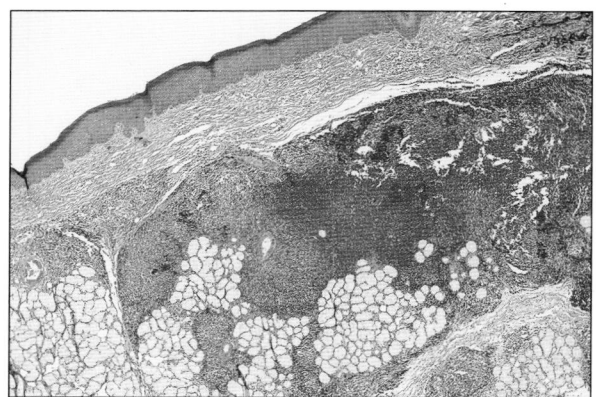

Fig 19-5 Extranodal non-Hodgkin lymphoma of the palate will show lymphoma cells infiltrating the submucosa and effacing the minor glands but leaving a clear zone (grenz zone) between the infiltrated area and the surface epithelium.

DIAGNOSTIC WORK-UP AND PROCEDURES ▶

unilateral or bilateral fused lymph node masses that give the patient a so-called bull-neck appearance (Fig 19-3). In others, the patient will present with enlarged but discrete lymph nodes and weight loss, giving the individual a cachectic appearance (Fig 19-4).

When the oral and maxillofacial specialist suspects lymphoma based on the presentation, a biopsy is indicated. Although laboratory studies will add to the database, only a tissue biopsy of the extranodal site or of a lymph node will be diagnostic. Because the patient will require a clinical staging work-up that may affect numerous tests, such as computed tomography (CT) scans, magnetic resonance imaging (MRI) scans, gallium scans, lymphangiography, and sometimes staging abdominal laparotomies or bone marrow biopsies, his or her treatments are often delayed. Delaying the diagnosis for the purpose of laboratory testing is not warranted and only further delays treatments that may affect the prognosis. Even if infectious diseases (such as tuberculosis, actinomycosis, or cat-scratch disease) or other immune-based diseases (such as sarcoidosis) are part of the differential diagnosis, a lymph node biopsy will usually either confirm them or rule them out. If the biopsy result is positive for a disease other than lymphoma, it nonetheless establishes that diagnosis. If the biopsy result is completely normal, it will give the patient peace of mind and direct the clinician to look elsewhere for a diagnosis. If the biopsy identifies a lymphoma, the staging can be scheduled and prompt treatment delivered.

Straightforward laboratory tests may include a complete blood count with Wintrobe indices and a differential white blood cell count. Serum electrolytes and blood chemistries are also useful, particularly determination of lactic dehydrogenase (LDH). No blood picture is diagnostic of lymphoma. Most early diagnosed cases and many cases of longer standing will have relatively normal peripheral blood values. A normochromic normocytic anemia is the most common abnormality, with hemoglobins in the range of 8 to 10 mg/dL and hematocrits in the range of 26% to 30%. These are termed *anemias of chronic disease*. Occasionally Hodgkin disease will show an eosinophilia above 8% or a mature neutrophilia greater than 80%. This should be distinguished from a "shift to the left" in which immature neutrophiles (band and stab cells) are seen and are indicative of acute inflammation. In the occasional Hodgkin lymphoma with a neutrophilia, there are few or no immature neutrophiles. In most lymphomas, alkaline phosphatase, lactic dehydrogenase, serum copper, and the erythrocytic sedimentation rate (ESR) are elevated and are consistent with and enhance the suspicion of lymphoma. However, these blood values are more useful in monitoring treatment response.

Lymphomas at extranodal sites are diagnosed with a deep incisional biopsy. Lymphomas limited to a lymph node chain are diagnosed via a lymph node biopsy. In those cases where an extranodal site and a lymph node chain are involved, biopsies of both sites are recommended.

Biopsies of an extranodal site such as the palate should include some overlying mucosa and should be of sufficient depth to include muscle or periosteum. This is because the lymphoma cells will usually infiltrate within the submucosa, leaving a characteristic clear zone between the basement membrane of the surface epithelium and the lymphoma cells. Some texts have referred to this as the *grenz zone* (Fig 19-5).

Biopsies of cervical lymph nodes are best accomplished with the support of intravenous sedation or general anesthesia. Before performing a cervical lymph node biopsy, the clinician should make an effort to rule out metastatic squamous cell carcinoma. This can be accomplished by a thorough oral examination, an indirect or direct laryngoscopy or fiberoptic nasopharyngoscopy, and a fine-needle biopsy of the mass. This preliminary work-up is necessary to avoid violating the anatomic planes if squamous cell carcinoma is found in the neck. Removing a lymph node involved with metastatic carcinoma and treating the disease appropriately after such biopsies have not been shown to promote recurrences or reduce survival; however, it is better to avoid the potential for seeding tumor cells in the neck, thereby committing the patient to radiotherapy as well. If no primary carcinoma focus is found and the fine-needle biopsy fails to show atypical epithelial cells, a cervical mass/lymph node biopsy is indicated.

The goal of a cervical lymph node biopsy is to provide the pathologist with a large, representative specimen with an intact capsule that is well fixed to avoid autolysis; a touch preparation; and a culture specimen. The surgeon should choose the largest and deepest lymph node if several are involved (Fig 19-6a). Smaller superficial lymph nodes are too often reactive nodes overlying the actual area of pathology. The use of intravenous sedation or general anesthesia is recommended so that the largest and deepest lymph node can be removed without tearing the capsule and introducing artifacts into the specimen. Before biopsy, a courtesy call to the receiving pathologist is advised. Some pathologists prefer to receive the specimen fresh or fresh frozen and will make arrangements for shipping or courier delivery. If not, the pathologist should be asked if he or she wants the specimen or a portion of the specimen placed in a particular fixative. Some pathologists request 95% alcohol for best preservation of lymph node architecture, Michel's medium or B-5 for fine cytologic organelle and nuclear preservation, or glutaraldehyde for electron microscopy. If there is no preference, 10% neutral-buffered formalin is a good all-purpose choice.

The surgeon will need to remove the lymph node using a dissection that is deep to the platysma. The diseased lymph node will be doughy or rubbery and usually oblong in shape. The lymph node, which will lie on or adjacent to the internal jugular vein, should be removed with a pericapsular dissection (Fig 19-6b). The surgeon should have an electrocautery available to coagulate small vessels to control bleeding that may obscure the surgeon's view during the dissection. The main reasons lymph node specimens are returned by the pathologist as nondiagnostic are lack of hemorrhage control and insufficient anesthesia. In these cases, the surgeon often damages the specimen because of obscured vision and a desire to expedite the procedure.

After the lymph node is removed (Fig 19-6c) and assuming that the pathologist did not request the specimens fresh or fresh frozen, the surgeon should first do a touch preparation by slicing the lymph node specimen in half through its smaller circumference (see Chapter 1). Like a rubber stamp, the cut edge is pressed lightly on a dry glass slide while avoiding any twisting motion (Fig 19-6d). Two such imprints can be placed on one slide. The slide is then placed into either formalin or 95% alcohol. The touch preparation will provide a monolayer of cells and thus allow the pathologist a better visualization of cellular and nuclear detail. The remaining specimen is sliced like a loaf of bread into 2-mm-thick sections (Fig 19-6e). A central section is further divided into smaller sections for various cultures. The remaining

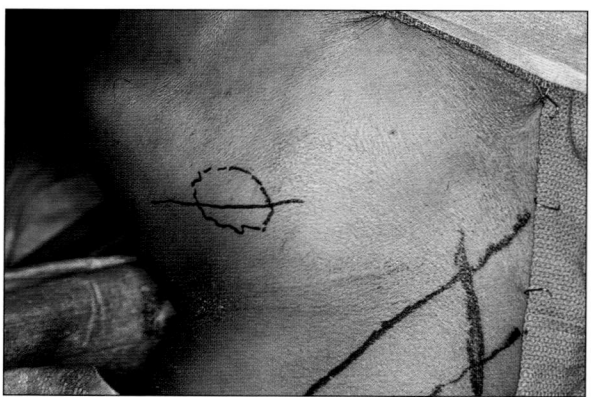

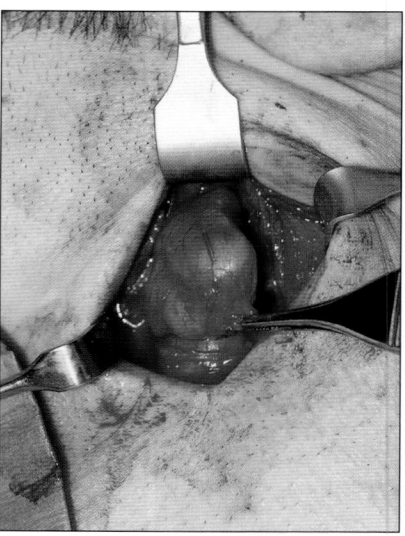

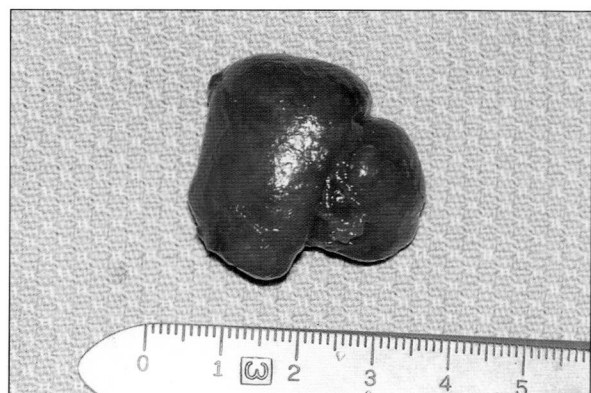

Fig 19-6a Lymph node biopsies are best approached under intravenous sedation or general anesthesia. The incision location is best placed over the mass and parallel to the mandible or within a convenient skin crease.

Fig 19-6b The lymph node should be removed without entering the node and with the capsule intact. Tissue forceps should engage the pericapsular fat rather than the capsule.

Fig 19-6c Pathologic lymph nodes are oblong rather than the normal oval shape. It is common for two diseased lymph nodes to be fused together, as seen here.

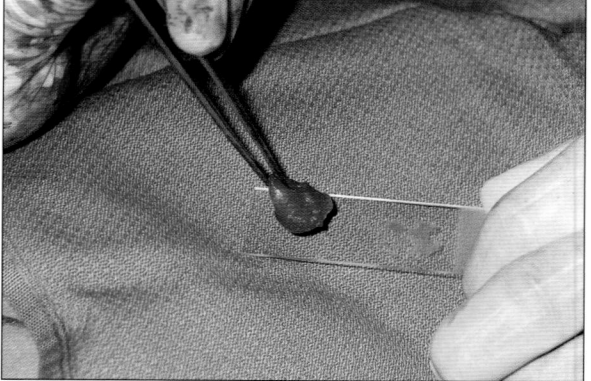

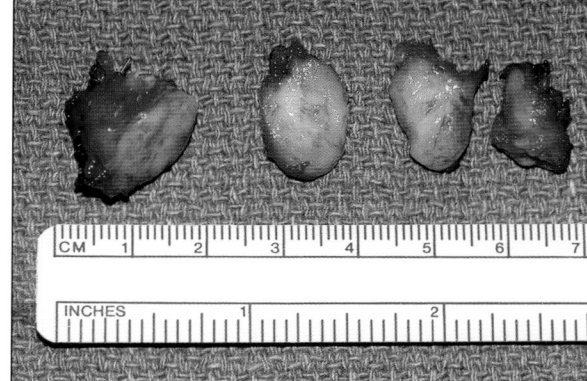

Fig 19-6d A "touch prep" can be accomplished by sectioning the lymph node and imprinting the cut edge on a clean, dry glass slide.

Fig 19-6e It is best to slice lymph nodes into 2-mm-thick sections. One section should be subdivided and sent for various cultures and the others placed into the fixative or fixatives preferred by the pathologist.

sections can then be placed into the requested fixative. The fixative volume should be 10 times the volume of the specimen. Lymph nodes have very little stroma and therefore are prone to autolysis, which can make the specimen nondiagnostic. Cutting 2-mm sections and using a high fixative-to-specimen volume ratio will prevent this.

Specimens removed and submitted in this manner will allow for a more rapid and unequivocal diagnosis and, therefore, early treatment. The need to rebiopsy lymph nodes can be virtually eliminated. Because the newer classifications of lymphoma rely heavily on cytologic detail, nuclear shape, and cell membrane markers, fresh or well-preserved representative tissue specimens are especially critical.

Once the diagnosis of a lymphoma is made, it is best to refer the patient to a medical oncologist/hematologist, who will develop and organize the staging work-up and treatment course. It is important that the oral and maxillofacial specialist continue to follow the patient through the treatment course and the follow-up period to offer a trained eye for potential treatment failures or new disease foci and to manage some of the treatment complications.

Hodgkin Lymphomas

Until recently, the classification for Hodgkin lymphoma had not changed dramatically since the Rye classification of 1966, which in turn was based on the Lukes-Butler classification. The histogenesis of the Reed-Sternberg cell and its variants, which are considered to be the malignant component of Hodgkin lymphoma, is still not entirely clear. While accepted as being of lymphoid origin, their lineage may be B cells or T cells or both. The majority of the cell population represents a reactive proliferation of immune and inflammatory cells rather than malignant cells, and in fact the classification depends essentially on the nature of the reactive component. The REAL and WHO (World Health Organization) classifications have instituted a significant change, however. These classifications separate nodular lymphocyte-predominant Hodgkin lymphoma (NLPHL) from the other types, which are defined as classic Hodgkin lymphoma (CHL). NLPHL is clinically, morphologically, and immunophenotypically distinct from the CHLs and has a far better prognosis.

The diagnosis of HL depends on the identification of characteristic neoplastic cells (Reed-Sternberg cells and its variants) against the proper cellular background. It is now recognized that the Reed-Sternberg cell is indeed a lymphoid cell and most frequently a B cell that is clonal. The unique nature of HL is the paucity of neoplastic cells that are found against an inflammatory, reactive background. The background is of considerable importance, for not only is its nature pivotal to the proper classification within HL, but because Reed-Sternberg–like cells may be seen in reactive lymphoid proliferations other than HL (eg, infectious mononucleosis), it becomes essential to the basic diagnosis. It is also apparent that the specific background and the morphology of the neoplastic cells are interrelated. In evaluating HL on morphologic grounds, there are three elements that must be considered: the neoplastic cells (Reed-Sternberg cells and its variants), the reactive inflammatory cells, and the stromal component.

The classic Reed-Sternberg cell is a giant cell (about 60 to 80 µm; a normal lymphocyte is 12 to 16 µm) with a bi- or multilobed nucleus that has a large eosinophilic nucleolus surrounded by a clear zone and a prominent nuclear membrane. It has a mirror-image appearance and is often said to resemble the eyes of an owl (Fig 19-7a). The cytoplasm is eosinophilic. It is this type of cell that has been required for the initial diagnosis of HL. However, more recently this has been questioned, particularly in cases of NLPHL. The neoplastic variants include the following:

- The Hodgkin cell, which is mononuclear but otherwise resembles the classic Reed-Sternberg cell with its large nucleolus (Fig 19-7b).
- Lacunar cells, which are multilobed with abundant cytoplasm and nucleoli that are far less conspicuous than those in the classic Reed-Sternberg cell. They appear to lie in spaces or "lacunae," which are actually the consequence of formalin fixation. Their appearance can be variable, depending on the background (Fig 19-7c).
- Lymphocytic and histiocytic (L&H) cells, which have multilobed, convoluted nuclei; small, peripherally placed nucleoli; and no perinucleolar halos. They are called "popcorn" cells because of this appearance (Fig 19-7d).

While the Reed-Sternberg cell and the Hodgkin cell appear to be fully neoplastic, the lacunar and L&H cells may actually represent transformed or aberrant cells that have the potential to transform into neoplastic Reed-Sternberg cells. The variable quantities of these cells in the different types of HL correlate with the aggressiveness of the tumor.

The background component includes lymphocytes, which are usually small with nuclei that are round and regular. The majority are T cells. In addition, there may be histiocytes, which can include epithelioid histiocytes, eosinophils, neutrophils, and plasma cells, along with fibroblasts. Acellular collagen and cellular noncollagenous fibrous tissue may be found. It is likely that much of what occurs in HL is the consequence of action by cytokines produced by the neoplastic cells. The presence of necrosis and a signifi-

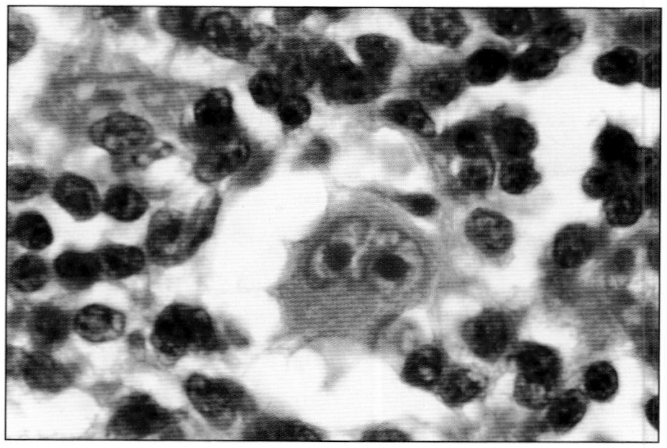

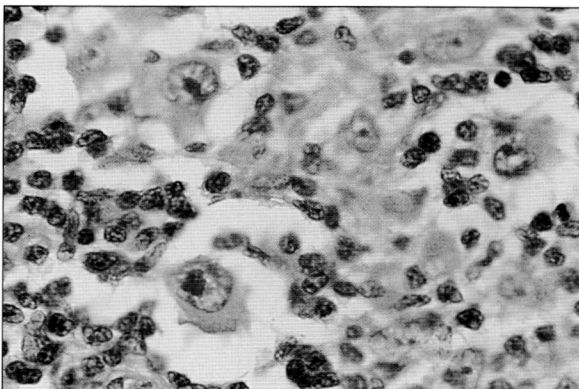

Fig 19-7a Classic Reed-Sternberg cell with a bilobed nucleus and very large nucleoli.

Fig 19-7b Hodgkin cell has a single nucleus and a large nucleolus.

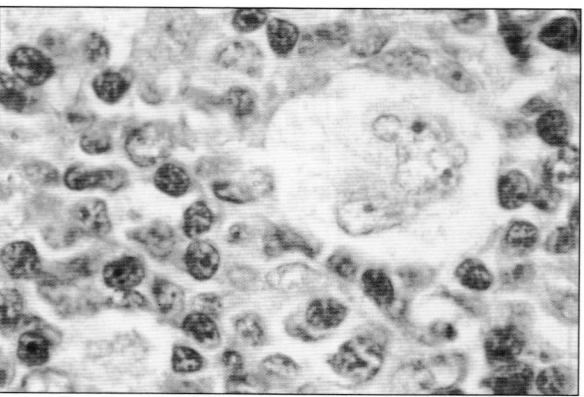

Fig 19-7c Lacunar cell with a multilobed nucleus and relatively small nucleoli. The cell appears to be floating in space.

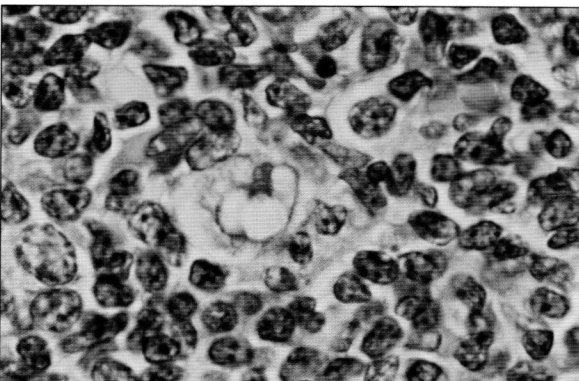

Fig 19-7d Lymphocytic and histiocytic cells (L&H cells) resembling popcorn, thus giving rise to the term *popcorn cells*.

cant neutrophilic component correlates with the presence of systemic symptoms such as fevers and night sweats.

The classification of HL is based on the reactive component, exemplified by the quantity of lymphocytes; the quality of the fibrosis; the quantity of the classic Reed-Sternberg cells; and the quality of the aberrant cells (lacunar and L&H cells). Favorable prognosis is associated with rare classic Reed-Sternberg cells, abundant lymphocytes, and birefringent collagen. A poorer prognosis is associated with abundant Reed-Sternberg cells, depleted lymphocytes, and non-birefringent fibrosis.

HISTOPATHOLOGY AND CLINICAL CORRELATIONS SPECIFIC TO HODGKIN LYMPHOMA TYPES

Nodular Lymphocyte-Predominant Hodgkin Lymphoma

NLPHL, which is not considered classic Hodgkin lymphoma, shares with other forms of Hodgkin lymphoma the finding of relatively few atypical cells in a background of inflammatory cells. It has significant differences, however. The classic Reed-Sternberg cell is absent or rare. L&H cells are present in a background of monotonous lymphocytes (Fig 19-8). Typically, there is a nodular pattern, although there may be diffuse areas. Clusters of epithelioid cells may be found.

Immunophenotype separates NLPHL from all other forms of HL, since the atypical cells are CD45 positive, and they express B-cell–associated antigens (CD19, CD20, CD22, CD79A) and epithelial membrane antigen, but they lack CD15 and CD30. They differ from B-cell non-Hodgkin lymphomas because

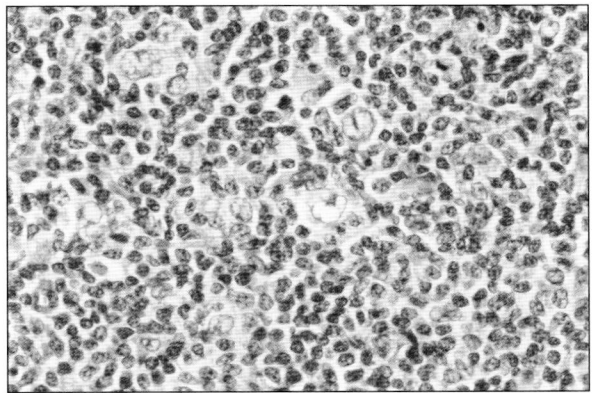

Fig 19-8 Nodular lymphocyte-predominant Hodgkin lymphoma showing sheets of small lymphocytes. At least two popcorn-like L&H cells can be seen.

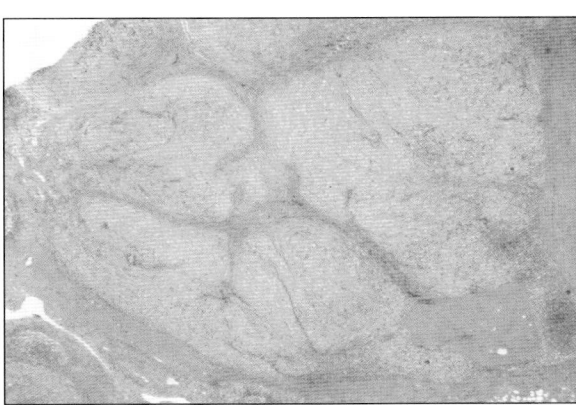

Fig 19-9a Nodular sclerosing Hodgkin lymphoma showing collagen bands forming a nodular pattern.

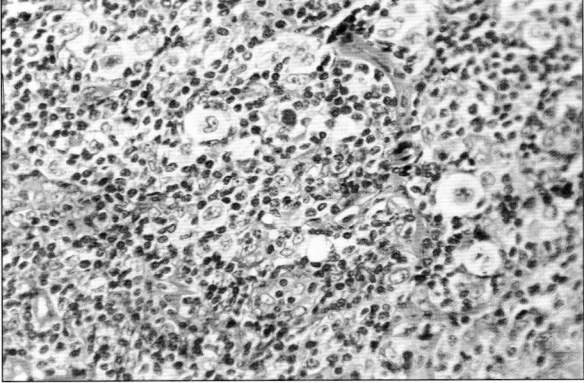

Fig 19-9b Nodular sclerosing Hodgkin lymphoma with lacunar cells in a cellular background that includes, most prominently, lymphocytes.

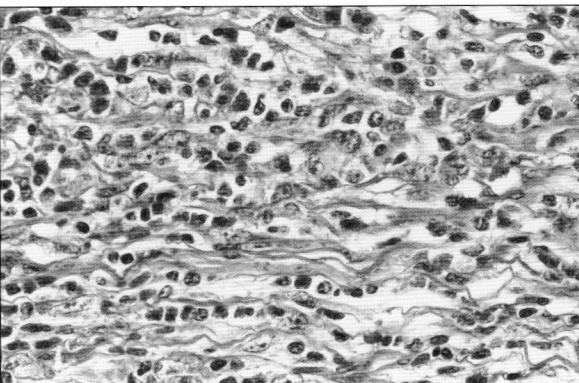

Fig 19-9c An area in a nodular sclerosing Hodgkin lymphoma showing numerous eosinophils together with lymphocytes and histiocytes in a fibrillar stroma.

they are usually immunoglobulin (Ig) negative. The nodules represent altered follicles. In contrast to classic HL, B cells predominate.

Clinically, about 5% of HLs are NLPHLs; they can occur at any age but are more frequent in adults, and they do not exhibit the bimodal age distribution. NLPHL involves peripheral lymph nodes. Eighty percent of patients are diagnosed in stages I or II; 90% are alive at 10 years. Late relapse is common, and 2% to 3% develop large B-cell lymphoma.

Nodular Sclerosing Hodgkin Lymphoma

Histologically, a distinguishing feature of nodular sclerosing Hodgkin lymphoma (cNSHL) is a nodular pattern with bands of collagenous tissue that surround the nodules and are continuous with the thickened capsule of the lymph node. These are often called "C" bands because of their shape (Fig 19-9a). Their birefringence with polarized light confirms their collagenous nature. There may also be diffuse areas. The characteristic cell is the lacunar cell, which is frequently numerous. Classic Reed-Sternberg cells may also be seen but are uncommon. Lymphocytes, histiocytes, eosinophils, neutrophils, and plasma cells may all be present, as may necrotic foci (Figs 19-9b and 19-9c).

A grading system distinguishes grade I tumors, which are more frequent and have a more favorable prognosis, from grade II tumors. Grade I tumors have fewer Reed-Sternberg cells and show less atypia.

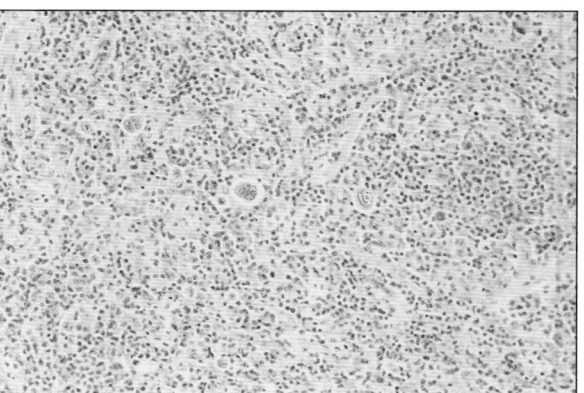

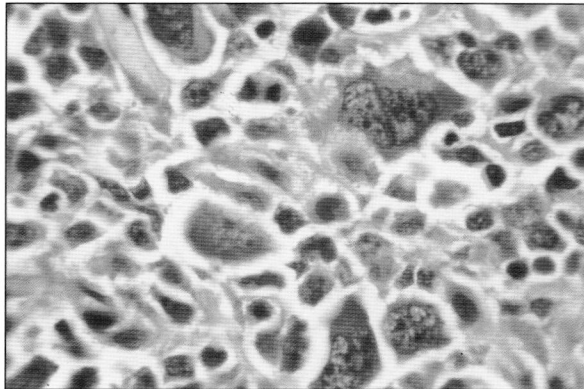

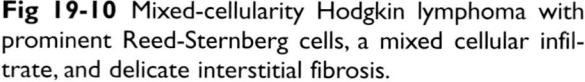

Fig 19-10 Mixed-cellularity Hodgkin lymphoma with prominent Reed-Sternberg cells, a mixed cellular infiltrate, and delicate interstitial fibrosis.

Fig 19-11 Lymphocyte-depleted Hodgkin lymphoma showing bizarre sarcomatous multinucleated cells.

Clinically, this is the most frequently occurring HL, constituting 60% to 80% of cases. Adolescents and young adults are most commonly affected, and it is seen almost equally in females and males, with a slight predilection for females. Presentation is most often in the mediastinum. Patients tend to be from a high socioeconomic background. Survival is approximately 80%. Stage and bulk of the disease have the greatest prognostic significance.

Mixed-Cellularity Hodgkin Lymphoma

Histologically, classic Reed-Sternberg cells are readily seen in mixed-cellularity Hodgkin lymphoma (cMCHL). Mononuclear (Hodgkin) cells are prominent, and there may be occasional lacunar cells. A pleomorphic infiltrate of lymphocytes, epithelioid histiocytes, eosinophils, neutrophils, and plasma cells is present, and fine interstitial fibrosis may be seen (Fig 19-10).

Clinically, cMCHL constitutes 15% to 30% of all HLs. It occurs in adults but lacks the usual bimodal distribution of other cHLs. Abdominal nodes and the spleen are most likely to be involved; thus late-stage presentation is often the case.

Lymphocyte-Depleted Hodgkin Lymphoma

Histologically, the infiltrate is diffuse and Reed-Sternberg cells occur in large numbers and often in bizarre sarcomatous forms in classic lymphocyte-depleted Hodgkin lymphoma (cLDHL) (Fig 19-11). Lymphocytes and other inflammatory cells are sparse. When the cellular element occurs in sheets (reticular subtype of cLDHL [formerly known as Hodgkin sarcoma]), the tumor resembles anaplastic large cell lymphoma (ALCL), which is a non-Hodgkin lymphoma. Absence of the t2:5 translocation that frequently occurs in ALCL may be helpful in identifying cLDHL. The diffuse fibrosis type of LDHL shows a diffuse, disorganized fine fibrosis with few classic Reed-Sternberg cells and a lymphocyte-depleted background. The fibrosis here is non-birefringent and noncollagenous. There may be necrosis.

Clinically, LDHL comprises only about 1% of all HLs. It is seen most frequently in older adults, in HIV-positive individuals, and in the populations of underdeveloped countries. Presentation is often without peripheral lymphadenopathy, but with abdominal, lymph node, bone marrow, spleen, and liver involvement. Diagnosis usually is made at a late stage.

Table 19-2 Ann Arbor Staging System for Hodgkin lymphoma

Stage	Clinical criteria
I	Involvement of single lymph node region (I) or of single extranodal organ or site (I$_E$)
II	Involvement of $\geq$ 2 lymph node regions on same side of the diaphragm alone (II) or with involvement of limited, contiguous extralymphatic organ or tissue (II$_E$)
III	Involvement of lymph node regions on both sides of diaphragm (III), which may include spleen (III$_S$), or limited, contiguous extralymphatic organ or site (III$_E$), or both (III$_{ES}$)
IV	Multiple or disseminated foci of involvement of $\geq$ 1 extralymphatic organs or tissues, with or without lymphatic involvement

Lymphocyte-Rich Hodgkin Lymphoma

Histologically, classic lymphocyte-rich Hodgkin lymphoma (cLRHL) has a diffuse pattern. Classic Reed-Sternberg cells are infrequent and lacunar cells may be seen. L&H cells are not present. Lymphocytes are numerous, but there are more eosinophils and plasma cells than in NLPHL, from which it can be readily separated by immunophenotype.

Clinically there is typically an early stage presentation with no fever or weight loss (B symptoms) or mediastinal disease. There is male dominance, and the median age is greater than in NLPHL and NSHL.

CLINICAL PRESENTATION ▶

Approximately 7,500 new cases of Hodgkin lymphoma are diagnosed each year. The average age of individuals is 27 years and the classic bimodal peak of age ranges at greatest risk (15 to 34 years and older than 50 years) is consistent throughout all studies but not in all histologic types. A male preponderance of 1.4 to 1 is also seen.

For the oral and maxillofacial specialist, the most common clinical presentation of Hodgkin lymphoma is that of a young adult who has recently noted an asymptomatic lymph node enlargement in the neck. In providing a detailed history, many of these individuals will identify the characteristic symptoms of fever, night sweats, pruritus, fatigue, or weight loss. As a result, it is often confused with some type of infection. Fevers in Hodgkin lymphomas are often cyclical and may increase and build to a peak over several days. This pattern has been termed *Pel-Ebstein fever*, but it is not pathognomonic of Hodgkin disease, since other lymphomas and infectious diseases may demonstrate such a pattern as well. Pain is not usually associated with Hodgkin lymphoma. However, pain is brought about by even a small amount of alcohol ingestion. This peculiar and somewhat specific association can even be used as a test. Ingestion of alcohol will often produce pain within minutes at the site of the Hodgkin lymphoma and may pinpoint a location not detected by other studies.

In general, Hodgkin lymphoma presents in two basic clinical forms: one is overt and almost obvious, producing numerous symptoms, while the other is occult. The occult form will resemble an infectious disease proper or may even be written off as malingering, depression, or "growing pains." Regardless of the general presentation, most patients will have occult disease beyond that which is diagnosed (see Figs 19-3 and 19-4).

CLINICAL STAGING ▶

The oral and maxillofacial specialist should become familiar with the clinical staging system for Hodgkin lymphoma because it is straightforward, will guide the treatment selections by the medical oncologist, and relates to prognosis. The accepted clinical staging system for patients with Hodgkin lymphoma is the four-stage system from the Ann Arbor conference of 1974 (Table 19-2). In this system, stage

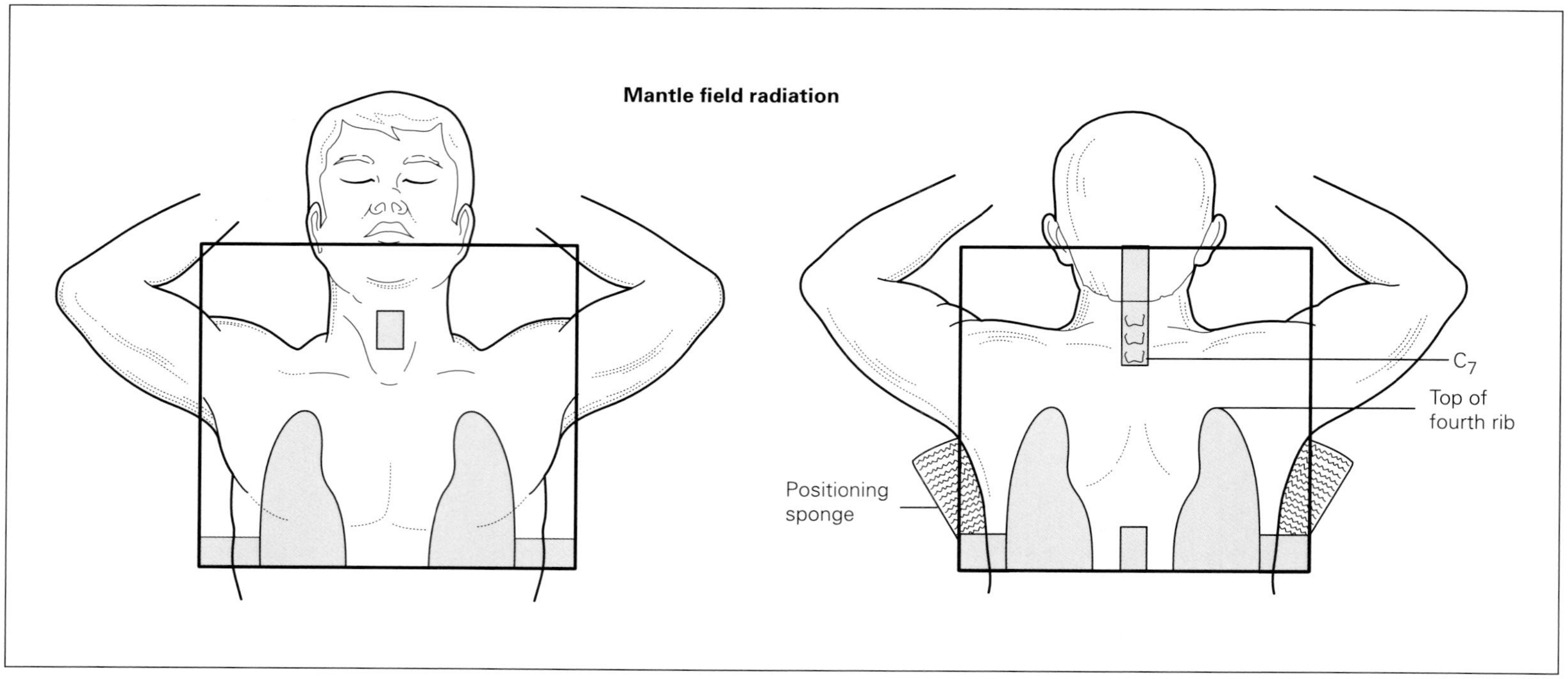

Mantle field radiation

C_7

Top of fourth rib

Positioning sponge

Fig 19-12 Traditional mantle field radiotherapy ports include the cervical lymphatic chains and the mandible, as well as the axillary and mediastinal lymphatic chains.

I is the involvement of one lymph node chain or one extranodal site, which would then be designated as stage I_E. Stage II is the involvement of two lymph node chains on the same side of the diaphragm. An extranodal site would be equivalent to a lymph node chain. If one of the involvements is a lymph node chain and the other an extranodal site, it would be designated as stage II_E. Stage III indicates involvement of lymph node chains or extranodal sites, including the spleen on both sides of the diaphragm. If one of the involvements is an extranodal site, it is designated as stage III_E. If one of the involvements is the spleen, it would be designated as stage III_S. If both an extranodal site and the spleen are involved, it is designated as stage III_{ES}. Stage IV indicates diffuse multiorgan involvement, usually implying bone marrow, lung, spleen and other sites, which may include lymph node chains. Each stage may be further subclassified according to symptoms. Some clinicians may add the designation A (ie, stage II_A or stage III_{ESA}) to note the absence of symptoms or the designation B (ie, stage II_B or stage II_{EB}) to note the presence of symptoms. In general use, these B symptoms refer to fever or to weight loss of at least 10%.

TREATMENT ▶

Treatment of Hodgkin lymphoma will depend on the stage of the disease. For most cases diagnosed in the head and neck region as stage I_A or stage II_A, mantle field radiotherapy of 4,000 cGy to 4,400 cGy over 4 to 5 weeks is used as a single modality (see Chapter 8). The mantle field refers to a square field of radiotherapy that includes the lymph node chains of the neck, axilla, and lungs. The mandible below the lingula is included in this field, as is the occiput (Fig 19-12).

Treatment for Hodgkin lymphoma stage I_B or stage II_B is more controversial. However, because of the B symptoms, it is felt that occult disease is present at sites other than those that are clinically apparent. Therefore, although a few centers may still use mantle field radiotherapy alone, most will use multidrug chemotherapy either alone or combined with mantle field radiotherapy of the clinically apparent sites.

Treatment of stage III_A may also be controversial. However, if no B symptoms exist and a staging laparotomy shows smaller nodes (less than 4 cm), specific nodal chain radiotherapy (mantle field plus a second field) of 4,000 cGy to 4,400 cGy over 4 to 5 weeks is often used. As an alternative, multidrug chemotherapy alone or combined with the same radiotherapy may be used.

Stage III$_B$ and stage IV Hodgkin lymphoma are almost always treated with multidrug chemotherapy as a single modality.

In the past, multidrug chemotherapy for Hodgkin lymphoma generally referred to MOPP (mechlorethamine [mustargen], oncovin, procarbazine, and prednisone). This regimen, followed over a period of 6 months to 1 year, produces a cure rate of 50% for nonrecurrent stage III$_B$ or stage IV disease. However, the toxicity of MOPP is significant and includes hair loss, nausea, vomiting, peripheral neuropathies, and often sterility or inducement of leukemia. Therefore, today, a regimen of actually superior response and cure rates together with reduced toxicity has either replaced MOPP altogether or is used in alternating cycles with MOPP. This regimen is ABVD (adriamycin, bleomycin, vinblastine, and dacarbazine). In particular, ABVD seems to have eliminated sterility and the inducement of secondary leukemias.

Management of Complications Related to Hodgkin Lymphoma or Its Treatment

Hodgkin lymphoma is a disease of the immune system; therefore, individuals with this disease are by definition immunocompromised. Some will develop specific infections before, during, or after treatment. Of these, herpes zoster is the most common. This infection usually affects one of the three divisions of the trigeminal nerve, particularly the ophthalmic division, which may be treated with acyclovir, 800 mg by mouth five times daily; famciclovir (Famvir, SK Beecham), 500 mg by mouth three times daily; or valacyclovir (Valtrex, GlaxoSmithKline), 1 g three times daily, until all lesions are crusted and no exudate remains. In cases where lesions are slow to regress or where the patient is severely immunocompromised, intravenous acyclovir, 10 mg/kg three times daily, or intravenous foscarnet (Foscavir, AstraZeneca), 40 mg/kg three times daily, may be required. Other patients may develop recurrent pneumococcal pneumonias, particularly if the spleen is involved or if a splenectomy has been accomplished. These are treated with antibiotics empirically chosen to cover *Streptococcus pneumonia* or *Haemophilus influenzae* such as the fluoroquinolones, doxycycline, and the macrolides.

More specific to the oral and maxillofacial specialist are the dental abscesses, pericoronitis, and advancement of periodontal disease that commonly affect such patients. For example, acute pericoronitis in a young individual with Hodgkin lymphoma should be treated without delay. Cultures should be taken, the pericoronitis debrided, and the offending tooth removed. During the procedure the patient should be given 3 g intravenous ampicillin with sulbactam (Unasyn, Pfizer US) or 1 g intravenous erythromycin if the patient is penicillin allergic. Either one should be followed by an oral form of the same antibiotic for a 10-day period. Should such a clinical situation develop after mantle field radiotherapy, the treatment approach would be identical provided that the radiotherapy dose did not exceed 5,000 cGy. If the radiotherapy dose exceeded 5,000 cGy, the standard protocol of hyperbaric oxygen, as published by the Undersea and Hyperbaric Medical Society, would be required (see Chapter 8). This protocol requires 20 sessions of hyperbaric oxygen at 2.4 atmospheres of absolute pressure (ATA) for 90 treatment minutes of 100% oxygen prior to surgery followed by 10 such sessions after surgery.

Some individuals develop a severe mucositis during or immediately following radiotherapy or chemotherapy. They will report pain and dysphagia and exhibit hypersalivation; drooling; and multiple raw, ulcerated areas with a yellow fibrinous coating. This is a nonspecific mucositis that is caused by direct cytotoxicity from the chemotherapy or direct cellular injury from the radiotherapy, compounded by secondary infection. The patient should first be given reassurance that this complication is self-limiting and usually lasts less than 1 month. It is treated with systemic oral antibiotics using one of the penicillins, tetracycline, or erythromycin. Topical agents should also be used to relieve the pain and to reduce the hypersalivation and drooling. As a standard, 2% viscous lidocaine (Xylocaine, AstraZeneca) oral swish and

Table 19-3 Working Formulation of non-Hodgkin lymphomas for clinical usage

Low grade

Malignant lymphoma, small lymphocytic/consistent with chronic lymphocytic leukemia/plasmacytoid
Malignant lymphoma, follicular/predominantly small cleaved cell/diffuse areas/sclerosis
Malignant lymphoma, follicular, mixed small cleaved and large cell/diffuse areas/sclerosis

Intermediate grade

Malignant lymphoma, follicular/predominantly large cell/diffuse areas/sclerosis
Malignant lymphoma, diffuse/small cleaved cell/sclerosis
Malignant lymphoma, diffuse, mixed small and large cell/epithelioid cell component/sclerosis
Malignant lymphoma, diffuse, large cell/cleaved cell/noncleaved cell/sclerosis

High grade

Malignant lymphoma, large cell, immunoblastic/plasmacytoid/clear cell/polymorphous/epithelioid cell component
Malignant lymphoma, lymphoblastic/convoluted cell/nonconvoluted cell
Malignant lymphoma, small noncleaved cell/Burkitt/follicular areas

Miscellaneous

Composite lymphomas
Mycosis fungoides
Histiocytic lymphomas (composed of actual malignant histiocytes)
Extramedullary plasmacytoma
Unclassifiable
Other

spit remains an effective topical agent. As an alternative, a combination of 12.5 mg of Benadryl (Warner Lambert) and 4 g of Carafate (Aventis) in 30 mL of Mylanta, called Magic Mouthwash (Johnson and Johnson/Merck), swish and swallow, provides excellent topical relief as well.

Non-Hodgkin Lymphomas

CLASSIFICATION ▶

Non-Hodgkin lymphoma (NHL) is a large and complex group of malignant diseases of the immune system composed of two broad groups: B-cell lymphomas and T-cell lymphomas. These are much more numerous and diverse than the Hodgkin lymphomas and in general have a poorer prognosis. They also differ from Hodgkin lymphomas in that their incidence increases with age, they frequently present in extranodal sites, and many are associated with leukemias. Classification of these lymphomas has changed frequently over the years as newer knowledge and newer biotechnologies have allowed us to learn more about their histogenesis and malignant potentials. The most recently applied biotechnology, *immunotyping*, identifies specific cell membrane antigens. Like fingerprints, these surface proteins are specific to each cell and can therefore be used to identify an individual cell or cell population.

Early classifications for NHL, such as the one devised by Rappaport, were essentially based on morphology: tumors with follicular (nodular) patterns were distinguished from those with a diffuse pattern because the former appeared to be more indolent. Tumors were classified according to the cells they resembled; hence, small cells were "lymphocytic" and larger cells were "histiocytic." The closer the resemblance to these cells, the better the "differentiation."

The Lukes-Collins classification of 1974 was an immunologic-based classification with morphologic considerations. It recognized that lymphomas could be of B-, T-, or null-cell origin and that there was often a cytologic resemblance to follicle center cells of normal lymph nodes. It recognized that lymphocytes undergo changes secondary to antigenic stimulation, such that they may morphologically resemble histiocytes or immature cells. Thus the terms *histiocytic* and *well* or *poorly differentiated* were inappropriate. The Kiel classification is also immunologic-based but includes grades of malignancy and has found less favor in the US, although it is widely used in Europe. Cell size appeared to correlate with the clinical course and prognosis of many lymphomas; thus large cells generally indicated a more aggressive course. For this purpose, the size of lymphoma cell nuclei are compared to that of normal histiocyte or endothelial cell nuclei.

In light of the large number of classification systems in use, the Working Formulation was devised to allow for translation between them. However, this classification quickly achieved acceptance in its own right and became the most widely used classification in the United States. The Working Formulation divided tumors into low-, intermediate-, and high-grade tumors, at the same time maintaining the distinction between nodular (follicular) and diffuse types as well as the concept of cell size. However, not only did it lack immunologic and genetic markers, but as many as 20% of NHLs did not fit into this classification (Table 19-3). In 1994, the Working Classification was superseded by the Revised European American Lymphoma (REAL) Classification, which listed all of the definable diseases that could be recognized by the clinical, morphologic, immunologic, and genetic parameters available at that time. It was born of the need to more clearly define homogeneous biologic entities so that treatment modalities could be developed to target their unique aberrations. The REAL classification also recognized that many distinct lymphomas themselves varied in terms of histologic grade and aggressiveness. The most recent WHO classification of neoplastic diseases of the hematopoietic and lymphoid tissue adopted this REAL classification of lymphoid neoplasms with some modifications. Obviously, modifications of even the most recent classification can be anticipated (Table 19-4).

Discussion of specific non-Hodgkin lymphomas in this text has been limited to those entities that occur most frequently in the population or have a predilection for extranodal sites in the head and neck area.

Small B-Cell Low-Grade Lymphomas

Small Lymphocytic Lymphoma/Chronic Lymphocytic Leukemia

CLINICAL PRESENTATION ▶ Small lymphocytic lymphoma (SLL)/chronic lymphocytic leukemia (CLL) primarily affects individuals older than 60 years and shows a predilection for males. It accounts for 4% of all NHL cases. Most individuals present with an asymptomatic lymphadenopathy or extranodal site (Fig 19-13a); a few present with symptoms. An abdominal examination will usually reveal some degree of hepatosplenomegaly. If the bone marrow is minimally involved, the peripheral blood will not show the CLL picture. If the bone marrow is significantly involved and malignant small B lymphocytes spill into the peripheral blood above the arbitrary level of 5×10^8 g/dL of blood, a leukemic process and CLL is diagnosed.

HISTOPATHOLOGY ▶ Involved lymph nodes show a diffuse effacement of nodal architecture by a monomorphic population of small round lymphocytes (Fig 19-13b). When there is palatal involvement, as is often the case in extranodal lymphomas, the mucous glands will be effaced and show no reactive change, as would occur in an inflammatory process (see Fig 19-5). To distinguish SLL/CLL deposits in the jaws from the more common inflammatory processes associated with periodontal and apical dental infections, a careful study of the cell types is necessary. An inflammatory process will consist of a variety of different inflammatory cells with numerous capillaries and some fibroblasts. However, an SLL/CLL focus will show a monotony of identical-looking small regular lymphocytes (Figs 19-13c and 19-13d). Scattered among the small lymphocytes may be larger cells that will produce a pseudofollicular pattern. Immunochemistry will identify these cells as mainly B cells that are CD5 positive, CD23 positive, and CD43 positive.

TREATMENT AND PROGNOSIS ▶ In older patients who are asymptomatic, often no treatment is the management provided; if the lymph nodes further enlarge or symptoms develop, individuals are treated with chlorambucil (Leukeran, Glaxo-

---

Table 19-4 Current (2001) WHO classification of lymphoid neoplasms: Major categories

B-cell neoplasms

Precursor B-cell neoplasm
- Precursor B-lymphoblastic leukemia/lymphoma (precursor B-cell acute lymphoblastic leukemia)

Mature (peripheral) B-cell neoplasms
- B-cell chronic lymphocytic leukemia/small lymphocytic lymphoma
- B-cell prolymphocytic leukemia
- Lymphoplasmacytic lymphoma
- Splenic marginal zone B-cell lymphoma (+/– villous lymphocytes)
- Hairy cell leukemia
- Plasma cell myeloma/plasmacytoma
- Extranodal marginal zone B-cell lymphoma of MALT type
- Nodal marginal zone B-cell lymphoma (+/– monocytoid B cells)
- Follicular lymphoma
- Mantle cell lymphoma
- Diffuse large B-cell lymphoma
    Mediastinal large B-cell lymphoma
    Primary effusion lymphoma
- Burkitt lymphoma/Burkitt cell leukemia

T- and NK-cell neoplasms

Precursor T-cell neoplasm
- Precursor T-lymphoblastic lymphoma/leukemia (precursor T-cell acute lymphoblastic leukemia)

Mature (peripheral) T-cell neoplasms
- T-cell prolymphocytic leukemia
- T-cell granular lymphocytic leukemia
- Aggressive NK-cell leukemia
- Adult T-cell lymphoma/leukemia (HTLV1+)
- Extranodal NK-/T-cell lymphoma, nasal type
- Enteropathy-type T-cell lymphoma
- Hepatosplenic $\gamma\delta$ lymphoma
- Subcutaneous panniculitis-like T-cell lymphoma
- Mycosis fungoides/Sézary syndrome
- Anaplastic large cell lymphoma, T-/null-cell, primary cutaneous type
- Peripheral T-cell lymphoma, not otherwise characterized
- Angioimmunoblastic T-cell lymphoma
- Anaplastic large cell lymphoma, T-/null-cell, primary systemic type

Hodgkin lymphoma (Hodgkin disease)
- Nodular lymphocyte-predominant Hodgkin lymphoma
- Classic Hodgkin lymphoma
    Nodular sclerosis Hodgkin lymphoma (grades 1 and 2)
    Lymphocyte-rich Hodgkin lymphoma
    Mixed-cellularity Hodgkin lymphoma
    Lymphocyte-depleted Hodgkin lymphoma

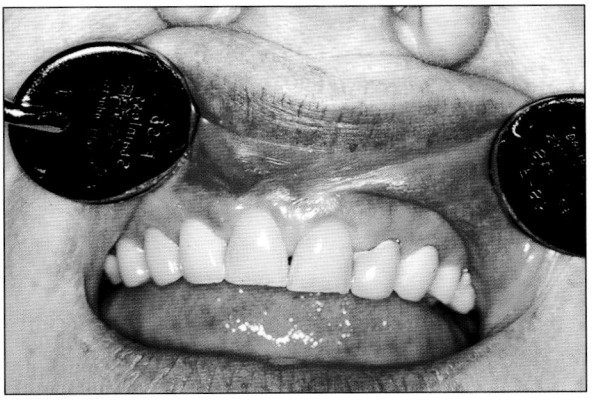

Fig 19-13a This asymptomatic, doughy, nonulcerated mass within the submucosa represented an extranodal presentation of small lymphocytic lymphoma (SLL). At this time, a leukocytosis of 18,000 was present with 90% lymphocytes, indicative of a CLL picture as well.

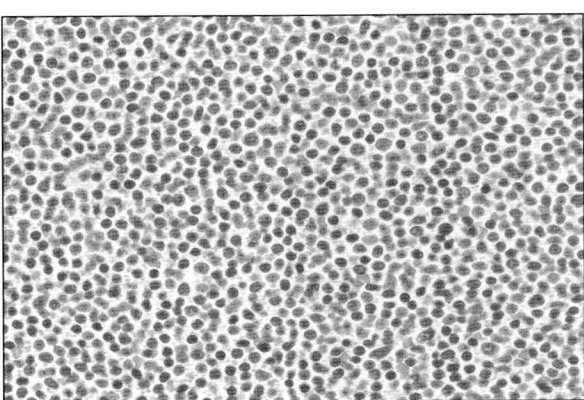

Fig 19-13b Small lymphocytic lymphoma with regular, monotonous, small round cells.

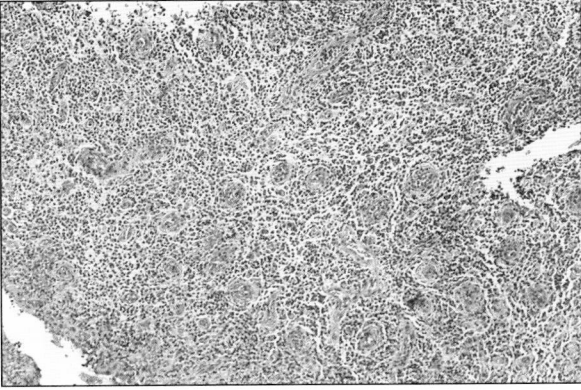

Fig 19-13c Periapical lesion in a patient with chronic lymphocytic leukemia, showing a typical inflammatory process with numerous capillaries and an infiltrate of a variety of inflammatory cells.

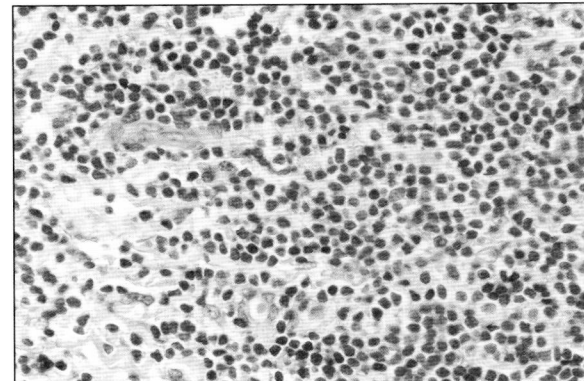

Fig 19-13d The same lesion shown in Fig 19-13c except this field shows a monotony of small, regular lymphocytes, consistent with CLL.

SmithKline) as a single agent. This treatment and all others to date are merely palliative; no curative therapy has been found. Most patients respond to chlorambucil, but the response may last for only 12 to 18 months. However, retreatment with chlorambucil usually induces another response. The median survival of patients with this disease and treatment is 10 years, partly because of deaths from other diseases in this age group and partly because about 15% transform into a high-grade large cell lymphoma. This transition is termed *Richter syndrome*, following the original case report of this phenomenon by Maurice Richter in 1928.

In younger individuals (that is, those younger than 60 years), experimental protocols using the purine analogues 2-deoxycoformycin, 2-chlorodeoxyadenosine (2-CdA), and fludarabine (Fludara, Berlex) have shown promising results with up to 70% complete remission. However, no data relating the long-term reliability of these results are available.

Extranodal Marginal Zone B-Cell Lymphoma (MALT Lymphoma)

CLINICAL PRESENTATION ▶ MALT lymphomas are of special importance to the oral and maxillofacial specialist because of their association with the oral and pharyngeal mucosa and with pre-existing diseases of chronic immune system

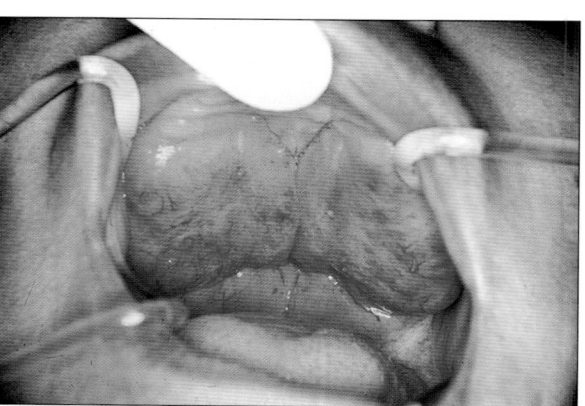

Fig 19-14 Extranodal marginal zone B-cell lymphoma (MALT lymphoma) presenting as a soft fleshy enlargement of the maxillary mucosa without ulcerations.

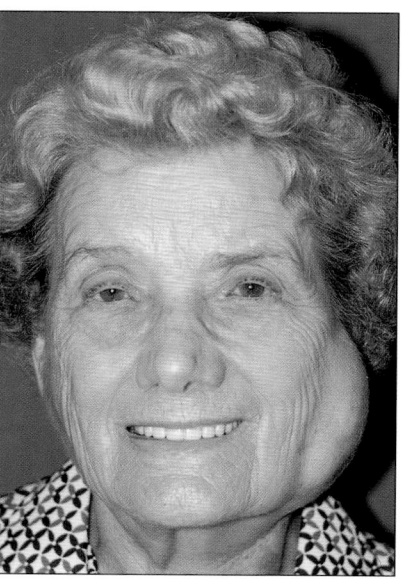

Fig 19-15a This lymphoma in the left parotid gland developed in a long-standing Sjögren syndrome and is considered one of the MALT lymphomas.

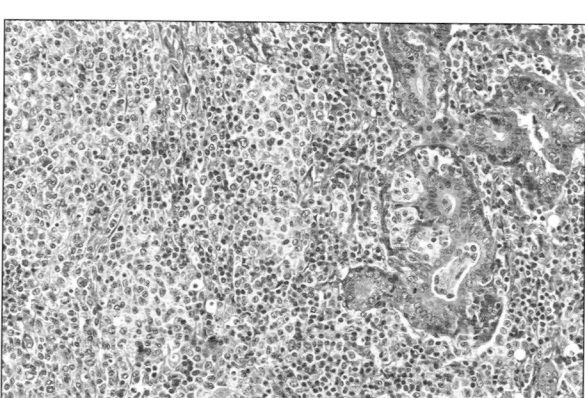

Fig 19-15b MALT lymphoma showing infiltration of epithelial structures. The infiltrate consists of centrocytic and centroblastic cells.

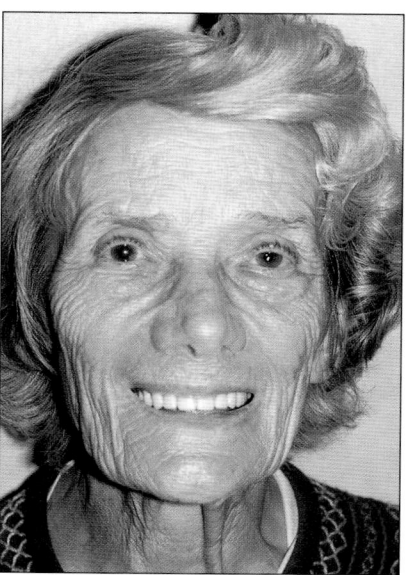

Fig 19-15c Individual with the MALT lymphoma shown in Fig 19-15a survived in a disease-free state after 4,500 cGy of radiotherapy.

stimulation, such as Sjögren syndrome, Hashimoto thyroiditis, and even the chronic gastritis caused by infection with *Helicobacter pylori*. They are primarily low-grade B-cell lymphomas that present in adults as extranodal tissue infiltrates within the glands of the submucosa from the oral cavity to the intestines. This infiltration of malignant B cells produces a fleshy tissue enlargement that is rarely ulcerated and is usually nonpainful. However, it can displace teeth, produce tooth mobility, or alter the fit of a denture (Fig 19-14). Infiltration into the parotid gland can produce a primary lymphoma of the parotid or a transformation of the chronically stimulated lymphocytes in a pre-existing Sjögren syndrome to produce the well-known secondary lymphomas in a long-standing Sjögren syndrome (Fig 19-15a).

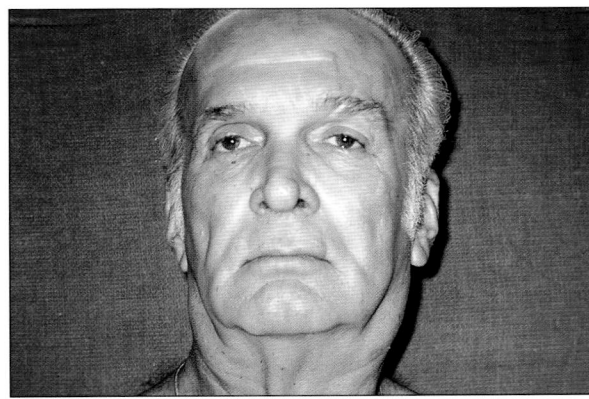

Fig 19-16a Follicular lymphoma with bilateral asymptomatic cervical lymph node enlargements, plus other lymph node enlargements in the mediastinum and axillas (not shown).

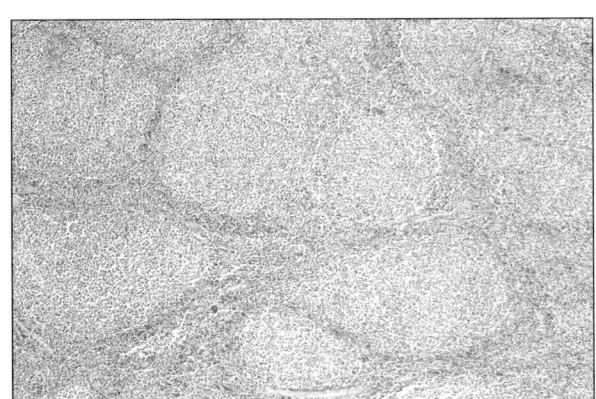

Fig 19-16b Follicular lymphoma with a distinctly nodular (follicular) pattern.

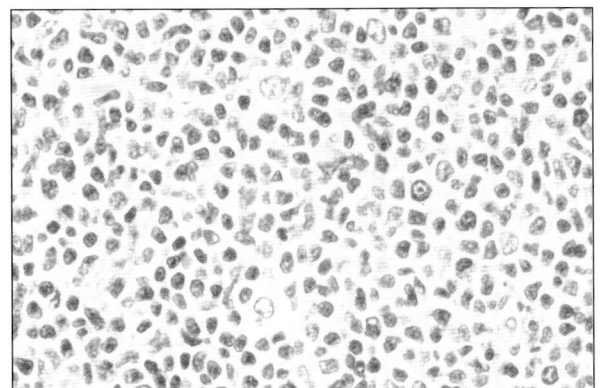

Fig 19-16c Follicular lymphoma showing a mixture of small and large lymphocytes.

HISTOPATHOLOGY ▶

Most MALT lymphomas remain localized and respond well to localized treatment. However, about 30% are disseminated at the time of diagnosis or later become disseminated, requiring systemic therapy.

MALT lymphomas are characterized by a heterogeneous cellular composition consisting of marginal zone cells, centrocyte-like (small, cleaved) cells, monocytoid B cells, small lymphocytes, and plasma cells. Some large cells (Fig 19-15b) and some reactive follicles may also be seen. Within the submucosa or the parotid marginal zone, cells will infiltrate epithelial structures, such as epimyoepithelial cells and ducts. The cells in MALT lymphomas are CD5 negative, distinguishing them from SLL/CLL cells and mantle cell lymphomas, both of which are CD5 positive. MALT lymphomas are also CD10 negative, whereas follicle center lymphomas are CD10 positive.

TREATMENT AND PROGNOSIS ▶

MALT lymphoma is one of the few types of lymphoma for which surgical excision significantly contributes to a cure or to control. Therefore, excision is recommended whenever feasible. Otherwise, radiotherapy of 4,000 cGy to 4,500 cGy to the involved tissues and to the adjacent lymph node chain is recommended. Only in cases of disseminated disease or transformation into a high-grade large-cell lymphoma is chemotherapy considered. In cases where the disease remains localized, treatment with radiotherapy has a good prognosis and a 60% long-term survival probability (Fig 19-15c).

Follicular Lymphomas

CLINICAL PRESENTATION ▶

Follicular lymphomas are the most common low-grade B-cell type of lymphoma, comprising 40% of all NHLs. Men and women are affected equally at a median age of 55 years. The course of follicular lymphoma is the prototype for all the low-grade B-cell lymphomas: Although it is treatable for palliation and undergoes regression, it will nonetheless recur and progress, and most patients will die either from it or from its treatment.

Follicular lymphoma will usually present with a diffuse asymptomatic lymphadenopathy (Fig 19-16a). Most individuals are stage III or stage IV at the time of presentation. It rarely forms in extranodal sites or does so only with concomitant lymph node involvement.

HISTOPATHOLOGY ▶

Follicular lymphomas have the most recognizable and consistent histopathology of all the NHLs. The normal nodal architecture is disrupted by follicular aggregates composed of a mixture of cleaved (centrocytes) and noncleaved (centroblasts) follicle center cells (Figs 19-16b and 19-16c). Although mostly follicular, diffuse effacement of portions of the node is also seen. Grading of these tumors according to the number of large cells (centroblasts) per high-power field is recommended, with 1 to 5 representing grade I and more than 15 grade III. As with the other low-grade B-cell lymphomas, more large cells and progression to a more diffuse pattern are ominous signs. Progression to a diffuse, large, B-cell lymphoma

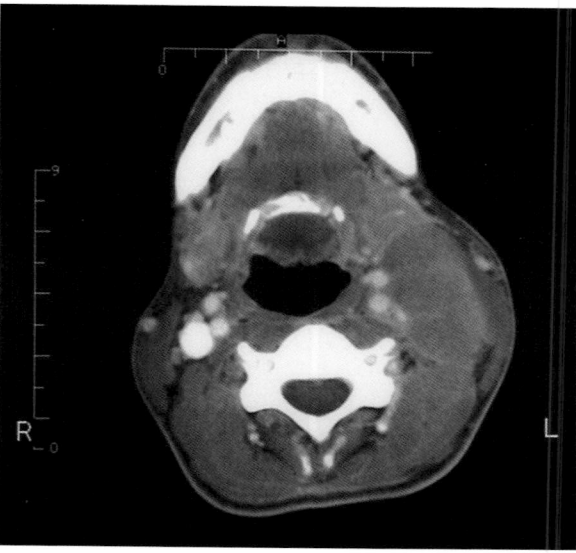

Fig 19-17 Enlarged cervical lymph node from a mantle cell lymphoma that also was associated with extranodal sites in the buccal mucosa and pharynx.

can occur and is almost always a terminal event. These tumors are CD10 positive (distinguishing them from marginal zone lymphoma), CD5 negative and CD43 negative (distinguishing them from mantle cell lymphoma), and they express B-cell leukemia/lymphoma-2 (BCL-2) protein (distinguishing them from reactive follicles). A nonrandom cytogenic translocation t(14;18) occurs and produces the BCL-2 gene rearrangement in 70% to 95% of cases. Since the normal BCL-2 gene is thought to induce or regulate programmed cell death, the BCL-2 gene dysfunction is thought to confer immortality to a cell line.

TREATMENT AND PROGNOSIS ▶

Follicular lymphoma is a terminal disease with or without treatment. The basic tenet of treatment is not to cure the disease but to make the patient feel better and live longer. Therefore, in asymptomatic and normally functioning individuals, no treatment—often termed *expectant treatment*—is the rule. However, if the lymphoma is symptomatic, compromises a vital organ, has bulky lymphadenopathy, is clinically progressive, or begins a large-cell transformation, treatment is instituted and has been shown to extend life. Treatment can vary greatly depending on the amount of the disease, presence of symptoms, and the health and wishes of the patient. A low-intensity therapy that will nonetheless induce a regression is chlorambucil. Moderately intensive therapy using CHOP (cyclophosphamide, hydroxydaunomycin, Oncovin [vincristine], and prednisone) is the next step, followed by a combination of doxorubicin, vincristine, and prednisone. In addition, experimental therapy with fludarabine and 2-chlorodeoxyadenosine (cladribine), interferon, interleukin-2, and even DNA vaccinations is available in various research trials.

Mantle Cell Lymphoma

CLINICAL PRESENTATION ▶

Mantle cell lymphoma is so named because the tumor is histologically characterized by expansion of the mantle zone, a homogeneous population of neoplastic small lymphocytes that surrounds the germinal centers. It represents yet another of the low-grade B-cell lymphomas. To describe these lymphomas as low grade is somewhat misleading, however, since all of the so-called low-grade B-cell lymphomas, particularly the mantle cell lymphoma, have a poor prognosis, and most progress to a terminal outcome.

Mantle cell lymphoma occurs in older adults and usually presents with a generalized lymphadenopathy, predominantly in men. However, these lymphomas frequently involve bone marrow and usually are not diagnosed until they have advanced to stage III or stage IV. Of pertinence to the oral and maxillofacial specialist, they frequently present with concomitant extranodal involvement that focuses on the gastrointestinal tract, including the oral cavity (Fig 19-17).

HISTOPATHOLOGY ▶

As noted, the neoplastic small cells populate the mantle zone surrounding the germinal center. They continue to proliferate until they efface the germinal center and produce a truly diffuse-patterned B-cell lymphoma. Therefore, early cases may have incomplete germinal center effacement and show residual germinal centers.

The neoplastic cells are small- to medium-sized with irregular (cleaved) or round nuclei and scant cytoplasm. Scattered histiocytes sometimes produce a "starry sky" appearance more commonly associated with Burkitt lymphoma. These tumors are CD23 negative, distinguishing them from B-cell SLL/CLL, and CD5 positive, distinguishing them from both follicular lymphoma and marginal zone lymphoma.

The cytogenetics of this tumor is identified to be a chromosome translocation on chromosomes 11 and 14, noted as t(11;14)(q13;q32). This chromosome aberration causes an overexpression of the protein cyclin D1 and parathyroid adenomatosis-1 (PRAD-1), which are the probable oncogenes for this tumor.

TREATMENT AND PROGNOSIS ▶ Mantle cell lymphoma is not curable by any currently available treatment. Patients die as a consequence of developing resistance to therapeutic drugs. Some cases transform into large B-cell lymphomas and rapidly succumb to this even higher-grade tumor.

Although treatments induce a response and partial regression of the tumor, the clinical course is one of reversal to disease progression and a downhill course to death, with median survivals of 2.5 to 4 years.

Small B-Cell Low-Grade Versus Large B-Cell High-Grade Lymphomas

As this chapter transitions from a group of lymphomas that has been called low-grade to a group that is considered high-grade, it is important to note an apparent paradox: small B-cell lymphomas are considered low grade and yet most progress to death with little hope for a cure; large B-cell lymphomas are considered high-grade, and yet, with accurate clinical staging and treatment regimens, they are curable, with 5-year survival rates ranging from 26% for high-risk advanced disease to as much as 87% for low-risk early disease. This paradox arises from the fact that a designation of low or high grade refers to the natural histories of untreated disease and not their response to treatment. Small B-cell lymphomas are described as low grade because the neoplastic cell is a more mature cell in the multistaged maturation sequence of a lymphocyte. Indeed, it resembles the size and shape of a non-neoplastic lymphocyte more closely than it does a large undifferentiated cell. Small B-cell lymphomas, however, do not respond completely to treatment. Therefore, their natural disease course—a slow but relentless progression usually leading to death—is minimally altered by treatment. Large B-cell lymphomas, on the other hand, are considered high grade because the neoplastic cell is a more primitive cell in the multistaged maturation sequence of a lymphocyte. It is closer to a blast cell, hence the often-used term *immunoblastic lymphoma*. The natural course of a large B-cell lymphoma is one of rapid progression and dissemination; however, for an as-yet unknown reason, the neoplastic cells are very sensitive to certain chemotherapeutic drugs to the point of total lysis, leading to many cures.

Large B-Cell High-Grade Lymphomas

Diffuse Large B-Cell Lymphoma

CLINICAL PRESENTATION ▶ Diffuse large B-cell lymphoma is one of the more common NHLs, accounting for 30% to 40% of all NHLs. It is a disease of middle-aged and older adults and has a median age of 56 years. Although they soon become widely disseminated, 40% are in stage I or stage II at diagnosis and 40% present with an extranodal involvement, which may include the oral or pharyngeal mucosa (Fig 19-18a). Because of its curability, this tumor in particular requires a representative biopsy specimen, an experienced hematopathologist, and an accurate, complete clinical staging (Fig 19-18b).

HISTOPATHOLOGY ▶ This lymphoma is indeed comprised of large cells in which the nuclei are at least twice the size of small lymphocytes and usually larger than a macrophage nucleus. The nucleus is vesicular with prominent nucleoli and basophilic cytoplasm (Fig 19-18c). Most often there is a combination of large noncleaved

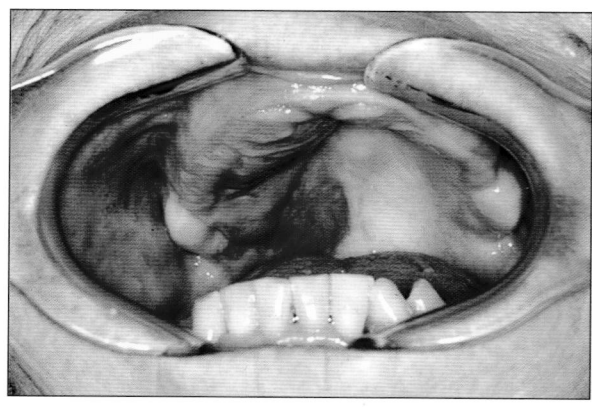
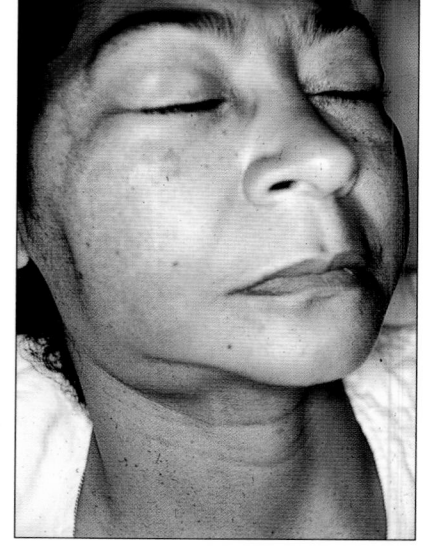
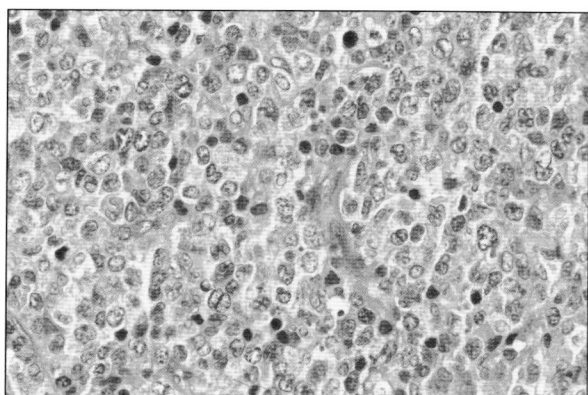

Figs 19-18a and 19-18b This large B-cell lymphoma presented with a soft, fleshy enlargement of the palatal and maxillary alveolar mucosa without ulceration and a single nodal involvement of an ipsilateral submandibular lymph node.

Fig 19-18c Large-cell lymphoma. There are also some small lymphocytic cells in the field. These lymphocytes are described as small because their nuclei are smaller than the nuclei of histiocytes, which are typically used as a reference.

(centroblast) and immunoblast-like cells, but large cleaved or multilobed and anaplastic large cells may also be seen. Some tumors have numerous T cells along with the neoplastic B cells (T-cell–rich, large B-cell lymphoma). To date, no cytogenetic abnormality is known as the oncogene for this tumor.

TREATMENT AND PROGNOSIS ▶ Because the curability of this lymphoma depends on the initial chemotherapy protocol, selection of the proper protocol is of critical importance. Therefore, the Ann Arbor Staging System (see page 841) is essential, along with a work-up to identify the patient's risk factors. The work-up includes: (*1*) a complete blood count and serum chemistries; (*2*) a chest radiograph and a chest CT scan; (*3*) a CT scan of the abdomen and pelvis; and (*4*) bilateral iliac crest bone marrow biopsies. Assessment of these risk factors allows the clinician to stratify patients into one of five risk groups.

Five pretreatment prognostic factors known to correlate well with outcome are graded:

1. Age in years ($\leq$ 60 vs $>$ 60)
2. Tumor stage (stage I or II vs stage III or IV)
3. Number of extranodal sites ($\leq$ 1 vs $\geq$ 2)
4. Patient performance to a doxorubicin-based combination chemotherapy trial (0 or 1 vs $\geq$ 2)
5. Serum lactic dehydrogenase (LDH) levels (normal vs abnormal)

From this grading, risk factors of low (0 or 1), low intermediate (2), high intermediate (3), and high (4 or 5) are determined. Cure rates correlate with the grading as follows: 5-year cure rates for low are 87%, for low intermediate are 57%, for high intermediate are 44%, and for high are 26%.

This selection of protocols and chemotherapy agents represents a myriad of possible combinations and is the province of the medical oncologist. The CHOP (cyclophosphamide, hydroxydaunomycin, Oncovin [vincristine], and prednisone) protocol is the one used most commonly. Radiotherapy is no longer used for this tumor.

Burkitt Lymphoma (Small Noncleaved Cell Lymphoma)

CLINICAL PRESENTATION ▶ Burkitt lymphoma is a very aggressive but potentially curable childhood-to-early-adult B-cell lymphoma that was brought to prominence by the Irish surgeon Denis Burkitt, who observed what he thought were

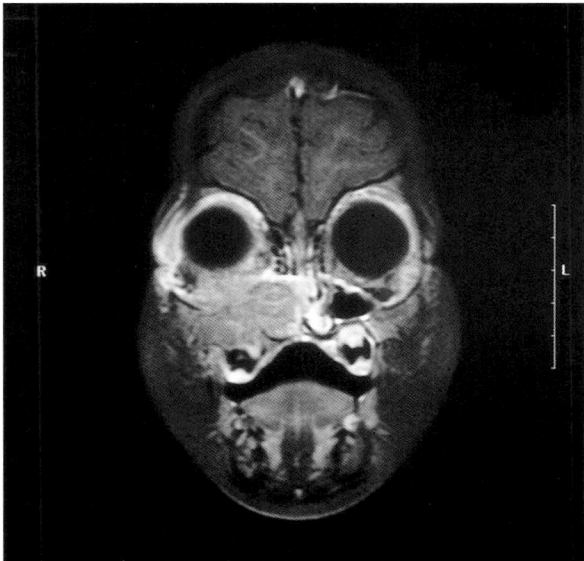

Fig 19-19 African type of Burkitt lymphoma with extensive involvement of the maxilla. Note the presence of the developing first molar teeth, which are thought to be associated with the stimulation of this tumor's growth.

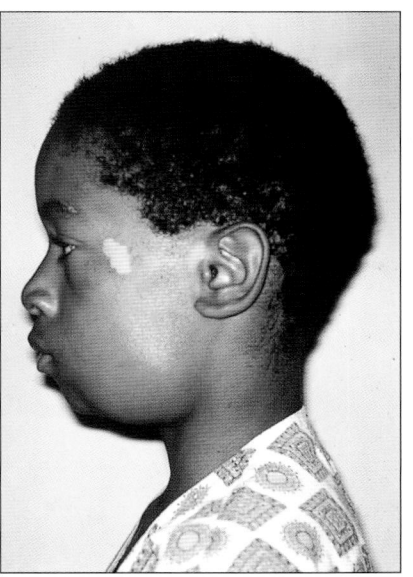

Fig 19-20 Burkitt lymphoma of the mandible in a 5-year-old. The incidence of Burkitt lymphoma involving either jaw drops from 75% at 5 years of age to 25% at 14 years of age.

sarcomas in the jaws of East African children. The same jaw tumors had previously been observed by the missionary physician Albert Cook in Uganda in 1897. Today, Burkitt lymphoma is still much more common in equatorial Africa, where it has a different presentation than in the United States. In equatorial Africa, Burkitt lymphoma has an incidence of 5 to 15 per 100,000 children and a predilection for the jaws and is related to the warm, humid climate areas. In the United States and elsewhere in the world, it has an incidence of only 2 or 3 per 100,000 children, a predilection for the abdomen (particularly the right lower quadrant), and is unrelated to climate

African Type

In the African type, individuals develop the well-known jaw tumors associated with this disease. However, the jaw tumors are age dependent and appear to be associated with the development of permanent molar teeth (Fig 19-19). Seventy-five percent of children 5 years or younger with Burkitt lymphoma have jaw tumors, whereas only 25% of Burkitt lymphoma patients older than 14 years have jaw tumors (Fig 19-20). This suggests a stimulatory effect from growth factors associated with tooth or jaw development. Maxillary tumors occur twice as often as those in the mandible, and multiquadrant tumors are common.

American Type

In the American type, individuals develop abdominal tumors in 90% of cases, from which they suffer pain, nausea, vomiting, and constipation. Occasionally, bleeding, appendicitis, and intestinal perforation cause significant distress and the need for emergency care. Jaw involvement may occur instead of or concomitantly with abdominal tumors but is seen in only 15% to 20% of the cases.

HISTOPATHOLOGY ▶ Burkitt lymphoma is composed of sheets of medium-sized B cells with nuclei that are equal to or smaller than the nuclei of benign histiocytes. They are uniform and round with two or three nucleoli and basophilic cytoplasm. They often have a squared-off appearance that makes the cells seem to be cohesive. Mitotic activity is high, and there is considerable apoptosis (cell death). Consequently, there are in-

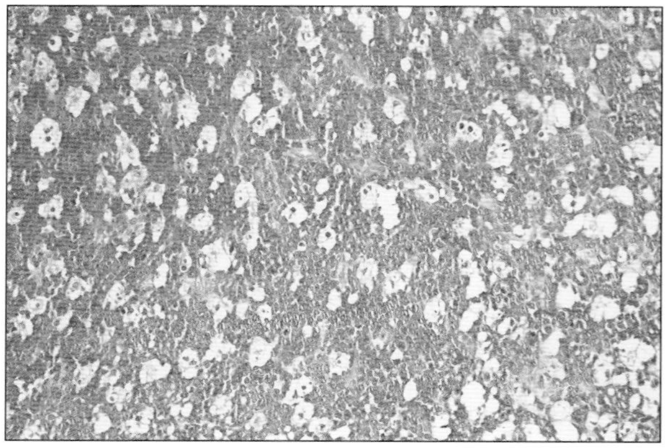

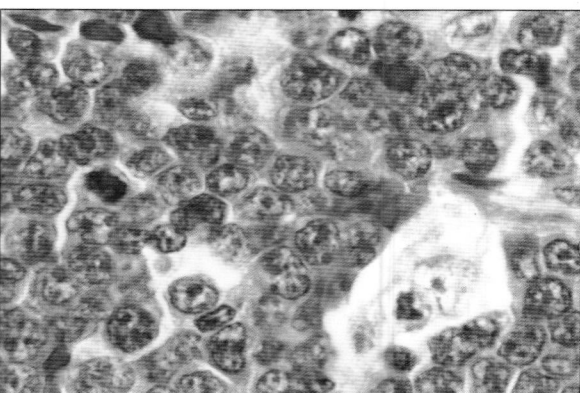

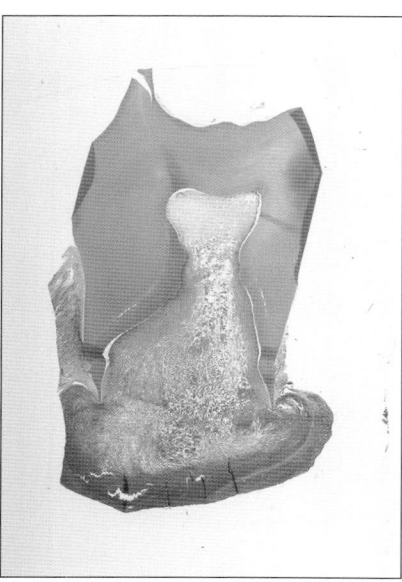

Fig 19-21a Burkitt lymphoma with a so-called starry sky pattern.

Fig 19-21b At 1,000× magnification, the squared-off, cohesive pattern of the dark-staining neoplastic cells can be appreciated. Several mitotic figures can be seen. The light-staining macrophage can be seen phagocytosing a necrotic tumor cell.

Fig 19-22 Burkitt lymphoma invading the pulpal tissue.

terspersed non-neoplastic macrophages that ingest necrotic cells. The appearance of these pale-staining macrophages against the darkly stained background of neoplastic B cells produces the well-known "starry sky" appearance of Burkitt lymphoma (Figs 19-21a and 19-21b). When the jaws are involved, there is a propensity for the neoplasm to invade dental pulps (Fig 19-22).

Burkitt lymphomas have a known chromosome t(8:14) translocation where the c-myc oncogene is juxtaposed to a heavy chain immunoglobulin gene sequence or as a variation to a light chain immunoglobulin sequence. This c-myc dysregulation seems to be the defining abnormality that eventuates into a Burkitt lymphoma. In addition, about 37% have a mutation in the p53 tumor suppression gene, and there is a 20% to 30% association with Epstein-Barr virus in the United States.

TREATMENT AND PROGNOSIS ▶

The treatment protocol and principles for a Burkitt lymphoma consist of multidrug chemotherapy, intensive short-term therapy, and prophylaxis of lymphoma spread into the central nervous system (CNS) using intrathecal methotrexate and cytarabine. This approach is used for all stages and all sites. Surgery is not effective beyond biopsy and the debulking of tumors to relieve symptoms or life-threatening obstructions. Radiotherapy also is of little benefit.

Burkitt lymphoma is staged based on the number of masses rather than the number of lymph node chains, as it is in the Ann Arbor Staging System. Stage I or II refers to one or two masses on the same side of the diaphragm. Stage III refers to multiple masses on either side of the diaphragm. Stage IV refers to the involvement of bone marrow on aspiration and to the presence of 5% to 25% malignant cells in the aspirate. If malignant noncleaved B cells comprise greater than 25% of the aspirate, it is considered a Burkitt type of B-cell acute lymphocytic leukemia (B-cell ALL).

The choice of chemotherapy agents is the province of medical oncologists. Of the many protocols used, cyclophosphamide, Oncovin (vincristine), methotrexate, and prednisone (COMP) is the centerpiece around which other various drug combinations are made.

With the intensive therapy used today, cases diagnosed in the early stages have a cure rate between 90% and 100%, and later stages have a cure rate between 80% and 90%.

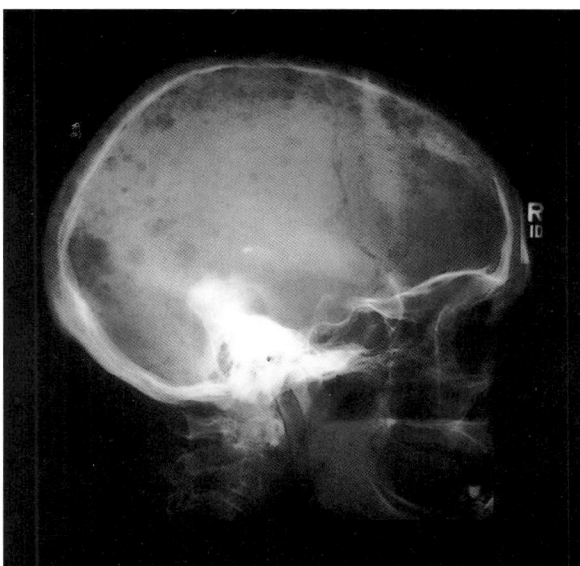

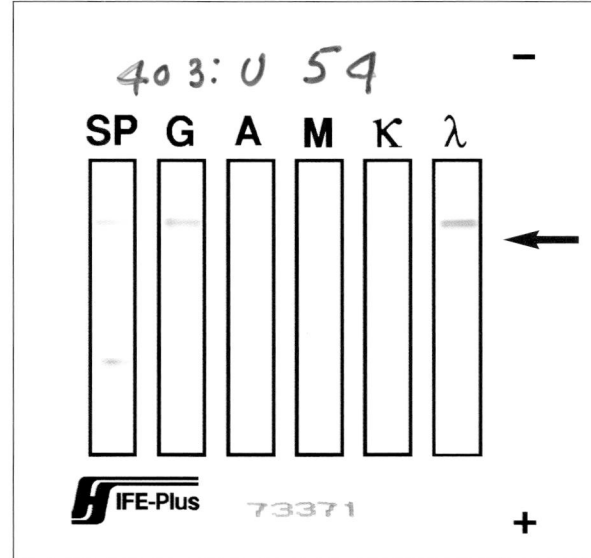

Fig 19-23a Multifocal osteolytic lesions of the skull in an individual with multiple myeloma.

Fig 19-23b A monoclonal gamma spike (shown here) or a beta spike in a serum protein electrophoresis is diagnostic for multiple myeloma.

Plasmacytomas/Multiple Myeloma

Multiple Myeloma and Plasma Cell Dyscrasias

CLINICAL PRESENTATION AND PATHOGENESIS ▶

Multiple myeloma is a monoclonal malignant neoplastic proliferation of plasma cells that involves multifocal sites of the bone marrow and occasionally involves extraskeletal sites as well.

Multiple myeloma is one of the more frequently occurring hematopoietic malignancies, accounting for 1% of all malignancies in whites and 2% of those in blacks. It is the most frequently occurring malignancy in bone. The incidence of multiple myeloma increases with age beginning at 40 years; 90% of patients are older than 40 years.

The clinical presentation is a triad of clinical signs: (*1*) multifocal osteolytic lesions, of which the skull (Fig 19-23a), vertebrae, pelvis, and the proximal portions of long bones are the most frequent locations; (*2*) proliferation in these lesions of atypical plasma cells; and (*3*) a serum monoclonal gammopathy (Fig 19-23b). These signs may in turn produce pain (particularly in the weight-bearing areas of the vertebrae), anemia, hypercalcemia, renal failure, proteinuria, and an increased incidence of infections. In the vast majority of individuals, an increased level of monoclonal immunoglobulins, called the *M component,* can be detected in the serum. This M component is of the IgG class in 50% of cases, of the IgA class in 25%, and rarely of the IgM or IgE classes. These immunoglobulins will produce a monoclonal spike usually in the gamma or beta regions on serum protein electrophoresis, and every 0.5 g/dL measured reflects 10 g of neoplastic plasma cells.

Like all malignancies, multiple myeloma results from genetic alterations. The most frequent altered chromosomes are 1, 11, and 14, with an apparent translocation of chromosomes t(11;14) as the specific oncogene.

RADIOGRAPHIC FINDINGS ▶

The earliest and most pronounced radiographic changes are the classic "punched out" radiolucencies in the skull, ribs, vertebrae, and pelvis. The oral and maxillofacial specialist may become aware of these findings when reviewing radiographs related to trauma or in routine preoperative chest radiographs. Occasionally, these same radiolucencies are noted in the jaws (Fig 19-24). In any location, they are due

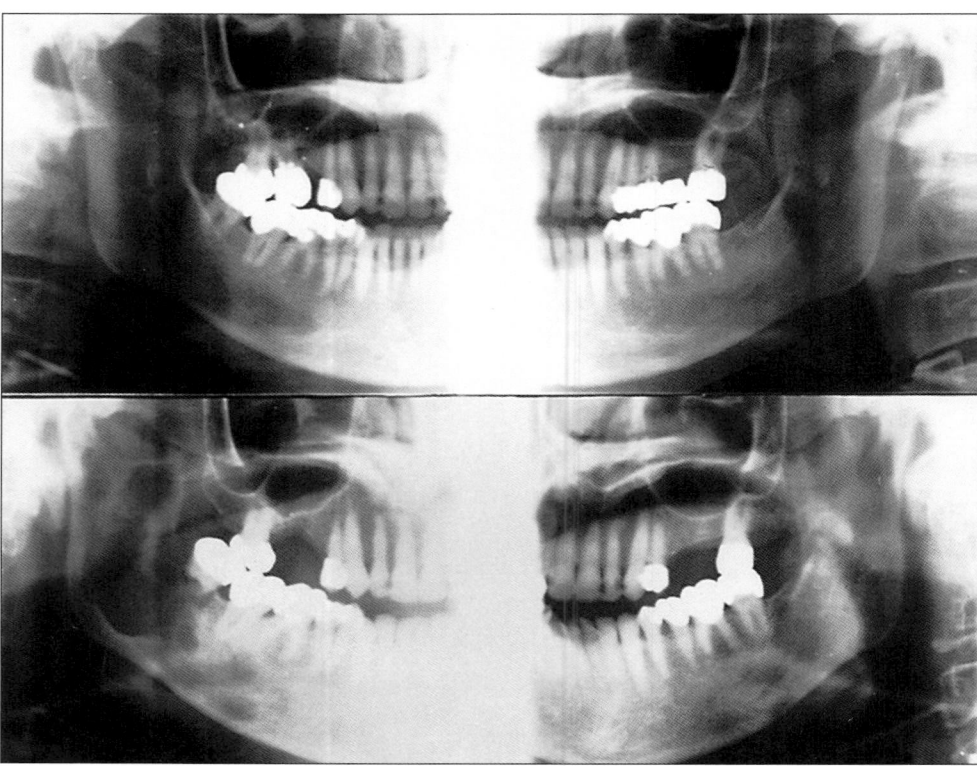

Fig 19-24 Two panoramic radiographs taken 1 year apart showing the development of multiple radiolucencies in the mandible due to multiple myeloma.

to the elaboration by neoplastic cells of an osteoclast-activating factor and proliferation of these cells in the larger resorption cavity created by the osteoclastic bone resorption.

DIAGNOSTIC WORK-UP ▶ Suspicion for multiple myeloma may arise from the incidental finding of punched-out radiolucencies, from a biopsy that shows a monotonous sheet of plasma cells, or from a finding of unexplained hypercalcemia. In such cases, the diagnostic study that will confirm or rule out multiple myeloma is a serum protein electrophoresis. Once the characteristic monoclonal gamma or beta spike is identified, it is reasonable to accomplish a complete serum chemistry study, including serum calcium and renal function tests. The determination of Bence Jones protein, which has been the subject of much discussion, is of little value today. This is a specific laboratory maneuver that identifies an excess of light chain immunoglobulins in the urine. It has not been of diagnostic significance since the use of protein electrophoresis in the mid-1970s. However, the identification of Bence Jones protein does imply a more severe renal dysfunction and therefore a poorer prognosis. Bence Jones protein is seen in only 20% of multiple myeloma patients. The test involves heating the urine sample to 55°C, where Bence Jones proteins and other urinary proteins may precipitate out. Bence Jones protein will then redissolve in the urine when it is heated beyond 60°C, which is unique and thus identifies its presence.

HISTOPATHOLOGY ▶ All of the clinical forms of multiple myeloma and plasmacytic tumors present the same histology. There is a monotonous proliferation of plasma cells showing varying degrees of differentiation, but the plasmacytic nature of the cells is usually apparent with the eccentricity of the nucleus and clumped chromatin. Binucleated cells and some mitoses may be present, although the latter are not numerous (Figs 19-25a and 19-25b). There is little supporting stroma, and the fibrovascular component associated with inflammatory lesions, as well as the pleomorphic mix of an inflammatory infiltrate, are absent. To confirm that these cells are plasma cells, methyl green–pyronin stain may be employed, since the ribonucleic acid within the cytoplasm reacts with pyronin and stains red. In addition, the monoclonality of the infiltrate

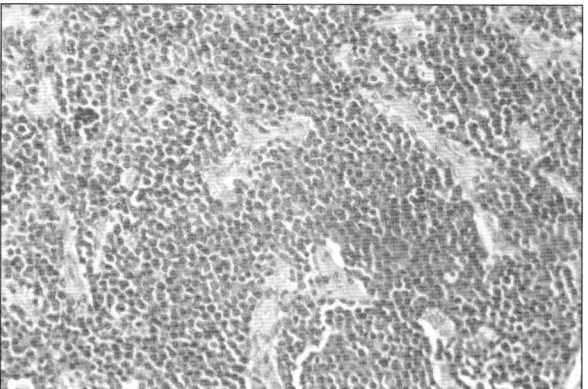

Fig 19-25a Sheets of abnormal plasma cells with little stroma. The histologic diagnosis is plasmacytoma. The patient, however, was found to have multiple myeloma.

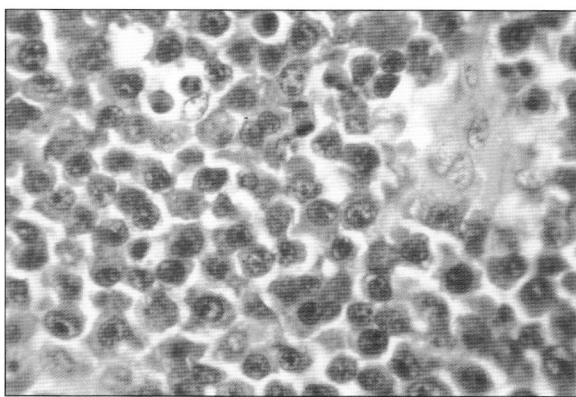

Fig 19-25b High-power view of Fig 19-25a showing a uniform proliferation of abnormal plasma cells with their eccentric nuclei.

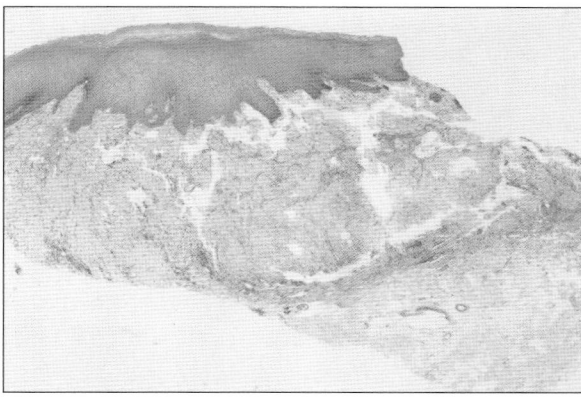

Fig 19-26a Amyloid in the buccal mucosa. The patient also had bilateral aggregates of amyloid in the tongue. This discovery led to the diagnosis of multiple myeloma.

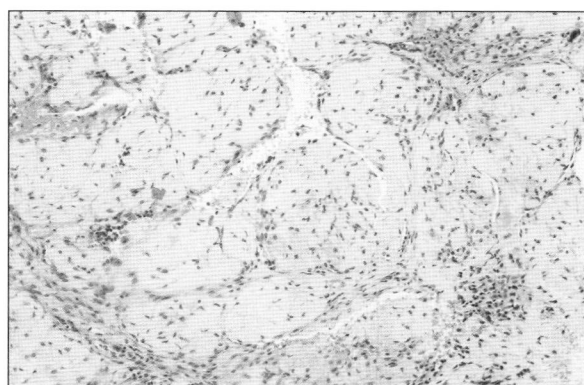

Fig 19-26b High-power view of Fig 19-26a showing amyloid compressing blood vessels.

may be demonstrated by immunocytochemistry to demonstrate the presence of a single type (kappa or lambda) of immunoglobulin light chain.

Significant deposits of amyloid are seen in about 10% of patients with multiple myeloma. Histologically, these appear as masses of pale homogeneous eosinophilic material within the soft tissue, which may compress blood vessels (Figs 19-26a and 19-26b). The amyloid can be identified by Congo red stain, which shows an apple-green birefringence with polarized light or by immunofluorescent stain with thioflavin T. Crystal violet stain may also be used, but this nonpermanent stain fades rapidly.

TREATMENT AND PROGNOSIS ▶

Although fully developed multiple myeloma is fatal, patients today live longer (4 to 10 years) than they did in the mid-1990s (2 to 4 years), mostly because of improved management of hypercalcemia and renal dysfunction. Chemotherapy protocols vary, but the combination of vincristine-adriamycin-dexamethasone (VAD) along with pamidronate (Aredia, Novartis) to treat hypercalcemia is the most common. This protocol may be combined with focal radiotherapy of 3,000 cGy to 4,500 cGy in areas of vertebral compression fractures or where large plasma cell collections compress vital structures. Renal failure is the most common cause of death, followed by infection. Therefore, peritoneal dialysis and standard dialysis have been factors in increasing the survival times.

With longer survival times, more patients develop complications of multiple myeloma or its treatment. Two complications are of special significance to the oral and maxillofacial specialist. The first is a relatively

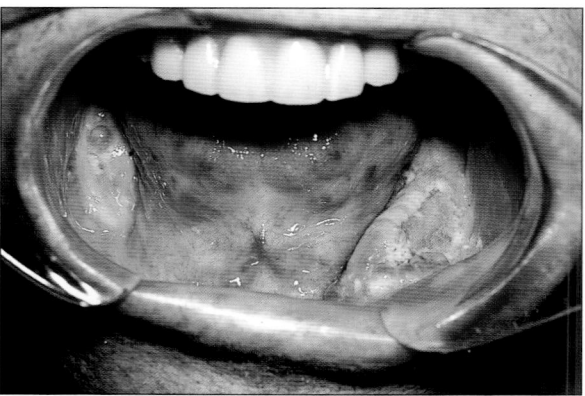

Fig 19-27 Exposed nonvital bone due to pamidronate (Aredia) therapy used in multiple myeloma to treat hypercalcemia.

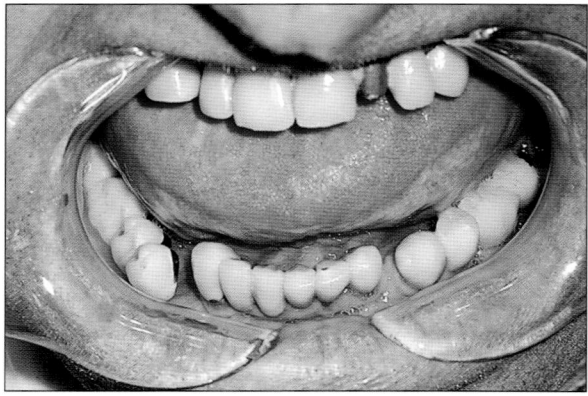

Fig 19-28 Amyloidosis secondary to multiple myeloma produced a firm enlargement of the tongue (macroglossia) that mobilized and buccally splayed the dentition.

recently recognized complication of avascular necrosis of the jaws, which is clinically manifested as exposed nonvital alveolar bone in edentulous areas or around periodontally diseased teeth (Fig 19-27). The presentation will resemble that of osteoradionecrosis or osteopetrosis. Related to multiple myeloma, it is caused by the anti-osteoclastic function of pamidronate (Aredia), which prevents bone cell renewal by the normal resorption-remodeling mechanism. In such cases, pamidronate must be discontinued for 2 months before a debridement and advancement flap closure can be attempted. A more thorough discussion of Aredia-induced avascular necrosis of the jaws is presented in Chapter 2.

The second complication is a well-known complication of multiple myeloma itself: secondary amyloidosis. Significant amyloidosis occurs in 15% to 25% of multiple myeloma cases. In the oral and maxillofacial area, this is most commonly seen as a firm symmetric macroglossia that may be of sufficient size to splay teeth and/or create tooth mobility (Fig 19-28). It can also affect speech, eating, or swallowing, and in severe cases may obstruct the upper airway, necessitating reduction and/or a tracheostomy.

The macroglossia is caused by an interstitial deposit of amyloid protein within and replacing the tongue musculature. These are specific lambda chain (light chain) deposits. The amyloid deposits in multiple myeloma are referred to as amyloid (AL) proteins and are the product of the malignant plasma cells. The amyloid deposits in idiopathic primary amyloidosis are referred to as AA proteins.

Variant Forms of Myeloma

The following four variations of classic multiple myeloma represent either precursers to so-called systemic multiple myeloma or lower-grade versions of multiple myeloma.

Solitary Myeloma

This is a single-bone focus of malignant plasma cells in an individual in whom the remaining marrow is normal. In 75% of these individuals, there is no M component in the serum, and in the remaining 25% there is less than 1.5 g/dL. However, about 70% of solitary myeloma cases progress to full systemic multiple myeloma within 3 years, supporting the concept that it represents a precurser to multiple myeloma. If only one bony focus is confirmed and no M component is present, radiotherapy of 3,500 cGy to 4,500 cGy is the treatment of choice.

Extramedullary Plasmacytoma

Approximately 5% of all myelomas originate in an extraskeletal site, and those sites are frequently within the mucosa of the oral cavity and pharynx. Such extramedullary plasmacytomas in the head and neck area have been associated with a favorable prognosis, as evidenced by a 70% 10-year survival rate. As with most solitary myelomas, the M component is either absent or less than 1.5 g/dL. This variation also is treated with radiotherapy of 3,500 cGy to 4,500 cGy.

Nonsecretory Myeloma

About 14% of systemic multiple myelomas with numerous bony lesions have no demonstrable M component. These are believed to be true multiple myeloma cases with the only difference being that the malignant cells do not secrete their monoclonal immunoglobulins. Because of this, nonsecretory myelomas have fewer disease-related complications, particularly renal impairment, and therefore a better prognosis. However, because it represents a true multiple myeloma, chemotherapy and anti-osteoclastic drugs are the usual therapies.

Plasma Cell Leukemia

Multiple myeloma becomes plasma cell leukemia when more than 20% of the peripheral white blood cell count represents malignant plasma cells or when the absolute count exceeds 2×10^{10}/dL. This diagnosis is an ominous sign and almost always represents a terminal finding. It may develop as a complication of an existing multiple myeloma (1% of cases) or arise de novo as a particularly aggressive form of multiple myeloma. It is treated with the VAD protocol but with little response.

T-Cell Lymphomas

Extranodal Natural Killer/T-Cell Lymphoma, Nasal Type (Angiocentric Lymphoma)

CLINICAL PRESENTATION ▶ The oral and maxillofacial specialist will recognize extranodal natural killer/T-cell lymphoma more by its older and less accurate name, *midline lethal granuloma*. Once thought to represent an overexuberant granulomatous disease, this entity has now been confirmed to represent one of several types of peripheral T-cell lymphomas, this one with a predilection for the nasal cavity and palate and for Latin Americans and Asians (Fig 19-29a).

The nomenclature *peripheral T-cell lymphoma* does not refer to its extranodal presentation but rather to the immaturity of the T cell. That is, the T cell does not arise directly from the thymus or the center of a lymph node but at the lymph node periphery, where immature T-lymphocytes exist. It therefore distinguishes itself from cutaneous lymphomas such as mycosis fungoides and HIV-related T-cell lymphomas. However, there is a strong correlation to Epstein-Barr virus, approaching 100% in some studies.

Patients are usually between 25 and 50 years of age and present with nasal stuffiness or palatal ulcers. Pain is common but not present in every case. The course is rapid and will often progress to an oronasal communication in a few days to a few weeks. Radiographs or CT scans will identify an irregular palatal bone destruction without the presence of a large tissue mass (Fig 19-29b).

DIFFERENTIAL DIAGNOSIS ▶ Palatal ulcerations that may or may not be painful but appear without any apparent cause should bring to mind several specific entities. The oral and maxillofacial specialist may immediately think of *Wegener granulomatosis*, in which the soft tissue appearance is nearly identical. However, Wegener granulomatosis does not destroy bone and will not create an oronasal communication. Fungal lesions such as *coccidiomycosis*, *histoplasmosis*, *aspergillosis*, and *mucormycosis* may also involve the palate and nasal cavities with similar lesions. Of these, mucormycosis is the most likely to mimic the destruction of an angiocentric lymphoma and produce an oronasal fistula. In addition, an *aggressive squamous cell carcinoma* or a *high-grade mucoepidermoid carcinoma* may show an aggressive destruction of the palate and nasal vault. Finally, rare cases of *tertiary syphilis* that have not been treated have been reported to erode through the palate.

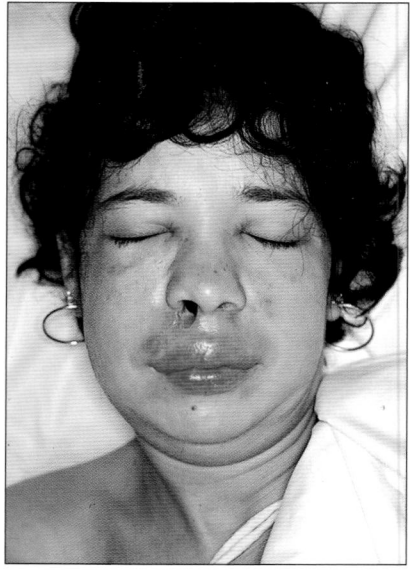

Fig 19-29a Young individual debilitated and in pain from an extranodal natural killer/T-cell lymphoma. Note the upper lip edema and the erosion of the right alar base.

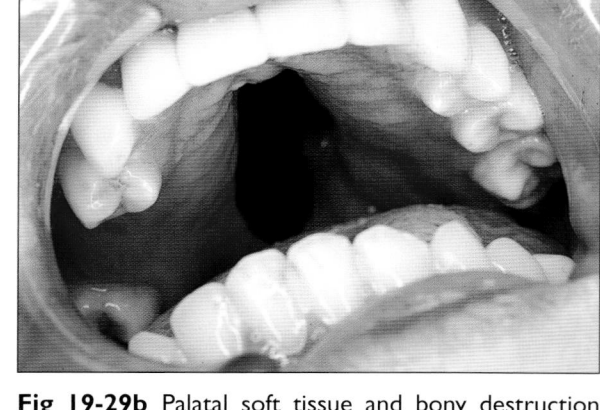

Fig 19-29b Palatal soft tissue and bony destruction produced this oronasal communication at the midline in the individual shown in Fig 19-29a. This typical presentation together with previously high mortality rates gave rise to the outdated term *midline lethal granuloma*.

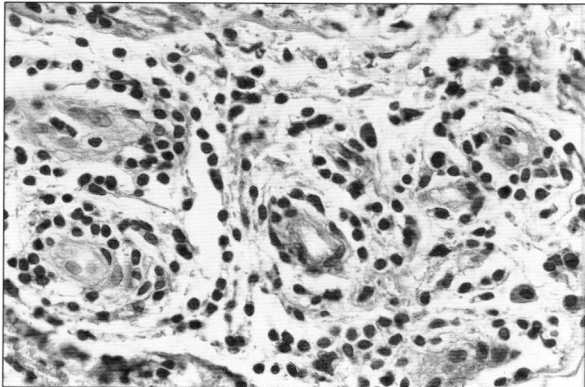

Fig 19-29c Peripheral natural killer T-cell lymphoma showing angiocentricity. Small lymphocytes can often be seen.

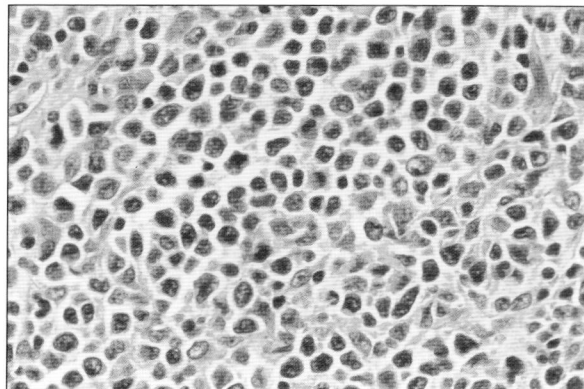

Fig 19-29d Peripheral natural killer T-cell lymphoma with a pleomorphic population. Some mitoses can be seen.

DIAGNOSTIC WORK-UP ▶

Biopsy of a non-necrotic soft tissue component of this lesion will be diagnostic. Because of the differential diagnosis of this presentation, cultures for fungi and a periodic acid–Schiff (PAS) stain to highlight fungi also are recommended.

HISTOPATHOLOGY ▶

Histologically, these tumors usually have an angio-invasive and angiodestructive growth pattern that results in ischemic necrosis of neoplastic cells and normal tissue. The cytologic composition is variable with normal-appearing small lymphocytes, atypical lymphoid cells, and immunoblasts, as well as eosinophils, histiocytes, and plasma cells (Figs 19-29c and 19-29d). This pleomorphic and variable histology explains why these lesions were so long overlooked as representing lymphomas.

TREATMENT AND PROGNOSIS ▶

This peripheral T-cell lymphoma, once thought to be universally fatal (hence the previous name, midline lethal granulomas), is now treated to a 3-year overall survival rate of about 50%. Early localized cases are treated with external beam radiotherapy of 5,000 cGy to 6,400 cGy. More extensive lesions are often treated with a six-drug chemotherapy protocol consisting of cyclophosphamide, Adriamycin (doxorubicin), procarbazine, bleomycin, vincristine, and prednisone, with or without adjunctive radiotherapy.

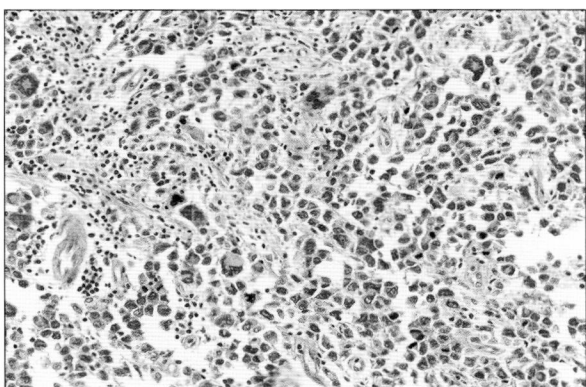

Fig 19-30 Anaplastic large-cell lymphoma showing large pleomorphic cells.

Anaplastic Large-Cell Lymphoma

CLINICAL PRESENTATION AND PATHOGENESIS ▶

While a name such as anaplastic large-cell lymphoma would suggest a disease with uniformly aggressive behavior, this is not necessarily the case because two different forms exist. The primary cutaneous form, which occurs in adults, may actually regress spontaneously but is otherwise slowly progressive and incurable. The systemic form is aggressive and rapidly progressive; however, like most high-grade lymphomas, it is much more responsive to treatment and is therefore curable. This form often involves extranodal sites in and around the head and neck area but may also involve lymph nodes and skin and is seen in children. In years past, this presentation may have been referred to as *Letterer-Siwe disease* because it was thought to represent an aggressive form of what was then termed *histiocytosis X* (see Chapter 20).

The primary cutaneous form is CD30 positive, cutaneous lymphocyte antigen positive (CLA+), and epithelial membrane antigen negative (EMA–). The systemic form is CD30 positive and EMA positive and frequently can be demonstrated to exhibit a chromosome translocation, t(2:5).

Both forms of this disease are known to be related to other lymphomas, particularly Hodgkin lymphoma and mycosis fungoides.

HISTOPATHOLOGY ▶

Histologically, these tumors have large anaplastic cells. The nuclei are pleomorphic and often multiple (Fig 19-30). Nucleoli may be multiple or single and prominent. Cells are usually larger than in large B-cell lymphomas and may resemble Reed-Sternberg cells. The cytoplasm is typically abundant. Macrophages may be present and can be prominent.

TREATMENT AND PROGNOSIS ▶

The primary cutaneous form is slowly progressive but relentless, even in the face of therapy. Early or localized disease may not require treatment or may be treated by 3,500 cGy to 4,500 cGy of radiotherapy in a field that includes the first echelon of lymph nodes. More widespread disease may be treated for relief of symptoms and palliation, most commonly with the chemotherapy protocol of cyclophosphamide, hydroxydaunomycin, Oncovin (vincristine), and prednisone (CHOP) or prednisone, methotrexate, Adriamycin (doxorubicin), cyclophosphamide, and etoposide (PRO-MACE). The systemic form is curable with intensive chemotherapy using CHOP or PRO-MACE.

Mycosis Fungoides and the Sézary Syndrome

CLINICAL PRESENTATION AND PATHOGENESIS ▶

Mycosis fungoides is a cutaneous T-cell lymphoma in which the oral and maxillofacial specialist can play a significant role in recognition and diagnosis. Although its name implies a fungal infection or a disease resembling a fungal infection, the French dermatologist Albert Sézary, who first described it in 1906, actually was relating the mushroom shape of its lesions in the tumor stage.

Mycosis fungoides often goes undiagnosed for several years because of its resemblance to nonspecific skin conditions or contact allergies. Because of its early presentation with plaque-like skin lesions

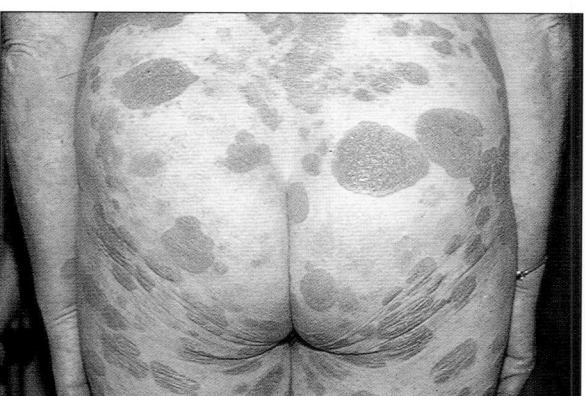

Fig 19-31 The plaque stage of mycosis fungoides with numerous red and white lesions.

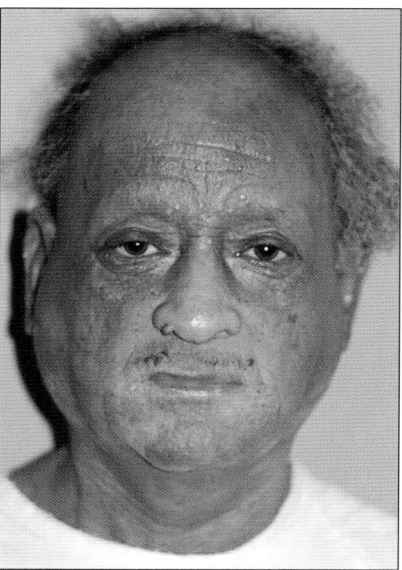

Fig 19-32 The diffuse erythrodermic stage of mycosis fungoides with violaceous pruritic and scaly skin as well as a parotid enlargement due to infiltration into the parotid gland and skin.

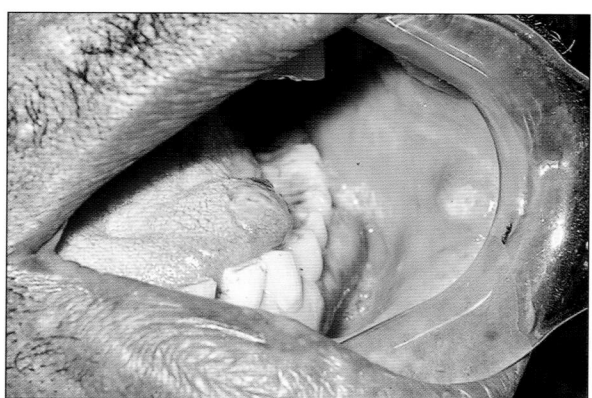

Fig 19-33a A white striaform appearance of the buccal mucosa resembling lichen planus in an individual with mycosis fungoides.

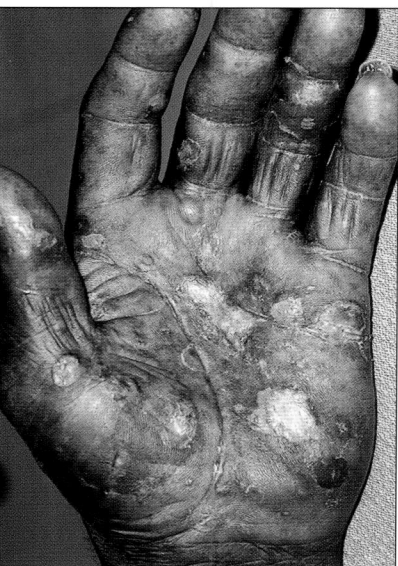

Fig 19-33b Thickened white plaques on the palms of the hands in the same individual.

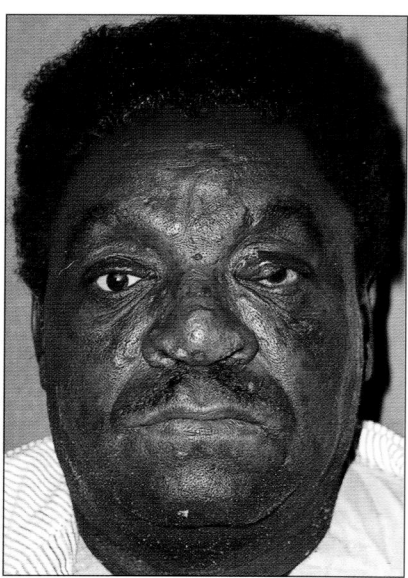

Fig 19-33c This individual also developed thickened plaques of his facial skin, which mimicked leprosy and discoid lupus erythematosis.

and significant pruritus, many are incorrectly diagnosed as psoriasis or lichen planus. In fact, mycosis fungoides classically progresses over 3 to 10 years before a final leukemic phase, known as the *Sézary syndrome*, develops. The three progressive stages are an initial plaque stage of red/white eczematous lesions (Fig 19-31), a tumor stage of nodules with possible ulcerations and lymph node enlargements, and a diffuse erythrodermic stage in which pruritus and cold intolerance develop over a majority of the skin surface area (Fig 19-32).

Along with the skin, the oral mucosa in the plaque stage will resemble striaform lichen planus or a diffuse clinical leukoplakia (Fig 19-33a). In the tumor stage, submucosal nodules are seen. Both can be readily biopsied and will usually identify the characteristic Pautrier microabscesses and the cerebriform nucleus of the abnormal T cells that infiltrate all levels of the submucosa without the grenz zone that is seen in other lymphomas.

Mycosis fungoides is a rare lymphoma occurring in adults older than 35 years. It has no known etiologic factors or chromosomal translocations, but a viral etiology is suspected. Most cases go undiagnosed for at least 5 years. Characteristic features that my lead the clinician to suspect mycosis fungoides are the combination of large surface areas of skin eczema and oral mucosal white plaques together with pruritus, alopecia, and a symmetric thickening of the palms and soles (Fig 19-33b). In addition, thickening of the facial skin is also frequently seen (Fig 19-33c).

DIFFERENTIAL DIAGNOSIS ▶

The early, nonspecific presentation of pruritic skin lesions and white oral patches will suggest *contact allergies*, *drug allergies*, *psoriasis*, and *skin lichen planus*. Although psoriasis and skin lichen planus may also have pruritus and alopecia, as does mycosis fungoides, psoriasis does not usually have oral lesions, and when it does they are not white patches but a thickening of the attached gingiva, and skin lichen planus rarely occurs concomitantly with oral lichen planus. Involvement of the facial skin may give the appearance of *leprosy* or *discoid lupus erythematosis*.

DIAGNOSTIC WORK-UP ▶

Cases suggestive of mycosis fungoides should undergo an oral biopsy of any nodules or white patches, a skin lesion biopsy, and a lymph node biopsy of any enlarged lymph nodes. In addition, a thorough physical examination with attention to abdominal masses, a CT scan of the chest and abdomen, and a complete blood count are needed for an accurate staging.

The staging system used for mycosis fungoides is the tumor, node, metastasis, blood (TNMB) system (Tables 19-5 and 19-6). The T stage represents the type and extent of skin involvement and closely correlates with survival. The N stage relates uninvolved to completely involved lymph nodes as determined both clinically and by histopathology of at least one biopsied lymph node. The M stage identifies the absence or presence of visceral involvement. The B stage signifies the absence or presence of 5% or more of abnormal circulating T lymphocytes.

HISTOPATHOLOGY ▶

Mycosis fungoides evolves through three stages. The initial plaque stage involves the epidermis and the papillary dermis. In the plaque and tumor stages there is proliferation in the reticular dermis. There may be subsequent dissemination to lymph nodes and viscera. In the initial plaque stage, lymphocytes sparsely infiltrate the epidermis and papillary dermis, which is fibrotic, while the epidermis usually shows a psoriasiform hyperplasia. The lymphocytic nuclei have irregular contours and are arranged linearly above the basement membrane. There is little in the way of vacuolar change. Diagnosis at this stage is often difficult and is primarily architectural. There is a resemblance to psoriasis and lichen planus.

In the fully developed plaque stage, the papillary dermis contains a denser band-like infiltrate of lymphocytes, but in addition the reticular dermis contains a lymphocytic infiltrate that may be perivascular or diffuse (Fig 19-33d). Cytologic atypia is more apparent. Aggregates of cells within intraepidermal vacuoles (Pautrier microabscesses) may occur (Fig 19-33e).

In the tumor stage, a dense infiltrate of neoplastic cells is present in the reticular dermis, and there is a decrease in the epidermotropism of the earlier stages. The cells are usually small with convoluted, cerebriform nuclei, but some larger cells may also be present (Fig 19-33f). These can compress the overlying epithelium and cause ulceration. These anaplastic cells may circulate in the blood (Sézary syndrome) and involve the paracortex of lymph nodes. Phenotypically these are CD4-positive cells. Eosinophils, plasma cells, Langerhans cells, and interdigitating cells may also be present.

TREATMENT AND PROGNOSIS ▶

There are several therapies available to treat mycosis fungoides: topical steroids, phototherapy, topical chemotherapy, radiotherapy, and systemic chemotherapy. The selection of therapy is based on the staging evaluation.

Early stages and minor asymptomatic cases initially can be managed with topical steroids such as 0.05% fluocinonide cream (Lidex, Medicis Dermatologics) or 0.25% desoximetasone cream (Topicort, Aventis).

Table 19-5 Tumor, node, metastasis, blood (TNMB) classification for mycosis fungoides

Classification	Description
T (skin)	
T1	Limited plaques, papules, or eczematous lesions covering < 10% of the skin surface
T2	Generalized plaques, papules, or eczematous lesions covering > 10% of the skin surface
T3	Tumors
T4	Generalized erythroderma
N (nodes)	
N0	No clinically abnormal peripheral lymph nodes; biopsies (if performed) are negative
N1	Clinically abnormal peripheral lymph nodes
N2	No clinically abnormal peripheral lymph nodes, but biopsy specimens show involvement by mycosis fungoides
N3	Clinically abnormal peripheral lymph nodes; pathologic findings positive for mycosis fungoides
M (viscera)	
M0	No visceral involvement
M1	Visceral involvement (biopsy documented)
B (blood)	
B0	Atypical circulating cells not present in peripheral blood (< 5%)
B1	Atypical circulating cells present (> 5%)

Table 19-6 Staging classification for mycosis fungoides

Stage	T (Skin)	N (Nodes)	M (Viscera)
IA	1	0	0
IB	2	0	0
IIA	1–2	1	0
IIB	3	0–1	0
IIIA	4	0	0
IIIB	4	1	0
IVA	1–4	2–3	0
IVB	1–4	0–3	1

Most symptomatic patients in stage I or stage II are treated with psoralen plus ultraviolet light-A (PUVA), similar to psoriasis therapy. Psoralen binds to DNA in the presence of ultraviolet light-A (UVA), which is in the 320- to 400-nm range, forming complexes that inhibit DNA synthesis. Since UVA penetrates to a depth only into the upper dermis, it is ideally suited to treat mycosis fungoides. Treatment with PUVA is two to three times per week for 6 months and is usually followed by maintenance with one treatment monthly.

Topical chemotherapy with nitrogen mustard (mechlorethamine or HN2) is another effective and convenient treatment for mycosis fungoides. The HN2 is mixed with water or in an ointment in a concentration of 10 to 20 mg/dL and is applied to skin lesions once or twice daily. This treatment also lasts about 6 months, after which time a monthly maintenance application is used.

Radiation therapy is the most effective therapy for mycosis fungoides and can be used in most stages. Individual plaques or nodules can be treated with small-field irradiation with minimally penetrating elec-

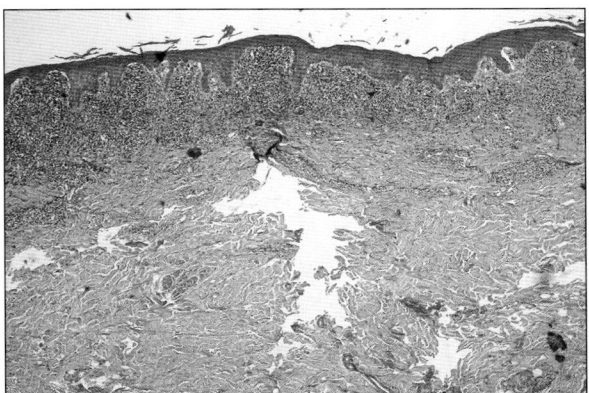

Fig 19-33d Mycosis fungoides showing the band-like infiltrate subjacent to the epithelium as well as some deeper focal infiltrates.

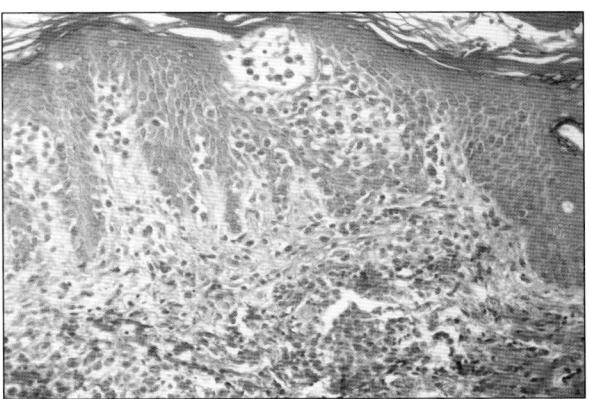

Fig 19-33e Epidermotropism, a characteristic feature of mycosis fungoides, can be seen here. A Pautrier micro-abscess is also present.

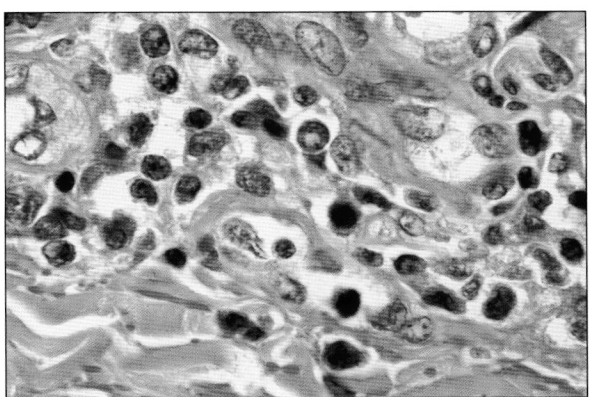

Fig 19-33f The neoplastic infiltrate shows small atypical cells as well as some larger cells. Some have convoluted or cerebriform nuclei.

tron beam radiotherapy of 1,500 cGy to 2,500 cGy. Electron beam is the preferred radiotherapy source because its voltage is ≤ 6 MeV, as compared to traditional beta particle photons, which have a voltage of ≥ 10 MeV as well as a deeper penetration and more side effects. However, large lymph nodes in advanced stages and deeply located tumor deposits may require such photon therapy up to 4,000 cGy.

Systemic chemotherapy using a variety of protocols and interferon have been disappointing and are generally used only in desperate situations involving the leukemic Sézary syndrome.

The median survival time of mycosis fungoides patients whose case begins with skin involvement is 10 years. However, once they reach the stages of extracutaneous involvement of viscera or lymph nodes, median survival is only 12 to 15 months.

Leukemias

PATHOGENESIS ▶

As noted at the beginning of this chapter, leukemias are malignancies of bone marrow. In all leukemias, the cell of origin is the pluripotential hematopoietic stem cell. The process begins with a clonal proliferation at one of the stages of hematopoietic stem cell maturation, when further maturity is arrested and the cell is partially differentiated toward a lymphoblast, a lymphocyte, a monocyte, a metamyelocyte, a promyelocyte, etc, giving rise to one of the many possible leukemias. For the purpose of this chapter and its pertinence to a clinician's understanding of leukemias, only the four basic types of leukemias will be discussed: acute lymphoblastic, chronic lymphocytic, acute myeloblastic, and chronic myelogenous.

The common pathogenesis of all leukemias is the proliferation of leukemia cells in the bone marow, which soon spill over into the blood, where they are seen in large numbers. These cells may also infiltrate the spleen, liver, lymph nodes, and at times even the gingiva. It is important to remember that in children the jaws are much more hematopoietic than in adults and may therefore form symptomatic collections, particularly in the mandible in acute lymphoblastic leukemia. It should also be remembered that, although extreme leukocytosis is one hallmark, leukemias are primarily a disease of bone marrow and may not spill neoplastic white cells into the blood, or may not have done so by the time of presentation. Therefore, some leukemias will show the characteristic blast cells in a bone marrow biopsy but actually have a peripheral blood leukopenia, the so-called aleukemic leukemia.

Acute leukemias are characterized by very immature blast cells and will progress rapidly to a fatal outcome if left untreated. As described in the quintuplets analogy at the beginning of this chapter, these cells are arrested at an early stage in their development and take over the population of the bone marrow with their immature behavior. This is underscored by their suppression of the other cell lines in bone marrow, leading to reductions in red blood cells (anemia), platelets (thrombocytopenia), and mature granulocytes (agranulocytosis, which leads to recurrent infections, etc). On the other hand, chronic leukemias are associated, at least initially, with cells that are somewhat more differentiated. Again, as in the quintuplets analogy, these cells are arrested further along in their maturation sequence and are therefore more mature. They do indeed proliferate but at a slower rate, and they have fewer effects (ie, a better behavior) on the other cell lines in the bone marrow. Consequently, they are not rapidly fatal if left untreated, and because they allow the other cell lines to mature and proliferate, anemia, thrombocytopenia, and agranulocytosis are not usually seen.

Acute Lymphoblastic Leukemia

CLINICAL PRESENTATION ▶

Acute lymphoblastic leukemia (ALL) represents the classic picture of childhood leukemia, of which it accounts for 80%. It usually has an onset of 3 months or less and produces significant symptoms, including fatigue mainly due to anemia, fever, bone pain (including in the jaws), an increased susceptibility to bruising, spontaneous ecchymosis, and petechiae. In addition, splenomegaly and a generalized lymphadenopathy may be present. Headache or vomiting may be frequent as well. The gingiva may be infiltrated with leukemic cells, creating a soft, friable enlargement that bleeds easily, but many cases of ALL do not have this sign (Fig 19-34).

DIFFERENTIAL DIAGNOSIS ▶

Before the results of any laboratory studies are known, a child with headache, vomiting, and bone pain may seem to have a common flu (influenza) or meningitis. If laboratory studies identify an anemia and the white blood cell count is not extremely high (ie, less than 25,000/μL) the picture may still represent meningitis or some other systemic infection. In addition, childhood anemia such as sickle cell anemia and thalassemia intermedia should be considered.

DIAGNOSTIC WORK-UP ▶

The diagnosis of any leukemia requires a bone marrow biopsy. On the rare occasions when the mandible is expanded, the biopsy can be accomplished by the oral and maxillofacial surgeon (Figs 19-35a and 19-35b). This amounts to a direct decortication of the expanded area and curettage of what will appear to be a friable white or red tissue representative of cellular marrow (Figs 19-35c and 19-35d). Biopsy of enlarged gingiva, when present, is not very diagnostic because of the superimposition of inflammation.

White blood cell counts over 25,000/μL should be viewed as suspicious for leukemia, since even severe infections such as a major appendicitis, peritonitis, or a head and neck cellulitis rarely produce such a leukocytosis.

HISTOPATHOLOGY ▶

The diagnosis of leukemia is dependent on peripheral blood studies and examination of a bone marrow biopsy, although cellular infiltration of other tissue may suggest the possibility of leukemia. Romanowsky stains (the prototype of eosin–methylene blue stains, which include Wright and Giemsa) as well as cytochemical stains are frequently employed.

The cells of acute lymphoblastic leukemia are usually small with round or convoluted nuclei and scant cytoplasm. The cells are slightly larger than small lymphocytes (see Fig 19-35d).

Most cases of ALL show chromosome abnormalities in the early precursors of B cells. About 70% will have hyperploidy, with 50 to 60 chromosomes present rather than the normal 46. About 5% to 10% have the Philadelphia chromosome abnormality, which carries a poor prognosis. A translocation of chromosomes 8 to 14 also confers a poor prognosis.

TREATMENT AND PROGNOSIS ▶

Treatment involves intensive chemotherapy and consideration of a bone marrow transplantation. Today ALL has a favorable prognosis. Over 90% of children achieve a complete remission, and more than 60% are cured. Adults who develop ALL, those cases that transform from a chronic lymphocytic leukemia or a small-cell lymphocytic lymphoma, and those with either the Philadelphia chromosome or the t(8:14) translocation, have a far less favorable prognosis.

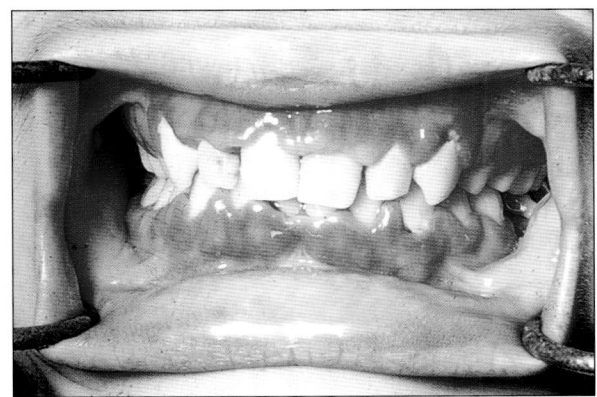

Fig 19-34 Acute lymphoblastic leukemia and other leukemias infiltrate the gingiva to produce a soft, friable, easily bleeding gingival enlargement.

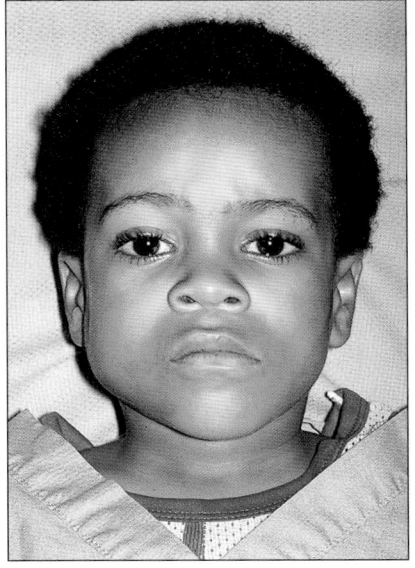

Fig 19-35a Acute lymphoblastic leukemia may produce marrow expansion of the mandible. In such situations, the jaw can serve as a convenient site for a diagnostic bone marrow biopsy.

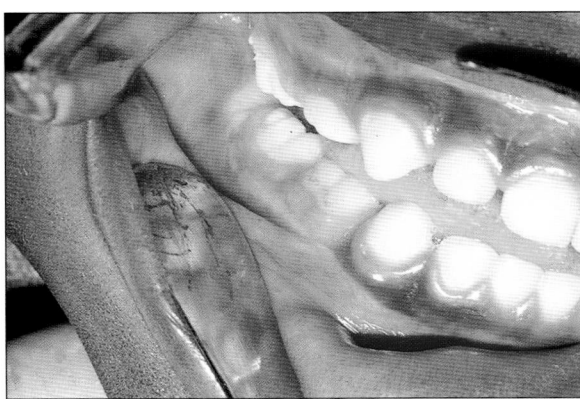

Fig 19-35b In this individual with ALL the mandibular ramus was expanded but there was no leukemic gingival infiltrate.

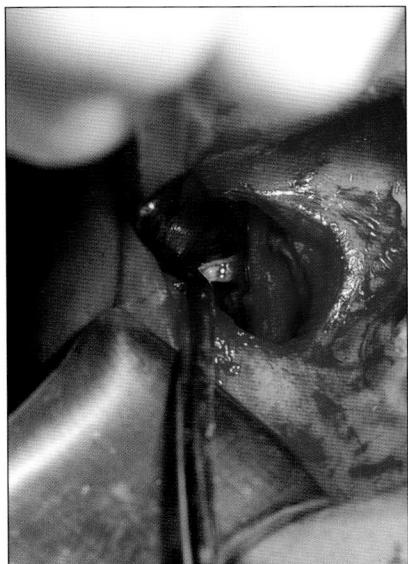

Fig 19-35c A diagnostic bone marrow biopsy was obtained from the ramus of the mandible.

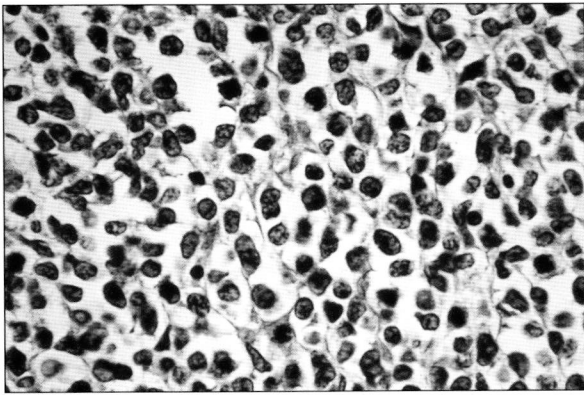

Fig 19-35d A collection of nearly identical lymphoblasts with dark-staining, convoluted nuclei consistent with ALL was obtained from the mandibular marrow biopsy.

Acute Myeloblastic Leukemia

CLINICAL PRESENTATION AND PATHOGENESIS ▶

Acute myoblastic leukemia (AML) is actually a heterogeneous group of leukemias arising from the pluripotential marrow stem cells that have seven separate partial differentiations and hence seven different diagnostic names: acute myeloblastic leukemia without differentiation (M-1); acute myeloblastic leukemia with differentiation (M-2); acute promyelocytic leukemia (M-3); acute myelomonocytic leukemia (M-4); acute monocytic leukemia (M-5); acute erythroleukemia (M-6); and acute megakaryocytic leukemia (M-7).

All of these forms of acute myeloblastic leukemia are progressive and devastating forms that primarily affect the 15- to 40-year age group. For the oral and maxillofacial specialist, one of the more common presentations is that of a severe pericoronitis in a lethargic, febrile teenager. This sign might be the initial presentation of AML, or it might not occur until after diagnosis. In either case it is a serious event since it poses the risk of cellulitis and osteomyelitis as a result of the effects of AML on normal white cell functions.

DIFFERENTIAL DIAGNOSIS ▶

If the presentation to the oral and maxillofacial specialist is a *pericoronitis* or other *odontogenic infection*, it may be assumed to be only that. However, continued infection, fatigue, and lethargy may be clues that the original infection was secondary to an AML and would suggest blood studies.

DIAGNOSTIC WORK-UP ▶

Only a bone marrow biopsy will confirm a suspected diagnosis of AML. In contrast to ALL, the mandible and maxilla are not sufficiently infiltrated by leukemic AML cells to provide the uncommon opportunity to accomplish a marrow biopsy in the jaws. Instead, bone marrow biopsies are accomplished in the sternum, iliac crest, or tibial plateau.

HISTOPATHOLOGY ▶

The cells of AML are myeloblasts and varying numbers of more differentiated cells. Nuclei are round to oval with distinct nucleoli and cytoplasm that may contain azurophilic granules and/or Auer rods. The latter are seen only in AML but are present only in up to 40% of cases. They represent aberrant primary lysosomes and are red to purple cytoplasmic bodies with Wright stain. They are derived from azurophilic granules. Further delineation of cells and subclassification usually require cytochemistry, immunophenotyping and/or cytogenic studies.

When masses of myeloblasts and promyelocytes develop in bone, soft tissue, or lymph nodes, the tumors are known as *granulocytic sarcomas* or *chloromas*. The latter name reflects the greenish color that may be brought on by the production of myeloperoxidase.

TREATMENT AND PROGNOSIS ▶

Treatment with various chemotherapy protocols usually results in a temporary remission only to lead to a relapse in less than 2 years, eventuating in death. Only about 10% to 15% experience a long-term, disease-free survival. More recently, however, the addition of bone marrow transplantation during a chemotherapy-induced remission has resulted in longer remissions and improved survival rates.

Chronic Myelogenous Leukemia

CLINICAL PRESENTATION AND PATHOGENESIS ▶

Chronic myelogenous leukemia (CML) is a disease affecting adults between 25 and 70 years of age; most occur in individuals in their 40s and 50s. The onset of CML is slow and may initially be asymptomatic but will soon lead to nonspecific symptoms, such as easy fatigability, weight loss, lymphadenopathy, and weakness that many attribute to "old age" (Fig 19-36a).

CML is specifically associated with the Philadelphia chromosomal abnormality Ph-1, a translocation between chromosomes 9 and 22 (t[9:22]) that appears in all seven forms (M-1 to M-7) of myelogenous leukemia. Because it is a chronic leukemia, normal marrow components are not suppressed and, along with leukemic cells, may be found in both the bone marrow and the peripheral blood.

DIAGNOSTIC WORK-UP ▶

The first and easiest diagnostic test to accomplish is a complete blood count. Chronic myelogenous leukemia will often have extremely high white blood cell counts of over 75,000/μL. Most are neutrophils and metamyelocytes. In addition, 50% of individuals with CML will have thrombocytosis. Of particular diagnostic value is the fact that CML cells lack alkaline phosphatase, which is abundant in normal granulocytes. This finding following a peripheral blood smear will focus on a diagnosis of CML and will distinguish it from a leukemoid reaction, which is a reactive outpouring of nonleukemic granulocytes.

Bone marrow biopsy for cytogenetic studies to identify the Philadelphia chromosome is the most specific diagnostic test.

HISTOPATHOLOGY ▶

In chronic myelogenous leukemia, the granulocytes proliferate at varying stages of development. Eosinophilic and basophilic granules may be seen.

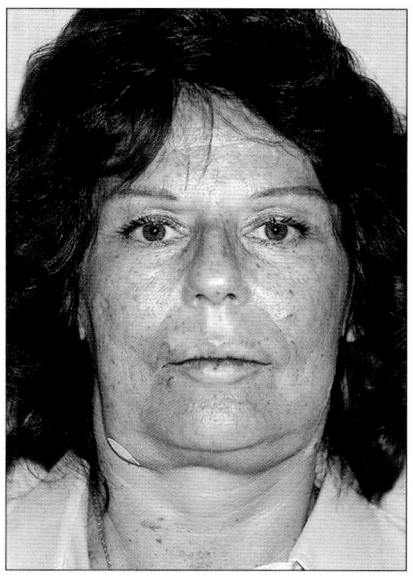

Fig 19-36a Diffuse lymphadenopathy and fatigue were the initial presenting signs and symptoms of this CML.

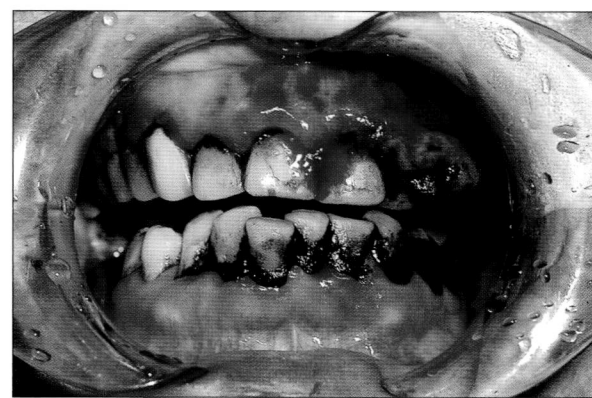

Fig 19-36b A rapid proliferation of a less-differentiated CML clone (blast crisis) will cause anemia and thrombocytopenia. Here the thrombocytopenia caused spontaneous gingival bleeding.

The cells of monocytoid leukemia are monoblasts and other monocytoid cells. The nuclei are round, indented, or folded with moderate amounts of blue-grey cytoplasm that may contain granules.

TREATMENT AND PROGNOSIS ▶ The course of CML is slowly progressive, permitting 2- to 3-year survivals even without treatment. Use of various chemotherapy protocols may induce a further remission in 50% of cases. In the 50% of individuals who do not respond to chemotherapy, a "blast crisis" abruptly develops. The 50% who do respond to chemotherapy will undergo a gradually reduced response that will finally end altogether and will lead to a slow lapse into a blast crisis. The blast crisis represents a rapid proliferation of a less-differentiated clone, which takes over the population of CML cells as well as the remainder of normal marrow and leads to severe anemia and thrombocytopenia and to death (Fig 19-36b).

Chemotherapy may extend survival to 3 to 4 years. However, younger patients with CML who receive bone marrow transplants have an improved prognosis, and some have even been cured. Therefore, at the time of this writing bone marrow transplantation is an encouraging treatment addition and is certainly indicated in the first year of this disease. Also at the time of this writing, the promising drug imatinib mesylate (Gleevec, Novartis), which specifically targets diseases in which there is a Philadelphia chromosome abnormality, has been introduced. Recent research has documented a high percentage of remissions in response to this drug.

Chronic Lymphocytic Leukemia

CLINICAL PRESENTATION AND PATHOGENESIS ▶ Chronic lymphocytic leukemia (CLL) is the slowest-progressing leukemia and is linked to small-cell lymphocytic lymphoma. A disease affecting adults older than 50 years, it accounts for 30% of all leukemias in the United States and is most common among the Asian population.

Chronic lymphocytic leukemia is a B-cell leukemia and, like all B cells, the leukemic cells express CD19 and CD20 antigens. However, they also express the T-cell–associated antigen CD5, which is identical to small cell lymphocytic lymphoma. Since the leukemic cells fail to respond to antigenic stimulation, hypogammaglobulinemia is a prominent feature of CLL. Paradoxically, 15% of CLL patients also have an

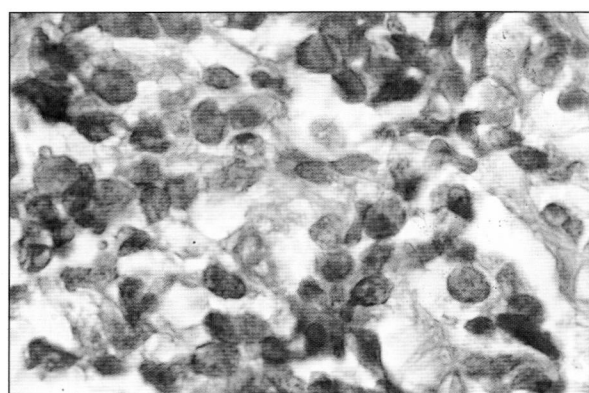

Fig 19-37a Low-power view of a palatal infiltration in chronic lymphocytic leukemia. Note the depth of the infiltrate and the grenz zone (zone of fibrous tissue devoid of neoplastic cells between the infiltrate and the epithelium).

Fig 19-37b High-power view of Fig 19-37a showing the poorly differentiated lymphocytic cells.

autoimmune hemolytic anemia, in which the CLL cells produce antibodies that are directed against red blood cell membranes.

As with CML, CLL is often asymptomatic initially and then slowly produces nonspecific symptoms such as easy fatigability, weight loss, and weakness. Because of the hypogammaglobulinemia, bacterial infections (skin infections, pneumonias, and advanced periodontitis) may be seen. A generalized lymphadenopathy is common, as is splenomegaly. White blood cell counts range widely from an aleukemic picture (normal white blood cell count) to one over 200,000/µL.

DIAGNOSTIC WORK-UP ▶ Certainly a complete blood count is the initial test to accomplish (see page 845). However, because of the variable leukocytosis seen in CLL and the near-normal appearance and staining of the nonfunctional B lymphocytes of CLL, the peripheral blood smear is not as suspicious for a leukemia as it is for CML. Therefore, unless the white blood cell count is over 25,000/µL, CLL may not be suspected. Bone marrow biopsies thus become the most reliable test.

HISTOPATHOLOGY ▶ CLL has been discussed under non-Hodgkin lymphoma. There is a proliferation of small uniform lymphocytes (Figs 19-37a and 19-37b). Peripheral blood counts are necessary to distinguish the leukemia from the lymphoma. On blood smears, "smudge" cells are characteristic because the fragile neoplastic cells often rupture.

TREATMENT AND PROGNOSIS ▶ CLL can be conceptualized as the accumulation of long-lived nonfunctional B lymphocytes that infiltrate bone marrow, blood, lymph nodes (small lymphocytic lymphoma), and other tissues including the gingiva. Many individuals with CLL live for more than 10 years with or without chemotherapy. The median survival time is 6 to 8 years. Unlike CML, CLL rarely transforms into an acute leukemia with a blast crisis and rapid death.

Langerhans Cell Histiocytosis

CLINICAL PRESENTATION AND PATHOGENESIS ▶ Langerhans cell histiocytosis (LCH) is a true neoplastic proliferation of cells of the immune system owing to its histogenesis from the ubiquitous dendritic antigen–processing and –presenting cells, termed *Langer-*

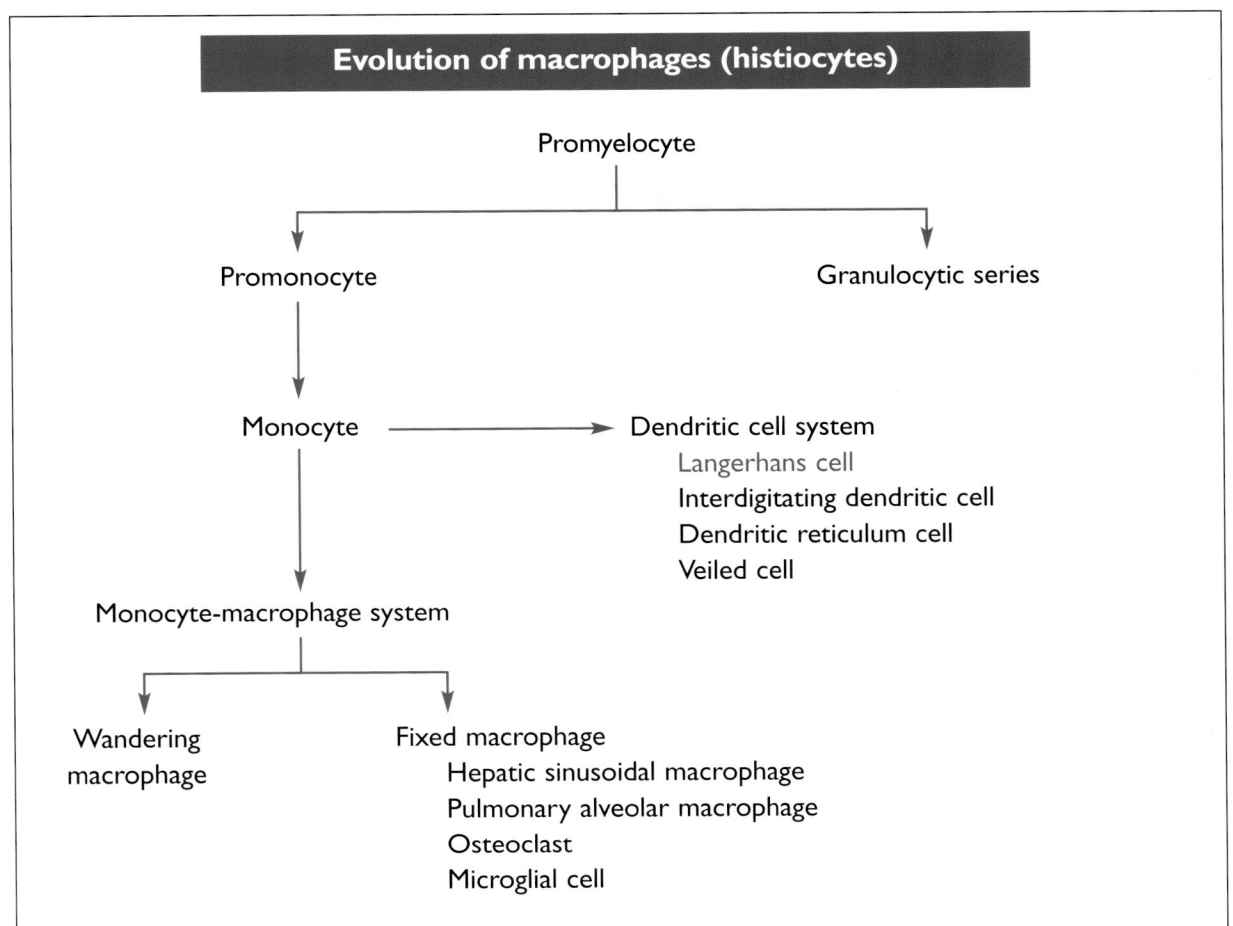

Fig 19-38 The monocyte differentiates in the bone marrow, circulates in the peripheral blood, and enters the tissues as a macrophage or histiocyte.

hans cells. Langerhans cells themselves are a type of macrophage (histiocyte). They arise from marrow precursor cells and are part of the monocytic series (Fig 19-38). Langerhans cell histiocytosis was formerly referred to as histiocytosis X based on the appearance of these cells under light microscopy (see Chapter 20).

Langerhans cells are found in every organ, but they are somewhat more numerous in bone marrow, the lungs, mucosa, and skin. Therefore, LCH may have unifocal or multifocal presentations in any bone, most commonly the skull (Fig 19-39), facial bones, proximal femur, and ribs, but also the lungs and either skin or mucosa, usually around the oral cavity (Fig 19-40) and genitals.

Historically, many confusing and incorrect terms have been used to describe this disease. Many of us can recall the educational mantra repeated on examinations of Letterer-Siwe disease, Hand-Schüller-Christian disease, and eosinophilic granuloma. Today, although our understanding is by no means complete, we recognize that Letterer-Siwe disease is not part of LCH but rather an anaplastic peripheral large T-cell lymphoma with positive epithelial membrane antigens (EMA+) and a t(2:5) chromosome translocation, as described earlier in this chapter. Hand-Schüller-Christian disease is indeed part of LCH, but it affects only the sphenoid bone and produces symptoms by its presence there and its involvement of the pituitary-hypothalamic axis. Therefore, the old Hand-Schüller-Christian triad of skull lesions, diabetes insipidus, and exophthalmos was based mostly on location. The term *eosinophilic granuloma* denotes the common low-grade biology of most LCH lesions and may be either unifocal or multifocal. The

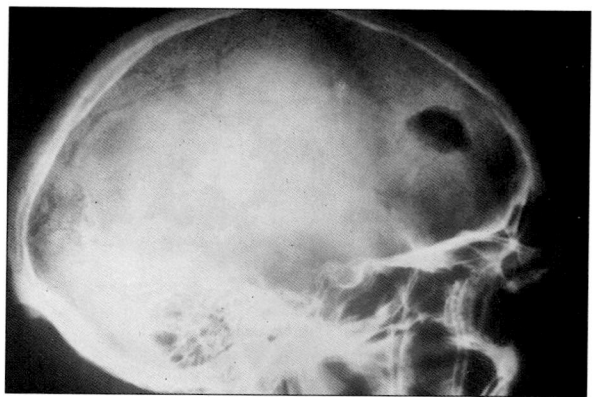

Fig 19-39 This radiolucency in the skull was a focus of LCH together with mandibular involvement as part of a multifocal LCH presentation.

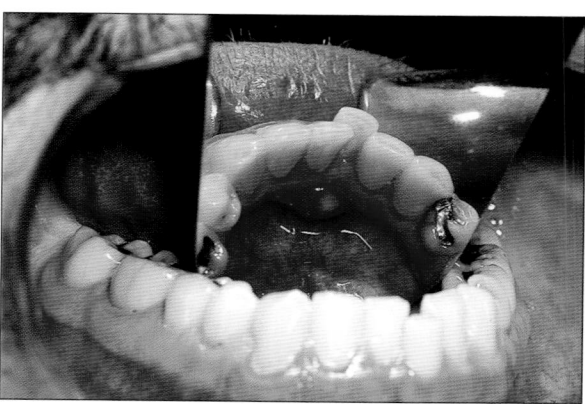

Fig 19-40 This small single focus of LCH was limited to the soft tissues of the lingual gingiva in an adult.

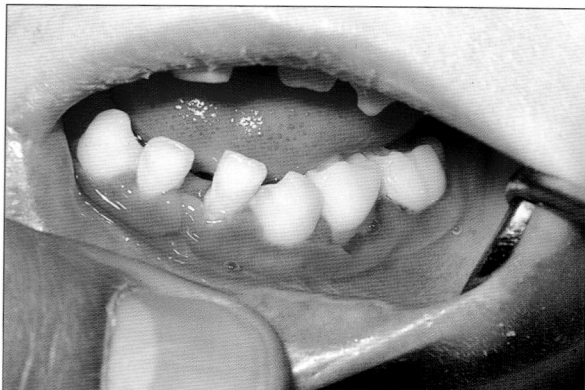

Fig 19-41 Mobile teeth due to alveolar bone loss in a child may be the initial clinical presentation of LCH.

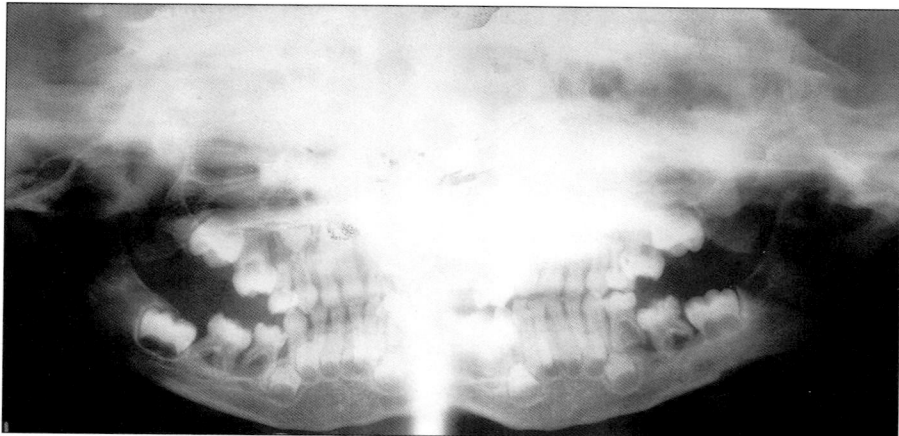

Fig 19-42a Alveolar bone loss around the primary molar teeth due to LCH.

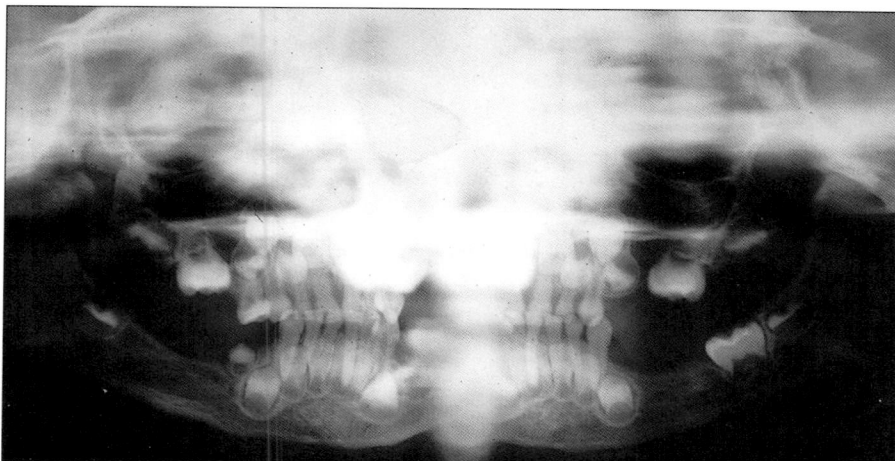

Fig 19-42b Resolution of the LCH and alveolar bone regeneration after removal of the involved teeth and curettage of the LCH.

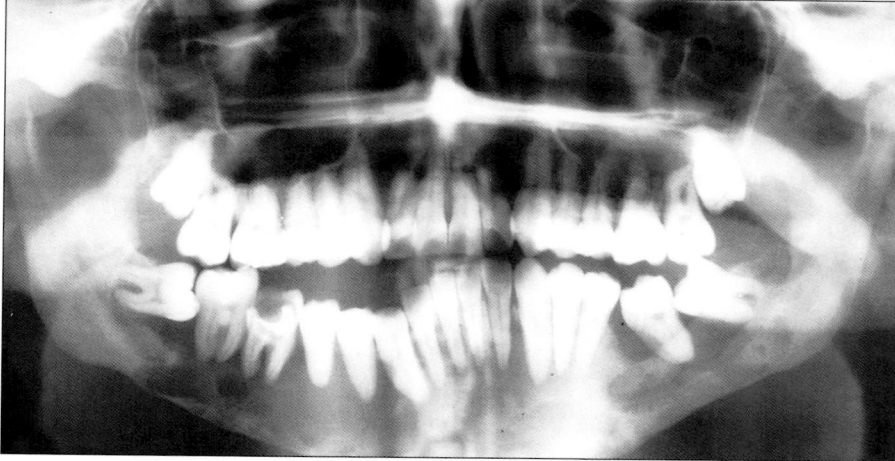

Fig 19-43a Extensive unifocal LCH involvement of the mandible in a young adult.

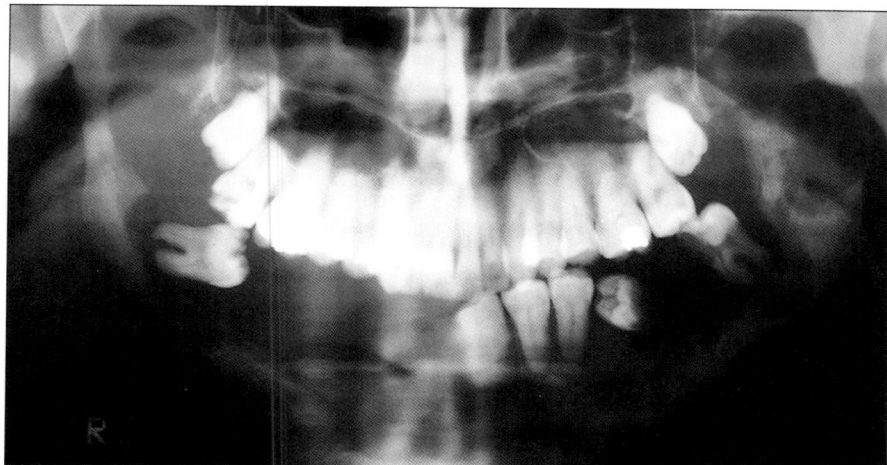

Fig 19-43b Untreated LCH slowly infiltrated and resorbed nearly the entire mandible over 3 years. During this time, no foci of LCH developed in any other location.

histopathology is seen to contain reactive eosinophils drawn to the lesion presumably from growth factors secreted by the Langerhans cells. Eosinophils are not part of the neoplastic process, and the lesions represent not a granuloma but a low-grade malignancy. (For further discussion of these differences, see Chapter 20.)

Pertinent to the oral and maxillofacial specialist are cases presenting in the jaws, facial bones, or head and neck soft tissues. In the jaws, where about 7% of bony lesions occur, oral and maxillofacial specialists mostly see LCH in children, teenagers, or young adults (Fig 19-41). However, it is important to remember that bony lesions occur in this young age group in any part of the skeleton, but soft tissue and particularly lung lesions occur between the ages of 20 and 40 years.

Jaw lesions may present with the classic picture of alveolar bone loss and mobile teeth, producing the "floating tooth" picture (Figs 19-42a, 19-42b, 19-43a, and 19-43b). However, others may present in the rami at the inferior border of the mandible or in other facial bones, mimicking an osteomyelitis, a sarcoma, or an odontogenic neoplasm. Some may even present with a multilocular radiographic appearance. Jaw lesions do not usually produce significant symptoms other than mild bone pain, tooth mobility, and at times expansion. Of course, sphenoid lesions often produce diabetes insipidus, exophthalmos, and diplopia, while pulmonary lesions produce dyspnea, chronic cough, and fatigue.

DIFFERENTIAL DIAGNOSIS ▶

The presentation of alveolar bone loss with loose teeth in a child represents a classic differential in oral and maxillofacial surgery. Other entities that may produce this same picture are *juvenile periodontitis, acute lymphocytic leukemia*, the juvenile periodontitis associated with *Papillon-Lefèvre syndrome, nonspecific periodontitis associated with juvenile-onset diabetes mellitus, osteomyelitis*, and a variety of sarcoma or sarcoma-like diseases such as *osteosarcoma, fibrosarcoma*, and *aggressive fibromatosis*.

In the rami or other non–tooth-bearing areas of the jaws, the facial bones, or the soft tissues of the head and neck, the periodontal diseases would not be considerations, although the infectious diseases, including *cellulitis* and *neoplastic disease*, would.

DIAGNOSTIC WORK-UP ▶

A presentation suspicious for LCH requires a biopsy that should include the removal of involved teeth to gain an adequate tissue specimen. The involved teeth are not salvageable since the alveolar bone will not regenerate.

If a biopsy is taken, it is advisable to alert the pathologist that LCH is one of the considerations and to recommend immunostaining for the CD1a glycoprotein cell membrane antigen, which is specific for LCH, and for S-100 protein, which is nonspecific but usually positive. This is important since oral LCH biopsies may appear to be very similar to nonspecific periodontal inflammation and accepted as such without a closer review and/or pursuit of these specific tests. In difficult cases, electron microscopy of even formalin-fixed paraffin-embedded specimens (glutaraldehyde or Karnofsky fixative is preferred) that identify Birbeck granules will be pathognomonic.

HISTOPATHOLOGY ▶

The low-power view often suggests an inflammatory process (Fig 19-44a). It is characterized, however, by the proliferation of Langerhans cells, which have abundant ill-defined cytoplasm and oval or indented nuclei that often have a central groove, giving it a coffee bean appearance. Inflammatory cells are also present and may include lymphocytes and neutrophils, but eosinophils predominate (Fig 19-44b). There may be infiltration of overlying epithelium. Giant cells and necrosis may be present, but mitoses are very uncommon. The histologic appearance does not seem to correlate with behavior (Fig 19-45a). The recognition of Birbeck granules in the lesional cell by electron microscopy is also pathognomonic. Birbeck granules are cytoplasmic structures that are rod-shaped and have periodic striations that resemble a zipper. One end may be dilated (Fig 19-45b). The impracticality of these latter techniques has been overcome by the use of the CD1a mouse monoclonal antibody 010, which can be employed on routinely processed paraffin-embedded tissue and has made this the diagnostic test of choice. Therefore, definitive diagnosis is achieved by light microscopy and positivity for the CD1a antigen by immunostaining.

TREATMENT AND PROGNOSIS ▶

Langerhans cell histiocytosis is generally responsive to a variety of treatments, each of which provides a cure or long-term palliation; only rare cases are unresponsive and progress to death. Therefore, many treatment modalities have been suggested, including surgical curettage, resection, radiotherapy, chemo-

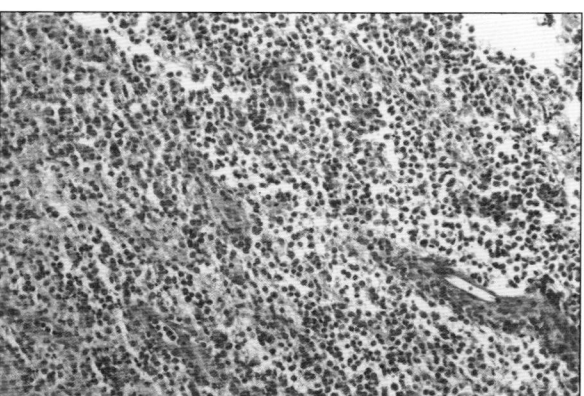

Fig 19-44a Langerhans cell histiocytosis can mimic inflammatory tissue.

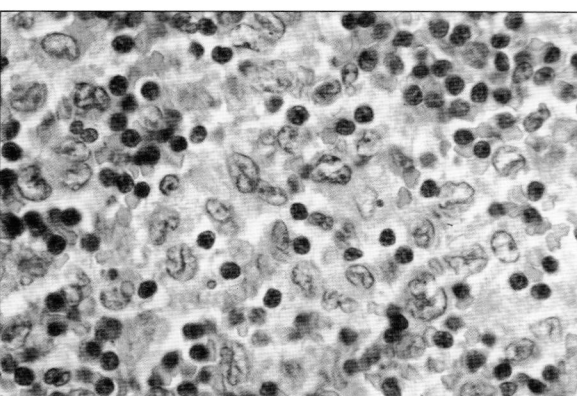

Fig 19-44b High-power view of Langerhans cell histiocytosis showing the altered Langerhans cells, which often have a grooved or coffee bean nucleus, and numerous eosinophils.

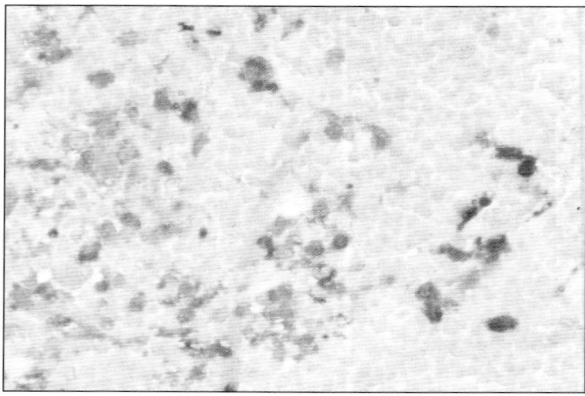

Fig 19-45a An S-100 protein stain showing positivity of the Langerhans cells.

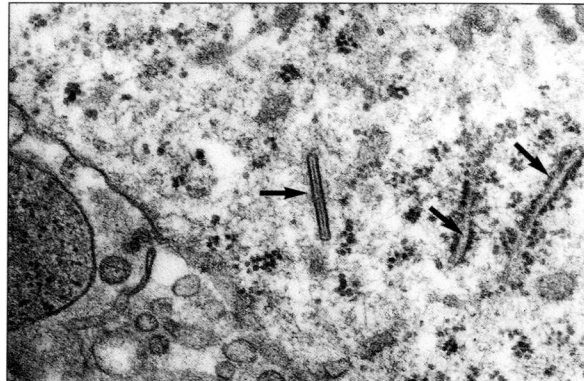

Fig 19-45b Electron photomicrograph of a Langerhans cell histiocytosis showing Birbeck granules (*arrows*).

therapy, intralesional steroids, and systemic steroids. However, surgical curettage or a peripheral resection with 3- to 5-mm margins is the most curative and predictable and is recommended for all accessible jaw and facial bone lesions, including those in the skull (Figs 19-46a to 19-46f). For lesions that are not accessible or have recurred in spite of surgery, radiotherapy of 1,200 cGy to 1,800 cGy is the next line of therapy.

For widespread lesions involving the jaws/facial bone areas and particularly the lung or lymph nodes, systemic chemotherapy becomes a necessary part of the treatment protocol. In such cases, vinblastine or 6-mercaptopurine (Purinethol, GlaxoSmithKline) as single agents have been shown to be the most effective with the least side effects. Of course, in LCH that produces a diabetes insipidus, long-term hormone replacement with desmopressin acetate (DDAVP, Aventis), 10 to 40 mg nasally at bedtime, is required.

The prognosis of LCH is generally very good because of its slow natural progression and its responsiveness to therapy. Both unifocal and multifocal lesions respond well to therapies selected for their particular presentation so that an overall 80% cure rate is achieved. However, about 20% of patients seem to develop a more aggressive multi-organ involvement requiring repeated therapies, leading to an overall LCH death rate of 9%. The majority of the refractory cases and the life-threatening involvements are those involving the lungs. By contrast, LCH with isolated bone involvements has a 97% cure rate.

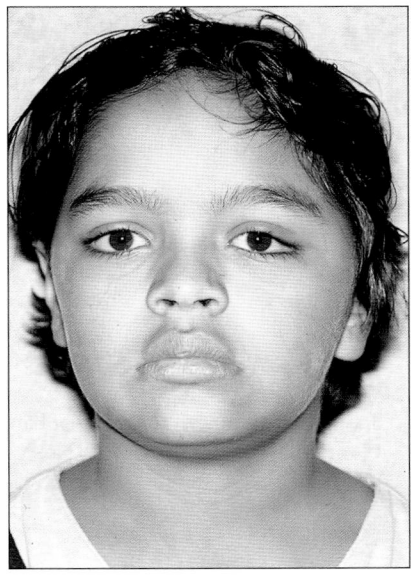

Fig 19-46a Expansion of the left zygoma and left temporalis muscle due to LCH. This LCH was referred after failure of two chemotherapy protocols.

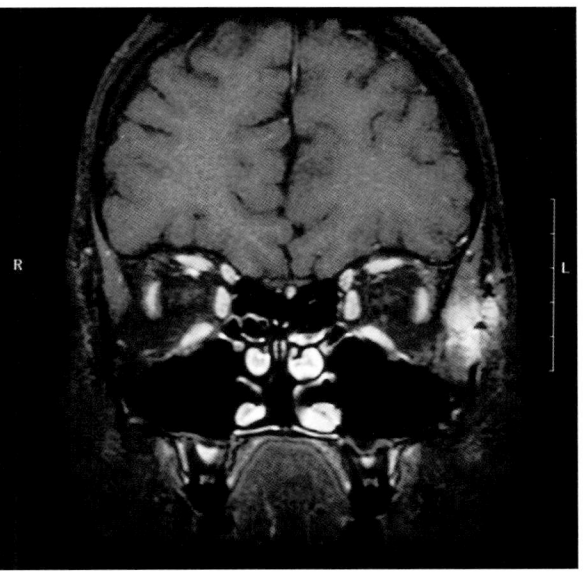

Fig 19-46b T-2–weighted MRI scan showing high signal density and identifying unencapsulated LCH in the zygoma with a diffuse infiltration into the temporalis muscle.

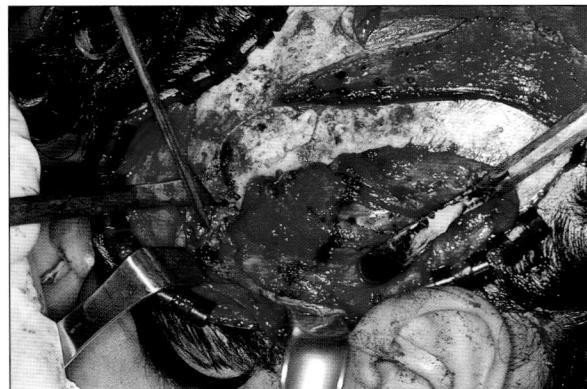

Fig 19-46c The location of this LCH required a resection of the left zygoma and the anterior portion of the temporalis muscle through a bicoronal flap access.

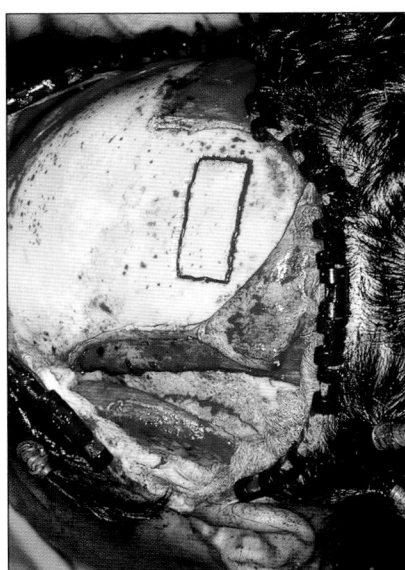

Fig 19-46d A split calvarial (outer table) graft was harvested to reconstruct the zygoma and lateral orbital rim. The calvarial donor site defect was reconstructed with hydroxyapatite cement (Bone Source, Stryker Leibinger).

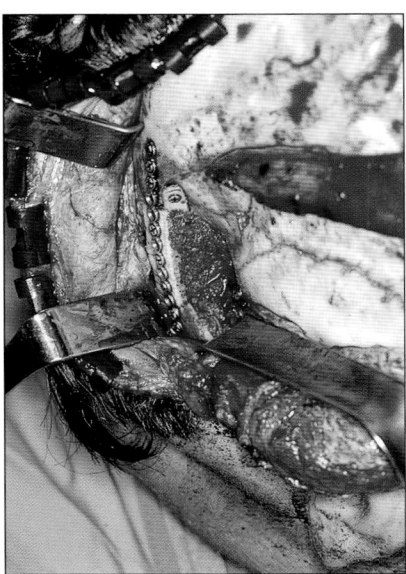

Fig 19-46e The outer table calvarial graft was fixated with 1.5-mm titanium fixation plates.

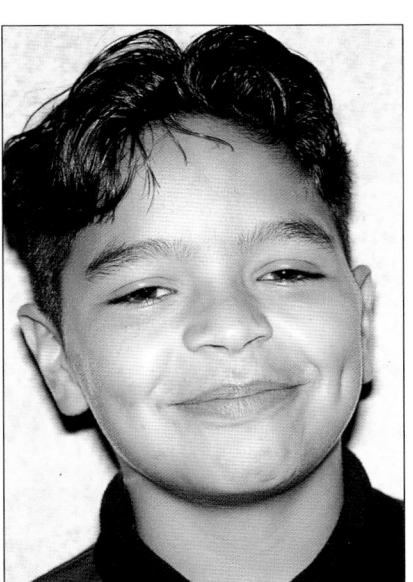

Fig 19-46f The LCH was resolved with this local resection-reconstruction approach.

Where Have All the Great Terms Gone?

▶ "The difficulty lies not in new ideas but in escaping old ones."
—*John Keynes*

Disease terminology should be simple, descriptive, and most of all, representative of our most up-to-date knowledge and information. Consequently, disease names undergo perpetual change, and with good reason. Nomenclature is like a chrysalis: necessary for development and advancement to a new stage but easily discarded when no longer necessary or appropriate. It has been the express intention of this book to simplify each disease name to a single accurate and descriptive term and in the process to eliminate multiple names and those that do not relate the true nature of the disease.

Today we find numerous inaccurate or misleading terms in oral and maxillofacial surgery and pathology. Some identify the person or persons who first described or recognized a particular condition; many of these names should and will be allowed to continue as a means of honoring such individuals. Other disease names were once appropriate but now bear changing to reflect newer data or more accurate findings. Some names represent well-meaning but flawed attempts to be descriptive, and still others reveal attempts at self aggrandizement or an advancement in academic rank. Regardless of their origins, if they are inaccurate, these terms must be corrected. This chapter focuses on those terms obviously requiring change and explains the rationale behind the update. It also provides some historical insight into bygone terms and names that may seem strange by today's standards. The authors of this textbook recognize that the terms we have used may also be imperfect and are subject to future change as new findings and studies give us a clearer picture of the disease mechanism.

Outdated Term

Updated Term

Adenoameloblastoma and Adenomatoid Odontogenic Tumor (AOT)

Adenomatoid Odontogenic Cyst (AOC)

The term *adenoameloblastoma* appeared in the literature in 1950 in an article by German and Tiecke. It described what they concluded to be a histologic variant of the ameloblastoma. This tumor was considered to be an ameloblastoma because of its similar behavior and because at that time both were treated with only simple enucleation.

In 1957, Lucas questioned the relationship of this tumor to the ameloblastoma. Through increased knowledge of its behavior and clinical presentation, it became apparent that the "adenoameloblastoma" was indeed a separate entity, with a younger age propensity and a more specific location. Even more significantly, the adenoameloblastoma was an encapsulated, cystic structure that was curable by enucleation, whereas the ameloblastoma was infiltrative and curable only by resection. In fact, the former represents a cyst and the latter a true neoplasm.

In 1958, Gorlin and Chaudry, in their discussion of adenoameloblastoma, emphasized the inappropriateness of this term and pointed out the distinct differences between the two lesions. To distance the adenomatoid lesion from the ameloblastoma, the terms *odontogenic adenomatoid tumor* and *adenomatoid odontogenic tumor* were introduced. Over time, the catchy abbreviation AOT prevailed, which unfortunately also is incorrect.

Today we recognize that the adenomatoid odontogenic tumor is not a tumor but rather a cyst that has a hamartomatous intraluminal proliferation of epithelial cells derived from Hertwig epithelial root sheath. While at times this proliferation may fill the lumen to give the impression of a solid tumor, a close inspection will reveal its emergence from an epithelial lining. The calcifications seen in these cysts, which represent attempts of the root sheath epithelium to induce root dentin, have been identified as dentinoid material. Therefore, the more appropriate term is adenomatoid odontogenic cyst or AOC, which has been introduced in this text and can be found in Chapter 13 covering cysts.

Outdated Term	Updated Term

Bowen's Disease

Carcinoma in Situ

In 1912, John Bowen published an article on precancerous skin lesions in which he described two cases of so-called chronic atypical epithelial proliferation. Both patients had long-standing skin lesions, one of the buttock, the other of the calf, which were slightly raised, reddish with papillary areas, some crusting, and sharp borders. The histology was described as "showing" marked proliferation of the rete Malpighii, along with much evidence of karyokinetic division and amitoses with peculiar clumping of the nuclei and vacuolation of the cells.

Bowen's disease is now generally considered to be synonymous with carcinoma in situ; its relationship to visceral malignancy is one of coincidence and age. There is little reason to retain the term *Bowen's disease*.

In 1914, Darier referred to these lesions as "Bowen's precancerous dermatosis" (*la dermatose precancereuse de Bowen*) or "Bowen's disease" (*la maladie de Bowen*). Reports of these lesions occurring on the genitalia, larynx, and conjunctiva, as well as on oral and nasal mucosa, also appeared. In 1950, Gorlin presented a series of oral Bowen's disease and reviewed the literature, describing the prevailing concept of the process as "a lateral spreading intraepithelial type of superficial epithelioma" with a low incidence of invasion.

In 1959, Graham and Helwig reported an association of internal malignancy in patients with Bowen's disease. Of 35 patients who had the disease and died, 20 (57%) had carcinomas of internal organs, 4 (11.5%) had lymphoma or leukemia, and 4 (11.5%) had squamous cell carcinoma or melanoma of the skin. Callen and Headington found no such correlation, and other studies have shown no significant increase in associated malignancy overall. Bowen's disease was characterized histologically by markedly disorganized growth, the presence of large hyperchromatic nuclei, and multinucleated cells as well as individually keratinized cells and mitotic figures. This is identical to what is today described as various degrees in the spectrum of dysplasia up to carcinoma in situ. However, the term *Bowen's disease* has become sufficiently ingrained, especially in dermatopathology, that sun damage–related lesions showing similar changes may still be called *Bowenoid actinic keratosis* and lesions induced by human papillomavirus *Bowenoid papulosis*.

Cementoma

Periapical Cemento-Osseous Dysplasia

Students of the 1960s were taught that cementomas are found in the periapical area of the mandibular anterior teeth in women of African heritage around the age of 40 years; that they underwent a series of three stages, from competely radiolucent to mixed radiolucent-radiopaque to completely radiopaque; and that the teeth remained vital.

Today this disease is recognized as a genetically related, disorganized product of the bone–periodontal membrane–cementum complex and is more correctly termed *periapical cemento-osseous dysplasia*.

True Cementoma

Cementoblastoma

During the same era, students were taught that a so-called true cementoma represented a benign proliferation of cementoblasts into a mass confluent with the lower half of the roots of premolar and molar teeth.

Today this is more correctly termed a *cementoblastoma* to reflect its true nature as a benign, slow-growing neoplastic proliferation of cementoblasts.

Gigantiform Cementoma

Ossifying Fibroma

Rare cases of large, round, radiopaque masses were termed *gigantiform cementomas*.

These turned out to be large ossifying fibromas with mature ossifications, thus eliminating the third disease that had come to be known as a cementoma.

Outdated Term

Updated Term

Cemento-Ossifying Fibroma

Ossifying Fibroma

Although the term *cemento-ossifying fibroma* is still in common usage today, it is scientifically inaccurate because it refers to a clinical presentation and histopathology that also occurs in areas where there is no cementum, such as the skull, femur, tibia, etc. These are all ossifying fibromas; those that happen to occur in the jaws should not be called cemento-ossifying fibromas simply because of the presence of teeth. Moreover, there is no histologic or biochemical difference between cementum and bone. We recognize a bone-like mineralized tissue to be cementum only if it clings to the dentin of a tooth root. If it is not on a tooth root surface, one cannot distinguish cementum from bone. What has fueled the retention of the term *cemento-ossifying fibroma* is that the dysmorphic round basophilic bone particles that can be seen within ossifying fibromas have arbitrarily been called *cementicles*. However, these so-called cementicles are not from cementum, but instead represent a dysmorphic product of this tumor analogous to the keratin pearls that are a dysmorphic product of squamous cell carcinomas.

The term *ossifying fibroma* more simply and accurately describes this tumor, which is a benign neoplasm of mesenchymal cells that sufficiently differentiate to produce both collagen and bone.

Central Giant Cell Reparative Granuloma and Aneurysmal Bone Cyst

Central Giant Cell Tumor

Central giant cell reparative granuloma is an old term that has survived because many in our profession are reluctant to call it a giant cell tumor for fear of confusing it with a malignancy first described in long bones. The so-called giant cell reparative granuloma does indeed contain osteoclastic-looking multinucleated giant cells, but it is destructive rather than reparative and it is not a granuloma (that is, a specific reaction to an infectious or inflammatory agent), but rather a proliferation of osteoclasts in a fibroblastic stroma. In fact, the giant cells in these lesions are indeed osteoclast precursors because they develop the ruffled borders typical of osteoclasts when explanted and exposed to parathyroid hormone, and they resorb bone just like an osteoclast.

Like the central giant cell reparative granuloma, the *aneurysmal bone cyst* is a contradiction in terms since it is neither aneurysmal nor a cyst. In fact, it is nothing more than a central giant cell tumor with large blood-filled spaces that lack an endothelial lining and are not under arterial pressure. It is not truly aneurysmal because the blood-filled spaces contain young fibroblasts rather than endothelium; and it is not a cyst because there is no epithelial lining to these blood-filled spaces. Clearly, the term *aneurysmal bone cyst* is not an accurate description of the pathology of this tumor and should be discontinued.

Giant cell tumors identical to those that occur in the jaws are also found in long bones, representing one of the most common benign tumors treated by orthopedic surgeons. In long bones they are usually treated with curettage or local resection; they have the same clinical bleeding during surgery; and they recur at the same rate as those found in the jaws. Though aggressive and sometimes quite large, these tumors are nonetheless benign. The present reluctance to describe this as a giant cell tumor stems from a 1962 report by Hutter et al, which characterized benign and malignant giant cell tumors in long bones. Since that time, oral pathology texts and many publications have accepted Hutter's assertion that giant cell tumors in bone are malignant. Yet a careful review of so-called malignant giant cell tumors reveals that nearly all of them are osteosarcomas with numerous osteoclasts, probably induced to resorb bone by cytokines secreted by the osteosarcoma. In fact, squamous cell carcinomas that invade the jaws are known to secrete osteoclast-activating factors that induce osteoclasts to resorb bone, yet these are not called giant cell tumors.

In addition, it is not beyond reason also to suspect that in rare instances the osteoclast precursors that produce this benign giant cell tumor can undergo a malignant genetic alteration as well and produce a true malignant giant cell tumor.

Today, the preponderance of evidence shows that the lesion once recognized as a central giant cell reparative granuloma is actually a benign tumor of osteoclast precursors and therefore more accurately termed a *central giant cell tumor*.

Similarly, the lesion once termed an *aneurysmal bone cyst* can be conceptualized as a rapidly proliferating variant of a central giant cell tumor because it has macroscopic rather than microscopic blood-filled spaces. Therefore, significant hemorrhage can arise from this tumor, since all central giant cell tumors have a venous pressure bleeding quality, and those with larger blood-filled spaces will exhibit a greater bleeding tendency.

Outdated Term	Updated Term

Chronic Diffuse Sclerosing Osteomyelitis

Chronic diffuse sclerosing osteomyelitis (CDSO) is at once inaccurate and accurate. It is inaccurate when applied to the entity that develops multiple-quadrant radiopacities associated with teeth roots and alveolar bone, a condition that is seen almost exclusively in women of African heritage and today is termed *florid cemento-osseous dysplasia*. It is somewhat more accurately applied to the painful condition of the mandible that causes endosteal sclerosis with the formation of small pockets of radiolucency and often cultures positive for *Actinomyces* organisms and *Eikenella corrodens*. This entity is a true infection of bone that is sclerotic rather than suppurative in the marrow space and is diffuse because it is not limited to the alveolar bone.

The confusion over this term originated with the classic oral pathology textbook by Shafer-Hine and Levy, which was first published in 1958 and reprinted multiple times through 1969. In each edition of this text, the multiple-quadrant radiopacities were conceptualized as representing chronic periodontal infection, which stimulated sclerotic bone. The strong racial predilection was not recognized at that time, and the occasional secondary infections that resulted from the exposure of this dense, poorly vascularized, sclerotic bone fueled this concept. In 1980, Melrose and Abrams first identified this entity as a dysplasia (in this sense, a dysmorphogenesis, not a premalignant dysplasia) of the products from the cementum–periodontal membrane–bone complex and recognized that these dense avascular masses were a bony product related not to an infection but to a genetic alteration. Consequently, either of the terms *florid osseous dysplasia* or *florid cemento-osseous dysplasia* would be accurate.

Florid Cemento-Osseous Dysplasia

Florid cemento-osseous dysplasia is preferred since bone and cementum are indistinguishable and this disease is limited to the tooth-forming areas of the jaws, where the lamina dura and cementum develop in association with the periodontal membrane.

Eagle Syndrome

In 1937, an otolaryngologist named Eagle reported two cases of neck pain associated with an elongated styloid process. He followed this in 1948 with a report of several additional cases, and declared that they represented a new syndrome. These cases and the ones seen today all have what appears to be an elongated styloid process and neck pain, particularly on rotation and flexion and on swallowing. However, careful radiographic review will reveal a radiolucent separation between the original styloid process and what seems to be a calcified stylohyoid ligament sometimes all the way to the lesser horn of the hyoid bone. Since Eagle's original description, many of these "calcified" stylohyoid ligaments have been removed (something Eagle did not do) and found to be ossified with mature bone. In addition, if neck C-spine radiographs are taken (something else Eagle did not do) or a CT scan is taken, one can see that nearly all of the intervertebral ligaments also are ossified. Indeed, in most of these individuals a careful history will identify paresthesias or pain in their arms, hands, or fingers consistent with a cervical nerve root radiculopathy.

Because the focus of oral and maxillofacial specialists and of other specialists is on the neck pain complaints and a panoramic radiograph will reveal a long styloid process, the concept of Eagle syndrome has prevailed.

Diffuse Intraosseous Skeletal Hypertrophy (DISH) Syndrome

This symptom complex is now recognized as only one part of a total body syndrome known as *diffuse intraosseous skeletal hypertrophy*, or DISH syndrome. DISH syndrome is suspected to be a reactive immune-based disease similar to myositis ossificans but targeting only ligaments.

Erythroplasia of Queyrat

In 1911, Queyrat reported on four patients who had chronic, painless, red, shiny plaques of the glans penis, which over time developed into carcinoma. Coincidentally, the patients in this series were serologically positive for syphilis. Since these lesions demonstrated behavior similar to those that had been called *leukoplakia* (*leucoplasie*), Queyrat suggested the term *erythroplasia of the glans* (*erythroplasia du gland*).

Carcinoma in Situ

This entity, like Bowen's disease, is nothing more than the spectrum of premalignant dysplasias leading up to carcinoma in situ and an eventual advancement into squamous cell carcinoma. As we now recognize, red lesions (erythroplasia) are even more concerning for dysplasia than are white lesions (leukoplakia).

Outdated Term	Updated Term

From a histologic standpoint, these lesions, like the tissue in so-called Bowen's disease, actually represent carcinoma in situ. Bowen's disease and erythroplasia of Queyrat are two older terms describing the same disease process.

In a report by Darier et al concerning the development of cancers of the oral mucosa, the term *erythroplasia of Queyrat* was used to identify oral erythroplasia, and for many years it continued to be employed in this context. However, while certainly of historic interest, this term today serves no purpose except to confuse the already overburdened nomenclature.

Globulomaxillary Cyst

Throughout the 1960s and through most of the 1970s, the term *globulomaxillary cyst* was used to describe a so-called classic fissural cyst that was said to be caused by entrapment of epithelium between the embryonic median nasal process and the maxillary process. Cysts would then develop after the teenage years and in later adult life between the permanent maxillary canine and the lateral incisor teeth, ostensibly due to spontaneous activation of these entrapped epithelial cells. The concept seemed to be reasonable and went unchallenged until embryologists pointed out that neither these processes nor most bony primordia are separated by epithelium. At the same time, Wysocki published the results of a review of 37 so-called globulomaxillary cysts and confirmed the observations of many others that most cysts in this location represent either another entity or a cyst or tumor from a different etiology, that is, a radicular cyst from nonvital lateral incisors, a primordial odontogenic keratocyst, a giant cell tumor, an ameloblastoma, an adenomatoid odontogenic cyst, etc.

Today, it is recognized that epithelium does not become entrapped in this location and therefore the notion of a globulomaxillary cyst is inaccurate.

Granular Cell Myoblastoma

Granular cell myoblastoma once seemed to be a reasonable name for a benign tumor of the tongue or floor of the mouth that contained granular cells and at times produced a pseudoepitheliomatous hyperplasia. The term denoted a muscle origin, and the tongue is composed mostly of striated muscle. In addition, light microscopy showed that the tumor seemed to arise indistinguishably from muscle. However, electron microscopy has identified the granules to be lysosomal vesicles, which are seen mostly in Schwann cells and in cells of neural origin. Immunohistochemistries have also shown the granular cells to be negative for muscle actin and positive for S-100 protein, further supporting a neural histogenesis.

Granular Cell Tumor

The term *granular cell myoblastoma* has been shown by more sophisticated medical technology to be an inaccurate term and has been replaced by the more generic term *granular cell tumor*.

Hand-Schüller-Christian Disease, Letterer-Siwe Disease, Eosinophilic Granuloma, and Histiocytosis X

In 1893, Hand reported the case of a 3-year-old child with diabetes insipidus, hepatosplenomegaly, petechiae over the abdomen, and a scabies-like eruption. At autopsy, an area of soft bone was found in the skull and "small rounded infiltrates" were found in the liver, spleen, and kidney. In 1906, Kay reported the case of a 7-year-old boy with bone defects, exophthalmos, and polyuria. In 1915, Schüller presented two cases with the same triad, one a 16-year-old boy and the other a 14-year-old girl. In 1920, Christian collected Schüller's two cases and added a similar one of his own involving a 5-year-old girl. At this time Hand-Schüller-Christian disease was established as an entity manifested by punched-out lesions in the skull, exophthalmos, and polyuria.

By 1928, Rowland had interpreted these cases as a xanthomatosis caused by lipid storage or lipid cell hyperplasia involving the reticuloendothelial system. He likened it to Niemann-Pick disease and Gaucher disease as a manifestation of a disturbance in lipid metabolism. Subsequently, Mallory

Langerhans Cell Histiocytosis (LCH)

While the etiology remains unknown, the dominant "histiocytic" cell has been identified as the antigen-processing Langerhans cell. The disease is now known as *Langerhans cell histiocytosis* (LCH), which describes a low-grade malignant proliferation of these ubiquitous cells. Like other immune cell malignancies, such as lymphomas, LCH may involve localized tissues, several tissues, or multiple organs. The term *Letterer-Siwe disease* actually describes a clinical situation rather than a specific pathologic entity and has included a variety of diseases. Some of these cases have actually been anaplas-

Outdated Term	Updated Term

pointed out that the basic histologic pattern of a granulomatous process with fibrosis could not be stimulated by cholesterol storage, either experimentally or in familial xanthomatosis. Thus, Hand-Schüller-Christian disease was classified as a nonlipid reticuloendotheliosis.

In 1924, Letterer reported the death of a 6-month-old infant with cutaneous petechiae, lymphadenopathy, low-grade fever, and hepatosplenomegaly; evidence of reticuloendothelial proliferation was found at autopsy. In 1933, Siwe described several similar cases, along with that of a 16-month-old child as a specific clinical pathologic syndrome consisting of lymphadenopathy, hepatosplenomegaly, purpura, progressive anemia, normal or decreased white blood cell counts with normal differentials and platelets, and a diffuse, nonlipid reticuloendothelial proliferation. In 1936, Abt and Demenholz coined the term *Letterer-Siwe disease* for this aggressive symptom complex that usually led to death.

In 1940, Otani and Ehrlich presented seven cases of what they called "solitary granuloma of bone," in which "granulomas of histiocytes, leukocytes, eosinophils and osteoclasts were present with necrosis, hemorrhage and bone repair." This was followed almost immediately by Lichtenstein and Jaffe's report of their own cases, to which they applied the term *eosinophilic granuloma of bone*.

As early as 1937, cases suggesting a transition between these diseases had been reported. Many felt that the granuloma-like proliferations of Hand-Schüller-Christian and Letterer-Siwe diseases were different facets of the same disease process, the more virulent form occurring in younger children and the milder form occurring in older children. When Farber subsequently included eosinophilic granuloma in this concept, the three diseases came to represent variations in degree, stage of involvement, and localization of the same basic disease. In 1953, Lichtenstein proposed uniting these three entities under the term "histiocytosis-X," to indicate that the basic disease process was of unknown etiology. Thus, eosinophilic granuloma came to be known as the localized form, Hand-Schüller-Christian disease as the chronic disseminated form, and Letterer-Siwe disease as the acute disseminated form.

tic T-cell lymphomas unrelated to Langerhans cell histiocytosis.

Juvenile Melanoma

In 1947, Spitz described an entity that she called *melanoma of childhood* based on her belief that it was analogous to the adult melanoma but had a benign behavior in children. The lesion was subsequently referred to as a *juvenile melanoma* and then as a *benign juvenile melanoma*. What now appears to be a contradiction in terms can be explained by Spitz's original concept of a melanoma that displayed a different biologic behavior in children. Later, the terms *Spitz nevus* and *epithelioid and spindle cell nevus* were applied, either of which is preferable to *juvenile melanoma*.

Spitz Nevus

Spitz nevus honors the name of this fine pathologist, whereas *epithelioid and spindle cell nevus*, though histologically correct, does not. The major problem with a Spitz nevus is that histologically it may resemble a true melanoma, and at times the diagnosis may be very difficult. But a Spitz nevus is indeed just a nevus and a benign lesion. To imply that it is a melanoma is misleading.

Juvenile Periodontosis

From the 1950s to the mid-1970s, *gingivosis* and *periodontosis* were common catch-all terms used to describe severe gingival or periodontal destruction that could not be explained by the paradigm of "local irritants." The terms implied some hidden defect in the periodontal tissue apart from inflammation that led to its loss. Since then, immune testing has shown that there was indeed a hidden defect in the tissues in the form of a macrophage and/or neutrophil loss of one or several cell membrane proteins that assist normal microorganism binding to their cell membranes and their engulfment for digestion. Collectively, these genetic defects in certain immune cells are called *leukocyte-adherence deficiencies*, but they are not limited to leukocytes per se since the macrophage may possess this deficiency as well.

Leukocyte-Adherence Deficiency Periodontitis

Today the spectrum of prepubertal periodontitis, rapidly progressing periodontitis, and juvenile periodontitis, which were all once termed *periodontosis*, all seem to have this dual association with a leukocyte-adherence deficiency and *A actinomycetemcomitans*.

Outdated Term	Updated Term

Many of these cell-surface deficiencies are specific to certain microorganisms and therefore will not be associated with systemic infections such as recurrent pneumonias and multiple skin infections. In particular, *Actinobacillus actinomycetemcomitans* is a gram-negative bacillus that seems to be resistant to leukocyte deactivation and macrophage engulfment by this mechanism and is the causative agent in what is known as *juvenile periodontitis*, and was formerly known as *periodontosis*.

Leontiasis Ossea

Leontiasis ossea is an obselete term that, literally translated, means "lion-like bone" and refers to facial features that may resemble the face of a lion. It was consistently used to describe the facies of individuals with Paget disease and fibrous dysplasia, although at times a good deal of imagination was needed to see the lion in it, particularly as it pertained to fibrous dysplasia since it is most always unilateral in the maxilla. This term was used so frequently throughout the 1950s and 1960s that it was thought to represent a specific form of each of these diseases. Today, of course, it is no longer used.

No term need be used other than the correct diagnosis that may produce this facial appearance.

Lymphoproliferative Disease of the Palate/Follicular Lymphoid Hyperplasia of the Palate

The term *lymphoproliferative disease of the palate* is misleading, both for the clinician and for the pathologist. It attempts to isolate low-grade lymphomas that occur in the palate as a separate entity without stating that they are actually lymphomas. This effort, which began in the late 1970s and gained some acceptance through the 1980s, fortunately failed. The recommendations of those in support of this term and its concept were to observe rather than to treat these conditions, which were actually dangerous lymphomas.

An illogical term for what was interpreted as a benign proliferation in the palate was proposed. *Follicular lymphoid hyperplasia of the palate* would be valid if it were associated with a definitive inflammatory focus, traumatic event, or infection and were seen in some inflammatory fibrous hyperplasias. In other parts of the mouth lymphoid hyperplasias resolve when the inflammatory focus and the tissue are removed, particularly if it is associated with a denture flange as in epulis fissuratum (see Chapter 2). However, as a nonlymphoma diagnosis on the palate without a source of inflammation, this term cannot be accepted. Unfortunately, too many real lymphomas have been overlooked or dismissed by this term.

Part of the argument that has been advanced for using this term to describe a nonlymphoma is that the B lymphocytes are polyclonal rather than monoclonal and that the mantle zone has both mature and immature B cells. However, as noted in Chapter 19, malignant lymphoid proliferations are originally monoclonal, but they become mixed with and/or cause a reactivity of the other lymphoid cells and may therefore appear polyclonal. Polyclonality should not be the sole criterion for ruling out a lymphoma; using this unproven diagnostic term can adversely affect treatment and prognosis.

Low-Grade B-Cell Lymphoma

In truth, all diseases termed *lymphoproliferative disease of the palate* are lymphomas, and most are low-grade B-cell lymphomas. As noted in the discussion of low-grade B-cell lymphomas in Chapter 19, these lymphomas are slowly progressive but deadly due to incomplete treatment responses. Initially, lymphoproliferative diseases of the palate were not considered to be true lymphomas because they remained clinically unchanged for months or years. However, as is consistent with low-grade B-cell lymphomas, these lesions eventually revealed their true nature as a malignant disease—that is, a true lymphoma—but even then it was conjectured that the so-called lymphoproliferative disease of the palate had merely transformed into a lymphoma or that it represented a benign precursor of lymphoma. The answer is no. These are lymphomas from their first appearance, and it is only their initial slow progression that may lead some to believe otherwise. To invent a term such as *lymphoproliferative disease of the palate* for what is really a lymphoma is as absurd as calling squamous cell carcinoma of the tongue epithelial proliferative disease of the tongue.

Today it is recognized that such follicular lymphoid proliferations in the palate are low-grade B-cell lymphomas that present in a follicular rather than in a diffuse pattern.

Outdated Term	Updated Term

Median Mandibular Cyst

An extremely rare midline cyst of the mandible had been attributed to entrapped epithelium during fusion of the bilateral mandibular arches and therefore was classified as another fissural cyst. Again, embryologic data indicated that epithelial entrapment was impossible, and a review of even the rare cases that were reported raised suspicions that primordial odontogenic cysts more accurately explained a cyst in this location. Today the median mandibular cyst is not recognized and, together with the globulomaxillary cyst and the median palatal cyst, is regarded as an invalid embryologic concept.

No term need be used other than the correct diagnosis of a cyst in this location.

Melanoameloblastoma/Retinal Anlage Tumor

Melanoameloblastoma is a term once applied to the melanotic neuroectodermal tumor of infancy. Throughout the 1950s and 1960s, many jaw tumors were labeled as ameloblastomas or as variants of an ameloblastoma on the assumption that a jaw tumor is a type of ameloblastoma until proven otherwise. Like ameloblastomas, the melanotic neuroectodermal tumor of infancy grows to impressive sizes, and since odontogenic epithelium is sometimes trapped within these tumors, it is easy to understand how they could have been interpreted as melanin-containing ameloblastomas. Similarly, the term *retinal anlage tumor* emerged through an effort to explain the presence of a large number of pigmented cells. The pigmented cells of the retina presented an obvious, convenient, and nearly singular source of pigment, lending some credibility to the concept that this tumor arose from retinal cell precursors.

Melanotic Neuroectodermal Tumor of Infancy

Since these older terms were introduced, our understanding of neuroectodermal and neural crest derivatives has been refined. Today, the *melanotic neuroectodermal tumor of infancy* has taken the place of these terms because it more accurately reflects its origin from neural crest remnants more densely located in the anterior maxilla and more numerous during infancy, after which these rests involute.

Monomorphic Adenoma

In the 1950s and 1960s, there was a dispute over the existence of a pure adenoma of salivary gland and a reluctance by some to separate this lesion from the pleomorphic adenoma, of which it was considered to be a variant. In 1967, Kleinsasser and Klein defined basal cell adenoma as a distinct tumor with a monomorphic histology, emphasizing its separateness and distinguishing it from the pleomorphic adenoma. Subsequently, Ranch, Seifert, and Gorlin classified all benign salivary gland tumors as either pleomorphic or monomorphic adenomas, the latter encompassing all other benign epithelial salivary gland tumors. One such tumor was basal cell adenoma, which included solid, tubular, canalicular, and basophilic variants.

The World Health Organization classification of 1972 used the same approach. The term *monomorphic* was used to designate a tumor with a regular, glandular pattern that lacked mesenchyme-like tissue or histologic features diagnostic of pleomorphic adenoma. Thus again, monomorphic adenoma was a broad designation applied to any benign epithelial tumor of salivary gland origin that was not a pleomorphic adenoma, including adenolymphoma (Warthin tumor), oxyphilic adenoma (oncocytoma), basal cell adenoma, trabecular adenoma, tubular adenoma, clear cell adenoma, and sebaceous lymphadenoma. This concept was perpetuated in the second Armed Forces Institute of Pathology (AFIP) fascicle.

In 1977, Batsakis redefined the monomorphic designation to include myoepithelioma and basal cell adenoma as well as glycogen-rich, clear cell, and membranous adenomas and to remove Warthin tumor and oncocytoma. In 1981, however, they were restored to the monomorphic adenoma grouping, and this time the "basal cell" or basaloid adenoma had solid, trabecular-tubular, and canalicular variants, confirming the confusion and the lack of consensus that all of these name changes signified.

At some point during the development of salivary gland tumor classifications, the monomorphic adenomas were equated with basal cell adenoma. In fact, Youngberg and Rao stated that "monomorphic adenoma (basal cell adenoma) of the salivary gland is now accepted as a definite entity," and the

Basal Cell or Canalicular Adenoma
(as per histopathology)

While *monomorphic adenoma* was initially a useful term to classify any benign tumor that was not a pleomorphic adenoma, it is not a specific entity. *Basal cell adenoma* and *canalicular adenoma* refer to separate tumors with their own biologic potentials. Thus, for the sake of clarity, the term *monomorphic adenoma* should be retired from current use and the terms *basal cell adenoma* and *canalicular adenoma* should be used to describe each respective tumor.

Outdated Term

Updated Term

two terms were often used synonymously. Many pathologists believed that the basal cell adenoma and the canalicular adenoma (a tumor that had actually predated basal cell adenoma in the literature) were variants of the same tumor. Further adding to the confusion, the designations "monomorphic adenoma, basal cell type" and "monomorphic adenoma, canalicular type" were often used, and both terms were frequently used synonymously. Based on ultrastructural studies, Chen and Miller showed that basal cell and canalicular adenomas were distinct and separate entities as evidenced by their individual clinicopathologic features.

Neuralgia-Inducing Cavitational Osteonecrosis (NICO)

The abbreviation NICO purportedly refers to *neuralgia-inducing cavitational osteonecrosis*, but we prefer to think of it as *nonexistent idiotic concept of osteopathology* because it is truly a bogus disease term. First published by Bouquet, NICO is simply the revival of a long-abandoned concept once termed *Ratner's bone cavities*. In NICO, patients with jaw pain are said to have hollow defects in the mandible or maxilla that induce painful neuralgias. The concept emerged when an autopsy of a single patient who was said to have facial neuralgias revealed several marrow defects. A cause-and-effect relationship was established, and shortly thereafter patients with pain, mostly older women, were diagnosed with NICO.

What was overlooked in this explanation is the fact that cadavers undergo significant marrow autolysis, leading to the formation of marrow cavities. Moreover, many older individuals, especially postmenopausal women, have hollow marrow cavities composed either of fatty marrow or a space created by fatty marrow degeneration; however, all such individuals do not have facial pain. Facial pains may have a myriad of possible causes, and to attribute them all to a hollow marrow cavity is extremely presumptuous. This author (REM) had the opportunity over a 1-week period to examine and work up 11 patients diagnosed with NICO by previous biopsies, the reports of which described nonvital bone (osteonecrosis). All 11 patients were women over 45 years of age, and each one brought their CT scans with them to show proof of their marrow cavities. The marrow cavities were indeed in evidence, but they were in the form of anatomic foramen, postsurgical defects, and osteoporosis defects common to age- and sex-matched CT scans of others. In 7 of these individuals a bona fide source of pain was found, ranging from pulpitis to abscessed teeth to infections around a foreign body, to one individual who had even suffered a nonunion fracture of C-2 from a garage door that hit her in the head 7 years earlier.

A review of the histologic slides purporting dead bone with "empty lacunae" showed that 40% of lacunae were indeed "empty." This, however, is normal bone histology. Most adult bone biopsies will show 15% to 40% empty lacunae due to the fact that an osteocyte lacuna is about 25 μm, the osteocyte itself is about 12 μm, the nucleus of the osteocyte (what appears in the histology) is only 4 μm, and histology sections are routinely cut at 6 μm. Consequently, many microtome cuts will section through a lacunar space without sectioning through an osteocyte or more particularly through a nucleus, and will thus give the false impression of being an empty lacuna.

Many NICO patients undergo repetitive surgeries to pack these mystical bone cavities, creating even more pain. The 11 patients reviewed had on average 8 teeth removed and 5 surgeries each related to the diagnosis of NICO, and yet they still had their original pain, and most of them had mutilated jaws from repetitive surgeries. NICO is not a term to be used and is not a disease.

No such disease exists. Normal marrow spaces in individuals with pain in the jaws are two separate, unrelated findings.

Outdated Term

Updated Term

Neurilemmoma, Neurinoma, Neurolemmoma, and Neurolemoma

The roots of the above terms are from the Greek: *neuron* meaning nerve, *lemma* meaning a husk or covering, and *eilema*, meaning a closely adhering sheath. Consequently, a tumor of a peripheral nerve might logically be called by any of these terms. Today we recognize two major groups of benign peripheral nerve sheath tumors: neurofibroma and the neurilemomma variations. Initially, Verocay introduced the term *neurinoma* to identify the latter entity, but this is inappropriate since it is a tumor of the Schwann cells around the nerve and not the nerve fiber or the nerve sheath. In 1932, Masson referred to these tumors as *schwannomas*, and in 1935 Stout, who believed this tumor included the nerve sheath, wrote of *neurilemmomas* to describe the same entity, and thus began the confusion.

Orthokeratinizing Keratocysts

Orthokeratinizing keratocyst is an unnecessary and confusing term that appears even in some World Health Organization publications. However, each time it appears, it is accompanied by an explanation that orthokeratinizing keratocysts are not as aggressive as so-called regular or parakeratinizing keratocysts and do not have their high recurrence rates. The reason is that orthokeratinizing keratocysts are not keratocysts at all, but cysts that produce keratin. True keratocysts have both a specific biologic behavior and a specific histopathology—that is, prominent basophilia of the basal cells, which are cuboidal to columnar with palisaded nuclei, and a corrugated parakeratinized surface. While many cysts—including dentigerous cysts, radicular cysts, calcifying epithelial odontogenic cysts, and even epidermoid cysts of the skin—will produce keratin, it is inaccurate to use the production of keratin as the sole diagnostic criterion for a keratocyst. The term *orthokeratinizing keratocysts* is essentially a nonentity and actually refers to any one of a number of cysts found to produce keratin at the time of their removal.

Periadenitis Necrotica Recurrens/Periadenitis Mucosa Necrotica Recurrens

The first report of periadenitis necrotica recurrens was by the dermatologist Richard Sutton in 1911. He described the disease as "a chronic recurring necrotic granulomatous affection of the lingual and buccal mucosa," characterized histologically by "an intense inflammatory process in the periglandular tissue with ensuing necrosis and separation of the central part of the affected area." He speculated that the disease was of tuberculous origin and presented a single case. He applied the term *periadenitis necrotica recurrens* to describe this condition because it had been used extensively in the dermatologic literature. *Periadenitis mucosa necrotica recurrens* is another inaccurate name because its emphasis on glandular structures distorts the pathologic process. The histologic picture will frequently include a "periadenitis," but the salivary glands do not have a primary role in the disease. Because the inflammatory process extends deep into the tissue, causing subsequent scarification, minor salivary glands in the area are often secondarily engulfed by the process.

Schwannoma

Schwann had shown that the nerve covering was composed not only of Schwann cells but also of an outer membrane, which subsequently became known as the *neurilemma*. This has been identified ultrastructurally as the Schwann cell membrane, basal lamina, and connective tissue ground substance with collagen fibrils external to the basal lamina. The neoplasm under consideration is composed only of a proliferation of Schwann cells that does not include the basal lamina or other components of the neurilemma. Therefore, *schwannoma* is a more scientifically correct term than neurilemmoma.

Besides being more accurate histologically, *schwannoma* also honors the name of Theodor Schwann (1810–1882), a German professor of anatomy whose many contributions include founder of the cell theory, on which all histology is based.

Keratinizing Odontogenic Cyst

This term indicates that any type of odontogenic cyst may undergo keratinization and that this is not a specific histopathologic entity.

Major Aphthae

Major aphthae is short, concise, and the preferred term to describe this disease.

Outdated Term	Updated Term

Postmenopausal Desquamative Gingivitis, Chronic Diffuse Desquamative Gingivitis, and Gingivosis

In 1894, Tomes and Tomes wrote of gingival lesions occurring in middle-aged women in which the tissue took on a red, smooth, polished appearance. In 1932, Prinz first used the term *chronic diffuse desquamative gingivitis* to describe a process that he characterized as desquamative, erythematous, erosive, and sometimes vesiculobullous in nature, noting that the majority of patients were female and of menopausal age. It became generally accepted that this specific entity could be identified histologically as a degeneration of connective tissue with fragmentation of fibrous tissue and formation of hyaline, granular material. Foss and coworkers preferred the term *gingivosis* to denote its degenerative as opposed to inflammatory process.

Although the etiology was still unclear, Ziskin and Zegarelli observed some improvement in these patients following the topical use of estrogen, and since, as noted above, a large proportion were postmenopausal-aged woman, they drew an assumptive but inaccurate conclusion that this condition represented a degenerative process resulting from female hormone depletion; this belief persisted for many years.

In 1953, Glickman suggested that chronic desquamative gingivitis may be a rare clinical manifestation common to a variety of disorders. In a study of its histopathology, Glickman and Smulow noted two main histologic patterns: bullous and lichenoid. In 1960, McCarthy et al concluded from their studies that chronic desquamative gingivitis was not a distinct entity but rather a manifestation of several disease processes. Hormonally related desquamative gingivitis was actually found to be uncommon.

Following the development of immunopathology, it became apparent that the majority of patients with desquamative gingivitis indeed suffered from a specific immune-based disease, the most frequent cause of which was mucosal pemphigoid followed by lichen planus. Of the 174 cases examined by Nisengard and Rogers, 48.9% were diagnosed with pemphigoid, 23.6% with lichen planus, and 2.3% with pemphigus, while 24.6% showed no significant immunoreactivity.

No term need be used other than the specific immune-based disease that produced this sign in the individual patient.

Reiter Syndrome

There are several reasons why *Reiter syndrome* should be replaced with the more appropriate term *reactive arthritis*. One reason is that Hans Reiter (1881–1969) was an individual who should not be honored and memorialized. An adjunct professor and Nazi physician in Rostock, Germany, he taught "hygienics" from a strictly racist point of view. Moreover, he was a major proponent of "racial hygiene," a fanatic anti-Semite, and a loyal supporter of Adolf Hitler. He rapidly advanced in medical and social circles through this association and enjoyed a spectacular career to become a leader in German medicine. He was involved in decisions for medical experimentation in the concentration camps and reportedly sent numerous Jews to their deaths. After the war and following his release from an American internment camp, he continued to practice medicine in Germany, served as a consultant to several American medical organizations, and enjoyed a revered reputation.

Reactive Arthritis

Equally important, the disease entity known as Reiter syndrome is in fact a reactive arthritis, and it was described in 1818 by Benjamin Collins Brodie. It is appropriate to remove Reiter's name, not only to acknowledge his inhumanity but also to redress an undeserved credit. *Reactive arthritis* is a scientifically more correct term because this disease is an immune-based complex of signs and symptoms provoked by any one of several infectious diseases.

Traumatic Bone Cyst

A traumatic bone cyst is yet another contradiction in terms. It is an empty space found in the mandible unrelated to trauma; and since it does not have an epithelial lining it is therefore not a cyst.

Idiopathic Bone Cavity

Because it persists as a cavity in bone containing no specific diagnostic elements, the term *idiopathic bone cavity* is an unembellished description that is appropriate for now.

Outdated Term

Updated Term

Unicystic Ameloblastoma

Ameloblastoma in Situ or Invasive Ameloblastoma *(as per histopathology)*

Few terms have resulted in more recurrences than the term *unicystic ameloblastoma*. First introduced in 1977 by Robinson and Martinez and popularized by Gardner in 1983, this term has created confusion between a cyst and a tumor and how each should be treated.

The terms *mural ameloblastoma in situ* and *intraluminal ameloblastoma in situ* are used to describe noninvasive ameloblastomas. The terms *intramural ameloblastoma* and *transmural ameloblastoma* describe microinvasive ameloblastomas, and the terms *solid ameloblastoma* and *multicystic ameloblastoma* are used to describe invasive ameloblastomas. These terms are preferred because they link the histopathology to clinical behavior and can be correlated with treatment. The terms referring to various unicystic ameloblastomas should be dropped from use.

Today we recognize that ameloblastomas and odontogenic cysts may each arise from the same set of odontogenic epithelium: rests of Serres, rests of Malassez, inner and outer enamel epithelium, etc. Thus, an ameloblastoma may arise from a cyst lining by undergoing a genetic change. We also recognize that ameloblastomas form internal cystic spaces by degeneration within the stellate reticulum. Consequently, the term *unicystic ameloblastoma* creates confusion for the clinician about whether it represents a dentigerous cyst that is developing an ameloblastoma from its lining, either in an intramural or intraluminal fashion, or whether it represents an invasive ameloblastoma with a single internal cystic space. In its purest sense, the term *unicystic ameloblastoma* describes the commonly recognized invasive ameloblastoma that happens to have a single lumen. Yet this term has often been used to describe cysts with ameloblastoma proliferations in their lining, implying a need for treatment by enucleation procedures. The result has been the enucleation and subsequent recurrence of invasive ameloblastomas.

In this text we introduce the terms *ameloblastoma in situ* and *microinvasive ameloblastoma,* which we apply in a manner analogous to the nomenclature used in the oral mucosal spectrum of dysplasia–carcinoma in situ–verrucous carcinoma–microinvasive carcinoma—invasive squamous cell carcinoma. In this spectrum, an odontogenic cyst is just a cyst, analogous to a normal mucosal epithelial surface, and is curable by enucleation. An odontogenic cyst with a focal mural ameloblastoma proliferation confined to the lining of an odontogenic cyst is analogous to dysplasia or carcinoma in situ, and it too is curable by enucleation. An odontogenic cyst with a focal intraluminal ameloblastoma without invasion through the connective tissue wall of the cyst is analogous to a verrucous carcinoma; therefore, it is not invasive and is also curable by enucleation. An odontogenic cyst showing at any point in its lining an ameloblastoma proliferation that invades into or through the connective tissue wall is an invasive ameloblastoma requiring a resective approach; this is analogous to a clinical erythroleukoplakia with various areas of dysplasia but one or more areas of invasive carcinoma, which of course requires a more extensive surgery. In addition, any ameloblastoma identified histopathologically, whether solid, multicystic, unicystic, or of any histopathologic subtype (follicular or plexiform) is an invasive benign tumor requiring a type of resection for cure.

Bibliography

Chapter 2

Adal KA, Cockerell CJ, Petri WA Jr. Cat-scratch disease, bacillary angiomatosis and other infections due to *Rochialimaea*. N Engl J Med 1994;330:1509–1515.

Brown JR. Human actinomycosis: A study of 181 subjects. Human Pathol 1973;4:319–330.

Buchner A, Hansen LS. The histomorphologic spectrum of peripheral ossifying fibroma. Oral Surg Oral Med Oral Pathol 1987;63:452–461.

Carithers HA. Cat-scratch disease: An overview based on a study of 1,200 patients. Am J Dis Child 1985;139:1124–1133.

Chaudhry Z, Barret AW, Corbett E, French PD, Zakrzewska JM. Oral mucosal leishmaniasis as a presenting feature of HIV infection and its management. J Oral Pathol Med 1999;28:43–46.

Chue PWY. Gonorrhea: Its natural history, oral manifestations, diagnosis, treatment and prevention. J Am Dent Assoc 1975;90:1297–1301.

Eng HL, Lu SY, Yang CH, Chen WJ. Oral tuberculosis. Oral Surg Oral Med Oral Pathol Oral Radiol Endod 1996;81:415–420.

English CK, Wear DJ, Margileth AW, Lissner CR, Walsh GP. Cat-scratch disease: Isolation and culture of the bacterial agent. JAMA 1988;259:1347–1352.

Fiumara NJ, Lessel S. Manifestations of late congenital syphilis: An analysis of 271 patients. Arch Dermatol 1970;102:78–83.

Flanagan AM, Tinkler SMB, Horton MA, Williams DM, Chambers TJ. The multinucleated cells in giant cell granulomas of the jaw are osteoclasts. Cancer 1988;62:1139–1145.

Frey L. Le syndrome du ners auriculo-temporal. Rev Neurol (Paris) 1923;2:97–104.

Katsikeris N, Kakarantza-Angelopoulos E, Angelopoulos AP. Peripheral giant cell granuloma: A clinicopathologic study of 224 new cases and review of 956 reported cases. Int J Oral Maxillofac Surg 1988;17:94–99.

Marx RE, Carlson ER, Smith BR, Toraya N. Isolation of *Actinomyces* species and *Eikenella corrodens* from patients with chronic diffuse sclerosing osteomyelitis. J Oral Maxillofac Surg 1994;52:26–33.

Meyer I, Shklar G. The oral manifestations of acquired syphilis: A study of 81 cases. Oral Surg Oral Med Oral Pathol 1967;2:45–61.

Nortje CJ, Wood RE, Grotepass F. Periostitis ossificans versus Garré's osteomyelitis. Part II: Radiologic analysis of 93 cases in the jaws. Oral Surg Oral Med Oral Pathol 1988;66:249–260.

Plauth M, Jenss H, Meyle J. Oral manifestations of Crohn's disease: An analysis of 79 cases. J Clin Gastroenterol 1991;13:29–37.

Praetorius-Clausen F. Histopathology of focal epithelial hyperplasia: Evidence of viral infection. Tandlaegebladet 1969;73:1013–1022.

Scully C. Orofacial herpes simplex virus infections: Current concepts in the epidemiology, pathogenesis, and treatment, and disorders in which the virus may be implicated. Oral Surg Oral Med Oral Pathol 1989;68:701–710.

Sedano HO, Carlos R, Koutlas IG. Respiratory scleroma. A clinicopathologic study. Oral Surg Oral Med Oral Pathol Oral Radiol Endod 1996;81:665–671.

Tozman ECS. Sarcoidosis. Br J Hosp Med 1991;3:155–159.

Wood RE, Nortje CJ, Grotepass F, Schmidt S, Harris AM. Periostitis ossificans versus Garré's osteomyelitis. Part I. What did Garré really say? Oral Surg Oral Med Oral Pathol 1988;65:773–777.

Chapter 3

Anhalt GJ, Kim SC, Stanley JR, Korman NJ, Jabs DA, Kory M, et al. Paraneoplastic pemphigus: An autoimmune mucocutaneous disease, associated with neoplasia. N Engl J Med 1990;323:1729–1735.

Brown RS, Bottomley WK, Puente E, Lavigne GJ. A retrospective evaluation of 193 patients with oral lichen planus. J Oral Pathol Med 1993;22:69–72.

Burrows NP, Lockwood NW. Antineutrophil cytoplasmic antibodies and their relevance to the dermatologist. Br J Dermatol 1995;132:173–181.

Church LF, Schosser RH. Chronic ulcerative stomatitis associated with stratified epithelial specific antinuclear antibodies. A case report of a newly described disease entity. Oral Surg Oral Med Oral Pathol 1992;73:579–582.

Cohen DM, Bhattacharyya I, Zunt SL, Tomich CE. Linear IgA disease histopathologically and clinically masquerading as lichen planus. Oral Surg Oral Med Oral Pathol Oral Radiol Endod 1999;88:196–201.

Devaney KO, Travis WD, Hoffman G, Leavitt R, Lebovics R, Fauci AS. Interpretation of head and neck biopsies in Wegener's granulomatosis. A pathologic study of 126 biopsies in 70 patients. Am J Surg Pathol 1990;14:555–564.

Domloge-Hultsch N, Anhalt GJ, Gammon WR, Lazarova Z, et al. Antiepiligrin cicatricial pemphigoid. A subepithelial bullous disorder. Arch Dermatol 1994;130:1521–1529.

Eisen D. The vulvovaginal-gingival syndrome of lichen planus. Arch Dermatol 1994;130:1379–1382.

Eversole LR. Immunopathology of oral mucosal ulcerative, desquamative and bullous diseases. Oral Surg Oral Med Oral Pathol 1994;77:555–571.

Gell PGH, Coombs RRA. Section IV. The allergic state as responsible for clinical hypersensitivity and disease. In: Clinical Aspects of Immunology, second ed. Gell PGH (ed). Oxford: Blackwell Science.

Hamideh F, Prete PE. Ophthalmologic manifestations of rheumatic diseases. Semin Arthrit Rheum 2001;30:217–241.

Horn TD, Anhalt GJ. Histologic features of paraneoplastic pemphigus. Arch Dermatol 1992;128:1091–1095.

International Study Group for Behçet's Disease. Criteria for diagnosis of Behçet's disease. Lancet 1990;335:1078–1080.

Lewis JE, Beutner EH, Rostami R, Chorzelski TP. Chronic ulcerative stomatitis with stratified epithelium: Specific antinuclear antibodies. Int J Dermatol 1996;35:272–275.

Marcos O, Cebrecos AI, Prieto A, Sancho de Salas M. Tongue necrosis in a patient with temporal arteritis. J Oral Maxillofac Surg 1998;56:1203–1206.

Mignogna MD, Muzio LL, Mignogna RE, Carbone R, Ruoppo E, Bucci E. Oral pemphigus: Long term behaviour and clinical response to treatment with deflazacort in sixteen cases. J Oral Pathol Med 2000;29:143–152.

Patten SF, Tomecki JT. Wegener's granulomatosis: Cutaneous and oral mucosal disease. J Am Acad Dermatol 1993;28:710–718.

Pindborg JJ, Gorlin RJ, Asboe Hansen G. Reiter's syndrome: Review of the literature and report of a case. Oral Surg Oral Med Oral Pathol 1963;16:551–560.

Roujeau JC. Stevens-Johnson syndrome and toxic epidermal necrolysis are severity variants of the same disease which differs from erythema multiforme. J Dermatol 1997;24:726–729.

Rzany B, Hering O, Ockenhaupt M, Schroder, et al. Histopathological and epidemiological characteristics of patients with erythema multiforme exudativum multiforme major, Stevens-Johnson syndrome and toxic epidermal necrolysis. Br J Dermatol 1996;135:6–11.

Savage NW, Ishir T, Seymour GJ. Immunopathogenesis of oral lichen planus. J Oral Pathol Med 1990;19:389–396.

Savage NW, Seymour GJ, Kruger BJ. T-Lymphocyte subset changes in recurrent aphthous stomatitis. Oral Surg Oral Med Oral Pathol 1985:60;175–181.

Scully C, Carrozzo M, Gandolfo S, Puiatti P, Monteil R. Update on mucous membrane pemphigoid: A heterogenous immune-mediated subepithelial blistering entity. Oral Surg Oral Med Oral Pathol Oral Radiol Endod 1999;88:56–68.

Van der Meij EH, Schepman KP, Smeele LE, Van der Wal JE, Bezemer PD, van der Waal I. A review of the recent literature regarding malignant transformation of oral lichen planus. Oral Surg Oral Med Oral Pathol Oral Radiol Endod 1999;88:307–310.

Zhang L, Michelson C, Cheng X, Zeng, Priddy R, Rosin MP. Molecular analysis of oral lichen planus: A premalignant lesion? Am J Pathol 1997;151:323–327.

Chapter 4

Ghaffar KA, Zahran FM, Fahmy HM, Brown RS. Papillon-Lefevre syndrome: Neutrophil function in 15 cases from 4 families in Egypt. Oral Surg Oral Med Oral Pathol Oral Radiol Endod 1999;88:320–325.

Haitjema T, Westermann CJ, Overtoom TT, Timmer R, et al. Hereditary hemorrhagic telangiectasia (Osler-Weber-Rendu disease): New insights in pathogenesis, complications, and treatment. Arch Inter Med 1996;156:714–719.

Levin LS, Wright JM, Byrd DL, et al. Osteogenesis imperfecta with unusual skeletal lesions: Report of three families. Am J Med Genetics 1985;21:257–269.

Poswillo D. The pathogenesis of the Treacher Collins syndrome (mandibulofacial dysostosis). Br J Oral Surg 1975;13:1–26.

Prindiville DE, Stern D. Oral manifestations of Darier's disease. J Oral Surg 1976;34:1001–1006.

Sadeghi EM, Witkop CJ. Ultrastructural study of hereditary benign intraepithelial dyskeratosis. Oral Surg Oral Med Oral Pathol 1977;44:567–577.

Chapter 5

Hyams VJ. Papillomas of the nasal cavity and paranasal sinuses: A clinicopathologic study of 315 cases. Ann Otol Rhinol Laryngol 1971;80:192–206.

Nowparast B, Howell FV, Rick GM. Verruciform xanthoma: A clinicopathologic review and report of fifty-four cases. Oral Surg Oral Med Oral Pathol 1981;51:619–625.

Chapter 6

Coppola D, Catalano E, Tang CK, Elfenbein IB, Harwick R, Mohr R. Basaloid squamous cell carcinoma of floor of mouth. Cancer 1993;72:2299–2305.

Marks VJ. Actinic keratosis: A premalignant skin lesion. Otolaryngol Clin North Am 1993;26:23–35.

Miller SJ. Biology of basal cell carcinoma (Part I). J Am Acad Dermatol 1991;24:1–13.

Miller SJ. Biology of basal cell carcinoma (Part II). J Am Acad Dermatol 1991;24:161–175.

Murti PR, Bohnsle RB, Gupta PC, Daftary DK, Pindborg JJ, Mehta FS. Etiology of oral submucous fibrosis with special reference to the role of areca nut chewing. J Oral Pathol Med 1995;24:145.

Pindborg JJ, Reibel J, Holmstrup P. Subjectivity in evaluating oral epithelial dysplasia, carcinoma in situ and initial carcinoma. J Oral Pathol 1985;14:698–708.

Rice RD Jr, Chonkich GD, Thompson KS, Chase DR. Merkel cell tumor of the head and neck. Five new cases with literature review. Arch Otolaryngol Head Neck Surg 1193;119:782–786.

Rook A, Whimster I. Keratoacanthoma: A thirty-year retrospective. Br J Dermatol 1979;100:41–47.

Silverman S, Gorsky M, Lozada F. Oral leukoplakia and malignant transformation: A follow up study of 257 patients. Cancer 1984;53:563–568.

Strutton GM. Pathological variants of basal cell carcinoma. Australas J Dermatol 1997;38 (Suppl I):S31–S35.

Wain SL, Kier R, Vollmer RT, Bossen EH. Basaloid-squamous carcinoma of the tongue, hypopharynx and larynx: Report of 10 cases. Human Pathol 1986;17:1158–1166.

Zakrzewska JM, Lopes V, Speight P, Hopper C. Proliferative verrucous leukoplakia. A report of ten cases. Oral Surg Oral Med Oral Pathol Oral Radiol Endod 1996;82:396–401.

Zhang L, Cheung KJ, Lam WL, Cheng X. Increased genetic damage in oral leukoplakia from high risk sites. Potential impact on staging and clinical management. Cancer 2001;91: 2148–2155.

Chapter 7

Bocca E, Pignataro O. A conservation technique in radical neck dissection. Ann Otol Rhinol Laryngol 1967;76:975–987.

Bolande RP. The neurocristopathies. A unifying concept of disease arising in neural crest maldevelopment. Human Pathol 1974;5:409–429.

Breslow A. Thickness, cross-sectional areas, and depth of invasion in the prognosis of cutaneous melanoma. Ann Surg 1970;172:902–908.

Campbell WM, McDonald TJ, Unni KK, Laws ER, Jr. Nasal and paranasal presentation of chordoma. Laryngoscope 1980; 90:612–618.

Chauvin PJ, Wysocki GP, Daley TD, Pringle GA. Palisaded encapsulated neuroma of oral mucosa. Oral Surg Oral Med Oral Pathol 1992;73:71–74.

Clark WH Jr, From L, Bernadino EA, Mihm MC. The histogenesis and biologic behavior of primary human malignant melanomas of the skin. Cancer Res 1969;29:705–727.

Doll R, Peto R. Mortality in relation to smoking: 20 years' observations on male British doctors. Br Med J 1976;2: 1525–1536.

Doll R, Peto R. Cigarette smoking and bronchial carcinoma: Dose and time relationships among regular smokers and lifelong non-smokers. J Epidemiol Commun Health 1978; 32:303–313.

Geist JR, Gander DL, Stefanac SJ. Oral manifestations of neurofibromatosis types I and II. Oral Surg Oral Med Oral Pathol 1992;73:376–382.

Heffelfinger MJ, Dahlin DC, MacCarty CS, Beabout JW. Chordomas and cartilaginous tumors at the skull base. Cancer 1973;32:410–420.

Kern WH, McCray MK. The histopathologic differentiation of keratoacanthoma and squamous cell carcinoma of the skin. J Cutan Pathol 1980;7:318–325.

Mirchandani R, Sciubba JJ, Mir R. Granular cell lesions of the jaws and oral cavity: A clinicopathologic, immunohistochemical, and ultrastructural study. J Oral Maxillofac Surg 1989;47:1248–1255.

Muhm M, Polterauer P, Gstottner W, et al. Diagnostic and therapeutic approaches to carotid body tumors. Review of 24 patients. Arch Surg 1997;132:279–284.

O'Connell JX, Renard LG, Liebsch NJ, Efird JT, Munzenrider JE, Rosenberg AE. Base of skull chordoma: A correlative study of histologic and clinical features in 62 cases. Cancer 1994; 74: 2261–2267.

Peto J, Doll R. Passive smoking. Br J Cancer 1986;54:381–383.

Sciubba JJ, D'Amico E, Attie JN. The occurrence of multiple endocrine neoplasia type IIb, in two children of an affected mother. J Oral Pathol 1987;16:310–316.

Shapiro SD, Abramovitch K, Van Dis ML, et al. Neurofibromatosis: Oral and radiographic manifestations. Oral Surg Oral Med Oral Pathol 1984;58:493–498.

Sobel HJ, Marquet E. Granular cells and granular cell lesions. Pathol Annual 1974;9:43–79.

Tang CK, Toker C. Trabecular carcinoma of the skin: An ultrastructural study. Cancer 1978;42:2311–2321.

Toker C. Trabecular carcinoma of the skin. Arch Dermatol 1972;105:107–110.

Williams HK, Cannell H, Silvester K, Williams DM. Neurilemmoma of the head and neck. Br J Oral Maxillofac Surg 1993;31:32–35.

Chapter 8

Bhattacharyya I, Williamson A, Cohen D, Bever JL. Metastatic neuroblastoma with ganglioneuromatous differentiation and mandibular involvement. Oral Surg Oral Med Oral Pathol Oral Radiol Endod 1999;88:586–592.

Bras J, Batsakis JG, Luna MA. Rhabdomyosarcoma of the oral soft tissues. Oral Surg Oral Med Oral Pathol 1987;64: 585–596.

Conley J, Healey WV, Stout AP. Fibromatosis of the head and neck. Am J Surg 1966;112:609–614.

DeWever I, Dal Cin P, Fletcher CDM, Mandahl N, Mertens F, Mitelman F, et al. Cytogenetic, clinical and morphologic correlations in 78 cases of fibromatosis: A report from the CHAMP study group. Mod Pathol 2000;13:1080–1085.

Ducatman BS, Sheithauer BW, Piepgras DG, Reiman HL, Ilstrup DM. Malignant peripheral nerve sheath tumors: A clinicopathologic study of 120 cases. Cancer 1986;57:2006–2021.

Eden BV, Debo RF, Larner JM, et al. Esthesioneuroblastoma. Long term outcome and patterns of failure: The University of Virginia experience. Cancer 1994;73:2556–2562.

Ficcara G, Berson A, Silverman S, Quivey JM, et al. Kaposi's sarcoma of the oral cavity: A study of 134 patients with a review of the pathogenesis, epidemiology, clinical aspects and treatment. Oral Surg Oral Med Oral Pathol 1988;66: 543–550.

Friedman-Kien AE, Saltzman BR. Clinical manifestations of classical, endemic African, and epidemic AIDS-associated Kaposi's sarcoma. J Am Acad Dermatol 1990;22:1237–1250.

Gagari E, Kabani GT. Intraoral liposarcoma: Case report and review of the literature. Oral Surg Oral Med Oral Pathol Oral Radiol Endod 2000;89:66–72.

Glick M, Cleveland DB. Oral mucosal bacillary epithelioid angiomatosis in a patient with AIDS associated with rapid alveolar bone loss: A case report. J Oral Pathol Med 1993; 22:235–239.

Hollowood K, Fletcher CDM. Rhabdomyosarcoma in adults. Sem Diag Pathol 1994;11:47–57.

Lieberman PH, Brennan MK, Kimmel M, Erlandson RA, Garin-Chesa P, Fleching BY. Alveolar soft part sarcoma: A clinicopathologic study of half a century. Cancer 1989;63:1–13.

Marx RE, Carlson ER, Smith BR, Toraya N. Isolation of *Actinomyces* species and *Eikenella corrodens* from patients with chronic diffuse sclerosing osteomyelitis. J Oral Maxillofac Surg 1994;52:26–33.

Mills SE, Frierson HF. Olfactory neuroblastoma. Clinicopathologic study of 21 cases. Am J Surg Pathol 1985;9:317–327.

Neville BW, Hann J, Narang R, Garen P. Oral neurofibrosarcoma associated with neurofibromatosis type I. Oral Surg Oral Med Oral Pathol 1991;72:456–461.

Peters E, Cohen M, Altini M, Murray J. Rhabdomyosacroma of the oral and paraoral regions. Cancer 1989;63:963–966.

Shmookler BM, Enzinger FM, Rannon RB. Orofacial synovial sarcoma: A clinicopathologic study of 11 new cases and review of the literature. Cancer 1982;50:269–276.

Tsokos M. The diagnosis and classifiaction of childhood rhabdomyosarcoma. Sem Diag Pathol 1944;11:26–38.

Chapter 9

Brannon RB, Fowler CB, Hartman KS. Necrotizing sialometaplasia: A clinicopathologic study of sixty nine cases and review of the literature. Oral Surg Oral Med Oral Pathol 1991;72:317–325.

Daniels TE. Labial salivary gland biopsy in Sjögren's syndrome; Assessment as a diagnostic criterion in 362 suspected cases. Arthritis Rheum 1984;27:147–156.

Daniels TE. Salivary histopathology in diagnosis of Sjögren's syndrome. Scand J Rheumatol 1986;61(suppl):36–43.

Donath K, Seifert G. Ultrastructural studies of the parotid glands in sialadenosis. Virchows Arch (A) 1975;365:119–135.

Eveson JW. Superificial mucoceles: Pitfall in clinical and microscopic diagnosis. Oral Surg Oral Med Oral Pathol 1988;66: 318–322.

Jordan RC, Speight PM. Lymphoma in Sjögren's syndrome: From histopathology to molecular pathology. Oral Surg Oral Med Oral Pathol Oral Radiol Endod 1996;81:308–320.

Marx RE, Hartmann KS, Rethman KV. A prospective study comparing incisional labial to incisional parotid biopsies in the detection and confirmation of sarcoidosis, Sjögren's disease, sialosis and lymphoma. J Rheumatol 1988;15: 621–629.

Melzack R, Wall PD. Pain mechanisms: A new theory. Science 1965;150:971–979.

Vitali C, Bombardieri S, Moutsopoulos HM, Coll J, et al. Assessment of the European classification criteria for Sjögren's syndrome in a series of clinically defined cases: Results of a prospective multicentre study. Ann Rheum Dis 1996;55:116–121.

Vitali C, Bombardieri S, Moutsopoulos HM. Preliminary criteria for the classification of Sjögren's syndrome: Results of a prospective concerted action supported by the European community. Arthritis Rheum 1993;36:340–347.

Chapter 10

Abrams AM, Melrose RJ. Acinic cell tumors of minor salivary glands origin. Oral Surg Oral Med Oral Pathol 1978; 48:220–233.

Auclair PL, Ellis GL. Atypical features in salivary gland mixed tumors: Their relationship to malignant transformation. Mod Pathol 1996;9:652–657.

Auclair PL, Goode RK, Ellis GL. Mucoepidermoid carcinoma of intraoral glands. Evaluation and application of grading criteria in 143 cases. Cancer 1992;69:2021–2030.

Brannon RB, Sciubba J, Giulani M. Ductal papillomas of salivary gland origin: A report of 19 cases and a review of the literature. Oral Surg Oral Med Oral Pathol Oral Radiol Endod 2001;92:68–77.

Ellis GL, Corio RL. Acinic cell carcinoma: A clinicopathologic analysis of 294 cases. Cancer 1983;52:542–549.

Eveson JW, Cawson RA. Salivary gland tumors: A review of 2,410 cases with particular reference to histologic types, site, age and sex distribution. J Pathol 1985;146:51–58.

Eveson JW, Cawson RA. Warthin's tumor (cystadenolymphoma) of salivary glands. A clinicopathologic investigation of 278 cases. Oral Surg Oral Med Oral Pathol 1986;61:356–362.

Goode RK, Auclair PL, Ellis GL. Mucoepidermoid carcinoma of the major salivary glands. Clinical and histopathologic analysis of 234 cases with evaluation of grading criteria. Cancer 1998;82:1217–1224.

Jensen OJ, Poulsen T, Schiodt T. Mucoepidermoid tumors of salivary glands. A long term follow-up study. APMIS 1988; 96:421–427.

Nascimento AG, Amaral AL, Prado LAF, Kligerman J, Silveira TRP. Adenoid cystic carcinoma of salivary glands. A study of 61 cases with clinicopathologic correlation. Cancer 1986; 57:312–319.

Perzin KH, Gullane P, Clairmont AC. Adenoid cystic carcinoma arising in salivary glands: A correlation of histologic features and clinical course. Cancer 1978;42:265–282.

Spiro RH. Salivary neoplasms: An overview of a 35 year experience with 2,807 patients. Head Neck Surg 1986;8:177–184.

Vincent SD, Hammond HL, Finkelstein MW. Clinical and therapeutic features of polymorphous low-grade adenocarcinoma. Oral Surg Oral Med Oral Pathol 1994;77:41–47.

Waldron CA, El-Mofty SK, Gnepp DR. Tumors of the intraoral minor salivary glands: A demographic and histologic study of 426 cases. Oral Surg Oral Med Oral Pathol 1088; 66:323–333.

Waldron CA, Koh ML. Central mucoepidermoid carcinoma of the jaws: Report of 4 cases with analysis of the literature and discussion of the relationship to mucoepidermoid, sialodontogenic and glandular odontogenic cysts. J Oral Maxillofac Surg 1990;48:871–877.

Chapter 11

Altini M, Shear M. The lateral periodontal cyst: An update. J Oral Pathol Med 1992;21:245–250.

Brannon RB. The odontogenic keratocyst: A clinicopathologic study of 312 cases. Part I: Clinical features. Oral Surg Oral Med Oral Pathol 1976;42:54–72.

Brannon RB. The odontogenic keratocyst: A clinicopathologic study of 312 cases. Part II: Histologic features. Oral Surg Oral Med Oral Pathol 1977;43:233–255.

Buchner A. The central (intraosseous) calcifying odontogenic cyst: An analysis of 215 cases. J Oral Maxillofac Surg 1991; 49:330–339.

Crowley TE, Kaugars GE, Gunsolley JC. Odontogenic keratocysts: A clinical and histologic comparison of the parakeratin and orthokeratin variants. J Oral Maxillofac Surg 1992; 50:22–26.

Forssell K, Forssell H, Kahnberg KE. Recurrence of keratocysts: A long-term follow-up study. Int J Oral Maxillofac Surg 1988;17:25–28.

Gardner DG, Gullane PJ. Mucoceles of the maxillary sinus. Oral Surg Oral Med Oral Pathol 1986:62;538-543.

Gardner DG. Pseudocysts and retention cysts of the maxillary sinus. Oral Surg Oral Med Oral Pathol 1984:58;561-567.

Gorlin RJ. Nevoid basal cell carcinoma syndrome. Medicine 1987;66:98–113.

Greer RO, Johnson M. Botryoid odontogenic cyst: A clinicopathologic analysis of ten cases with three recurrences. J Oral Maxillofac Surg 1988;46:574–579.

Hong SP, Ellis GL, Hartman KS. Calcifiying odontogenic cyst: A review of ninety two cases with re-evaluation of their nature as neoplasms, the nature of ghost cells and subclassification. Oral Surg Oral Med Oral Pathol 1992;72:56–64.

Hussain K, Edmondson HD, Rowne RM. Glandular odontogenic cysts. Diagnosis and treatment. Oral Surg Oral Med Oral Pathol Oral Radiol Endod 1995;79:593–602.

Katz AD, Hachigian M. Thyroglossal duct cysts: A thirty-year experience with emphasis on occurrence in older patients. Am J Surg 1988;155:741–744.

King RC, Smith BR, Burk JL. Dermoid cyst in the floor of the mouth. Review of the literature and case reports. Oral Surg Oral Med Oral Pathol 1994;78:567–576.

Kpponag HS, Johannessen S, Haugen LK, Haanaes HR, Solheim T, Donath K. Glandular odontogenic cyst (sialo-odontogenic cyst): Report of two cases and literature review of 45 previously reported cases. J Oral Pathol Med 1998;27: 455–462.

Manor Y, Buchner A, Peleg M, Taicher S. Lingual cyst with respiratory epithelium: An entity of debatable histogenesis. J Oral Maxillofac Surg 1999;57:124–127.

Marx RE, Hartman KS, Rethman KV. A prospective study comparing incisional labial to incisional parotid biopsies in the detection and confirmation of sarcoidosis, Sjögren's disease, sialosis and lymphoma. J Rheumatol 1988;15: 621–629.

Philipsen HP, Reichert PA, Zhang KJ, Nikai H, Yu QX. Adenomatoid odontogenic tumor: Biologic profile based on 499 cases. J Oral Pathol Med 1991;20:149–158.

Shear M. Developmental odontogenic cysts: An update. J Oral Pathol Med 1994;23:1–11.

Swanson KS, Kugars GE, Gunsolley JG. Nasopalatine duct cyst: An analysis of 334 cases. J Oral Maxillofac Surg 1991;49:268–271.

Wysocki GP, Brannon RB, Gardner DG, Sapp P. Histogenesis of the lateral periodontal cyst and the gingival cyst of the adult. Oral Sur Oral Med Oral Pathol 1980;50:327–334.

Chapter 12

Ackermann GI, Altini M, Shear M. The unicystic ameloblastoma: A clinicopathologic study of 57 cases. J Oral Pathol 1988;17:541–546.

Byrne MN, Session DG. Nasopharyngeal craniopharyngioma. Case report and literature review. Ann Otol Rhinol Laryngol 1990;99:633–639.

Corio RL, Goldblatt LI, Edwards PA, Hartman KS. Ameloblastic carcinoma: A clinicopathologic study and assessment of eight cases. Oral Surg Oral Med Oral Pathol 1987;64:570–576.

Franklin CD, Pindborg JJ. The calcifying epithelial odontogenic tumor: A review and analysis of 113 cases. Oral Surg 1976;42:753–774.

Gardner DG. Peripheral ameloblastoma: A study of 21 cases including five reported as basal cell carcinoma of the gingiva. Cancer 1970;39:1625–1633.

Handlers JP, Abrams AM, Melrose RJ, Danforth R. Central odontogenic fibroma: Clinicopathologic features of 19 cases and review of the literature. J Oral Maxillofac Surg 1991;49:46–54.

Kaffe I, Buchner A, Taicher S. Radiologic features of desmoplastic variant of ameloblastoma. Oral Surg Oral Med Oral Pathol 1993;76:525–529.

Kaugers GE, Miller ME, Abbey LM. Odontomas. Oral Surg Oral Med Oral Pathol 1989;67:172–176.

Krolls SO, Pindborg JJ. Calcifying epithelial odontogenic tumor: Survey of 23 cases and discussion of histomorphologic variations. Arch Pathol 1974;98:206–210.

Li TJ, Wu YT, Yu SF, Yu GY. Unicystic ameloblastoma: A clinicopathologic study of 33 Chinese patients. Am J Surg Pathol 2000;24:1385–1392.

Muller S, Parker DC, Kapadia SB, Budnick SD, et al. Ameloblastic fibrosarcoma of the jaws. A clinicopathologic and DNA analysis of five cases and review of the literature. Oral Surg Oral Med Oral Pathol 1995;79:469–477.

Philipsen HP, Reichart PA. Squamous odontogenic tumor (SOT), a benign neoplasm of the periodontium. A review of 36 reported cases. J Clin Periodontol 1996;23:922–926.

Robinson L, Martinez MG. Unicystic ameloblastoma: A prognostically distinct entity. Cancer 1977;40:2278–2285.

Slabbert H de V, Altini M. Peripheral odontogenic fibroma: A clinicopathologic study. Oral Surg Oral Med Oral Pathol 1991;72:86–90.

Slootweg PJ. Cementoblastoma and osteoblastoma: A comparison of histologic features. J Oral Pathol Med 1992;21:385–389.

Ulmansky M, Hjorting-Hansen E, Praetorius F, Haque MF. Benign cementoblastoma: A review and five new cases. Oral Surg Oral Med Oral Pathol 1994;77:48–55.

Waldron CA, El Mofty SM. A histopathologic study of 116 ameloblastomas with special reference to the desmoplastic variant. Oral Surg Oral Med Oral Pathol 1987;63:441–451.

White DK, Chen SY, Mohnac AM, Miller AS. Odontogenic myxoma: A clinical and ultrastructural study. Oral Surg Oral Med Oral Pathol 1975;39:901–917.

Chapter 13

Brandwein MS, Rothstein A, Lawson W, et al. Sinonasal melanoma. Arch Otolaryngol Head Neck Surg 1997;12:290–296.

Buchner A, Hansen LS. Pigmented nevi of the oral mucosa: A clinicopathologic study of 36 new cases and review of 155 cases from the literature. Part I: A clinicopathologic study of 36 new cases. Oral Surg Oral Med Oral Pathol 1987;63:566–572.

Buchner A, Hansen LS. Pigmented nevi of the oral mucosa: A clinicopathologic study of 36 new cases and review of 155 cases from the literature. Part II: Analysis of 191 cases. Oral Surg Oral Med Oral Pathol 1987;63:676–682.

Clark WH, Elder DE, Guerry D IV, Epstein MN, Greene MH, Van Horn M. A study of tumor progression: The precursor lesions of superficial spreading and nodular melanoma. Human Pathol 1984;15:1147–1165.

Dehner LP, Sibley RK, Sauk JJ, et al. Malignant melanotic neuro-ectodermal tumor of infancy. Cancer 1979;43:1389–1410.

Heasley DD, Toda S, Mihm MC. Pathology of malignant melanoma. Surg Clin North Am 1996;76:1223–1255.

Kapadia SB, Frisman DM, Hitchcock CL, Popek EJ. Melanotic neuroectodermal tumor of infancy. Am J Surg Pathol 1993;17:566–573.

Kaugars GE, Heise AP, Riley WT, Abbey LM, Svirsky JA. Oral melanotic macules: A review of 353 cases. Oral Surg Oral Med Oral Pathol 1993;76:59–61.

Kilpatrick SC, White WL, Browne JD. Desmoplastic malignant melanoma of the oral mucosa: An unrecognized diagnostic pitfall. Cancer 1996;78:383–389.

Rapini RP, Golitz LE, Greer RO, Krekorian EA, Poulson T. Primary malignant melanoma of the oral cavity cancer. A review of 177 cases. Cancer 1985;55:1543–1551.

Skelton HG, Smith KJ, Laskin WB, McCarthy WF, et al. Desmoplastic malignant melanoma. J Am Acad Dermatol 1995;32:717–725.

Chapter 14

Brannon RB, Fowler CB, Carpenter WM, Corio RL. Cementoblastoma: An innocuous neoplasm? A clinicopathologic study of 44 cases and review of the literature with special emphasis on recurrence. Oral Surg Oral Med Oral Pathol Oral Radiol Endod 2002;93:311–320.

Davies ML, MacPherson P. Fibrous dysplasia of the skull: Disease activity in relation to age. Br J Radiol 1991;64:576–579.

Melrose RJ, Abrams AM, Mills BG. Florid osseous dysplasia: A clinical pathologic study of 34 cases. Oral Surg Oral Med Oral Pathol 1976;41:62–82.

Pindborg JJ. On dentinomas. Acta Pathol and Microbiol 1955;105(suppl):135.

Su L, Weathers DR, Waldron CA. Distinguishing features of focal cemento-osseous dysplasias and cemento-ossifying fibromas. Part I: A pathologic spectrum of 316 cases. Oral Surg Oral Med Oral Pathol Oral Radiol Endod 1997;84:301–309(A).

Su L, Weathers DR, Waldron CA. Distinguishing features of focal cemento-osseous dysplasias and cemento-ossifying fibromas. Part II: A clinical and radiologic spectrum of 316 cases. Oral Surg Oral Med Oral Pathol Oral Radiol Endod 1997;84:540–549(B).

Summerlin DJ, Tomich CE. Focal cemento-osseous dysplasia: A clinicopathologic study of 221 cases. Oral Surg Oral Med Oral Pathol 1994;78:611–620.

Thomas DW, Shepherd JP. Pagets disease of bone: Current concepts in pathogenesis and treatment. J Oral Pathol Med 1994;23:12–16.

Vickers RA, Gorlin RJ. Ameloblastoma: Delineation of early histopathologic features of neoplasia. Cancer 1970;26:699–710.

Waldron CA, Giansanti JS. Benign fibro-osseous lesions of the jaws. Part I: Fibrous dysplasia of the jaw. Oral Surg Oral Med Oral Pathol 1973;35:190–201.

Waldron CA. Fibro-osseous lesions of the jaws. J Oral Maxillofac Surg 1993;51:828–835.

Younai F, Eisenbud L, Sciubba JJ. Osteopetrosis: A case report including gross and microscopic findings in the mandible at autopsy. Oral Surg Oral Med Oral Pathol 1988;65:214–221.

Chapter 15

de Lange J, Rosenberg AJWP, van den Akker HP, Koole R, Wirds JJ, van den Bergh H. Treatment of giant cell granuloma of the jaw with calcitonin. Int J Oral Maxillofac Surg 1999;28:372–376.

Eversole LR, Leider AS, Nelson K. Ossifying fibroma: A clinicopathologic study of sixty four cases. Oral Surg Oral Med Oral Pathol 1985;60:505–511.

Inwards CY, Unni KK, Beabout JW, Sim FH. Desmoplastic fibroma of bone. Cancer 1991;68:1978–1983.

Johnson LC, Yousefi M, Vinh T, et al. Juvenile active ossifying fibroma: Its nature, dynamics and origin. Acta Otolaryngol (Suppl) 1991;488:1–40.

Kaffe I, Arkedian L, Taicher S, Littner MM, Buchner A. Radiologic features of central giant cell granulomas of the jaw. Oral Surg Oral Med Oral Pathol Oral Radiol Endod 1996;81:720–726.

Kransdorf MJ, Sweet DE. Aneurysmal bone cyst: Concept, controversy, clinical presentation and imaging. Am J Roentgenol 1995;164:573–580.

Peters TED, Oliver DR, McDonald JS. Benign osteoblastoma of the mandible. Report of a case. J Oral Maxillofac Surg 1995;53:1347–1349.

Sciubba JJ, Younai F. Ossifying fibroma of the mandible and maxilla: Review of 18 cases. J Oral Pathol Med 1989;18:315–321.

Slootweg PJ, Panders AK, Koopmans R, et al. Juvenile ossifying fibroma. An analysis of 33 cases with emphasis on histopathological aspects. J Oral Pathol Med 1994;23:385–388.

Su L, Weathers DR, Waldron CA. Distinguishing features of focal cemento-osseous dysplasias and cemento-ossifying fibromas. Part I: A pathologic spectrum of 316 cases. Oral Surg Oral Med Oral Pathol Oral Radiol Endod 1997;84: 301–309(A).

Su L, Weathers DR, Waldron CA. Distinguishing features of focal cemento-osseous dysplasias and cemento-ossifying fibromas. Part II: A clinical and radiologic spectrum of 316 cases. Oral Surg Oral Med Oral Pathol Oral Radiol Endod 1997;84:540–549(B).

Terry BC, Jacoway JR. Management of central giant cell lesions. An alternative to surgical therapy. Oral Maxillofac Surg Clin North Am 1994;6:579–600.

Waldron CA, Giansanti JS. Benign fibro-osseous lesions of the jaws: A clinical-radiologic-histologic review of sixty-five cases. Part II: Benign fibro-osseous lesions of periodontal membrane origin. Oral Surg Oral Med Oral Pathol 1973; 35:340–350.

Whitaker SB, Waldron CA. Central giant cell lesion of the jaw: A clinical, radiologic and histopathologic study. Oral Surg Oral Med Oral Pathol 1993;75:199–208.

Chapter 16

Batsakis JG, MacKay B, El-Naggar AK. Ewing's sarcoma and peripheral primitive neuroectodermal tumor: An interim report. Ann Otol Rhinol Laryngol 1996;105:838–843.

Bennett JH, Thomas G, Evans AW, Speight PM. Osteosarcoma of the jaws: A 30-year retrospective review. Oral Surg Oral Med Oral Pathol Oral Radiol Endod 2000;90:323–333.

Dehner LP. Primitive neuroectodermal tumor and Ewing's sarcoma. Am J Surg Pathol 1993;12:1–13.

El-Mofty S. Psammomatoid and trabecular juvenile ossifying fibroma of the craniofacial skeleton: Two distinct clinicopathologic entities. Oral Surg Oral Med Oral Pathol Oral Radiol Endod 2002;93:296–304.

van Es RJ, Keus RB, van der Waal I, Koole R, Vermey A. Osteosarcoma of the jaw bones. Long-term follow up of 48 cases. Int J Oral Maxillofac Surg 1997;35:357–362.

Garrington GE, Collett WK. Chondrosarcoma I: A selected literature review. J Oral Pathol 1988;17:1–11.

Garrington GE, Collett WK. Chondrosarcoma II: Chondrosarcoma of the jaw: Analysis of 37 cases. J Oral Pathol 1988;17:12–20.

Garrington GE, Scofield HH, Cornyn J, Hooker SP. Osteosarcoma of the jaws: Analysis of 56 cases. Cancer 1967;20: 377–391.

Ha PK, Eisele DW, Frassica FJ, Zahurak ML, McCarthy EF. Osteosarcoma of the head and neck: A review of the Johns Hopkins experience. Laryngoscope 1999;109:964–969.

Hirshberg A, Leibovich P, Buchner A. Metastatic tumors to the jawbone: Analysis of 390 cases. J Oral Pathol Med 1994;23: 337–341.

Makek M. Clinical Pathology of Fibro-Osteo-Cemental Lesions of the Cranio-Facial Skeleton and Jaw Bones. Basel (Switzerland): Karger, 1983.

Millar BG, Browne RM, Flood TR. Juxtacortical osteosarcoma of the jaws. Br J Oral Maxillofac Surg 1990;28:73–79.

Siegal GP, Oliver MD, Reinus WR, et al. Primary Ewing's sarcoma involving the bones of the head and neck. Cancer 1987:60:2829–2840.

Vencio EF, Reeve CM, Unni KK, Nascimento AG. Mesenchymal chondrosarcoma of the jaw bones. Clinicopathologic study of 19 cases. Cancer 1998;82:2350–2355.

Worth HM, Stoneman DW. Osteomyelitis, malignant disease, and fibrous dysplasia. Some radiologic similarities and differences. Dent Radiogr Photogr 1977;50:1–8,12–15.

Younai F, Eisenbud L, Sciubba JJ. Osteopetrosis: A case report including gross and microscopic findings in the mandible at autopsy. Oral Surg Oral Med Oral Pathol 1988;65:214–221.

Chapter 18

Arico M, Egeler RM. Clinical aspects of Langerhans' cell histiocytosis. Hematol Oncol Clin North Am 1998;12:247–259.

Banks PM, Isaacson PG. MALT lymphomas in 1997. Where do we stand? Am J Clin Pathol 1999;111(suppl 1):S75–S83.

Bataille R, Sany J. Solitary myeloma: Clinical and prognostic features of a review of 114 cases. Cancer 1981;48:845–851.

Corwin J, Lindberg RD. Solitary plasmacytoma of bone vs. extramedullary plasmacytoma and their relationship to multiple myeloma. Cancer 43;1979:1007–1013.

Dimopoulos MA, Kiamouris C, Moulopoulos LA. Solitary plasmacytoma of bone and extramedullary plasmacytoma. Hematol Oncol Clin North Am 1999;13:1249–1257.

Eisenbud L, Sciubba J, Mir R, Sachs SA. Oral presentations in non-Hodgkin's lymphoma; A review of 31 cases. Part 1: Data analysis. Oral Surg Oral Med Oral Pathol 1983;56: 151–156.

Epstein JB, Epstein JD, Le ND, Gorsky M. Characteristics of oral and paraoral malignant lymphoma: A population-based review of 361 cases. Oral Surg Oral Med Oral Pathol Oral Radiol Endod 2001;92:519–525.

Foucar K. Chronic lymphoid leukemias and lymphoproliferative disorders. Mod Pathol 1999;12:141–150.

Fukada Y, Ishida T, Fujimoto M, Ueda T, Aozasa K. Malignant lymphoma of the oral cavity: Clinicopathologic analysis of 20 cases. J Oral Pathol 1987;16:8–12.

Grogan TM, Miller TP, Fisher RI. A Southwest Oncology Group perspective on the Revised European-American Lymphoma classification. Hematol Oncol Clin North Am 1997;11: 819–844.

Hanna E, Wanamaker J, Adelstein D, Tubbs R, Lavertu P. Extranodal lymphomas of the head and neck. A 20 year experience. Arch Otolaryngol Head Neck Surg 1997;12: 1318–1323.

Harris NL, Jaffe E, Stein H, Banks PM, et al. A Revised European-American Classification of lymphoid neoplasms: A proposal from the International Lymphoma Study Group. Blood 1994;84:1361–1392.

Harris, NL. Hodgkin's disease: Classification and differential diagnosis. Mod Pathol 1999;12:159–176.

Kapadia SB, Desai U, Cheng VS. Extramedullary plasmacytoma of the head and neck: A clinicopathologic study of 20 cases. Medicine 1982;61:317–329.

Kilpatrick SE, Wenger DE, Gilchrist GS, Shives TC, Wollan PC, Unni KK. Langerhans cell histiocytosis (histiocytosis X) of bone. A clinicopathologic analysis of 263 pediatric and adult cases. Cancer 1995;76:2471–2484.

Koeppen H, Vardiman JW. New entities, issues and controversies in the classification of malignant lymphoma. Semin Oncol 1998;25:421–434.

Kyle RA. Monoclonal gammopathy of undetermined significance: Natural history in 241 cases. Am J Med 1978;64: 814–826.

Kyle RA. Multiple myeloma: Review of 869 cases. Mayo Clin Proc 1975;50:29–40.

Lieberman PH, Jones CR, Steinman RM, Erlandson RA, et al. Langerhans cell (eosinophilic) granulomatosis: A clinicopathologic study encompassing 50 years. Am J Surg Pathol 1996;20:519–552.

Meis JM, Butler JJ, Osborne BM, Ordonez NG. Solitary plasmacytomas of bone and extramedullary plasmacytomas: A clinicopathologic and immunohistochemical study. Cancer 1987;59:1475–1485.

Shindoh M, Takami T, Arisue M, Yamashita T, Saito T, Notani K, et al. Comparison between submucosal (extra-nodal) and nodal non-Hodgkin's lymphoma (NHL) in the oral and maxillofacial region. J Oral Pathol Med 1997;26:283–289.

Sirois DA, Miller AS, Harwick RD, Vonderheid EC. Oral manifestations of cutaneous T-cell lymphoma. A report of eight cases. Oral Surg Oral Med Oral Pathol 1993;75:700–705.

Smoller BR, Bishop K, Glusac E, Kim YH, Hendrickson M. Reassessment of histologic parameters in the diagnosis of mycosis fungoides. Am J Surg Pathol 1995;19:1423–1430.

Wax MK, Yun KJ, Omar RA. Extramedullary plasmacytomas of the head and neck. Otolaryngol Head Neck Surg 1993;109: 877–885.

Chapter 19

Lukes RJ, Collins RD. New approaches to the classification of the lymphomata. Br J Cancer 1975;31:1–28.

Rappaport H. New concepts in the classification of malignant hemopathies. Bull Cancer 1974;61:11–22.

Glossary

Acantholysis (*acantha*–Gr thorn; *lysis*–Gr loosening) Loss of cohesion between epithelial cells.

Acanthosis Increased thickness of prickle cell layer or stratum Malphigii.

A fibers Nerve fibers that are large (20 to 25-μm diameter), are myelinated, and have fast conduction velocities (20 to 100 m/sec).

Allogeneic Tissue transplant from one genetically unrelated member of a species to another member of the same species.

ANA Antinuclear antibody. Circulating antibody with a receptor site specific to antigens in the nucleus. It is used as a screening blood test for many immune-based diseases.

Anaplasia (*ana*–Gr backwards; *plassein*–to form) Loss of differentiation of cells and loss of cellular orientation.

ANCA Antineutrophil cytoplasmic antibodies. Circulation antibodies with a receptor site specific for antigens in the cytoplasm of neutrophils. C-ANCA antibodies are directed against various cytoplasmic components in the cytoplasm. P-ANCA antibodies are directed against myeloperoxidase in the perinuclear cytoplasm.

Anlage A primordial structure.

Apocopation (*apokope*–Gr cutting off, amputation) Process by which melanin is transferred from the dendrite of the melanocyte to the keratinocyte.

Apoptosis (*apo*–Gr off; *ptosis*–Gr fall) Programmed cell death (cells fall off into dermis).

Artifact Tissue that has been physically altered from its natural state by processing.

Bone morphogenetic protein An acid-inoculable morphogen growth factor that promotes cell migration and bone differentiation in the embryo and reforms bone after osteoclastic resorption in the adult.

Bosselated An intact surface that has numerous round eminences.

Bossing The development of a rounded enlargement of a surface area.

Bulla Space within or beneath epithelium that contains serous or seropurulent fluid and is greater than 5 mm in circumference.

CD Cluster designation. This is a system for classifying cell surface markers that are expressed by leukocytes. These markers are used to distinguish cell lineages, stages of development, and functional subsets. The system is based on computer analysis of monoclonal antibodies against human leukocyte antigens with antibodies having similar specificity characteristics grouped together and assigned a number (eg, CD1, CD4, etc).

Chvostek sign A spasm of the facial muscles resulting from tapping the muscles or branches of the facial nerves; seen in hypercalcemia and tetany. Also may be called *Chvostek-Weiss sign*.

Civatte bodies Apoptotic cells.

Clavulanate potassium A competitive inhibitor of bacterial penicillinase. It is added to various penicillins to extend their spectrum to include bacteria with penicillinase.

Comedo A plug of dried sebum in the excretory duct of the skin.

Cytokine A cellular product with an active biologic function. Mostly refers to protein growth factors, which promote certain cellular responses.

Desmoplasia (*desmos*–Gr band or ligament) Formation and development of fibrous tissue.

Desmosome Dense circular body that is the site of attachment between some epithelial cells, and particularly in stratified squamous epithelium of skin and mucosa.

Dinitrochlorobenzene (DNCB) An organic compound used to test the cellular immune response. Injected intradermally, it will provoke an erythema at the injection site in 48 hours if the individual's cellular immunity is functioning normally.

Diplopia The visual perception of two images when viewing a single object; double vision.

Down-regulation, down regulate The reduction of a biologic activity. It mostly refers to a decrease in the expression of a gene.

Dysplasia (*dys*–Gr abnormal, disordered; *plassein*–Gr to form) Abnormality in organization, size, and shape of adult cells.

Erosion (*erosio/erodere*–L to eat out) Loss of epidermis only; no scarring occurs.

Erythema nodosum An acute inflammatory skin response produced by various diseases, particularly hypersensitivity and autoimmune diseases, which is marked by tender red nodules due to exudation of inflammatory cells, blood, and/or serum and accompanied by intense itching and burning.

Exudate A tissue fluid that has a high protein content or cell count.

Fascicle (L *fascis*) A bundle.

Forme fruste A mild or incomplete form of an anomaly, disease entity, or syndrome.

FTA-ABS Fluorescent treponemal antibody absorption. A confirmatory serum test for syphilis that tests for anti-treponemal antibodies by using killed treponema with a fluorescent tag as the antigen. It also absorbs nonsyphilitic treponemal antibodies from the test.

Furuncle A painful nodule formed in the skin by bacteria, which enter through the hair follicle and produce an intense inflammation around a central core.

Ghon focus A round or bean-shaped density that represents the primary lesion of tuberculosis in the lungs; seen in a chest radiograph. Named after the Czechoslovakian pathologist Anton Ghon.

Granuloma Aggregates of macrophages that accumulate for the purpose of phagocytosis.

Grenz zone A narrow tumor-free space between the epithelium and a subepithelial lesion.

Hemidesmosome Site of attachment between basal surface of basal epithelial cell and the basement membrane.

HLA Human lymphocyte antigen. One of many lymphocyte cell surface antigens specific to an individual. It is used in tissue typing and is thought to indicate vulnerability to certain diseases and conditions.

Hyalin (*hyalos*–Gr glass) Homogeneous eosinophilic material, which ultrastructurally represents excessive amounts of basement membrane material.

Intra-articular Within the space of a joint.

Keratinocyte Epidermal cells other than dendritic cells. They have the potential to form keratin.

Koilocytotic A deformity in the shape of a cell; usually has a concave or hollow appearance.

Langerhans cell Dendritic cells present in the upper prickle cell layers. They appear clear with the light microscope. They are antigen-presenting cells and are distinguished by the presence of Birbeck granules, which are seen ultrastructurally in the cytoplasm. They lack tonofilaments and desmosomes.

Lymphokine An active biologic product of a lymphocyte; usually refers to an enzyme, destructive chemical, or inflammatory mediator.

Lysosome (*soma*–Gr body; *lysis*–dissolution) Membrane-bound organelles containing hydrolytic enzymes, which are involved in intracellular digestion. They are present in many types of cells.

Macule A discolored spot that is not raised above the surface.

Metaplasia (*meta*–Gr after beyond, over; *plassein*–to form) Changing of one type of adult tissue into another type of adult tissue that is not normal for that tissue.

Microtia Hypoplasia or aplasia of the pinna of the ear, together with an absent or incomplete external auditory meatus.

Monostotic Affecting a single bone.

Myoepithelium (*mys/myos*–Gr muscle) A type of epithelium with contractile qualities.

Omphalocele Congenital protrusion of part of the intestine through a large defect in the abdominal wall at the umbilicus, the protruding bowel being covered only by a thin transparent membrane of amnion and peritoneum.

Oncogene A gene that causes neoplasia. A "good gene gone bad."

Orthokeratosis (*ortho*–Gr normal, correct) Keratinization in which nuclei are not present.

P53 A specific protein from a tumor suppressor gene that bypasses cells with abnormal DNA; it is thought to resist or prevent tumors by this action.

Papule Small, circumscribed solid raised portion of skin or mucosa.

Parakeratosis (*para*–Gr to, at, from the side of) Incomplete keratinization whereby nuclei are retained in the stratum corneum and the granular cell layer is absent or minimal. This process is normal in oral and vaginal mucosa.

PDGF Platelet-derived growth factor. Three isomers of a protein growth factor found mainly in platelets, macrophages, and embryonic stem cells that initiate cellular activities associated with healing and development.

Proto-oncogene A gene that has a high incidence of transforming into a gene that causes neoplasia.

Pustule Vesicle or bulla containing numerous neutrophils or eosinophils.

Sanguineous Pertaining to or resembling blood.

Schaumann bodies Red-brown nodules in sarcoidosis.

Sulbactam A competitive inhibitor of bacterial penicillinase. It is added to various penicillins to extend their spectrum to include bacteria with penicillinase enzyme–producing capability.

Suppurative Producing pus or associated with the formation of pus.

Syncytium An interdigitation or merging of cells.

TGF-beta Transforming growth factor–beta. A "super family" of numerous protein growth factors that initiate and modulate connective tissue healing. The thirteen known bone morphogenetic proteins are within the family of TGF-betas, which has been described to have 47 or more growth factors.

Thenar The prominence on the palm at the base of the thumb.

Theque A round or oval collection, or nest, of melanin-containing nevus cells occurring at the dermal-epidermal junction of the skin or in the dermis proper.

Translocation Attachment of a fragment of one chromosome to a nonhomologous chromosome. The short arm of the chromosome is designated p and the long arm q.

Transudate A tissue fluid that has no or low protein content and cell count.

Tumor suppressor gene A gene that produces a protein that resists, suppresses, or lyses cells that have abnormal DNA and would lead to neoplasia.

Ulcer (*ulcus*–L sore, ulcer) The epidermis and part of the dermis are absent, leading to scarring.

Vesicle A bulla that is less than 5 mm in circumference.

Villi (L tuft of hair) Elongated papillae covered by a single layer of epithelium and extending into a bulla, vesicle, or lacuna.

Wormian Immature or dysmorphic bones of the skull that take on an appearance of the cranial sutures.

Index

GREYSCALE

BIN TRAVELER FORM

Cut By_____W.King_____ Qty__23___ Date__3/3_____

Scanned By_____ Qty_____Date_____

Scanned Batch IDs

_____ _____ _____

Notes / Exception

_____

_____

_____

_____

_____